Family Practice Examination & Board Review

NOTICE

Medicine is an ever-changing science. As new research and clinical experience broaden our knowledge, changes in treatment and drug therapy are required. The authors and the publisher of this work have checked with sources believed to be reliable in their efforts to provide information that is complete and generally in accord with the standards accepted at the time of publication. However, in view of the possibility of human error or changes in medical sciences, neither the authors nor the publisher nor any other party who has been involved in the preparation or publication of this work warrants that the information contained herein is in every respect accurate or complete, and they disclaim all responsibility for any errors or omissions or for the results obtained from use of the information contained in this work. Readers are encouraged to confirm the information contained herein with other sources. For example and in particular, readers are advised to check the product information sheet included in the package of each drug they plan to administer to be certain that the information contained in this work is accurate and that changes have not been made in the recommended dose or in the contraindications for administration. This recommendation is of particular importance in connection with new or infrequently used drugs.

Family Practice Examination & Board Review

Third Edition

Editors

Jason K. Wilbur, MD

Clinical Associate Professor
Department of Family Medicine
Roy J. and Lucille A. Carver College of Medicine
University of Iowa
Iowa City, Iowa

Mark A. Graber, MD

Clinical Professor
Departments of Family Medicine and Emergency Medicine
Roy J. and Lucille A. Carver College of Medicine
University of Iowa
Iowa City, Iowa

McGraw Hill Medical

New York Chicago San Francisco Lisbon London Madrid Mexico City Milan
New Delhi San Juan Seoul Singapore Sydney Toronto

The McGraw-Hill Companies

Family Practice Examination & Board Review, Third Edition

1 2 3 4 5 6 7 8 9 0 2WCK/QVR 17 16 15 14 13 12

ISBN 978-0-07-178185-5
MHID 0-07-178185-4

This book was set in Janson by Aptara, Inc.
The editors were Christine Diedrich and Robert Pancotti.
The production supervisor was Catherine H. Saggese.
Project management was provided by Ruchira Gupta, Aptara, Inc.
The cover designer was Ty Nowicki.
Front cover image: © Jim Craigmyle/Corbis.
Quad/Graphics was printer and binder.

This book is printed on acid-free paper.

Library of Congress Cataloging-in-Publication Data

Family practice examination & board review / editors, Jason K. Wilbur,
Mark A. Graber.—3rd ed.
p. ; cm.—(McGraw-Hill specialty board review)
Family practice examination and board review
Includes bibliographical references and index.
ISBN 978-0-07-178185-5 (pbk. : alk. paper)
1. Family medicine—Examinations, questions, etc. I. Wilbur, Jason K. II. Graber, Mark A., MD.
III. Title: Family practice examination and board review. IV. Series: McGraw-Hill specialty board review.
[DNLM: 1. Family Practice—Examination Questions. WB 18.2]
RC58.F346 2012
610.76–dc23

2012017850

To Gary and Carol Wilbur. Thanks Mom and Dad for everything!
—JKW

To Everybody (that means you!). And to the Family Medicine Team in Jogjakarta, Indonesia at Gadjah Mada University.
—MAG

Contents

Contributors

Azeemuddin Ahmed, MD
Clinical Associate Professor
Department of Emergency Medicine
Roy J. and Lucille A. Carver College of Medicine
University of Iowa
Iowa City, Iowa
Emergency Medicine

Olivia E. Bailey, MD
Clinical Assistant Professor
Department of Emergency Medicine
Roy J. and Lucille A. Carver College of Medicine
University of Iowa
Iowa City, Iowa
Emergency Medicine

David Bedell, MD
Clinical Associate Professor
Department of Family Medicine
Roy J. and Lucille A. Carver College of Medicine
University of Iowa
Iowa City, Iowa
Patient-Centered Care

Christopher T. Buresh, MD
Clinical Associate Professor
Department of Emergency Medicine
Roy J. and Lucille A. Carver College of Medicine
University of Iowa
Iowa City, Iowa
Emergency Medicine

Bogdan Cherascu, MD
Clinical Assistant Professor
Division of Rheumatology
Department of Internal Medicine
Roy J. and Lucille A. Carver College of Medicine
University of Iowa
Iowa City, Iowa
Rheumatology

Dustin DeYoung, MD
Resident
Departments of Psychiatry and Family Medicine
Roy J. and Lucille A. Carver College of Medicine
University of Iowa
Iowa City, Iowa
Substance Use Disorders

Alex Ellison, MD
Resident
Department of Neurology
Roy J. and Lucille A. Carver College of Medicine
University of Iowa
Iowa City, Iowa
Neurology

Mark A. Graber, MD
Clinical Professor
Departments of Family Medicine and Emergency Medicine
Roy J. and Lucille A. Carver College of Medicine
University of Iowa
Iowa City, Iowa
Emergency Medicine; Cardiology; Allergy and Immunology; Nephrology; Hematology and Oncology; Gastroenterology; Infectious Diseases; Endocrinology; Obstetrics and Women's Health; Ophthalmology; Otolaryngology; Care of the Surgical Patient; Psychiatry; Nutrition and Herbal Medicine; Substance Use Disorders; Ethics; Evidence-Based Medicine; Final Examination

Philip Gregory, PharmD, FACN
Prescriber's Letter
Stockton, California
Nutrition and Herbal Medicine

Sailesh C. Harwani, MD, PhD
Fellow, Division of Cardiology
Department of Internal Medicine
Roy J. and Lucille A. Carver College of Medicine
University of Iowa
Iowa City, Iowa
Cardiology

Christopher P. Hogrefe, MD
Clinical Assistant Professor
Department of Emergency Medicine
Roy J. and Lucille A. Carver College of Medicine
University of Iowa
Iowa City, Iowa
Emergency Medicine

Karol Z. Krements, MD
Fellow, Division of Pulmonary, Critical Care, and Occupational Medicine
Department of Internal Medicine
Roy J. and Lucille A. Carver College of Medicine
University of Iowa
Iowa City, Iowa
Pulmonary

Jason Maxfield, MD
Resident
Department of Neurology
Roy J. and Lucille A. Carver College of Medicine
University of Iowa
Iowa City, Iowa
Neurology

Andrew Peterson, MD
Clinical Assistant Professor
Department of Pediatrics
Roy J. and Lucille A. Carver College of Medicine
University of Iowa
Iowa City, Iowa
Pediatrics

Jason Powers, MD
Associate
Department of Family Medicine
Roy J. and Lucille A. Carver College of Medicine
University of Iowa
Iowa City, Iowa
Adolescent Medicine

Sandra Rosenfeld-O'Tool, MD
Clinical Assistant Professor
Department of Family Medicine
Roy J. and Lucille A. Carver College of Medicine
University of Iowa
Iowa City, Iowa
Obstetrics and Women's Health

Benjamin Shepherd, MD
Family Medicine and Psychiatry
Private Practice
Mount Morris, Illinois
Psychiatry

Jack T. Stapleton, MD
Professor
Division of Infectious Diseases
Department of Internal Medicine
Roy J. and Lucille A. Carver College of Medicine
University of Iowa
Iowa City, Iowa
HIV/AIDS

Janeta F. Tansey, MD, PhD
Private Practice, Psychiatry
Iowa City, Iowa
Ethics

Jon Van Heukelom, MD
Clinical Assistant Professor
Department of Emergency Medicine
Roy J. and Lucille A. Carver College of Medicine
University of Iowa
Iowa City, Iowa
Orthopedics and Sports Medicine

Michelle Weckmann, MS, MD
Clinical Assistant Professor
Departments of Family Medicine and Psychiatry
Roy J. and Lucille A. Carver College of Medicine
University of Iowa
Iowa City, Iowa
End-of-Life Care

Jason K. Wilbur, MD
Clinical Associate Professor
Department of Family Medicine
Roy J. and Lucille A. Carver College of Medicine
University of Iowa
Iowa City, Iowa
Allergy and Immunology; Nephrology; Hematology and Oncology; Gastroenterology; Adolescent Medicine; Men's Health; Dermatology; Ophthalmology; Otolaryngology; Care of the Older Patient; Psychiatry; Patient-Centered Care; Final Examination

Regina Won, MD
Fellow, Infectious Diseases
Department of Internal Medicine
Roy J. and Lucille A. Carver College of Medicine
University of Iowa
Iowa City, Iowa
HIV/AIDS

Kelly Wood, MD
Clinical Assistant Professor
Department of Pediatrics
Roy J. and Lucille A. Carver College of Medicine
University of Iowa
Iowa City, Iowa
Pediatrics

Preface

Welcome to the third edition of *Family Practice Examination & Board Review*. So how does this edition compare with the second edition? All of the science has been updated. And there are new cases in almost every chapter. Plus, the jokes are better . . . really.

With all of the board review books out there, why should you choose our text? **There are two crucial differences between this book and other board review books on the market.** First, we have written this book not only to help you pass the boards but also to broaden your knowledge of family medicine. The majority of questions contain a detailed explanation not only of why an answer is right but also why the other answers are wrong. **If the current "state of the art" differs substantially from the answers that will be on the boards (which generally reflect information that is 2–3 years out of date), we have made a note of that and have given you the "state-of-the-art" information as well.**

The second difference is that we are not boring. You will find (sometimes feeble) attempts at humor throughout the book. There is no reason that studying has to be an exercise in tedium and endurance. It should be enjoyable and provide a surprise every now and again. We have noticed that an occasional reader does not appreciate our sense of humor. Oh well. . . .

We have tried to make this book as broad and as comprehensive as possible. In addition to its use as a board review book for family medicine, it can be employed as a general review for primary care physicians, physician assistants, and nurse practitioners. Medical students studying for Step 3 of the licensing exam should find the book helpful as well. However, no board review book can possibly cover the entire scope of family medicine. Use these questions as a guide: what areas are you strong in and in what areas do you need further study? We have provided a 149-question "final exam" so you can gauge what you have learned. Each answer of the "final exam" is referenced in the book so you can go back and review any topic that you might have missed.

In this book, the use of eponymous medical terms such as Crohn disease, Wegner disease, and Wilson disease reflects the current American Medical Association recommendations for these and similar terms.

We enjoyed writing this book and we hope that you enjoy using it. If you have suggestions or complaints (OK, maybe all of our jokes aren't politically correct), do not hesitate to write us at mark-graber@uiowa.edu or jason-wilbur@uiowa.edu. We take your comments seriously as we endeavor to make studying for the board exam more efficient and more fun.

Mark would like to thank all of the authors for their contributions . . . sometimes "a bit" over deadline but you know who you are. . . . Thanks also to my family: Hetty, Rachel, and Abe (as always). But not to the dogs, Nietzsche and Dante. They need to learn to stay either in or out of the house. No more of this back and forth. Finally, thanks to my bicycle (for keeping me sane . . . although some would argue this point), Buckethead, Yoko Kanno, and the soundtrack from "Noir" (the anime) for keeping me awake in the wee hours when text begins to swim across the screen (doing the side stroke, I think).

Jason thanks his wife, Deb, who has shown great patience during the writing of this book (look . . . he lives!), and his boys, Ken and Ted, who seem to have changed more than medicine since the second edition. And then there are the growers, producers, and roasters of fine coffee, without whom there would be no fuel for this endeavor. Who would I be without coffee? I get a chill down my spine just thinking about it.

1

Emergency Medicine

Azeemuddin Ahmed, Olivia E. Bailey, Christopher T. Buresh, Christopher P. Hogrefe, and Mark A. Graber

CASE 1

You get a call from a panicked mother because her 4-year-old took some of her theophylline. She thinks it may have been as many as 10 pills but is not clear on the actual number. She is about 35 minutes from the hospital.

Your advice to her is:

A) Give ipecac to promote stomach emptying and reduce theophylline absorption.
B) Do not give ipecac and proceed directly to the hospital.
C) Call poison control and then proceed to the hospital.
D) None of the above.

Discussion

The correct answer is "B." Do not give ipecac but proceed to the hospital. "A" is incorrect for a couple of reasons. First, ipecac is not a particularly effective method of emptying gastric contents. More importantly, if the patient should start to seize while vomiting as a result of the ipecac, she could aspirate the vomitus causing an aspiration pneumonitis. "C" is incorrect because you do not want to delay definitive treatment. You can call poison control while the patient is on the way in.

HELPFUL TIP: Ipecac is ineffective and possibly harmful. It causes myopathy and cardiac problems when used chronically (such as in those with anorexia nervosa).

* *

The patient arrives in your emergency department (ED). She is alert but with a tachycardia of 160 beats per minute and a stable blood pressure (BP). The ingestion occurred about 2.5 hours ago. You decide that the next step is gastrointestinal (GI) decontamination.

Which of the following statements is true about gastric lavage?

A) Except in extraordinary circumstances it should only be done in the first 1.5 hours after an overdose.
B) Patients who have had gastric lavage have higher incidence of pulmonary aspiration than patients who have not.
C) The maximum volume that should be used is 5 L.
D) It can push pill fragments beyond the pylorus.
E) All of the above are true.

Discussion

The correct answer is "E." All of the options are true. Generally, the efficacy of gastric lavage is limited. Outcome data do not support the use of gastric lavage after the first 1–1.5 hours. In a particularly severe overdose or in an overdose that is likely to delay gastric emptying (e.g., anticholinergics such as diphenhydramine or tricyclic antidepressants), you might want to try lavage beyond the 1.5 hours, but such circumstances are unusual. Gastric lavage increases the risk of aspiration, can push pill fragments beyond the pylorus, and 5 L is the maximum volume that should be used.

The next best step to take in this patient is to:

A) Check blood theophylline levels and refer for hemodialysis if markedly elevated.
B) Administer 1 g/kg of charcoal with sorbitol.
C) Prophylactically treat this patient for seizures using lorazepam.
D) Prophylactically treat this patient for seizures using phenytoin.

Discussion

The correct answer is "B." Giving charcoal is indicated in almost all overdoses. "A" is incorrect because the patient's situation could deteriorate by the time blood levels return. "C" and "D" are incorrect because seizure prophylaxis is not indicated in this patient. Although seizures are a major manifestation of theophylline toxicity, they are more likely to occur in patients who take theophylline chronically and have toxic blood levels. Acute ingestions are less worrisome.

> HELPFUL TIP: Although standard of care, charcoal has limited or no effect on outcomes. It reduces absorption by about 30% if given within 1 hour of ingestion and likely has no benefit after 1 hour.

For which of these overdoses is charcoal NOT indicated?

A) Acetaminophen.
B) Aspirin.
C) Iron.
D) Digoxin.
E) Opiates.

Discussion

The correct answer is "C." Charcoal will not bind iron. Some of you may have answered "A." Theoretically, charcoal could interfere with the action of *N*-acetylcysteine, the antidote for acetaminophen ingestion by absorbing it. However, this is more of a theoretical concern than an actual one. First, the drugs should be used at different times. Charcoal should be given immediately while *N*-acetylcysteine is given only after 4-hour levels are available. Second, the doses of *N*-acetylcysteine recommended are quite high, and you can give a higher dose if you will be using it with charcoal. Finally, intravenous (IV) *N*-acetylcysteine is available and is obviously not affected by charcoal. "B," "D," and "E" are all incorrect. While we do have antidotes for digoxin and opiates (Digibind, naloxone), charcoal is still indicated to reduce absorption.

Objectives: Did you learn to . . .

- Manage a patient with an acute ingestion?
- Describe the appropriate use of gastric lavage and charcoal administration?
- Identify situations where charcoal may not be indicated?

QUICK QUIZ: BIOTERRORISM

Oh no. Godzilla is attacking Tokyo. And this time it is with weapons of mass destruction. Which of the following properly describes the isolation requirements of a patient with pulmonary anthrax?

A) No isolation necessary. The patient may be in the same room with an uninfected patient.
B) Respiratory isolation only.
C) Respiratory and contact isolation.
D) Negative pressure room (such as with tuberculosis) + contact isolation.

Discussion

The correct answer is "A." Pulmonary anthrax is not transmitted person to person. Contact isolation is indicated in those with cutaneous anthrax and GI anthrax (where diarrhea may be infectious).

Godzilla is not done yet . . . Which of the following drugs should be used as prophylaxis against inhaled anthrax should exposure to aerosolized spores be documented?

A) A first-generation cephalosporin.
B) Trimethoprim/sulfamethoxazole.
C) Ciprofloxacin.
D) A third-generation cephalosporin.

Discussion

The correct answer is "C." Fluoroquinolones are the drugs of choice when treating those exposed to anthrax. Doxycycline may also be used. Cephalosporins and TMP/SMX are not active against anthrax.

* Fluroquinolones are often used for UTI and also for hospital acquired infections due to urinary catheters.

Godzilla, frustrated by his failed anthrax attack, is now spreading smallpox. Which of the following is NOT true about smallpox?

A) Isolation is best done at home if possible.
B) The patient is infectious until he or she becomes afebrile.
C) All lesions are generally in the same stage of evolution, unlike what is seen in varicella.
D) Smallpox immunization causes an encephalitis in 1:300,000 of which 25% of cases are fatal.

Discussion
The correct answer is "B." The patient is infectious until all lesions crust over and (infectivity has nothing to do with the presence or absence of fever.) "A" is true. Isolation is best done at home since this will limit spread (those in the household have likely already been exposed). "C" is also true; all lesions are in a similar state of evolution. Finally, "D" is correct and is the reason we do not currently immunize against smallpox.

CASE 2

A 22-year-old female presents to the ED with an overdose. She has a history of depression, and there were empty bottles found at her bedside. The bottles had contained clonazepam and nortriptyline. The patient is unconscious with diminished breathing and is unable to protect her own airway.

The BEST next step is to:

A) Intubate the patient.
B) Begin gastric lavage and administer charcoal.
C) Administer flumazenil, a benzodiazepine antagonist, to awaken her and improve her respirations.
D) Administer bicarbonate.
E) Any of the above.

Discussion
The correct answer is "A." This patient should be intubated. Remember in any emergency situation that the ABCs (airway, breathing, and circulation) are the priority. "B" is incorrect because, as noted earlier, patients who are lavaged have a higher incidence of pulmonary aspiration—an even greater concern in the obtunded patient. In fact, airway protection is MANDATORY before undertaking lavage. "C" is incorrect. Flumazenil *will* reverse the benzodiazepine. However, we know from experience that seizures in patients who have had flumazenil are particularly difficult to control. This would be particularly problematic in a patient with a mixed overdose, such as with a tricyclic, where seizures are common. Thus, it is recommended that flumazenil be used only as a reversal agent after procedural sedation in patients who are not on chronic benzodiazepines.

* *

You notice that the patient begins to have an abnormal ECG tracing.

Which of the following findings would you expect to find in a tricyclic overdose?

A) Normal QRS complex.
B) Second- and third-degree heart block.
C) Widened QRS complex.
D) Sinus tachycardia.
E) Any of the above.

Discussion
The correct answer is "E." All of the above findings can be seen with a tricyclic overdose. In fact, the most common presenting rhythm is a narrow-complex sinus tachycardia. As toxicity progresses, you can get a prolonged PR interval, a widened QRS complex, and a prolonged QT interval. Heart blocks (second and third degree) herald a poor outcome and may be seen late in the course. Asystole is not a primary rhythm in tricyclic overdose and tends to reflect the end stage of another arrhythmia.

* *

YIKES!! The patient becomes unresponsive and you look at the monitor. You obtain an ECG (Figure 1–1).

What is the patient's rhythm?

A) Monomorphic ventricular tachycardia.
B) Sinus tachycardia with a bundle branch block.
C) Paroxysmal supraventricular tachycardia.
D) Torsade de pointes.
E) None of the above.

Discussion
The correct answer is "D." This is torsades de pointes (literally "twisting of the points"), which is a subtype of polymorphic ventricular tachycardia. It can be recognized by the varying amplitude of the complex in a somewhat regular pattern. "A" is incorrect because the complexes are not monomorphic. "B" is incorrect for two reasons. First, there are no P waves visible.

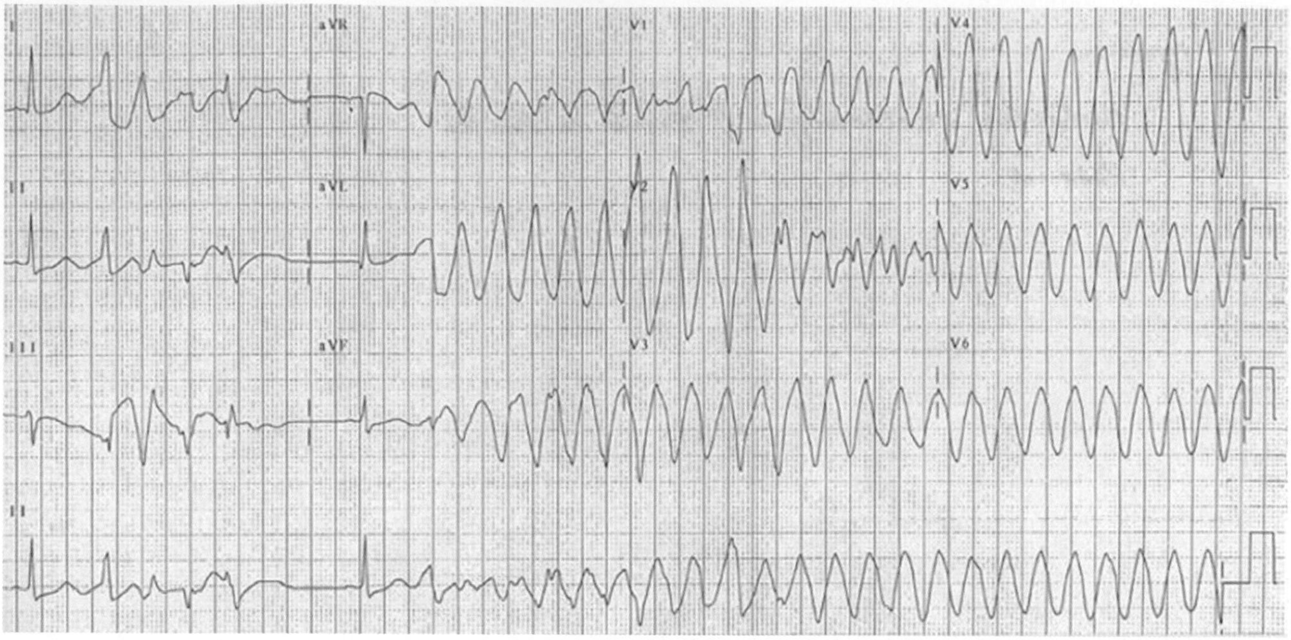

Figure 1–1

Second, sinus tachycardia should not have varied amplitude. "C" is incorrect because, again, there are no P waves and the complexes are polymorphic.

This patient needs treatment *post haste*. After taking care of the ABCs, what is the ONE BEST drug for the treatment of this arrhythmia in a patient with a tricyclic overdose?

A) Beta-blockers.
B) Lidocaine.
C) Sodium bicarbonate.
D) Procainamide.
E) Amiodarone.

Discussion
The correct answer is "C." The treatment of choice for arrhythmias in patients with a tricyclic overdose is sodium bicarbonate. Raising the pH and administering sodium seem to "prime" the sodium channels in the heart reversing the toxicity of the tricyclic. Procainamide and quinidine should not be used because they act in similar fashion to tricyclics and may worsen the problem. Lidocaine can be used as can amiodarone, but they are not the best choices. Beta-blockers can worsen hypotension and should be avoided.

* *

This is not your patient's lucky day. She begins to seize after the administration of the bicarbonate.

The treatment of choice for this seizing patient is:

A) Lorazepam.
B) Repeat the bolus of sodium bicarbonate and start a bicarbonate drip.
C) Phenytoin (Dilantin).
D) Fosphenytoin (Cerebryx).
E) None of the above.

Discussion
The correct answer is "A." Benzodiazepines are the treatments of choice in tricyclic-induced seizures. While most seizures are self-limited, it is important to control seizures because the resultant acidosis can worsen tricyclic toxicity. "B" is incorrect. This patient is already alkalinized, and sodium bicarbonate is not particularly effective in tricyclic-induced seizures. Choice "C," phenytoin, can be used, but benzodiazepines and phenobarbital should be administered first if possible. Phenytoin is not a particularly good antiepileptic drug in tricyclic overdose. "D" is incorrect for two reasons. First, since fosphenytoin is metabolized to phenytoin, the concern about efficacy applies. Second, fosphenytoin is a prodrug and requires adequate circulation and renal and hepatic function to be converted into active drug. If our patient becomes hypotensive with poor liver and renal perfusion, adequate drug levels might not be achieved. Finally, both phenytoin and fosphenytoin can cause hypotension—not what you need in this unstable patient.

* *

The patient's seizures stop and she is admitted to the intensive care unit.

HELPFUL TIP: A patient who is entirely asymptomatic 6 hours after a tricyclic overdose is unlikely to have any serious consequences from the ingestion. They can be "medically cleared" at that point for admission to psychiatric unit. Note that "symptomatic" may just be tachycardia or mild confusion. We mean the *entirely* asymptomatic patient.

Objectives: Did you learn to . . .

- Describe the role of flumazenil in toxicologic emergencies?
- Manage a tricyclic overdose?
- Recognize ECG findings in a tricyclic overdose?
- Recognize torsades de pointes and its treatment?

QUICK QUIZ: DESIGNER AND CLUB DRUGS

An 18-year-old male presents after a party. He is having alternating episodes of combative behavior interspersed with episodes of coma. He becomes almost apneic during the episodes of coma. He has alternating bradycardia (while in coma) and tachycardia when awake. The patient is also having myoclonic seizures. His serum alcohol level is zero.

The most likely drug causing this is:

A) Ecstasy (MDMA).
B) GHB (gamma-hydroxybutyrate aka "liquid ecstasy").
C) Methamphetamine.
D) LSD (lysergic acid diethylamine aka "acid").
E) Opiate overdose.

Discussion

The correct answer is "B." The episodic coma and bradycardia interspersed with episodes of extreme agitation are almost pathognomonic of GHB overdose. "A" is incorrect because MDMA causes an amphetamine-like reaction with agitation, hypertension, hyperthermia, tachycardia, etc. "C" is incorrect for the same reason. "D" is incorrect because LSD rarely (if ever) causes coma. "E" is incorrect because patients with opiate overdoses are generally somnolent or comatose without interspersed episodes of agitation.

* *

GHB is odorless and has slight salty taste. It has become a drug of choice for "date rape." The toxicity tends to be self-limited and can be treated with intubation if needed along with tincture of time. The half-life is only 27 minutes.

QUICK QUIZ: TOXIDROMES

A patient presents to the hospital with a diphenhydramine overdose.

Which of the following signs and symptoms are you likely to find in this patient?

A) Bradycardia, dilated pupils, flushing.
B) Bradycardia, pinpoint pupils, flushing.
C) Tachycardia, dilated pupils, diaphoresis.
D) Tachycardia, dilated pupils, flushing.
E) Tachycardia, pinpoint pupils, flushing.

Discussion

The correct answer is "D." This patient has an anticholinergic TOXIDROME. Toxidromes are symptom complexes associated with a particular overdose that should be immediately recognized by the clinician. Common toxidromes are listed in Table 1–1.

CASE 3

A patient presents to your office with neck pain after a motor vehicle accident. He was restrained and the airbag deployed. He notes that he had some lateral neck pain at the scene. He continues to have lateral neck pain.

Which of the following IS NOT a criterion for clearing the cervical spine clinically?

A) Absence of all neck pain.
B) Normal mental status including no drugs or alcohol.
C) Absence of a distracting injury (such as an ankle fracture).
D) Absence of paralysis or another "hard" sign that could be caused by a neck injury.
E) All of the above are needed to clear the cervical spine clinically.

Table 1–1 TOXIDROMES

Drug Class	Examples	Signs and Symptoms
Anticholinergic	Tricyclics, diphenhydramine, scopolamine, loco weed (jimson weed), some mushrooms, etc.	Tachycardia, flushing, dilated pupils, low-grade temperature, and confusion. **Mnemonic:** Dry as a bone, red as a beet, mad as a hatter, blind as a bat
Opiates	Morphine, heroin, codeine, oxycodone, etc.	Pinpoint pupils, hypotension, hypopnea, coma, hypothermia
Cholinergic	Organophosphate or carbamate pesticides, some mushrooms	Lacrimation, salivation, muscle weakness, diarrhea, vomiting, miosis. **Mnemonic:** SLUDGE BBB (salivation, lacrimation, urination, diarrhea, GI upset, emesis . . . Bradycardia, bronchorrhea, bronchospasm).
Sympathomimetic	Cocaine, ecstasy, methamphetamine	Tachycardia, hypertension, elevated temperature, dilated pupils (mydriasis)
Gamma-hydroxybutyrate (GHB)	GHB, liquid ecstasy, etc.	Alternating coma with agitation, hypopnea while comatose, bradycardia while comatose, and myoclonus.

Discussion

The correct answer is "A." Patients can have lateral neck pain and still have their cervical spines cleared clinically. However, no one will fault you for obtaining radiographs in patients with lateral muscular (e.g., trapezius) neck pain. Patients with central neck pain (e.g., over the spinous processes) DO NEED radiographs to clear their cervical spine. All of the other criteria are required in order to clinically clear the cervical spine (Table 1–2).

HELPFUL TIP: The most common cause of missed fractures is an inadequate series of radiographs. An adequate series of radiographs for the cervical spine includes an AP film, a lateral film including the top of T-1, and an odontoid film. CT should be done if radiographs are negative and there is still clinical suspicion of a fracture. Flexion–extension views add little and should be avoided.

Table 1–2 CLEARING THE CERVICAL SPINE CLINICALLY

No central neck pain on questioning or palpation
No distracting, painful injury (e.g., bone fracture)
No symptoms or signs referable to the neck (paralysis, stinger-type injury, etc.)
Normal mental status including no drugs or alcohol. This includes any retrograde amnesia, etc.

The patient's daughter, aged 4 years, was in the same motor vehicle accident and also had her cervical spines cleared by radiograph. However, you get a call from the ED 48 hours after the initial accident that she is paralyzed from just above the nipple line down (never a good thing. . . . can the lawyers be far behind?). You review the initial radiographs with the radiologist, which are negative as is a CT of the cervical spine bones done after the onset of the paralysis.

The most likely cause of this patient's paralysis is:

A) Missed transection of the thoracic cord.
B) Conversion reaction from the psychological trauma of the accident.
C) Subarachnoid hemorrhage.
D) SCIWORA syndrome.

Discussion

The correct answer is "D." This likely represents SCIWORA syndrome (**s**pinal **c**ord **i**njury **w**ithout **r**adiologic **a**bnormality). This occurs from stretching of the cord secondary to flexion/extension-type of movement in an accident. Patients with SCIWORA syndrome may be paralyzed at the time of initial presentation (in the event of cord transection) or may have a delayed presentation up to 72 hours after the injury. Answer "A" is incorrect because a cord transection would present with paralysis immediately at the time of injury. Answer "B" is incorrect because this child is 4 years old, and conversion reaction is unlikely in children. Additionally, conversion reaction **IS ALWAYS** a diagnosis of exclusion. Answer "C" is incorrect because this is not the presentation of a subarachnoid hemorrhage (headache, stiff neck, perhaps focal neurologic symptoms).

The next step in the management of this patient is:

A) IV methylprednisolone to reduce cord edema.
B) Fluid restriction and diuretics to reduce cord edema.
C) Mannitol to reduce cord edema.
D) Neurosurgical intervention to decompress the cord.
E) None of the above.

Discussion

The correct answer is "A." Patients with a cord injury should be treated with IV methylprednisolone 30 mg/kg bolus (3 g in an adult!) followed by a 5.4 mg/kg drip for 24 hours. The efficacy of this therapy in spinal cord injury is limited, and its efficacy in SCIWORA is unknown. However, it is currently considered the standard of care. Neither diuretics nor mannitol will be useful in this situation. Answer "D" is incorrect because the process of SCIWORA involves stretching of the cord (and subsequent dysfunction) rather than cord compression such as would be seen with a bony injury.

The father is, understandably, irate that his child is now paralyzed. You can tell him that the natural history of SCIWORA syndrome in THIS CHILD is likely to be the following:

A) Continued paralysis with the necessity of long-term, permanent adaptation to the injury.
B) Progression of the injury over the next week to include further paralysis in an ascending fashion.
C) Resolution of paralysis and sensory symptoms over the next several months.
D) Resolution of all symptoms except sensory symptoms of the next several months.
E) Large lawsuit payout on the way. Do not pass go, do not collect $200, adjusted for inflation.

Discussion

The correct answer is "C." Generally, patients with SCIWORA syndrome regain their strength and sensory abilities over time. **However, this depends on when they present with symptoms!** Patients who present with paralysis right after the accident may have complete cord transection and thus will not regain function. For this reason, it is important to obtain an MRI on all patients with SCIWORA syndrome (and any trauma induced paralysis for that matter).

Objectives: Did you learn to . . .

- Clinically "clear" the cervical spine and decide when to order cervical spine radiographs?
- Describe causes of missed cervical spine fractures?
- Understand the physiology, natural history, and management of SCIWORA syndrome?

CASE 4

A hard-core alcoholic presents to the ED after drinking a bottle of automobile winter gas treatment (Rothschild Vintage 1954). He is intoxicated, has a headache, and describes a "misty" vision, such as might be seen during a snowstorm (if you live in southern Florida or California, call one of us in Iowa for a description). He is tachycardic and tachypneic. You start an IV and administer saline. You obtain a blood gas, which shows a mild metabolic acidosis.

A metabolic acidosis is consistent with all of the following ingestions EXCEPT:

A) Ethylene glycol.
B) Methanol.
C) Ethanol (e.g., vodka, gin).
D) Petroleum distillates (e.g., nonalcohol-containing gasoline products).

Discussion

The correct answer is "D." Ethylene glycol, methanol, and ethanol can all cause a metabolic acidosis. Hydrocarbons (e.g., gasoline products) do not cause a metabolic acidosis. The main manifestation of hydrocarbon toxicity is secondary to the inhalation of the hydrocarbon and the resulting pneumonitis.

* *

This patient's electrolytes are as follows: sodium 135 mEq/L, bicarbonate 12 mEq/L, chloride 108 mEq/L, BUN 12 mg/dL, Cr. 1.0 mg/dL.

This patient's anion gap is:

A) 13.
B) 15.

C) 23.
D) Unable to calculate the anion gap with the information provided.

Discussion
The correct answer is "B." By convention, the anion gap is calculated without using a major cation, potassium. Thus, the anion gap is calculated as follows:

sodium − (chloride + bicarbonate).

In this patient, the anion gap = 135 − (108 + 12) = 15.

The normal gap is 12 or less.

HELPFUL TIP: In methanol ingestions, the severity of acid–base disturbance is generally a better predictor of outcome than serum methanol levels.

All of the following are causes of an anion gap acidosis EXCEPT:

A) Lactic acidosis.
B) Diabetic ketoacidosis.
C) Renal tubular acidosis.
D) Uremia.
E) Ingestions such as methanol.

Discussion
The correct answer is "C." See Table 1–3 for more on causes of anion gap acidosis.

Which of the following findings IS NOT frequently seen in patients with methanol ingestion?

A) Hypopnea.
B) Optic disk abnormalities.
C) Abdominal pain and vomiting.
D) Basal ganglia hemorrhage.
E) Meningeal signs, such as nuchal rigidity.

Discussion
The correct answer is "A." Hypopnea is not commonly seen in methanol poisoning until the patient is close to death. In fact, the reverse is true. Tachypnea is a frequent finding in methanol overdose. This makes sense. The patient is trying to compensate for a metabolic acidosis by blowing off CO_2. Optic disk abnormalities, abdominal pain and vomiting, basal ganglia hemorrhage, and meningeal signs are all seen as part of methanol toxicity. It is thought that many of these signs and symptoms are secondary to central nervous system (CNS) hemorrhage.

* *

You can test for ethanol at your hospital but do not have a test for methanol on a stat basis and want to be sure that this patient is not just saying he has a methanol ingestion in order to obtain alcohol (a treatment for methanol ingestion—break out the single malt scotch!).

What test is most likely to help you determine if the patient has methanol ingestion?

A) Complete blood cell count (CBC).
B) BUN/creatinine.
C) Liver enzymes.
D) Serum osmolality.
E) Amylase and lipase.

Discussion
The correct answer is "D." With a measured serum osmolality, you can calculate the osmolar gap. What is done here is to subtract the total *measured* serum osmoles from the osmoles known to be due to ethanol (each 100 mg/dL of ethanol accounts for approximately 22 osmoles). If there is an elevated osmolar gap, it is evidence of a circulating, unmeasured osmole. In this case, it would be methanol. So, for example:

Measured serum osmolality = 368.

Blood alcohol = 200 mg/dL or about 44 osmoles.

Calculated osmolality = 2(Na) + BUN/2.8 + glucose/18 = 280 + 6 + 8 = 294.

So, osmolar gap = 368 − (294 + 44) = 30.

Table 1–3 CAUSES OF ACIDOSIS

Causes of an **elevated** anion gap acidosis	Lactic acidosis Diabetic ketoacidosis Ingestions such as ethanol, methanol, etc. Uremia Alcoholic ketoacidosis
Causes of a **normal** anion gap acidosis	GI bicarbonate loss (e.g., chronic diarrhea) Renal tubular acidosis (types I, II, and IV) Interstitial renal disease Ureterosigmoid loop Acetazolamide and other ingestions Small bowel drainage

This means that there are 30 unmeasured osmoles that could, in this case, represent methanol. Thus, we know that the patient is not simply drunk.

* *

You decide that there is sufficient evidence that this patient has ingested methanol to institute treatment.

Appropriate treatment(s) for this patient include:

A) Fomepizole (4-MP).
B) Cimetidine.
C) Ethanol.
D) A and C.
E) All of the above.

Discussion

The correct answer is "D." Both Fomepizole (4-MP) and ethanol are used for methanol ingestion. The idea is to slow down the metabolism of the methanol. The toxicity of methanol is caused by formic acid, which is a by-product of methanol metabolism. Ethanol is metabolized by alcohol dehydrogenase, the same enzyme that breaks down methanol. Thus, methanol metabolism is competitively inhibited by ethanol. The same holds true for fomepizole, which is a competitive inhibitor of alcohol dehydrogenase. Fomepizole and ethanol can both be used for ethylene glycol ingestion as well. "B" is incorrect. While cimetidine does reduce alcohol metabolism, the effect size is so small as to be negligible.

HELPFUL TIP: Hemodialysis should be available for any patient who has ingested methanol. Indications for hemodialysis include methanol level >50 mg/dL, severe and resistant acidosis, and renal failure.

Objectives: Did you learn to . . .

- Recognize manifestations of alcohol ingestion?
- Identify causes of metabolic acidosis with elevated and normal anion gaps?
- Use the osmolar gap to narrow down the differential diagnosis of metabolic acidosis?

QUICK QUIZ: BETA-BLOCKER OVERDOSE

Which of the following has been shown to be useful in beta-blocker overdose when conventional, adrenergic pressors are ineffective?

A) Calcium Chloride.
B) Glucagon.
C) Milrinone.
D) All of the above.

Discussion

The correct answer is "D." In beta-blocker overdoses, the following findings may be observed: bradycardia, AV block, hypotension, hypoglycemia, bronchospasm, nausea, and emesis. When an overdose has been identified, the usual treatments are employed (e.g., pressure support, airway protection, charcoal). If conventional pressors have failed, glucagon in a dose of 3–5 mg IV bolus and a drip at 1–5 mg/hr may be effective in treating beta-blocker overdose. It is generally preferred over atropine in this situation. Milrinone and other phosphodiesterase inhibitors may also be used but are considered third-line agent. Likewise, calcium is considered a third-line agent in beta-blocker overdose. Calcium chloride may potentiate the action of glucagon.

QUICK QUIZ: TOXICOLOGY

The best therapy for seizures secondary to isoniazid ingestion is:

A) Lorazepam.
B) Phenytoin.
C) Pyridoxine.
D) Thiamine.
E) Phenobarbital.

Discussion

The correct answer is "C." Isoniazid is a B-6 antagonist. Thus, pyridoxine (in massive doses!!) is the drug of choice in isoniazid-induced seizures. These seizures are often resistant to conventional therapy. Look for this type of overdose in patients who are being treated for tuberculosis (either active or latent disease).

QUICK QUIZ: TOXICOLOGY

Which of the following can be used to increase the metabolism of alcohol in an intoxicated patient?

A) IV fluids.
B) Charcoal.
C) Forced diuresis.

D) GABA antagonists such as flumazenil.
E) None of the above.

Discussion
The correct answer is "E." The rate of alcohol metabolism is fixed with zero-order kinetics at lower doses (fixed metabolic rate) and first-order kinetics at higher doses (rate proportional to levels). In general, this rate is in the range of 9–36 mg/dL/hr with 20 mg/dL/hr being the accepted norm. At this point, there are no available agents to increase the metabolism of ethanol. "B" is incorrect because ethanol is too rapidly absorbed for charcoal to be of any benefit.

CASE 5

A family of four comes into your ED after being exposed to carbon monoxide (CO). They were in an idling car and were running the engine and heater to stay warm. You want to get a carboxyhemoglobin level on the whole family but cannot get a blood gas from the youngest child.

What is your response?

A) Check an oxygen saturation, and if the oxygen saturation is normal, be reassured.
B) Check a venous carboxyhemoglobin level.
C) Check a venous carboxyhemoglobin and correct for the difference between venous and arterial samples.
D) None of the above.

Discussion
The correct answer is "B." A venous carboxyhemoglobin is just as accurate as an arterial carboxyhemoglobin—in fact, no correction is needed, which is why "C" is wrong—and it is much less painful to draw. "A" is incorrect because the pulse oximeter does not reflect hypoxia in carbon monoxide poisoning. Thus, pulse oximetry is useless in determining the carboxyhemoglobin level.

When determining which patients need hyperbaric oxygen on the basis of a carboxyhemoglobin level, the level to rely upon is:

A) The carboxyhemoglobin level on arrival to the ED.
B) The carboxyhemoglobin level at 4 hours after exposure.
C) The carboxyhemoglobin level projected to "time zero" (e.g., at the time of exposure).
D) None of the above.

Discussion
The correct answer is "C." A major consideration regarding the initiation of hyperbaric oxygen therapy is the patient's clinical situation. More severely ill patients with CO poisoning (e.g., severe acidosis, unconscious, unresponsive) should be considered candidates for hyperbaric oxygen. Also, treatment should be based on the carboxyhemoglobin level projected to time zero. This is the level that gives the most accurate information about the degree of exposure. The rest of the answers are incorrect.

* *

The father has a headache and a time zero carboxyhemoglobin level of 12%. The mother, who is pregnant, is asymptomatic and has a carboxyhemoglobin level of 16%, and one of the children, age 6, has a level of 18% while another has a carboxyhemoglobin level of 23% and was asymptomatic at the scene.

The first step in the treatment of these patients is:

A) Start an IV and administer saline.
B) Start *N*-acetylcysteine, which is a free radical scavenger.
C) Start continuous positive airway pressure (CPAP) to maximize airflow by keeping the airways from collapsing.
D) Administer 100% oxygen.
E) Intubate the most severe patient, 100% oxygen for the others.

Discussion
The correct answer is "D." Because CO competitively binds to hemoglobin in place of oxygen and in fact has greater affinity for hemoglobin than oxygen, high-flow 100% oxygen is the cornerstone of treating CO poisoning. Thus, *the first step in CO poisoning is to administer 100% oxygen*. The rest of the answers are incorrect. If the patient is not ventilating well and requires intubation, this would be appropriate. However, in our patients who are breathing well, there will be no advantage (and a substantial downside) to intubation.

Which of the following can be seen with carbon monoxide poisoning?

A) Rhabdomyolysis.
B) Cardiac ischemia.

C) Long-term neurologic sequelae, including dementia.
D) Pulmonary edema.
E) All of the above.

Discussion

The correct answer is "E." All of the above can be seen with carbon monoxide poisoning. Additional findings include acidosis, seizures, syncope, and headache. "C" deserves a bit more discussion. Long-term neurologic sequelae can develop from days to months after the exposure and include cognitive deficits, focal neurologic deficits, movement disorders, and personality changes. It appears that using hyperbaric oxygen in the appropriate patient can reduce long-term neurologic sequelae.

* *

Your closest diving chamber is about 90 minutes away and will hold only one patient at a time. You need to make a decision about who to send for hyperbaric oxygen.

Which patient will benefit most from hyperbaric oxygen therapy?

A) Asymptomatic pregnant mother, time zero carboxyhemoglobin of 16%.
B) Asymptomatic 6-year-old, time zero carboxyhemoglobin of 18%.
C) Asymptomatic 8-year-old, time zero carboxyhemoglobin of 23%.
D) Adult male with mild headache only, time zero carboxyhemoglobin level of 12%.

Discussion

The correct answer is "A." Generally accepted criteria for hyperbaric oxygen include mental status changes, carboxyhemoglobin level >25%, acidosis, cardiovascular disease, and age >60. Obviously, these are relative criteria. An otherwise normal 61-year-old with a mild exposure need not have HBO. *Pregnancy is an indication for HBO therapy* because fetal hemoglobin has a high affinity for carbon monoxide and the fetus is highly susceptible to carbon monoxide.

All of the following are well-established consequences of hyperbaric oxygen EXCEPT?

A) Seizures.
B) Psychosis.
C) Myopia.
D) Ear and pulmonary barotraumas.
E) Direct pulmonary oxygen toxicity.

Discussion

The correct answer is "B." All of the rest are found as a result of hyperbaric oxygen. "C," myopia, is actually found in up to 20% of patients being treated with hyperbaric oxygen. It is due to direct toxicity of oxygen on the lens and usually recovers within weeks to months.

Objectives: Did you learn to . . .

- Diagnose and manage patients with carbon monoxide poisoning?
- Describe complications of carbon monoxide poisoning?
- Identify patients who may benefit from hyperbaric oxygen therapy?
- Describe the complications of hyperbaric oxygen therapy?

CASE 6

A 50-year-old immigrant from a country in the developing world is brought to your ED after being bitten by a stray dog. The bite was unprovoked and is on the abdomen. The patient has no other health history of note and has not taken antibiotics for over a year. You irrigate the wound and are deciding about closure. There is a 3-cm laceration on the abdomen.

All of the following are true about dog bites EXCEPT:

A) They tend to be primarily crush-type injuries.
B) In general, the infection rate is similar to a laceration from any other mechanism (e.g., knife cut), except on the hands and feet.
C) A common organism in infected dog bites is *Staphylococcus aureus*.
D) Primary closure of dog bite wounds is an acceptable option (except perhaps on the hands and feet).
E) They always require antibiotics.

Discussion

The correct answer is "E." All of the rest are true statements. Dog bites (except for those from little poodles named Fifi) tend to be crush injuries (as contrasted with cat bites, which are primarily puncture wounds). The infection rate is about the same as other lacerations. Bites on the hands and feet tend to have a higher rate of infection. Most dog bite infections are polymicrobial with *S. aureus* playing a large role, and *Pasteurella* and *Capnocytophaga* playing a smaller but significant roles. Other organisms include *Streptococcal* species and gram-negative species. Dog bites do not generally require antibiotic prophylaxis, except under certain circumstances (e.g., present >9 hours after bite, immunocompromised, large or complicated wound).

You are concerned about rabies prophylaxis. Which of the following is the best next step?

A) Isolate the suspect animal for 3 days.
B) Sacrifice the suspect animal and examine the liver.
C) Administer rabies immune globulin IM.
D) Administer rabies immune globulin IV followed by rabies vaccination series.
E) Administer rabies immune globulin by infiltrating it around the wound followed by rabies vaccination series.

Discussion

The correct answer is "E." You should infiltrate rabies immune globulin around the wound and then begin the rabies vaccination series. As much of the immune globulin as possible should be infiltrated around the wound and the rest should be given IM at a different site. "A" is incorrect because animals need to be isolated for *10 days*, not 3. "B" is incorrect. The animal can be sacrificed but the brain should be examined—not the liver. "C" and "D" are both incorrect methods of administering the vaccine/immune globulin.

Which of the following requires rabies prophylaxis in all cases?

A) Stray rabbit bites.
B) Stray rat bites.
C) Stray bat bites.
D) Stray squirrel bites.
E) Stray snake bites.

Discussion

The correct answer is "C." All bats should be considered rabid unless available for observation and testing. See Table 1–4 below for detailed recommendations. Also see the CDC Web site for information about rates of infection in wild animals in your area.

Table 1–4 GUIDELINES FOR RABIES PROPHYLAXIS

General Rule	Animals
Always assume rabid unless available for testing	Foxes, bats, raccoons, skunks, dogs, cats, ferrets, other carnivores
Judge on an individual basis	Rodents (rats, mice, etc.), lagomorphs (rabbits, etc.), squirrels
Never require rabies prophylaxis	Nonmammals (snakes, lizards, etc.)

HELPFUL TIP: Patients should receive a tetanus booster every 10 years. For a contaminated wound, the tetanus booster should be documented within the last 5 years. Patients should receive at least one dose of Tdap (tetanus, diphtheria, and acellular pertussis) between ages 11 and 18 and a single dose between ages 18 and 64. In addition, health-care workers and those >65 years of age who will be around infants should receive a single dose of Tdap.

HELPFUL TIP: If a patient at risk for tetanus has not had a primary series of tetanus immunizations, administer tetanus immune globulin *and* start the primary tetanus series.

* *

You have irrigated this patient's wound.

Which of the following statements is true about irrigating a wound and subsequent risk of wound infections?

A) Povidone-iodine as a 50% irrigation solution (e.g., Betadine) in the wound will decrease the infection rate.
B) Irrigation with normal saline is the only recommended method of cleaning a wound.
C) Irrigation with normal saline and irrigation with tap water are equally effective in reducing wound infection rates.
D) Use of epinephrine with lidocaine in a wound increases the rate of infection.

E) Irrigation of a wound with either alcohol or hydrogen peroxide will reduce the rate of wound infection.

Discussion

The correct answer is "C." Infection rates are the same whether the wound is irrigated with normal saline or tap water. **We are not recommending that you start using tap water as an irrigation solution!** This is **not** standard of care although it is just as effective. "A" is incorrect. Povidone-iodine is toxic to tissue and polymorphonuclear leukocytes and actually may **increase** infection rates unless a solution of 1% or less is used. Full strength povidone-iodine **can** be used on intact skin as a cleanser but should not be used in a wound. "B" is incorrect because other solutions (poloxamer 188, balanced salt solutions, etc.) can be used but are more expensive and do not offer any benefit in reduction in infection rates. "D" and "E" are both incorrect. As with povidone-iodine, alcohol may be used for cleaning skin but should be kept out of the wound. It is toxic to tissue and acts a fixative. Hydrogen peroxide is also toxic to tissue and should not be used in open wounds.

How long after a laceration occurs can the wound be closed primarily?

A) 6 hours.
B) 12 hours.
C) 18 hours.
D) 24 hours.
E) Any of the above can be correct depending on the wound.

Discussion

The correct answer is "E." There is no arbitrary time limit to when a wound can be closed. Facial wounds may be closed up to 24 hours after injury for cosmetic reasons, while you may not want to close other, contaminated wounds more than 12 hours after injury. Some wounds you may not want to close at all (e.g., bites to the hand, wounds contaminated with grease, wounds contaminated with manure), rather allowing them to close by secondary intention.

Objectives: Did you learn to . . .

- Describe the indications for rabies prophylaxis?
- Recognize the issues that arise with animal bites and indications for closure and/or prophylactic antibiotics?
- List recommendations for tetanus prophylaxis?
- Use various wound irrigation solutions for cleansing wounds?
- Decide upon the time frame for wound closure?

CASE 7

A 52-year-old male presents to your ED via ambulance complaining of a headache after a fall. He was working and fell approximately 10 feet. He notes no injury except for head and neck pain. A quick survey reveals that he has a BP of 128/86, pulse 100, and respirations 12. There was no loss of consciousness at the scene. He "saw stars" and was clumsy, dazed, and slow at the scene without any focal neurologic deficit. He is now back to his baseline.

A concussion is defined as:

A) Any neurologic symptoms (e.g., clumsy, dazed, or slow) after head injury.
B) Loss of consciousness followed by return to baseline.
C) Loss of consciousness with continued neurologic symptoms.
D) Requires confusion after head trauma regardless of whether the patient lost consciousness or not.
E) Any traumatic injury to the head.

Discussion

The correct answer is "A." A concussion is defined as *any* neurologic symptom after head trauma. Note that a concussion does not require a loss of consciousness. For this reason, "B" and "C" are incorrect. "D" is incorrect because manifestations of concussion are not limited to confusion but also include protracted vomiting, transient amnesia, slowed mentation, "dizziness," and other neurologic symptoms. "E" is incorrect because by definition, a concussion requires neurologic symptoms.

* *

Your patient opens his eyes on his own, follows commands, answers all orientation questions correctly, but appears unsteady when ambulating.

His Glasgow Coma Scale (GCS) is:

A) 5.
B) 10.
C) 14.
D) 15.
E) 20.

Table 1–5 GLASGOW COMA SCALE

Eye opening Mnemonic: "4 eyes"	Spontaneous = 4 To speech = 3 To pain = 2 No response = 1
Verbal response Mnemonic: "Jackson 5"	Alert and oriented = 5 Disoriented conversation = 4 Nonsensical speech = 3 Moaning = 2 No response = 1
Motor response Mnemonic: "Six cylinders"	Follows commands = 6 Localizes pain = 5 Withdraws from pain = 4 Decorticate flexion = 3 Decerebrate extension = 2 No response = 1

Discussion

The correct answer is "D." The GCS is a scale used to indicate the severity of neurologic dysfunction and is often applied to victims of head trauma. Remember, however, that it does not predict mortality or morbidity but is only used as a descriptive scale of the patient's current state. Only the maximum score of 15 is considered a normal GCS. There are three components to the GCS, listed in Table 1–5.

HELPFUL TIP: My chair and refrigerator each have a GCS of 3. Remember that *nothing* can have a GCS less than 3.

Independent of other factors, an entirely normal GCS score of 15 indicates that:

A) The patient does not require a head CT scan.
B) There is essentially no possibility that this patient has an intracranial injury requiring surgical intervention.
C) There is little or no possibility that this patient has any focal intracranial bleed.
D) There is up to a 4% chance this patient will need neurosurgical intervention.
E) None of the above.

Discussion

The correct answer is "D." In appropriately selected patients (e.g., those with a significant mechanism of injury), about 18% with a GCS of 15 will have some intracranial lesion, and up to 4% will eventually require neurosurgical intervention. These are generally patients who have a depressed skull fracture but a normal GCS. "A" is incorrect since a normal GCS in and of itself does not allow one to forgo head CT in patients with a significant mechanism of injury. "B" and "C" are also incorrect for the reasons noted earlier. Remember that the GCS is *not* linear; a GCS of 14 is bad. Patients with a GCS of 14 *must* have a CT scan—unless another factor in the clinical decision making dictates otherwise (e.g., dementia, the finding is preexisting).

In an adult patient with a significant head injury, which of the following is NOT an indication for a head CT scan?

A) Intoxication with drugs or alcohol.
B) Vomiting once or more.
C) Amnesia or memory deficit.
D) Age greater than 40.
E) Seizure.

Discussion

The correct answer is "D." Older patients are at greater risk of developing serious intracranial injuries, but the age of 60 years or greater is usually used as an indication. While there is no "upper limit of normal" for vomiting after head trauma, the best data available suggest that any vomiting after head trauma in an *adult* indicates the need for a head CT scan. The currently recommended criteria for a CT of the head in various age groups are listed in Table 1–6.

* *

You are going to transfer this patient for neurosurgical intervention to drain the subdural hematoma. It is about a 4-hour drive by ambulance to the nearest facility that has a neurosurgeon.

Which of the following is indicated as prophylaxis against increased intracranial pressure in this patient?

A) Hyperventilation after intubation.
B) IV mannitol.
C) Keeping the head of the bed elevated at 30 degrees.
D) IV dexamethasone.
E) None of the above.

Discussion

The correct answer is "E." None of the above is indicated as prophylaxis for increased intracranial pressure. "A" is incorrect for two reasons. First, this patient does not need to be intubated. Second,

Table 1–6 INDICATIONS FOR HEAD CT SCAN BY AGE

Patient Age	Indications for Head CT Scan After Trauma with a Significant Mechanism
Adult	• Intoxication • Age >60 • Any memory deficit • Vomiting (number of times undefined) • Seizure • Headache
Children >2 yr	• Loss of consciousness • Amnesia • Seizure • Headache • Persistent vomiting • Irritability • Behavioral changes
Children <2 yr, >3 mo	Any of the above as well as: • Any unusual behavior • Large scalp hematoma
Children <3 mo	Any of the above as well as: • A significant mechanism • Any scalp hematoma

routine hyperventilation as prophylaxis for increased intracranial pressure is of no benefit. This has been well studied. What happens is that hyperventilation *does* cause vasoconstriction reducing intracranial blood flow and therefore intracranial pressure. However, hyperventilation also causes ischemia around the area of the injury and may worsen outcomes. "B" is incorrect because prophylactic mannitol, like prophylactic hyperventilation, confers no benefit. "C" is incorrect. Elevating the head of the bed not only reduce intracranial pressure but also reduces perfusion pressure and is therefore a wash; there is no discernible benefit. "D" is incorrect since steroids are not useful acutely in *head trauma* (vs. spinal cord trauma). However, steroids are useful in cerebral edema secondary to tumor.

HELPFUL TIP: About two-thirds of patients with a mild head injury (not deemed severe enough to obtain a CT scan) will have some measurable decrement in function at 1 month secondary to postconcussion syndrome (*J Emerg Med* 2011;40:262).

Objectives: Did you learn to . . .

- Use the GCS?
- Recognize which patients with head trauma are appropriate for head CT scan?
- Manage patients presenting with potential intracranial injuries?

CASE 8

A 23-year-old male is in a bar fight. He only had two beers and was just standing there minding his own business when he was jumped by those infamous "2 dudes" (yeah, right!). He presents to you about 1 hour after the event with facial trauma. His vitals are normal and he is mentating well (with the exception of some impaired judgment secondary to the alcohol). His blood alcohol level is 150 mg/dL, showing that he is legally intoxicated. On exam, you notice that the patient has some epistaxis and a quite swollen nose. Additionally, there is one avulsed tooth and one tooth that is displaced.

The best way to transport an avulsed tooth is:

A) In sterile water.
B) In the buccal mucosa after thorough washing with soap.
C) In a glass of milk.
D) Wrapped in saline-soaked gauze.
E) Under a pillow.

Discussion

The correct answer is "C." The best way to transport an avulsed tooth is either (1) in a glass of milk or (2) in the buccal mucosa or under the tongue in a patient in whom the risk of aspiration is not a concern. "A" is incorrect because sterile water is hypotonic and may damage the tooth root decreasing the success rate of reimplantation. "B" is incorrect because *washing the tooth with soap* is not appropriate. Again, you want to maintain the viability of the root if possible. "D" is incorrect as well. If this is the only option available to you, it is better than nothing, but a glass of milk or under the buccal mucosa is preferred. "E" is fine only if you are a tooth fairy.

* *

You call the dentist who is (of course) out of town. A dentist will not be available for at least 12 hours.

Your best course of action at this point is:

A) Continue to keep the tooth viable in a glass of milk.
B) Continue to keep the tooth viable in the buccal mucosa.
C) Clean the tooth and keep it sterile and dry for reimplantation in 12 hours realizing that a bridge will probably be needed to hold the tooth in position.
D) Reinsert the tooth into the socket yourself.

Discussion

The correct answer is "D." If there is going to be any delay in reimplantation by a dentist, the best course of action is to reinsert the tooth into the socket yourself. "A," "B," and "C" are all incorrect because they will reduce the rate of successful reimplantation.

> HELPFUL TIP: **Primary teeth should not be reinserted into the socket!** They ankylose to the bone preventing the eruption of the permanent tooth and cause a cosmetic deformity.

> HELPFUL TIP: Any patient who is in the ED, says he only had three beers, and was minding his own business is probably not telling the truth on either account...

* *

You now turn your attention to this patient's nose. You are trying to decide whether or not to do a radiograph of the patient's nose.

The BEST timing for a radiograph of the nose is:

A) As soon as possible after the trauma once other injuries are stabilized and more important problems are addressed.
B) As soon as possible to assure that there are no bone fragments threatening the brain.
C) There is no need for a radiograph acutely. You can wait for 3 or 4 days.
D) There is never any indication for nasal radiographs.

Discussion

The correct answer is "C." There is no need for radiographs acutely except in extraordinary circumstances. The reasons for a radiograph are to document a fracture *and* to assist in reduction. Because of swelling, it is difficult to get a good cosmetic result reducing a nasal fracture acutely. Thus, a radiograph is indicated in 3–4 days *only* if there is evidence of nasal deformity once swelling has resolved. If there is good cosmesis and the patient can breathe through his (they are almost always male...) nose, a radiograph is unnecessary just to document a fracture. "A" and "B" are incorrect because, as noted earlier, there is no reason to do a radiograph at all unless there is evidence of deformity once the swelling is resolved. "D" is incorrect for the reasons noted earlier.

You get the epistaxis stopped and examine the nasal mucosa. Which one of these is considered an emergency?

A) Closed nasal fracture.
B) Septal hematoma.
C) Trauma to Kiesselbach plexus.
D) A deviated septum.

Discussion

The correct answer is "B." A septal hematoma is considered an emergency. The problem is that the perichondrium, which supplies nutrition to the septum, is no longer in contact with the septum because of the intervening hematoma. Thus, the septal cartilage can necrose leading to a perforated septum. Septal hematomas should be drained acutely and the nose packed to keep the perichondrium in contact with the septal cartilage. "A" is incorrect (see previous question). "C" is incorrect. Kiesselbach plexus is in the anterior nose and is a venous plexus. Bleeding is easily controlled and generally is self-limited. "D," a deviated septum, may indicate an underlying fracture but in and of itself is not an emergency.

* *

You continue to evaluate this patient and note that he has the loss of upward gaze in the right eye, the side on which he was hit. All of the other extraocular motions are intact.

The most likely diagnosis in this patient is:

A) Blowout fracture with entrapment of the inferior rectus.
B) Blowout fracture with dysfunction of the superior rectus.

C) Injury to cranial nerve III, which controls the superior AND inferior rectus muscles.
D) Volitional refusal to perform upward gaze on the right side in this intoxicated patient.

Discussion

The correct answer is "A." The most likely diagnosis is blowout fracture with entrapment of the inferior rectus. The force of a blow to the globe is transmitted to the inferior orbital wall, which is the weakest point in the orbit. This can cause entrapment of the contents of the inferior orbit, including the inferior rectus, causing an inability to perform upward gaze. Due to disconjugate gaze, patients with entrapment of the inferior rectus muscle from a blowout fracture may complain of diplopia. "B" is incorrect because a blowout fracture generally refers to the inferior orbital wall, which would not entrap the superior rectus. Additionally, patients with an entrapped superior rectus would have difficulty with downward gaze. "C" is incorrect because it is unlikely that being hit in the face would cause an injury to CN III. Additionally, a CN III lesion would affect all extraocular muscles except for the lateral rectus (CN VI) and the superior oblique (CN IV). "D" is incorrect because it is impossible to move the eyes independently of one another unless you are a chameleon or particularly talented.

> HELPFUL TIP: Fluid in the maxillary sinus on radiograph is considered presumptive evidence of a blowout fracture given the proper clinical scenario. You may also see fat and other tissue herniated into the sinus in the area of the fracture even if the fracture itself is not visible. If there is any question, CT scan should resolve the issue.

* *

The patient has had a long night of partying, and it is 3:00 Saturday morning when you call your consultant about the blowout fracture. The consultant is not happy about being called for an intoxicated patient at 3:00 AM and refuses to see the patient acutely. He wants you to send him to the office in 3 days (Tuesday morning).

Your response is:

A) To call another consultant; a blowout fracture should be attended to immediately.
B) Do nothing; evaluation in 2–3 days for a blowout fracture, even with inferior rectus entrapment, is appropriate.
C) Start steroids to reduce muscle edema to facilitate the spontaneous release of the entrapped muscle.
D) Start antibiotics and hospitalize the patient so that he can be seen in the morning when the consultant makes rounds.
E) Stick pins in a voodoo doll of your consultant.

Discussion

The correct answer is "B." While blowout fractures with muscle entrapment require close follow-up, there is no need to intervene acutely. In fact, a decision to operate may be delayed for up to 14 days. If the entrapment spontaneously resolves when the swelling goes down (not uncommon) and there is no diplopia or other complicating symptoms, surgery is not needed. The other answers are all incorrect because acute intervention is not required in this patient. "E," however, may be of some benefit... depending on your voodoo skills.

> HELPFUL TIP: **Caveat to the above: In the pediatric population, immediate surgical repair should be undertaken in trapdoor fractures.** A trapdoor fracture is one in which there is significant entrapment of the inferior rectus muscle. If the muscle is left entrapped in the pediatric population, restriction and fibrosis may occur, so immediate evaluation by a surgeon is warranted. **Oral steroids** at a dose of 1 mg/kg may decrease edema in the first 7 days limiting ultimate fibrosis. In patients with significant sinus disease, antibiotics may be considered, usually a penicillin or cephalosporin.

* *

The patient mentioned above has a friend who was also in the altercation. He, too, was just minding his business—like everyone in the bar—until there was a gentleman's disagreement that could only be resolved with a broken bottle. He has a simple laceration of the chin, which you repair. This patient has a blood alcohol level of 150 mg/dL (the legal limit in most states is 80 mg/dL). Since he is intoxicated, the nurses are reluctant to allow the patient to leave because of liability issues. He seems initially very cooperative and competent. However, the nurse manager reminds you of the legal issues. The patient is getting more agitated; he wants to go home.

Your response is:

A) Sedate the patient with haloperidol and observe him until sober.
B) Sedate the patient with a benzodiazepine and observe him until sober.
C) Call the police to remove this patient from your ED.
D) Use restraints on the patient and observe him until sober, as sedative drugs may prolong time in the ED.
E) Let the patient leave the ED with a competent adult.

Discussion

The correct answer is "E." The patient was initially cooperative and competent. Competence *is not* based on a blood alcohol level but rather on your judgment of the patient's ability to make rational decisions. We allow patients on narcotics to make decisions about their care all of the time despite having narcotics on board. There are patients who will be competent and safe at a blood alcohol of 200 mg/dL and others who may be impaired at 80 mg/dL. So, judge competence individually.

Objectives: Did you learn to . . .

- Treat acute dental trauma?
- Diagnose and manage nasal and periorbital trauma?
- Care for the intoxicated patient with minor trauma?

CASE 9

A 17-year-old female fell asleep with her contact lenses in her eyes last evening. This morning she notes quite a bit of eye pain and photophobia. You evert the eyelids (something that should be done in all cases) and find no evidence of a foreign body. When you stain her eye, you find a corneal ulcer.

The treatment for this patient is:

A) Debridement with a burr and systemic antibiotics.
B) Debridement with a cotton swab and systemic antibiotics.
C) Topical antibiotics, cycloplegia, and referral to ophthalmology.
D) Copious irrigation, systemic antibiotics, and cycloplegia.

Discussion

The correct answer is "C." This is an ophthalmologic emergency that requires topical antibiotics, cycloplegia (for pain control), and referral to an ophthalmologist. These ulcers can become quite deep and result in a ruptured globe.

* *

You consult with your ophthalmologist who would like you start a cycloplegic agent in this patient prior to transfer.

The drug you would choose for a cycloplegic agent is:

A) Pilocarpine eye drops.
B) Timolol eye drops (e.g., Timoptic).
C) Tetracaine eye drops.
D) Cyclopentolate eye drops.

Discussion

The correct answer is "D." Cyclopentolate is the only cycloplegic agent listed above. Cycloplegic agents paralyze the ciliary muscle so the eye cannot accommodate. Pilocarpine is a miotic agent. Timolol is a beta-blocker used in the treatment of glaucoma. Tetracaine eye drops are a topical anesthetic. Thus, "D" is the only correct answer. **Other cycloplegic agents include homoatropine and atropine. However, these have a prolonged effect.**

If your patient just had a simple corneal abrasion, you would not have had to think so hard! Regarding corneal abrasions, you realize that:

A) Patching an eye after a corneal abrasion reduces pain and promotes healing.
B) If a topical antibiotic is needed after a large corneal abrasion, gentamicin ophthalmic ointment is the drug of choice.

C) Tetracaine is a good topical anesthetic and should be considered for home use in patients with a painful corneal abrasion.
D) Patients should avoid wearing contact lenses until the eye has been healed for at least a week.

Discussion

The correct answer is "D." "A" is incorrect because patching an eye may actually increase pain and decrease healing. Whether or not to use a patch should be a matter of patient comfort only. "B" is incorrect because gentamicin ophthalmic ointment (as well as other topical aminoglycosides) actually reduces healing of the cornea, and antibiotics are not necessary unless there are signs of infection. "C" is incorrect because patients should never be sent home with a topical anesthetic. They reduce healing and can lead to further injury if the patient, whose eyes are now insensate, continues a harmful activity, rubs his/her eyes, etc.

> HELPFUL TIP: To differentiate a topical ophthalmologic problem from iritis, put in some tetracaine. If the pain resolves, it is likely, **but does not prove,** that the problem is superficial (e.g., corneal abrasion). Posttraumatic iritis is manifested by ciliary flare, anterior chamber cells, and marked photophobia. These patients really need a slit lamp exam.

Objectives: Did you learn to . . .

- Recognize a corneal ulceration and treat it appropriately?
- Treat corneal abrasions?
- Understand the proper use of cycloplegic agents?

QUICK QUIZ: EYE TRAUMA

You are on call for your group and a welder who was welding and grinding presents at 2:00 AM with severe bilateral eye pain. When he left work at 5:00 PM the day before, he did not notice any problem. He notes that he was wearing his dark goggles some of the time while he was welding but did quite a bit of work without goggles as well.

The most likely diagnosis in this patient is:

A) Foreign body.
B) Ultraviolet (UV) keratitis.
C) Globe penetration secondary to the welding and a foreign body.
D) Iritis.

Discussion

The correct answer is "B." This patient likely has UV keratitis. The others are not likely because they generally present unilaterally. Additionally, in the cases of "A" and "C," they should present directly after the event rather than 9 hours later, as in our patient.

* *

UV keratitis is found in patients who are welders or have been out in the sun for an extended period of time (at the beach, skiing ("snow blindness"), tanning bed, etc.). UV keratitis generally presents as severe, bilateral, eye pain about 6–10 hours following the activity. It is treated with cycloplegic agents and pain medication, often requiring narcotics.

> HELPFUL TIP: Patients who have a foreign body in the eye following a high-speed injury (e.g., grinding wheel) should be assumed to have a globe perforation until proven otherwise.

QUICK QUIZ: ORTHOPEDIC EMERGENCIES

Which of the following is most commonly associated with significant vascular injury?

A) Pubic ramus fracture.
B) Knee dislocation.
C) Shoulder dislocation.
D) Elbow dislocation.
E) Ankle dislocation.

Discussion

The correct answer is "B." Knee dislocations (*not patellar dislocations*) are highly associated with injury to the popliteal artery. *All* patients who have had a dislocated knee should have an angiogram to document vascular integrity since vascular injury is a major cause of limb loss and morbidity. "A" is incorrect because pubic ramus fractures are relatively minor injuries without vascular involvement, requiring only pain control. Shoulder dislocations are commonly associated with injury to the axillary nerve. Elbow dislocations can be associated with injury to the median nerve and brachial artery. However, arterial injuries are much less common than with knee dislocations. Ankle dislocations are rarely associated with vascular injury.

CASE 10

A 55-year-old male farmer is injured by a cow that pins him against a fence. His leg was trapped against the fence for a several minutes. Being a typical midwestern farmer, he ignores the injury until later that afternoon when he presents to your office complaining of severe pain in the calf area. A radiograph is normal, and the patient has normal distal pulses. The calf (his leg, not the cow) is tender with increased pain on passive stretch. His pain seems to be out of proportion to his injury.

Which of the following is true?

A) Since the patient has excellent pulses, a compartment syndrome is not likely.
B) Compartment syndrome is defined as compartment pressure >30 mm Hg.
C) Compartment syndrome is only associated with significant crush injuries or fractures.
D) Pain out of proportion to the injury is a red flag for compartment syndrome.
E) His calf (the leg, not the cow) likely has mad cow disease.

Discussion

The correct answer is "D." Pain out of proportion to the injury is a red flag for compartment syndrome. "A" is incorrect because pulses can be maintained until there is significant increase in compartment pressures and significant injury to muscle and nerves. "B" is incorrect because it is difficult to define a specific cut off for compartment syndrome. Some patients tolerate higher pressures and others cannot tolerate 30 mm Hg (normal compartment pressure is zero). However, when the pressure gets above 20–30 mg Hg, strong consideration should be given to the presence of compartment syndrome. "C" is incorrect. Compartment syndrome can be due to a number of factors including electrical injury, excessive muscle use, tetany, reperfusion after ischemia, etc.

HELPFUL TIP: The classic findings of arterial insufficiency (the "5 Ps" being pulselessness, paresthesia, pallor, pain, and paralysis) are often considered necessary for there to be compartment syndrome. This is incorrect. Of these, pain is often the only symptom; the second most frequent would be paresthesia. If your patient has compartment syndrome with the 5 Ps present, there is likely extensive injury.

* *

You decide that it is likely that this patient has a compartment syndrome.

Which of the following labs will be the most helpful in guiding treatment for this patient?

A) CBC.
B) Urinalysis.
C) Glucose.
D) Sodium.
E) PT/PTT.

Discussion

The correct answer is "B." One of the major complications of compartment syndrome is rhabdomyolysis. This will manifest itself as a urine which is dipstick positive for blood but with a negative microscopic exam for red blood cells. The positive dipstick is picking up myoglobin in the urine. This can be confirmed by a serum CPK. CBC, glucose, sodium, and coagulation studies may be appropriate depending on the clinical situation but are not useful in establishing the presence of myoglobinuria.

HELPFUL TIP: Myoglobin can be measured in the urine. However, many laboratories have stopped doing this test favoring the positive dipstick/negative microscopic exam approach. **There can be heme positive dipstick findings.** Thus, check a CPK as well if rhabdomyolysis is a consideration.

* *

The patient has a positive dipstick for blood with no red blood cells on microscopic exam (presumptive myoglobinuria). His serum CPK is 32,000, which is well above five times the upper limit of normal, so you make the diagnosis of rhabdomyolysis.

The most common adverse consequence and greatest danger of rhabdomyolysis is:

A) Disseminated intravascular coagulation.
B) Acute renal failure.
C) Seizure from hypocalcemia.
D) Acute gout from hyperuricemia.
E) Cardiac arrhythmia from hyperkalemia.

Discussion

The correct answer is "B." Myoglobin precipitates in the renal tubules causing acute renal failure. "A," DIC, can occur but is rare. "C," seizures from hypocalcemia, has not been reported in this condition, nor has "D," gout. The potassium elevation from rhabdomyolysis generally does not reach a level sufficient to cause arrhythmias.

The primary treatment for rhabdomyolysis is:

A) Mannitol infusion.
B) Saline infusion.
C) Furosemide.
D) Dialysis.

Discussion

The correct answer is "B." The most important treatment for rhabdomyolysis is saline infusion with alkalinization of the urine (using sodium bicarbonate). "A," mannitol, can be used to increase urine flow, but this is really a treatment that is secondary to good hydration and urine alkalinization. "C," furosemide, is not used in rhabdomyolysis. Loop diuretics will actually acidify the urine and are contraindicated. "D," dialysis, is what we are trying to avoid using saline.

> HELPFUL TIP: In patients with rhabdomyolysis, try to maintain urine output of 200–300 cc/hr for an adult. Alkalinize the urine using sodium bicarbonate. Remember that in order to alkalinize the urine you have to maintain an adequate serum potassium level, otherwise the body will reabsorb potassium in exchange for hydrogen ions causing urine acidification.

* *

The patient is able to maintain urine output after you institute saline.

What treatment are you going to suggest for the underlying compartment syndrome?

A) Fasciotomy.
B) Immobilization and traction.
C) Hot packs and elevation of the affected limb.
D) Ice and elevation of the affected limb.

Discussion

The correct answer is "A." The treatment of compartment syndrome is fasciotomy. A rapid surgical or orthopedic consultation is critical in the treatment of compartment syndrome.

* *

The patient does well and everyone is happy ... except for the cow who finds his way onto the table as the centerpiece of Christmas dinner.

Objectives: Did you learn to . . .

- Recognize manifestations of compartment syndrome and understand that compartment syndrome can be present with pain alone?
- Identify patients at risk for compartment syndrome and rhabdomyolysis?
- Manage compartment syndrome?
- Diagnose and treat rhabdomyolysis?

CASE 11

A 24-year-old African American male presents to the ED complaining of fever, chills, and dyspnea. He has chest pain that is respirophasic ("pleuritic") in nature. He is noted to be tachypneic with a respiratory rate of 36 and an oxygen saturation of 90%. He has a history of sickle cell disease and has had a number of sickle cell crises in the past. He is up to date on immunizations, including *Streptococcus pneumoniae* and *Haemophilus influenzae* vaccines.

The patient's current symptoms are MOST suggestive of:

A) Pneumothorax.
B) Pulmonary embolism.
C) Acute chest syndrome.
D) Sickle cell–related pericarditis.

Discussion

The correct answer is "C." This patient likely has acute chest syndrome, which is associated with sickle cell anemia *and may be indistinguishable from pneumonia*. Acute chest syndrome is characterized by pleuritic chest pain, fever, cough, chills, dyspnea, rales, and rhonchi. The etiology is unknown, but it may be secondary to infarction of the lung and/or fat emboli.

All of the following are recommended in the initial treatment of acute chest syndrome EXCEPT:

A) Hydroxyurea.
B) Oxygen.
C) IV normal saline.
D) Morphine.

Discussion

The correct answer is "A." Hydroxyurea, while useful for the chronic treatment of sickle cell anemia, is not indicated for the treatment of acute chest syndrome. However, it can reduce the incidence of acute chest syndrome by 50% when used chronically. Other treatments include IV antibiotics to cover for community-acquired pneumonia (although acute chest syndrome is *not bacterial*). It is prudent to cover these patients with antibiotics because they are de facto splenectomized and the initial presentation of acute chest syndrome can be easily confused with pneumonia.

* *

The patient continues to be hypoxic despite your therapy. His CBC shows a slight elevation in the WBC count and a hemoglobin of 11 g/dL. A chest radiograph indicates progression of infiltrates.

The next step in treating this patient is:

A) Fresh frozen plasma.
B) Pentoxifylline.
C) Packed red blood cells.
D) Exchange transfusion.

Discussion

The correct answer is "D." Patients with acute chest syndrome who remain hypoxic with progressing infiltrates are candidates for exchange transfusion to bring the level of HbS to <30% of the total. Simply administering blood ("C") will not resolve the problem because HbS will still be present in significant amounts. If this patient had a more significant anemia, packed red cell transfusion would be a more viable option. "A" and "B" are also incorrect. Fresh frozen plasma has no role in the treatment of acute chest syndrome, nor does pentoxifylline.

* *

Your patient recovers from this episode. He has had numerous pain crises in the past, as well as hospitalizations for other reasons. You have an opportunity to provide some patient education. You answer a few of your patient's questions and then review potential manifestations of sickle cell disease.

Which of the following may be a manifestation of sickle cell disease?

A) Joint and bone pain.
B) Acute abdominal pain.
C) Acute sequestration syndrome.
D) Aplastic crisis.
E) All of the above.

Discussion

The correct answer is "E." All of the above can be associated with sickle cell anemia (keep reading for additional information . . .).

Which of the following infections is a common cause of aplastic crisis in sickle cell anemia?

A) Parvovirus B-19.
B) Influenza virus.
C) CMV virus.
D) Parainfluenza virus.
E) None of the above.

Discussion

The correct answer is "A." Patients with sickle cell anemia can develop aplastic anemia in response to a parvovirus B-19 infection. Also, Epstein–Barr virus and some bacteria have also been reported to cause aplastic crisis in patients with sickle cell anemia.

Acute sequestration syndrome is a manifestation of sickle cell anemia. In which group does acute sequestration syndrome occur?

A) Younger than 5 years.
B) 5–12 years old.
C) 12–25 years old.
D) Older than 25 years.

Discussion

The correct answer is "A." Acute sequestration syndrome occurs when the spleen sequesters red blood cells, leading to a drop in hemoglobin. The presentation can be quite dramatic with severe left upper quadrant pain, splenomegaly, and profound anemia, sometimes resulting in hypovolemic shock and death. Because it requires a functional spleen, it is most common in children younger than 5 years. Patient with sickle cell anemia who are older than 5 years generally do not have a functioning spleen; most often it has infarcted so that acute sequestration syndrome no longer occurs. The mortality is 15% per episode and 50% recur.

Objectives: Did you learn to . . .

- Recognize acute chest syndrome?
- Manage a patient with acute chest syndrome?
- Use exchange transfusion in a patient with sickle cell anemia?
- Recognize various other manifestations of sickle cell anemia?

CASE 12

A 52-year-old truck driver presents to your ED after being out in subzero (Fahrenheit) temperatures for several hours trying to repair his truck. He is hypothermic when you use a rectal thermometer with appropriate calibration ("Thanks for getting the most accurate temperature, doc!"). His initial core temperature is noted to be 28°C. He has a pulse of 24, a BP of 70/30, and slow mentation. He is awake, however, thus able to joke about a thermometer in his rectum.

The appropriate first-line treatment for this patient's profound bradycardia is:

A) Atropine.
B) Epinephrine.
C) Dopamine.
D) Lidocaine.
E) None of the above.

Discussion

The correct answer is "E." The hypothermic heart is generally resistant to drugs. Thus, the best treatment for this patient is rewarming. If the patient has poor perfusion, rapid rewarming with CPR if indicated is the treatment of choice.

All of the following are acceptable methods of rewarming THIS patient EXCEPT:

A) Active external rewarming (e.g., hot packs).
B) Immersion in 40°C water.
C) Passive external rewarming (e.g., blankets).
D) Heated, humidified oxygen.
E) Thoracic lavage with warm fluids.

Discussion

The correct answer is "C." Patients with a temperature of below 30°C generally do not have enough endogenous heat production to effectively rewarm themselves. Thus, external or internal *active* rewarming is indicated. All of the other options are acceptable methods of rewarming this patient. Extracorporeal blood warming is also effective. Heated lavage fluids (e.g., gastric and rectal) are generally not very effective because of the limited surface area involved and can cause large electrolyte shifts. Thoracic cavity lavage via chest tubes is especially effective.

Rapid rewarming of the extremities is associated with:

A) Alkalosis, hypokalemia.
B) Acidosis, hypokalemia.
C) Acidosis, hyperkalemia.
D) Alkalosis, hyperkalemia.
E) None of the above.

Discussion

The correct answer is "C." Rewarming of the extremities can lead to return of cold blood to the core leading to a paradoxical drop in body temperature. Additionally, hypothermia causes lactic acidosis with hyperkalemia in the extremities; as the peripheral blood is rewarmed and mobilized, systemic metabolic acidosis with hyperkalemia may result.

Which of the following is NOT associated with an increased risk of hypothermia?

A) Diabetes mellitus.
B) Obesity.
C) Alcohol use.
D) Old age.
E) Chronic illness.

Discussion

The correct answer is "B." In Iowa, we start to work on our winter fat layer in October for just this reason. Obese patients have a smaller body mass to surface area ratio and do not have an increased risk of hypothermia. "C," alcohol use, causes patients to be relatively insensate to cold (thus the term "liquid jacket") and also causes a peripheral vasodilatation, increasing heat loss. Thermoregulation is impaired as we age. Thus, "D," old age, is associated with a greater propensity toward hypothermia. Diabetes ("A") and any chronic illness ("D") can also predispose to hypothermia.

* *

The patient's mental status clears and he complains that his fingers and toes, which were numb and cold, are now quite painful. You note that there is probably freezing of tissue (frostbite).

The BEST method of rewarming the frostbite is:

A) Slowly in tepid water.
B) Rapidly in the hottest water he can stand (tested by you, of course, to ensure that there will be no burns).
C) Using a hot air source such as a hair dryer.
D) Using moist heat via a heating pad.

Discussion

The correct answer is "B." Frostbitten parts should be rewarmed as quickly as possible in hot water between 37°C and 40°C. Water cooler and hotter than this can lead to incomplete thawing and increased tissue loss. The other methods "A," "C," and "D" are not recommended. *Do not rewarm parts that may become frozen again* (e.g., if you are in the field). Refreezing will cause additional damage.

* *

The patient has a lot of pain after thawing and reperfusion. You control the pain with morphine.

Which of the following is the most appropriate dose of morphine in this 100-kg male?

A) 2 mg IV.
B) 4 mg IV.
C) 6 mg IV.
D) 8 mg IV.
E) 10 mg IV.

Discussion

The correct answer is "E." The correct dose of IV morphine is 0.1 mg/kg or 10 mg in this 100-kg male. Similarly, the correct dose of fentanyl is 0.1 μg/kg (100 μg in an adult) and the dose of hydromorphone is 0.015 mg/kg. However, there really is no "fixed" dose of narcotic pain medication in the ED. Titrate the dose until you obtain pain relief—with the patient is still breathing.

* *

It is 2 days later. The patient is noted to have black eschar on the multiple fingers and toes. There is no obvious perfusion to these areas.

The best course at this point is:

A) Debridement of the nonviable tissue.
B) Skin grafting over open areas after debridement.
C) Observation for a number of weeks despite the black eschar.
D) Amputation of the nonviable distal digits.

Discussion

The correct answer is "C." It can take weeks for the proper demarcation line for debridement and grafting to become apparent. Thus, aggressive intervention at this point is counterproductive and may lead to additional tissue loss. For this reason, "A" and "D" are incorrect. Skin grafting is also not appropriate at this time because debridement of the eschar is not appropriate.

Objectives: Did you learn to . . .

- Identify severe bradycardia in hypothermia and treat it appropriately?
- Manage a patient with hypothermia?
- Use methods of rewarming and identify complications of rewarming?
- Recognize risk factors for hypothermia?
- Diagnose and manage frostbite?

QUICK QUIZ: TOXICOLOGY

Which of the following is true about the ingestion of household bleach?

A) Patients who drink household bleach are at a high risk of esophageal and gastric burns.
B) Oral burns are a good predictor of esophageal burns.
C) All patients who ingest household bleach should be referred for gastroscopy to rule out burns.
D) Household bleach ingestions are generally benign and require no treatment if the patient is not symptomatic.

Discussion

The correct answer is "D." Most **household** bleach ingestions are benign and need no therapy if the patient is asymptomatic. However, **this does not extend to industrial bleach or drain cleaner.** There is a high risk of esophageal and gastric burns with industrial bleach. "B" is incorrect. The oral mucosa may be normal in **industrial bleach or drain cleaner** ingestion and there may still be significant esophageal and gastric burns. For this reason, all patients with **drain cleaner or industrial bleach ingestion** should have gastroscopy. "C" is incorrect; patients with household bleach ingestions do not require gastroscopy.

CASE 13

A 26-year-old male was working outside in the heat and humidity. The outside temperature reached 105°F with 90% humidity. He usually lives in northern Canada and works as a penguin herder—which is weird since penguins are native to the southern hemisphere—but he is here on a job detasseling corn. (Don't believe it? Look at www.teamcorn.com.) His friends noticed that he became confused, complained of a headache and muscle cramps, and became lightheaded. On arrival to your ED, he is not sweating and is lethargic. His rectal temperature is 41.5°C.

All of the following are indicated in the treatment of this patient EXCEPT:

A) Pack the patient in ice to reduce core temperature.
B) IV fluids.
C) Use a fan on the patient to promote evaporative cooling.
D) Administer glucose if the patient is hypoglycemic.

Discussion

The correct answer is "A." Packing patients in ice is contraindicated. Total body immersion in ice water is useful but packing the person in ice actually reduces cooling for two reasons. First, it causes cutaneous vasoconstriction reducing cooling. Second, it does not allow conductive cooling such as would be seen in ice water submersion: solid ice does not have as much skin contact as water or the circulation to conduct away the heat. Remember that submersion in ice is also associated with causing HYPOthermia. The appropriate treatment of heat exhaustion/heat stroke (heat stroke being defined as CNS dysfunction with a change in the level of consciousness) is cool water–soaked blankets and towels with fans aimed at the patient. This allows evaporative cooling and also conductive heat loss (to the water in the towels). Antipyretics are generally not effective because by this point, the patient's endogenous thermoregulation is kaput.

Which of the following IS NOT a contributing factor to heat exhaustion/heat stroke?

A) Use of stimulants such as ephedra or amphetamines.
B) Dehydration.
C) Anticholinergic drugs.
D) Thin body habitus.
E) Extremes of age.

Discussion

The correct answer is "D." This is why Iowans start to work on their swimsuit figure in April—it's a matter of life-or-death, not narcissism. A thin body habitus is not a risk factor for heat stroke/exhaustion; the opposite is true. Obesity predisposes to heat stroke/exhaustion because there is less evaporative surface area per kilogram of weight. All of the others predispose to heat-related illness. "A" and "C" reduce sweating and, in the case of "A," increase metabolic rate. Both of these predispose to heat-related disease. Of particular note is "E." Small children, while thin, sweat less readily than do adults. This predisposes them to heat-related disease, but makes them less stinky than adults. The elderly do not have the same compensatory ability as younger people.

HELPFUL TIP: Up to 80% of patients with heat stroke will not have a prodrome of nausea, lightheadedness, confusion, headache, etc., which is seen in heat exhaustion. Make sure you check hepatic enzymes in patients in whom you suspect heat stroke. They are almost uniformly elevated and normal liver enzymes should cause you to question your diagnosis. But they may take several hours to rise.

Objectives: Did you learn to . . .

- Recognize and manage heat exhaustion/heat stroke?
- Recognize risk factors for heat exhaustion/heat stroke?
- Locate penguin habitats? (Penguins do not live at the North Pole, so the patient could not have been working as a penguin herder, but corn detasseling does occur in Iowa.)

CASE 14

A 19-year-old female presents to the ED with complaints of wheezing. She has a history of asthma and you have been following her since her eighth birthday. In general, she has mild asthma not requiring an inhaled steroid. However, over the past several months, things have accelerated so that she now uses her rescue inhaler daily. On exam, she is tachypneic, using accessory muscles of respiration, with a respiratory rate of 30 and wheezing in all fields. Her oxygen saturation is 95% and pulse is 110 with a normal BP. Her blood gas is as follows: pH 7.40, CO_2 40 mm Hg, O_2 80 mm Hg, and HCO_3 24 mEq/L.

A normal blood gas in this patient suggests that:

A) This is a mild exacerbation and should respond well to therapy.
B) She has a respiratory acidosis.
C) She has a respiratory alkalosis.
D) This is a severe exacerbation that will require aggressive therapy.
E) None of the above.

Discussion

The correct answer is "D." A pH of 7.4 with a CO_2 of 40 mm Hg in a patient who is asthmatic and tachypneic is a bad sign. The CO_2 *should* be low in a tachypneic patient because they will be blowing off CO_2. Thus, a normal CO_2 and normal pH indicate that the patient is retaining CO_2. This is just another case where looking at the patient is more important than looking at the labs. "B" and "C" are both incorrect, since the blood gas indicates neither an acidosis nor alkalosis.

Which of the following tests are indicated in routine evaluation of a patient with an asthma exacerbation?

A) Chest x-ray.
B) CBC.
C) Arterial blood gas.
D) All of the above.
E) None of the above.

Discussion

The correct answer is "E." None of the above tests are indicated in the routine evaluation of an asthma exacerbation. A chest x-ray should be reserved for those patients in whom pneumonia or other pulmonary process is suspected. A CBC is not going to change your therapy in the routine asthma exacerbation and is not indicated. Likewise, an ABG is unnecessary in most asthma exacerbations. It can be used to assist in your clinical evaluation to determine whether or not the patient is retaining CO_2; however, even in the "crashing patient," an ABG is not necessary because **intubation is a clinical decision and should not be based on the blood gas.**

You decide to initiate therapy for this patient. Of the following options, the *initial* treatment of this patient is:

A) Subcutaneous epinephrine.
B) Albuterol MDI (metered-dose inhaler) with spacer.
C) Nebulized ipratropium.
D) Oral steroids.
E) IV steroids.

Discussion

The correct answer is "B." The initial treatment for this patient—and any patient presenting with an asthma exacerbation—is a bronchodilator, and a beta-agonist is preferred, in this case albuterol. It makes little difference whether this is via nebulizer or MDI, as long as one uses adequate doses. One albuterol nebulization is equal to about 8–10 puffs of an albuterol MDI with a spacer. "A" is incorrect because subcutaneous epinephrine is second or third line in the treatment of asthma. "C" is incorrect. While ipratropium *is* effective in asthma, it is secondary to albuterol in the treatment of asthma. "D" and "E" are incorrect. Steroids are indicated, but bronchodilator therapy is the primary treatment in acute asthma exacerbations.

* *

There is no albuterol MDI available to you in your ED, so the patient receives nebulized albuterol. However, she continues to wheeze.

How many albuterol treatments can this patient safely receive?

A) One every other hour.
B) One per hour.
C) Two per hour.
D) Three per hour.
E) Continuous nebulization of albuterol is safe.

Discussion

The correct answer is "E." Albuterol can be administered via nebulizer continuously if needed, even in the pediatric age group. Tachycardia, one of the main side affects of albuterol treatment, will often **improve** with continuous albuterol. This occurs because the patient's tachycardia is often driven by hypoxia. Once the asthma is adequately treated, oxygenation improves, and the pulse comes down.

* *

The patient does not respond well to albuterol alone, so you request the addition of ipratropium. At this point, you also want to order steroids.

Which of the following statements about steroids is true?

A) IV steroids are superior to PO steroids in the treatment of asthma.
B) All patients who are steroid dependent should have additional steroids even if they have already taken their dose for the day.
C) The effective dose range for steroids in asthma is well established.
D) Only patients requiring admission should have oral or parenteral steroids.

Discussion

The correct answer is "B." All patients who are steroid dependent should get steroids if they present to the ED with an acute exacerbation of asthma. "A" is incorrect. IV steroids and oral steroids have the same efficacy in acute asthma exacerbations. Thus, the choice of route depends mostly on convenience and cost. "C" is incorrect. Multiple steroid dosing regimens and ranges of doses have been used in asthma with success. "D" is incorrect. Discharged patients who have anything more than a minor asthma exacerbation should receive steroids.

HELPFUL TIP: When compared with oral steroids, IV steroids *may increase* hospitalizations, cost, and treatment failure in those with chronic obstructive pulmonary disease. Use oral steroids whenever possible; the bioavailability is high (*JAMA* 2010;303(23):2359–2367. doi: 10.1001/jama.2010.796).

Which of the following is true about the role of theophylline in the treatment of acute asthma?

A) Theophylline/aminophylline should be used in cases unresponsive to two to three doses of nebulized albuterol since it has added benefits when used with an inhaled beta-agonist.
B) Patients who get theophylline/aminophylline have more side effects than do patients who get continuously nebulized albuterol and get no benefit from the drug.
C) If you choose to use theophylline/aminophylline, the therapeutic goal is a serum level of 150 μg/dL.
D) None of the above is correct.

Discussion

The correct answer is "B." Patients who are treated with theophylline have more side effects, including tachycardia, nausea, and arrhythmias, than do patients who get continuously nebulized albuterol. Theophylline/aminophylline has essentially no role in the treatment of acute asthma exacerbations. There is no benefit to theophylline or aminophylline over *optimal* beta-agonist therapy (e.g., continuous nebulized albuterol if required). "C" is incorrect because if used at all, the therapeutic goal for theophylline is a serum level of 15 μg/dL.

HELPFUL TIP: Magnesium sulfate (2 g over 10 minutes in adults, 25 mg/kg in children) can be used in patients with status asthmaticus. Magnesium is a direct smooth muscle relaxant. Not all patients will respond, and in patients who will respond, you can expect a 60–90-minute effect. Avoid using magnesium in patients with renal failure since they may become toxic.

* *

The patient responds to nebulizers and steroids. You decide to send her home.

Which of the following is true?

A) You should discharge the patient on 2 puffs of an albuterol MDI via spacer to be used PRN.
B) You should place the patient on a steroid taper.

Discussion

The correct answer is "E." Testicular torsion is characterized by acute onset of unilateral testicular pain, often during activity such as running. It has a bimodal age distribution, during the first year of life and again during puberty. The differential diagnosis is dependent on the patient's age. If the patient is younger than 15 years, the differential consists of testicular torsion, epididymitis, torsion of appendix testis/appendix epididymis, orchitis, hydrocele, and varicocele. In patients older than 15 years, the differential includes all of these diagnoses plus testicular tumor. However, testicular tumors are generally painless.

What is the most reliable method for diagnosing testicular torsion?

A) Doppler (Duplex color).
B) Radionuclide scan.
C) Surgical exploration.
D) Checking the cremasteric reflex.
E) MRI.

Discussion

The correct answer is "C." *Every patient with suspected testicular torsion should have surgical exploration of the scrotum.* All of the other studies are adjunctive. For example, radionuclide scan has a false-negative rate of about 20%. Ultrasound has a sensitivity as low as 82%. Surgical exploration is the only definitive diagnostic tool. The window of opportunity for surgery is about 6 hours, after which the testicle may not be salvaged. Orchiopexy should be performed on the involved and uninvolved sides to prevent torsion.

Objectives: Did you learn to . . .

- Examine a patient presenting with acute scrotal pain?
- Generate a differential diagnosis for scrotal pain based on the patient's age?
- Evaluate a patient with suspected testicular torsion?

QUICK QUIZ: UROLOGY

What is the most common agent causing epididymitis in a 21-year-old male?

A) *Escherichia coli.*
B) *Neisseria gonorrhoeae.*
C) *Chlamydia trachomatis.*
D) *Pseudomonas* species.
E) *Ureaplasma urealyticum.*

Discussion

The correct answer is "C." In young males, epididymitis is usually the result of sexually transmitted diseases. Of these, *C. trachomatis* is currently the most common etiologic agent. *N. gonorrhoeae* is second most common in this age group. It is therefore essential to treat for both agents when the diagnosis of epididymitis is suspected.

QUICK QUIZ: UROLOGY

What is the most common agent causing epididymitis in a 55-year-old male?

A) *E. coli.*
B) *N. gonorrhoeae.*
C) *C. trachomatis.*
D) *Pseudomonas* species.
E) *U. urealyticum.*

Discussion

The correct answer is "A." Gram-negative rods are the most common cause of epididymitis in older men. Of these, *E. coli* is the most common etiologic agent, followed by *Klebsiella* and *Pseudomonas* species.

CASE 17

A 22-year-old white female college student presents to the ED with dysuria and urinary frequency of 2 days duration. She denies any abdominal/pelvic pain, flank pain, hematuria, fever, chills, vaginal discharge, nausea, vomiting, or diarrhea. Her LMP was 2 weeks ago and she is not sexually active. She is on oral contraceptives to treat menstrual cramps and denies any allergies. Her past medical history is negative. She states she has never been sexually active.

A urine beta-HCG is NOT indicated for which of the following patients who presents with abdominal pain?

A) A 32-year-old female who has had a tubal ligation.
B) A 16-year-old female who by history has never been sexually active.

C) A 25-year-old female who has had a normal period 1 week ago and states she couldn't possibly be pregnant.
D) A 24-year-old, married, professional female who is taking oral contraceptives and had a normal last menses.
E) A 25-year-old male.

Discussion

The correct answer is "E." Of course males do not need a pregnancy test (although the HCG may be elevated in testicular cancer). All female patients of reproductive age, except for those who have had a hysterectomy, must have a pregnancy test as part of the evaluation of abdominal pain. There are several reasons for this position. First, many patients may not be candid about their sexual activity. In fact, in one study, almost one-third of patients who said "they could not possibly be pregnant," including one who denied ever having intercourse, were pregnant. Second, the failure rate of tubal ligation is up to 3% over 10 years depending on the technique used (laparoscopic tubal ligation is the least reliable). To raise your concern a little higher, almost all of the pregnancies in patients who have had a tubal ligation are ectopic.

> HELPFUL TIP: When examining a patient whose history is consistent with vulvovaginitis, remember that a KOH preparation is only 65–80% sensitive for *Candida* and treatment based on symptoms and physical findings is certainly reasonable.

* *

You get a urinalysis (UA) on this patient, mostly out of habit. The UA shows 5–10 WBCs/HPF, 2+ bacteria, 2+ leukocyte esterase, and 1+ nitrite.

Which of the following antibiotic regimens IS NOT indicated for the treatment of simple cystitis?

A) 3-day course of trimethoprim–sulfamethoxazole (TMP–SMX).
B) 3-day course of a fluoroquinolone.
C) 7-day course of nitrofurantoin.
D) Single dose of fosfomycin.
E) Single dose of cephalexin.

Discussion

The correct answer is "E." The usual causative agents for uncomplicated cystitis are gram-negative organisms such as *E. coli*. In areas that have high rates of resistance to TMP–SMX ($>30\%$ or more of isolated *E. coli* bacteria resistant), it is wise to use a quinolone as the first-line agent; however, quinolones are more costly and quinolone resistance is rising. All of the above regimens are usually effective for treating cystitis except a single dose of cephalexin. Cephalexin is effectively used in pregnant females, although a 7-day course is recommended. Fosfomycin has a lower cure rate than the other regimens and is more expensive; therefore, it is not generally recommended.

> HELPFUL TIP: A false-negative UA is common in women with uncomplicated cystitis. Empiric treatment of urinary tract infection (UTI) is reasonable in a female of childbearing years presenting with one or more typical symptoms (urgency, frequency, dysuria) and no vaginal discharge.

All of the following patients with pyelonephritis should be admitted EXCEPT:

A) 22-year-old G1 P0 female <24 weeks pregnant, but hemodynamically stable.
B) 22-year-old female unable to tolerate PO fluids or medications.
C) 22-year-old female with unreliable social situation and/or compliance.
D) 22-year-old female with an unclear diagnosis or extreme pain.

Discussion

The correct answer is "A." The old adage that all pregnant patients with pyelonephritis must be admitted has gone out of favor. It is safe to send patients home who are <24 weeks of gestations, compliant, have stable vital signs, and are accessible by telephone. Patients should be given clear instructions to return for any complications. All of the other situations require in-hospital care.

Objectives: Did you learn to . . .

- Decide which patients should have a urine beta-HCG in the ED?

- Provide appropriate antibiotic treatment to a patient with an uncomplicated UTI?
- Identify patients with pyelonephritis who require hospital admission?

CASE 18

A 63-year-old male presents to the ED with a 2-day history of fever, urinary frequency, dysuria, and difficulty initiating the urinary stream. He also relates having some perineal pain. On exam, his vitals are stable except for a temperature of 102°F. His rectal exam is remarkable for a tender, warm, edematous prostate. There are no perirectal masses and the stool is heme negative. He has no penile lesions, discharge, scrotal masses, or tenderness. He does not exhibit any costovertebral angle tenderness. His UA is positive for 10 WBCs/HPF, 1+ nitrite, 1+ leukocyte esterase.

What is the most likely diagnosis in this patient?

A) Pyelonephritis.
B) Perirectal abscess.
C) Epididymitis.
D) Acute prostatitis.
E) Cystitis.

Discussion
The correct answer is "D." This patient's symptoms most closely fit those of someone with acute prostatitis. Although his UA is also consistent with pyelonephritis or cystitis, his exam findings are more suggestive of acute prostatitis; he lacks costovertebral angle tenderness (pyelonephritis), and he has a significant temperature that argues against a simple cystitis. In the past, prostatic massage was recommended when obtaining a urine specimen; this practice is to be avoided since it is quite painful and bacterial seeding into the bloodstream may occur. In the absence of scrotal tenderness, epididymitis is also quite unlikely.

What should be included in the treatment regimen for this patient?

A) Oral fluoroquinolone or TMP–SMX for 21–30 days.
B) Instructions for hydration, sitz baths, stool softeners, and non-steroidal anti-inflammatory drugs (NSAIDs).
C) Admission for IV antibiotics if he appears toxic or hemodynamically unstable.
D) Foley or suprapubic catheter if urinary retention is a problem.
E) All of the above.

Discussion
The correct answer is "E." Patients with acute prostatitis should be treated for 21–30 days with PO antibiotics to prevent chronic prostatitis. Treatment should be initiated with a quinolone while urine cultures are pending, since sulfa resistance is high in some areas of the country.

* *

While this patient is still in the ED, he develops acute urinary retention. A Foley catheter is placed without difficulty and 300 cc of slightly cloudy urine is obtained. Your patient feels much better and thanks you for alleviating his pain. You decide to discharge him home with the Foley catheter and a leg bag after discussion with a urologist and follow-up arrangement.

Which of the following IS NOT a cause of urinary retention?

A) Phimosis, urethral stricture, benign prostatic hyperplasia (BPH), calculi.
B) Anticholinergics, sympathomimetics, narcotics, antipsychotics.
C) Psychogenic.
D) Cauda equina syndrome, diabetes, spinal cord injuries, herpes.
E) All of the above can cause urinary retention.

Discussion
The correct answer is "E." All of the above can cause urinary retention in men. The most common cause of acute urinary retention by far is BPH. The categories of acute urinary retention may be divided into neurogenic (spinal cord injuries, cauda equina syndrome, diabetes, syringomyelia, herpes, etc.), obstructive (BPH, phimosis, paraphimosis, calculi, urethral stricture, etc.), pharmacologic (anticholinergics, antihistamines, narcotics, antipsychotics, tricyclics, etc.), and psychogenic, which is a diagnosis of exclusion.

> HELPFUL TIP: Sending patients home on an alpha-blocker (e.g., doxazosin, tamulosin) *may* reduce the need for recatheterization after the catheter is removed.

Objectives: Did you learn to . . .

- Recognize the clinical presentation of prostatitis?
- Treat a patient with prostatitis?
- Identify causes of urinary retention in a male?

QUICK QUIZ: UROLOGY

Which of the following is characterized by a swollen, painful foreskin that cannot be reduced back to its normal position?

A) Phimosis.
B) Paraphimosis.
C) Balanoposthitis.
D) Meatal stenosis.

Discussion

The correct answer is "B." Paraphimosis is a condition in which the foreskin is retracted, swollen, and unable to reduce into its normal position. Ice and steady manual compression often permits reduction. Surgery is indicated if manual reduction fails. "A," phimosis, is a condition in which the distal foreskin is too tight to be retracted to allow exposure of the glans. It is often confused with penile adhesions in those younger than 2 years. "C," balanoposthitis, is a form of cellulitis involving the foreskin and glans in the uncircumcised male, associated with poor hygiene. Treatment is with warm soaks, antibiotics, and possible circumcision. "D," meatal stenosis, is common in circumcised males, associated with an inflammatory reaction involving the meatus. Symptoms that indicate the need for surgical treatment include spraying of the urine stream or dorsal deflection of the stream.

QUICK QUIZ: UROLOGY

Until what age is it normal to have adhesions between the glans and foreskin in uncircumcised males?

A) Adhesions are always abnormal.
B) Age 6 months.
C) Age 1 year.
D) Age 2 years.
E) Age 3 years.

Discussion

The correct answer is "E." Some adhesions are normal in young children. However, the foreskin should be fully retractable in uncircumcised males by the age of 3–5 years. Before this, no action need be taken.

CASE 19

A 20-year-old female presents to your ED complaining of lower quadrant abdominal pain. She is on "the patch" for contraception and has been faithfully using it. She has had regular menses and has not noticed any change in her pattern of menses. Her pain had a sudden onset but is not associated with any vaginal bleeding. On vaginal exam, you find marked cervical motion tenderness but no palpable adnexal mass.

Based on this information you decide that:

A) The absence of an adnexal mass effectively rules out ectopic pregnancy.
B) If a patient becomes pregnant, all forms of contraception reduce the risk of ectopic pregnancy.
C) The fact the patient has had normal periods effectively rules out an ectopic pregnancy.
D) Cervical motion tenderness effectively clinches the diagnosis of pelvic inflammatory disease.
E) None of the above is true.

Discussion

The answer is "E," none of the above. "A" is incorrect because only 10% of patients with an ectopic pregnancy will have a palpable mass in the adnexa. "B" is incorrect because both intrauterine device and tubal ligation *increase* the risk of ectopic pregnancy if the patient becomes pregnant. "C" is incorrect because 15–20% of patients with ectopic pregnancy have no history of missed menses. "D" is incorrect because cervical motion tenderness can be present not only in pelvic inflammatory disease but also in other illnesses such as ovarian torsion, ectopic pregnancy, etc.

Risk factors for ectopic pregnancy include all of the following EXCEPT:

A) Prior ectopic pregnancy.
B) History of pelvic inflammatory disease.
C) Treatment for infertility.
D) Current intrauterine device use.
E) Oral contraceptive use.

Discussion

The correct answer is "E." All of the others increase the risk of an ectopic pregnancy. Other risk factors include cigarette smoking, recent elective abortion, previous tubal surgery, and tubal ligation.

* *

You decide that this patient may have an ectopic pregnancy. A urine HCG test is positive for pregnancy.

The significance of a positive pregnancy test is that:

A) An ultrasound will be able to detect an ectopic pregnancy if one is present.
B) The serum level of HCG is *at least* 1000 mIU/mL.
C) Combined with the patient's abdominal pain and cervical motion tenderness, it effectively rules in an ectopic pregnancy.
D) The urine HCG is 98% sensitive for pregnancy 7 days after implantation.

Discussion

The correct answer is "D." "A" is incorrect. The pregnancy test is positive very early and ultrasound may not be positive by an experienced operator until 6 weeks of pregnancy. "B" is incorrect. The urine may be positive at serum HCG levels of 25–50 IU/L. Patients may not have an HCG level of 1000 IU/L until 6 weeks of pregnancy. "C" is incorrect because patients with a normal pregnancy may also have abdominal pain and cervical motion tenderness.

* *

The patient's serum HCG is 440 IU/L. You order an ultrasound and find no evidence of an intrauterine OR ectopic pregnancy.

Your next step is to:

A) Reassure the patient that she does not have an ectopic pregnancy.
B) Recheck the HCG in 48 hours.
C) Refer for a laparoscopy to rule out ectopic pregnancy.
D) Recheck an HCG in 1–2 weeks.
E) Follow the patient clinically.

Discussion

The correct answer is "B." The HCG should double in a normal pregnancy every 1.8–3 days. If the HCG *is not* doubling in this time frame, it is likely an ectopic pregnancy. Remember, the fact that you did not see an ectopic pregnancy on ultrasound is irrelevant. The HCG is generally *at least* 1500 IU/L before anything is seen on ultrasound. By an HCG of 6500 IU/L, you should certainly be able to see a pregnancy on ultrasound. "A" is incorrect because of the above. "C" is incorrect. This is invasive and not needed. "D" is incorrect because of the time frame; the HCG should be rechecked in 24–48 hours. An ectopic may well rupture within 1–2 weeks. "E" is incorrect. If you follow the patient clinically, you are basically saying that you will wait until the ectopic ruptures before addressing the problem.

You recheck the HCG in 48 hours and it is now 1000 IU/L (prior level 440 IU/L). Your interpretation is that:

A) This patient does not likely have an ectopic pregnancy.
B) This patient has a molar pregnancy.
C) This patient has a blighted ovum.
D) The patient has fetal demise of an intrauterine pregnancy.
E) All of the above are possible.

Discussion

The correct answer is "A." Since the HCG doubled normally, it is **not** likely that this is an ectopic pregnancy, a blighted ovum ("C") or intrauterine fetal demise ("D"). In all of these conditions, the HCG would not double. "B" is also not likely because in a molar pregnancy, the HCG would rise dramatically.

Objectives: Did you learn to . . .

- Evaluate a fertile female with pelvic pain?
- Diagnose and manage an ectopic pregnancy?

QUICK QUIZ: GYNECOLOGY

Which of the following is typical of ovarian torsion?

A) Periumbilical pain gradually migrating to both the right and left quadrants.
B) Sudden onset of colicky abdominal pain in one of the lower quadrants.
C) Sudden onset of colicky abdominal pain with vaginal bleeding.
D) All of the above can be presentations of ovarian torsion.

Discussion

The correct answer is "B." Patients with ovarian torsion present with sudden onset of severe lower abdominal pain. The pain is frequently colicky. Since only one ovary is involved, the pain is located in one side or the other. Spontaneous torsion/detorsion may also occur so that the pain may remit spontaneously. Ovarian torsion can be diagnosed by Doppler ultrasound that examines flow to the ovaries.

CASE 20

A middle-aged unresponsive, disheveled patient is brought by emergency medical services (EMS) to your ED. They had been called by his girlfriend who had seen him lying in the grass outside his home this morning. He has spontaneous respirations and has a pulse shallow respirations of 20 per minute and a weak but palpable pulse at 110 beats per minute.

What should be your first steps in assessment and treatment?

A) Oxygen by non-rebreather mask, stat serum glucose, naloxone.
B) Oxygen by non-rebreather mask, ECG, head CT.
C) Oxygen by non-rebreather mask, intubate, ECG, head CT.
D) Intubate, ECG, head CT.

Discussion

The correct answer is "A." There are several causes of unresponsiveness that can be immediately corrected. A helpful algorithm to recall in the initial treatment for an unresponsive patient is "DON'T": Dextrose, Oxygen, Naloxone, Thiamine. Answer "A" is correct because naloxone and oxygen are administered and a glucose is checked. If rapid blood sugar is unavailable, empirical administration of dextrose would be appropriate. Rapid treatment of hypoxia, hypoglycemia, and narcotic overdose can improve mental status and thus avoid intubation. ECG and head CT may be indicated later in the evaluation.

* *

The patient is found to be hypothermic, hypoglycemic, and hypoxic. He is placed on oxygen and given warm normal saline, an amp of D50W, and naloxone. The patient now is saturating at 98% on non-rebreather mask (NRB). He is responding to painful stimuli by moaning and withdrawing his extremities but is not opening his eyes; he still has no gag reflex.

What is your next step?

A) Intubate.
B) Obtain head CT.
C) Obtain ECG.
D) Continue on a non-rebreather mask.
E) Obtain an ABG.

Discussion

The correct answer is "A." Although the patient has improved and has a normal oxygen saturation, his level of consciousness is still too low to protect his airway. Thus, he should be intubated before further diagnostic studies are performed. A simple method to determine the need for intubation is the GCS (Table 1–5). Patients with a GCS of 8 or less should be intubated, as they cannot protect their airway from aspiration of oral secretions and/or emesis. The rhyme "GCS of 8, intubate" assists in recollection of this rule. This patient has a GCS of 7 (eyes 1, verbal 2, movement 4) and therefore should be intubated before other studies or interventions. "D" is incorrect because he cannot protect his airway. "E" is incorrect **because the decision to intubate is a clinical one and not tied directly to the blood gas!**

* *

The girlfriend arrives and gives further history that the patient is an alcoholic and had told her he had quit drinking 2 days ago. She states he has had a seizure in the past when he stops drinking. He starts to seize before your eyes.

What should you do now?

A) Give lorazepam and admit for probable delirium tremens (DTs).
B) Give lorazepam, obtain a head CT, blood cultures, and ECG.
C) Give lorazepam, extubate, and admit for probable DTs.
D) Give phenytoin and admit for probable DTs.
E) Give lorazepam, obtain head CT, and ECG.

Discussion

The correct answer is "B," give lorazepam to abort the seizure. Even though it is easy to assume that the patient had a seizure from DTs, which may have resulted in hypoxia, hypothermia, and hypoglycemia, this kind of thinking can lead to errors. It is still possible that the patient has a spontaneous or traumatic brain hemorrhage, thus the need for a head CT. It is also possible that the patient is septic; remember that hypothermia can be seen with sepsis. Thus, blood cultures should be obtained and possibly an LP performed. Finally, an ECG can show a myocardial infarction or arrhythmia that may also result in seizure. "D" is incorrect because phenytoin is not the drug of choice for an actively seizing patient; a benzodiazepine such as lorazepam should be administered. Answer "C" is incorrect; the patient still has a GCS of less than 8 and is unable to protect his airway so he should not be extubated.

Objectives: Did you learn to . . .

- Rapidly assess and treat an unresponsive patient?
- Use the GCS to determine need for intubation?
- Assess and treat a seizing patient?

CASE 21

You are working in a rural ED and get a call that the volunteer ambulance service is bringing an unresponsive, adult male patient status post-MVC. They bring the patient on a backboard with a c-collar.

The primary survey of a trauma patient includes all of the following EXCEPT:

A) Check for pulses.
B) Immobilize the c-spine, evaluate the airway, and listen for breath sounds.
C) GCS.
D) Abdominal exam.
E) Unclothe the patient.

Discussion

The correct answer (and what you do not want to do in the primary survey) is "D." The primary survey is the initial evaluation performed on every trauma patient by the algorithm ABCDE. A: Airway assessment includes c-spine immobilization; opening the airway by jaw thrust/chin lift; and, when indicated, bag-valve mask, intubation, or cricothyrotomy. B: Breathing includes listening for breath sounds, administering oxygen, and treating pneumothoraces. C: Circulation requires assessment of BP by checking pulses and treatment of hypotension and tachycardia with crystalloids and blood. D: Disability is the rapid neurologic exam for potential cord injury and GCS. E: Exposure involves disrobing the patient and rolling them to assess any injury to the back.

* *

On the primary survey, the patient was not protecting his airway and was intubated with an 8-Fr endotracheal tube (ETT) with rapid sequence intubation (RSI). The patient is noted to have breath sounds on the right but no breath sounds on the left.

What is the next best step in evaluation and treatment of this patient?

A) Remove the ETT; you must be in the esophagus.
B) Get a chest x-ray to confirm tube placement.
C) Do needle decompression of left chest.
D) Insert a left chest tube.
E) Check ETT for depth at the teeth and position.

Discussion

The correct answer is "E." This patient has breath sounds on the right; therefore, esophageal intubation is unlikely, making answer "A" incorrect. The most likely and easily recognizable source of absent breath sounds on the left is a right main stem intubation. Thus, looking at the depth of placement of the ETT at the teeth (answer "E") is the initial evaluation indicated. The ETT should be placed at about three times the size of the ETT (i.e., $3 \times 8 = 24$ cm) assuming that the size of ETT was correctly chosen. This is an important calculation to remember, as it also applies to pediatric patients. A chest x-ray can also evaluate for right main stem intubation but should not be the first step. A pneumothorax may be the cause of unilateral breath sounds, but right main stem intubation should be considered first.

You now note that there is an open chest wound to the left lateral rib cage. Funny . . . you didn't notice that before. What is the initial treatment of this new finding?

A) Needle thoracostomy.
B) Chest tube placement.
C) Occlusive dressing.
D) Chest x-ray.

Discussion

The correct answer is "C." This patient has an open "sucking" chest wound. Each time the patient inspires, air can be sucked into the chest cavity acting as a one-way valve. This can result in a tension pneumothorax. Thus, apply an occlusive dressing to the wound (e.g., such as petrolatum gauze).

* *

The patient continues to have absence of breath sounds on the left, is hypotensive, and has distended neck veins. The presumed diagnosis is a tension pneumothorax.

What should you do now?

A) Chest x-ray.
B) Chest tube placement through wound.
C) Chest tube placement through separate site.
D) Remove occlusive dressing.

Discussion

The correct answer is "D." The occlusive dressing itself may cause a tension pneumothorax, so its placement should be immediately followed by chest tube placement. If a tension pneumothorax develops before the tube is placed, removing the dressing (answer "D") can usually alleviate the tension component. Emergency medical technicians will often place a dressing that is closed only on three sides to serve as a release valve and avoid this possibility. The diagnosis of tension pneumothorax is clinical. The time required to obtain a chest x-ray may result in the death of the patient. When placing a chest tube in a patient with an open wound, never pass the tube through the wound, as it is likely to follow the path of the initial penetration into lung parenchyma.

HELPFUL TIP: Needle thoracostomy is also useful in a tension pneumothorax and is the treatment in most cases.

* *

The patient now has a chest tube in place but remains hypotensive. Two large bore (18 gauge or larger) IVs were established. No external source of bleeding is identified. When should blood be administered?

A) Immediately.
B) If persistent hypotension after 1 L of normal saline.
C) If persistent hypotension after 2 L of normal saline.
D) If persistent hypotension after 4 L of normal saline.
E) If FAST exam shows intra-abdominal free fluid.

Discussion

The correct answer is "C." If a patient arrives hypotensive with no signs of external bleeding, 2 L of crystalloid (normal saline) should be given immediately. If the patient continues to be hypotensive, packed red blood cells should be started along with additional normal saline. The FAST exam is a rapid bedside ultrasound to identify free fluid in the trauma patient's abdomen and pericardial sac. Persistent hypotension with positive FAST exam is an indication for emergent exploratory laparotomy.

Which of the following findings is a contraindication to placing a Foley catheter in this male trauma victim?

A) Rectal blood.
B) Blood at the urethral meatus.
C) Penile erection.
D) All of the above are contraindications.

Discussion

The correct answer is "B." Contraindications to Foley placement in the trauma patient include high riding, soft boggy prostate; blood at the urethral meatus; and perineal hematoma. A retrograde urethrogram should be performed prior to Foley placement to assess urethral injury. Penile erection is not a contraindication and is suggestive of a spinal cord injury. Rectal blood and vaginal bleeding do not indicate urethral injury but should be noted in the secondary survey.

Objectives: Did you learn to . . .

- Employ the primary assessment of a trauma patient?
- Treat an open chest wound?
- Resuscitate an unstable trauma patient?
- Describe the contraindications to Foley placement in a trauma patient?

QUICK QUIZ: CHEST PAIN

A 54-year-old female presents to your ED with a chief complaint of chest pain. She states it came on suddenly while she was working in her garden. She describes it as "sharp" and it radiates through to her back. She reports difficulty breathing. Her past medical history is pertinent for hypertension, breast cancer, and obesity. She is a smoker. Based on this history, what diagnosis can be excluded from your differential?

A) Acute myocardial infarction.
B) Aortic dissection.
C) Pulmonary embolism.
D) Pneumothorax.
E) None of the above.

Discussion

The correct answer is "E." The patient's history is most suggestive of pulmonary embolism with her complaint of sharp chest pain, trouble breathing, cancer history, and smoking. However, at this point in time, all of the etiologies listed—and more—must be considered. Women often have atypical presentations of cardiac chest pain. In addition, patients often use the term "sharp" to describe "intense" or "strong" pain.

QUICK QUIZ: AORTIC DISSECTION

In aortic dissection, the BP is different between the extremities in only 15% of cases.

What limb should you use to guide BP management?

A) Right arm.
B) Left arm.
C) Either lower extremity.
D) The limb with the highest BP.
E) The limb with the lowest BP.

Discussion

The correct answer is "D." An aortic dissection may impair the blood flow to certain extremities due to the false lumen. The BP should be maintained at a systolic BP of 100–120 mm Hg (or a bit lower) in the extremity with the highest BP. This will decrease the forces propagating the dissection.

> HELPFUL TIP: Patients with an aortic dissection should be started on a beta-blocker and vasodilator drip (nitroglycerin, nitroprusside) to control BP and minimize stress to the aortic wall.

CASE 22

A mother brings her 3-year-old child into the ED. She states that the child has been vomiting and complaining of abdominal pain all afternoon. He has had between 8 and 10 episodes of emesis; the last two have contained small amounts of bright red blood. He has had a little nonbloody diarrhea. He has not been tolerating fluids. On exam, you find the child to be moderately ill appearing with normal color, but he seems less interactive than you would expect. His vitals reveal a temperature of 36.5°C, a pulse of 170, a respiratory rate of 28, and a BP of 98/58.

His abdomen is slightly and diffusely tender. He has dry mucous membranes.

In general (not specifically in this patient) what is the initial treatment of a moderately dehydrated child?

A) 20 cc/kg bolus of D5 1/2 NS.
B) 10 cc/kg bolus of isotonic crystalloid fluid.
C) Oral challenge of a small amount of electrolyte solution.
D) 12.5 mg promethazine suppository.

Discussion

The correct answer is "C." Many children who are vomiting and have diarrhea will be able to tolerate small (5 cc) sips of fluid administered every few minutes. Oral fluids should be attempted prior to IV therapy. In children who are severely dehydrated, as evidenced by altered mental status or change in skin turgor, IV fluid resuscitation should begin immediately.

If IV rehydration is considered appropriate, use normal saline in 20 cc/kg aliquots. Therefore, answers A and B are not correct. Promethazine (answer "D") is an antiemetic that has been used in children in the past. However, promethazine has received a "black box" warning from the FDA for children younger than 2 years, as there is a risk of respiratory depression.

* *

You obtain some lab work and notice that the child has normal renal function but low serum bicarbonate, indicating a possible metabolic acidosis. In speaking with his mother, you discover that earlier in the day, he was playing unsupervised in the bathroom, where she keeps her prenatal vitamin. Upon questioning the child, he states that he ate a bunch of "candy" in the bathroom (about 3 hours ago).

What component of prenatal vitamins is most concerning for toxicity?

A) Folic acid.
B) Iron.
C) Calcium.
D) Vitamin D.

Discussion

The correct answer is "B." Folic acid, calcium, and vitamin D are all tolerated well in high doses, as their absorption from the GI tract is limited. Iron, however, can continue to be absorbed while it remains in the GI tract. Iron is a direct irritant to the GI mucosa (therefore, the bloody emesis and diarrhea) and interferes with the electron transport chain and aerobic metabolism.

The nurse asks if you should add on an iron level to the blood that was drawn 3 hours after the ingestion. You respond:

A) "No thanks. Iron levels are not helpful."
B) "No thanks. It's too early. We need to wait until at least 12 hours have elapsed."
C) "Yes, please. If it's normal, we don't need any further treatment."
D) "Yes, please. It may help us determine the severity of toxicity."

Discussion

The correct answer is "D." The iron level between 2 and 4 hours after ingestion is the most accurate; beyond this period, the majority of the iron is moving intracellularly and cannot be measured. For slow-release iron, serum concentrations should be measured at 6–8 hours after ingestion. These measures will give you a peak serum iron concentration that correlates well with the severity of toxicity. However, a low serum level of iron does not mean the symptomatic patient is OK. Treatment is based on clinical findings and NOT on serum iron levels. Once the iron moves into the periphery, the serum levels will be low despite significant toxicity.

How do patients with iron toxicity present?

A) Abdominal pain, vomiting, and diarrhea.
B) Hematemesis, shock, and coma.
C) Relatively asymptomatic.
D) All of the above.

Discussion

The correct answer is "D." Patients who have had an iron overdose classically pass through five different stages. The first stage is characterized by nausea, vomiting, diarrhea, and abdominal pain. There may be hematemesis and hematochezia as the GI mucosa becomes irritated. The second phase is a relatively asymptomatic period as the GI symptoms resolve. During this quiet phase, iron is absorbed and transported to the periphery where it causes the interruption of aerobic metabolism. In the next (third) phase, patients become hypotensive, acidotic, and can develop multisystem organ failure and coma. It is this shock that is the usual cause of death in iron toxicity. The fourth phase is heralded by hepatic necrosis. Liver failure, which does not occur in all patients, is the second most frequent cause of death in cases of iron toxicity. Finally, the patient may develop bowel obstructions 2–4 weeks or longer after the ingestion due to stricture at the site of mucosal irritation.

Abdominal films reveal radiopaque pills in the stomach. What is the best next step in treatment for this patient?

A) Whole bowel irrigation with polyethylene glycol solution.
B) Gastric lavage.
C) Activated charcoal.
D) Syrup of ipecac.

Discussion

The correct answer is "A." Gastric lavage and vomiting induced by syrup of ipecac both are treatments that entail a fair amount of risk and neither has been shown to be beneficial. In addition, there is the risk of aspiration and subsequent pneumonitis. Therefore, answers B and D are not correct. Iron, lithium, and lead will not adsorb to activated charcoal; therefore, it is of no benefit in such cases, and answer C is incorrect. Treatment for iron toxicity involves whole bowel irrigation with polyethylene glycol solution to flush the iron out of the GI tract. There are various doses and rates of administration published, but 10–15 mL/kg/hr, up to 2000 cc/hr, seems to be a reasonable place to start. This requires the placement of a nasogastric tube. If a patient does not tolerate the volume of the infusion, the rate should be decreased by 50%. The irrigation should continue until the rectal effluent is clear and there are no visible pill fragments. If follow-up radiographs demonstrate persistent iron tablets in the stomach, consider the possibility of a bezoar having formed, which may require endoscopic or surgical intervention for removal.

HELPFUL TIP: Patients who are entirely asymptomatic from the time of supposed iron ingestion to 6 hours afterwards *and* do not have any radiographic evidence of iron in the GI tract are not at risk for toxicity. They can be safely discharged with close follow-up. The caveat is that chewable multivitamins are not radiopaque and will not show up on x-ray (Table 1–7).

Table 1–7 MANIFESTATIONS OF IRON TOXICITY

First (or early) phase	Hours 0–6 (rarely >6 hr)	Vomiting and diarrhea, often bloody Metabolic acidosis Shock
Second (or quiescent) phase	3–48 hr (time variable)	Resolving acidosis Resolving hypovolemia Frequently, asymptomatic
Third phase	12–48 hr (time variable)	GI hemorrhage Lethargy, coma, shock Cardiovascular collapse Metabolic acidosis Renal failure (variable)
Fourth phase	2 days or more	Hepatotoxicity Hepatic necrosis Coma
Fifth phase	2–4 weeks	GI obstruction due to strictures and scarring

The patient is symptomatic (vomiting and diarrhea) and also has an iron level 650 μg/dL, which puts him at significant risk for toxicity. What is your next step?

A) Correction of acid–base disturbance and aggressive fluid resuscitation.
B) EDTA.
C) Deferoxamine.
D) A and B.
E) A and C.

Discussion

The correct answer is "E." In addition to symptoms and acidosis, an iron level >500 μg/dL or ingestion of more than 60 mg/kg of elemental iron are considered high-risk situations, and chelation with deferoxamine is warranted. Deferoxamine is used to chelate iron, while EDTA is a chelation treatment for lead poisoning. Fastidious supportive care, with correction of the patient's volume and acid–base disturbances, is imperative. Ensuring that the patient is euvolemic is especially important when using chelation therapy, given that the major side effect of deferoxamine is hypotension. The dose of deferoxamine is 15 mg/kg/hr for 24 hours, but may be slowed down if the patient becomes hypotensive.

HELPFUL TIP: Dialysis does not remove iron from the blood stream nor the intracellular space, where the majority of it will be found.

Dialysis may be indicated to treat renal failure or persistent profound acidosis.

HELPFUL TIP: The much touted "deferoxamine challenge" to see if there is free iron in the blood is not an accurate predictor of toxicity. The test is done by giving an individual a single challenge dose of deferoxamine and seeing if the urine changes to a "vin rosé" color reflecting circulating free iron. However, this again does not predict who needs therapy, since the iron may already be working its evil in the periphery.

Objectives: Did you learn to . . .

- Rehydrate a child with GI symptoms?
- Recognize the manifestations of iron poisoning?
- Manage a child with an iron ingestion?

CASE 23

A 25-day-old female newborn is brought to the ED by her parents. They state that she has not been breast feeding well this morning and has felt warm. They measured her axillary temperature as 100.6°F with an axillary digital thermometer at home. They have not noticed any rhinorrhea, cough, or rashes. The baby is having five to six wet diapers per day and five to six yellow seedy stools per day. The child has not had any sick contacts. She slept normally last night, but was a little hard to wake up from her morning nap today. The baby was the 7 lb 8 oz product of an uncomplicated term gestation, born via normal spontaneous vaginal delivery to a group B *streptococcus* (GBS)-negative mother. There were no complications in the early neonatal period and the baby was discharged with the mother at 2 days of life after receiving routine neonatal care. At her 2-week weight check, she seemed to be gaining weight well and her doctor had no concerns.

Which of these is NOT a common cause of serious infections in children younger than 1 month?

A) *Listeria monocytogenes.*
B) *Neisseria meningitides.*
C) GBS.
D) *Pseudomonas aeruginosa.*

Discussion

The correct answer is "D." "A," *L. monocytogenes*, is an obligate intracellular anaerobe that is transmitted transplacentally from mother to child. "B," *N. meningitides*, is a gram-negative diplococcus that colonizes the respiratory tract of up to 15% of healthy individuals. It is usually spread through close contact. "C," GBS, is a gram-positive organism that colonizes the genital tract of normal healthy women. GBS may be the most common cause of bacterial infection in the newborn. The peak incidence of GBS disease is in the first 7 days of life, but there may be a delayed presentation out to 30 days. *Pseudomonas* infections are not commonly seen in the neonatal period.

HELPFUL TIP: Look carefully for cold sores or other vesicular lesions on children with rashes. Also try to get a history of any close contacts between the patient and people with cold sores. Herpes virus infection can be devastating to the newborn, and they may require treatment with antiviral medication.

* *

The child is seen in her father's arms. She appears to have normal color and tone. She is sleeping, but arouses after some stimulation. She seems fussy, but can be consoled by her parents. Vitals: temperature 38.7°C rectally, pulse 165, and respiratory rate 32. She appears to be well hydrated, and otherwise has a completely normal physical exam.

What further evaluation is indicated now?

A) CBC, blood cultures, catheterized urine for analysis and culture.
B) CBC, blood cultures, bag urine for analysis and culture.
C) CBC, blood cultures, chest radiograph, catheterized urine for analysis and culture.
D) CBC, blood cultures, catheterized urine for analysis and culture, lumbar puncture, and chest radiograph.

Discussion

The correct answer is "D." It is important that a complete evaluation and septic workup be performed on all children younger than 2 months without a definite source of infection. This includes CBC, blood cultures, catheterized urine specimens for analysis and culture, and a lumbar puncture. A chest x-ray need not be done in the patient without respiratory symptoms but is highly recommended. LP is mandatory. Even if you suspect a pneumonia or UTI, a lumbar puncture should still be considered, as it is impossible to tell if the bacteria have spread hematogenously to the meningeal space.

HELPFUL TIP: Do not delay antibiotic therapy to obtain a lumbar puncture. Lumbar punctures performed within 2–4 hours of receiving antibiotics should still yield valid results.

HELPFUL TIP (AND CONTROVERSY): Some would argue that a bag urine should be done as the initial urine exam. While not as specific as a cath urine, it is more sensitive for UTI. If the bag UA comes back positive, a cath specimen should be sent for culture.

You are awaiting lab results. Should you play World of Warcraft or start antibiotics? You decide to start antibiotics. Which antibiotics are most appropriate for empiric therapy in this patient?

A) Ampicillin and gentamicin.
B) Ceftriaxone.
C) Valacyclovir.

D) Amoxicillin with or without clavulanate.
E) Any of the above are equally valid choices.

Discussion

The correct answer is "A." Ampicillin and gentamicin cover all of the common causes of serious bacterial infection in the newborn, and both antibiotics penetrate into the cerebrospinal fluid (CSF) well. Ceftriaxone also penetrates the CSF well, but is highly bound to albumin and may displace bilirubin that has already bound. There have been case reports of kernicterus following the administration of ceftriaxone in newborns, so its use is not recommended in children younger than 1 month. If there is concern for a herpes virus infection, acyclovir IV would be preferred over valacyclovir, but neither of these is used on an empiric basis routinely. Amoxicillin, with or without clavulanate, does not penetrate the CSF as well as ampicillin and is thus not preferred when meningitis is a possibility.

What is the appropriate disposition for this child?

A) Admission to the general pediatrics floor.
B) Admission to the pediatric intensive care unit.
C) Monitor for 3 hours in the ED, and decide based on laboratory results.
D) Discharge with 24-hour follow-up.

Discussion

The correct answer is "A." This child does not look toxic and can probably be managed appropriately on a general pediatrics floor instead of an intensive care unit. This child should be admitted, regardless of what the laboratory results demonstrate. Some experienced practitioners will discharge a nontoxic febrile child from the ED if he or she is older than 3 months and has followed-up within 24 hours. However, there is some risk inherent in this practice—namely, that deterioration in the patient's condition may go unrecognized at home and that the family will fail to follow up. The standard of care is to admit all children who have a fever when they are 1 month old or younger.

HELPFUL TIP: With the advent of the polyvalent pneumococcal vaccine and the implementation of universal screening for GBS, the incidence of occult serious bacterial infection is falling. It may be that in the near future, the way in which febrile infants younger than 3 months are evaluated and treated will change. However, the practice outlined in Table 1–8 represents the current standard of care.

HELPFUL TIP: Even when present, otitis media **is not** considered a source of fever when evaluating the neonate. You should continue with your clinical and laboratory evaluation as if you did not even see the ears!

Objectives: Did you learn to . . .

- Describe common infections in the early neonatal period?
- Evaluate the febrile newborn?
- Manage the febrile newborn?

CASE 24

A 6-month-old male is brought to the ED by his father. He has had a little bit of rhinorrhea for the last 36 hours but no fevers. A few hours ago, he began coughing and seemed to be having some difficulty breathing. He has been taking his bottle and rice cereal well. His father states that there have been no changes in his stools. He is fully vaccinated, has no significant past medical history, and has had no known sick contacts.

What is the *most common* cause of respiratory distress in a 6-month-old (and not necessarily the diagnosis in this child)?

A) Pneumonia.
B) Foreign body aspiration.
C) Bronchiolitis.
D) Second-hand smoke exposure.

Discussion

The correct answer is "C." Bronchiolitis is very common, especially in the winter months. It is usually caused by the respiratory syncytial virus, but can also be caused by parainfluenza, influenza, and human metapneumovirus. Bronchiolitis is usually associated with profuse rhinorrhea, bronchospasm, and mucus plugging of the bronchiole tree. Although, "A," pneumonia is a serious cause of respiratory problems, it is not terribly common in infants. "B," foreign body aspiration, is something that must be always considered in an infant, especially a 6-month-old who is

Table 1–8 CURRENT RECOMMENDATIONS FOR EVALUATING THE FEBRILE CHILD

Age <28 days
- These neonates are assumed to have bacteremia and potential seeding of the CSF, even if a source is discovered.
- Workup should include cultures of blood, urine, CSF, and stool (if GI symptoms present) and CXR (if respiratory symptoms present).
- CBC and/or CRP can be obtained, but the decision about whether or not to proceed with evaluation should not be based on these results!
- The child should be admitted for IV antibiotics until cultures are negative.

Age 1–3 months
- It is safest to assume they are still unable to contain bacterial infections at this age.
- Patients at low risk of having a serious bacterial infection have the following labs:
  - WBC >5000, <15,000/mm^3 with band count <1500/mm^3
  - Normal urinalysis
  - Normal CSF
  - Stool microscopy <5 WBC/HPF if diarrhea present
- If no source is found on exam, it is reasonable for patients meeting these low-risk criteria to be managed with intramuscular ceftriaxone in the ED/clinic—if follow-up can be arranged to receive a second dose in 24 hours.
- It should be emphasized that these infants are still vulnerable to dissemination of bacterial infections. Therefore, those with an obvious source, those who appear clinically ill, or those who do not meet the low-risk criteria should be cultured and admitted for IV antibiotics until cultures are negative.

Age 3–36 months
- Management of fever in this group is somewhat controversial, as the advent of Prevnar (pneumococcal vaccine) and continued use of HIB vaccine will presumably reduce the risk of invasive bacterial disease.
- It is generally accepted that well-appearing children with fevers less than 39°C do not require further evaluation or antibiotics.
- Up to 5% of children with temperature >39°C who appear clinically well will have positive blood cultures (occult bacteremia), putting them at risk for serious infections. One approach is to obtain screening WBC on those with fevers >39°C. If WBC <5000 or >15,000/mm^3 or bands >1500/mm^3, then further evaluation of blood, urine, and CSF should be considered.

becoming more mobile (and to whom everything looks like food. . . .). Second-hand smoke exposure can cause chronic irritation to the respiratory tract and can exacerbate bronchospasm, but it is infrequently the sole cause of respiratory distress.

* *

As you examine the child, you note that he is mildly tachypneic with some suprasternal, subcostal, and intercostal retractions. He makes a wheezing whistling sound on inspiration (stridor) that seems to get worse the harder he breathes. He also has a brassy-sounding cough that does not seem to be productive.

What is the most likely diagnosis at this point?

A) Pneumonia.
B) Croup.
C) Laryngomalacia.
D) Asthma.

Discussion

The correct answer is "B." Croup, or laryngotracheobronchitis, is a common infection of the upper and lower respiratory tract. It is most commonly caused by parainfluenza virus, but may also be caused by influenza and respiratory syncytial virus. Classically, this affects children younger than 5 years, although it is occasionally seen in older children. As the glottis swells, children develop a wheeze/whistle on inspiration (inspiratory stridor) and a characteristic brassy "seal-like" barking cough. The vast majority of cases are mild. Occasionally, however, children may require control of the airway due to hypoxia. "A," pneumonia, is an infection of the lower airways that can be either bacterial or viral in nature. These children generally have a fever and productive cough. They may be tachypneic and have an increased work of breathing, but they usually do not have inspiratory stridor. "C," laryngomalacia, is a congenital disorder of unknown etiology; it may be due to supraglottic edema from reflux, hypotonia of the supraglottic tissues, etc. These children usually develop symptoms at a few weeks of age and present with inspiratory stridor that gets worse with crying. It tends to be a little better when the child is calm and in the supine position.

Laryngomalacia resolves spontaneously in the majority of children as the larynx becomes more firm and the airway diameter increases, but some children will require surgical intervention to facilitate feeding and growth. The child in this vignette is presenting with a new problem, as opposed to a chronic one, so this is not laryngomalacia. "D," asthma, is another disease of the lower airways, and wheezing is expiratory in nature.

* *

You decide to do a radiograph of this child's neck to aid in the diagnosis (although this is certainly not necessary nor advocated in most cases—but this is a board review book, not real life).

You are most likely to see which of the following on cervical radiograph?

A) Thumb sign.
B) Sign of Leser-Trélat.
C) Spine sign.
D) Retropharyngeal space swelling.
E) Steeple sign.

Discussion

The correct answer is "E." Radiographs in croup show the "steeple sign," which is a subglottic narrowing of the trachea from edema, giving it a steeple-like appearance. "A," the thumb sign, is seen in epiglottitis. "B," the sign of Leser-Trélat, is the sudden development of numerous seborrheic keratoses in a patient with internal malignancy—it's rare, not seen in children, and nearly useless knowledge . . . but that is what you are paying us for! "C," the spine sign, is loss of progressive radiolucency of the spine on lateral chest radiograph. This is seen when something—classically an infiltrate indicative of pneumonia—is overlaying the lower thoracic spine making the vertebral bodies appear more dense. Finally, "D," retropharyngeal space swelling, is seen in retropharyngeal abscess.

What is the most appropriate definitive therapy for this patient at this time?

A) Epinephrine 0.01 mg SQ.
B) Nebulized albuterol.
C) Dexamethasone 0.6 mg/kg PO/IM/IV.
D) High flow oxygen and prepare to intubate.

Discussion

The correct answer is "C." Corticosteroids help to decrease the glottic edema. One dose of dexamethasone 0.3–0.6 mg/kg (maximum of 10 mg) can be given via multiple routes (PO/IM/IV) and is usually sufficient to improve the airway swelling enough to allow the child to breathe comfortably. The advantage of dexamethasone over prednisone or another corticosteroid is that its long half-life obviates the need for further dosing at home. *While waiting for the dexamethasone to work, racemic epinephrine is commonly administered via nebulizer.* This usually leads to significant clinical improvement and gives time for the steroid to begin to take effect. Subcutaneous epinephrine is usually unnecessary. Albuterol, while helpful for bronchospasm, does not do anything to treat the glottic edema that is causing the majority of the respiratory distress. Intubation is not indicated at this point if the child is not in impending respiratory failure, hypoxic, or minimally responsive.

> HELPFUL TIP: While classically we have used racemic epinephrine, the "d" isomer is inactive. Additionally, racemic epinephrine is more expensive and must be kept refrigerated if a multidose vial is used. L-epinephrine, 5 cc of 1:1000, delivered by nebulizer is as—if not more—effective, than racemic epinephrine, is cheaper, and (our favorite since we can't do simple math!) is the same dose for everyone.

* *

You administer the appropriate dose of dexamethasone to the child along with a treatment of nebulized epinephrine. He improves markedly. You watch him for 2 hours. He is able to tolerate oral fluids well, and is active and playful. He still has a brassy cough, but no inspiratory stridor.

What should his disposition be?

A) Admit for 23 hours of observation.
B) Administer second dose of racemic epinephrine and reevaluate.
C) Discharge to home with close outpatient follow-up.
D) Administer albuterol and reevaluate.

Discussion

The correct answer is "C." After administering dexamethasone and epinephrine, it is imperative to observe children for at least 2 hours. If a child redevelops stridor at rest, he/she should receive a second dose of epinephrine. Any child who needs a second treatment has more severe croup, is at higher risk of having complications, and should be considered for hospital admission. If the child is free of stridor while at rest, he can be safely discharged with close outpatient follow-up (within 24 hours) as long as the parents are reliable, able to monitor the child, comfortable with the plan, and able to return if the child's condition should deteriorate.

HELPFUL TIP: Remember that an oxygen saturation of less than 95% is singularly abnormal in a child.

Objectives: Did you learn to . . .

- Describe common causes of respiratory distress in children?
- Manage pediatric airway problems?
- Treat children with croup?

QUICK QUIZ: FOREIGN BODY

A 3-year-old boy and his 5-year-old sister were being silly, avoiding bedtime, and jumping on their parent's bed. He had a nickel in his mouth that he'd found on the floor. When their mother walked in to wrangle them into their pajamas, they predictably collided in mid-air and both fell off the bed and onto the floor. She was unable to find the nickel after the incident. Coincidentally, the 3-year-old feels like he has something stuck in his throat.

When the family arrives in your office, he takes liquids without much trouble, but won't take anything solid. He says his "throat hurts." He's not drooling or having any trouble breathing.

How do you confirm that the coin is not in the airway?

A) CT of the larynx and chest without IV contrast.
B) CT of the larynx and chest with IV contrast.
C) AP and lateral plain films of the neck.
D) Direct laryngoscopy.
E) Call a pulmonologist for emergent fiberoptic bronchoscopy.

Discussion

The correct answer is "C." Fortunately coins are radiopaque. Some plastic toys legally contain barium and are radiopaque while others are inadvertently radiopaque (like those made in China contaminated with lead . . . a mixed blessing at best!). The esophagus tends to collapse from anterior to posterior when there is nothing in the lumen. Therefore, a coin in the esophagus should look round on an AP x-ray. By contrast, the trachea is supported by cartilaginous rings around most of its circumference. The anterior part of the trachea, however, abuts the esophagus and has no cartilage. Therefore, coins that fall into the trachea have an end-on appearance on AP radiographs and look like a disc on a lateral film.

* *

The coin fell into the stomach on the way to x-ray and the little boy feels better.

What foreign bodies in stomach need to be removed emergently?

A) A button battery.
B) A paperclip that is folded in its original form.
C) Two small magnets.
D) A doll's shoe.

Discussion

The correct answer is "C." Two magnets can attract each other through opposing loops of bowel, causing bowel necrosis and perforation. One magnet should not cause any trouble, but two should be taken seriously. **Batteries lodged in the esophagus need to be removed emergently. However, once a battery transitions to the stomach, it will likely pass without causing any difficulty. However, it should be removed if it remains in the stomach for more than 48 hours or is ≥15 mm.** Other smooth or rounded objects are unlikely to cause any trouble. Even small sharp objects (pushpins) generally pass without causing perforation or other significant damage.

CASE 25

A 67-year-old female with a history of dialysis presents slumped over and complaining of generalized weakness. By the time she is in a room, her eyes are closed, she is nonverbal, and she withdraws from painful stimuli and does not follow commands but has a palpable pulse at 80 beats per minute.

Your next step is:

A) Get a STAT potassium.
B) Check code status.
C) Check a stat bedside glucose or administer an amp of D50.
D) Start CPR.

Discussion

The correct answer is "C." Hypoglycemia is a common cause of altered mental status that is readily reversible. In a patient with a low GCS such as this one, preparation for intubation is always indicated. However, do not overlook easily reversible causes of mental status changes and give the "coma cocktail" (dextrose, oxygen, narcan, and thiamine) first. The other actions are all important but secondary. Starting CPR is not a good idea in a patient who responds (albeit to painful stimuli) and who has a pulse. However, you could add a little drama to your day this way.

> HELPFUL TIP: Many patients with narcotic overdose *do not have* pinpoint pupils. Give the naloxone regardless of pupil size. Remember the "coma cocktail": dextrose, thiamine, naloxone, and oxygen.

* *

The patient's blood sugar is 211. The patient's husband states that dialysis was not performed today. The patient also missed her last dialysis appointment 2 days ago because she felt ill at home. Her mental status is unchanged after the "coma cocktail"; she is unable to protect her airway. Husband confirms patient is full code. You decide to proceed with intubation.

The best medications to use in this patient are (induction agent/paralytic agent):

A) Etomidate/succinylcholine.
B) Etomidate/ketamine.
C) Etomidate/rocuronium.
D) An induction agent and a paralytic are unnecessary in this patient since she is only responsive to deep stimuli.

Discussion

The correct answer is "C." Rocuronium would be the paralytic of choice in this patient. In a patient with end-stage renal disease on hemodialysis, assume the presence of hyperkalemia until proven otherwise. Succinylcholine may cause hyperkalemia (and cardiac arrest) so it is contraindicated in patients with a high likelihood of hyperkalemia. Succinylcholine should also be avoided in crush injuries, neurologic injuries/myopathies, and burn patients where it may cause malignant hyperthermia. A sedative should be used for induction to prevent pain and either etomidate or ketamine may be used.

* *

You secure the airway. A STAT potassium returns at 7.9. You look at the monitor and notice the QRS is looking a little wide. While you are waiting for an ECG to be obtained, you let your nurse know to grab what first:

A) Kayexalate.
B) Sodium bicarbonate.
C) Calcium gluconate.
D) Insulin/glucose.
E) Albuterol nebulizer.

Discussion

The correct answer is "C." In hyperkalemia with evidence of ECG changes (peaked T waves, wide QRS, sine wave), calcium needs to be administered immediately. The calcium stabilizes cardiac cell membranes within 1 minute. Calcium gluconate 1 g or calcium chloride 1 g may be given. Calcium chloride is irritating to veins and may cause necrosis if it extravasates: central line administration is preferred. All of the other answers do lower potassium levels (including continuously nebulized albuterol), but when there is evidence of ECG changes, giving calcium is your top priority. The other agents may take as long as 30–60 minutes to act. As a note, bicarbonate may not be particularly effective in patients with end-stage renal disease, another reason to use calcium first in this patient.

> HELPFUL TIP: Continue administering calcium every 5 minutes until ECG changes resolve. However, **in a patient with digitalis toxicity and hyperkalemia, DO NOT give calcium. Treat with digoxin-specific antibodies (Fab fragments) along with the rest of the treatments listed . . . just avoid calcium that increases digoxin binding to the heart.**

* *

After two doses of calcium gluconate, the QRS narrows and you want to get the excess potassium out of your patient's body.

Which of the following removes potassium from the body?

A) Hemodialysis.
B) Insulin/glucose.
C) Kayexalate.
D) Albuterol.
E) A and C.

Discussion
The correct answer is "E." Both hemodialysis and kayexalate will remove potassium from the body. Insulin/glucose will drive it intracellularly in 30–60 minutes but does not rid the body of potassium. Be careful: kayexalate exchanges sodium for potassium and thus may worsen congestive heart failure.

* *

The patient does well and, in the future, knows to avoid "light" salt (KCl) (of course, "light" is now spelled "lite" for some unknown reason).

Objectives: Did you learn . . .

- The contraindications of succinylcholine in intubation?
- The treatment of hyperkalemia in the acute situation?
- The use of the "coma cocktail" and what that entails?
- A bit about RSI?

CASE 26

A 24-year-old male presents to your ED complaining of "dental pain." He reports a long history of poor dental hygiene and has not seen a dentist in several years. He smokes two packs of cigarettes per day (and proudly wears a "Marlboro" hat) and admits drinking a 2-L bottle of "My Sugary Pop" every day at work (it includes a free coupon for dental service after 100 bottles, but he has never availed himself of this). The pain is described as constant and throbbing in nature located in the right lower jaw area.

What findings during your examination would raise your concern regarding the patient's clinical condition?

A) Large amounts of secretions.
B) Decreased ability to open his mouth for the examination.
C) Swollen and elevated tongue.
D) Pain and decreased range of motion of the neck.
E) All of the above.

Discussion
The correct answer is "E." If a patient is having trouble swallowing secretions ("A"), it should raise concern for swelling in the posterior pharynx which can compromise not only the ability to swallow one's saliva but can also signal a high risk for upper airway occlusion secondary to swelling. Trismus ("B") is also concerning because it may indicate deeper infection involving the muscles of mastication. "C," a swollen and elevated tongue, may indicate the development of Ludwig angina, a life-threatening infection of the floor of the mouth, which can spread to the deeper tissues of the submandibular and submaxillary spaces. "D," pain and decreased range of motion of the neck, could indicate the possibility of a retropharyngeal abscess.

> **HELPFUL TIP:** Adult epiglottitis often presents with sore throat and neck tenderness. So, if the patient has neck tenderness out of proportion to what you would expect, consider epiglottitis or a retropharyngeal abscess.

* *

Luckily, the patient is otherwise clinically stable aside from the focal dental pain. Your examination shows the tissues around tooth no. 29 to be swollen and inflamed with signs of fluctuance and severe tenderness on palpation. An orthopantogram shows a periodontal abscess.

Which antibiotic is NOT an appropriate choice for this clinical condition?

A) Penicillin VK.
B) Clindamycin.
C) Amoxicillin/clavulanate.
D) Trimethoprim–sulfamethoxazole.

Discussion
The correct answer is "D." Penicillin VK, clindamycin, and amoxicillin/clavulanate all provide good coverage for anaerobic bacteria and gram-negative cocci, which are the main culprits in dental infections. TMP–SMX has some gram-negative coverage but lacks the anaerobic coverage needed to treat infections of the oral cavity.

* *

The same gentleman returns to you 3 weeks later complaining of a sore throat. On exam, he looks toxic and has fever, chills, dyspnea/cough, and unilateral neck swelling. His throat looks similar to a streptococcal tonsillitis. However, the neck is tender *and this guy really looks sick*. Pulse is 130 and BP is 80/50. He was seen last week by someone else for a mild sore throat and given a "Z-Pack" (azithromycin—mostly on a whim). He has gotten progressively worse. Chest x-ray shows infiltrates.

Your presumptive diagnosis is:

A) Mononucleosis.
B) *Fusobacterium*.
C) *Arcanobacterium heamolyticum*.
D) Viral URI.

Discussion

The correct answer is "B." *Fusobacterium* is an anaerobic infection that has been found with increasing frequency in adolescent/college age patients. It can initially present similarly to a strep throat but may go on to "Lemierre syndrome," which is a septic thrombophlebitis of the internal jugular vein. This can then lead to septic emboli to the lungs, sepsis, and multiorgan failure. The point here is that penicillin is still the drug of choice for strep throat, and it covers *Fusobacterium*, which the macrolides do not. As for the other answers, this is not likely mononucleosis ("A"), since the neck swelling is unilateral and patients with mono usually are not this toxic nor have infiltrate on chest x-ray. "C," *A. heamolyticum*, is also common in college age students and is initially indistinguishable from strep throat. However, 50% of patients will have a maculopapular or scarlatiniform rash starting on the extremities and involving the trunk and back but sparing the head. It rarely causes invasive disease such as pneumonia or meningitis. It also will respond to erythromycin or clindamycin. "D" is obviously incorrect and if you chose this one, back to medical school for you!

* *

The patient spends 3 weeks in the ICU and eventually succumbs to his disease. Not good.

Objectives: Did you learn . . .

- About *Fusobacterium* and *Arcanobacterium*?
- A bit about the treatment of dental abscesses?
- Warning signs of impending badness in those with head and neck infections?

BIBLIOGRAPHY

ACEP Clinical Policies Committee; Clinical Policies Subcommittee on Seizures. Clinical policy: Critical issues in the evaluation and management of adult patients presenting to the emergency department with seizures. *Ann Emerg Med*. 2004;43:605-625.

Carraro S, et al. Bronchiolitis: From empiricism to scientific evidence. *Minerva Pediatr*. 2009;61:217-225.

Frithsen IL, Simpson WM Jr. Recognition and management of acute medication poisoning. *Am Fam Physician*. 2010;81:316-323.

Herz AM, et al. Changing epidemiology of outpatient bacteremia in 3- to 36-month-old children after the introduction of the heptavalent-conjugated pneumococcal vaccine. *Pediatr Infect Dis J*. 2006;25:293-300.

Isbister GK, Kumar VV. Indications for single-dose activated charcoal administration in acute overdose. *Curr Opin Crit Care*. 2011;17:351-357.

Leung AKC, Sigalet DL. Acute abdominal pain in children. *Am Fam Physician*. 2003;67:2321-2326.

Marx JA, et al. *Emergency Medicine: Concepts and Clinical Practice*. 7th ed. Elsevier Health Sciences; 2010; Mosby, St Loius, MO.

Mokhlesi B, et al. Adult toxicology in critical care: Part II: Specific poisonings. *Chest*. 2003;123:897-922.

Nikkanen H, Skolnik A. Diagnosis and management of carbon monoxide poisoning in the emergency department. *Emerg Med Pract*. 2011;13:1-14.

Panju AA, et al. Is this patient having a myocardial infarction? *JAMA*. 1998;280:1256.

Rogers RL, McCormack R. Aortic disasters. *Emerg Med Clin North Am*. 2004;22:887-908.

Steiner RW. Treating acute bronchiolitis associated with RSV. *Am Fam Physician*. 2004;69:325-330.

Touger M, et al. Relationship between venous and arterial carboxyhemoglobin levels in patients with suspected carbon monoxide poisoning. *Ann Emerg Med*. 1995;25(4):481-483.

Yucesoy K, Yuksel KZ. SCIWORA in MRI era. *Clin Neurol Neurosurg*. 2008;110:429-433.

2

Cardiology

Sailesh C. Harwani and Mark A. Graber

CASE 1

A 35-year-old female presents with a 1-hour history of chest pain, which resolved spontaneously. The pain is described as a chest pressure radiating to both arms. The patient is a smoker but has no other risk factors (no family history of cardiac disease, hypertension, diabetes, hyperlipidemia, etc.). The patient is diaphoretic and has a normal blood pressure. Physical exam reveals that the patient has tenderness to palpation of the anterior chest wall that reproduces the chest pressure. She is now otherwise chest pain free, and serologies, including cardiac enzymes, are normal.

Which of the following is true about this patient's physical findings and history?

A) Pain radiating to both arms makes it unlikely that this patient's pain is cardiac.
B) The physical findings that are most highly associated with an acute myocardial infarction (AMI) include hypotension, diaphoresis, and a new S3 gallop.
C) The absence of risk factors makes it unlikely that this patient has cardiac disease.
D) The fact that the pain is reproducible on palpation of the chest wall effectively rules out cardiac disease.
E) Based on the information available, further cardiac evaluation is unnecessary.

Discussion

The correct answer is "B." The findings that are most likely to be associated with an AMI are hypotension, diaphoresis, and a new S3 gallop. "A" is not true because pain radiating to both arms can still be associated with cardiac disease. In fact, compared with left arm radiation, right arm radiation or bilateral arm radiation increases the likelihood of the pain being cardiac. Women with AMI often present atypically and may experience more chest pain radiating to the right arm/shoulder and the anterior neck as compared with men. "C" is incorrect. The absence of risk factors is only one consideration in the evaluation of this patient. Smoking, hypertension, family history, etc., do not change the prior probability of cardiac disease enough to allow them to be used to rule out or rule in cardiac disease. However, male gender and diabetes do increase the pretest probability of coronary artery disease (CAD). "D" is incorrect. It is true that chest pain reproduced by palpation of the chest wall makes cardiac disease less likely. However, 15% of patients with cardiac disease and 17% of patients with a pulmonary embolism (PE) will have their pain reproduced by chest wall pressure. This does not mean that you are making their cardiac pain worse. It is likely because of the patient's inability to discriminate between the types of pain (cardiac vs. chest wall).

* *

You decide that further testing is warranted, including an ECG and cardiac enzymes.

Which of the following statements is TRUE?

A) A normal initial ECG in the emergency department (ED) effectively rules out cardiac disease.

B) The serum troponin is more sensitive than the CPK-MB in the first 6 hours after a myocardial infarction.
C) Serum troponin is an unreliable marker of cardiac ischemia in patients with renal failure.
D) The serum troponin is 100% specific for myocardial infarction.
E) A normal troponin and CPK in the ED cannot be used to make decisions about who to admit.

Discussion

The correct answer is "E." Except in cases where the chest pain has been continuous for over 12 hours, normal cardiac enzymes (troponin, CPK-MB) do not rule out cardiac disease. If they did, we would not admit patients for a "rule out" but would rather rely on the single level drawn in the ED. "A" is incorrect since 9% of patients with AMI will have a normal initial ECG in the ED. In fact, only about 50% of those with AMI have a diagnostic ECG in the ED. **Even a normal ECG obtained during chest pain does not reliably rule out AMI** (Acad Emerg Med 2009;16:495). "B" is incorrect since the CPK-MB is more sensitive in the first 6 hours than is the troponin (about 84% vs. 74%). However, at least one of them will be positive in 80% of patients within 2–3 hours ED arrival **(but of course, 80% is not good enough when you are dealing with a potential AMI)**. "C" is incorrect. Patients with renal disease may have a mildly elevated troponin at baseline due to poor clearance, but troponin can still be useful in these patients if it continues to rise. It is useful to have knowledge of the patient's baseline troponin. "D" is incorrect because we now know that other processes, such as PE, can elevate the serum troponin.

> HELPFUL TIP: Elevated troponin levels may be due to conditions other than AMI, including CHF, PE, burns, sepsis or other critical illness, stroke, and others.

> HELPFUL TIP: The new ultra-sensitive troponin May be positive within 3 hours. You need to know what test your hospital is doing.

All of the following statements are true EXCEPT:

A) All myocardial infarctions present with chest pain.
B) Dyspnea may be the only presenting symptom of myocardial infarction.
C) Patients with myocardial infarction can present with syncope.
D) Females, the elderly, and diabetic patients are more likely to present with atypical symptoms of myocardial infarction.

Discussion

The correct answer is "A." This statement is not true. Many elderly and diabetic patients will present with painless or "silent" myocardial infarctions. In fact, up to 30% of myocardial infarctions are pain free. "B" is a correct statement because, especially in the elderly, dyspnea may be the only presenting symptom due to left ventricular failure secondary to ischemia. "C" is a correct statement because syncope (as well as lightheadedness and fatigue) can be presenting symptoms of a myocardial infarction. "D" is correct because the elderly and diabetic patients may present with atypical symptoms.

* *

Her ECG shows nonspecific ST-T changes.

Which of the following drug(s) is/are indicated in the initial management of this patient?

A) Aspirin.
B) Thrombolytic such as tPA or streptokinase.
C) Heparin.
D) A and B.
E) A and C.

Discussion

The correct answer is "A." Immediate therapy in the ED requires ASA 325 mg orally (chewed). Since we are not sure that this patient has AMI or unstable angina, there is no indication for thrombolytic therapy or heparin. Additionally, since she is currently pain free, heparin carries more of a risk than a benefit at this juncture. However, all patients with possible angina or an AMI should have aspirin unless they are truly allergic (hives, anaphylaxis). "B" is incorrect because thrombolytics are indicated for acute ST elevation myocardial infarctions (STEMI).

> HELPFUL TIP: Should "MONA (morphine, oxygen, nitroglycerin, aspirin) greet all patients," as the editors learned in med school? The efficacy of oxygen in AMI has been questioned and may even be detrimental in those

with a normal oxygen saturation (94% or greater). (*Cochrane Database of Systematic Reviews* 2010, Issue 6. Art No.: CD007160. DOI: 10.1002/14651858.CD007160.pub2.).

HELPFUL TIP: Current use of warfarin or aspirin should **not** preclude the administration of aspirin in the ED for a patient with chest pain that may be cardiac in origin. You never know whether the patient is actually taking it or not. So, unless there is a real allergy to aspirin, it must be given to chest pain patients in the ED.

* *

The patient tells you that she is allergic to aspirin, which causes hives and bronchospasm. She can, however, take other nonsteroidal anti-inflammatory drugs (NSAIDs) without difficulty. Oh, great. Now you need to go to plan B.

Which of the following is an acceptable substitute for aspirin in this situation?

A) Dipyridamole.
B) Clopidogrel (Plavix).
C) Ibuprofen or naproxen
D) Celecoxib (Celebrex)
E) Salsalate.

Discussion
The correct answer is "B." Clopidogrel in a loading dose of 600 mg can be used as a substitute for aspirin in the setting of unstable angina or AMI. "A" is incorrect because dipyridamole (in combination with aspirin) is indicated only for stroke prevention. It is a relatively weak platelet inhibitor. "C" is incorrect because neither ibuprofen nor naproxen has been shown to be of benefit in angina/AMI and they are reversible platelet inhibitors that do not give adequate platelet inhibition. Additionally, both can block the effect of aspirin by making binding sites on platelets unavailable (Catella-Lawson et al., 2001). In fact, stopping NSAIDs in any patient being admitted for possible CAD is considered good practice. "D" and "E" are both incorrect because neither drug inhibits platelets to a significant degree and thus would be of no use in this situation.

HELPFUL TIP: Note that the loading dose of clopidogrel has been increased to 600 mg from 300 mg. But either is likely an acceptable answer on the board exam (and in practice).

* *

Well, not all chest pain is cardiac, and this patient may have another cause for hers.

Which of the following is TRUE?

A) Giving a "GI cocktail" (e.g., Maalox and lidocaine) can reliably differentiate cardiac from esophageal/GI causes of chest pain.
B) A normal chest radiograph and symmetrical pulses in the upper extremities reliably rules out a thoracic aortic dissection.
C) Most patients with a spontaneous pneumothorax should be treated with a chest tube.
D) If nitroglycerin relieves the chest pain, then the pain is certainly cardiac.
E) Pain is a finding in only approximately 60% of patients with a PE.

Discussion
The correct answer is "E." Only a small majority (59%) of PEs have pain as a feature. "A" is incorrect because about 20% of patients with cardiac pain will have their pain relieved by a GI cocktail. Conversely, "D" is incorrect because nitroglycerin can relieve pain from esophageal spasm. "B" is incorrect because only 50% of patients with an aortic dissection will have unequal pulses and blood pressures, and only 75% will have an abnormal chest x-ray. The consideration of an aortic dissection mandates a chest CT scan, transesophageal echo, or angiogram. Remember that about 20% of the population will have unequal blood pressures in the upper extremities at baseline. "C" is incorrect because most patients with spontaneous pneumothorax can be treated with a "pigtail" catheter with a Heimlich valve. This type of treatment reduces the morbidity associated with a chest tube.

HELPFUL TIP: Chest x-ray findings in patients with thoracic aortic dissection may include widened mediastinum, obliterated aortic knob, pleural "capping," tracheal deviation, depression of left main stem bronchus, esophageal deviation, and loss of the paratracheal stripe

* *

The patient's pain recurs in the ED. You suspect that the patient is having a myocardial infarction, but do not yet have unequivocal proof such as ECG changes or elevated enzymes. The patient becomes markedly hypotensive in response to another dose of sublingual nitroglycerin.

Which of the following is TRUE?

A) Intravenous nitroglycerin is contraindicated in this patient.
B) Hypotension caused by nitroglycerin is usually unresponsive to IV saline.
C) Hypotension caused by nitroglycerin may be indicative of a right ventricular infarction, which is most commonly associated with an inferior wall MI.
D) Hypotension caused by nitroglycerin is diagnostic of cardiogenic shock, suggesting that this patient will have a poor outcome.

Discussion

The correct answer is "C." Hypotension in response to nitroglycerin may be indicative of a right ventricular infarct, which is most commonly associated with an inferior wall MI. Since the right ventricle is dependent on filling pressure (preload), nitroglycerin, which drops the preload, will frequently result in hypotension in those with a right ventricular infarct. "A" is incorrect because hypotension from sublingual nitroglycerin is not a contraindication to additional nitrates *once the patient's blood pressure is stable.* A typical sublingual dose is 400 μg (0.4 mg). A typical IV dose starts at 20 μg/min. Thus, the sublingual dose is quite a bit larger than the IV dose. In such a situation, you could consider starting IV nitroglycerin at 10–20 μg/min and titrating up as the blood pressure allows. "B" is incorrect because hypotension from nitroglycerin will generally respond to a saline bolus. "D" is incorrect. Certainly, patients with cardiogenic shock will be hypotensive, but hypotension with nitroglycerin is a common result of the drug itself and does not define cardiogenic shock.

HELPFUL TIP: Consider holding beta-blockers in inferior wall acute MI (IAMI), as these patients often have bradycardia and heart block. Also, beware of atypical presentations of IAMI such as nausea, vomiting, and other GI symptoms.

Which of the following is TRUE of patients with an inferior wall myocardial infarction?

A) They will likely continue to have problems with right ventricular functioning in the future.
B) They will need to increase their salt intake in order to increase preload and right ventricular filling pressure.
C) Their right ventricular function should return to normal or close to normal following her infarction.
D) A and B.

Discussion

The correct answer is "C." Most patients will have return of right ventricular functioning following a myocardial infarction. "B" is incorrect because there will be no need to increase right ventricular filling pressure (which is what IV saline does acutely) once right ventricular function returns to normal.

* *

The patient's pain continues despite treatment with nitroglycerin, and you obtain another ECG (Figure 2–1).

Which of the following is TRUE regarding this ECG?

A) This injury pattern on ECG is most consistent with an anterior wall MI.
B) In this situation, intervention in the cath lab with percutaneous transluminal coronary angioplasty (PTCA) and stent placement is superior to tPA or other thrombolytic.
C) This injury pattern on ECG is most consistent with pericarditis.
D) This injury pattern on ECG proves that this patient does not have an aortic dissection.
E) This pattern on ECG is totally fine. What, me worry?

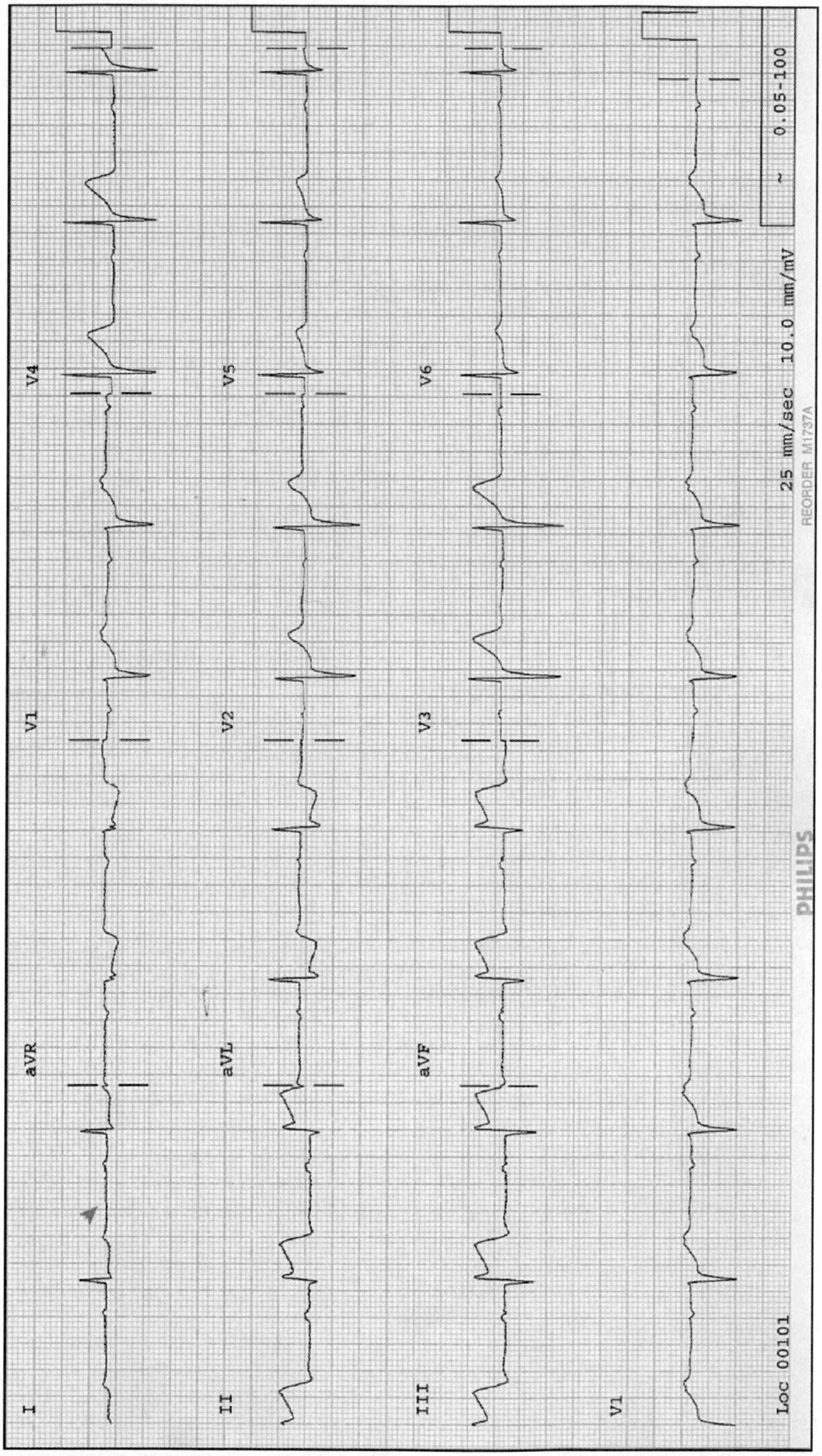

I
aVR
V1
V4
II
aVL
V2
V5
III
aVF
V3
V6
V1
Loc 00101
PHILIPS
25 mm/sec 10.0 mm/mV
REORDER M1737A
~ 0.05-100

Figure 2–1

Discussion

The correct answer is "B." Intervention in the cath lab with PTCA and/or stent placement is superior to thrombolytic therapy in the treatment of MI, provided that the "door to balloon" time is 90 minutes or less. In cases where the patient is located in a facility without a cardiac catheterization laboratory, the patient may receive thrombolytic therapy. "A" is incorrect because this pattern is indicative of an **inferior wall**, not an anterior wall, MI. You will note that this ECG shows ST elevations in leads II, III, and aVF (inferior leads) along with reciprocal ST segment depression in leads V1 and V2. An anterior wall MI is defined by ST elevations in leads V3, V4, and V5, and an anteroseptal MI shows ST elevations in leads V1, V2, and V3. "D" is incorrect because patients with pericarditis should have ST elevations in all leads (although an ECG is only 80% sensitive for pericarditis). "D" is incorrect because patients with an aortic dissection can present with an abnormal ECG that looks similar to an infarct pattern. So, ECG changes do not prove that the patient does not have an aortic dissection. "E" is just plain wrong.

* *

You now have all the evidence that you need to show that this patient is indeed having an ongoing myocardial infarction. Since your rural hospital is "just around the corner from nowhere," you decide to initiate thrombolytic therapy.

All of the following are true statements EXCEPT:

A) Patients who are candidates for thrombolytics must have at least 1 mm of ST-segment elevation in at least 2 contiguous limb leads or at least 1–2 mm of ST-segment elevation in at least 2 contiguous precordial leads.

B) Patients who are candidates for thrombolytics must have an absence of prior history of hemorrhagic stroke within the past year.

C) Patients who are candidates for thrombolytics should have no active bleeding, including menstrual bleeding.

D) Patients who are candidates for thrombolytics should have no history of recent head trauma.

E) Patients who are candidates for thrombolytics should not be pregnant.

Discussion

The correct answer is "C." While active internal bleeding is a contraindication to the use of thrombolytics, menstrual bleeding is not. While there are no controlled trials, anecdotal evidence suggests that thrombolytics are safe with menstrual bleeding. "A" is correct. In addition to these ECG criteria, the presence of a new complete bundle branch block with characteristic MI pain also indicates that the patient will benefit from thrombolysis. Patients with only ST-segment depression or a normal ECG, even with symptoms, do **not** benefit. "B," "D," and "E" are all true statements. Patients are not candidates for thrombolytics if they have recent head trauma, are pregnant, or have had a hemorrhagic stroke in the last year. There are additional criteria for and contraindications to the use of thrombolytics. See Tables 2–1a and 2–1b.

Table 2-1a ACC/AHA GUIDELINES FOR THE MANAGEMENT OF PATIENTS WITH ST-ELEVATION MYOCARDIAL INFARCTION

Class 1 recommendations for the use of thrombolytics in myocardial infarction include any ONE of the following three ECG findings:

- $\geq$1 mm of ST-segment elevation in at least 2 contiguous limb leads
- 1–2 mm of ST-segment elevation in at least 2 contiguous precordial leads
- **New** complete bundle branch block that obscures the ST segment analysis plus a history suggestive of MI

And

- 12 hours since the onset of pain, age <75 years (although treating those >75 years of age is still a class 2 recommendation below)

Class 2 recommendations for the use of thrombolytics in myocardial infarction include any ONE of the following:

- $\geq$1 mm of ST-segment elevation in at least 2 contiguous limb leads and age >75 years OR presenting 12–24 hours after onset of infarction
- 1–2 mm of ST-segment elevation in at least 2 contiguous precordial leads and age >75 years OR presenting 12–24 hours after the onset of infarction
- Blood pressure of >180 systolic and >100 diastolic in a patient with a "high-risk" myocardial infarction (e.g., the high risk of the MI mitigates the warning about thrombolytic use in uncontrolled hypertension)

Reproduced from Antman EM, et al. ACC/AHA guidelines for the management of patients with ST-elevation myocardial infarction—executive summary. *J Am Coll Cardiol.* 2004;44(3): 671-719. Copyright 2004, with permission from Elsevier.

HELPFUL TIP: "Facilitated PCI," that is, use of PCI within 2+ hours of giving thrombolytics has very mixed (and mostly negative) data.

Outcomes are worse (and not just because PCI is a "rescue" technique at this point). It certainly is not standard of care. If facilitated PCI is being considered, it is worth contacting the cardiologist at the cath center to determine whether she would like thrombolytics before transfer.

HELPFUL TIP: Remember to repeat the ECG **after** thrombolytics to prove that ST elevations have resolved.

* *

After conferring with your closest cath center, you give a thrombolytic—and cross your fingers. Unfortunately, the patient develops a new left bundle branch block (LBBB). Additionally, the ECG shows evidence of a first-degree heart block (a prolonged PR interval), although the heart rate remains normal at 80 bpm.

Table 2-1b ACC/AHA GUIDELINES FOR THE MANAGEMENT OF PATIENTS WITH ST-ELEVATION MYOCARDIAL INFARCTION

Class 3 "Absolute" contraindications to the use of thrombolytic therapy in MI

- Previous hemorrhagic stroke at any time or stroke within the last 12 months
- Known intracranial neoplasm
- Active internal bleeding (but not menstrual bleeding)
- Suspected aortic dissection

Relative contraindications to the use of thrombolytic therapy in MI

- Uncontrolled hypertension (>180/110) at the time of presentation.
- History of bleeding diathesis, ongoing anticoagulation (INR >2–3)
- Trauma, including traumatic CPR within 2–4 weeks, major surgery within 3 weeks
- Noncompressible vascular punctures (e.g., subclavian line)
- Internal bleeding within the last 2–4 weeks
- Pregnancy
- Peptic ulcer disease (bleeding or not)
- Severe, chronic hypertension

Reproduced from Antman EM, et al. ACC/AHA guidelines for the management of patients with ST-elevation myocardial infarction—executive summary. *J Am Coll Cardiol.* 2004;44(3): 671-719. Copyright 2004, with permission from Elsevier.

Table 2-2 TYPE OF HEART BLOCK ASSOCIATED WITH INFARCTION

Anterior myocardial infarction	Bundle branch blocks Mobitz type II second-degree heart block
Inferior myocardial infarction	Bradycardia from: • Mobitz type I second-degree heart block • Third-degree heart block

The proper response to this is to:

A) Insert a Swan-Ganz catheter to monitor central pressures.
B) Insert a temporary pacemaker regardless of the heart rate.
C) Administer atropine to this patient.
D) Administer isoproterenol to this patient.
E) Do nothing, other than observe this patient.

Discussion

The correct answer is "B." For patients with an AMI, a transvenous pacemaker should be inserted if she develops (1) complete heart block, (2) 2nd degree heart block type II (Mobitz II), or (3) new LBBB with first-degree AV block. See Tables 2–2 and 2–3 for more on arrhythmia and pacemakers in the setting of AMI. "A" is incorrect because a Swan-Ganz catheter will be of no help in arrhythmias. "C" is incorrect because atropine is indicated for symptomatic bradycardia and not for just a bundle branch block. "D" is incorrect for the same reason as "C." Additionally, isoproterenol is arrhythmogenic and is no longer recommended. "E" is incorrect because the patient may rapidly progress into a complete heart block. Of note, the placement of a transvenous pacemaker should not delay catheterization since a pacemaker may be placed in the cath lab.

Table 2-3 CLASS I INDICATIONS FOR PACEMAKER IN PATIENTS WITH AN ACUTE MYOCARDIAL INFARCTION

New left bundle branch block + first-degree AV block
New right bundle branch block + left anterior or posterior fascicular block + first-degree AV block
Mobitz type II heart block
Third-degree heart block
Symptomatic bradycardia unresponsive to atropine.

* *

The patient requires heparin with the thrombolytic that you choose.

Which of the following dosing regimens is the best accepted for use in AMIs?

A) Enoxaparin 30 mg SQ every 12 hours.
B) Enoxaparin 1 mg/kg SQ every 12 hours.
C) Heparin 5000 units bolus and a drip at 1000 units per hour.
D) Heparin 100 unit/kg bolus with a drip at 25 unit/kg/hr.
E) None of the above represents the best dosing option in this situation.

Discussion

The correct answer is "B." For anticoagulation in AMI, the dose of enoxaparin is 1 mg/kg SQ every 12 hours. "A" is incorrect since 30 mg SQ every 12 hours is the dose for DVT prophylaxis, not for anticoagulation. "C" is incorrect. This is the classic way that heparin has been dosed but it **is not** the best option listed. "D" is incorrect as well. The **correct** dose for heparin **when given with a thrombolytic is** 60 U/kg bolus (maximum of 4000 units) with a drip of 15 units/kg/hr (maximum dose of 1000 units/hr). The bottom line here is that either enoxaparin or heparin can be used in this setting, and they are more or less equivalent. If you choose to use heparin, do not use fixed dose heparin but rather weight-based dosing.

> HELPFUL TIP: Did you know that for ST-elevation MI, an initial dose of 30 mg of **IV enoxaparin** (that's right—intravenous) should be given with the **first (and only the first)** SQ dose for those age <75 years. Do it.

* *

The patient receives her thrombolytic, enoxaparin, and transvenous pacing, and she is admitted to the hospital to a monitored bed. You get a call from the nursing staff 5 hours later. The rhythm strip shows 3 PVCs per minute. Your patient remains pain free and is hemodynamically stable.

The nurse (who has more than a few gray hairs) would like an order for lidocaine. Your response is:

A) "Do it. Give the lidocaine."
B) "Give amiodarone—it works better than lidocaine."
C) "Give no antiarrhythmic at this point in time."
D) "Check labs including potassium and magnesium."
E) C and D.

Discussion

The correct answer is "E." The use of lidocaine in this setting incurs no benefit and is proarrhythmic. The same is true for prophylactic amiodarone, which can cause torsades de pointes. In the setting of AMI, antiarrhythmics may be indicated only for complex arrhythmias (PVC couplets, triplets, nonsustained ventricular tachycardia [<30 seconds], or >10 PVCs per minute). More than 90% of patients will have isolated PVCs in the peri-infarct period, and there is no association with increased mortality. Correcting hypokalemia and hypomagnesemia can help to reduce arrhythmias, and checking these labs is prudent.

* *

The patient remains pain free while in the hospital. She is ready to be discharged 4 days later.

Which of the following tests is the most appropriate for this patient prior to discharge?

A) Coronary angiography.
B) Submaximal stress test.
C) Full Bruce protocol, symptom limited, stress test.
D) Spiral CT to assess for coronary artery calcification.

Discussion

The correct answer is "B." Submaximal stress testing is considered the standard of care. Patients with a positive submaximal stress test should be referred for catheterization. Patients with a borderline stress test can be sent for a radionuclide study. Coronary angiography **is not** routinely recommended for all patients who have had a myocardial infarction unless they are considered to be at high risk (continued symptoms, positive screening test such as submaximal stress test, CHF, etc.). "C" is incorrect because a symptom-limited, full-protocol stress test should be done only 14–21 days after an infarction. Finally, spiral CT to assess for coronary artery calcification has no role in risk stratification after a myocardial infarction... their risk is 100%!

The patient passes her stress test with flying colors. Patients after a myocardial infarction should be routinely discharged on all of the following medications EXCEPT:

A) Aspirin.
B) Beta-blocker.
C) Continuous nitroglycerin (e.g., patch or isosorbide).
D) Lipid lowering agent, if appropriate.
E) Sublingual nitroglycerin for PRN use.

Discussion

The correct answer is "C." There is no benefit to scheduled nitrates unless needed for a specific indication (e.g., recurrent angina). **All postmyocardial infarction patients should be discharged on aspirin, beta-blocker, statin (in most cases), nitroglycerin PRN, and an angiotensin-converting enzyme (ACE) inhibitor (if tolerable, of course).**

* *

This patient had a STEMI (or "Q-wave" MI).

Which of the following statements is TRUE?

A) Patients with a non-STEMI have the same or perhaps a bit worse outcomes long term than do patients with a STEMI.
B) Patients with a non-STEMI have worse in-hospital outcomes when compared with patients with a STEMI.
C) Unstable angina and non-STEMI can be readily differentiated from one another on presentation.
D) None of the above is true.

Discussion

The correct answer is "A." Patients with a non-STEMI actually have the same or perhaps even slightly worse outcomes long term as do patients with a STEMI. This makes sense; there is still myocardium left to infarct after a non-STEMI. As to the other answers, patients with a STEMI do have worse in-hospital outcomes, and unstable angina and non-STEMI look similar on ECG with T-wave inversion, etc., but without the ST elevations that are classically seen in a transmural infarction.

* *

Two months later, the patient presents with her sister, who wants to know what risk factors you consider when determining a patient's cholesterol goal for primary prevention.

The following are all considered cardiac risk factors when calculating target cholesterol EXCEPT:

A) Male >45 years old.
B) First-degree female relative with CAD >65 years old.
C) Smoking.
D) Hypertension.
E) HDL cholesterol of <40 mg/dL.

Discussion

The correct answer is "B." It should be female relative with CAD at <65 years of age, not >65 years of age. See Table 2–4 for a complete listing of cardiac risk factors. Just to be complete, if the patient has an HDL >60 mg/dL, this counts as a protective factor and "cancels out" one of the risk factors. Also, this is a mental exercise. None of this applies to the patient who has already had an AMI.

* *

The patient remembers reading something about risk factors that are considered equivalent to having CAD when deciding whether or not to start lipid-lowering therapy.

All of the following are *automatically* considered "CAD equivalents" when determining whether or not to start a statin EXCEPT:

A) Diabetes mellitus.
B) Symptomatic carotid disease.
C) Peripheral vascular disease.
D) Severe, sustained hypertension (>180/110).
E) A and D.

Table 2-4 RISK FACTORS FOR CORONARY ARTERY DISEASE

- First-degree male relative with CAD at age <55 or first-degree female relative with CAD at age <65
- Smoking
- HDL <40 mg/dL
- Hypertension
- Age: males >45, females >55
- Elevated LDL

Discussion

The correct answer is "E." Severe hypertension and diabetes **are not** considered CAD equivalent risk factors when deciding whether a patient should be started on lipid-lowering therapy. In addition to symptomatic carotid disease and peripheral vascular disease, other CAD equivalent risk factors include abdominal aortic aneurysm and multiple risk factors that elevate the risk of CAD to $>20\%$ in the next 10 years (see Table 2–5).

> HELPFUL TIP: So what about this diabetes thing not being considered a CAD equivalent? Diabetes essentially adds 15 years to the patient's age in terms of cardiac risk. So, a 30-year-old diabetic patient has the cardiac risk of a 45-year-old without diabetes. **Over age 50, diabetes becomes a CAD equivalent in terms of MI risk.** (*Lancet* 2006; 368:29–36)

* *

The patient actually wants to know about something she read about "crap" and cardiac disease. A light bulb goes off and you realize she wants to know about C-reactive protein (CRP).

Which of the following best represents the role of CRP in cardiac disease in 2012?

A) CRP should be measured in all patients in whom cardiac disease is suspected.
B) CRP should be measured only in patients with intermediate cardiac risk factors (e.g., those with a 10-year risk of CAD of 10–20%).
C) CRP should be measured in patients with known heart disease in order to monitor inflammation and risk.
D) CRP should be measured in low-risk ($<10\%$ risk of CAD in next 10 years) patients who have no known cardiac disease. An elevated CRP suggests that these patients should be treated with a lipid-lowering therapy.
E) CRP has not been shown to be useful and does not contribute significantly to cardiac risk stratification.

Discussion

The correct answer is "E." Although, high-sensitivity CRP (hsCRP) was initially thought to be a possible biomarker for cardiac risk assessment, it has been shown to be of marginal benefit. The use of hsCRP led to a minimal reclassification of patients (Patel and Budoff, 2010). The Class IIa recommendation to use hsCRP was published by the AHA in 2003, prior to further studies that have questioned its usefulness.

> HELPFUL TIP: We don't do hsCRP. However, if its use is appropriate at all, it would be in the intermediate-risk patients.

* *

The next day, you obtain fasting labs. The patient has normal electrolytes and the following cholesterol panel: LDL 110 mg/dL, HDL 35 mg/dL, TRG 150 mg/dL. You review the ATP III (Adult Treatment Panel III, National Cholesterol Education Panel) guidelines to determine your next step in the treatment of this patient based on these labs.

Given the lipid profile mentioned above, you:

A) Consider the LDL to be too high and start an HMG-CoA reductase inhibitor ("statin").
B) Consider the lipid profile to be in the normal range, so that no further intervention should occur.
C) Consider the LDL to be too high and recommend diet and other lifestyle modifications.
D) Repeat the lipid profile because this patient clearly was not fasting and the LDL cannot be relied upon since her triglycerides are so high.

Discussion

The correct answer is "C." At this point, the first step is to change lifestyle and diet. This includes exercise, weight loss if indicated, and a low-fat diet. Even in patients with cardiac disease, statins are not mandatory for patients with an LDL between 100 and 130 mg/dL unless 6 months of dietary modifications have failed to reduce the LDL to <100 mg/dL. Although there is not a firm recommendation to start statins with a normal LDL in those who have had a recent myocardial infarction, there is some data that suggest benefit to the use of statins even in those with a normal LDL. "A" is incorrect because life style modification for 6 months is indicated before starting a drug. "B" is incorrect because for a patient with cardiac disease, this LDL is **not** considered optimal. "D" is incorrect.

Table 2-5 CALCULATING 10-YEAR CORONARY ARTERY DISEASE RISK IN MEN AND WOMEN

Estimate of 10-Year Risk for Men

(Framingham Point Scores)

Age	Points
20–34	–9
35–39	–4
40–44	0
45–49	3
50–54	6
55–59	8
60–64	10
65–69	11
70–74	12
75–79	13

Total Cholesterol	Points				
	Age 20–39	Age 40–49	Age 50–59	Age 60–69	Age 70–79
<160	0	0	0	0	0
160–199	4	3	2	1	0
200–239	7	5	3	1	0
240–279	9	6	4	2	1
≥280	11	8	5	3	1

	Points				
	Age 20–39	Age 40–49	Age 50–59	Age 60–69	Age 70–79
Nonsmoker	0	0	0	0	0
Smoker	8	5	3	1	1

HDL (mg/dL)	Points
≥60	–1
50–59	0
40–49	1
<40	2

Systolic BP (mm Hg)	If Untreated	If Treated
<120	0	0
120–129	0	1
130–139	1	2
140–159	1	2
≥160	2	3

Point Total	10-Year Risk %
<0	<1
0	1
1	1
2	1
3	1
4	1
5	2
6	2
7	3
8	4
9	5
10	6
11	8
12	10
13	12
14	16
15	20
16	25
≥17	≥30

10-Year Risk ____ %

Estimate of 10-Year Risk for Women

(Framingham Point Scores)

Age	Points
20–34	–7
35–39	–3
40–44	0
45–49	3
50–54	6
55–59	8
60–64	10
65–69	12
70–74	14
75–79	16

Total Cholesterol	Points				
	Age 20–39	Age 40–49	Age 50–59	Age 60–69	Age 70–79
<160	0	0	0	0	0
160–199	4	3	2	1	1
200–239	8	6	4	2	1
240–279	11	8	5	3	2
≥280	13	10	7	4	2

	Points				
	Age 20–39	Age 40–49	Age 50–59	Age 60–69	Age 70–79
Nonsmoker	0	0	0	0	0
Smoker	9	7	4	2	1

HDL (mg/dL)	Points
≥60	–1
50–59	0
40–49	1
<40	2

Systolic BP (mm Hg)	If Untreated	If Treated
<120	0	0
120–129	1	3
130–139	2	4
140–159	3	5
≥160	4	6

Point Total	10-Year Risk %
<9	<1
9	1
10	1
11	1
12	1
13	2
14	2
15	3
16	4
17	5
18	6
19	8
20	11
21	14
22	17
23	22
24	27
≥25	≥30

10-Year Risk ____ %

There is no reason to suspect that the patient was not fasting, and the triglyceride level is not too high to calculate LDL (generally with a TRG >400 LDL cannot be reliably calculated). Note that ATP IV is due to be released in 2012, so the recommendations you have just read may change (and probably will).

If you choose to start this patient on a statin, what will your goal be?

A) LDL <130 mg/dL.
B) LDL <100 mg/dL.
C) LDL <110 mg/dL.
D) HDL >40 mg/dL.
E) Triglycerides <150 mg/dL.

Discussion

The correct answer is "B." The LDL goal is <100 mg/dL in those with a history of CAD or those with >20% risk of a cardiac event in the next 10 years. Other goals set forth by ATP III include LDL <130 mg/dL in patients with two or more risk factors for cardiac disease and LDL <160 mg/dL in patients with 0 or 1 risk factor (see Table 2–6). HDL and triglycerides are not targets, making choices "D" and "E" wrong.

* *

She tries diet and exercise, but her lipids do not change. If you are not surprised, are you pessimistic or just realistic? You start a statin on this patient, and her liver enzymes (AST and ALT) rise to twice the upper limit of normal. You recheck them in 2 weeks, but they remain the same.

The proper response at this point is to:

A) Stop the statin because of the elevated liver enzymes.
B) Start a different statin since this is not a "class effect."
C) Continue the statin. These elevated liver enzymes are not a problem.
D) Add cholestyramine to help ease the burden on the liver.
E) Consider a liver biopsy to rule out other causes of elevated liver enzymes.

Discussion

The correct answer is "C." Statins can be continued as long as the elevation of liver enzymes is **less than three times the upper limit of normal**. However, the liver enzymes should be monitored. In general, the elevation in liver enzymes will resolve with discontinuation of the medication if this is what you choose to do. **However, never assume that this is a drug effect if there is a reason to believe that the patient could have another disease, such as hepatitis C**. "A" is incorrect since the levels are only two times normal. "B" is incorrect for two reasons. First, there is no need to act to change the drug at this point. Second, elevated liver enzymes are a class effect. "D" is incorrect because you do not need to add another drug at this time, and cholestyramine will do nothing to ease the burden on the liver. "E" is incorrect. If you want to check for other causes of elevated LFTs, biopsy certainly is not the next step!

Table 2-6 LDL CHOLESTEROL GOALS AND OUTPOINTS FOR THERAPEUTIC LIFESTYLE CHANGES (TLC) AND DRUG THERAPY IN DIFFERENT RISK CATEGORIES

Risk Category	LDL Goal (mg/dL)	LDL Level at Which to Initiate Therapeutic Lifestyle Changes (TLC) (mg/dL)	LDL Level at Which to Consider Drug Therapy
CHD or CHD risk equivalents (10-year risk >20%)	<100	≥100	≥130 mg/dL (100–129 mg/dL: drug optional)[a]
2+ risk factors (10-year risk ≤20%)	<130	≥130	10-year risk 10–20%: ≥130 mg/dL 10-year risk <10%: ≥160 mg/dL
0–1 risk factor[b]	<160	≥160	≥190 mg/dL (160–109 mg/dL: LDL-lowering drug optional)

[a] Some authorities recommend use of LDL-lowering drugs in this category if an LDL cholesterol <100 mg/dL cannot be achieved by therapeutic lifestyle changes. Others prefer use of drugs that primarily modify triglycerides and HDL, e.g., nicotinic acid or fibrate. Clinical judgment also may call for deferring drug therapy in this subcategory.

[b] Almost all people with 0–1 risk factor have a 10-year risk <10%; thus, 10-year risk assessment in people with 0–1 risk factor is not necessary.

In patients on statin therapy who are *not* having problems with liver enzymes, how often should you check liver enzymes?

A) Initially, then every 12 weeks.
B) Initially, at 12 weeks, then every 3 months.
C) Initially, at 12 weeks, then annually.
D) Initially, at 8 weeks, then every 6 months.

Discussion

The correct answer is "C." This is currently the recommendation. The other answers are incorrect.

> HELPFUL TIP: The FDA changed the recommendation for liver enzyme monitoring in 2012. It turns out that liver damage from statins is an idiosyncratic reaction and that monitoring liver enzymes does not help. The new recommendations are to check an initial set of enzymes and as clinically indicated thereafter. We don't know which answer will be correct on the test.

* *

You start a statin and the patient returns to your office in 2 months for a recheck. This patient did not meet her LDL goal with just one drug. In fact, her LDL went up a bit. You decide that the patient needs a second drug.

Which of the following is the *safest* drug to add to a statin in order to control this patient's LDL?

A) Niacin.
B) Gemfibrozil.
C) Cholestyramine.
D) Probucol.

Discussion

The correct answer is "C." Cholestyramine is the safest of the drugs listed above. It is not systemically absorbed and has very few side effects (constipation being the primary one). "A" is incorrect because niacin can elevate liver enzymes, can cause rhabdomyolysis, and has other side effects such as insulin resistance and diabetes. Additionally, although niacin has been shown to increase the HDL, it has not been shown to have any positive clinical benefits, and there is a hint of additional strokes (N Engl J Med 2011;365:2255–2267). Thus, niacin has fallen out of favor. Gemfibrozil and probucol can reduce triglycerides and LDL. However, probucol is no longer available because it may increase mortality, and the combination of gemfibrozil and a statin can cause rhabdomyolysis (as can the use of a statin alone).

> HELPFUL TIP: The best option is to bump up the dose of the statin! This is the only class that has shown a "real-life" benefit (in terms of improved cardiovascular endpoints).

Which of the following is classified as a bile acid sequestrant?

A) Ezetimibe.
B) Colestipol.
C) Colesevelam.
D) B and C.
E) All of the above.

Discussion

The correct answer is "D." Ezetimibe (Zetia) is not a bile acid sequestrant but rather reduces cholesterol absorption by blocking at the brush border of the small intestine. This is a mechanism that is different from any of the other lipid-lowering agents. It is relatively safe but expensive and less potent than the statins. Even in combination with statins, the additional lowering of LDL is on the order of 15–18%. "B" and "C" bind bile acids to reduce serum cholesterol.

> HELPFUL (BUT YET ANOTHER UNFORTUNATE) TIP: Ezetimibe (Zetia) *has not* been shown to reduce arterial plaque formation. Thus, it should really not be used. (N Engl J Med 2008;358:1431–1443). Similar to niacin, ezetimibe was a good idea that didn't pan out.

> HELPFUL RANT: Don't feel obligated to "just do something." Since niacin and ezetimibe don't have any clinical benefit, you don't need to use them—even if you are not meeting LDL goals. Just "doing something" to address numbers is not always the best policy.

Side effects of ezetimibe include which of the following?

A) Diarrhea.
B) Arthralgia.
C) Angioedema.
D) Liver enzyme elevation.
E) All of the above.

Discussion

The correct answer is "E." "C" deserves special mention. As with ACE inhibitors, angioedema has been reported with the use of ezetimibe during postmarketing research. The rate of occurrence is not known. However, it can be life threatening although no deaths have been reported to date. All of the other side effects are known to occur at a rate greater than with placebo.

* *

Due to GI side effects, she is unable to tolerate bile acid sequestrants. Since you had not yet read this book, you decide to start this patient on niacin to lower her LDL and elevate her HDL. She returns to your office in 2 weeks complaining of muscle aching and weakness. She has also some depressive symptoms such as anhedonia and sleep disturbance. You want to evaluate the patient to make sure that she does not have myopathy secondary to the medications she is taking. Her CPK and aldolase are normal.

From this you can conclude that:

A) She does not have myopathy since her CPK and aldolase are within normal limits.
B) Her fatigue and aches are a manifestation of her depression and sleep disturbance.
C) You can continue her statin and niacin since the CPK is normal.
D) She still may have statin-related myopathy despite a normal CPK and aldolase.

Discussion

The correct answer is "D." She still may have statin-induced myopathy despite a normal CPK and aldolase, so "A" is incorrect. There are several crossover trials that demonstrate myopathy in patients with normal muscle enzymes. The mechanism is thought to be a mitochondrial dysfunction. "B" is incorrect, and the reverse may actually be true (myopathy causing poor sleep and anhedonia). "C" is incorrect because she may indeed have a myopathy, and a trial off one or both drugs is warranted.

* *

You stop her medications and her symptoms improve over the course of several weeks. Everybody is happy... except the manufacturers of atorvastatin, niacin, and ezetimibe. They would have liked this case to end with the patient taking their drugs... twice a day if possible.

> HELPFUL TIP: Metamucil or other psyllium products are useful in reducing serum cholesterol and provide a "non-drug" alternative. At least 7 g of soluble fiber daily are required.

Objectives: Did you learn to...

- Define the accuracy of the initial history, ECG, and labs in the diagnosis of cardiac disease in the ED or office?
- Recognize the role and significance (or lack thereof) of risk factors, such as diabetes, family history, smoking, and hypertension, in the decision of whether or not to admit a patient to the hospital for chest pain?
- Generate a differential diagnosis of chest pain?
- Identify the roles of various diagnostic tests in the evaluation of chest pain?
- Treat a patient with an AMI?
- Describe the role of lipid-lowering therapy in the treatment of cardiac disease and as prophylaxis?
- Identify some of the potential side effects of lipid-lowering medications?

QUICK QUIZ: CORONARY CALCIUM

You are seeing a 47-year-old male patient. His presenting complaint is chest pain. The chest pain is right sided and is not associated with exertion. The patient looks well conditioned and admits (well, beams... the jerk) he exercises daily without any chest pain. On clinical exam, you find that the chest pain is reproducible on palpation of the anterior chest wall. He smokes one pack of cigarettes per day and has a blood pressure of 135/87, a total cholesterol of 179 mg/dL, and HDL of 30 mg/dL. He takes no medication.

Which of the following is TRUE regarding the role of a coronary calcium score in this patient (hint: calculate his risk score from the tables above)?

A) Coronary calcium score is a helpful tool in the evaluation of this patient **in combination with** the Framingham risk score.
B) Coronary calcium score is a helpful tool in the evaluation of this patient **independent** of the Framingham risk score.
C) Coronary calcium score is only useful in evaluating this patient once he has had an echocardiogram.
D) Coronary calcium score cannot provide useful information regarding cardiac function.

Discussion

The correct answer is "A." The patient presented with a Framingham risk score of 13% which places him in the intermediate risk category for 10-year cardiac risk. Coronary calcium score **may** be useful in those with an intermediate risk. (JAMA 2010 28;303:1610). It certainly is not useful as a screening tool (despite the TV commercials).

QUICK QUIZ: HYPERTENSION

According to JNC 7, a blood pressure of 120/80 is classified as:

A) Normal.
B) Prehypertension.
C) Hypertension.
D) Posthypertension.
E) Pseudohypertension.

Discussion

The correct answer is "B." The others are not correct. See Table 2–7 for the JNC 7 classification scheme for hypertension. By the time you are reading this, we hope you will be able to refer to JNC 8 (a long time coming!).

Table 2–7 JNC 7 CLASSIFICATION OF HYPERTENSION

<120/80: normal
120/80–139/89: prehypertension
140/90–159/99: stage 1 hypertension
>160/100: stage II hypertension

HELPFUL TIP: There are new recommendations for treating hypertension in the elderly. The goal is still less than 140/90 but with a systolic pressure of **greater than** 115 mm Hg. In those older than 80 years, a blood pressure of 140–145 mm Hg is considered adequate.

QUICK QUIZ: GIIb/IIIa INHIBITORS

You are seeing a patient in the ED with chest pain. The ECG shows elevated ST segments in leads V1, V2, and V3 with reciprocal changes inferiorly. You have run through the "standard" medications, but the patient continues to have pain. You consult a cardiologist who suggests the use of a glycoprotein IIb/IIIa inhibitor.

Which of the following is true about the glycoprotein IIb/IIIa inhibitors?

A) They are best used in patients who are not candidates for PTCA and stenting.
B) They cause no increase in the rate of intracranial bleeding.
C) They are useful in all groups of patients with acute coronary syndrome.
D) They are most effective in patients going to PTCA and/or stenting.

Discussion

The correct answer is "D." The glycoprotein IIb/IIIa inhibitors are most effective in patients who are undergoing PTCA or stenting. The GUSTO V trial showed **no** difference in 30-day mortality in patients **who were not** scheduled for catheterization. Thus, "A" is incorrect. "B" is incorrect because glycoprotein IIb/IIIa inhibitors do increase rates of intracranial and other bleeding. "C" is incorrect because patients who have an acute coronary syndrome that is well controlled with other drugs (e.g., heparin, metoprolol, and ASA) are not likely to benefit from glycoprotein IIb/IIIa inhibitors.

CASE 2

A 53-year-old male with a history of hypertension and smoking, but no family history of cardiac disease, presents to your office complaining of a chest pain. The pain is substernal, radiates to his left arm, and is associated with exertion. The patient notes that this same pain has been going on for the last 6 months and has not changed at all in duration, intensity, or characteristic. It generally lasts 5 minutes or so and resolves with rest.

You tell the patient that:

A) Without doing any test, you know that the probability that this pain is cardiac is greater than 85%.
B) If his ECG in the office is normal, his pain is unlikely to represent cardiac disease.
C) Even with risk factors, his probability of having CAD with "typical angina" is still only 50% or so.
D) The only intervention indicated at this point are life style modifications (e.g., stop smoking) and addressing his cholesterol and hypertension.
E) It is likely that he has unstable angina.

Discussion

The correct answer is "A." A 50-year-old male with "classic" angina symptoms has **greater than a 90%** probability of having CAD. "B" is incorrect because patients with angina who are pain free may have a normal electrocardiogram (as will many patients with active angina or even a myocardial infarction). Thus, his pain could still be cardiac in origin. "C" is incorrect because, based on demographic data, his risk of CAD is much higher than 50%. "D" is incorrect because he needs a further evaluation and treatment of his chest pain. "E" is incorrect since this pain represents "stable angina." There has been no change in quality, duration, amount of exertion required to bring on symptoms, etc., eliminating unstable angina as a diagnosis.

HELPFUL TIP: Know your pretest probability of cardiac disease before embarking upon testing for chest pain. This varies by age and type of chest pain. An approximation of the probability of cardiac disease is as follows:

Male: Atypical Angina:

age 30–39–34%, age 40–49–51%, age 50–59–65%, age 60–69–72%

Male: Typical Angina:

age 30–39–76%, age 40–49–87%, age 50–59–93%, age 60–69–94%

Female: Atypical Angina:

age 30–39–12%, age 40–49–22%, age 50–59–31%, age 60–69–52%

Female: Typical Angina:

age 30–39–26%, age 40–49–55%, age 50–59–73%, age 60–69–86%

* *

You send the patient home on aspirin with a prescription for sublingual nitroglycerin for PRN use and arrange for a stress test.

All of the following are considered absolute contraindications to exercise stress testing EXCEPT:

A) LBBB.
B) Presence of severe CHF.
C) Critical aortic stenosis.
D) Myocarditis.
E) Unstable angina.

Discussion

The correct answer is "A." An LBBB is a relative—not absolute—contraindication to stress testing. There are already repolarization abnormalities that limit the usefulness of the stress test. One should add an imaging modality, such as myocardial perfusion scanning in cases of LBBB. The rest are all "absolute" contraindications to exercise stress testing. See Table 2–8 for a list of contraindications.

Exercise stress testing is best suited to which group of individuals?

A) Men with an intermediate probability of cardiac disease.
B) Women with a high risk of cardiac disease.
C) Men at a high risk of cardiac disease.
D) Men at a low risk of cardiac disease.
E) Women with a low risk of cardiac disease.

Discussion

The correct answer is "A." Stress testing is best suited to patients with an intermediate pretest probability of cardiac disease (between 25% and 75%). "B" and "C" are incorrect since patients with a high risk of cardiac disease should go directly to another study,

Table 2–8 CONTRAINDICATIONS TO EXERCISE STRESS TESTING

Absolute contraindications	• Acute myocardial infarction within 2 days • Dissecting aneurysm • Recent pulmonary embolism • Active thrombophlebitis • BP >200/120 • Hemodynamically significant arrhythmias • Severe CHF • Severe aortic stenosis • Active myocarditis, pericarditis, or endocarditis • Inability to complete test
Relative contraindications	• Left bundle branch block • Moderate aortic stenosis • Hypertrophic cardiomyopathy • Electrolyte disturbance • High grade AV block • Tachyarrhythmias or bradyarrhythmias including uncontrolled atrial fibrillation

such as thallium testing and stress echocardiography. "D" and "E" are incorrect since these are not the best groups in whom to use exercise stress testing. There will be a greater proportion of false-positive results in these low-risk patients. Exercise stress testing in these groups is best used to allay patient fears that they do not have cardiac disease, not to prove they do have cardiac disease. **However, a false-positive stress test may lead to other unnecessary invasive testing!**

* *

You decide to do an exercise stress test on this patient. It turns out to be negative.

Your next step is to:

A) Reassure the patient that he does not have cardiac disease.
B) Suggest a chest CT scan to rule out possible aortic aneurysm.
C) Schedule the patient for another cardiac test such as stress echocardiogram, exercise thallium test, or angiography.
D) Schedule the patient for endoscopy to rule out gastroesophageal disease as a cause of these symptoms.
E) Start an anxiolytic to treat the panic disorder, which is the underlying cause of his chest pain.

Discussion

The correct answer is "C." This patient who is in his 50s and who has a "classic" history for angina has greater than a 90% pretest probability of cardiac disease. Thus, it is likely that the negative stress test is a false negative. In fact, male patients >40 years of age and women >60 years of age who have classic angina have a pretest probability of cardiac disease of 87% and 91%, respectively. **Thus, a stress test probably should not have been done in this patient in the first place, since a negative test just leads to further testing (as would have a positive test, probably resulting in angiography).** For this reason, "A" is incorrect. "B," "D," and "E" are incorrect. Initiating evaluation and management for another cause of chest pain is premature, since we still have not proven that this patient does not have cardiac disease.

* *

You are considering whether to do a thallium stress test or a stress echocardiogram.

Which of the following is true?

A) Stress echocardiography is more sensitive for cardiac disease than is a thallium test.
B) Stress echocardiography is more specific than is stress thallium.
C) Thallium testing is more specific for cardiac disease than is stress echocardiography.
D) None of the above is true.

Discussion

The correct answer is "B." Stress echocardiography is more specific for cardiac disease than is thallium testing. Alternatively, thallium testing is more sensitive. Table 2–9 summarizes this data. Remember that

Table 2–9 OVERALL SENSITIVITY AND SPECIFICITY OF NONINVASIVE CARDIAC TESTING

	Sensitivity (%)	Specificity (%)
Exercise stress testing	45–68	77
Thallium stress testing (SPECT)	88	77
Stress echocardiography	76	88

positive and negative predictive values of these tests will vary depending on the pretest probability of disease in the patient **and** severity of disease. Numbers given above are overall.

* *

You decide to send the patient for a thallium stress test. However, since his exercise capacity is limited, you choose to stress him chemically. The patient is taking theophylline for chronic obstructive pulmonary disease (COPD) (a pox on the doctors still prescribing that drug!).

The LEAST desirable method of stressing this patient is:

A) Adenosine.
B) Dobutamine.
C) Dipyridamole.
D) All of the above are equally acceptable methods of chemically stressing this patient.
E) Neither A nor C is desirable.

Discussion

The correct answer is "E." Theophylline (and caffeine) interact with both adenosine and dipyridamole, attenuating their effect; thus, neither is a good choice for stressing this patient. Dobutamine is an acceptable method of chemically stressing those on theophylline or caffeine (like us).

HELPFUL TIP: An LBBB is a relative contraindication to stress echo testing. There is already a wall motion repolarization abnormality. This makes a stress echo particularly difficult to interpret.

The patient's thallium stress test shows a nonreversible defect. The best interpretation of this is that it indicates:

A) Attenuation artifact from breast tissue.
B) Prior myocardial infarction.
C) Angina.
D) Anomalous cardiac circulation.
E) It is not significant and therefore adds no value to this test.

Discussion

The correct answer is "B." A nonreversible defect suggests prior myocardial infarction. A reversible defect suggests inducible ischemia. "A" is incorrect since breast attenuation occurs mostly in women. "C" is incorrect since angina is manifested by a reversible deficit.

* *

Since a reversible defect was not found on the thallium stress test, you conclude that there is no myocardium currently at risk. However, the patient continues to have chest pain and now at an increasing frequency with less exertion. He is asymptomatic when he presents to your office. He was noted at the last visit to have an elevated glucose at 350 mg/dL.

What is the next step in the evaluation or treatment of this patient?

A) Stress echocardiogram to document what segments are involved.
B) Start the patient on insulin to control his blood sugars.
C) Proceed directly to cardiac catheterization.
D) Since there were no reversible deficits on thallium stress, schedule the patient to see a gastroenterologist.
E) Give a trial of NSAIDs to help differentiate chest wall pain from other causes.

Discussion

The correct answer is "C." "A" is incorrect since we already have done a noninvasive test. We already know what segment has previously been infarcted, as noted on the thallium stress test. "B" is incorrect for two reasons. First, addressing his diabetes will not address the immediate problem of what you must presume is unstable angina. Second, insulin is not necessarily the first drug to use in this patient who presumably has type 2 diabetes. Certainly, the blood glucose needs to be addressed and so does the chest pain. Which is going to kill him first? "D" is incorrect. The sensitivity of thallium testing is in the 88% range (see Table 2–9), so it will miss 12% of disease. Thus, we still have not proven in this high-risk patient that he does not have treatable cardiac disease causing his chest pain. "E" is incorrect for the same reason.

* *

The patient has a catheterization done that shows three-vessel disease including left main CAD. The cardiologist calls you with the report the next day and suggests PTCA with stenting, since, in his opinion, "this is the best modality for diabetics and diabetics are high-risk candidates when it comes to surgery."

Your opinion is that:

A) Patients generally have better outcomes in terms of control of angina with stenting when compared with coronary artery bypass grafting (CABG).
B) Diabetic patients do particularly well with stenting when compared with CABG.
C) Medical control of symptoms is indicated as the best management in this diabetic patient with three-vessel disease.
D) You would like to send this patient for CABG.
E) None of the above.

Discussion

The correct answer is "D." This patient should probably have surgery for his three-vessel disease because diabetic patients generally have **worse** outcomes with stenting than do non-diabetic patients. "A" is incorrect because a proportion of patients with stents have to go on to have an open CABG. "B" is incorrect. Diabetic patients do particularly poorly with stents when compared with other patients. Diabetic patients have a much higher rate of secondary occlusion. "C" is incorrect. The indications for CABG are significant left main CAD (>50%) or three-vessel disease with evidence of LV dysfunction (ejection fraction <50%). This patient has left main vessel disease and thus medical control is **not** the best option for this patient.

HELPFUL TIP: Drug-eluting stents decrease reocclusion rates in diabetic patients and others compared with bare metal stents. Women who have multiple stents and multivessel disease are at a higher risk of restenosis, as are patients with a small poststenting lumen size. **Early reocclusion secondary to thrombosis is higher with drug-eluting stents. This is because it takes the body longer to cover these stents with fibroblasts. Thus, clopidogrel, prasugrel (not our favorite), or ticagrelor should be used for a full year in patients who have a drug-eluting stent inserted. They should be used for at least 3 months in those with bare metal stents.**

HELPFUL TIP: A plea from your editors. Don't continue clopidogrel, etc., outside of the time frame in which they have been shown to be useful (3 months for a bare metal stent, 1 year for a drug-eluting stent). The bleeding risk is increased for no benefit. Continue aspirin indefinitely, of course.

* *

Your patient has a CABG and comes into your office complaining of chest pain and fever 3 weeks after the surgery. He has had the pain and fever for 4 days and does not seem to be getting any better. He has no cough, no sputum production, and the pain seems to be worse when he breathes or lies down. He reports no dyspnea and has 97% oxygen saturation on room air. The wound from the surgery is well healed, and a chest radiograph shows no evidence of abnormalities.

Which of these studies is LEAST likely to be abnormal in this patient?

A) ECG.
B) V/Q scan.
C) Echocardiogram.
D) Sedimentation rate.

Discussion

The correct answer is "B." A V/Q scan is not likely to be positive in this patient. This patient is unlikely to have a PE given the duration of symptoms, the fact that the patient has chest pain that worsens with inspiration (found in only 59% of those with PE), and that he is febrile, reports no dyspnea, and has a normal oxygen saturation. Certainly, this **could** still be a PE, but it would be less likely than other, more plausible, explanations. The most likely diagnosis in this patient, given the lack of other symptoms, is postpericardotomy syndrome. This is similar to Dressler syndrome, which occurs after a myocardial infarction and presents with fever and chest pain several days to weeks after the inciting event. The white blood count is often elevated, as is the sedimentation rate. The ECG can also be helpful as can an echocardiogram.

* *

You obtain an ECG on this patient that shows a pattern consistent with pericarditis.

Which of the following patterns can be seen in a patient with pericarditis?

A) Diffuse ST segment elevation.
B) Normal ECG.
C) LBBB.
D) A and B.
E) All of the above.

Discussion

The answer is "D." Both diffuse ST segment elevations and a normal ECG can be seen with pericarditis. The initial ECG is only 80% sensitive for pericarditis. Small (low voltage) QRS complexes or electrical alternans can also be seen with pericarditis. "C" is incorrect since bundle branch blocks have nothing to do with pericarditis. You will have a chance to look at an ECG of pericarditis later in the chapter.

* *

You decide to treat this patient for pericarditis based on echocardiogram and an ECG consistent with this diagnosis.

Which of the following drugs might be helpful in this patient?

A) Heparin.
B) Warfarin.
C) Furosemide.
D) Indomethacin.
E) None of the above.

Discussion

"D" is correct. You must prescribe an anti-inflammatory in this patient. You can use aspirin, an NSAID, or steroids. Generally, indomethacin or aspirin are considered first-line drugs with steroids being reserved for those who fail NSAID therapy. Do not use anticoagulation, either heparin or warfarin, in patients with pericarditis. This can cause bleeding into the pericardial space and tamponade. Thus, "A" and "B" are incorrect. "C" is incorrect because furosemide will likely make this patient worse. Patients with increased pericardial pressures are dependent on circulating preload volume in order to fill the right heart. Decreasing the preload may worsen this patient's dyspnea.

* *

The patient returns the next day and is feeling more short of breath. On exam, you notice JVD and peripheral edema.

The best initial treatment of this patient is:

A) Furosemide.
B) Nitroglycerin.
C) IV saline.
D) Morphine.

Discussion

The correct answer is "C." This patient is in "pure" right heart failure secondary to cardiac tamponade. He is preload dependent. The treatment is to increase his preload by using IV saline. All the other options reduce the preload and will worsen this patient's symptoms.

* *

You give a bolus of IV saline, but he remains dyspneic with elevated neck veins and has a pulsus paradoxus of 14 mm Hg (normal <10 mm Hg).

The *next step* for this patient is:

A) Change the patient to steroids from indomethacin.
B) Perform a pericardiocentesis.
C) Start a positive inotrope (e.g., dopamine) to improve right heart function.
D) Start an afterload reducer to reduce cardiac demand.

Discussion

The correct answer is "B." The patient is clearly not doing well if he is getting more short of breath and not responding to your treatment. The pulsus paradoxus is 14 mm Hg. This is indicative of possible cardiac tamponade, but it may be seen in constrictive pericarditis, severe asthma, or anything else that reduces right heart filling (e.g., tension pneumothorax). This patient's clinical picture is consistent with decompensated cardiac tamponade, and drastic action is indicated to relieve the symptoms of right heart failure. The definitive treatment is pericardiocentesis. "A" is incorrect because more drastic action is required. You would be correct to change the patient to prednisone if he were failing an NSAID but was not decompensated. "C" is incorrect since an inotrope will do little to help this problem. "D" is incorrect for two reasons: the first is that this is a right heart problem and reducing afterload (systemic vascular resistance) will not help the right heart, which pumps against pulmonary resistance; second, most drugs that reduce systemic vascular resistance will also decrease preload to some degree, worsening the symptoms of tamponade.

> HELPFUL TIP: One thing to be aware of is that only up to 75% of patients with cardiac tamponade have an elevated pulsus paradoxus. So, a normal pulsus paradoxus does not rule out cardiac tamponade.

> HELPFUL TIP: Measuring pulsus paradoxus: deflate BP cuff slowly and listen for the first Korotkoff sound heard **only** during expiration; continue slowly deflating until you hear the Korotkoff sounds with inspiration as well. The difference is the pulsus paradoxus.

* *

You perform a pericardiocentesis and the patient gets better. Of course, a good outcome never protected anyone from a lawsuit...

Objectives: Did you learn to ...

- Evaluate a patient with typical anginal chest pain?
- Describe the test characteristics of various types of noninvasive cardiac testing?
- Become familiar with the interpretation of noninvasive cardiac testing?
- Recognize various indications for PTCA with stent placement versus CABG?
- Understand the physiology, presentation, and treatment of postpericardotomy syndrome?
- Treat pericarditis and cardiac tamponade?

QUICK QUIZ: HYPERTENSION

According to JNC 7, the blood pressure goal in a patient with diabetes is:

A) <100/50.
B) <110/70.
C) <130/80.
D) <140/90.
E) None of the above.

Discussion

The correct answer is "C." The goal for a diabetic patient (or any patient with underlying renal disease) is 130/80 or lower.

> HELPFUL TIP: Tight control of BP (<120 mm Hg systolic) in those with preexisting type 2 diabetes mellitus and CAD has **not** been shown to be any better than keeping the systolic BP <140 mm Hg. So, we are interested to see what JNC 8 will say. Stay tuned...

CASE 3

A 24-year-old male presents to your clinic with a 50-hour history of an irregular heart rate. He is generally well but has a history of hypertension (too many super-jumbo burgers... with bacon... he's been "supersized"), which he has been trying to control with exercise and diet (he switched to tofu burgers yesterday). There is no prior history of cardiac disease or palpitations. He did "have a bit to drink" celebrating... well, whatever, just celebrating... who needs a reason! He was embarrassed about his drinking and thus waited 2 days to seek care. There is no family history of heart disease and the patient does not smoke. Vital signs reveal an irregular pulse of 130 bpm and a blood pressure of 160/100 mm Hg. The patient is afebrile and has normal respirations. He has no heart murmur. The ECG is shown below (Figure 2–2).

The most appropriate diagnosis is:

A) Multifocal atrial tachycardia.
B) Wandering atrial pacemaker.
C) Atrial fibrillation.
D) Ventricular tachycardia.
E) Accelerated junctional rhythm.

Discussion

The correct answer is "C," atrial fibrillation. This is characterized by the lack of P waves and an irregularly irregular rhythm. "A" and "B" are incorrect. While both multifocal atrial tachycardia and a wandering atrial pacemaker are irregularly irregular, both have P waves. "D" is incorrect. Ventricular tachycardia is a wide complex tachycardia and is regular. "E"

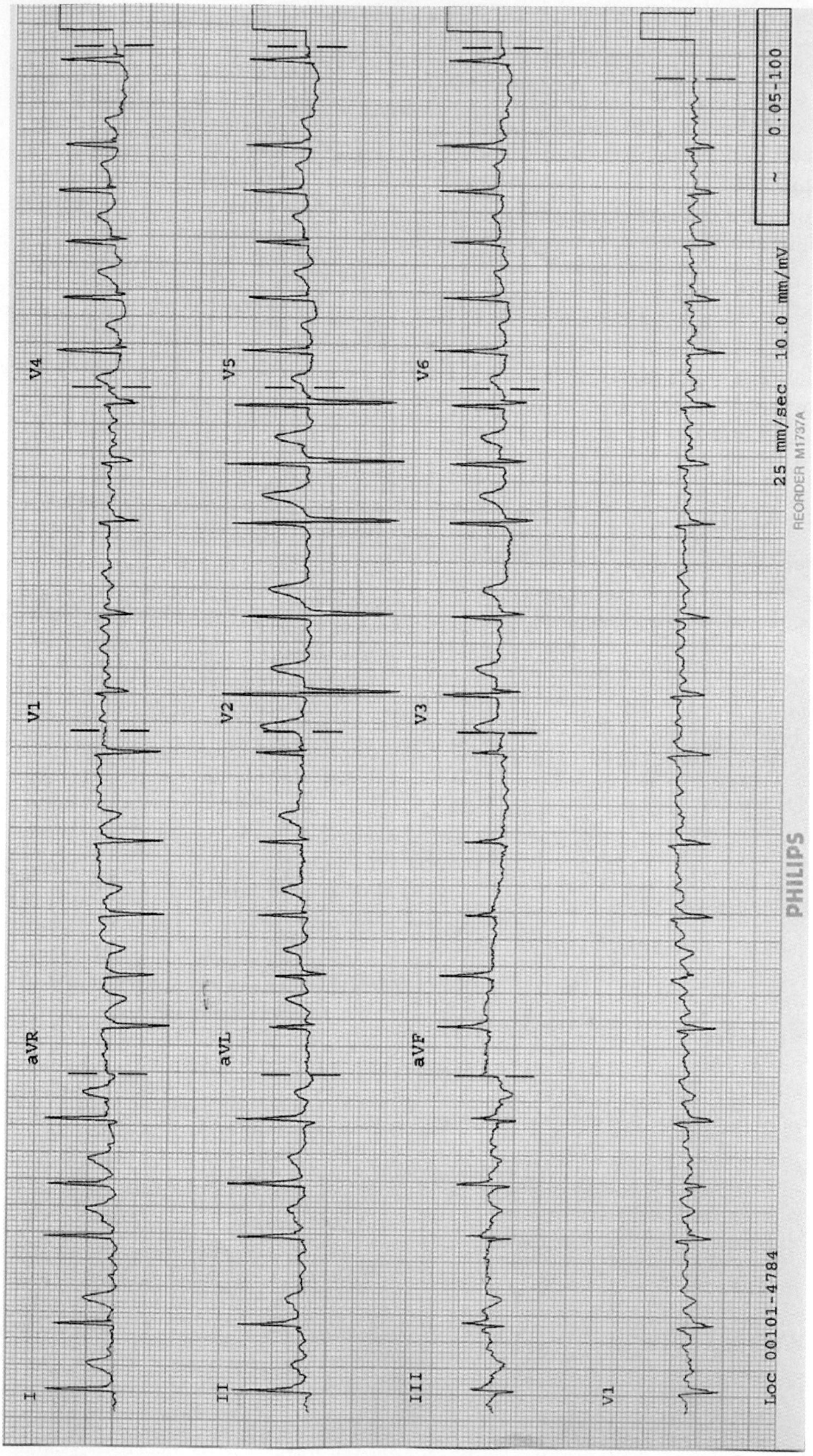
I
aVR
V1
V4
II
aVL
V2
V5
III
aVF
V3
V6
V1
Loc 00101-4784
PHILIPS
25 mm/sec 10.0 mm/mV
~ 0.05-100
REORDER M1737A

Figure 2–2

is incorrect. While there are no P waves in an accelerated junctional rhythm, it should be a regular, organized rhythm.

What is the most likely cause of this patient's dysrhythmia?

A) Congenital prolonged QT syndrome.
B) Hypertrophic cardiomyopathy.
C) Alcohol.
D) Marijuana use.
E) Ischemic cardiac disease.

Discussion
The correct answer is "C." The most likely cause of atrial fibrillation in this 24-year-old is alcohol. This is also known by the moniker "holiday heart." It occurs after episodes of significant alcohol intake. The underlying mechanism is not known. "A" is incorrect because prolonged QT typically causes polymorphic ventricular tachycardia (torsades de pointes). "B," hypertrophic cardiomyopathy, is unlikely since the patient has never had a murmur, and hypertrophic cardiomyopathy generally presents with signs of aortic outlet obstruction (syncope or angina with exercise). "D" is incorrect because marijuana is not implicated in causing atrial fibrillation, and "E" is incorrect because a patient who is 24 years old is unlikely to have ischemic cardiac disease.

Other states that can cause atrial fibrillation include all of the following EXCEPT:

A) Valvular disease, especially mitral disease.
B) Hyperthyroidism.
C) Stroke.
D) CHF.
E) Acute PE.

Discussion
The correct answer is "C." Stroke does not generally cause atrial fibrillation. Certainly, stroke and other intracranial injuries can be associated with arrhythmias. However, these are generally isolated PVCs. Stroke may also be associated with CHF and ischemic changes on the ECG, but it is rarely an isolated cause of atrial fibrillation. Valvular heart disease, hyperthyroidism, CHF, and PE are all causes of atrial fibrillation. Valvular heart disease, CHF, and PE all have a similar mechanism: stretching of the atrium leading to atrial irritability. Atrial fibrillation is found in 10–20% of those with hyperthyroidism, especially in the elderly.

* *

The patient confides that he was indeed at a bachelor party several days ago and had a bit too much to drink. This is quite unusual for the patient. He generally drinks 2–3 beers per week (hmm... we're wondering). The patient's pulse increases to 160, but he remains asymptomatic.

The INITIAL goal for this patient with 50 hours of atrial fibrillation is:

A) Anticoagulation.
B) Immediate cardioversion.
C) Transesophageal echocardiogram to rule out vegetations.
D) Rate control.
E) Blood pressure lowering

Discussion
The correct answer is "D." Since this patient has had >48 hours of atrial fibrillation, rate control is the goal. If the onset of atrial fibrillation is indeterminate or >48 hours, one should withhold cardioversion. For those with <48 hours of atrial fibrillation, cardioversion is a viable option.

* *

The patient's heart rate remains elevated at 160 bpm with occasional forays into the 170-bpm range.

Which of the following is the best drug to administer to this patient?

A) Digoxin.
B) Lidocaine.
C) Amiodarone.
D) Adenosine.
E) Verapamil or diltiazem.

Discussion
The correct answer is "E." "A" is incorrect. Digoxin will be of limited use since it takes at least 30 minutes to have an effect. It can be used in those with atrial fibrillation secondary to CHF but will still not help with rate control. "B" is incorrect because lidocaine is indicated for a wide complex tachycardia. "C" is incorrect. Amiodarone will work as a treatment of atrial fibrillation but is a second-line drug because it can cause torsades de pointes. It can be used in patients with atrial fibrillation and congestive failure, where verapamil or

diltiazem might be contraindicated. "D" is incorrect. Adenosine is ultra-short acting, blocks the AV node, and can be used to convert a paroxysmal supraventricular tachycardia (PSVT) or slow down the rate of the arrhythmia temporarily if you are not sure what the diagnosis is (e.g., a rapid atrial flutter vs. PSVT). However, adenosine will not reduce the ventricular rate in atrial fibrillation, since atrial fibrillation does not require the AV node to propagate. A beta-blocker could also be used in this situation.

* *

Being the astute clinician that you are, you realize that 50% of atrial fibrillation will spontaneously convert to normal sinus rhythm. A transthoracic echocardiogram was performed and did not demonstrate any structural heart disease. Thus, you choose to watch the patient. At 24 hours, he still is in atrial fibrillation, although the rate is controlled well with verapamil and he is now normotensive (must have been a bit anxious—were you wearing a white coat?).

If the patient desires cardioversion, the next step in the management of this patient is:

A) Start warfarin.
B) Start heparin and warfarin at the same time.
C) Start heparin and wait until the patient's PT/PTT/INR are stabilized before starting warfarin.
D) Start aspirin.

Discussion

The correct answer is "B." We may want to cardiovert this patient in the future. The rest are incorrect. We add heparin or low-molecular-weight heparin at initiation of anticoagulation because warfarin initially causes a hypercoagulable state by reducing protein C and protein S.

How long must you wait after the patient has been anticoagulated before cardioverting him?

A) 1 week.
B) 3 weeks.
C) 3 months.
D) Only until therapeutic on warfarin.
E) There is no need to wait before cardioversion in this patient.

Discussion

The correct answer is "B." If the patient has been in atrial fibrillation for more than 48 hours, one should wait until the patient has been anticoagulated (target INR 2–3) for 3 weeks before attempting cardioversion. This is based on recommendations from expert consensus. If atrial fibrillation has been present for less than 48 hours, you can proceed directly to cardioversion. Some physicians may order a transesophageal echocardiogram to assess for thrombus formation before cardioversion; this approach is acceptable. The patient will also need anticoagulation for 4 weeks after successful cardioversion.

HELPFUL TIP: Remember that both *Xarelto (rivaroxaban) and Pradaxa (dabigatran)* are approved for use in atrial fibrillation. But it seems as though dabigatran may **increase** the risk of **cardiac** (not stroke) events (*Arch Intern Med.* Published online January 9, 2012. doi:10.1001/archinternmed.2011.1666).

All of the following can be used to cardiovert atrial fibrillation EXCEPT:

A) Ibutilide.
B) Electrical cardioversion.
C) Quinidine.
D) Digoxin.
E) Procainamide.

Discussion

The correct answer is "D." Digoxin does not work to cardiovert atrial fibrillation. Digoxin may facilitate cardioversion in patients with CHF by reducing CHF and atrial stretching. However, it does not convert atrial fibrillation. All of the other answers are correct. Because of potential induction of arrhythmias with the other agents, electrical cardioversion is becoming the preferred method of restoring normal sinus rhythm.

Objectives: Did you learn to . . .

- Recognize the clinical and ECG presentation of atrial fibrillation?
- Use rate-controlling drugs to treat a patient with atrial fibrillation?

- Appropriately employ anticoagulation in atrial fibrillation for a patient undergoing cardioversion?
- Identify appropriate situations for cardioversion of atrial fibrillation?

QUICK QUIZ: ANTIHYPERTENSIVE AGENTS

A 70-year-old male complains of impotence and requests sildenafil (Viagra) for erectile dysfunction, which you believe is secondary to vascular disease.

Which of the following antihypertensive drugs can cause prolonged hypotension when used with sildenafil?

A) Peripheral alpha-blockers.
B) Calcium channel blockers.
C) An ACE inhibitor.
D) Diuretics.
E) Beta-blockers.

Discussion

The correct answer is "A." The peripheral alpha-blockers (doxazosin, prazosin, and tamsulosin) can cause symptomatic hypotension when combined with sildenafil or other drugs of this class (Cialis [tadalafil], Levitra [vardenafil]). This hypotensive effect is more severe when these drugs are combined with a nitrate. Nitrates should not be administered within 24 hours (or longer in patients with renal or hepatic dysfunction) of these drugs, as the combination has reportedly resulted in strokes. None of the other drugs ("B"–"E") cause this hypotensive effect when combined with sildenafil.

CASE 4

A 55-year-old male with a history of newly identified atrial fibrillation is referred to you for "medical clearance" for surgery. He has a history of hypertension and hypercholesterolemia (calculate his CHADS2 score, below). He has normal cardiac function otherwise with a normal ejection fraction and no valvular disease on echocardiogram. His atrial fibrillation has not been addressed since it was picked up by the surgeon at a preop visit. His heart rate is 80 bpm when you see him, his rhythm is irregularly irregular, and he has no signs of heart failure.

Table 2–10 CALCULATING THE CHADS2 SCORE

Criteria	Points	Scoring
History of stroke, TIA, or thromboembolic disease	2	0–1: Aspirin 100–300 mg 2: Aspirin or warfarin (or like drug)[a] >2: Warfarin (or like drug)[a]
Age ≥75	1	
Hypertension (treated or untreated)	1	
Diabetes	1	
CHF	1	

[a] Xarelto (rivaroxaban) and Pradaxa (dabigatran).

Which of the following options would be appropriate for this patient?

A) Anticoagulate the patient with warfarin and allow him to stay in atrial fibrillation.
B) Place the patient on aspirin and allow him to stay in atrial fibrillation.
C) Give digoxin to cardiovert the patient.
D) Strongly suggest cardioversion to this patient since sustained normal sinus rhythm yields the best long-term outcomes.
E) Add furosemide to prevent the development of CHF and edema.

Discussion

The correct answer is "B." This patient's CHAD2 score is "1" allowing him to take aspirin rather than being fully anticoagulated. A CHAD2 score of "1" is considered "lone atrial fibrillation." It is reasonable to allow the patient to remain in atrial fibrillation, as long as they are rate controlled. Outcomes of patients who stay in atrial fibrillation and are given appropriate therapy are the same as in patients in whom one tries to maintain sinus rhythm with drugs such as amiodarone, etc.

* *

The patient returns at age 75. He is older. You, however, have not aged a day 'cause doctors are immortal, right? He is now hypertensive, has diabetes, and he needs surgery to remove his gallbladder. His CHAD2 score is now 3 and he is on anticoagulation (warfarin, rivaroxaban, dabigatran . . . one or the other). Which of the following approaches is the best for controlling his anticoagulation given that he needs surgery?

A) Stop the warfarin several days before surgery to allow his INR to normalize. Restart the warfarin after surgery.
B) Hospitalize the patient a couple of days ahead of time and start heparin. Then stop his warfarin. Restart the warfarin after surgery.
C) Use low-molecular-weight heparin at home and stop the warfarin once this is started. Restart the warfarin after surgery.
D) Stop the warfarin several days before surgery to allow his INR to normalize. Start heparin after surgery and simultaneously restart warfarin.

Discussion

The correct answer is "A." For patients with atrial fibrillation who are undergoing surgery or invasive diagnostic procedures, it is reasonable to interrupt anticoagulation for up to 1 week without substituting heparin (assuming they haven't had a recent stroke or other thromboembolic event). "Bridge" therapy with IV heparin or low-molecular-weight heparin is not necessary. The risk of perioperative bleeding with heparin is actually greater than the risk of thromboembolism from atrial fibrillation. "B," "C," and "D" are incorrect because the patient does not need heparin.

* *

The 75-year-old patient has his surgery and returns to your clinic for a postoperative check-up 1 month after his surgery. You check his INR and it is noted to be 5.2. There is no active bleeding.

The most appropriate action at this point is to:

A) Hospitalize the patient for observation since he is at a high risk of bleeding.
B) Give the patient 5 mg of vitamin K orally.
C) Give the patient 2 units of fresh frozen plasma to reverse his anticoagulation.
D) Hold the next warfarin dose and reduce the maintenance dose.
E) A, B, and C.

Discussion

The correct answer is "D." The risk of bleeding in a relatively healthy patient with an INR of 5.2 is very low. Thus, simply holding the next one to two doses of warfarin and reducing the maintenance dose of warfarin is appropriate. "A" is incorrect because the patient does not need hospitalization. "B" is incorrect because it will be difficult to re-anticoagulate the patient after vitamin K is administered. "C" is incorrect because there is no active bleeding.

* *

The patient misunderstands your instructions and takes an **extra** dose of warfarin that evening and for the next 2 days. He returns to your clinic and his INR is now 13.

What is the best option for therapy at this point?

A) Vitamin K 10 mg IV × 1.
B) Fresh frozen plasma.
C) Vitamin K 1 mg PO × 1.
D) Vitamin K 5 mg PO × 1.
E) Vitamin K 10 mg IV × 1.

Discussion

The correct answer is "D." Giving this patient 5 mg of PO vitamin K is the best solution. This has been found to reduce the INR while still allowing the patient to be anticoagulated relatively easily after treatment. "B" is incorrect because there is no call for FFP in this asymptomatic patient. The other answers are incorrect because there is no advantage to higher doses of vitamin K in this patient, and the higher doses will make continued anticoagulation more difficult.

HELPFUL TIP:

- If the INR is 5 or less, simply hold the next dose of warfarin.
- If the INR is 5–9, you have several options. Either hold one or two doses or administer PO vitamin K (1 mg is generally recommended but up to 5 mg can be used).
- If the INR is 10–20, administer 5–10 mg of vitamin K PO.
- If the INR is over 20, rapid reversal of INR is indicated with FFP and vitamin K.
- Hospitalization, vitamin K, and FFP are appropriate regardless of the INR if there is **active bleeding** (e.g., intracranial hemorrhage) or if the patient will need an invasive procedure in the near future (e.g., a few hours).

Note: New 2012 Chest guidelines suggest simply holding warfarin for an INR of <10 without bleeding. . . .no Vit K! That was easy!

> **HELPFUL TIP:** (that you will also learn in the heme chapter): *Xarelto (rivaroxaban)* is a factor Xa inhibitor and can be reversed with prothrombin complex (and maybe factor VIIa). Sixty percent of *Pradaxa (Dabigatran)* can be dialyzed off.

Objectives: Did you learn to . . .

- Weigh the advantages and disadvantages of rate control versus rhythm control strategies for atrial fibrillation?
- Define "lone atrial fibrillation"?
- Manage anticoagulation and atrial fibrillation vis-à-vis surgery?
- Manage the over-anticoagulated patient?

CASE 5

A 62-year-old female presents to your office with a history of occasional palpitations that are of great concern to her. She notes that she feels a racing heart that lasts for a matter of seconds and occurs every 7 days or so. However, when she has the symptoms, she will generally get four to five episodes during that day. She neither has chest pain, dyspnea, lightheadedness, nor other associated symptoms. The event monitor shows that the patient is having nonsustained episodes of monomorphic ventricular tachycardia lasting less than 4 beats each.

The best approach at this point is to:

A) Start an antiarrhythmic such as quinidine or mexiletine to control the heart rhythm.
B) Refer the patient to a cardiologist for an EP study to determine the best drug to control this rhythm.
C) Implant an automatic defibrillator to prevent sudden death.
D) Implant a pacemaker.
E) Check serum potassium, magnesium, TSH.

Discussion

The correct answer is "E." The first step in determining the treatment of this patient is to make sure that there is not an underlying metabolic abnormality that could predispose to this rhythm abnormality.

* *

You check a panel of laboratory studies including thyroid function tests, electrolytes, magnesium, glucose, and CBC. They are all within normal limits. You suggest that the patient avoid potential triggers such as caffeine and sympathomimetics.

The next step for this patient is to:

A) Start an antiarrhythmic such as quinidine or mexiletine to control the heart rhythm.
B) Refer the patient to a cardiologist for an EP study to determine the best drug to control this rhythm.
C) Implant an automatic defibrillator to prevent sudden death.
D) Start a beta-blocker.
E) Order transthoracic echocardiogram to rule out structural heart disease.

Discussion

The correct answer is "E." Nonsustained ventricular tachycardia may have an adverse prognosis in the presence of structural heart disease such as hypertrophic cardiomyopathy or ischemic heart disease. An echocardiogram as well as stress test may be helpful in ruling them out. There is no evidence that nonsustained, asymptomatic ventricular tachycardia worsens outcomes **as long as the patient has no underlying cardiac disease.** In an otherwise healthy, asymptomatic patient, the risk of trying to use drugs to suppress ventricular ectopy leads to worse outcomes than doing nothing. Quinidine, mexiletine, amiodarone, and other antiarrhythmics all have proarrhythmic effects. In general, there is more sudden death in these patients if they are treated with drugs than if they are watched. Therefore, "A" is incorrect because these drugs will actually increase mortality. "B" is incorrect since the patient has asymptomatic, self-limited episodes. The reason to do an EP study is to see if there is an inducible arrhythmia and to determine treatment. This patient does not need treatment. "C" is incorrect because this patient has asymptomatic ventricular tachycardia. Thus, an implantable defibrillator is not indicated. After your evaluation is complete, you may prescribe a beta-blocker for symptomatic relief.

* *

The echocardiogram is normal, and the patient does well for the next 3 months but then becomes symptomatic with prolonged episodes of ventricular tachycardia. While all of the episodes are self-limited, the patient has had two episodes of syncope.

Which of the following is the next best step in treating this patient?

A) Sotalol.
B) Implantable defibrillator.
C) Amiodarone.
D) Electrophysiologic study.
E) Tocainide (an oral lidocaine equivalent).

Discussion

The correct answer is "D." An electrophysiologic study is indicated to induce and characterize the ventricular tachycardia. Certain types of ventricular tachycardia respond very well to radiofrequency ablation. **Some of you may have answered "B." This is true in patients with ischemic heart disease and left ventricular dysfunction and symptomatic ventricular tachycardia. These patients should get an implantable defibrillator.** However, this patient does not have any underlying CHF.

Objectives: Did you learn to . . .

- Evaluate a patient with palpitations?
- Manage nonsustained, asymptomatic, ventricular tachycardia?

CASE 6

A 22-year-old female presents to your office with a history of palpitations. You are able to capture the arrhythmia on the monitor in your office: the rhythm strip shows evidence of isolated premature atrial contractions (PACs). She is taking no medications, and there is no family history of heart disease.

All of the following are salient points of the history with regard to PACs EXCEPT:

A) Aged cheese consumption.
B) Caffeine use.
C) Tobacco use.
D) Alcohol use.
E) COPD.

Discussion

The correct answer is "A." Aged cheese **can** cause problems in combination with monoamine oxidase inhibitors (MAOIs). In combination with an MAOI, aged cheese and other sources of tyramine can cause a hypertensive emergency. However, this patient is not taking any medications. All of the other conditions and drugs listed can cause PACs. While there are conflicting data about the strength of the association, caffeine, COPD, tobacco, and alcohol can all cause an increase in sympathetic tone, leading to PACs. Neurologic abnormalities (e.g., stroke) can also be associated with PACs, as can some drugs (e.g., theophylline).

HELPFUL TIP: You have to eat 2 pounds of cheddar cheese in half an hour in order to develop a hypertensive crisis with an MAOI. In studies where there was free access to cheese, the maximum anyone was able to eat was 1.9 pounds in 2 hours. Believe it or not, someone studied this (probably somewhere in Wisconsin).

Which of the following statements about PACs is true?

A) Mitral valve prolapse is associated with PACs.
B) Mitral valve stenosis is associated with PACs.
C) Bicuspid aortic valve is associated with PACs.
D) None of the above is true.

Discussion

The correct answer is "B." Anything that can cause an increase in left atrial pressures (and therefore atrial wall stretching) is associated with an increase in the number of PACs. Mitral stenosis causes increased pressures in the left atrium, wall stretching, and enlargement and thus predisposes to PACs. "A" is incorrect. Even though multiple problems have been blamed on mitral valve prolapse, a study done as part of the Framingham study showed that the symptoms blamed on mitral valve prolapse (anxiety, PACs, tachycardia, etc.) are no more prevalent in those with mitral valve prolapse than in those without it. "C" is incorrect. A bicuspid aortic valve **may** cause PACs as a result of CHF when the patient decompensates and has increased left-sided heart pressures. However, a bicuspid aortic valve itself is not a source of PACs. Similarly, hypertrophic cardiomyopathy, other causes of CHF, drugs (e.g., theophylline and digoxin), and neurologic diseases can be associated with PACs.

* *

This patient is bothered by her PACs. She is rather aware of them and finds them disconcerting.

What is the best pharmacologic therapy to consider at this point?

A) Sotalol.
B) Metoprolol.
C) Trasylol.
D) Amiodarone.
E) Mountain Dew—lots of it.

Discussion

The correct answer is "B." A beta-blocker may help to reduce this patient's PACs. "A" is incorrect because, while sotalol can be used for both atrial and ventricular arrhythmias, it is proarrhythmic and can cause torsades de pointes. Thus, it should be reserved for those with severe arrhythmias. "C" is incorrect because Trasylol is the trade name for aprotinin, an enzyme that is used to reduce bleeding during surgical procedures. "D" is incorrect because, like sotalol, amiodarone is proarrhythmic, and its use should be limited to those with significant arrhythmias.

Objectives: Did you learn to . . .

- Recognize causes of PACs?
- Treat a patient with bothersome PACs?

QUICK QUIZ: VALVULAR DISEASE

Surgery is indicated in which of these patients with valvular disease?

A) An asymptomatic patient with severe mitral regurgitation and a left ventricular ejection fraction of less than 60%.
B) An asymptomatic patient with a bicuspid aortic valve.
C) Asymptomatic aortic regurgitation with a left ventricular ejection fraction of less than 50% on echocardiogram.
D) Only symptomatic valvular lesions should be approached surgically.
E) A and C.

Discussion

The correct answer is "E." Once patients with mitral regurgitation and aortic regurgitation become symptomatic, the morbidity and mortality increases significantly. Thus, these patients should be operated on **before** they become symptomatic. As noted in Table 2–12 (later in this chapter), patients should have routine echocardiography yearly if they have severe valvular disease. In addition to evaluating the valve, echocardiography allows you to evaluate ventricular function.

CASE 7

A 74-year-old male presents to your office with a chief complaint of a "long cold" with a cough for 5 months. He has also noticed that he gets up to urinate twice a night although he has no trouble with his urine stream, starting urination, or dribbling afterward. He has been a bit more tired lately and notices that his exercise tolerance has decreased to several blocks, limited mainly by shortness of breath. He has had no episodes of chest pain. He has no history of asthma or COPD and has not had any new exposures to drugs or chemicals. He has a history of hypertension and noncompliance with medical recommendations. In fact, he is taking no medications except for an aspirin a day. His pulse is 100 with a blood pressure of 160/95. He looks pretty well. On exam, you find only trace pitting edema of the lower extremities.

Which of the following is NOT a possible cause of cough in this patient?

A) CHF.
B) Asthma.
C) Deconditioning.
D) COPD.
E) GERD.

Discussion

The correct answer is "C." Deconditioning may cause dyspnea on exertion but should not cause a cough. The purpose of this question is to point out the fact that a "chronic cold" or "chronic cough" in an elderly person can be due to a myriad of causes, including "occult" CHF. Do not make the assumption that the patient's diagnosis (e.g., a "chronic cold"), is necessarily the correct diagnosis.

You decide that this patient may have CHF and decide to do an electrocardiogram in your office. The ECG shows no evidence of prior or ongoing ischemia. There are no signs of atrial enlargement or ventricular hypertrophy.

The proper conclusion from this is:

A) The patient does not have cardiac chamber enlargement or hypertrophy and therefore it is unlikely to have CHF.

B) The absence of evidence for an infarct makes CHF unlikely.
C) Regardless of the ECG results, clinical judgment alone is sufficient to make the diagnosis of CHF, being correct 85% of the time.
D) The patient's edema is likely from venous insufficiency.
E) Despite a normal ECG, further testing is needed in this patient to evaluate for CHF.

Discussion

The correct answer is "E." "A" is not correct because only 30–60% of moderate-to-severe left ventricular hypertrophy (LVH) is detectible on ECG. "B" is incorrect because patients with diastolic dysfunction (discussed later) may not have any evidence of prior ischemia or MI. "C" is incorrect. The clinical diagnosis of CHF is incorrect up to 50% of the time. For this reason, confirmation is required before embarking upon a therapeutic adventure for CHF. "D" is unlikely, since the patient has other symptoms of CHF (exertional dyspnea, etc.) that make simple venous insufficiency unlikely.

You decide on further testing. Assuming every test is easily available to you (which, of course, might not be the case depending on the setting in which you work), what is the *one best test* that you would use to determine if this patient has CHF?

A) Echocardiography.
B) Brain natriuretic peptide (BNP) level.
C) Chest radiograph looking for evidence of pulmonary edema (Kerley B lines, etc.).
D) SPECT thallium test.
E) Adenosine thallium testing.

Discussion

The correct answer is "A." Echocardiography is the procedure of choice for the diagnosis of CHF. This is for two reasons. First, you can assess left ventricular systolic function as well as look for diastolic dysfunction to determine if this is systolic or diastolic heart failure. Second, you can evaluate the potential causes of heart failure including valvular heart disease, ischemic heart disease, and pericardial disease. "B" is incorrect because the BNP will give you less information about the patient than will echocardiography. In this patient with a high pretest probability of CHF, BNP will most likely be elevated. "D" and "E" are incorrect because SPECT thallium and adenosine thallium testing are better used to diagnose ischemic cardiac disease.

> **HELPFUL TIP:** In a low-risk patient, a BNP of <100 pg/mL effectively rules out CHF. A BNP of 100–500 pg/mL is indeterminate and may not be related to cardiac disease. A BNP of >500 pg/mL is relatively specific for CHF.

> **(LESS) HELPFUL TIP:** Non-CHF causes of an elevated BNP include renal failure, ACS, sepsis/SIRS, pulmonary hypertension (PHTN), and COPD. Obesity causes a falsely low BNP. BNP-directed therapy **may** be useful in some patients <75 years of age (found in a subgroup analysis of a study). Unfortunately, a study to test this subgroup-based hypothesis has not been done.

* *

The patient has an echocardiogram that shows a left ventricular ejection fraction of 40% and regional wall motion abnormalities.

This is the most consistent with a diagnosis of:

A) CHF secondary to myocarditis.
B) CHF from systolic dysfunction secondary to ischemic disease.
C) Diastolic dysfunction.
D) CHF secondary to constrictive pericarditis.
E) Age-related changes and a normal variant.

Discussion

The correct answer is "B." Regional wall motion abnormalities suggest that this patient has infarcted or poorly perfused ("hibernating") myocardium is incorrect since those with myocarditis should have global hypokinesis. "C" is less likely to be true given low ejection fraction. Diastolic dysfunction is associated with a hypertrophied left ventricle and a **preserved** ejection fraction. Echocardiogram in constrictive pericarditis generally shows normal left ventricular systolic function. It may reveal pericardial thickening, dilated inferior vena cava or hepatic veins, abnormal septal motion, and abnormal mitral and tricuspid flow Dopplers. Therefore, "D" is incorrect.

> **HELPFUL TIP:** Methamphetamine and cocaine can cause a cardiomyopathy and should be considered as a possible etiology in the appropriate patient.

Which of the following is the most appropriate next strategy to workup this patient's CHF?

A) Cardiac MRI to assess myocardial viability.
B) Coronary angiogram.
C) Measure serial troponins to rule out acute coronary syndrome.
D) Electrophysiologic study to assess for inducible ventricular arrhythmia.
E) CT to assess calcium scores.

Discussion

The correct answer is "B." Ischemic heart disease is the most common etiology for heart failure associated with systolic dysfunction. Of all the options listed above, coronary angiogram remains the gold standard to evaluate for CAD. Coronary angiograms provide information about anatomy and feasibility of revascularization but do not predict recovery of function. This patient does not have chest pain or ECG changes to suggest acute cardiac ischemia; therefore, "C" is incorrect. "D" is incorrect, as there is no indication for an electrophysiologic study in the absence of any arrhythmia.

* *

The coronary angiogram shows diffuse CAD; no coronary lesions are considered to be amenable to angioplasty or bypass surgery. You decide to initiate medical therapy in this patient. In addition, you advise the patient regarding the nonpharmacologic therapies for heart failure treatment.

These include all of the following EXCEPT:

A) Fluid restriction of <2 L/day.
B) Sodium restriction of <2 g/day.
C) Dietary consultation.
D) Cardiac risk factor modification.
E) Monthly weight monitoring.

Discussion

The correct answer is "E." The keystone of an effective heart failure treatment regimen is sodium as well as fluid restriction. Frequently overlooked, these are the most common causes of heart failure exacerbation. It is imperative to get a dietary consultation for every patient with newly diagnosed heart failure. Cardiac risk factors including hypertension, diabetes, and hyperlipidemia need to be treated with the same aggressiveness as in a patient with an acute coronary syndrome. Patient should be advised about **daily** weight monitoring rather than monthly monitoring. A weight gain of more than 3–5 lb may necessitate additional doses of a diuretic.

* *

You wish to start an appropriate drug regimen for this patient's heart failure.

All of the drugs given below have been shown to reduce mortality in patients with CHF secondary to systolic dysfunction EXCEPT:

A) Digoxin.
B) Metoprolol.
C) ACE inhibitors.
D) Hydralazine and long-acting nitrates used in combination in patients intolerant of ACE inhibitors.
E) Spironolactone.

Discussion

The correct answer is "A." Digoxin has **not** been shown to increase survival and in fact may worsen outcomes, especially in women. Thus, if using digoxin in CHF, use 0.125 mg/day and not the old dose of 0.25 mg/day. Digoxin **does** reduce hospitalizations and improves symptoms in those with systolic dysfunction and can be appropriately used for symptom control if other treatments are not working. All of the others, including the combination of isosorbide dinitrate and hydralazine, have been shown to reduce mortality. However, hydralazine and isosorbide dinitrate are generally reserved for those patients who are unable to tolerate ACE inhibitors or angiotensin-receptor blockers (ARBs). Enalapril reduces mortality by 28% when compared with hydralazine and nitrates. Thus, hydralazine and nitrates are second line. None of the "traditional" loop diuretics such as furosemide, bumetanide, etc., have been shown to positively affect mortality.

* *

You start this patient on furosemide for diuresis and lisinopril for systolic dysfunction. You also decide to initiate metoprolol for its survival benefits. However, the patient's symptoms worsen.

Which of these is true about the use of metoprolol in CHF?

A) It is the only beta-blocker indicated for use in CHF.
B) The best use is in those patients who are still symptomatic since it will help to control symptoms.
C) It should only be initiated in patients with well-controlled CHF who are not currently having significant symptoms.
D) Beta-blockers can lead to significant hypokalemia when combined with diuretics, so potassium levels should be monitored closely.
E) Beta-blockers are contraindicated in patients who have a combination of COPD and CHF.

Discussion

The correct answer is "C." Beta-blockers **are not** indicated for patients who are significantly symptomatic. While they do reduce mortality, they can increase symptoms and exacerbate heart failure. Therefore, they are best initiated in the stable patient (think outpatient or at hospital discharge and on a stable drug regimen). Even then some patients cannot tolerate the introduction of beta-blockers without a worsening of symptoms, which may require additional diuresis, discontinuation of the beta-blocker, a reduction in dose, or other measures. "A" is incorrect. Other beta-blockers have been used in CHF, including carvedilol. "B" is incorrect because beta-blockers may actually worsen heart failure symptoms and thus should not be initiated in a patient who is symptomatic. "D" is incorrect since beta-blockers do not cause hypokalemia. "E" is incorrect. Beta-blockers can be used in patients with COPD with the same caveats that apply to any other patient: if the patient is becoming more symptomatic on the beta-blocker, reduce the dose or discontinue the drug. In fact, beta-blockers *may* improve survival in COPD (Short PM et al., *BMJ* 2011;342:d2549).

HELPFUL TIP: When starting a beta-blocker for CHF, start low and go slow!

* *

You reduce the dose of metoprolol and consider starting this patient on another medication.

Which of the following patients is/are good candidates for spironolactone therapy?

A) A patient with NYHA Class I and Class II CHF.
B) A patient with NYHA Class III and Class IV CHF.
C) Both A and B.
D) Neither A nor B.

Discussion

The correct answer is "B." Spironolactone has been shown to reduce mortality in patients with New York Heart Association (NYHA) Class III and Class IV CHF. It has not been studied in Class I and Class II failure. Serum potassium needs to be monitored closely after initiation of spironolactone, especially since it will generally be used with an ACE inhibitor or ARB, both of which can increase the serum potassium. This drug should be avoided in patients with renal insufficiency or patients with serum potassium >5 mEq/L. Eplerenone is another aldosterone inhibitor but is much more expensive with little, if any, advantage.

HELPFUL TIP: Aliskiren (Tekturna), a renin inhibitor, **is contraindicated** with an ARB or ACE inhibitor. It worsens outcomes and causes hyperkalemia.

* *

You treat this patient with metoprolol, lisinopril, furosemide, and aspirin. This regimen seems to help, and the patient's symptoms improve. However, a few weeks later, he presents to the ED with increased dyspnea. There have been no changes in his medications, and he assures you that he is taking his medications as directed. His exam reveals that he has elevated JVD, rales over the lower half of his lung fields bilaterally, and pedal edema.

Common causes of decompensation in patients with otherwise stable CHF include all of the following EXCEPT:

A) Inactivity.
B) Fever.
C) Arrhythmia.
D) Dietary indiscretion.
E) Ischemia.

Discussion

The correct answer is "A." Inactivity will not generally cause an exacerbation of CHF. The major causes of increased CHF include dietary indiscretion (increased salt intake—"Say, can you pass the potato chips?"—and increased fluid consumption), increased metabolic demand (from infection), anemia, medication noncompliance, arrhythmia, and ischemia. The inappropriate use of medications, such as some calcium channel blockers, and the institution of betablockers are also common causes of exacerbations of CHF.

* *

The patient notes that he did have some chest pain earlier in the day. You want to initiate therapy. You take his vitals, and his pulse is 100, blood pressure 140/95 mm Hg, oxygen saturation 89% on room air, and a respiratory rate 32.

Besides oxygen, the one best drug to initiate first in the ED to treat this patient with CHF is:

A) Furosemide.
B) Digoxin.
C) A positive inotrope, such as dobutamine.
D) Nitroglycerin.
E) An ACE inhibitor

Discussion

The correct answer is "D." This patient will benefit from nitroglycerin for several reasons. First, the patient has told you that he had chest pain earlier today. Thus, it is likely that this patient's CHF exacerbation is due to ischemic disease. Nitroglycerin will help this. The second reason is that the goal here is to restore normal cardiac function by causing vasodilation and decreasing preload and afterload. Nitroglycerin will do both of these. "A," furosemide, is also a good choice but not the one best choice. By inducing diuresis, furosemide will also significantly decrease preload and provide symptomatic relief. But remember not all CHF patients are fluid overloaded (such as with flash edema from ischemia). "B" is incorrect because it will take some time for digoxin to have a significant impact on this patient's symptoms. "C" is incorrect because dobutamine is a second-line drug reserved for those not responding to more conservative therapy. "E" is technically not incorrect, but it is not the best answer. There is ample evidence that ACE inhibitors can be used in acute CHF exacerbations either IV (e.g., enalapril) or sublingual (e.g., captopril). However, these drugs should be reserved as second-line therapy for patients who do not respond to more conservative measures.

* *

You treat the patient with nitroglycerin, he improves, and you admit him to the floor. While in the hospital, the patient develops some additional chest pain that lasts for 10 minutes and responds to additional sublingual nitroglycerin. His BNP is noted to be elevated. His hemoglobin (Hb) is 7.2 g/dL and hematocrit (HCT) is 20%. He is still in congestive failure. The pathologist tells you that there is blood available in the blood bank to transfuse this gentleman if you so choose. There is a problem, of course: he is in CHF and now is somewhat tachycardic at 110.

You tell the pathologist that:

A) The Hb of 7.2 g/dL is not an indication for transfusion.
B) Transfusing this gentleman is inappropriate since he is already in CHF and may become more fluid overloaded with a blood transfusion.
C) You would like to go ahead with transfusing this patient.
D) Making this patient's blood more viscous with a transfusion will increase the stress on his heart.
E) A and B.

Discussion

The correct answer is "C." This patient should be transfused. There are no official ACC/AHA recommendations regarding transfusion. However, the mortality at 30 days is increased if the Hb is <11 mg/dL in a patient with a non-STEMI. Whether or not transfusion will help this is not known: it may just be that patients with anemia are sicker at baseline. Patients with an HCT of <20–24% likely benefit from a transfusion while those with an HCT >27–30% do not. For 25–26% use your judgment. CHF is different. Blood transfusion should be reserved for patients with heart failure that are severely anemic and the transfusion be undertaken SLOWLY and with the concurrent use of diuretics to avoid volume overload (Garty et al., 2009). "A" and "B" are incorrect because this patient should be transfused carefully as noted above. "D" is incorrect since transfusing this patient to a normal Hb and HCT will not cause excess blood viscosity.

HELPFUL TIP: Nesiritide (Natrecor), a BNP analog, can be used for CHF but is expensive, contributes to renal failure, and likely increases mortality. Nesiritide can produce prolonged hypotension, which limits the dose that can be used. This is a therapy of last resort . . . and that may be too charitable. Just don't use it.

Objectives: Did you learn to . . .

- Recognize atypical presentations of CHF in the elderly?
- Describe the sensitivity and specificity of an ECG for LVH?
- Evaluate a patient with CHF?
- Manage a patient with CHF and understand the role of beta-blockers, ACE inhibitors, ARBs, digoxin, and spironolactone in the treatment of CHF?
- Describe the role of BNP measurement in the evaluation of CHF and of nesiritide in the treatment of heart failure?

CASE 8

Your patient with heart failure does well and is discharged from the hospital after a couple of days. You are just beginning to think that the authors are tired of writing questions about CHF . . . but you are wrong. The patient's 70-year-old wife shows up with shortness of breath. Her physical examination is consistent with heart failure. Since you have learned so much from this case already, you send her to get an echocardiogram. You also get the recommended tests: CBC, electrolytes, ECG, thyroid functions, etc. The results of the echocardiogram show a concentric thickening of the left ventricle with an ejection fraction of 75%. This is most consistent with:

A) Ischemic cardiomyopathy.
B) Diastolic dysfunction.
C) Viral cardiomyopathy.
D) Hypertrophic cardiomyopathy.
E) None of the above.

Discussion

The correct answer is "B," diastolic dysfunction. "A" is incorrect since there would be evidence of regional wall motion abnormality if there had been an old myocardial infarction. Also, this patient has a preserved ejection fraction, which is consistent with diastolic dysfunction rather than the decreased ejection fraction associated with ischemic cardiomyopathy. "C" is incorrect. Viral cardiomyopathy is associated with a dilated ventricle rather than a hypertrophic one, and there is a global dyskinesia with decreased ejection fraction. "D" is incorrect; hypertrophic cardiomyopathy is usually associated with asymmetric septal hypertrophy rather than concentric hypertrophy of the left ventricle. Hypertrophic cardiomyopathy may lead to diastolic dysfunction in addition to left ventricular outflow tract obstruction.

Diastolic dysfunction is associated with which of the following?

A) A prolonged history of untreated hypertension.
B) Poor relaxation of the ventricular wall.
C) Hemochromatosis.
D) A and B.
E) B and C.

Discussion

The correct answer is "D." Diastolic dysfunction is associated with long-standing hypertension as well as a stiff ventricular wall that does not relax to allow good filling during diastole (therefore "diastolic dysfunction"). "C" is incorrect because hemochromatosis produces a dilated cardiomyopathy rather than diastolic dysfunction.

Diastolic dysfunction represents approximately what percentage of CHF?

A) <5%.
B) Approximately 10%.
C) Approximately 25%.
D) Approximately 50%.
E) >75%.

Discussion

The correct answer is "D." Diastolic dysfunction represents between 40% and 60% of cases of CHF when looking at the population as a whole. The other answers are incorrect. The point here is that, as discussed earlier, patients with CHF need an echocardiogram to determine what type of heart failure they have.

HELPFUL TIP: Diastolic dysfunction occurs more commonly in elderly populations.

Which of the following drugs is the LEAST desirable in patients with diastolic dysfunction?

A) Diuretics.
B) ACE inhibitors.
C) Nitrates.
D) Digoxin.
E) Negative inotropes such as beta-blockers and calcium channel blockers.

Discussion
The correct answer is "D." Digoxin and other positive inotropes (milrinone) are not very useful in diastolic dysfunction. This makes sense. The problem here is not a lack of contractility but exactly the opposite—a lack of muscle relaxation. The goals of therapy are blood pressure control, the use of diuretics to relieve congestion and edema, treatment of ischemia, control of the heart rate and elimination of tachycardia. See Table 2–11 for more details.

Which of the following drugs is theoretically the best choice for the treatment of diastolic dysfunction?

A) ACE inhibitors.
B) Beta-blockers.
C) Diuretics.
D) Hydralazine.
E) ARBs.

Discussion
The correct answer is "B." Beta-blockers, especially metoprolol, are useful as initial therapy in diastolic dysfunction. Beta-blockers (1) slow down the heart to permit better filling during diastole and (2) help to relax the myocardium to promote a less restrictive filling pattern. If a patient fails beta-blockers, try calcium channel blockers (e.g., verapamil, diltiazem). Unlike systolic dysfunction, the treatments of diastolic dysfunction are not well established, and there is no convincing evidence that beta-blockers or ACE inhibitors reduce mortality.

Objectives: Did you learn to . . .

- Understand the pathophysiology of diastolic dysfunction?
- Treat a patient with diastolic dysfunction?

HELPFUL TIP: CHF is a terminal illness with a 5-year survival of only 50%. This is worse than many cancers.

CASE 9

Your "congestive heart failure couple," as they now call themselves, are doing so well that the wife refers her cousin to you. Her cousin, a 65-year-old male, arrives at your office and you immediately notice the smell of tobacco leaching from his clothing. The small burns in his clothing confirm to you that he smokes, and he informs you that he has smoked three packs per day "since birth." He recently has noticed some swelling in his feet and increased shortness of breath. He denies a history of cardiac disease. An ECG performed in the office shows right axis deviation and a right bundle branch block (RBBB). An echocardiogram shows that he has normal left ventricular function but a hypertrophied right heart with paradoxical bulging of the ventricular septum into the left ventricle.

This clinical picture is most consistent with which of the following?

A) Constrictive pericarditis.
B) Chronic mitral valve prolapse.
C) Cor pulmonale.
D) Old right ventricular infarction with subsequent dysfunction.
E) Atrial myxoma.

Discussion
The correct answer is "C." A typical picture of cor pulmonale is right ventricular hypertrophy with paradoxical bulging of the septum into the left ventricle, right axis deviation on ECG, and partial or complete RBBB. "A" is incorrect; constrictive pericarditis is associated with pericardial thickening, dilated inferior vena cava or hepatic veins, abnormal septal motion, and abnormal mitral and tricuspid flow Dopplers. "B" is incorrect because mitral valve prolapse in the absence of mitral regurgitation is not likely to be hemodynamically significant. "D" is incorrect because with a right ventricular infarct, you would expect to see a poorly functioning right ventricle. "E" is incorrect because an atrial myxoma is in the atrium and would not cause right ventricular hypertrophy.

Cor pulmonale (*not* right ventricular failure) may result from all of these disease processes EXCEPT?

A) Sickle cell anemia.
B) Left ventricular failure.
C) PE.

Table 2–11 PACEMAKER NOMENCLATURE

The first letter represents the chamber paced: A = Atrium, V = Ventricle, D = Dual (both atrium and ventricle). Thus, to maintain atrial function in a patient with a slow atrial rate, we will need a "D" as the first letter (pacing both atrium and ventricle). The second letter represents the chamber sensed. Again, A, V, and D stand for the same as above. Finally, the third letter is the response to sensing. This can be either "T" (triggered), "I" (inhibited) or "D" (triggered and inhibited). "I" means that if the pacer senses innate electrical activity it does not trigger the heart.

This is the mechanism of the original VVI pacer. If there are no ventricular beats sensed, the pacer fires. This keeps the patient from becoming bradycardic. Alternatively, if the ventricle is chugging along faster than the pacer is programed, the pacer senses this and does not fire (because it is inhibited).

DVI is an "A-V sequential" pacer. There is dual pacing. If there is a conducted beat in response to the atrial contraction, there is no ventricular pacing ("I" = inhibited). If there is no ventricular beat, the pacer fires in the ventricle. Thus, it is an A-V sequential pacer. However, the atrial rate is set, and there is no feedback since the atrium is not sensed. Thus, the pacer cannot respond to exercise. The atrial rate is fixed.

DDI pacer senses both atrium and ventricle. It fires if a minimum heart rate (atrial and ventricular) is not maintained. If there is intrinsic activity in both chambers, everything is fine. But, the minimum rate is fixed and as long as this is met, the pacer is inhibited (e.g., does not fire). Thus, it does not pace the ventricle in response to the **endogenous** atrial rate but only maintains a minimum ventricular rate. Thus, there is no response to exercise, etc. A DDD pacer can sense atrial activity and triggers ventricular activity in response. This is best for patients with a functional SA node but heart block. If the atrial rate increases in response to exercise, the ventricular rate is paced to keep up.

Cardiac Pacemaker Nomenclature

Position of letter	1st	2nd	3rd
What it represents	Chamber paced	Chamber sensed	Response to sensing
Possible options	0 = none A = atrium V = ventricle D = dual (atrium and ventricle)	0 = none A = atrium V = ventricle D = dual (atrium and ventricle	0 = none T = triggered I = inhibited D = dual

Examples:

DVI = Paces both atrium and ventricle, senses ventricle, in response to sensed ventricular firing, the pacer does not fire.

DDD = Can pace both atrium and ventricle, senses both atrium and ventricle, can trigger or be inhibited by sensing beats. So, for example, if it senses an atrial beat but not a ventricular beat the pacer will fire in the ventricle. If is senses both an atrial and ventricular beat, the pacer will be inhibited and will not fire. If it senses neither an atrial **nor** a ventricular beat, the pacer will trigger both atrial and ventricular contractions.

D) Chronic obstructive lung disease.
E) Interstitial lung disease.

Discussion
The correct answer is "B." Cor pulmonale is the term used for right heart failure caused by diseases primarily affecting the lungs and pulmonary vasculature. The resistance of the lung vasculature increases causing right ventricular hypertrophy and right-sided heart failure.

A possible finding on the ECG of this patient would include:

A) P-mitrale (an "m" shaped, notched P wave).
B) P-pulmonale (an enlarged, peaked, P wave).
C) Absent P waves.
D) Inverted P waves.
E) We give up. No more foils for this question.

Discussion
The correct answer is "B." Patients with cor pulmonale often have an enlarged and peaked P wave in lead II reflecting right atrial enlargement. "P-mitrale" is found in **left** atrial enlargement.

Besides stopping smoking, the best treatment of this patient's cor pulmonale and PHTN is:

A) Continuous prostacyclin infusion.
B) Continuous, low flow oxygen.
C) Calcium channel blockers.
D) Nitroglycerin.
E) Antibiotics to reduce pulmonary inflammation secondary to infection.

Discussion
The correct answer is "B." In this patient who is a smoker with cor pulmonale, the best drug is continuous, low-flow oxygen. This will help to reverse the pulmonary vasoconstriction caused by chronic hypoxia. It should go without saying that you must do everything you can to get him to **stop smoking**. His disease process will progress much faster if he continues to smoke. "A" is incorrect because prostacyclin infusion is useful in primary PHTN, not this type of cor pulmonale. "C" is incorrect. In some cases of **primary** PHTN, calcium channel blockers, PDE5 inhibitors (e.g., sildenafil), and several other medications, which serve as direct vasodilators to dilate the pulmonary vascular bed, can be useful. However, this is not the best choice for this patient with COPD. "D" is incorrect because patients with cor pulmonale are dependent on high right heart filling pressures to get blood through the pulmonary vasculature. Nitroglycerin will reduce preload, worsening this patient's symptoms. "E" is also incorrect. Antibiotics might be needed in this patient for pneumonia, bronchiectasis, etc., but they are not going to help with the treatment of cor pulmonale.

> HELPFUL TIP: Always remember sleep apnea as a cause of cor pulmonale. Nocturnal oxygen desaturation causes increased pulmonary vascular resistance causing right-sided failure.

Objectives: Did you learn to . . .

- Diagnose cor pulmonale?
- Describe causes of cor pulmonale?
- Treat a patient with cor pulmonale?

CASE 10

A 65-year-old male presents to your clinic for a complete history and physical exam. You notice that his abdominal exam reveals a pulsatile mass which you suspect may represent an aortic aneurysm. This finding is confirmed by ultrasound. The radiologist reports that the patient has a 3.5-cm abdominal aortic aneurysm without evidence of leak or thrombus formation.

The best advice to this patient is:

A) Have the aortic aneurysm fixed now while he is still healthy.
B) Have a follow-up ultrasound every 3 months.
C) Have a stent placed to prevent further aortic dilatation.
D) Have an angiogram in the next several days to rule out vascular disease below the aorta (femoral arteries, iliac arteries, etc.).
E) Have a repeat ultrasound at 1 year.

Discussion
The correct answer is "E." Patients with an abdominal aortic aneurysm less than 4 cm in diameter should have an ultrasound yearly to check progression. Those with an aneurysm 4–5 cm in diameter should have an ultrasound every 6 months. "A" is incorrect (see next question for an explanation). "C" is incorrect since a stent is not indicated at this point. "D" is incorrect. The only reason to do an angiogram at this point is if the patient is symptomatic or you are planning surgical intervention.

* *

The patient is really worried that this aneurysm will rupture and kill him. You let him know that the benefit of having the aneurysm repaired is greater than the risk of the surgery when the aneurysm reaches:

A) $\geq$4.5 cm.
B) 5.0–5.5 cm.
C) 5.5–6.0 cm.
D) $>$6.0 cm.
E) No repair is indicated until the patient becomes symptomatic.

Discussion

The correct answer is "B." The risk of the surgery outweighs the benefits until the aneurysm reaches somewhere between 5.0 and 5.5 cm. The rest are incorrect. It would be an especially bad idea to wait until an aneurysm is symptomatic, as a ruptured aortic aneurysm can be lethal in a matter of minutes.

* *

The patient goes to Texas (or Arizona or Florida—somewhere warmer than Iowa) for the winter as part of the reestablishment of human annual migration. When he returns, he calls you complaining of back pain that is somewhat sharp and radiating into his legs. You meet him in the ED and suspect that he is having a dissection of his aneurysm.

All of the following are true regarding aortic dissection EXCEPT:

A) A substantial number of patients will have palpable pulses below the level of the dissection.
B) Patients may have an elevated LDH and microangiopathic findings on RBC examination.
C) Blood pressure should be kept on the high side to ensure perfusion below the area of the aneurysm.
D) The pain may migrate down from the chest to the lower abdominal area over time.
E) The pain may be episodic.

Discussion

The correct answer is "C." One does **not** want to keep the blood pressure on the high side. In fact, reducing the blood pressure is the initial treatment of choice for a dissecting aneurysm. "A," "B," "D," and "E" are all correct statements. Patients may have an elevated LDH and microangiopathic findings on RBC smear as a result of trauma and cell lysis. "D" is a correct statement, but patients often do not have this "classic" migrating pattern of pain. "E" is often true of pain in aortic dissection—it may be episodic.

* *

The patient has a blood pressure of 160/105. Clearly, this is too high in a patient who has an ongoing dissection. You decide to treat this patient before transferring him to a tertiary care center where he can be surgically managed.

The best medication(s) to use in this patient to control his blood pressure is/are:

A) Sublingual nifedipine plus metoprolol.
B) Amlodipine.
C) Intravenous hydralazine.
D) Intravenous labetalol plus nitroprusside.
E) Intravenous nitroglycerin.

Discussion

The correct answer is "D." The goal of therapy here is not only blood pressure reduction but also control of shear forces on the aorta, which requires the prevention of tachycardia. Intravenous beta-blockers such as labetalol, propranolol, metoprolol, or esmolol are the first-line agents. Nitroprusside (or our favorite, IV nitroglycerin) can be added if the blood pressure control remains suboptimal even after beta-blockade. In this scenario, nitroprusside should never be given without beta-blockade, as it may cause tachycardia induced by vasodilation and thus further aortic shear stress. The same rationale is true for not using intravenous hydralazine in this scenario. "A" is incorrect for two very good reasons. First, nifedipine should **never** be used sublingually. Syncope, heart block, MI, stroke, and other serious adverse consequences have been reported. Second, nifedipine increases heart rate causing an increase in shear forces on the aorta. "B" is incorrect since amlodipine does nothing to reduce heart rate and is not titratable to any useful degree. "E" is incorrect because nitroglycerin alone causes reflex tachycardia.

HELPFUL TIP: Esmolol, a short-acting beta-blocker, plus either IV nitroglycerin or IV nitroprusside are optimal drugs for BP control in a dissecting aneurysm. All three are short acting and can be stopped should the patient become hypotensive.

HELPFUL TIP: Screen for an aortic aneurysm **once** in men age 65–75 who have ever smoked.

Objectives: Did you learn to . . .

- Identify the treatment options and timing of treatment of an abdominal aortic aneurysm?
- Manage a patient with a dissecting aneurysm?

CASE 11

A 60-year-old male presents with dizziness and palpitations. The patient has a blood pressure of 100/60 mm Hg and a pulse of 160. His ECG is shown in Figure 2–3.

Which of the following are appropriate options in the treatment of this patient?

A) Amiodarone, lidocaine, defibrillation, metoprolol.
B) Amiodarone, lidocaine, defibrillation, diltiazem.
C) Amiodarone, lidocaine, cardioversion, diltiazem.
D) Procainamide, lidocaine, adenosine, defibrillation.
E) Procainamide, lidocaine, cardioversion, amiodarone.

Discussion

The correct answer is "E." The rhythm is stable ventricular tachycardia. Procainamide, lidocaine, amiodarone, and *synchronized cardioversion* can all be used for ventricular tachycardia. "A" is incorrect for two reasons. The rhythm is ventricular tachycardia and is stable, and neither metoprolol nor defibrillation is appropriate. Defibrillation could be appropriate if the patient was unstable or pulseless. "B" is incorrect because of the inclusion of diltiazem and defibrillation. "C" is incorrect because of the inclusion of diltiazem. "D" is incorrect because adenosine, which is used for atrial arrhythmias, is included and because, again, defibrillation is inappropriate.

HELPFUL TIP: Procainamide is no longer in the ACLS protocols. It is still a really good drug if you have the time to load it.

* *

The patient does not respond to IV amiodarone and you choose to cardiovert him. Which of the following is the recommended energy (in joules) for an initial attempt at synchronized cardioversion?

A) 200 joules, monophasic.
B) 360 joules, monophasic.
C) 200 joules, biphasic.
D) 360 joules, biphasic.
E) None of the above.

Discussion

The correct answer is "A." For cardioversion of stable ventricular tachycardia, start with 100–200 joules for monophasic waveforms and 100 joules for biphasic waveforms. The rest are incorrect.

HELPFUL TIP: For **defibrillation**, escalating doses of electricity are out of the new protocols. Start with a single shock at 360 joules with a monophasic defibrillator or 150–200 joules if using a biphasic defibrillator.

* *

You cardiovert the patient, and the rhythm in Figure 2–4 is on the monitor. Is it getting hot here, or is it just you?

Of the following, what is the first step you will take (while maintaining good compressions and ventilations, of course)?

A) Re-shock the patient at the same energy level.
B) Check another lead to assure the readout is accurate.
C) Give epinephrine, 1 mg IV.
D) Give atropine, 1 mg.

Discussion

The correct answer is "B." This rhythm is asystole. It is important to check another lead and make sure that all of the leads are connected properly. "A" is incorrect

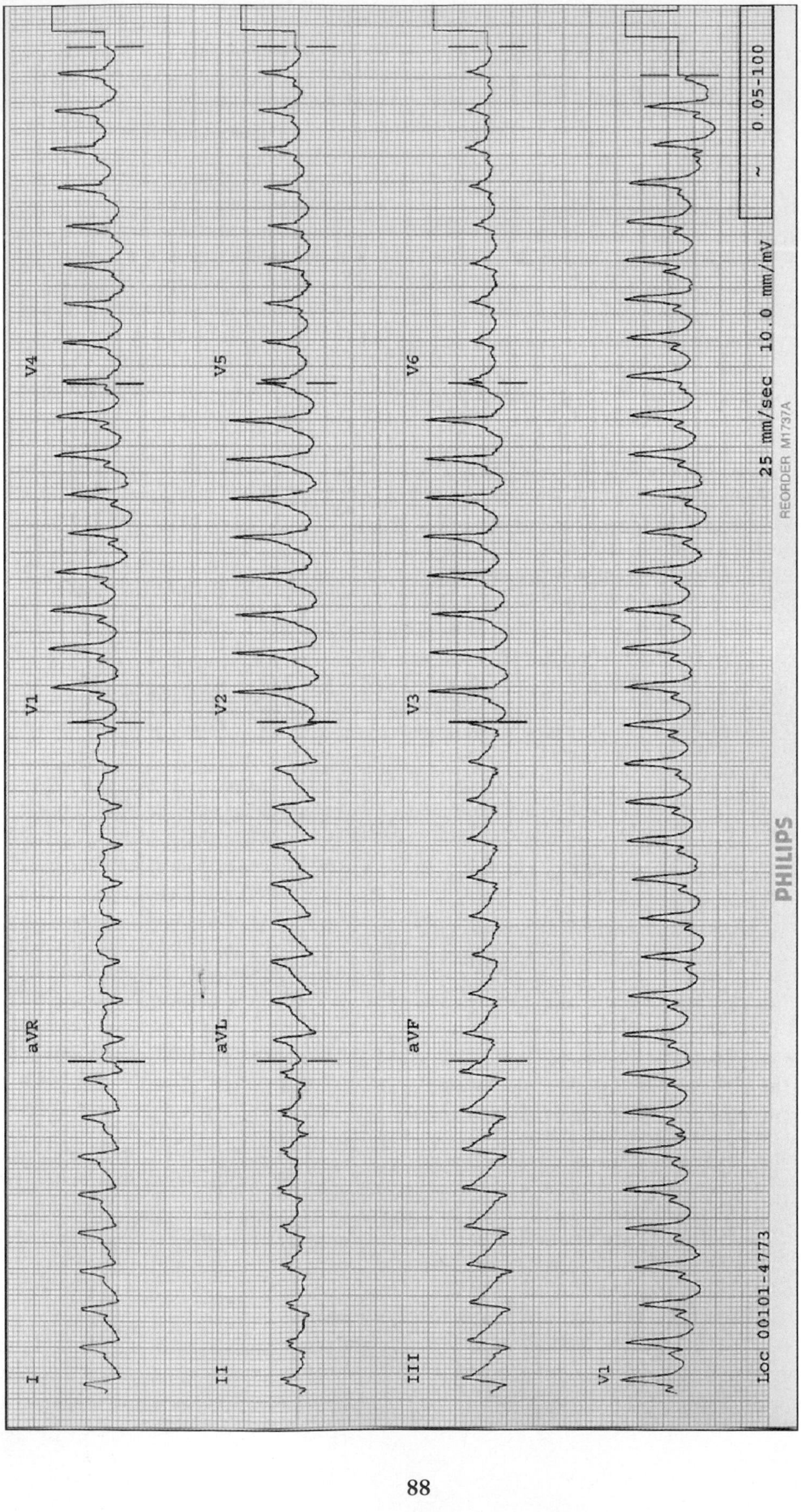
I
aVR
V1
V4
II
aVL
V2
V5
III
aVF
V3
V6
V1
Loc 00101-4773
25 mm/sec 10.0 mm/mV
~ 0.05-100
REORDER M1737A

Figure 2–3

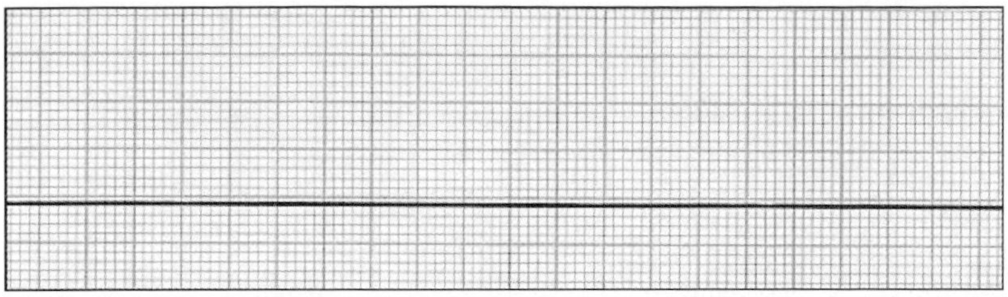

Figure 2–4

because cardioversion/defibrillation is not routinely indicated in the treatment of asystole. "C" and "D" are incorrect because it is important to ensure that the patient actually is in asystole.

> HELPFUL TIP: With regards to ACLS, doing compressions and ventilations are particularly important. There is no need to intubate the patient if he/she can be easily bagged. The correct number of ventilations (8/min) and compressions (100 bpm with 2 inches of depth) is important. The Bee-Gees "Staying Alive" has the correct rate for compressions. Queen's "Another One Bites the Dust" also has the correct rate but is considered less decorous in the code situation.

> HELPFUL (AND VERY IMPORTANT) TIP: The 2010 AHA guidelines for ACLS emphasize the importance of NEVER interrupting chest compressions during resuscitation (really that means minimizing interruptions—they feel that too often chest compressions are halted for less important interventions such as intubation, venous access, etc.).

The new lead placement continues to show asystole. Which of the following drugs and doses are considered appropriate in asystole?

A) Epinephrine 1 mg.
B) Atropine 0.5 mg.
C) Atropine 1 mg.
D) Epinephrine 10 mg.
E) A and C.

Discussion

The correct answer is "A." Atropine is no longer in the ACLS guidelines for asystole. Older ACLS recommendations for asystole included both epinephrine and atropine.

Objective: Did you learn to . . .

- Recognize and manage ventricular tachycardia and asystole?

CASE 12

A 75-year-old female presents to your office complaining of episodic palpitations with episodes of lightheadedness that are **not** concurrent with the palpitations. You perform an electrocardiogram in your office, and the rhythm is shown in Figure 2–5.

What rhythm does this represent?

A) First-degree heart block.
B) Second-degree heart block type I (Wenckebach).
C) Second-degree heart block type II.
D) Third-degree heart block.
E) Atrial flutter with variable block.

Discussion

The correct answer is "C." Your patient's ECG shows a second-degree heart block, type II (Mobitz II). This is characterized by a **fixed PR interval** with an intermittently nonconducting P wave and resultant dropped beats. "A" is incorrect. First-degree heart block is characterized by a prolonged PR interval without any blocked beats. The upper limit of normal of the PR interval is 0.2 seconds (and we admit that this one is darn close, but Mobitz II is the issue here). A second-degree heart block, Mobitz type I (Wenckebach), is defined by a progressively prolonged PR interval ending with a nonconducted P wave and a dropped beat. A third-degree heart block is characterized by no consistent pattern between the P waves and the QRS complex. "E" is incorrect because, by definition, atrial flutter is represented by a rapid atrial rate. In this patient, the rate is slow.

* *

By the time the patient arrives at the hospital, she is having a rapid, chaotic rhythm, which appears to be atrial fibrillation on the monitor. It seems as though there are also episodes of atrial flutter with 2:1 block.

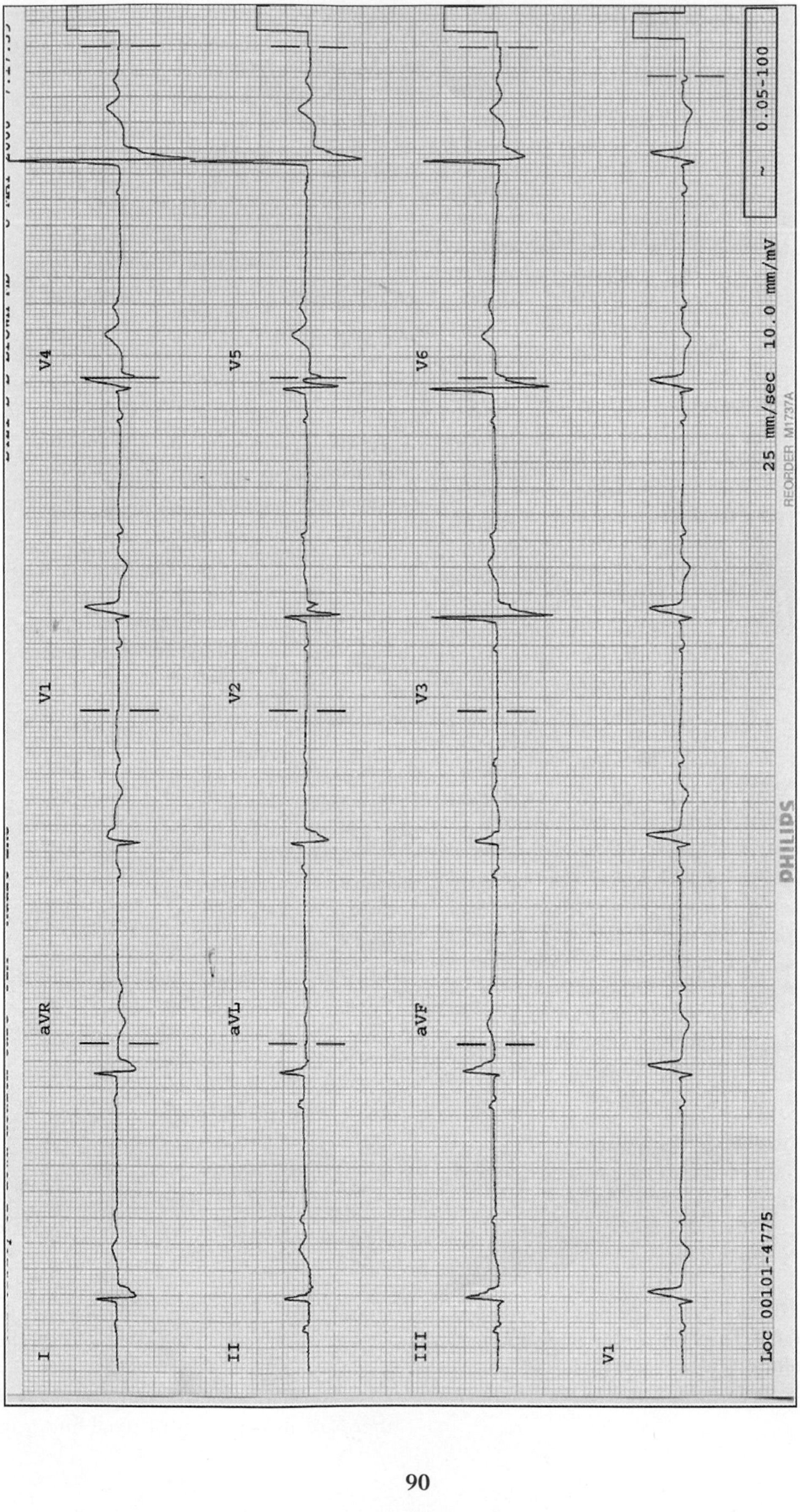
I
aVR
V1
V4
II
aVL
V2
V5
III
aVF
V3
V6
V1
Loc 00101-4775
25 mm/sec 10.0 mm/mV
~ 0.05-100
REORDER M1737A

Figure 2–5

The most likely diagnosis in this patient with varying rate is:

A) Sick sinus syndrome (bradycardia–tachycardia syndrome).
B) Hypothyroidism.
C) Hyperthyroidism.
D) Hyperkalemia.

Discussion

The correct answer is "A." The most likely diagnosis in this patient is "sick sinus syndrome," also known as "tachy–brady" syndrome and "bradycardia–tachycardia" syndrome. This syndrome is most common in elderly individuals and reflects the replacement of the SA node with fibrous tissue. "B" is incorrect because hypothyroidism should cause bradycardia without intermittent tachycardia. "C" is incorrect because hyperthyroidism should cause tachycardia without bradycardia. "D" is incorrect because hyperkalemia generally causes a widened QRS complex on ECG and eventually ventricular tachycardia.

Definitive treatment of this syndrome generally includes which of the following?

A) Mexilctine.
B) Hydralazine.
C) Quinidine.
D) Pacemaker.
E) Implantable defibrillator.

Discussion

The correct answer is "D." In general, patients with sick sinus syndrome become symptomatic because of the bradycardia episodes. Thus, pacing is necessary. "A" and "C" are incorrect because these two drugs are aimed primarily at ventricular arrhythmias; sick sinus syndrome is a problem with the SA node. "B" is incorrect because hydralazine is an afterload reducer with no direct effect on cardiac rhythm. "E" is incorrect because patients with sick sinus syndrome do not have ventricular fibrillation or ventricular tachycardia, and thus there is no need for a defibrillator.

> HELPFUL TIP: In addition to the pacemaker, it is often necessary to add a beta-blocker, digoxin, or a calcium channel blocker to address the tachycardia (e.g., PSVT or atrial fibrillation).

Objectives: Did you learn to . . .

- Identify and differentiate second-degree heart blocks?
- Diagnose and treat sick sinus syndrome?

CASE 13

A 58-year-old male smoker with a history of type 2 diabetes mellitus presents with complaints of easy fatigability and pain in his thighs when exerting himself. The thigh pain resolves after resting. The pain is no worse going downhill than uphill. He works as a carpenter, and the leg pain is now limiting his ability to work. He will not quit smoking ("It's the only thing I truly love, Doc"). The patient states that his symptoms are better when he hangs his leg over the side of the bed at night.

The etiology of this patient's leg pain is most likely:

A) Peripheral venous disease (e.g., venous insufficiency, varicose veins).
B) Spinal stenosis.
C) Diabetic neuropathy.
D) Peripheral arterial disease (e.g., arterial occlusion).
E) None of the above.

Discussion

The correct answer is "D." Intermittent claudication is the classic presenting symptom of peripheral vascular disease. When rest pain is present, relief of symptoms occurs by making the affected area dependent (e.g., hanging the legs over the side of the bed), letting gravity help increase blood flow. The pain associated with diabetic neuropathy begins distally, has a burning quality to it, and is not typically relieved with rest. In fact, patients often notice it more at rest (e.g., during the night). Patients with peripheral venous disease will often have worsening of their symptoms when the leg is dependent. Spinal stenosis is often made worse by walking downhill and better when walking uphill or leaning forward (a kyphotic position opens up the foramen).

* *

His exam shows decreased pulses in the lower extremities bilaterally. You would like to confirm your suspicion that this patient has peripheral vascular disease.

What is the first study you would order in this patient?

A) Spiral CT to confirm vascular calcification.
B) Ankle-brachial index (ABI).
C) Color Doppler to assess flow.
D) Arteriography.
E) None of the above is the recommended first test.

Discussion

The correct answer is "B." The ABI is sensitive and specific for peripheral arterial disease in the lower extremity. The pressure in the ankle should be higher than that in the brachial artery in a normal person. Highest sensitivity is achieved by measuring pressures in both brachial arteries, both dorsalis pedis, and both posterior tibial arteries. Neither spiral CT nor color Doppler are recommended tests for the diagnosis of peripheral vascular disease (although CT angiogram may be useful in the future to define the degree and location of narrowing). Arteriography is an option but should be reserved for patients in whom surgery is a consideration and who have the diagnosis of peripheral vascular disease.

* *

The ABI results are normal. However, you strongly suspect claudication.

The next step should be:

A) Arteriography.
B) Repeat ABI after an exercise stress test.
C) Magnetic resonance arteriography.
D) CT arteriography.
E) None of the above.

Discussion

The correct answer is "B." In patients in whom you strongly suspect peripheral vascular disease, ankle-brachial indices after exercise can be positive when a resting test is negative. This would be the least invasive and most cost-effective test of the options given.

* *

The postexercise ankle-brachial indices are as follows: 0.9 in the right leg, 0.4 in the left leg.

The proper interpretation of this information is:

A) 95% probability of some degree of occlusive disease in the right leg, advanced occlusive disease in the left.
B) No occlusive disease in the right leg, mild disease in the left.
C) Moderate occlusive disease on both sides.
D) None of the above.

Discussion

The correct answer is "A." A normal ABI should be 1.0 or greater. An ABI of 0.9 is 95% sensitive for finding **some** degree of occlusive disease on arteriography (although it may not be hemodynamically significant). An ABI of 0.41–0.9 represents disease that is usually associated with claudication, while an ABI of 0.4 represents advanced disease. Paradoxically, an ABI >1.30 represents noncompressible arteries and may be a marker for artery calcification. In these cases, a toe-brachial index should be measured (don't ask us . . . we don't know where to find a toe BP cuff either. Maybe you can use a full-sized gnome or pixie cuff. We'd love to sell you one).

* *

You decide to start the patient on a medication to help control his claudication.

Which of the following statements is correct?

A) Pentoxifylline is relatively contraindicated in heart failure.
B) Cilostazol is the best choice for claudication in patients with heart failure.
C) Beta-blockers are good arterial dilators and are thus useful in claudication.
D) The main mechanism of action of pentoxifylline and cilostazol is selective vasodilation.
E) None of the above is correct.

Discussion

The correct answer is "A." Cilostazol (Pletal) and pentoxifylline (Trental) are phosphodiesterase inhibitors. Their mechanism of action in improving walking distance is poorly understood. Other phosphodiesterase inhibitors (such as milrinone) increase mortality in patients with heart failure. Thus, pentoxifylline and cilostazol should be used with extreme caution, if at all, in patients with heart failure. Selective beta-blockers actually cause arterial constriction, not arterial dilation. "C" is also incorrect. The purported benefit of pentoxifylline is to increase RBC malleability and thus reduce the viscosity of blood in the microcirculation. It has no vasodilative effects. However, cilostazol does have some vasodilative effects. Therapeutic benefit with these drugs may take several weeks. A dedicated and supervised exercise program is of paramount importance and underutilized.

Pharmacologic therapy of PAD should include antiplatelet therapy and cardiovascular risk factor modification.

> HELPFUL TIP: Remember that peripheral artery disease is considered a CAD equivalent.

In and of themselves, indications for further intervention for peripheral artery disease (e.g., bypass, stenting) include all of the following EXCEPT:

A) Rest pain.
B) Persistent pain that interferes with day-to-day functioning.
C) Tissue loss.
D) 80% occlusion of the femoral artery.

Discussion

The correct answer is "D." Classic indications for invasive treatment of lower extremity PAD are (1) salvage of a threatened limb (rest pain, nonhealing ulceration, or gangrene) and (2) improvement in functional capacity. An 80% occlusion of the femoral artery, in and of itself, is not an indication for percutaneous or surgical revascularization in a patient who is asymptomatic.

* *

The patient sees the light, but does not go into it, and quits smoking. The case ends happily...

> HELPFUL TIP: No anticoagulation regimen seems to prevent reocclusion of lower extremity arteries after stenting. Patients should, however, continue on their current antithrombotic regimen as indicated for cardiovascular disease (ASA, warfarin, etc.).

Objectives: Did you learn to...

- Recognize symptoms and signs of peripheral vascular disease?
- Order appropriate diagnostic tests for a patient suspected of having peripheral vascular disease?
- Develop an understanding of the agents used to treat peripheral vascular disease?

CASE 14

A 75-year-old male presents to your office for a complete physical exam before prostate surgery. On exam, you notice a 3/6 midsystolic ejection murmur radiating to the neck. S1 and S2 are normal. An echocardiogram notes mild aortic stenosis. Currently he is asymptomatic.

The indications for valve replacement surgery include:

A) Grade 4/6 murmur.
B) Requirement for major, semielective surgery such as prostatectomy.
C) Severe aortic stenosis without symptoms.
D) Severe aortic stenosis in a patient undergoing coronary bypass grafting.
E) All of the above.

Discussion

The correct answer is "D." Mostly, aortic stenosis is repaired when it becomes symptomatic. Repair of asymptomatic severe aortic stenosis is indicated in the following scenarios: undergoing CABG or other valve or aorta surgery, LV EF <50%, hypotension in response to exercise, high likelihood of rapid progression, or surgery might be delayed at symptom onset. Answer "A" is incorrect because the loudness of the murmur does not always correlate with its functional significance. "B" is incorrect as well. As long as the lesion is not hemodynamically significant, the patient should tolerate prostate surgery. "C" is incorrect because surgery is not usually necessary even in severe valvular disease **without** symptoms.

The patient would like to know how often he should have a repeat echocardiogram given that he has mild disease. Your answer is:

A) Every 3–5 years.
B) Every year.
C) Every 6 months.
D) When he develops symptoms.
E) None of the above.

Discussion

The correct answer is "A." Patients with mild aortic stenosis who are asymptomatic can be followed by echocardiogram every 3–5 years. Patients with severe disease should have yearly echocardiography to evaluate for left ventricular dysfunction. See Table 2–12.

Table 2–12 RECOMMENDED INTERVALS FOR ECHOCARDIOGRAPHIC EVALUATION FOR VALVULAR DISEASE

Lesion	Mild Disease	Significant Disease
Aortic stenosis	Every 2 years (moderate disease) Every 3–5 years (mild disease)	Every year
Aortic regurgitation	Any change in symptoms	Every year
Mitral stenosis	No need for regular echocardiography Therapy based on symptoms	
Mitral regurgitation	Periodically[a]	Every 6–12 months

[a] Recommendations vary.

* *

Two years later, the patient returns for a checkup and states that he believes he has been having symptoms from his aortic stenosis.

All of the following can occur with symptomatic aortic stenosis EXCEPT:

A) Left-to-right intracardiac shunt.
B) Exertional dyspnea.
C) Syncope.
D) Angina.
E) None of the above.

Discussion

The correct answer is "A." Intracardiac shunts don't occur with aortic stenosis. If you got this one wrong, back to anatomy for you! An isolated, fixed valvular lesion as an adult cannot cause intracardiac shunting.

Which of the following statements about aortic valve disease is INCORRECT?

A) Aortic stenosis can be treated quite effectively with valvulotomy.
B) There are no known medical treatments that reduce the need for aortic valve replacement.
C) Risk factors for the development of aortic stenosis are similar to CAD.
D) Valve replacement surgery is the preferred treatment of symptomatic aortic stenosis.

Discussion

The correct answer is "A." Valvulotomy is not effective in the treatment of aortic stenosis and carries a high risk for cerebral embolism. Valve replacement surgery is preferred. The epidemiological risk factors for aortic stenosis and CAD are similar (as is their pathophysiology). Unfortunately, there are no drugs that are effective at reducing the need for valve replacement. You can provide symptomatic relief but that is all.

HELPFUL TIP: In patients who are not candidates for valve replacement, there is now a catheter-based approach for replacement of the aortic valve (transcatheter aortic valve implantation or "TAVI"). TAVI appears to reduce overall mortality compared with standard nonsurgical care but increases the risk of stroke.

Objectives: Did you learn to . . .

- Recognize symptoms of aortic stenosis?
- Manage a patient with aortic stenosis?
- Evaluate aortic valve disease and determine long-term follow-up vis-à-vis periodic echocardiograms?

CASE 15

A 35-year-old male presents to the office with upper respiratory symptoms. He is taking no medications except for a bit of pseudoephedrine for his cold. You notice when looking at his vital signs that his blood pressure is 180/106. Repeat measurement confirms that the blood pressure is elevated at 175/103. What is your initial approach to this patient?

A) Start a chronic antihypertensive since he is at risk for a stroke within the next couple of days with a blood pressure at this level.
B) Administer clonidine in the office to reduce the blood pressure to a safe level of about of 150/100.

C) Watch the patient over the next 2 weeks and get additional blood pressure readings before deciding what to do.
D) Schedule the patient for outpatient labs and electrocardiogram.
E) Fire the patient from your practice. He's messing up your quality measures.

Discussion

The correct answer is "C." The diagnosis of hypertension requires two elevated blood pressures on two different occasions. This patient's elevated blood pressure could be situational, related to decongestants, etc. Neither "A" nor "B" is correct because a blood pressure of 175/103 does not pose a risk of acute stroke, and the pressure need not be lowered acutely unless there is evidence of end-organ injury (e.g., angina, CHF, hypertensive encephalopathy). "D" is not correct because you cannot definitively establish that this patient has hypertension based on just one office blood pressure measurement. As for "E"... really? Is this why we went into medicine?

* *

The patient returns to your office with blood pressures measured six times over a period of 2 weeks at a local pharmacy. Only three of the six readings suggest that the patient is hypertensive. The patient states that the elevated blood pressures were while he was under stress at work.

Your best response at this point is to:

A) Start an antihypertensive.
B) Send the patient for a 24-hour ambulatory blood pressure measurement.
C) Don't worry about the blood pressure since the majority of the readings were within a normal range.
D) Get a nephrology consult to help in decision making.

Discussion

The correct answer is "B." One way to determine if a patient with contradictory readings is hypertensive is to perform 24-hour ambulatory blood pressure monitoring. This can be useful in patients who have elevated blood pressures in the office but not at home or vice versa. It can also be used if you do not trust the blood pressure readings taken outside of your office. "A" is incorrect since we have not yet established that this patient is hypertensive. "C" is incorrect since we have not yet established that this patient is not hypertensive. "D" is incorrect because you are smarter than that and should be able to work through this kind of case yourself!

The following are all well-accepted indications for 24-hour ambulatory blood pressure monitoring EXCEPT:

A) Suspected white-coat hypertension.
B) Patients with difficult-to-control hypertension.
C) Patients having hypotensive symptoms on their antihypertensive treatment.
D) Follow up after initiating antihypertensive treatment.
E) Evaluation of patient for autonomic dysfunction.

Discussion

The correct answer is "D." One need not do 24-hour ambulatory blood pressure monitoring to document response to antihypertensive therapy in patients in whom most or all measurements posttreatment are normal. All of the other answer choices are considered reasonable indications for 24-hour ambulatory blood pressure monitoring.

* *

Elevated blood pressure in response to stress (especially in the doctor's office) is called "white-coat hypertension."

Which of the following statements is true about white-coat hypertension?

A) As long as the majority of blood pressure readings are normal, the patient does not require treatment because there is no increased risk of adverse cardiac outcomes.
B) Patients with white-coat hypertension have an intermediate risk for adverse outcomes when compared with patients with normal blood pressure and those with chronically elevated blood pressure.
C) White-coat hypertension is more common in young patients.
D) Patients with white-coat hypertension have an elevated left ventricular mass when compared with patients with normal blood pressures.
E) B and D.

Discussion

The correct answer is "E." Patients with white-coat hypertension have outcomes that are intermediate between normotensive and hypertensive patients. Additionally, they have an elevated left ventricular mass. Surprisingly, white-coat hypertension is more common in the elderly.

According to the JNC 7 guidelines, hypertension is defined as an ambulatory 24-hour monitor *average* blood pressure of:

A) 135/85 during the day and 125/75 at night.
B) 140/90 during the day and 130/85 at night.
C) 130/85 over 24 hours.
D) 140/90 over 24 hours.

Discussion

The correct answer is "A." Patients with an average blood pressure of >135/85 during the day and >125/75 at night are defined by JNC 7 as being hypertensive. Another published criterion is a blood pressure of >140/90 more than 40% of the time.

* *

The ambulatory blood pressure monitor reveals that the patient is hypertensive (>140/90 more than 40% of the time).

The initial evaluation of the hypertension includes the following:

A) History, physical, CBC, urinalysis, glucose, BUN, creatinine, electrolytes, ECG, lipids.
B) History, physical, CBC, urinalysis, glucose, BUN, creatinine, electrolytes, lipids.
C) History, physical, CBC, urinalysis, glucose, BUN, creatinine, electrolytes, ECG, lipids, echocardiography.
D) History, physical, and labs only as indicated by history and physical.

Discussion

The correct answer is "A." History, physical, CBC, urinalysis, glucose, BUN, creatinine, electrolytes, ECG, and lipids are the generally agreed-upon initial workup of the hypertensive patient. Do we really need all of these? That is an interesting question, but we're just stating what is recommended by the experts. Answer "C" includes echocardiography, which is not recommended as part of the routine evaluation but may be indicated if signs of cardiac disease are present.

* *

The patient's ECG comes back showing evidence of LVH.

This finding suggests that:

A) You should initiate this patient's therapy with an ACE inhibitor since ACE inhibitors promote cardiac remodeling.
B) The patient has diastolic dysfunction.
C) You should recommend an echocardiogram for this patient.
D) You should order a B-natriuretic peptide (BNP) level to screen for LVH and early CHF.
E) None of the above

Discussion

The correct answer is "C." The sensitivity of ECG for LVH is only in the 30–60% range with a specificity of 80%. Thus, a "positive" ECG is not enough to embark on a therapeutic adventure for LVH. For this reason, an echocardiogram should be done to confirm the diagnosis of LVH. "A" is incorrect since an ACE inhibitor is not necessarily the first drug one would start. Additionally, we really don't know if this patient has LVH yet. "B" is incorrect. Certainly, longstanding hypertension and significant LVH can cause diastolic dysfunction. However, we cannot conclude that this patient has diastolic dysfunction on the basis of an ECG, especially in the absence of symptoms. "D" is incorrect since the sensitivity of the BNP as a screening tool in an asymptomatic population is poor.

* *

The echocardiogram is normal. You have decided to start this patient on treatment for his hypertension.

Based on outcome data, the BEST drug to start this patient on is:

A) An ACE inhibitor, such as lisinopril.
B) An alpha-blocker, such as doxazosin.
C) A beta-blocker, such as metoprolol.
D) A thiazide diuretic, such as chlorthalidone.
E) A calcium channel blocker, such as amlodipine

Discussion

The correct answer is "D." The ALLHAT study suggests that the one best drug to start for hypertension is a thiazide diuretic (specifically, chlorthalidone). This recommendation can be modified if there is a compelling reason for starting another agent (see next question).

Time to digress a bit. Which of the following drugs is the best choice as your initial agent for the treatment of hypertension in a patient with diabetes and known microalbuminuria?

A) Lisinopril.
B) Metoprolol.
C) Losartan.
D) Verapamil.
E) Amlodipine.

Discussion

The correct answer is "A." In a diabetic patient who has proteinuria, an ACE inhibitor is indicated to slow down the progression of renal disease. An ARB or nondihydropyridine calcium channel blocker (verapamil, diltiazem) are viable alternatives for those who cannot tolerate an ACE inhibitor. However, ACE inhibitors are still first line. These recommendations stem from the renal and cardiac benefits of ACE inhibitors.

> HELPFUL TIP: Although thiazide diuretics decrease the left ventricular diameter (due to diuresis), beta-blockers, calcium channel blockers, and ACE inhibitors **all** reverse LVH.

> HELPFUL TIP: Hydrochlorothiazide, the old standby, is falling out of favor. Chlorthalidone has a much longer duration of action and is the best studied of the diuretics with regard to outcomes. Hypokalemia **may** be a bit more frequent with chlorthalidone.

* *

Digressing a bit further... Which of the following drugs might you want to use as your initial agent for the treatment of hypertension in a 72-year-old male with a history of symptomatic benign prostatic hypertrophy?

A) Amlodipine.
B) Doxazosin.
C) Captopril.
D) Losartan.
E) Verapamil.

Discussion

The correct answer is "B." Doxazosin is an alpha-blocker that is useful in the treatment of symptomatic BPH. None of the other choices can be used for this indication. Of course, alpha-blockers are also antihypertensives, and thus serve a useful purpose by killing two birds with one stone (Why would you want to kill two birds? And why with stones? Isn't there something more efficient here?). *Note*: There is some evidence that alpha-blockers do not confer as much benefit for the hypertensive patient as other classes of drugs. Thus, alpha-blockers are not the best choice in general.

* *

The point of these digressions is that thiazides are recommended as initial therapy in most cases of hypertension unless there is a compelling reason to use another agent. Another example would be a patient with CAD and angina starting on a beta-blocker as initial treatment rather than a thiazide (since the beta-blocker may improve angina symptoms and is indicated for CAD).

> HELPFUL (AND IMPORTANT) TIP: Beta-blockers have fallen out of favor as a first-line choice for hypertension. They don't seem to confer as much survival benefit as other antihypertensive classes. The one exception is in patients with CAD.

* *

Remember the 35-year-old guy? You start him on chlorthalidone, but his blood pressure does not respond at a dose of 12.5 mg/day (have your patients cut the 25 mg tabs in half).

The best approach for such a patient is to:

A) Push his chlorthalidone to 50 mg daily before starting another medication.
B) Stop the chlorthalidone and start another medication.
C) Rely on exercise and diet to normalize the blood pressure.
D) Start a second drug **before** you have maximized the dose of the first drug.
E) Start a workup for secondary causes of hypertension.

Discussion

The correct answer is "D." Experts, and the JNC 7 guidelines, recommend a low dose of two drugs rather than pushing one drug to its maximum. This is for two reasons: (1) most patients will eventually require two or more drugs and (2) you can get good blood pressure control while minimizing the side effects seen at a higher dose of a single drug. "A" is incorrect because you get little if any additional blood pressure benefit with chlorthalidone doses above 25 mg per day. In fact, low-dose chlorthalidone (12.5 mg) provides the greatest blood pressure reduction per mg of drug. "B" is incorrect because a patient with this level of blood pressure elevation will generally require more than one drug to achieve a normalized blood pressure. "C" is incorrect because the majority of patients are unable to maintain an adequate diet or exercise regimen to effectively treat blood pressure. Exercise and dietary change are certainly laudable goals and should be encouraged in all patients. However, they are not likely to normalize blood pressure in most hypertensive patients. "E" is incorrect since this patient has not yet proven to be resistant to treatment.

* *

You decide to start this patient on diltiazem as a second agent.

Which of the following side effects is most characteristic of diltiazem and other calcium channel blockers?

A) Dehydration.
B) Cough.
C) Dependent edema.
D) Hypokalemia.
E) Elevated cholesterol.

Discussion

The correct answer is "C." As a class, calcium channel blockers tend to cause peripheral edema. Dehydration and hypokalemia can be caused by diuretics. Cough and hyperkalemia are characteristic of ACE inhibitors. Diuretics can also increase cholesterol, while beta-blockers can increase triglycerides.

* *

Despite the fact that the patient is on two medications, he remains hypertensive. In fact, the blood pressure has barely moved. With your thorough history taking, you have ruled out excess alcohol intake (often an "occult" cause of hypertension). The patient is compliant with his medications.

Table 2–13 CAUSES OF SECONDARY HYPERTENSION

Drugs, including over-the-counter medications
Sleep apnea
Endocrine: • Hyperaldosteronism • Pheochromocytoma • Thyroid disease • Cushing syndrome (innate or iatrogenic)
Vascular: • Renal artery stenosis • Coarctation of the aorta
Renal disease

Further investigations that might be helpful in determining the cause of hypertension in this patient include all of the following EXCEPT:

A) Checking the potassium level while the patient is taking his drugs to rule out hyperaldosteronism.
B) Assessing for renal artery stenosis.
C) Checking a 24-hour urine for glucocorticoids.
D) Checking a 24-hour urine for catecholamines.

Discussion

The correct answer is "A." Hypertension is secondary to another cause in about 1% of patients with mild hypertension but in 10–45% of those with severe, difficult to control hypertension. Secondary causes of hypertension include hyperaldosteronism, renal artery stenosis, pheochromocytoma, Cushing disease, sleep apnea, primary hyperparathyroidism, and others. "A" is the thing to avoid because when checking the serum potassium level for hyperaldosteronism, the patient must be off all diuretic medications and have an unrestricted salt intake. All of the others choices can be a part of a workup for secondary hypertension caused by renal artery stenosis ("B"), Cushing disease ("C"), and pheochromocytoma ("D"), respectively (see Table 2–13).

You decide to check this patient for renal artery stenosis. The most sensitive test for renal artery stenosis is:

A) Doppler ultrasound.
B) Captopril renal scan.

C) Serum renin level.
D) MR angiography.

Discussion

The correct answer is "D." When angiography is used as the gold standard, MR angiography is the most sensitive test for renal artery stenosis (90%), followed by captopril-enhanced Doppler ultrasound (63%), followed by captopril renal scan (33%). Frequently, renal artery stenosis is an incidental finding when the patient has angiography for another indication. In these cases, intervention is usually not needed so long as blood pressure control is adequate.

> HELPFUL TIP: Consider an evaluation for renal artery stenosis in a patient who has a "positive" clinical "captopril challenge." If you start an ACE inhibitor and see a dramatic decline in renal function in a few days, renal artery stenosis is the likely culprit.

* *

Your patient does not have any identifiable cause for secondary hypertension. You add a third agent, and his blood pressure comes under control. Sometimes, you just have to be persistent!

> HELPFUL TIP: Adding spironolactone to the regimen of a patient with difficult to control blood pressure can often be helpful even in the presence of another diuretic. Watch for hyperkalemia when used with ACE inhibitors, however. Eplerenone is an acceptable alternative but is much more expensive.

Objectives: Did you learn to . . .

- Evaluate a patient with initial high blood pressure readings?
- Select initial antihypertensive therapy?
- Appropriately tailor the treatment of hypertension, based on patient-specific characteristics?
- Use and interpret 24-hour ambulatory blood pressure monitoring?
- Understand the concept of white-coat hypertension?
- Generate a differential diagnosis and an appropriate evaluation of secondary hypertension?

CASE 16

You have a patient who is mildly hypertensive and decide to check baseline labs. The patient's potassium is low at 3.0 mEq/L. Being the good physician that you are, you recheck the potassium before getting too excited, and it is 2.9 mEq/L.

Of the following, the MOST LIKELY cause of low potassium in this patient is:

A) Hyperaldosteronism.
B) Hypoaldosteronism.
C) Spuriously low potassium because of an elevated glucose.
D) Metabolic acidosis.

Discussion

The correct answer is "A." **Hyper**aldosteronism can cause **hypo**kalemia and hypertension. Aldosterone increases the secretion of potassium, which leads to hypokalemia. "B" is incorrect because **hypo**aldosteronism, such as that seen with adrenal failure secondary to adrenal destruction, causes **hyper**kalemia and **hypo**tension. "C" is incorrect because elevated glucose does not result in a spuriously low potassium; if you answered "C," maybe you were thinking of sodium (the sodium goes down approximately 2 mEq/L for every 100 mg/dL increase in the glucose). Finally, "D" is incorrect because a metabolic acidosis should cause an elevated potassium rather than a low one.

> HELPFUL TIP: The serum potassium goes up by approximately 1 mEq/L for every 0.1 decrease in the pH from 7.4. Thus, the potassium would go from 4 to 6 mEq/L if the pH changes from 7.4 to 7.2.

* *

You suspect that the patient has hyperaldosteronism.

Which of the following is true?

A) Many patients with hyperaldosteronism have normal serum potassium.
B) In hyperaldosteronism, the plasma aldosterone-to-renin ratio is usually high.
C) All antihypertensives should be stopped before checking a plasma renin level.

D) If a confirmatory 24-hour urine is done, the urine potassium should be low to confirm the diagnosis of hyperaldosteronism.
E) A and B.

Discussion
The correct answer is "E." Many patients with hyperaldosteronism will have normal serum potassium levels. Additionally, the plasma aldosterone-to-renin level is usually high. "C" is incorrect because, although ACE inhibitors and spironolactone (and perhaps all diuretics) should be stopped before renin and aldosterone levels are drawn, other antihypertensives (e.g., calcium channel blockers) will have little effect on plasma renin levels. "D" is incorrect because hyperaldosteronism causes potassium wasting, so the urine potassium should be elevated.

* *

You diagnose this patient with hyperaldosteronism.

The most common cause of hyperaldosteronism is:

A) Adrenal adenoma.
B) Idiopathic.
C) Pituitary adenoma.
D) Aldosterone-secreting tumor such as small-cell carcinoma.
E) Renal artery stenosis.

Discussion
The correct answer is "A." Adrenal adenomas are the most common cause of hyperaldosteronism. The second leading cause is idiopathic.

Accepted approaches to the treatment of hypertension caused by hyperaldosteronism include all of the following EXCEPT:

A) Unilateral adrenalectomy in the case of adrenal adenoma.
B) Liberalized sodium intake.
C) Use of a potassium-sparing diuretic.
D) Use of a combination of amiloride and hydrochlorothiazide.

Discussion
The correct answer is "B." Liberalizing sodium intake will actually cause volume expansion, which is counterproductive and can lead to further hypokalemia. Once the patient is hypervolemic, there will be a spontaneous diuresis (the so-called aldosterone escape) leading to increased hypokalemia. The exact mechanism of aldosterone escape is not known, but it occurs after a weight gain of approximately 3 kg from fluid retention. If you want to sound smart just say it is "neurohumeral." You will probably be right and it makes you sound cool.

Objectives: Did you learn to . . .

- Identify laboratory abnormalities that occur in hyperaldosteronism?
- Evaluate a patient suspected of having hyperaldosteronism?
- Initiate treatment of hyperaldosteronism?

QUICK QUIZ

Which of the following side effects is/are associated with the use of ACE inhibitors?

A) Cough.
B) Dependent edema.
C) Hypokalemia.
D) Angioedema.
E) A and D.

Discussion
The correct answer is "E." Both chronic dry cough and angioedema (more common in blacks) are side effects of ACE inhibitors. Hyperkalemia is another potential concern. These side effects may not occur immediately. Hence, you should be wary of these symptoms in *any* patient on and ACE inhibitor for *any* period of time.

What is the rhythm on the rhythm strip shown in Figure 2–6?

A) Second-degree heart block, type I.
B) Second-degree heart block, type II.
C) Third-degree heart block with junctional escape rhythm.
D) Sinus rhythm with nonconducted PACs.

Discussion
The correct answer is "A." This is a Wenckebach block, also known as second-degree heart block type I or Mobitz type I AV block. Note the progressive prolongation of the PR interval before a nonconducted P wave on the rhythm strip in Figure 2–7 (*arrows* indicate P waves).

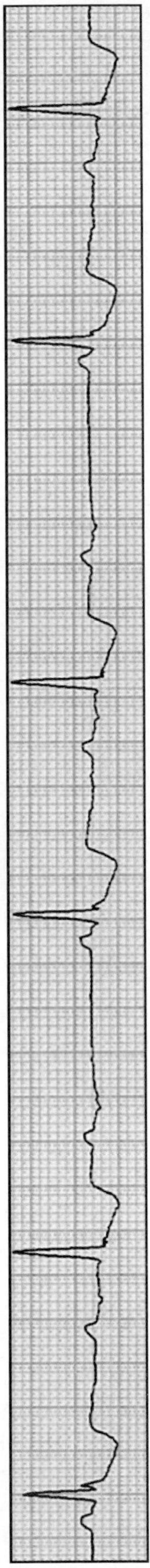

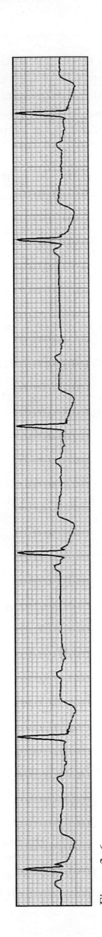

Figure 2–6

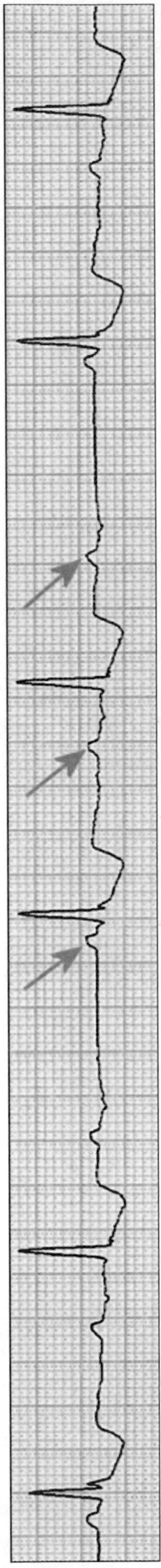

Figure 2–7

The proper treatment of an asymptomatic patient with this rhythm is:

A) Treat any underlying causes identified and observe.
B) Place temporary pacemaker followed by permanent pacemaker.
C) Give atropine followed by permanent pacemaker.
D) None of the above.

Discussion
The correct answer is "A." Wenckebach/second-degree heart block type I can be treated with observation as long as any underlying cardiac disease is treated. You should also stop any medications that might be contributing to this rhythm disturbance, such as digoxin and other AV node blocking agents. Pacemaker is appropriate for selected patients, usually those with symptoms. Atropine is used in the emergent setting for treatment of bradycardia.

What is the proper diagnosis of the ECG shown in Figure 2–8?

A) Anterior wall myocardial infarction.
B) Posterior wall myocardial infarction.
C) Pericarditis.
D) Hyperkalemia.
E) Inferior wall myocardial infarction.

Discussion
The correct answer is "E." This is an inferior wall MI. Note the ST elevations in leads II and III, and aVF with reciprocal changes in leads V2–V5 (see indicator *arrows* in Figure 2–9).

CASE 17

A patient presents with a history of lightheadedness when he stands and has the ECG shown in Figure 2–10.

What is the rhythm?

A) Atrial flutter with 4:1 block.
B) Atrial fibrillation with slow ventricular response.
C) Atrial tachycardia with third-degree heart block.
D) Mobitz type I (Wenckebach).

Discussion
The correct answer is "C." This is an atrial tachycardia with a third-degree heart block. The P wave preceding each QRS complex is indicated with an *arrow* on the ECG shown in Figure 2–11. Note that there is no consistent relationship between the P waves and the QRS complexes (i.e., the PR interval varies and there is no predictability), giving the diagnosis third-degree heart block.

The appropriate treatment of this patient with atrial tachycardia and third-degree block is:

A) Pacemaker.
B) Isoproterenol.
C) Lidocaine.
D) Atropine.

Discussion
The correct answer is "A." The treatment of a third-degree heart block is a pacemaker. Atropine will increase the atrial rate, but that is not the problem here. The problem is AV conduction. Isoproterenol will increase the ventricular rate but is arrhythmogenic and may cause hypotension. Lidocaine is not indicated in this patient.

> **HELPFUL TIP FOR THE RHYTHM CONNOISSEUR:** Atrial tachycardia with block is "classic" for digitalis intoxication. If this patient were on digoxin, you would treat with Digibind.

The drug of choice for the rhythm in Figure 2–12 is:

A) Atropine.
B) Procainamide.
C) Quinidine.
D) Metoprolol.
E) Lidocaine.

Discussion
The correct answer is "D." This is an **accelerated junctional rhythm** that generally occurs only in the setting of **cardiac ischemia**. Note the absence of P waves. Using a Class I antiarrhythmic can extinguish this rhythm, causing asystole (usually considered a bad outcome . . .). The patient also has inferior wall ischemia (see Figure 2–13, with indicator *arrows* showing depressed ST segments in the inferior

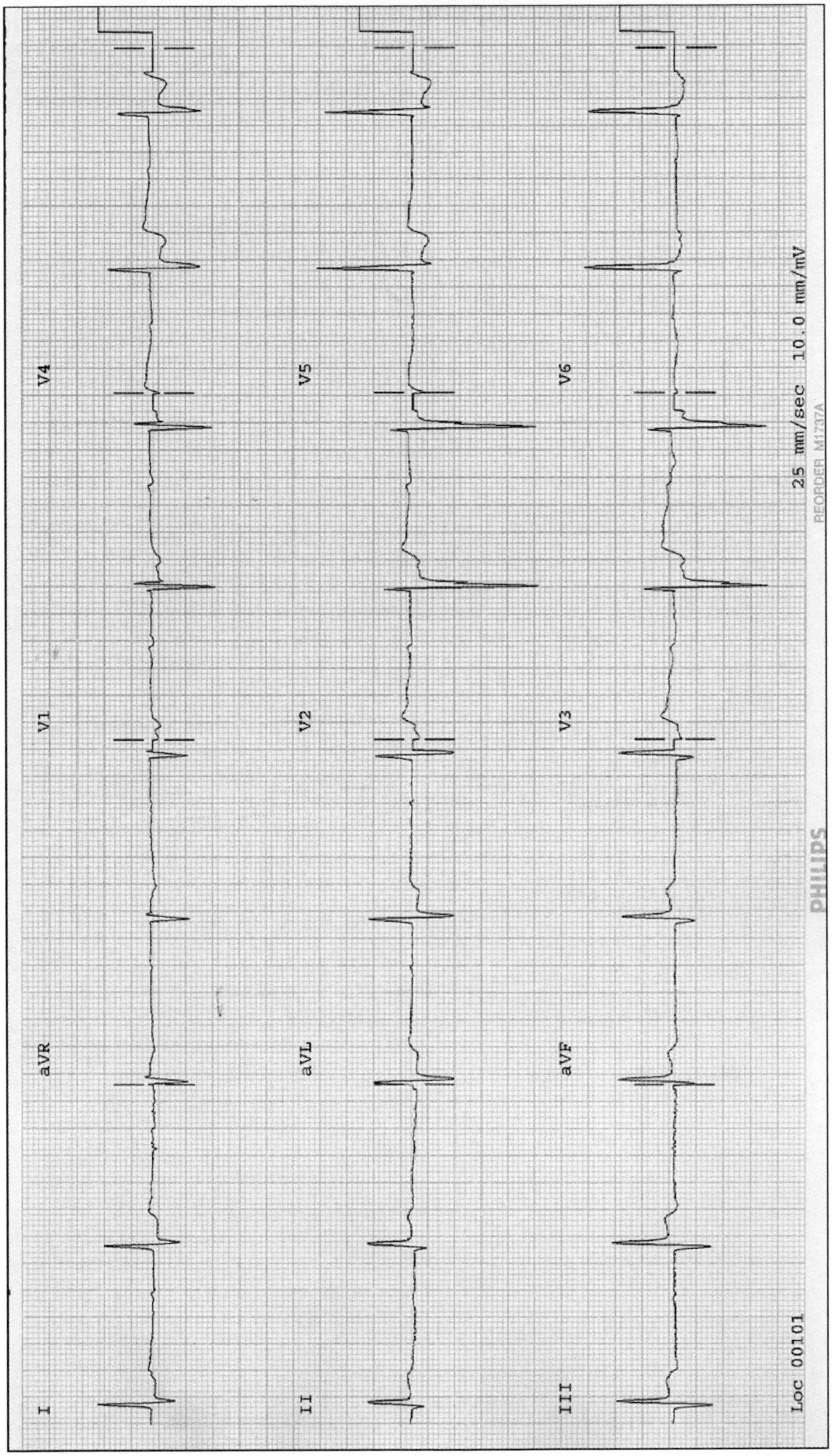
I
aVR
V1
V4
II
aVL
V2
V5
III
aVF
V3
V6
Loc 00101
25 mm/sec 10.0 mm/mV
REORDER M1737A

Figure 2–8

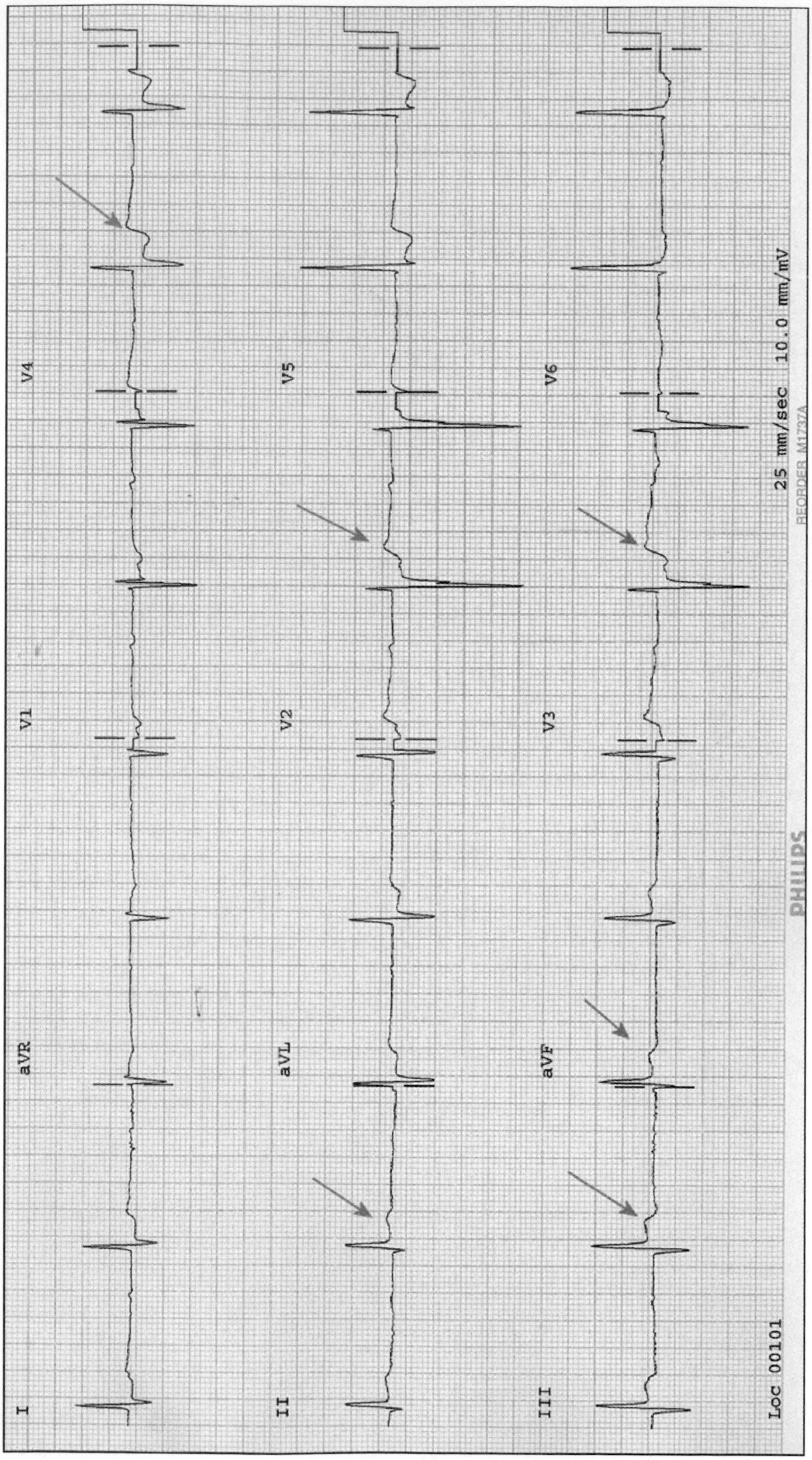
I
aVR
V1
V4
II
aVL
V2
V5
III
aVF
V3
V6
Loc 00101
25 mm/sec 10.0 mm/mV
PHILIPS
REORDER M1737A

Figure 2–9

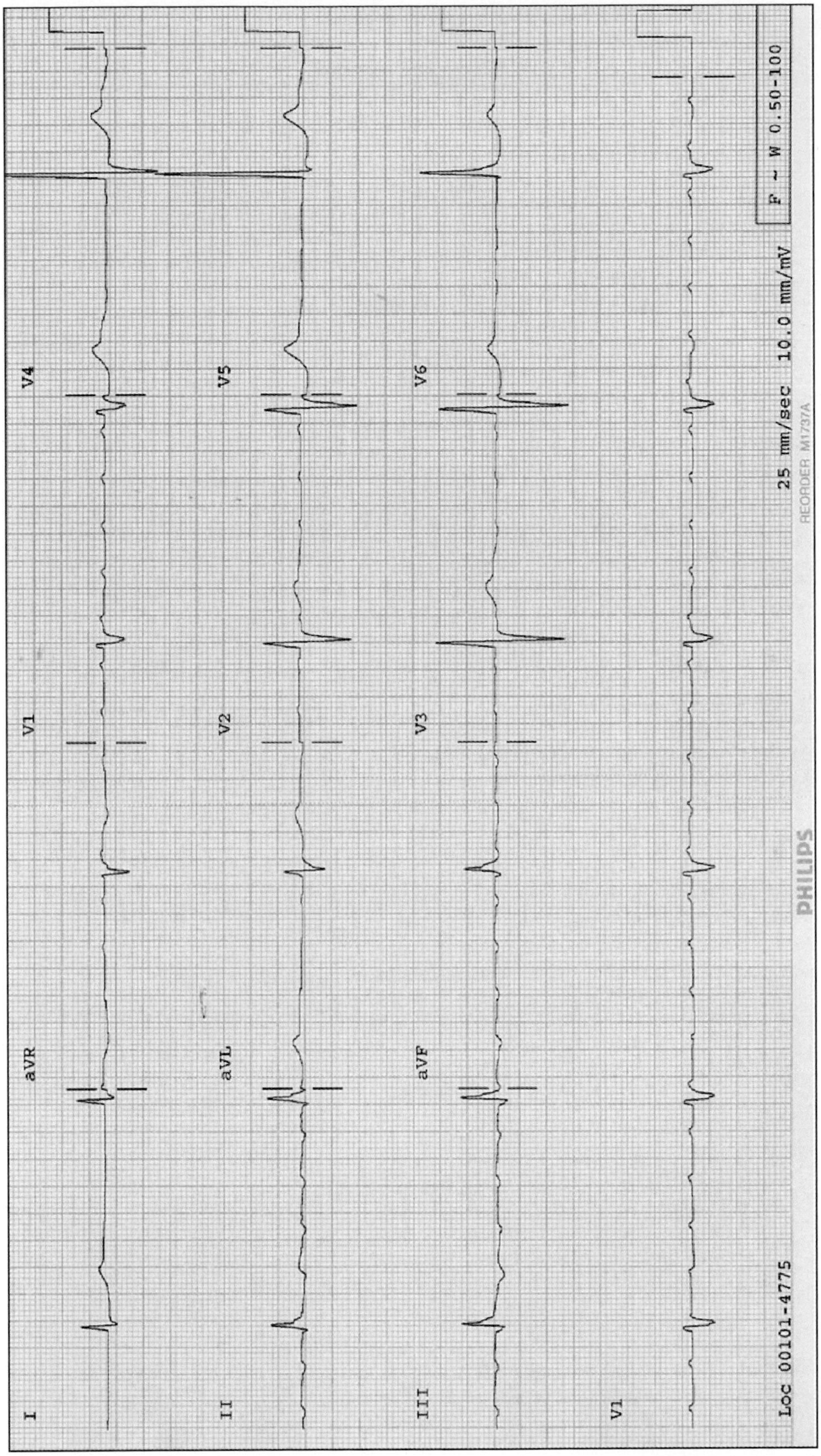
I
aVR
V1
V4
II
aVL
V2
V5
III
aVF
V3
V6
V1
Loc 00101-4775
25 mm/sec 10.0 mm/mV
F ~ W 0.50-100
REORDER M1737A

Figure 2–10

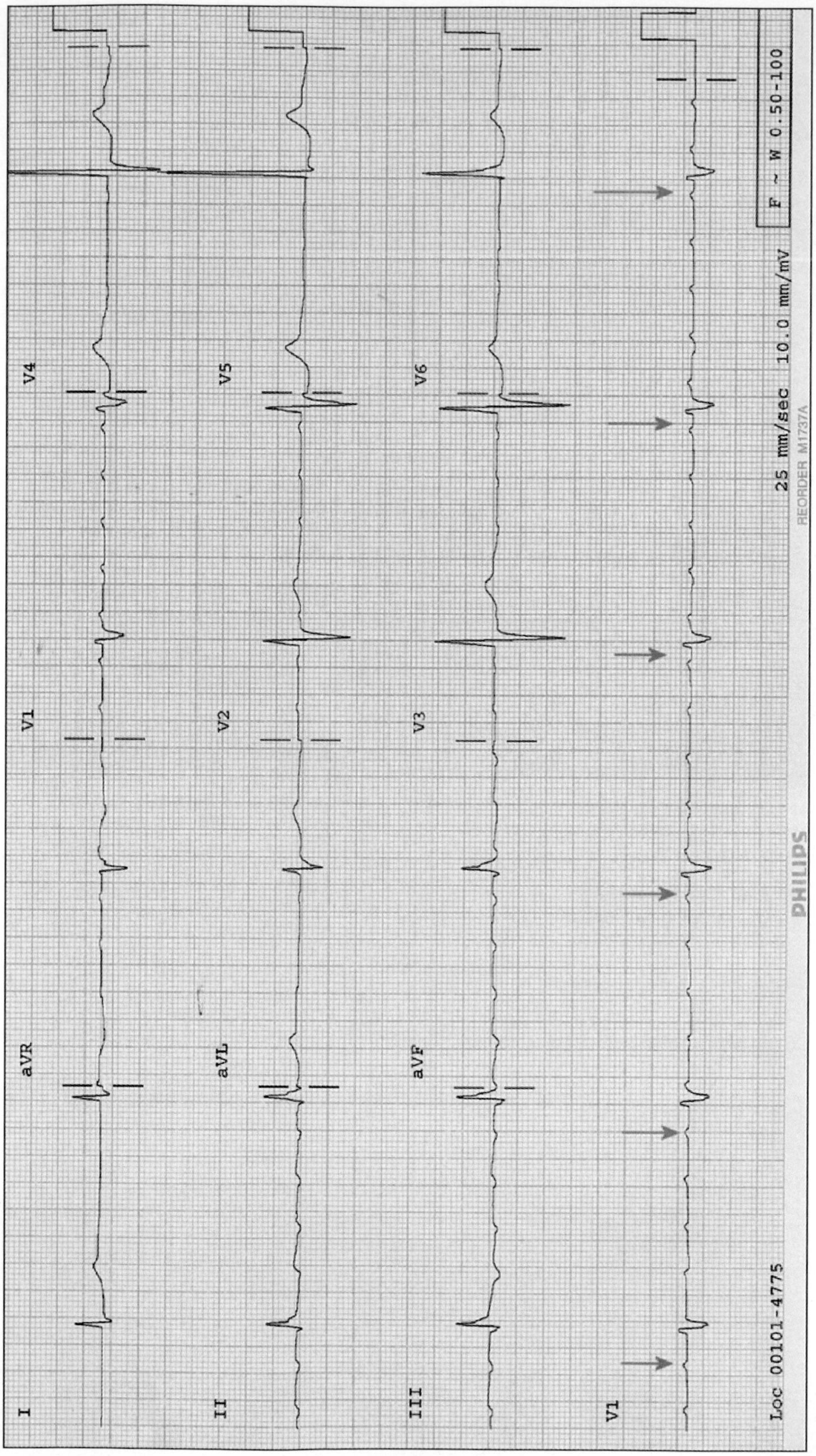
I
aVR
V1
V4
II
aVL
V2
V5
III
aVF
V3
V6
V1
Loc 00101-4775
25 mm/sec 10.0 mm/mV
F ~ W 0.50-100
PHILIPS
REORDER M1737A

Figure 2–11

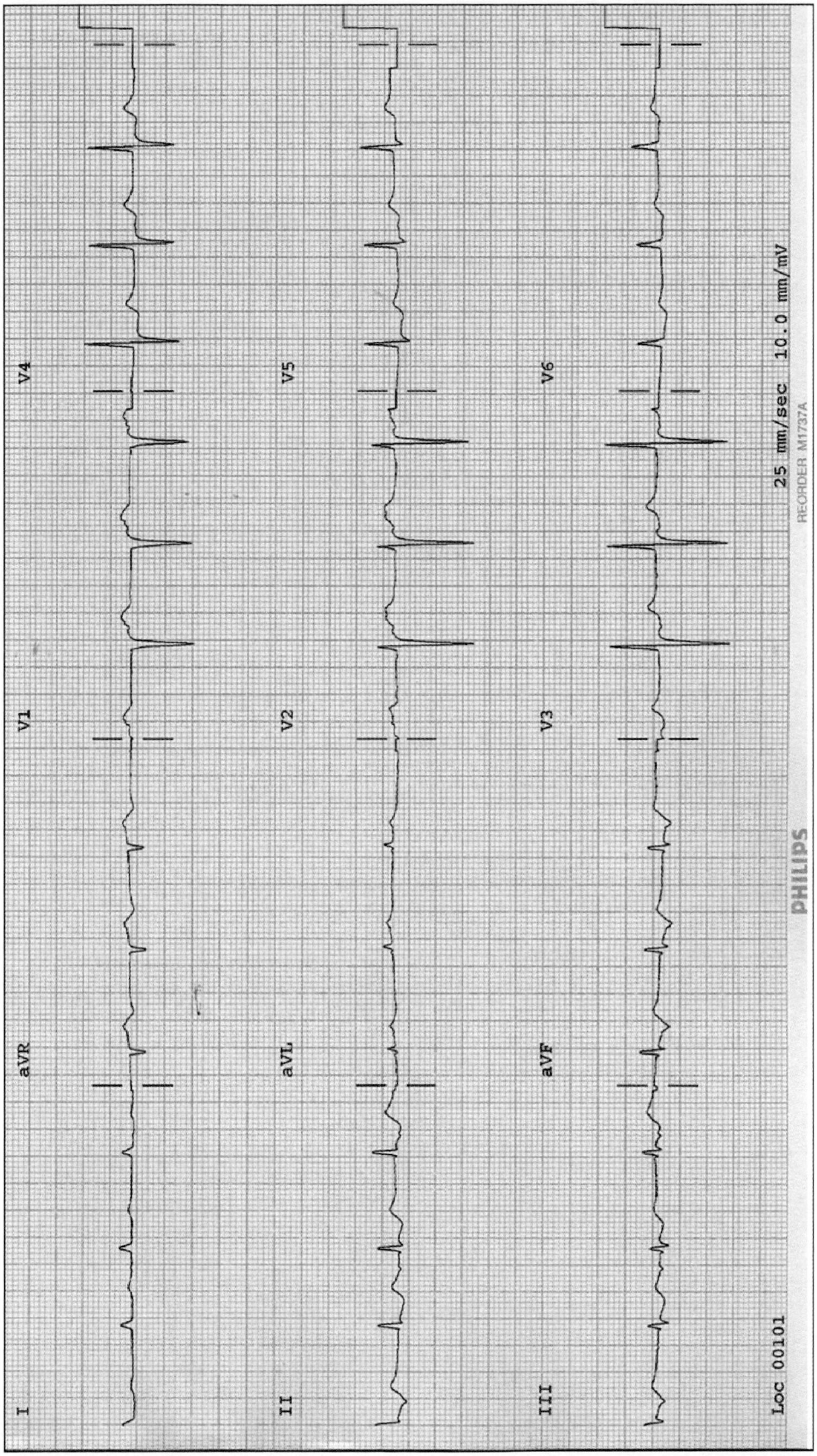
I
aVR
V1
V4
II
aVL
V2
V5
III
aVF
V3
V6
Loc 00101
25 mm/sec 10.0 mm/mV
REORDER M1737A

Figure 2–12

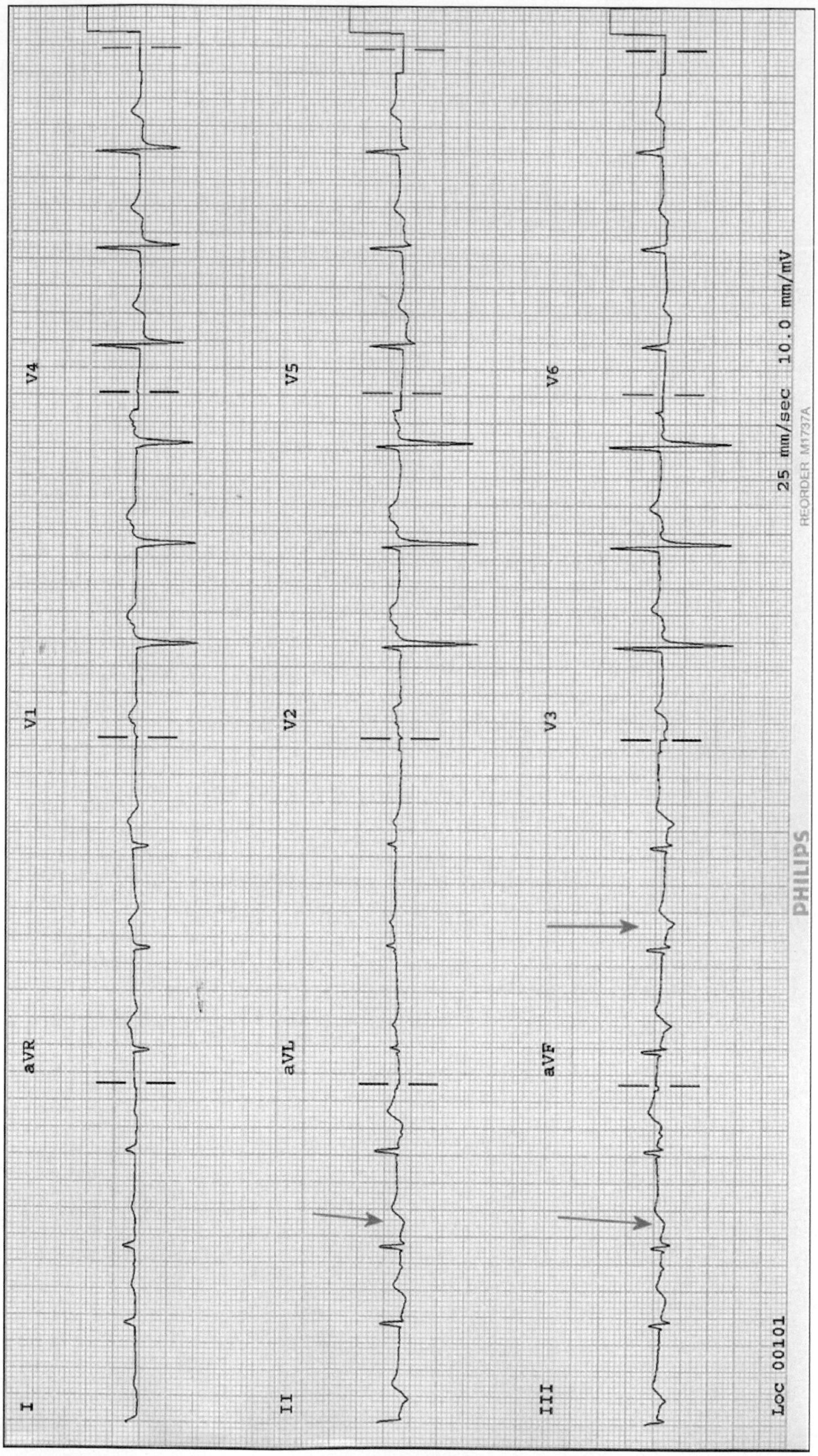
I
aVR
V1
V4
II
aVL
V2
V5
III
aVF
V3
V6
Loc 00101
PHILIPS
25 mm/sec 10.0 mm/mV
REORDER M1737A

Figure 2–13

leads). Slowing down this rhythm with metoprolol is acceptable, but you should treat the ischemia first. If the rhythm is not causing any problem, observation is good for now.

The rhythm shown in Figure 2–14 is best described as:

A) Atrial flutter with 2:1 block.
B) 2:1 second-degree heart block, Mobitz type II.
C) Sinus bradycardia.
D) Third-degree heart block.

Discussion
The correct answer is "B." This rhythm strip represents second-degree heart block, Mobitz type II. Notice that the PR interval is constant and there are dropped beats (see Figure 2–15, with indicator *arrows* showing P waves with no associated QRS complexes). This patient needs a pacemaker.

The electrocardiogram shown in Figure 2–16 is consistent with which of the following?

A) Pericardial effusion.
B) Pneumothorax.
C) PE.
D) Cardiac contusion.
E) None of the above.

Discussion
The correct answer is "A." This is an example of electrical alternans. Note the low QRS voltages that alternate in height from beat to beat. This type of pattern is seen with pericardial effusion. It is a late finding and one should be very concerned about tamponade.

The ECG in Figure 2–17 is consistent with which of the following?

A) Anterior myocardial infarction.
B) Anterolateral myocardial infarction.
C) Pericarditis.
D) Early repolarization.
E) Everywhere infarction

Discussion
The correct answer is "C." This ECG is consistent with pericarditis. This ECG demonstrates several findings that indicate pericarditis, including sinus tachycardia, diffuse ST elevations, and PR depression (see also Figure 2–18).

CASE 18

A 24-year-old female presents to the ED with a history of tachycardia and the rhythm strip shown in Figure 2–19. Her blood pressure is 115/70 with an oxygen saturation of 98% on room air. There are no associated symptoms of chest pain, dyspnea, etc.

The appropriate treatment of this patient is:

A) Adenosine 6 mg IV followed by 12 mg IV.
B) Diltiazem 5 mg/kg IV.
C) Verapamil 25 mg IV.
D) Digoxin 0.5 mg IV.
E) Defibrillation.

Discussion
The correct answer is "A." There are several treatment options for PSVT. These include adenosine, diltiazem, and verapamil. However, "B" and "D" are incorrect because the dose for diltiazem is 0.25 mg/kg IV, not 5 mg/kg, and the dose for verapamil is 2.5–5.0 mg IV, not 25 mg IV. While **cardioversion** is also an option in a hemodynamically stable patient, medication should be tried first. **Defibrillation** is never recommended for a perfusing rhythm.

* *

You treat the patient with adenosine but there is no response. Thus, you choose to try a calcium channel blocker. Unfortunately, the patient rapidly deteriorates with the calcium channel blocker and the heart rate actually increases, so you successfully cardiovert the patient. The ECG done after cardioversion is shown in Figure 2–20. This ECG represents:

A) Normal ECG.
B) Wolf–Parkinson–White (WPW) syndrome.
C) RBBB.
D) Right axis deviation.
E) LVH.

Discussion
The correct answer is "B." This is an ECG demonstrating WPW pattern. When combined with documented tachyarrhythmia, it is referred to as WPW syndrome. Note the short PR interval as well as the delta wave (Figure 2–21).

* *

Let's say this patient comes back to the ED with atrial fibrillation in the upcoming week. This time you suspect WPW and want to choose a rate-controlling

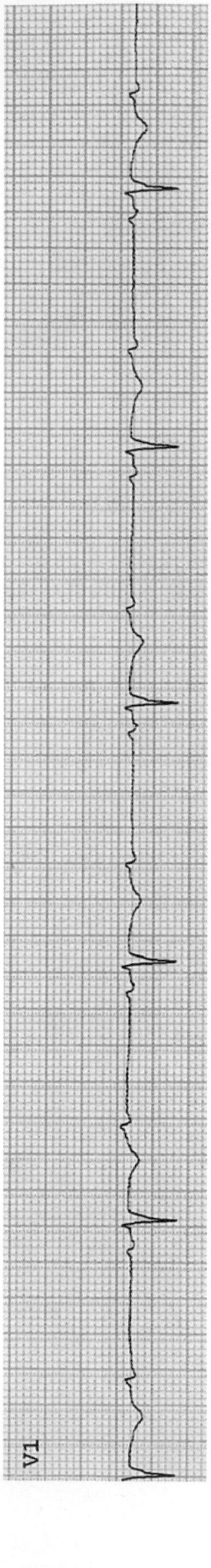

Figure 2–14

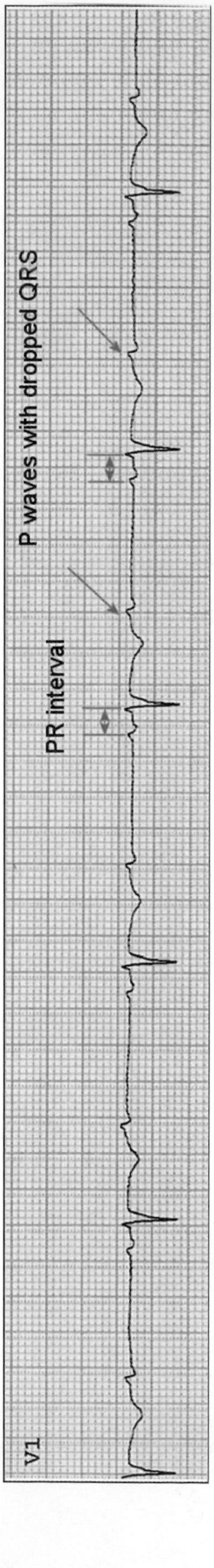

Figure 2–15

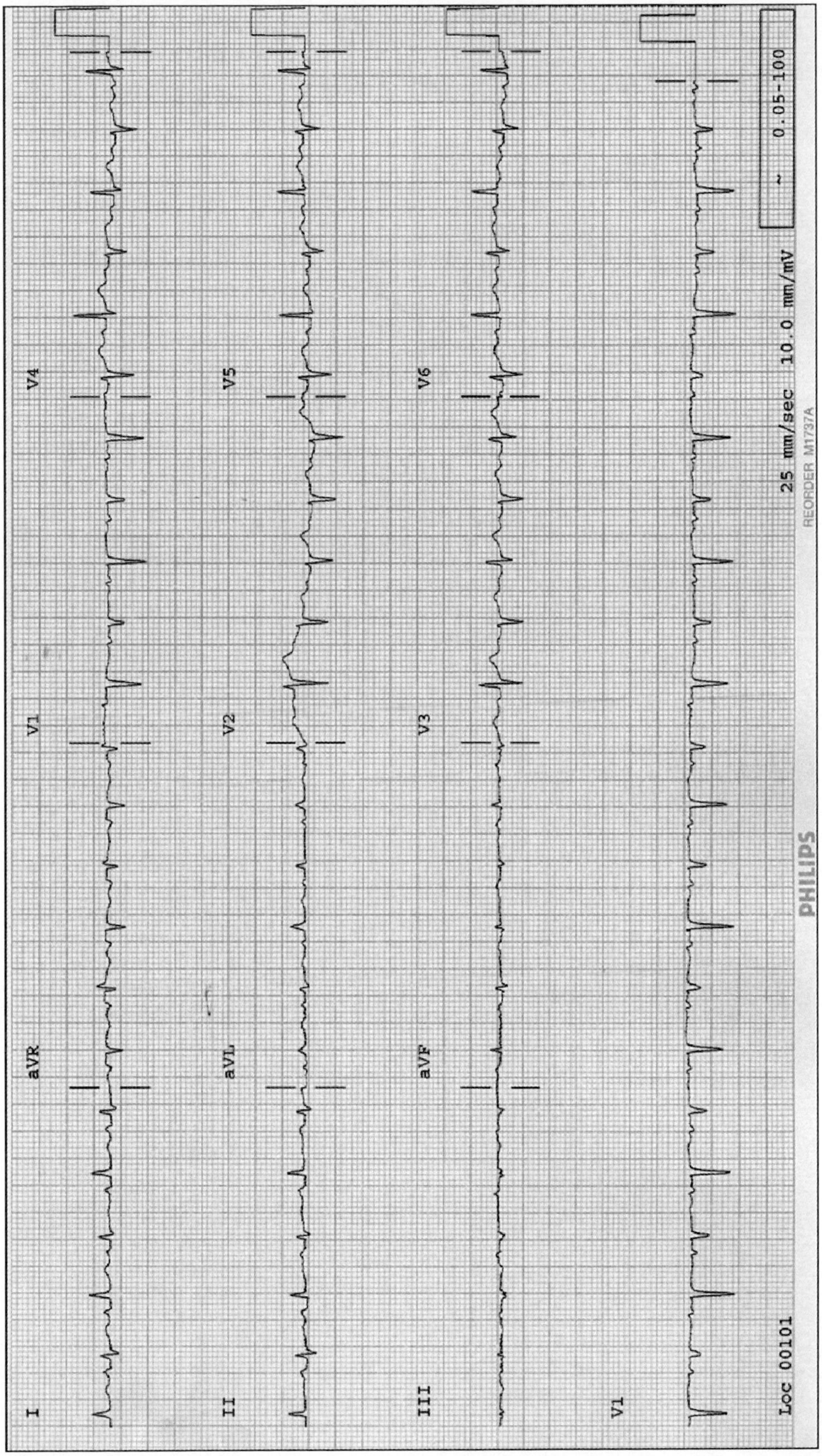
I
aVR
V1
V4
II
aVL
V2
V5
III
aVF
V3
V6
V1
Loc 00101
25 mm/sec 10.0 mm/mV
~ 0.05-100
PHILIPS
REORDER M1737A

Figure 2–16

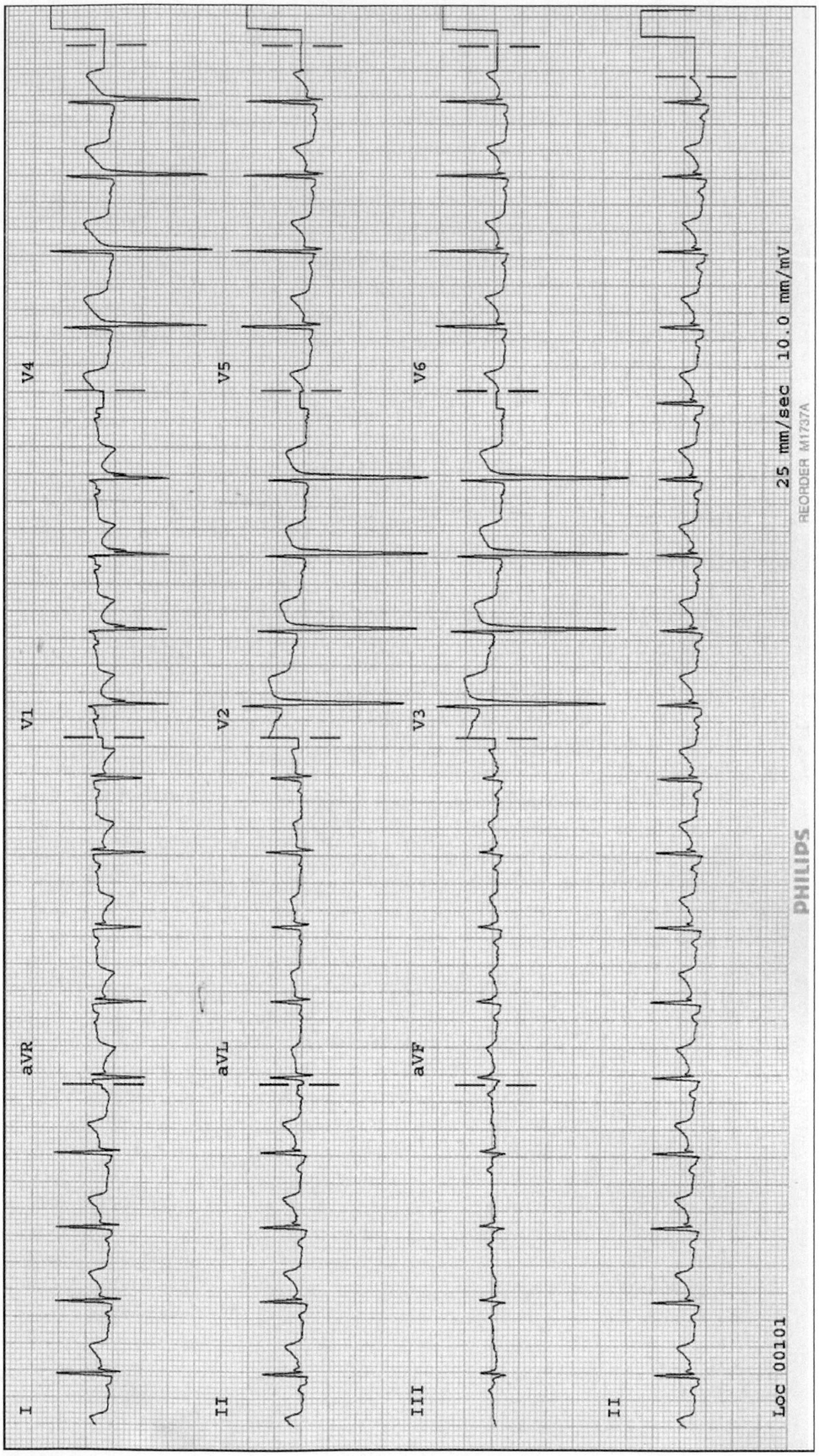
I
aVR
V1
V4
II
aVL
V2
V5
III
aVF
V3
V6
II
Loc 00101
25 mm/sec 10.0 mm/mV
REORDER M1737A

Figure 2–17

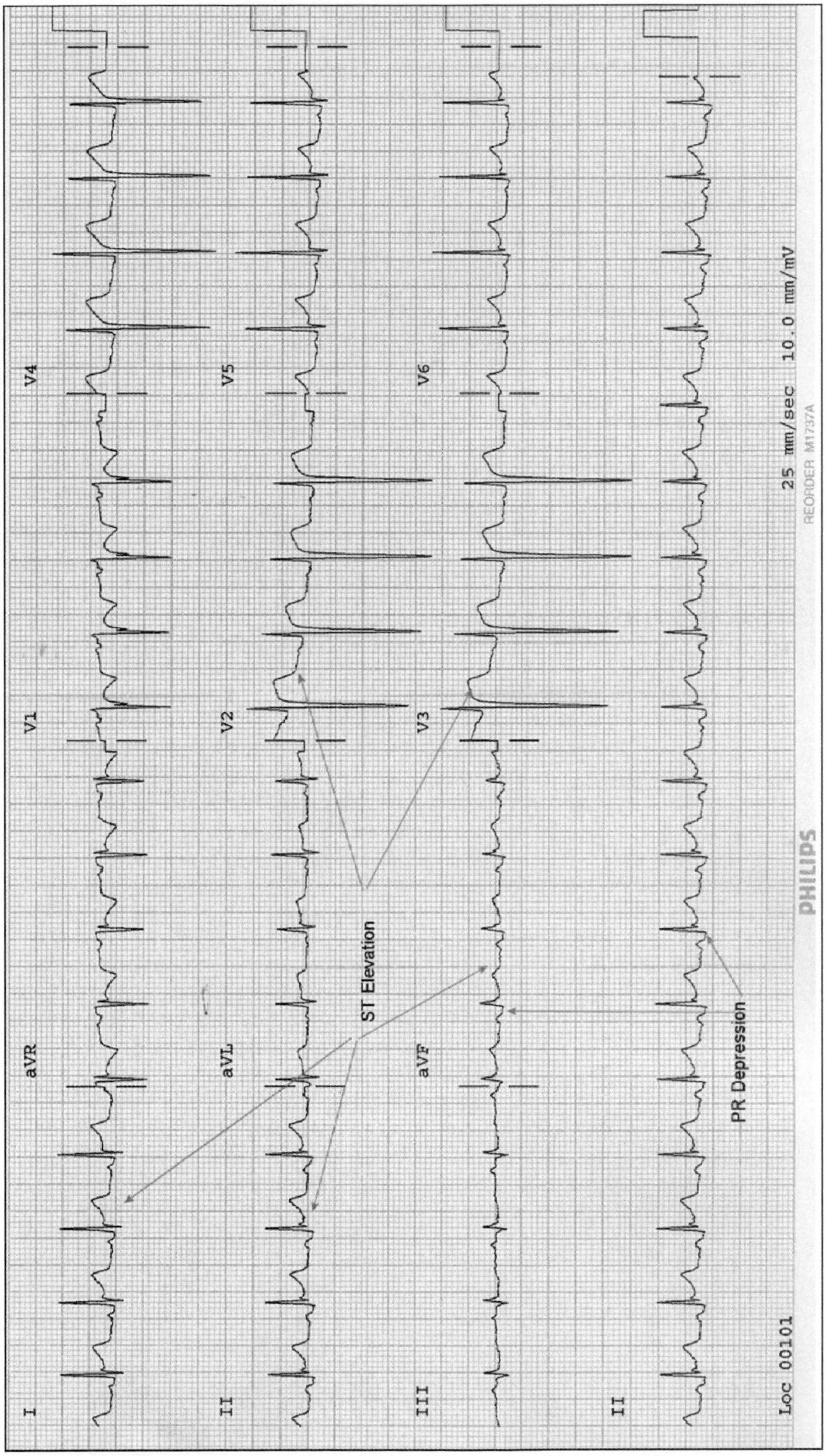

I
aVR
V1
V4
II
aVL
V2
V5
III
aVF
V3
V6
II
Loc 00101
ST Elevation
PR Depression
PHILIPS
25 mm/sec 10.0 mm/mV
REORDER M1737A

Figure 2–18

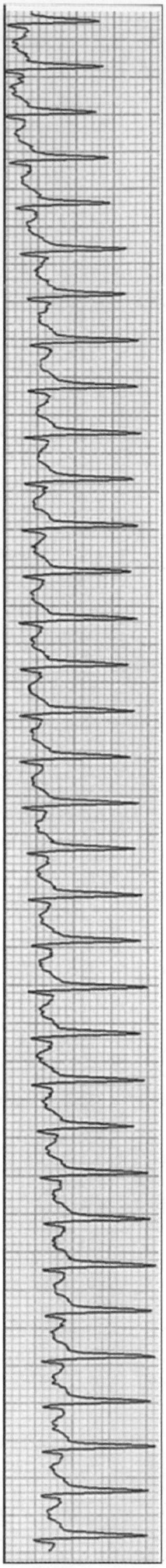

Figure 2–19

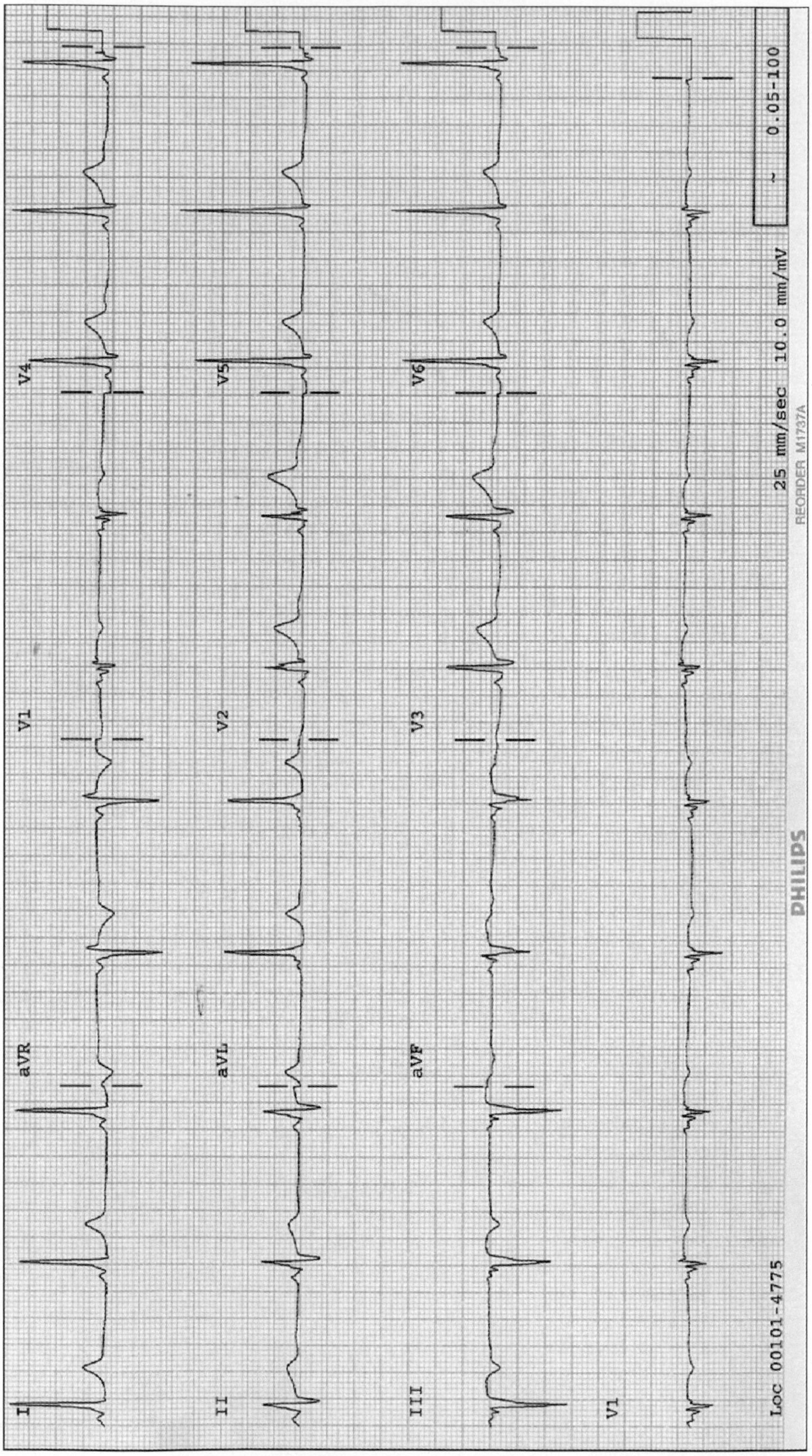

Figure 2–20

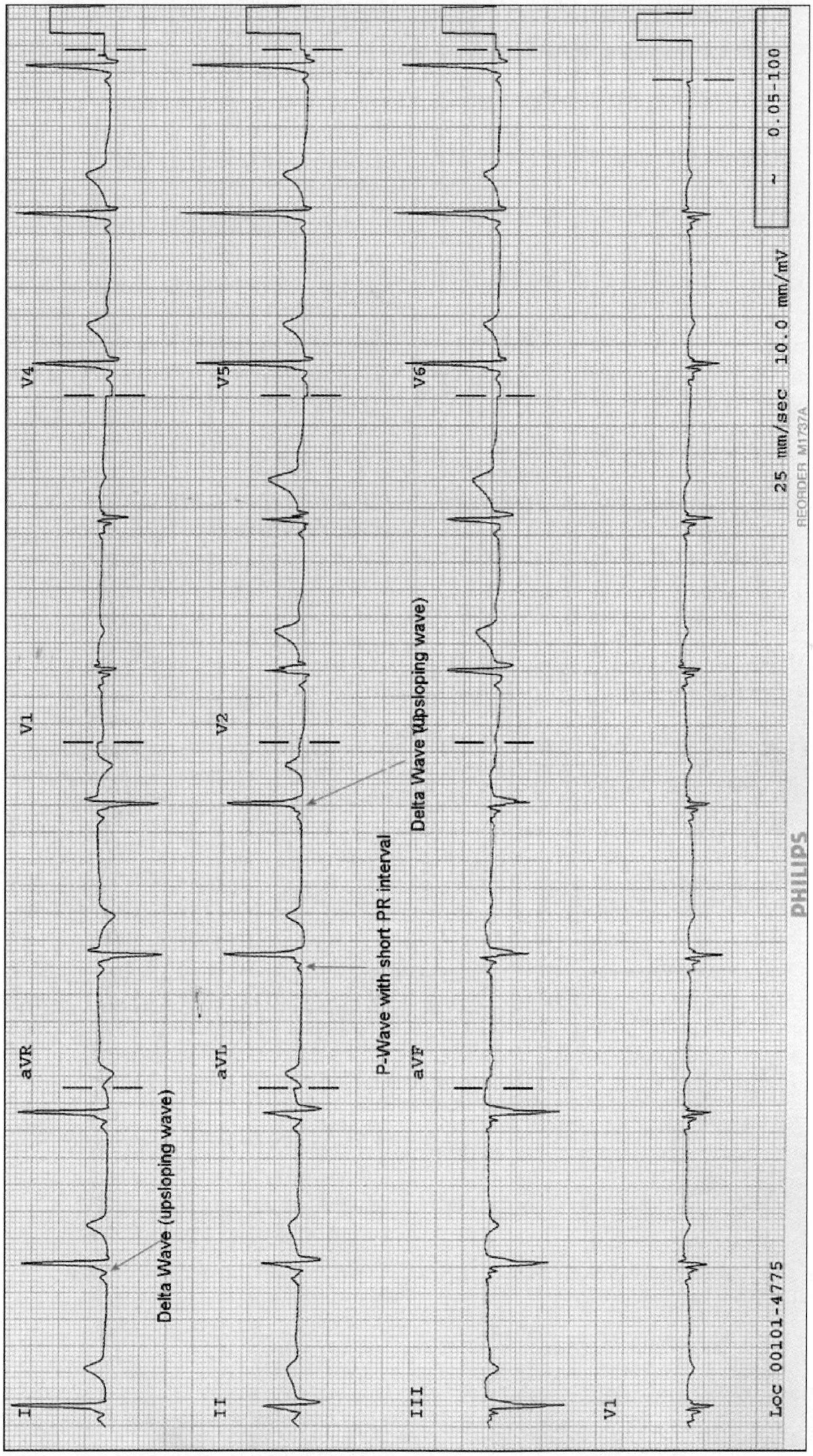
I
aVR
V1
V4
II
aVL
V2
V5
III
aVF
V6
V1
Delta Wave (upsloping wave)
P-Wave with short PR interval
Delta Wave (upsloping wave)
Loc 00101-4775
25 mm/sec 10.0 mm/mV
~ 0.05-100
REORDER M1737A
PHILIPS

Figure 2–21

medication. Which is the BEST medication choice for this patient in light of her diagnosis of WPW?

A) Procainamide.
B) Sotalol.
C) Diltiazem.
D) Verapamil.
E) Metoprolol.

Discussion

The correct answer choice is "A." Patients with WPW deteriorate with beta-blockers and calcium channel blockers (choices B–E). The drug of choice is procainamide in patients with WPW that presents with PSVT, including atrial fibrillation/flutter. The other alternative is ibutilide. The reason is that the AV node is protective since it helps block most reentrant conductions. If you block the AV node with beta-blockers or calcium channel blockers, the reentrant loop is allowed to go "wild" (Hey, maybe this can be a new reality show, "Rhythms Gone Wild"). The clues to look for to help identifying patients with WPW are a **young** patient with previous episodes of **palpitations**, rapid heart rate, or **syncope.**

The ECG shown in Figure 2–22 represents which of the following?

A) LBBB.
B) RBBB.
C) Left anterior fascicular block (LAFB).
D) Left posterior fascicular block.
E) None of the above.

Discussion

The correct answer is "C." For those of us who are visually challenged, any patient with a net negative force in lead II (i.e., left axis deviation) will have a LAFB. Also, look for net negative deflection in leads III and aVF. For those who like the numbers, LAFB is present when the QRS axis is -45° to -90°, there is an rS pattern (with small r waves) in leads II, III, and aVF and a qR pattern (with small q waves) in I and aVL. Because the QRS is narrow, neither LBBB nor RBBB can be correct. Left posterior block is quite uncommon due to the size of the posterior fascicle.

The ECG shown in Figure 2–23 represents which of the following?

A) LBBB.
B) RBBB.
C) Left anterior fascicular block.
D) Left posterior fascicular block.
E) None of the above.

Discussion

The correct answer is "A." This ECG represents an LBBB. Criteria include QRS width ≥ 0.12 ms, upright (monophasic) QRS in leads I and V6, and a mostly negative QRS in V1.

HELPFUL TIP: We don't suggest you to use this but... the R-R prime is on the **right** side of the ECG in an RBBB (V-1, 2, 3). The R-R prime is on the **left** side of the ECG in an LBBB (lead 1).

The ECG shown in Figure 2–24 represents which of the following?

A) First-degree block.
B) RBBB.
C) Left anterior fascicular block.
D) All of the above.
E) None of the above.

Discussion

The correct answer is "D." This ECG represents a first-degree AV block, an RBBB, and an LAFB. The RBBB is defined by a QRS width of ≥ 0.12 ms (>3 small blocks) and an rsR′ ("rabbit ears") in chest leads V1–V3. This patient also has an LAFB (see the ECG in Figure 2–22 for criteria).

CASE 19

A 75-year-old patient presents to your ED with the ECG shown in Figure 2–25.

What is the most likely electrolyte abnormality in this patient?

A) Hypokalemia.
B) Hyperkalemia.
C) Hyponatremia.
D) Hypermagnesemia.
E) Hypercalcemia.

Discussion

The correct answer is "B," hyperkalemia. Note the peaked T-waves across the precordium. Note also that the patient has early repolarization.

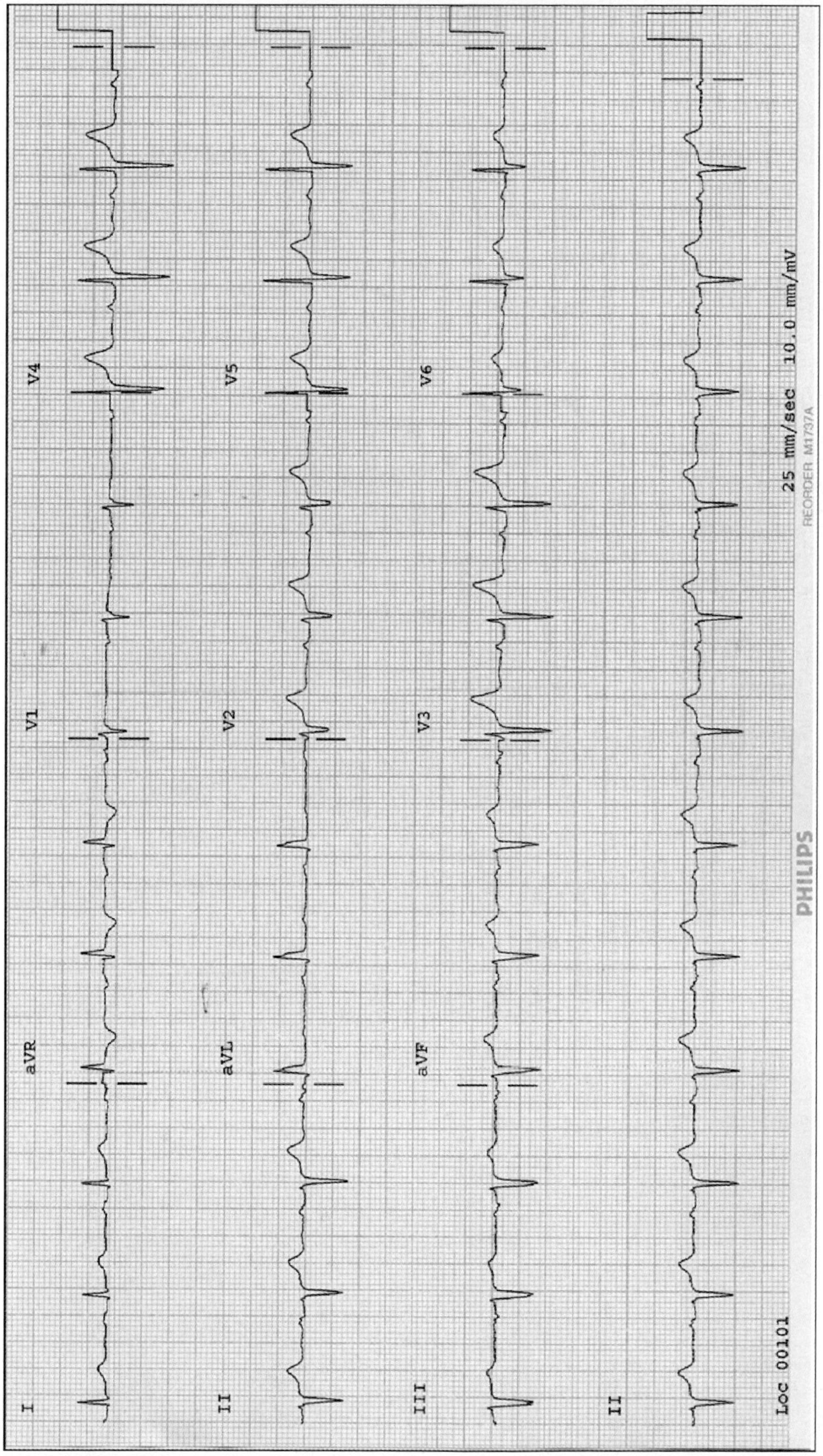
I
aVR
V1
V4
II
aVL
V2
V5
III
aVF
V3
V6
II
Loc 00101
25 mm/sec 10.0 mm/mV
PHILIPS

Figure 2–22

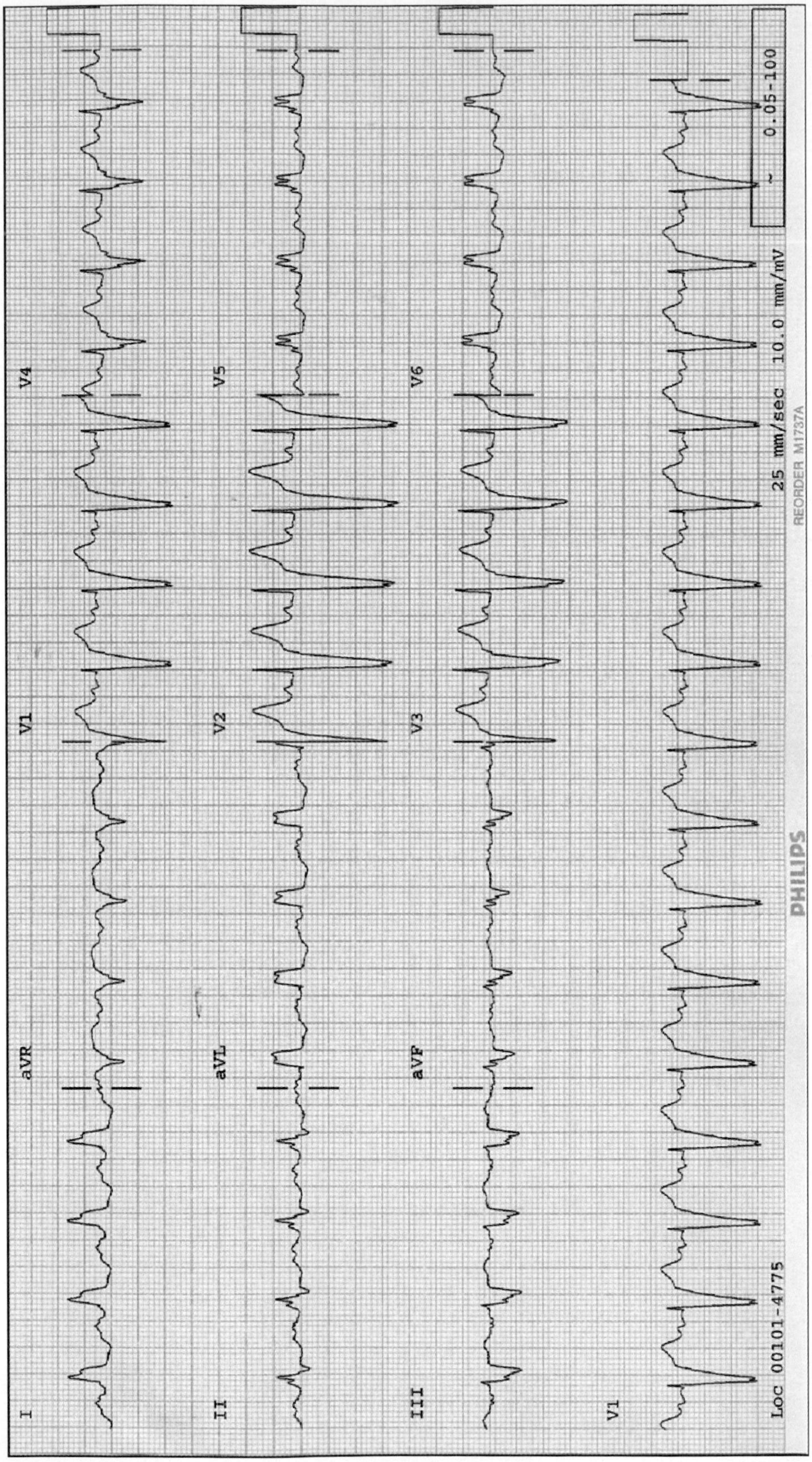

I
aVR
V1
V4
II
aVL
V2
V5
III
aVF
V3
V6
V1
Loc 00101-4775
PHILIPS
25 mm/sec 10.0 mm/mV
REORDER M1737A
~ 0.05-100

Figure 2–23

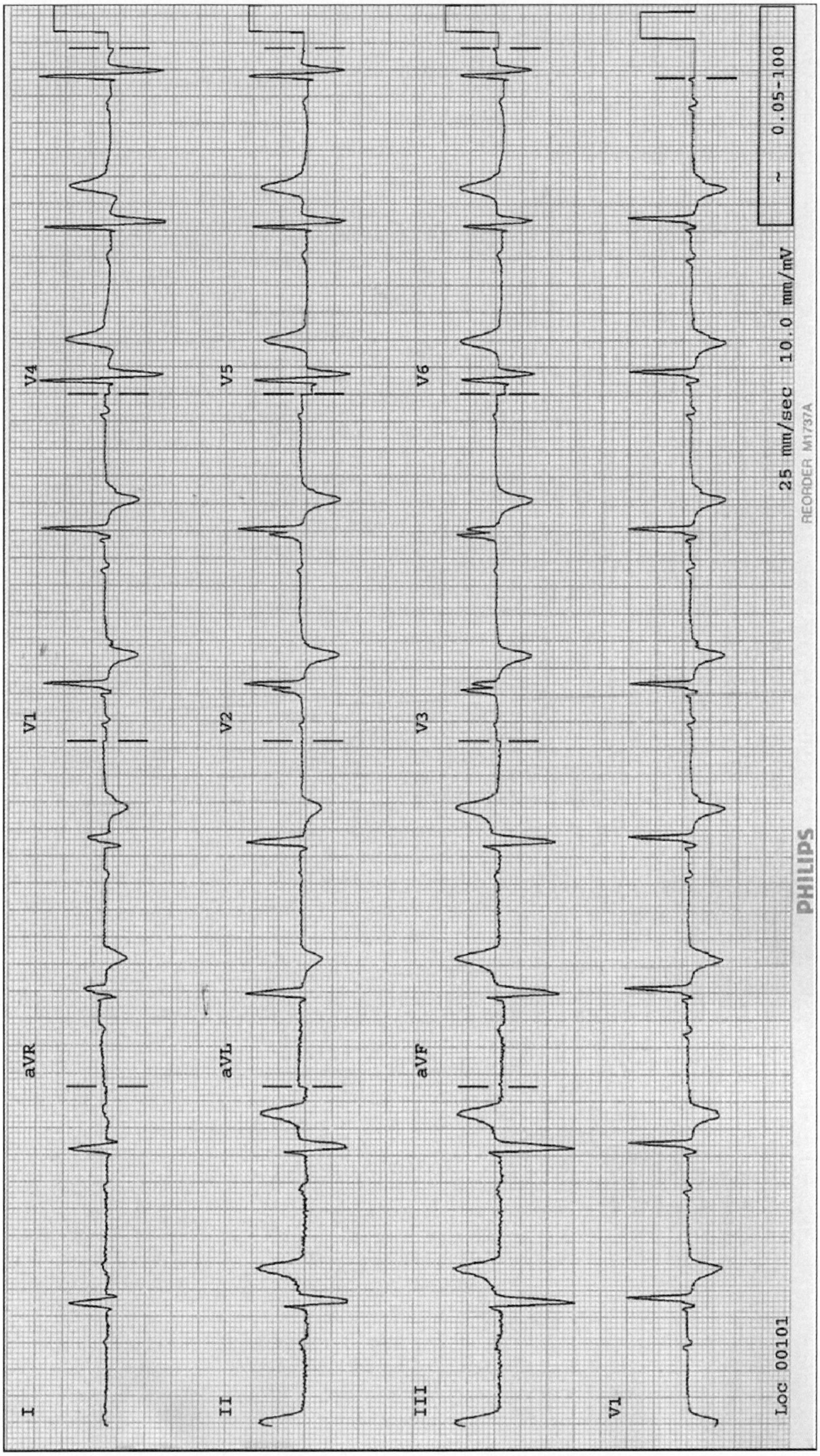
I
aVR
V1
V4
II
aVL
V2
V5
III
aVF
V3
V6
V1
Loc 00101
25 mm/sec 10.0 mm/mV
~ 0.05-100
REORDER M1737A

Figure 2–24

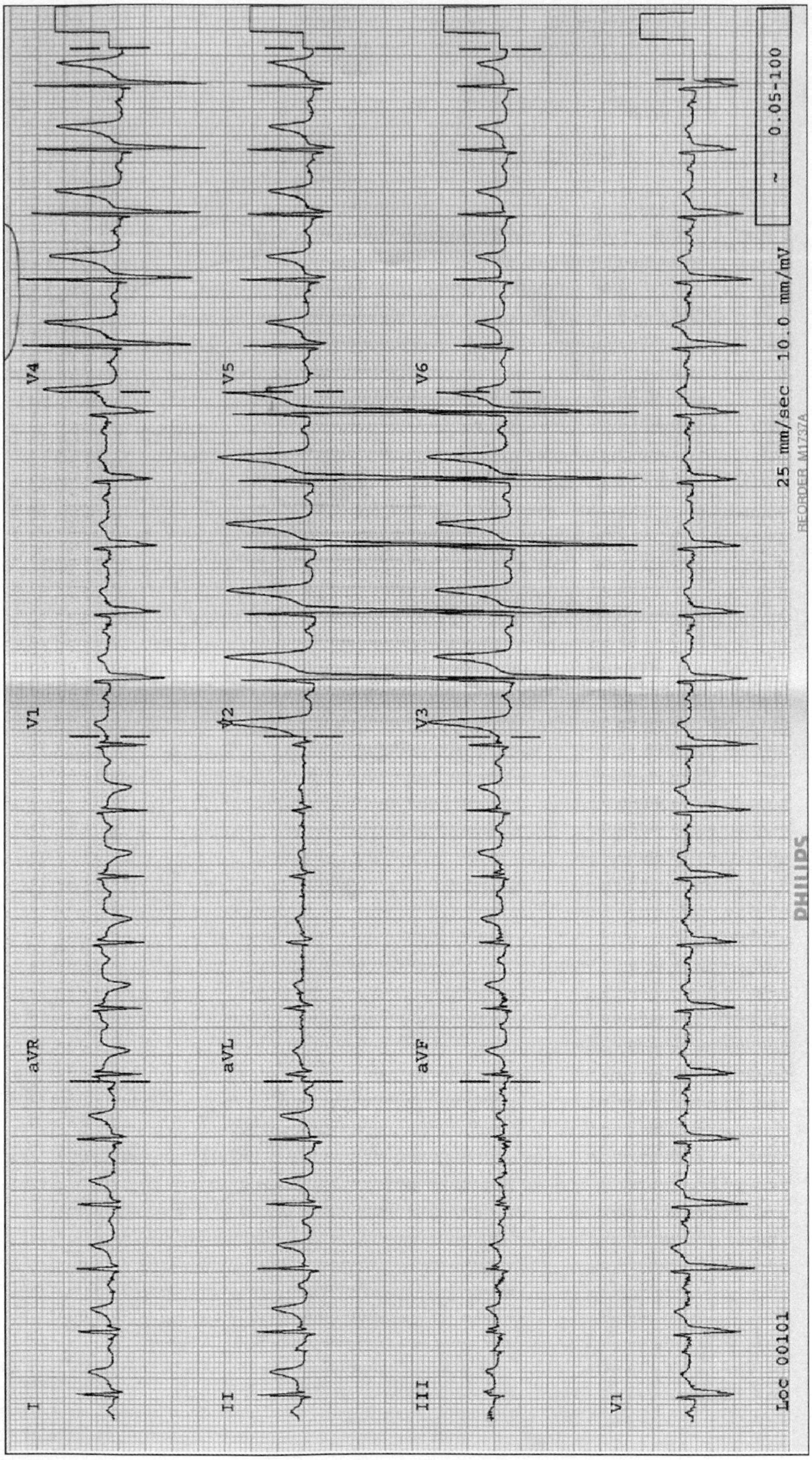
I
aVR
V1
V4
II
aVL
V2
V5
III
aVF
V3
V6
V1
Loc 00101
PHILIPS
25 mm/sec 10.0 mm/mV
REORDER M1737A
~ 0.05-100

Figure 2–25

All of the following are potential causes of this patient's hyperkalemia EXCEPT:

A) Metabolic acidosis.
B) ACE inhibitors.
C) ARBs.
D) Renal failure.
E) Furosemide.

Discussion

The correct answer is "E." Furosemide will cause hypokalemia rather than hyperkalemia. All the other answer choices are potential causes of hyperkalemia. Other causes of hyperkalemia include a potassium load from muscle breakdown (e.g., rhabdomyolysis, burns, transfusion of old blood) and other exogenous sources of potassium such as penicillin, potassium supplements, and water softeners. Consider also Addison disease and hypoaldosteronism. Digoxin toxicity is also a possibility.

What is the rhythm shown in Figure 2–26?

A) Atrial fibrillation.
B) Normal sinus rhythm with multiple PACs.
C) Third-degree heart block with rapid rate.
D) Multifocal atrial tachycardia.

Discussion

The correct answer is "D." This is a multifocal atrial tachycardia. Note the multiple morphologies of the P waves indicated by *arrows* in Figure 2–27. Here are helpful tips in diagnosing and treating multifocal atrial tachycardia: three or more different P-wave morphologies with varying PR intervals. Causes include theophylline, pulmonary disease, and abnormal electrolytes (K^+ or Mg^{2+}). Digoxin may worsen MAT!!! Just don't use it in this circumstance. AV nodal ablation with permanent pacing can be considered in refractory cases.

All of the following are treatments of multifocal atrial tachycardia EXCEPT:

A) Nondihydropyridine calcium channel blocker (verapamil, diltiazem).
B) Beta-blocker.
C) Magnesium.
D) Improving pulmonary function and reducing hypoxia.
E) Adenosine.

Discussion

The correct answer is "E." All of the others are indicated in the treatment of multifocal atrial tachycardia. Adenosine may slow down the rhythm temporarily but is not considered a treatment of this rhythm.

CASE 20

A 28-year-old woman with no significant past medical history presents to clinic with complaints of progressive shortness of breath; she becomes dyspneic with less activity than 1 year ago. If she exerts herself beyond a brisk walk, she becomes lightheaded, presyncopal, and feels tightness in her chest. She also notes generalized fatigue. Your examination discloses a heart rate of 105 bpm and normal blood pressure. Resting transcutaneous oximetry is 92% at rest. BMI is 24 kg/m^2. She has JVD but clear lungs. A grade 2/6 midsystolic murmur is heard over the left upper sternal border. Electrocardiogram is shown (Figure 2–28).

What is the most likely diagnosis?

A) CAD.
B) PHTN.
C) Asthma.
D) Congenital aortic stenosis.
E) Mitral valve prolapse.

Discussion

The correct answer is "B." The physical examination is consistent with right ventricular pressure overload. This is supported by the electrocardiogram demonstrating right atrial enlargement, right axis deviation, and right ventricular hypertrophy. CAD is almost unheard of in a woman younger than 30 years without any risk factors. Asthma may cause her symptom complex but is not supported by her examination. Aortic stenosis causes neither resting hypoxemia nor right ventricular hypertrophy.

* *

Note: Findings that suggest right ventricular hypertrophy on the ECG: right axis deviation, right atrial abnormality (P-wave >2.5 boxes tall in lead II), right ventricular hypertrophy (tall R in V1), and strain pattern in leads II and III. Often patients with pulmonary hypertension will have an intraventricular conduction delay with R-R′ in V1 (not shown on this cardiogram, Figure 2–29).

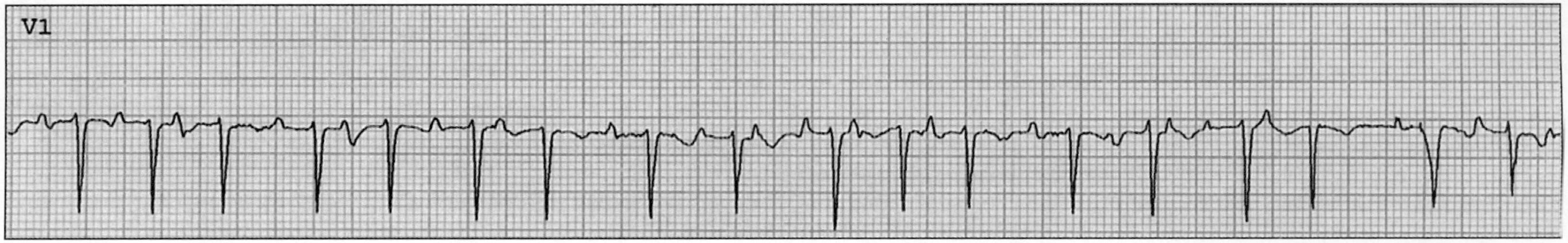

Figure 2–26

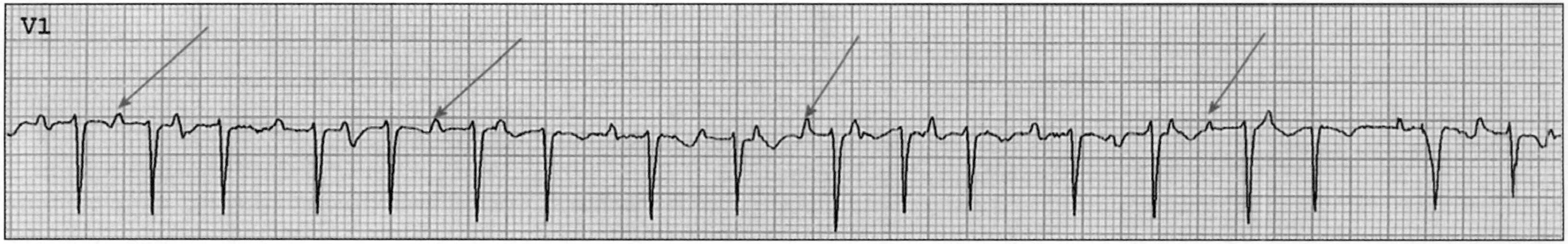

Figure 2–27

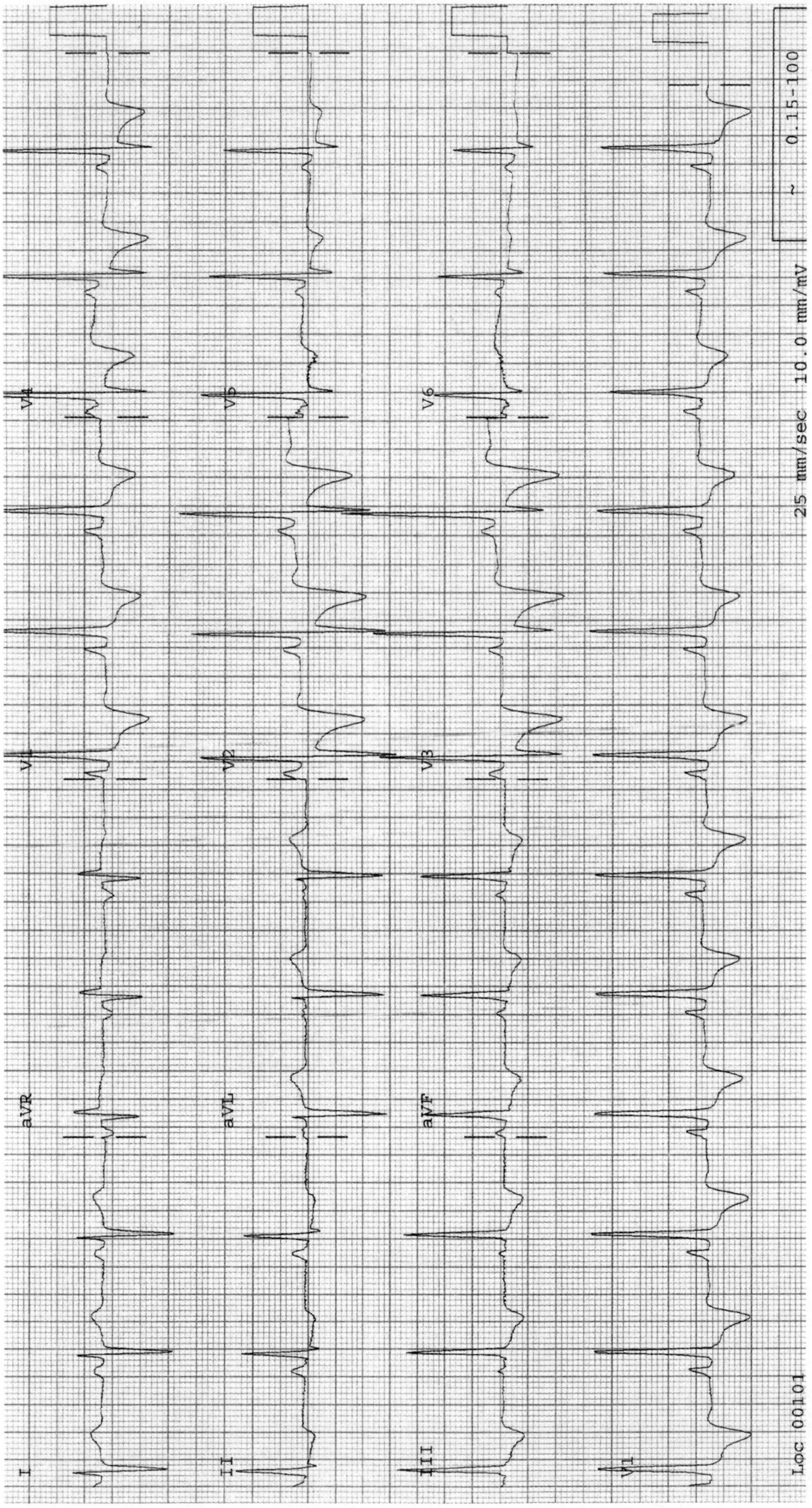
I
aVR
V1
V4
II
aVL
V2
V5
III
aVF
V3
V6
V1
Loc 00101
25 mm/sec 10.0 mm/mV
~ 0.15-100

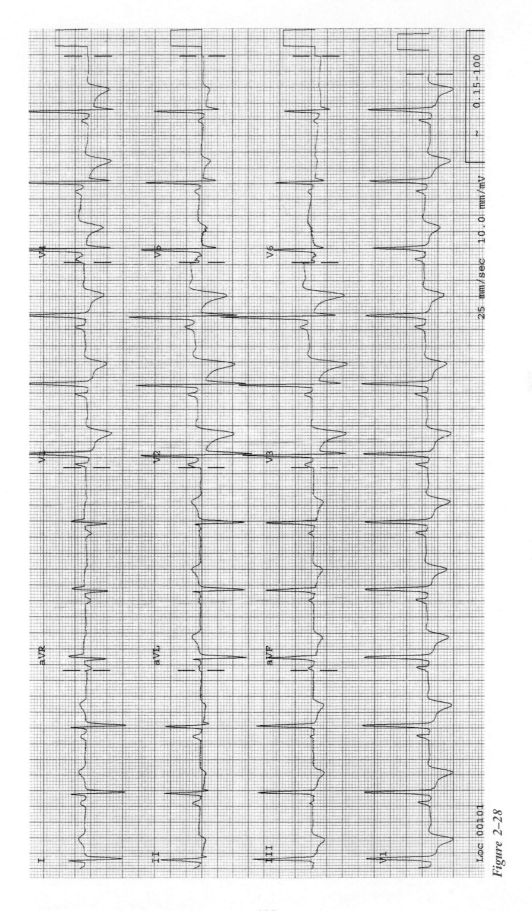

Figure 2–28

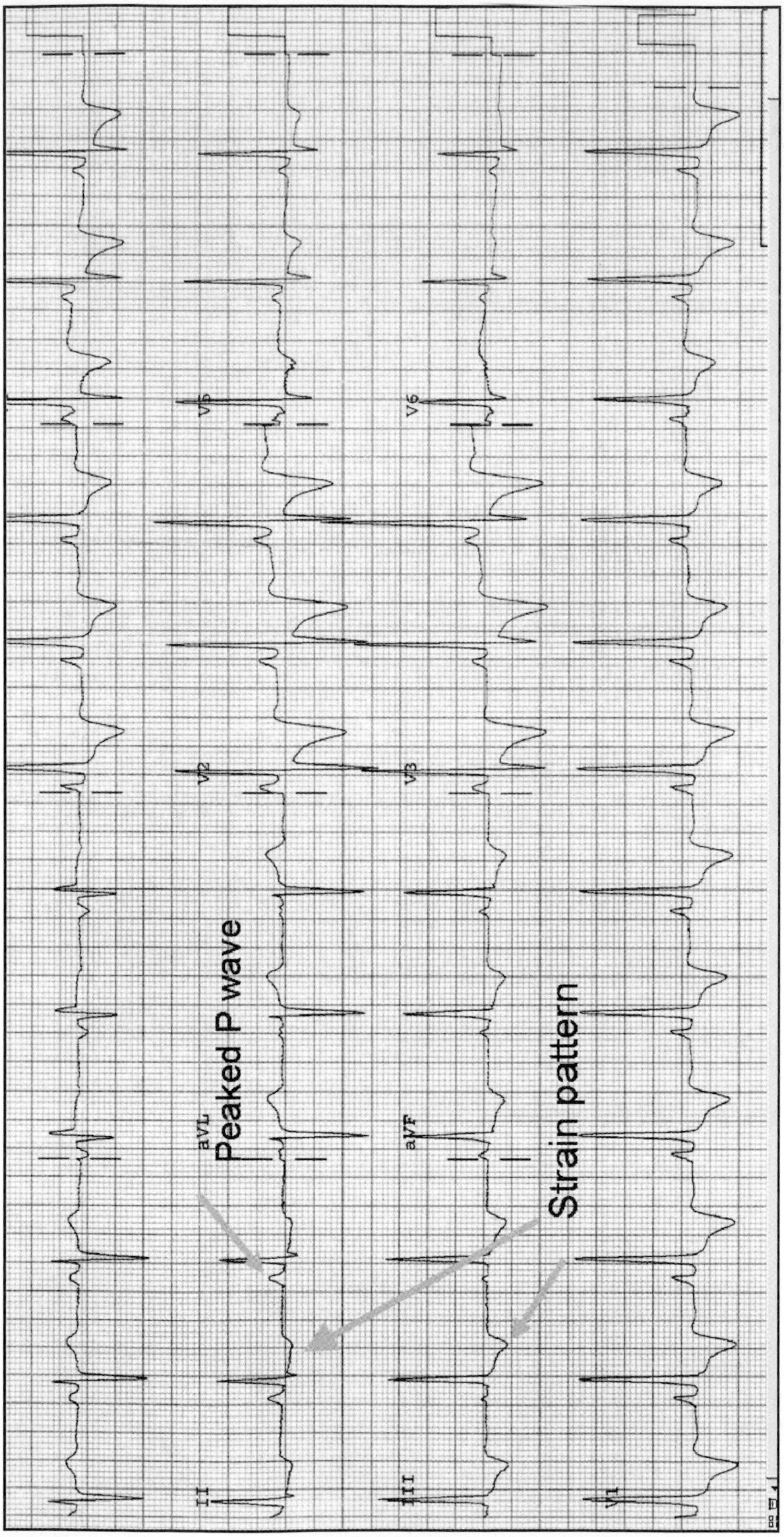

Figure 2–29

The following tests may be helpful in elucidating the cause of pulmonary hypertension EXCEPT:

A) Chest x-ray and pulmonary function studies.
B) CT scan.
C) ANA, HIV-1,2, and liver function studies.
D) Nasopharyngoscopy.
E) Polysomnogram.

Discussion

The correct answer is "D." An important part of the workup for pulmonary hypertension is defining the etiology and potentially reversible causes. There is no cook-book approach, and diagnostic workup should be tailored by the history and physical examination. Chest radiography and PFTs can identify chronic lung disease causing (or contributing to) pulmonary hypertension. A CT scan is done to exclude chronic thromboembolic pulmonary disease and to evaluate for fibrosis, sarcoid, etc. Connective tissue disease, HIV, and cirrhosis are known to cause pulmonary hypertension. Sleep apnea is an important, treatable cause of PHTN. Nasopharyngoscopy has no role in this workup.

* *

An echocardiogram confirms severe pulmonary hypertension and changes consistent with right ventricular pressure overload. No intracardiac shunt is identified. The remainder of her diagnostic workup fails to identify a secondary cause of pulmonary hypertension. A right heart catheterization confirms severe pulmonary hypertension but also fails to identify a shunt. A vasodilator challenge (with adenosine) is performed and no change in pulmonary pressure is elicited. She is given a diagnosis of idiopathic pulmonary arterial hypertension. The treatment of pulmonary hypertension is, in general, very specialized and a cardiologist should be involved. Exceptions include pulmonary hypertension from chronic hypoxia (smoking, sleep apnea) that are amenable to primary care management. Chronic PE can also be managed by the primary care practitioner.

> HELPFUL TIP: Additional therapy for pulmonary hypertension may include prostacyclin and phosphodiesterase inhibitors (e.g., sildenafil, tadalafil, vardenafil). Some patients require anticoagulation. Management is best done in conjunction with a specialist.

CASE 21

A 54 year old male presents to your clinic complaining of dyspnea and fevers. His temperature in the office is 38.5°C and heart rate is 113 bpm with pulse oximetry of 93%. On physical exam, you notice that he had nodules on his fingertips and notice a slight reddish discoloration under his fingernails. On further questioning, he tells you that he recently moved here from a major city and had used IV drugs in the past.

Your next step in management is:

A) Order a chest x-ray and start empiric levofloxacin.
B) Order a chest x-ray and start empiric ceftriaxone and azithromycin.
C) Order a chest x-ray, echocardiogram, draw blood cultures.
D) Order a chest x-ray and start empiric piperacillin and vancomycin (Zosyn).
E) Order a chest x-ray and do nothing, it is probably viral.

Discussion

The correct answer choice is "C." Although the chest x-ray is overkill for a case of endocarditis, overkill for a case of endocarditis, it may identify other causes of fever and help evaluate for CHF. The patient is presenting with IV drug use history, Osler nodes, and Janeway lesions (nail-bed hemorrhages), as well as fever. These easily meet three MINOR criteria—qualifying for a "possible diagnosis of endocarditis." Now what you need is one major criterion to definitively diagnose endocarditis. A positive echocardiogram or blood culture would qualify. Once the blood cultures are drawn, if your suspicion is high, you may start empiric antibiotics for endocarditis (Table 2–14).

Which valve(s) are most commonly affected by endocarditis?

A) Aortic valve.
B) Mitral valve.
C) Pulmonic valve.
D) Demonic valve.
E) A and B.

Discussion

The correct answer is "E." The aortic and mitral valves are most commonly affected. There is no demonic valve, we hope, but there is the tricuspid, of course.

Table 2–14 REVISED DUKE'S CRITERIA FOR ENDOCARDITIS (DEFINITIVE DIAGNOSIS: TWO MAJOR CRITERIA OR ONE MAJOR + THREE MINOR CRITERIA. POSSIBLE DIAGNOSIS: ONE MAJOR + ONE MINOR CRITERION OR THREE MINOR CRITERIA)

Major Criteria	Minor Criteria
Two positive blood cultures for organisms typical of endocarditis	Predisposing heart disorder
Three positive blood cultures for organisms consistent with endocarditis	IV drug abuse
Serologic evidence of *Coxiella burnetii*	Fever ≥38°C
Echocardiographic evidence of endocardial involvement:	Vascular phenomena: arterial embolism, septic pulmonary embolism, mycotic aneurysm, intracranial hemorrhage, conjunctival petechiae, or Janeway lesions
Oscillating intracardiac mass on a heart valve, on supporting structures, in the path of regurgitant jets, or on implanted material without another anatomic explanation; cardiac abscess; new dehiscence of prosthetic valve; or new valvular regurgitation	Immunologic phenomena: glomerulonephritis, Osler nodes, Roth spots, or rheumatoid factor
	Microbiologic evidence of infection consistent with but not meeting major criteria
	Serologic evidence of infection with organisms consistent with endocarditis

Which of the following organisms is most common in acute endocarditis?

A) *Staphylococcus aureus* and group B streptococci.
B) Alpha-hemolytic streptococci or enterococci.
C) Enterovirus.
D) Fungi.
E) *Elmo muppetl.*

Discussion

The correct answer is "A." Staph and group B strep are generally responsible for acute endocarditis while alpha-hemolytic streptococci and enterococci are more common with subacute endocarditis. Fungi may be present in IV drug abusers. As to *E. muppetl*, it is a new species recently described by us. We groveled it in Big Bird cultures.

Objectives: Did you learn to . . .

- Suspect pulmonary hypertension on the basis of history and physical?
- Order baseline studies for the evaluation of new onset pulmonary hypertension?
- Identify patients with PHTN appropriate for anticoagulation?
- How to identify and treat bacterial endocarditis?

BIBLIOGRAPHY

Adan V. Diagnosis and treatment of sick sinus syndrome. *Am Fam Physician*. 2003;67(8):1725.

Body R, et al. Do risk factors for chronic coronary heart disease help diagnose acute myocardial infarction in the emergency department. *Ann Emerg Med*. 2007;49: 145.

Bouknight DP. Current management of mitral valve prolapse. *Am Fam Physician*. 2000;61(11):3343.

Braunwald E, et al. Management of patients with unstable angina and non-ST-segment elevation myocardial infarction. *J Am Coll Cardiol*. 2002;40:1366.

Carabello BA, Crawford F. Valvular heart disease. *N Engl J Med*. 1997;337(1):32.

Catella-Lawson F, et al. Cyclooxygenase inhibitors and the antiplatelet effects of aspirin. *N Engl J Med*. 2001; 345(25):1809-1817.

Dahlof B, et al. Reversal of left ventricular hypertrophy in hypertensive patients. A metaanalysis of 109 treatment studies. *Am J Hypertens*. 1992;5(2):95-110.

Eagle KA, et al. Perioperative cardiac evaluation for noncardiac surgery update. 2002. Available at: www.acc.org/clinical/guidelines/perio/update/periupdate_index.htm.

Elkayam U. Pregnancy and cardiovascular disease. *Braunwald's Heart Disease: A Textbook of Cardiovascular Medicine*. Philadelphia, PA: Saunders, 2005.

Garty M, et al. Blood transfusion for acute decompensated heart failure–friend or foe? *Am Heart J*. 2009;158: 653-658.

Gibbons RJ, et al. Management of patients with chronic stable angina update. Available at: http://www.acc.org/clinical/guidelines/stable/update_index.htm.

Goyle KK. Diagnosing pericarditis. *Am Fam Physician*. 2002;66(9):1695.

Gregoratos G, et al. ACC/AHA/NASPE 2002 Guideline update for implantation of cardiac pacemakers and antiarrhythmia devices. Available at: www.acc.org/clinical/guidelines/pacemaker/incorporated/index.htm.

Harris GD. Heart disease in children. *Prim Care.* 2000; 27(3):767.

Hazinski MF, et al. *Handbook of Emergency Cardiovascular Care for Healthcare Providers.* Dallas, TX: American Heart Association; 2000.

Hebbar AK. Management of common arrhythmias: Part I. Supraventricular arrhythmias. *Am Fam Physician.* 2002; 65(12):2479.

Hebbar AK. Management of common arrhythmias: Part II. Ventricular arrhythmias in special populations. *Am Fam Physician.* 2002;65(12):2491.

Hirsh J, et al. American Heart Association/American College of Cardiology Foundation guide to warfarin therapy. *J Am Coll Cardiol.* 2003;41:1633.

Hunt SA, et al. Evaluation and management of heart failure. Available at: www.acc.org/clinical/guidelines/failure/hf_index.htm.

Koenig W, et al. C-reactive protein modulates risk prediction based on the Framingham score: implications for future risk assessment: Results from a large cohort study in southern Germany. *Circulation.* 2004;109(11): 1349-1353.

Laussen PC. Neonates with congenital heart disease. *Curr Opin Pediatr.* 2001;13(3):220.

McLaughlin VV, McGoon MD. Pulmonary arterial hypertension. *Circulation.* 2006;114:417-1431.

Moodie DS. Diagnosis and management of congenital heart disease in the adult. *Cardiol Rev.* 2001;9(5):276.

National Heart, Lung and Blood Institute. The Seventh Report of the Joint National Committee on Prevention, Detection, Evaluation, and Treatment of High Blood Pressure (JNC 7). Available at: www.nhlbi.nih.gov/guidelines/hypertension.

National Heart, Lung and Blood Institute. Third Report of the Expert Panel on Detection, Evaluation, and Treatment of High Blood Cholesterol in Adults (Adult Treatment Panel III). Available at: www.nhlbi.nih.gov/guidelines/cholesterol.

Patel AA, Budoff MJ. Screening for heart disease: C-reactive protein versus coronary artery calcium. *Expert Rev Cardiovasc Ther.* 2010;8(1):125-131.

Rector TS, et al. Evaluation by patients with heart failure of the effects of enalapril compared with hydralazine plus isosorbide dinitrate on quality of life. V-HeFT II. The V-HeFT VA Cooperative Studies Group. *Circulation.* 1993:87(6, Suppl):VI71-VI77.

Roden DM. Risks and benefits of antiarrhythmic therapy. *N Engl J Med.* 1994;331:785.

Ryan TJ, et al. ACC/AHA Guidelines for the management of patients with acute myocardial infarction. *Circulation.* 1999;100(9):1016.

Shammash JB. Perioperative assessment and perioperative management of the patient with nonischemic heart disease. *Med Clin North Am.* 2003;87(1):137.

Shipton B. Valvular heart disease: review and update. *Am Fam Physician.* 2001;63(11):2201.

Taylor AL, et al. Combination of isosorbide dinitrate and hydralazine in blacks with heart failure. *N Engl J Med.* 2004;351(20):2049-2057.

Van Gelder I, et al. A comparison of rate control and rhythm control in patients with recurrent persistent atrial fibrillation. *N Engl J Med.* 2002;347:1834-1840.

Wilson PW, et al. C-reactive protein and risk of cardiovascular disease in men and women from the Framingham Heart Study. *Arch Intern Med.* 2005;165(21): 2473-2478.

3 Pulmonary

Karol Z. Krements

CASE 1

A 42-year-old male who works in a hog confinement area presents to your office complaining of cough, fever, wheeze, and dyspnea. He and some other workers were cleaning the confinement area with high-pressure hoses (which aerosolized hog waste), and they *all* with the same symptoms, which started between 4 and 8 hours after work. On examination, he is febrile with a respiratory rate of 28. He is able to talk in complete sentences. There are slight crackles when you auscultate the lungs. His chest x-ray is normal.

The most likely diagnosis is:

A) "Farmer's lung" (hypersensitivity pneumonitis).
B) Organic dust toxicity syndrome.
C) Reactive airway disease.
D) Hydrogen sulfide poisoning.
E) Bronchiolitis obliterans.

Discussion

The correct answer is "B." Organic dust toxicity syndrome (ODTS) occurs when moldy or decomposed hay and other organic material (such as hog manure) is moved. Endotoxins are aerosolized and inhaled, leading to the symptoms. The tip off here is that everyone on the job site was affected. Since hypersensitivity pneumonitis ("A") is specific to the individual, generally only one worker at the site will have symptoms. Compared with ODTS, these patients may have an abnormal chest x-ray with micronodular or reticular opacities. "C" is incorrect because everyone is involved and febrile which is not consistent with reactive airway disease. "D" is not correct. Hydrogen sulfide poisoning presents as a toxic pneumonitis with pulmonary edema, dyspnea, hypoxia, and loss of consciousness. Hydrogen sulfide also acts as a direct cellular toxin that binds to cytochrome oxidase system, similar to cyanide. Additionally, hydrogen sulfide exposure comes when cleaning manure pits (as anyone in Iowa would know). Finally, "E," bronchiolitis obliterans, is a chronic illness rather than an acute one.

* *

Of note, a strong association between ODTS and development of chronic bronchitis has been identified.

Appropriate treatment for this patient includes:

A) Antibiotics.
B) Intubation and mechanical ventilation
C) Supportive care.
D) A and B.
E) A and C.

Discussion

The correct answer is "C." Supportive care is the usual treatment of ODTS. Antibiotics are not needed because the syndrome is mediated by endotoxins rather than direct infection. "B" is incorrect because this patient is not in significant respiratory distress.

HELPFUL TIP: Remember that other work exposures can cause fever, including "metal fume fever" caused by zinc (febrile by end of the week, resolves on the weekend only to recure on Wednesday or so), Teflon by-products, contaminated humidifier water, etc.

CASE 2

This patient's brother, who also works on a farm, notes that every time he unloads hay he has fever, cough, dyspnea, and sputum production. It tends to resolve in 2–5 days but reoccurs when he is reexposed to hay. None of the other workers on the farm are affected, and they are beginning to wonder if he is malingering. His exam reveals tachypnea and fine rales. There is no wheezing present. A chest radiograph shows bilateral interstitial opacities.

The most likely cause of this patient's symptoms is:

A) *Thermoactinomyces candidus* (an actinomyces species).
B) *T. sacchari.*
C) *Botrytis cinerea.*
D) *Cryptostroma corticale.*
E) None of the above.

Discussion
The correct answer is "A." This patient presents with classic symptoms of hypersensitivity pneumonitis or, in this case, "Farmer's lung." This is caused by exposure to the *Actinomyces* species. Acute findings include fever, chills, cough, dyspnea, and chest tightness. Occasionally, the radiograph is normal. High-resolution chest CT should then be obtained, which commonly show centrilobular micronodules and ground-glass opacification. "B," *T. sacchari*, is involved in hypersensitivity pneumonitis from sugarcane (so-called Bagassosis). "C," *Botrytis cinerea*, is involved in hypersensitivity pneumonitis from grapes (so-called Spatlese lung). Finally, "D," *Cryptostroma*, is involved in "Maple bark stripper's lung," another type of hypersensitivity pneumonitis.

The correct treatment for this patient with Farmer's lung includes:

A) Antibiotics.
B) Inhaled steroids.
C) Oral steroids.
D) Leukotriene inhibitors.
E) Bronchoalveolar lavage (BAL).

Discussion
The correct answer is "C." Oral steroids are effective in the treatment of hypersensitivity pneumonitis. However, neither antibiotics ("A") nor inhaled steroids ("B") are of any benefit. "E," bronchoalveolar lavage, is not a treatment. However, it can be used as a diagnostic tool. One would expect to see lymphocytes on BAL.

You would advise this patient to:

A) Get a new job.
B) Apply for disability.
C) Use a respirator at work and avoid exposure to this toxin if possible.
D) Sue the employer.
E) Take up worm farming or monoculture in rhubarb.

Discussion
The correct answer is "C." Wearing an appropriate respirator at work can be beneficial. Avoiding exposure is even better. As for the other answers, you are a doctor not a lawyer or career counselor. Stick with what you know!

* *

The patient is unable to change jobs or wear a respirator because it itches and he "keeps forgetting it." But he's persistent (or brave or thickheaded or unable to learn a new skill), and keeps farming. Three years later, he returns with a chronic cough, weight loss, dyspnea, fatigue, and clubbing of the fingers.

Further evaluation will most likely reveal:

A) Bronchogenic carcinoma.
B) Air space disease (e.g., a pneumonia-like picture).
C) Decreased carbon monoxide diffusing capacity (decreased DLCO).
D) Markedly abnormal BAL with lymphocytosis.
E) Obstructive changes on pulmonary function testing.

Discussion
The correct answer is "C." Hypersensitivity pneumonitis can become chronic if exposure is not limited. In these cases, patients will generally have systemic complaints such as fatigue and possibly weight loss; fever will be absent. Dyspnea and clubbing of the fingers are also generally noted, reflecting chronic pulmonary disease. Along with this finding, pulmonary fibrosis can occur and the DLCO may be decreased. "A" is incorrect. Hypersensitivity pneumonitis does not lead to lung cancer. "B" is incorrect. While acute hypersensitivity pneumonitis causes an alveolitis, chronic hypersensitivity pneumonitis causes

pulmonary fibrosis with an occasional micronodular pattern. "D" is incorrect. BAL in chronic hypersensitivity pneumonitis does not contain the markedly elevated lymphocyte count that is seen with *acute* hypersensitivity pneumonitis. Finally, "E" is incorrect. One would see a restrictive pattern on pulmonary function testing reflecting the fibrosis and not an obstructive pattern.

HELPFUL TIP: If you have a patient with recurrent "pneumonia," consider hypersensitivity pneumonitis. It has many causes in addition to farming, and it is idiopathic up to 25% of cases.

Objectives: Did you learn to . . .

- Recognize the clinical presentations of ODTS and hypersensitivity pneumonitis?
- Manage patients with lung disease related to agricultural exposures?

QUICK QUIZ: ASTHMA

All of the following populations are at increased risk for developing asthma EXCEPT:

A) Obese children.
B) Female children.
C) Children exposed to tobacco.
D) Children with atopy.
E) City children.

Discussion

The correct answer is "B." Male children have a greater prevalence of asthma. Interestingly, adult women "catch up" so that there is gender equity in young adulthood, and after age 40, the prevalence is higher in females. Of note, frequent respiratory infections seem to be *protective*. There is an inverse association between children living on farms and asthma incidence (another feather in the cap of Iowa) (Ege et al., 2011). Presumably, this is related to the greater variety of antigen exposure.

CASE 3

A 20-year-old woman with no significant past medical history presents with a 2-month history of episodic shortness of breath. These symptoms began with an upper respiratory tract infection. She has fits of coughing and trouble catching her breath with exertion. She states that her breath "sounds like whistles" at times. She tried a friend's albuterol inhaler with some improvement and wonders if she has asthma. On exam, she is breathing comfortably at 16 times per minute and her oxygen saturation is 96% on room air. Her lungs are clear to auscultation, and the remainder of her exam is unremarkable. You want to better categorize this patient's disease.

Which of the following tests is most appropriate to order now?

A) Spirometry.
B) Chest x-ray.
C) Arterial blood gas (ABG).
D) Methacholine challenge.
E) Chest CT.

Discussion

The correct answer is "A." Since this patient has symptoms of bronchospasm, spirometry will be essential in determining if there is objective evidence of obstructive lung disease. However, spirometry results are often normal in mild cases of asthma, especially when the patient is asymptomatic. Bronchoprovocation testing, with methacholine or histamine, may be useful in such cases, but should follow basic spirometry. Although chest radiography (x-ray or CT) may reveal an unsuspected process, it is not indicated in otherwise healthy patients with symptoms of bronchospasm. Bacterial pneumonia is a potential precipitant of bronchospasm that may be diagnosed on chest x-ray, but this patient has no constitutional symptoms (like fever) associated with serious bacterial infection. ABG levels may be helpful when a patient presents with respiratory distress but certainly not in the office setting.

HELPFUL TIP: A normal blood gas in a patient with an asthma exacerbation and tachypnea is an ominous sign that signals impending respiratory failure. The carbon dioxide ($PaCO_2$) should be low in a patient with tachypnea. Thus, a normal appearing ABG with a normal carbon dioxide level is an indication of respiratory muscle fatigue and early respiratory failure.

If this patient has mild asthma, which of the following pulmonary function test results would you expect to find?

A) Forced vital capacity (FVC) 50% of predicted.
B) Forced expiratory volume in 1 second (FEV_1) 100% of predicted.
C) FEV_1/FVC ratio <0.7.
D) Total lung capacity (TLC) 50% of predicted.
E) FEV_1/TLC <0.7.

Discussion

The correct answer is "C." Patients with asthma will have a decreased FEV_1. The FVC may fall as well, but FEV_1 falls first and to a greater degree as the lung becomes obstructed. The ratio of FEV_1/FVC is very sensitive to airflow limitations, and FEV_1/FVC <0.7 (not predicted, just the ratio of the two numbers) is generally considered diagnostic of obstructive airway disease. The rest are incorrect. TLC is not measured by spirometry (which is why "E" is incorrect).

Your patient's office spirometry shows the following:

Normal FVC.
FEV_1 82% predicted.
FEV_1/FVC 0.68.

These findings are most consistent with which of the following?

A) Normal spirometry.
B) Obstructive lung disease.
C) End-stage emphysema.
D) Interstitial fibrosis.

Discussion

The correct answer is "B." Always go first to the FEV_1/FVC ratio. In this case, it is <0.70, which is suggestive of airway obstruction. The information provided here lacks data regarding reversibility, so you could not really differentiate between chronic obstructive pulmonary disease (COPD) and asthma. But this is clearly not end-stage emphysema, so "C" is incorrect. "D" is incorrect. Interstitial fibrosis is generally marked by a restrictive pattern on spirometry and decreased TLC. Both flow rate (e.g., FEV_1) and FVC are decreased in interstitial lung diseases but in proportion to each other. Thus, the FEV_1/FVC is often normal or elevated. See Table 3–1 for more on interpreting spirometry results.

* *

Six months after you discuss her findings and prescribe inhaled beta-agonist therapy, she returns with complaints of continued wheezing and difficulty breathing. Her symptoms are brought on by cold weather and exercise and she uses her inhaler two times per week. She woke up two nights over the last 6 months with shortness of breath and coughing. Her albuterol still works for these symptoms, but she finds them bothersome and asks, "Why haven't I gotten over this?"

How would you categorize this patient's respiratory state?

A) Intermittent asthma.
B) Mild persistent asthma.
C) Moderate persistent asthma.

Table 3–1 GENERAL INTERPRETATION OF PULMONARY FUNCTION TESTS RESULTS COMPARING OBSTRUCTIVE AND RESTRICTIVE DISEASE (MAY NOT BE APPLICABLE FOR ALL FORMS OF LUNG DISEASE)

PFT Result	Obstructive Pattern	Restrictive Pattern
FEV_1	<80% predicted	Decreased in proportion to loss of lung volume
FVC	Decreased	<80% predicted
FEV_1/FVC	<0.7	>0.7
FEF_{25-75}	<60% predicted	Decreased in proportion to loss of lung volume
TLC	Normal or elevated	Decreased
DLCO	Normal or elevated in asthma; normal or decreased in COPD	Decreased in intrinsic restrictive lung disease; normal in neuromuscular or musculoskeletal restrictive disease

FEV_1, forced expiratory volume in 1 second; FVC, forced vital capacity; FEF_{25-75}, forced expiratory flow at 25–75% vital capacity; TLC, total lung capacity; DLCO, diffusing capacity of the lung for carbon monoxide; COPD, chronic obstructive pulmonary disease.

Table 3–2 CATEGORIZATION OF SEVERITY OF ASTHMA AND STEPWISE APPROACH TO THERAPY

Determine Severity When Initiating Therapy

	Components of Severity	Classification of Asthma Severity (≥12 years of age)			
		Intermittent	Persistent		
			Mild	Moderate	Severe
Impairment (Normal FEV_1/FVC*)	Symptoms	≤2 days/week	>2 days/week but not daily	Daily	Throughout the day
	Nighttime awakenings	≤2×/month	3–4×/month	>1×/week but not nightly	Often 7×/week
	SABA[†] use for symptom control (not prevention of EIB[‡])	≤2 days/week	>2 days/week but not daily and more than 1× on any day	Daily	Several times per day
	Interference with normal activity	None	Minor limitation	Some limitation	Extremely limited
	Lung function	• Normal EFV_1 between exacerbations • EFV_1 > 80% predicted • EFV_1/FVC normal	• EFV_1 > 80% predicted • EFV_1/FVC normal	• EFV_1 > 60% but <80% predicted • EFV_1/FVC reduced 5%	• EFV_1 < 60% predicted • EFV_1/FVC reduced > 5%
Risk	Exacerbations requiring oral systemic corticosteroids	0–1/year	≥2/year →		
		Consider severity and interval since last exacerbation. Frequency and severity may fluctuate over time for patients in any severity category. Relative annual risk of exacerbations may be related to FEV_1			
	Recommended step for initiating therapy. See bar chart in Figure 3–1 for treatment steps	Step 1	Step 2	Step 3 and consider short course of oral systemic corticosteroids	Step 4 or 5 and consider short course of oral systemic corticosteroids
		In 2–6 weeks, evaluate level of asthma control that is achieved and adjust therapy accordingly.			

*Short-acting inhaled beta$_2$-agonist; †Inhaled corticosteroid; ‡Leukotriene receptor antagonist.

Reproduced from: Guidelines for the Diagnosis and Management of Asthma. National Asthma Education and Prevention Program, National Institutes of Health. Expert Panel Report 3, pages 305–310, 343–345. http://www.nhlbi.nih.gov/guidelines/asthma.

D) Severe persistent asthma.
E) Recurrent lower respiratory tract infections.

Discussion

The correct answer is "A." According to the National Asthma Education and Prevention Program (2007 NHLBI/NAEPP guidelines; Table 3–2), your patient meets the criteria for intermittent asthma. In such patients, mild symptoms correspond to an FEV_1 (not an FEV_1/FVC ratio) that is greater than 80% predicted.

Which of the following is most appropriate for this patient given that she has intermittent asthma?

A) Add theophylline.
B) Add montelukast.
C) Continue albuterol as needed.
D) Schedule albuterol every 4 hours.
E) Prednisone 5 mg daily.

Discussion

The correct answer is "C." As already discussed, this patient appears to have intermittent asthma. She is in no respiratory distress, is oxygenating normally, and is still responding well to albuterol by her report. Although there is some debate about the role of inhaled steroids in intermittent asthma, the NAEPP and most experts do not recommend their use. Oral prednisone is certainly not indicated in this case. She should be continued on a short-acting inhaled beta-2 agonist, such as albuterol, without the addition of another medication. "D" is incorrect. Scheduled albuterol actually yields *less effective* symptom control than does PRN use.

* *

Your patient goes on to develop more frequent recurrent symptoms, such that she is using her albuterol inhaler more than three times per week, although her nighttime symptoms are rare.

Which medication is the most appropriate next step in treating this patient's asthma?

A) Inhaled triamcinolone.
B) Inhaled salmeterol.
C) Inhaled cromolyn sodium.

D) Inhaled ipratropium.
E) Oral montelukast.

Discussion

The correct answer is "A." Your patient now has mild persistent asthma and should be started on an inhaled steroid. When asthma symptoms become more persistent (i.e., when they occur >2 days per week or the patient awakens from sleep >2 times per month), the inflammatory component of the disease should be addressed while simultaneously treating the bronchospastic component with a short-acting beta-2 agonists. Anti-inflammatory drugs are the mainstay of chronic asthma therapy, and inhaled corticosteroids are the most efficacious with the fewest side effects. Although ipratropium, cromolyn sodium, and montelukast have a place in asthma treatment, none of these medications is a first-line agent. Ipratropium works through its bronchodilatory effects, while cromolyn sodium is a mast cell stabilizer. Montelukast is a leukotriene inhibitor. The long-acting inhaled beta-2 agonists, such as salmeterol, are only recommended at Steps 3 and higher of persistent asthma control (Table 3–2, Figure 3–1; NHLBI recommendations, 2007).

HELPFUL TIP: Remember the "rule of twos": any patient who has >2 asthma exacerbations per week requiring rescue medication or who wakes with nocturnal symptoms >2 times per month should be on an anti-inflammatory drug, preferably an inhaled corticosteroid. Asthma classification and treatment has gotten ridiculously complex at 74 pages in length (and this is the summary version!). See http://www.nhlbi.nih.gov/guidelines/asthma/asthsumm.htm for a summary of current diagnosis and treatment recommendations including younger children.

HELPFUL TIP: The leukotriene inhibitors (e.g., montelukast, zafirlukast) add little or nothing to maximize inhaled steroid therapy. In fact, they are clearly not as effective as inhaled steroids. They should be used only once a patient has failed inhaled steroids and should be added to the regimen; they are not a substitute for inhaled steroids.

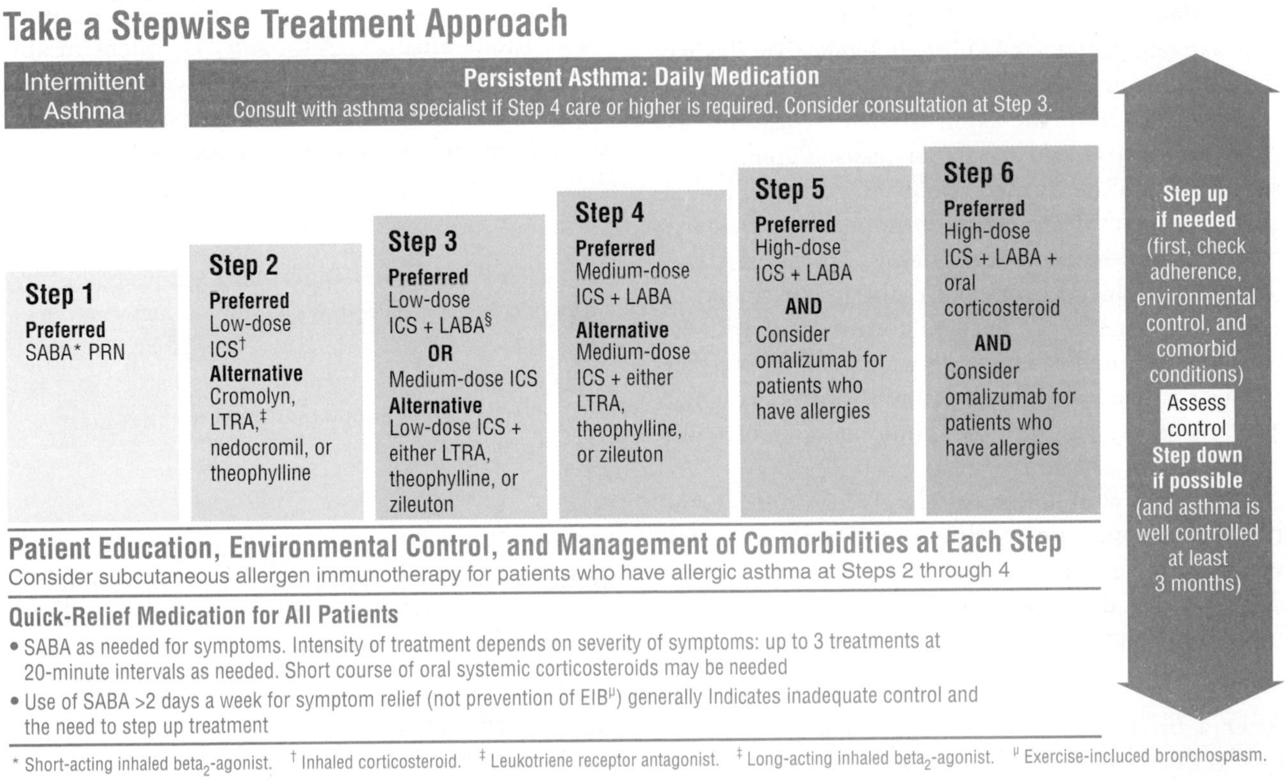

Take a Stepwise Treatment Approach
Intermittent Asthma
Persistent Asthma: Daily Medication
Consult with asthma specialist if Step 4 care or higher is required. Consider consultation at Step 3.
Step 1
Preferred
SABA* PRN
Step 2
Preferred
Low-dose ICS†
Alternative
Cromolyn, LTRA,‡ nedocromil, or theophylline
Step 3
Preferred
Low-dose ICS + LABA§
OR
Medium-dose ICS
Alternative
Low-dose ICS + either LTRA, theophylline, or zileuton
Step 4
Preferred
Medium-dose ICS + LABA
Alternative
Medium-dose ICS + either LTRA, theophylline, or zileuton
Step 5
Preferred
High-dose ICS + LABA
AND
Consider omalizumab for patients who have allergies
Step 6
Preferred
High-dose ICS + LABA + oral corticosteroid
AND
Consider omalizumab for patients who have allergies
Step up if needed (first, check adherence, environmental control, and comorbid conditions)
Assess control
Step down if possible (and asthma is well controlled at least 3 months)
Patient Education, Environmental Control, and Management of Comorbidities at Each Step
Consider subcutaneous allergen immunotherapy for patients who have allergic asthma at Steps 2 through 4
Quick-Relief Medication for All Patients
• SABA as needed for symptoms. Intensity of treatment depends on severity of symptoms: up to 3 treatments at 20-minute intervals as needed. Short course of oral systemic corticosteroids may be needed
• Use of SABA >2 days a week for symptom relief (not prevention of EIB‖) generally Indicates inadequate control and the need to step up treatment
* Short-acting inhaled beta2-agonist. † Inhaled corticosteroid. ‡ Leukotriene receptor antagonist. § Long-acting inhaled beta2-agonist. ‖ Exercise-incluced bronchospasm.

Figure 3–1 **Reproduced from: Guidelines for the Diagnosis and Management of Asthma. National Asthma Education and Prevention Program, National Institutes of Health. Expert Panel Report 3, pages 305–310, 343–345. http://www.nhlbi.nih.gov/guidelines/asthma.**

Your patient does quite well over the next year, having very few exacerbations. During one of her visits, you note slightly edematous nasal mucosa and nasal polyps. You prescribe intranasal steroids.

* *

One night when you are on call, she comes in severely dyspneic with audible wheezing. She talks in two- or three-word phrases and reports headache today, which she treated with aspirin (something she never takes but a friend gave her thinking it was acetaminophen). Her asthma attack started about an hour after the aspirin dose. She has been otherwise well. She denies fever, rhinorrhea, nasal congestion, and sore throat. Her respiratory rate is 40, heart rate 120, and oxygen saturation 88% on room air. She has poor air movement on auscultation of her lung fields.

Which of the following is the most likely reason for this patient's acute exacerbation of asthma?

A) Viral upper respiratory infection (URI).
B) Sinusitis.
C) Noncompliance with inhaled albuterol.
D) Sensitivity to aspirin.
E) Noncompliance with nasal steroids.

Discussion

The correct answer is "D." It is likely that this patient has aspirin sensitivity. Up to 10% of adults with asthma have the clinical triad of asthma, aspirin sensitivity, and nasal polyposis. Patients with asthma should be warned about the potential for exacerbations resulting from consumption of aspirin and nonsteroidal anti-inflammatory drugs (NSAIDs). The drug-induced bronchial constriction caused by these medications can have an abrupt onset with severe symptoms. Patients with aspirin sensitivity can be desensitized with daily administration of small amounts of aspirin, but this should be done carefully with close supervision.

Although viral URIs frequently cause exacerbations of asthma, your patient did not report antecedent symptoms of such an infection. Further discussion of the treatment of acute asthma can be found in Chapter 1, "Emergency Medicine."

* *

After a brief hospitalization, your patient recovers nicely. Prior to this incident involving aspirin, she had been free of exacerbations for about a month.

In addition to a short course of oral steroids, which of the following medication regimens do you prescribe for this patient with *aspirin-sensitive* asthma at discharge?

A) Inhaled triamcinolone and inhaled albuterol as a "rescue."
B) Inhaled triamcinolone, oral montelukast, and inhaled albuterol as a "rescue."
C) Oral montelukast and inhaled albuterol as a "rescue."
D) Inhaled albuterol as a "rescue."
E) Inhaled salmeterol and inhaled triamcinolone.

Discussion

The correct answer is "B." Leukotriene inhibitors (e.g., montelukast, zafirlukast) do not have a primary role in asthma management. However, these medications have demonstrated effectiveness in reducing symptoms and improving peak flow in patients with aspirin-sensitive asthma.

Leukotriene inhibitors should be used only in asthma patients who are already using a corticosteroid inhaler—or those who cannot tolerate inhaled corticosteroid therapy. Therefore, "C" is not an appropriate choice. "D" is incorrect because there is no anti-inflammatory. Although "E" offers an anti-inflammatory agent, there is no rescue inhaler, and patients with asthma must always have access to a short-acting inhaled bronchodilator.

HELPFUL TIP: Other NSAIDs have been implicated in "aspirin-exacerbated" asthma. The theory is that there is an imbalance between pro- and anti-inflammatory mediators that is exacerbated acutely by COX-1 inhibition.

Which of the following medications, when used alone as maintenance therapy in persistent asthma, is associated with an increased risk of asthma-related mortality?

A) Inhaled fluticasone.
B) Inhaled salmeterol.
C) Oral zafirlukast.
D) Oral prednisone.

Discussion

The correct answer is "B." Inhaled salmeterol, when used alone as a controller agent for asthma, has been associated with a two- to fourfold increase in the risk of death related to asthma or other respiratory conditions. Thus, the Food and Drug Administration (FDA) has mandated a "black box" warning be applied to salmeterol-containing products. It is not known whether inhaled steroid therapy is protective, but NHLBI/NAEPP guidelines recommend adding long-acting inhaled beta-agonists only after inhaled steroids are already in use.

HELPFUL TIP: The importance of patient education in asthma cannot be overstated. Patients diagnosed with asthma should receive a written plan of action, detailing when to increase beta-2 agonist use and when to start an oral steroid. While there is no proven benefit to home peak flow monitoring, this may serve to get patients more involved in management of their illness. A home peak flow meter can be used as a part of the educational process and to enhance communication between the healthcare practitioner and the patient.

Objectives: Did you learn to . . .

- Identify triggers of bronchospasm?
- Evaluate symptoms of wheezing and dyspnea?
- Classify asthma?
- Prescribe appropriate medications for intermittent and mild persistent asthma?
- Describe the triad of asthma, aspirin sensitivity, and nasal polyposis?

QUICK QUIZ: SPIROMETRY

A 60-year-old female who smokes two packs of cigarettes per day complains of shortness of breath and fullness in her throat. You obtain spirometry in the office and the results are given below along with the flow/volume loop (Figure 3–2).

How do you interpret these findings?

A) Chronic obstructive lung disease.
B) Restrictive lung disease.

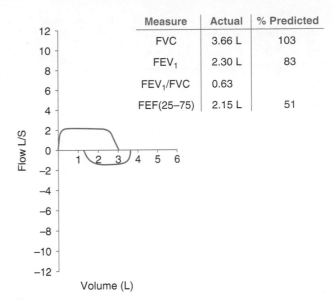

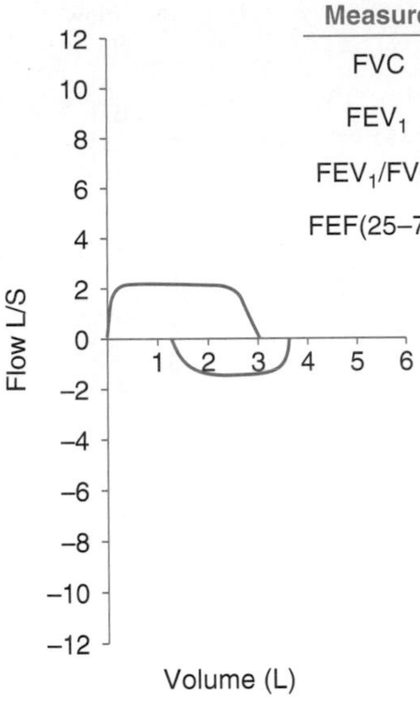

Measure	Actual	% Predicted
FVC	3.66 L	103
FEV_1	2.30 L	83
FEV_1/FVC	0.63	
FEF(25–75)	2.15 L	51

Figure 3–2

C) Fixed upper airway obstruction.
D) Poor patient effort.
E) Within normal range.

Discussion

The correct answer is "C." The flattened flow/volume loop is consistent with a fixed upper airway obstruction. In this case, FEV_1 and the FEV_1/FVC ratio may look like other obstructive diseases (i.e., asthma, COPD), so you have to look at the flow/volume loop (always a good idea). Some examples of flow/volume loops are given below (Figure 3–3).

CASE 4

You are seeing a 65-year-old male in the emergency department (ED) where he presented with complaint of increasing shortness of breath. He has obvious difficulty breathing and cannot speak in full sentences. However, you are able to elicit that he has been having increasing respiratory problems over the last 3–4 days. He has known COPD with FEV_1 of "less than one" (normal FEV_1 is about 4 L for a 50-year-old male and 3 L for a 50-year-old female. For the calculations based on age, etc., see www.hankconsulting.com/RefCal.html). He has been using his inhalers much more than usual but with minimal improvement. He has smoked one pack per day since age 18 (but proudly points out he quit 2 days

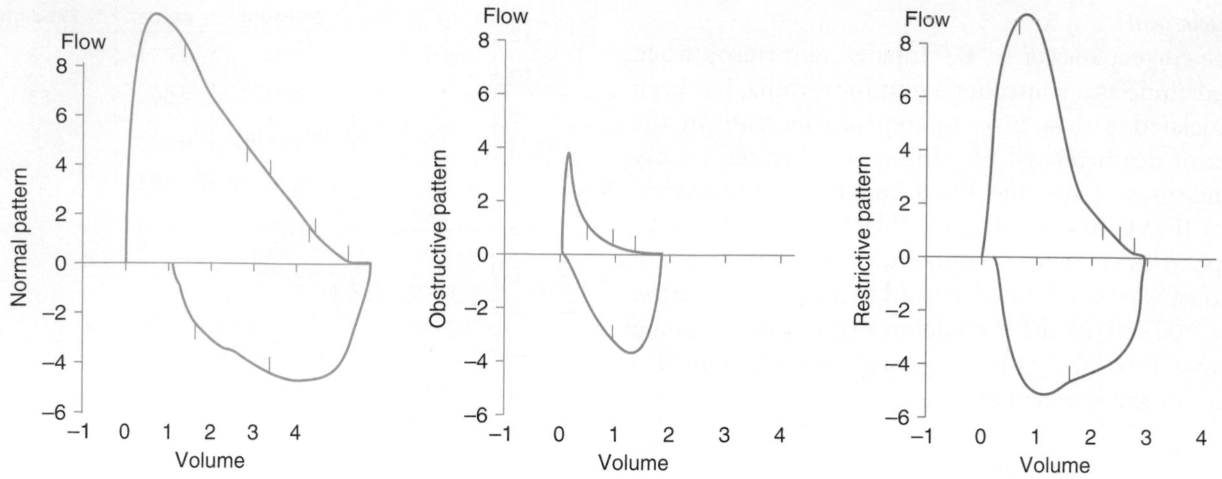

Figure 3–3 **Flow volume loops**

ago) and has a past medical history of high cholesterol, obesity, and hypertension.

On exam, he has a respiratory rate of 26–28, heart rate of 100, blood pressure of 130/90, and temperature of 37.7. His O_2 saturation is 84% on room air. On auscultation, you do not appreciate much due to his body habitus but you still manage to hear some wheezing. He has a normal cardiac exam and no lower extremity edema.

What is the next best step to help this patient?

A) Perform emergent endotracheal intubation.
B) Administer supplemental O_2 via nasal cannula.
C) Administer Solu-Medrol, 1 g IV.
D) Start antibiotics IV.
E) Obtain a chest x-ray.

Discussion

The correct answer is "B." This patient is hypoxic, and your first priority should be to improve his oxygenation. There exists a theory that oxygenating patients with COPD will suppress their respiratory drive. The classical teaching (mostly incorrect) is that COPD causes a switch from carbon dioxide levels driving respiration to oxygen levels driving respiration. While this may be partly true, further study has suggested that the main reason COPD patients are at risk of worsening hypercapnia is due to loss of hypoxic pulmonary vasoconstriction and worsening ventilation–perfusion mismatch that occurs with excess oxygen delivery. Regardless of that, you need to first worry about this patient's oxygenation.

* *

"A" is incorrect. The patient is protecting his airway and you have not attempted at improving his oxygenation with less invasive methods yet. Administering steroids, IV or PO, will have no immediate effect on his respiratory status. In fact, IV steroids *might* be worse than PO steroids (question of whether higher IV doses cause immunosuppression and subclinical myopathy). Antibiotics and a chest x-ray may be reasonable, but with low O_2 saturations, your priority is to quickly improve your patient's oxygen status.

When initiating supplemental oxygen by nasal cannula, you instruct the nurse to keep the patient's oxygen saturation:

A) Between 96% and 100%.
B) Between 90% and 95%.
C) Between 85% and 89%.
D) At whatever saturation he looks most comfortable.

Discussion

The correct answer is "B." The primary goal of supplemental oxygen is to reduce the risk of tissue hypoxia. Maintaining oxygen saturations above 90% (or PaO_2 60–65 mm) will ensure tissue oxygenation. Higher oxygen saturations may result in CO_2 retention and hypercapnia, as noted earlier. Also, aiming at 100% with excessive levels of O_2 supplementation takes away an important patient assessment parameter because now you cannot tell easily whether his O_2

needs are going up or down. "D" is of special note. Patients with COPD who look comfortable may be becoming hypercapnic and developing CO_2 narcosis. Thus, while comfort is a goal, it may not be the best judge of clinical status in patients with COPD exacerbations. To assess CO_2 levels, you will need an ABG or VBG.

* *

You obtain an ABG: pH 7.29, PCO_2 74 mm Hg, PO_2 58 mm Hg. The patient is awake and alert but says that he still feels "like dirt." He remains tachypneic, in obvious respiratory distress, with a respiratory rate of 28. Albuterol and ipratropium were given.

What is the best next step?

A) Clearly, he is failing therapy—emergently intubate.
B) Increase his O_2 to 100% via face mask.
C) Initiate noninvasive positive pressure ventilation (e.g., BiPAP).
D) Start IV antibiotics.
E) Obtain a chest CT with PE protocol (you're barking up the wrong bronchial tree).

Discussion

The correct answer is "C." This patient is retaining CO_2 despite tachypnea and is in impending respiratory failure. He is also not oxygenating well despite low-flow oxygen. Noninvasive positive pressure support (BIPAP) can relieve hypercapnia and improve oxygenation by decreasing work of breathing without requiring intubation and its associated morbidity. Often IV antibiotics are used for empiric therapy in severe exacerbations of COPD, but again, improving the respiratory status comes first. He is hypoxic, but his main problem is CO_2 retention—increasing his O_2 delivery will not alleviate that. Although his respiratory status is tenuous, he is not in imminent respiratory failure, and intubation is not warranted at this time. Chest CT can rule out a PE in this hypoxic patient and may confirm COPD changes including emphysema but will greatly delay treatment and would not change your immediate course of action.

* *

After several hours of noninvasive positive pressure ventilation, your patient is doing well and he is transferred out of the intensive care unit (ICU). When you see him the next day, his medications include inhaled bronchodilators, ceftriaxone, azithromycin, and prednisone. A chest x-ray shows no evidence of infiltrate. He is weaned from the positive pressure support and is now on 2 L/min of oxygen by nasal cannula. He appears comfortable, with a respiratory rate of 14 and an oxygen saturation of 95%.

Now you know that he has COPD, what would be the best treatment for him?

A) Inhaled long-acting beta-agonist (LABA) + albuterol.
B) Inhaled steroid + albuterol.
C) Inhaled steroid + LABA + albuterol as needed.
D) Albuterol.
E) Albuterol and theophylline.

Discussion

Correct answer is "C." This is a bit tricky, but due to the severity of his exacerbation, "C" is the best choice. Compared with patients with asthma, where LABA is not indicated as first-line therapy, COPD patients have a clear symptomatic benefit from long-acting bronchodilators. The two available choices are anticholinergics (e.g., tiotropium) or LABAs (e.g., salmeterol or formoterol). Either choice is fine. In patients with FEV_1 <60%, the combination of a LABA and an inhaled steroid decreases the rate of decline of the lung function. An inhaled steroid will reduce the frequency of exacerbations, but should not be used alone in a patient with COPD (unlike asthma).

> HELPFUL TIP: American Thoracic Society guidelines categorize obstructive airway disease based on the predicted FEV_1% of the patient. The response to bronchodilator is also categorized by ATS. To state that there was significant response to bronchodilator, there has to be increase of *both* 200 cc and an increase of at least 12% in the FEV_1.

* *

Holding his inhalers and smiling toothlessly, your patient asks, "Which of these is going to keep me alive—just in case I can't afford both?"

Which of the following medication regimens has demonstrated decreased mortality in the treatment of stable COPD?

A) Inhaled tiotropium (a long-acting anticholinergic).
B) Inhaled salmeterol.
C) Inhaled ipratropium (a short-acting anticholinergic).
D) Inhaled corticosteroid.
E) None of the above.

Discussion

The correct answer is "E." Aside from oxygen, no medical therapy has clearly demonstrated a mortality benefit for stable COPD. Inhaled tiotropium has the advantage of once daily dosing.

* *

Later that year, the same patient gets admitted to the hospital for community-acquired pneumonia. During his stay in the hospital, the hospitalist orders a CT chest "to rule out other things." The patient recovers from his infection and returns to you with the CD of his CT chest images. The reading of the CT chest describes a 2-cm pulmonary nodule in the right upper lobe *along with extensive subcarinal lymphadenopathy*.

What is the next best step in management of this patient?

A) Repeat CT chest in 3 months.
B) Repeat CT chest in 6 months.
C) Refer for bronchoscopy with endobronchial ultrasound-guided biopsy.
D) Refer to an oncologist.
E) Refer for a mediastinoscopy.

Discussion

The correct answer is "C." This patient probably has a malignant disease and tissue is needed to either diagnose it or rule it out. Bronchoscopy with EBUS (endobronchial ultrasound) guided fine needle biopsies is a minimally invasive procedure that can relatively safely obtain a tissue sample for the pathologist. There is good evidence that EBUS has good sensitivity and specificity compared with PET scanning. "A" and "B" are incorrect as this patient has a nodule that is larger than 1 cm along with mediastinal lymphadenopathy. This needs to be worked up and cannot wait 3–6 months. Answer "D" is incorrect. Your patient will likely need to see an oncologist, but you need to first provide a tissue diagnosis. "E," mediastinoscopy, would likely provide you with the diagnosis, but it is a far more invasive procedure than bronchoscopy and carries higher mortality and morbidity.

HELPFUL TIP: CATEGORIZING COPD

There are several scales to rate COPD including the GOLD, MMRC dyspnea scale, and the BODE index. The BODE index (*b*ody mass index, air-flow *o*bstruction, *d*yspnea, and *e*xercise capacity) incorporates functional capacity and is preferred by some. There are BODE and MMRC calculators available. The Global Initiative for Obstructive Lung Disease (GOLD) categorizes COPD as follows:

Stage 1 (mild COPD)—mild airflow obstruction with FEV_1/FVC <70% and FEV_1 >80% + cough and occasional sputum production.

Stage 2 (moderate COPD)—FEV_1/FVC <70% and FEV_1 50–79% + occasional exacerbations.

Stage 3 (severe COPD)—FEV_1/FVC <70% and FEV_1 30–49% + frequent exacerbations.

Stage 4 (very severe COPD)—FEV_1/FVC <70% and FEV_1 <30% or FEV_1 <50% + chronic respiratory failure.

HELPFUL TIP: Note that inhaled steroids should be used in those with moderate to severe COPD based on the GOLD guidelines. There is no benefit in patients with mild COPD and there is a downside (an increase in pneumonia).

* *

Your patient returns with increasing dyspnea now at rest. Despite both of you being blue in the face, he has not quit smoking.

Criteria for the use of continuous low-flow oxygen in those with COPD include all of the following EXCEPT:

A) PO_2 <55 mm Hg.
B) Oxygen saturation <88%.

C) PO_2 of <59 mm Hg with evidence of cor pulmonale.
D) Episodic sleep apnea–related desaturations at night.

Discussion
The correct answer is "D." Episodic sleep apnea–related oxygen desaturations, while a cause for concern and amenable to treatment (e.g., CPAP), is not one of the criteria for the use of continuous low-flow oxygen. The other choices are correct. "C" deserves some special attention. Evidence of cor pulmonale can include "p-pulmonale" on ECG, peripheral edema, or a hematocrit >55%.

Concerning hypoxemic patients with COPD, which of the following is true?

A) Patients on continuous, low-flow O_2 become oxygen dependent and cannot function without it.
B) Continuous low-flow O_2 used for at least 8 hours a day helps to reverse pulmonary hypertension.
C) Concurrent smoking is a contraindication to the prescribing continuous low-flow home O_2 because patients are spontaneously combusting right and left (like Spinal Tap drummers).
D) Low-flow O_2 used at least 15 hours a day significantly enhances survival.
E) None of the above.

Discussion
The correct answer is "D." Patients who use low-flow O_2 at home for 24 hours a day have an improved rate of survival. Patients should be encouraged to use O_2 at least 15 hours a day if possible. "B" is incorrect because patients need at least 15 hours of O_2 per day to have any significant benefit with regard to pulmonary hypertension. "C" is incorrect. Clearly, smoking while on O_2 is not a good idea, but patients can turn off their O_2 supply while smoking.

HELPFUL (AND IMPORTANT) TIP: Data suggests that up to 20% of patients hospitalized with a COPD exacerbation of unknown origin may actually have a PE.

Objectives: Did you learn to . . .

- Recognize a patient with COPD?
- Develop a plan to manage hypoxemia and hypercapnia?
- Manage medications for acute exacerbations of COPD?
- Direct therapy for chronic COPD?
- Identify causes of dyspnea other than COPD presenting in a patient with known COPD?

QUICK QUIZ: COPD

In a patient with COPD, a lung transplantation referral can be considered:

A) Once the patient requires oxygen.
B) When you feel you have run out of interventions.
C) Once insurance accepts your referral.
D) After the patient meets strict criteria for the referral.
E) If the patient's family keeps asking for the referral.

Discussion
The correct answer is "D." The International Society for Heart and Lung Transplantation created a set of criteria for when to consider transplantation and, more importantly, when should you consider *referral* for a lung transplant consultation. In COPD patients, the indication for *referral* is easy to remember and consists of BODE index >5. Criteria for *transplantation* in COPD are more complex and are beyond the scope of this book.

CASE 5

Ms. Sarah Bellum (if you're not smiling, try saying the name out loud or the joke is just lame . . .) is a 32-year-old Caucasian female who presents to your ED with shortness of breath. She just returned home after the International Conference of Coordination in London. Immediately after walking through her front door, she became acutely short of breath (not attributable to the Justin Bieber poster in her living room). This is associated with some moderately sharp chest pain located along the left side of her chest. The pain seems worse when she attempts to breathe deeply.

Which important question(s) do you next ask to Ms. Bellum?

A) Do you smoke cigarettes?
B) When was your last menstrual period?
C) Have you had surgery recently?
D) Do you have a history of kidney disease?
E) All of the above.

Discussion

The correct answer is "E." Each of these questions addresses risk factors associated with pulmonary embolism (PE) and/or deep vein thrombosis (DVT). Smoking cigarettes and recent surgery are strong risk factors, as is an active pregnancy. Addressing a patient's menstrual cycle serves as a natural segue to a discussion about the use of oral contraceptives, which, too, is a prominent risk factor. As for renal disease, nephrotic syndrome has been associated with an increased risk of PE.

* *

After further verbal probing, you discover that Ms. Bellum recently completed her menstrual cycle and the other presented questions turned up no risk factors. However, your smooth segue did reveal that she takes low-dose estrogen for birth control. During this discourse, you also learn that her aunt Erin had a blood clot in her leg once. She has no further details but does not think that her aunt (Aunt E. Bellum) had any further complications from this condition. Regardless, PE just took a violent leap to the top of your differential. You glance at her vitals (temperature 37.1°C, heart rate 92, blood pressure 129/68, respiratory rate 21, SpO_2 95% on room air) and notice that she appears mildly uncomfortable but is in no acute distress. Her physical exam is entirely unremarkable. You elect to secure an ECG on the patient to evaluate for potential cardiac etiologies for her symptoms.

Assuming Ms. Bellum does have a PE, what is her ECG most likely to show?

A) $S_1Q_3T_3$.
B) Nonspecific ST-T wave changes.
C) Sinus tachycardia.
D) Normal sinus rhythm.
E) Multifocal atrial tachycardia.

Discussion

The correct answer is "D." The most common ECG finding associated with the diagnosis of PE remains normal sinus rhythm. With that said, the most common *arrhythmia* found in patients with a PE is sinus tachycardia. But alas, Sarah had a normal heart rate. The other choices can certainly be found with this condition but are far less frequent. Of note, the "textbook" $S_1Q_3T_3$ ECG rarely occurs and historically traces back to a handful of patients in the 1930s that had massive pulmonary emboli. Even if you do spot this pattern on an ECG, it is not specific enough to confirm the diagnosis. In the end, the clinical signs attributed to pulmonary emboli (such as the shortness of breath and chest pain) are frequently more valuable than any abnormal ECG finding.

* *

As you attempt to rule out other potential etiologies for the patient's symptoms (e.g., pneumonia, atelectasis, and pneumothorax), you order a trusty chest radiograph.

What is the most common radiographic finding in a patient with a PE?

A) Pleural effusion.
B) No acute cardiopulmonary processes.
C) Westermark sign.
D) Hilar/Mediastinal enlargement.
E) Hampton hump.

Discussion

The correct answer is "B." Admittedly, this one is a bit tricky. Approximately 75% of the chest radiographs in the setting of PE are abnormal. However, there are numerous causes for these abnormalities and none of them individually surpass the frequency of the normal chest radiographs. Specifically, the "textbook" findings of Westermark sign (loss of peripheral vascular markings) and Hampton hump (a wedge-shaped opacity due to pulmonary infarction) are infrequent, and both have a low sensitivity and low specificity. In short, all the other options can be seen as the result of a PE but none are more frequent than a normal chest radiograph.

* *

ECG and chest radiograph in hand, you turn your attention toward ordering the appropriate laboratory tests to solidify your presumptive diagnosis.

Which test should you AVOID ordering?

A) CBC.
B) D-dimer.
C) PT/PTT.
D) Basic metabolic panel (Na^+, K^+, Cl^-, CO_2^-, BUN, Cr^-, and glucose).
E) Urine pregnancy test.

Discussion

The correct answer is "B." The D-dimer can be a blessing for some but is the bane of existence for others. In this patient, a D-dimer is not useful. This test has great sensitivity but poor specificity. It is positive in far more conditions than PE. Used as a "rule-out" test for PE, it only applies in low-risk patients. Ms. Bellum is not a low-risk patient as suggested by the pulmonary embolism rule-out criteria (PERC) rules (see Helpful Tip) due to her use of exogenous estrogen. The Wells criteria for PE place her in the moderate-risk group (16.2% risk of PE). As such, even a negative D-dimer in such a patient is insufficient for ruling out the diagnosis. As for the other tests, they all serve a valuable role in her evaluation. For instance, the CBC could provide evidence of anemia (a potential cause of chest pain), while the PT/PTT may reveal a coagulopathy. Assessing her renal function may be needed for her evaluation moving forward, and the same can be said for verifying her nongestational status. Plus, a urine pregnancy test is performed on almost every women in an ED... It might as well be part of the triage process.

* *

That pesky med student seemed to know a lot about the PERC rules and Wells criteria. But when he listed the Wells criteria, he got one wrong.

The Wells criteria for PE include all of the following EXCEPT:

A) Estrogen use.
B) Pulse >100.
C) Previous history of venothromboembolism.
D) Clinical symptoms and signs consistent with PE.
E) Hemoptysis.

Discussion

The correct answer is "A." While an important risk factor for PE, estrogen use is not included in the Wells criteria. All the others count in the Wells criteria, as well as a history of surgery or 3 days immobilization in the last 4 weeks and a history of malignancy treated in the last 6 months. Each of these criteria counts for a certain number of points, which add up to a percentage risk of having PE. Using a medical calculator Web site, such as www.medcalc.com, is most helpful.

> HELPFUL TIP: The PERC rules (pulmonary embolism rule-out criteria) are a validated set of rules that allow categorization of a patient into a low-risk group to rule out PE clinically. If the patient meets *all* of the following, PE is ruled out *assuming you believe the patient is low risk.*

PERC rules:

1) Age <50.
2) Heart rate <100.
3) SaO_2 >94%.
4) No unilateral leg swelling.
5) No hemoptysis.
6) No recent history of trauma or surgery.
7) No prior DVT or PE.
8) No hormone use.

> HELPFUL TIP: Remember not to get a D-dimer on *no-risk* patients. This simply increases the CT rate and exposure to unnecessary radiation. The *fatal* cancer rate in a 20-year-old female undergoing a 64-slice chest CT is 1:142 (really) (*JAMA* 2007;298:317-323)! See also *Lancet* 2009;374:1160 and *J Pediatr* 2009;154:912 among others.

* *

The CBC, coagulation studies, and basic metabolic panel all return within normal limits. Additionally, Ms. Bellum is not pregnant. Thus, you wish to (finally) solidify that diagnosis you have suspected for quite some time.

Since you do not put her in the low-risk category by your clinical judgment, what diagnostic study should you order?

A) VQ (ventilation–perfusion) scan.
B) CT scan of the chest without contrast.
C) CT scan of the chest with contrast.
D) Pulmonary angiogram.

Discussion

The correct answer is "C." The American College of Radiology (ACR) lists the CT scan of the chest with contrast (i.e., CT angiography or CTA) as the modality of choice in stable patients with a suspected PE. The CTA is considered to be the standard of care. Its benefits include the fact that it is noninvasive, cheaper than pulmonary angiography, and far more available than VQ scans. It should be noted that pulmonary angiography still remains the "gold standard" for diagnosing pulmonary emboli, but that is more of an academic point. As for VQ scans, they are not available in many locales and often return nondiagnostic. However, they can be used in a patient with a normal chest x-ray. A chest CT without contrast will not enhance the pulmonary arteries, making the diagnosis of a PE far more difficult, if not impossible.

> HELPFUL TIP: You may want to start with a lower extremity Doppler study. If this is positive, you are done. The patient needs anticoagulation and you can avoid the radiation of a CT scan and the risk of contrast.

> HELPFUL TIP: In pregnancy, chest CT is still an option according to 2011 guidelines published by the American College of Obstetrics and Gynecology (ACOG); V/Q scan is not necessarily preferred.

* *

As keenly suspected, Ms. Bellum's CTA of the chest reveals a moderate-sized pulmonary embolism in the left pulmonary artery. Her vital signs are still stable and her pain is well controlled with intravenous morphine. She is surprised by the diagnosis you give her but appears to be taking it in stride.

What is the optimal management plan for the patient moving forward?

A) Give her a bolus of unfractionated heparin (UFH), start her on oral warfarin, and discharge her to home.
B) Provide the patient with a dose of enoxaparin in the ED, provide education, and discharge the patient to home with primary care follow-up in the next 2–3 days.
C) Start the patient on low-molecular-weight heparin (LMWH), initiate oral warfarin therapy, and admit the patient to the family practice service.
D) Give her a bolus of UFH, initiate a UFH drip, and admit the patient to the family practice service.
E) Start her on oral warfarin and discharge her to home with primary care follow-up in the next 2–3 days.

Discussion

The correct answer is "C." Full anticoagulation is considered mandatory for all patients with a PE. *While discharging a patient with only a DVT is considered standard of care, this is not (yet) true for pulmonary embolism.* Thus, any plan that centers on a discharge to home is incorrect (although we are moving in that direction with stable patients; Jodang et al., 2011). With regard to selecting an anticoagulant, current evidence does not support the use of one agent over another; UFH, LMWH, and fondaparinux are all appropriate. Regardless of the selected anticoagulant, the current recommendations stipulate the initiation of warfarin at the time of diagnosis as well. The UFH, MMWH, or fondaparinux should be continued until the patient's INR has been 2.0 for at least 24 hours.

How long are you going to maintain this patient on anticoagulation?

A) 3 months.
B) 6 months.
C) 9 months.
D) Lifetime.

Discussion

The correct answer is "A." For a PE that has a reversible cause (oral contraceptive pills in this patient with a long airplane trip), 3 months of anticoagulation is adequate. For those with a second PE, lifetime anticoagulation is warranted. For those with a cryptogenic PE or PE from an unreversible cause (Factor V Leiden), recommendations are all over the place from 3 months to life. Nine months is likely adequate for a patient with a PE from an irreversible cause, *although patients go back to their pretreatment risk as soon as you stop anticoagulation.* And, a first PE trumps everything else in terms for risk factors for a second PE. So, finding that thrombophilia does not necessarily help your decision-making process.

> HELPFUL TIP: An elevated A–a gradient suggests a ventilation/perfusion mismatch and occurs in a number of conditions, including

atelectasis, a right-to-left shunt, acute respiratory distress syndrome (ARDS), air embolism, resolving severe asthma, COPD with oxygen treatment, and bronchiectasis with impaired gas exchange. Thus, an elevated A–a gradient is not specific for PE. Likewise, a normal A–a gradient and normal oxygen saturation do not rule out PE! In fact, in patients without underlying lung disease, the PIOPED study found no difference in the oxygen saturation and A–a gradient among patients with and without PE.

HELPFUL TIP: Only 88% of patients with a PE are hypoxic, 70% have dyspnea or tachypnea, 65% have pleuritic pain, and as few as 30% are tachycardic. The point here is to have a high clinical suspicion in the right situation despite the lack of the classic triad. To make things worse, the troponin and BNP can be elevated in patients with a PE.

HELPFUL TIP: Compressions stockings may prevent postphlebitic syndrome, the recurrent swelling, and edema often found after a DVT. Prescribe compression stockings routinely in these patients.

* *

Your patient does well, completes her course of warfarin, and has no further episodes over the next 2 years. She develops gallstones and plans to have an elective laparoscopic cholecystectomy. A surgeon colleague sends her back to see you for a preoperative evaluation. You find no evidence of cardiac, pulmonary, or hematologic disease. She is no longer on warfarin and is doing well.

Which of the following postoperative management strategies do you recommend?

A) Aspirin 81 mg PO daily.
B) Warfarin 5 mg PO daily.
C) UFH 5000 units subcutaneously daily.
D) Enoxaparin 40 mg subcutaneously daily.
E) No antiplatelet or anticoagulant drugs.

Discussion

The correct answer is "D." Even for a relatively minor surgical procedure, where anesthesia is used for 30 minutes or less and the postoperative recovery is usually quick, your patient is at moderate risk for venous thromboembolism. Her history of PE puts her in a higher risk category, and she requires prophylaxis. Of the choices available, enoxaparin would be the most appropriate. LMWH and UFH are both acceptable for prevention of DVT/PE in the postoperative period, but "C" is wrong because UFH must be dosed every 8–12 hours rather than daily. "A" is incorrect. Aspirin is sometimes used postoperatively, but the dose should be 160 mg/day or greater. Also, compared with heparin and its derivatives, aspirin is less efficacious in the prevention of thrombus. "B" is incorrect. Warfarin alone is not appropriate in this setting due to its slow onset of action.

HELPFUL TIP: The optimal length of time that patients require prophylaxis for venous thromboembolism after surgery is unknown. Arguments can be made for prophylaxis until the patient is ambulating several hundred feet per day.

Objectives: Did you learn to . . .

- Recognize risk factors for a PE?
- Understand the variability of symptoms and signs in PE?
- Appreciate the PERC rules and Wells criteria and how they can be used to rule out a PE without any testing?
- Implement treatment and prevention for PE?
- Understand the A–a gradient?

CASE 6

A 50-year-old male who is a heavy drinker with a history of squamous cell carcinoma of the neck presents to your office complaining of abdominal pain. He has been coughing and expectorating bloody sputum and notes a low-grade fever, chills, and mild dyspnea starting about 1 week ago. He denies nausea, emesis, and chest pain. His squamous cell carcinoma was treated with external beam radiation several years ago. Examination reveals an afebrile male in mild distress. His vital signs are normal, and his lungs sound clear. The abdominal exam reveals only mild epigastric tenderness.

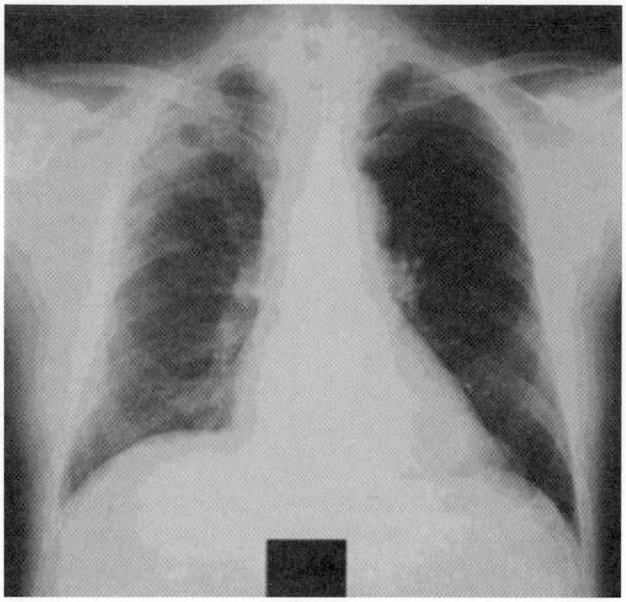

Figure 3–4

The chest x-ray is available for your review (see Figure 3–4). Your colleague, who is on call today, walks by and asks if you have any admissions for her.

You consider this 50-year-old with a cough and reply:

A) "Yes. This gentleman will need the ICU."
B) "Yes. This gentleman will need a respiratory isolation room."
C) "No. I'm sending this gentleman home with metronidazole."
D) "No. I'll work up this gentleman as an outpatient."

Discussion

The correct answer is "B." Because he is expectorating bloody sputum and has a cavitary lesion on chest x-ray (right upper lobe), this patient should be admitted to a respiratory isolation room until tuberculosis is ruled out. He will need further evaluation and possibly intravenous antibiotic therapy, both of which may be accomplished during his hospitalization. "A" is incorrect. There is no need to send this patient to the ICU based on his current picture. "C" is also incorrect. Metronidazole alone is not an appropriate therapy for this patient even if this is bacterial (see below).

What is the best next step in the diagnosis of this process?

A) Bronchoscopy.
B) Sputum cultures.
C) Blood cultures.
D) Chest CT.
E) Open lung biopsy.

Discussion

The correct answer is "D." The chest x-ray demonstrates a cavitary lesion in the right upper lobe. Chest CT is warranted for further characterization of the lesion. From history, exam, and chest x-ray, it is not possible to determine whether the lesion is an abscess or a malignant process. An indolent course with low-grade fever is characteristic of lung abscess. However, the preexisting squamous cell carcinoma has potential to have spread to the lungs, and squamous cell carcinoma is known to cause cavitations. Culture of sputum and blood, including evaluation of first morning sputum for AFB, will be an essential part of the assessment but may not yield as much information as chest CT, and sputum culture should be done in conjunction with cytology and Gram stain. Bronchoscopy should be postponed until CT results are available. Bronchoscopic biopsy is potentially detrimental if the lesion is an abscess since the airway could flood with pus if the entire cavity wall is penetrated.

* *

Chest CT further confirms a parenchymal abscess in the right upper lobe with cavitation and air within the cavity. Bronchoscopy reveals pus in the airway and extrinsic compression of the bronchi. A lavage sample is obtained, but biopsies are not taken due to the clinical impression that this is a lung abscess.

What organisms are most commonly isolated in lung abscesses?

A) Anaerobic bacteria.
B) Aerobic bacteria.
C) Tuberculosis.
D) Mixed aerobic/anaerobic bacteria.

Discussion

The correct answer is "A." Anaerobes are isolated most often, followed by mixed anaerobic/aerobic bacteria, followed by aerobic bacteria alone (especially staphylococci).

* *

Gram stain of sputum demonstrates gram-positive cocci and gram-negative rods. Cultures are pending. Tuberculin skin test is negative.

What is the most appropriate therapy for this patient?

A) Refer for surgical drainage.
B) Oral levofloxacin.
C) Intravenous clindamycin.
D) Intravenous metronidazole.
E) Intravenous ceftriaxone.

Discussion

The correct answer is "C." Most lung abscesses are polymicrobial, but the most important aspect in treatment appears to be the use of an antibiotic active against anaerobes. Intravenous clindamycin is the usual choice for lung abscess due to its coverage of anaerobes and *Streptococcus pneumoniae*. Metronidazole is less effective, failing in up to 50% of cases of putrid lung abscess. A beta-lactam with beta-lactamase inhibitor (e.g., piperacillin/tazobactam) is another good choice. Ceftriaxone and levofloxacin offer poor coverage of anaerobes. Surgical drainage of lung abscesses is needed in only 5–10% of cases. Most resolve with just antibiotics.

Objectives: Did you learn to . . .

- Recognize the presence of a cavitary lesion on chest x-ray?
- Identify the common causes of cavitary lesions?
- Decide when to place a patient in respiratory isolation?
- Manage a patient with a lung abscess?

CASE 7

A 53-year-old male is accompanied by his wife to your office and complains of a cough for 6 weeks. It is worse at night and any time he lies down. He denies sputum production, shortness of breath, chest pain, and wheezing. He takes an antacid once or twice per day to settle his stomach and notes very bad heartburn. He smoked three packs of cigarettes per day until 1 year ago, when he quit "cold turkey." He takes only hydrochlorothiazide for hypertension and a daily aspirin. He has no cardiac disorders. His wife reports that he snores at night, and she adds, "He's always hacking and clearing his throat—all night." The review of systems is negative. In order to sleep better, he has recently started having a shot of whiskey before going to bed.

What is the most likely cause for the cough?

A) Gastroesophageal reflux.
B) Lung cancer.
C) Antihypertensive medication.
D) Alcohol abuse.
E) Congestive heart failure (CHF).

Discussion

The correct answer is "A." This patient appears to have a chronic cough that is most likely due to gastroesophageal reflux disease (GERD). He takes antacids and exhibits throat clearing, which can be a subtle sign and is not typically identified by patients as reflux. Additionally, he drinks alcohol at bedtime, further predisposing to reflux. He has a history of smoking, which does place him at increased risk for developing a bronchogenic carcinoma, but a lung mass would not be a common cause for cough. Aspirin is associated with bronchospasm in some people, but it would not usually present as cough in a patient with no history of asthma. Hydrochlorothiazide is not known to cause cough (although angiotensin-converting enzyme [ACE] inhibitors are). Also, it is unlikely that symptoms would be isolated to nighttime if his cough was medication related.

HELPFUL TIP: Remember that ACE inhibitors may cause cough in 5–20% of patients taking them. For patients who develop a cough and are on an ACE inhibitor, a brief trial off the medication may save a costly workup for chronic cough. Usually, symptoms resolve within 1 week but may persist for 1 month. Cough due to an ACE inhibitor may first occur up to 6 months after starting the ACE inhibitor.

HELPFUL TIP: *Asymptomatic* reflux disease does not exacerbate asthma. So, don't blame asthma on *asymptomatic* nocturnal reflux (*Am J Respir Crit Care Med* 2009;180:809, *N Engl J Med* 2009;360:1487).

* *

On physical examination, you note a mildly overweight male in no distress. His vital signs are normal. His lungs are clear to auscultation. The nasal and oropharyngeal mucosae are intact, moist, and not inflamed. The remainder of the exam is unremarkable. Chest x-ray shows flattened diaphragms but is otherwise negative. You suspect GERD, but also entertain other diagnoses.

Which of the following is your next step in managing this patient's cough?

A) Start a proton pump inhibitor.
B) Start an inhaled steroid.
C) Order 24-hour esophageal pH monitoring.
D) Obtain spirometry.
E) Obtain a chest CT.

Discussion

The correct answer is "A." An empiric trial of an effective gastric acid–suppressing medication in this *symptomatic patient* is likely to relieve the cough if the diagnosis is accurate. The American College of Chest Physicians (ACCP) recommends starting therapy with a proton pump inhibitor rather than an H_2-blocker. The usual antireflux measures, such as avoiding fatty foods, alcohol, and food before bedtime, should be instituted as well. Prescribers must be aware that sometimes a complete resolution of cough takes months. A 24-hour pH monitor is invasive and often not necessary if an empiric trial of gastric acid suppression resolves the problem. Starting the evaluation of chronic cough with a chest x-ray is part of the ACCP recommendations, but CT scan is not indicated with a negative chest x-ray. If the cough does not resolve with empiric therapy, spirometry should be considered.

* *

He does not respond after 2 months of empiric treatment, and he is becoming more concerned. The examination is unchanged. Spirometry is normal with a normal flow volume loop.

Which of the following management options is LEAST likely to benefit this patient?

A) Combination antihistamine and decongestant.
B) Inhaled corticosteroid.
C) Inhaled beta-2 agonist.
D) Antibiotics.

Discussion

The correct answer is "D." This patient has no signs or symptoms of sinusitis or bacterial pulmonary infection, so treating with an antibiotic is inappropriate and unlikely to help. However, some form of empiric therapy might be tried. He could have postnasal drainage without signs on physical exam, and empiric therapy with combination antihistamine and decongestant may improve the cough. Inhaled corticosteroids and beta-2 agonists are the mainstay of chronic asthma therapy and may help relieve this patient's chronic cough. This patient could yet have "cough-variant asthma" despite normal spirometry results.

The three most common causes of chronic cough (cough lasting longer than 8 weeks) are:

A) Postnasal drip, asthma, GERD.
B) GERD, COPD, congenital lung disease.
C) Lung cancer, postnasal drip, COPD.
D) Obstructive sleep apnea, respiratory infections, asthma.

Discussion

The correct answer is "A." Epidemiologic studies have demonstrated that most cases of chronic cough are due to postnasal drainage, asthma, or SYMPTOMATIC GERD. Most cases of chronic cough seem to have only a single cause, although some will have more than one cause. Empiric therapy should be aimed at these top three causes. Of course, infection (pertussis in particular), malignancy, and other causes of cough are important to consider—and potentially rule out—as well.

The evaluation of chronic cough should proceed in a logical manner. Usually, history and physical exam will find the cause. If this is unrevealing, consider a stepwise evaluation including addressing each of the etiologies in Table 3–3 in a serial fashion. If this still does not give you an answer, consider a methacholine challenge test to see if you can reproduce the symptoms that would lead you to a presumptive diagnosis of asthma with normal spirometry.

Table 3–3 SELECTED COMMON CAUSES OF ACUTE AND CHRONIC COUGH

Acute	URI, pertussis, allergic rhinitis, COPD exacerbation, asthma, acute sinusitis
Chronic	GERD, postnasal drip, asthma, chronic sinusitis, allergic/vasomotor rhinitis, ACE inhibitors, eosinophilic bronchitis, chronic bronchitis, postinfectious, asthma

COPD, chronic obstructive pulmonary disease; GERD, gastroesophageal reflux disease; ACE, angiotensin-converting enzyme.

HELPFUL TIP: Look in the ears—cerumen impaction can cause a chronic cough and is often overlooked. Remember medications, especially ACE inhibitors (as above); other drugs that can cause cough include amiodarone, olanzapine, and some asthma medications (e.g., albuterol, montelukast).

Objectives: Did you learn to . . .

- Recognize the most common causes of chronic cough?
- Evaluate a patient with chronic cough?
- Develop a management plan for chronic cough?

CASE 8

You see a 38-year-old female in follow-up for a recent episode of sinusitis. The illness has been present for about 6 weeks and has not responded to 2 weeks of appropriate antibiotics. She continues to have intermittent nosebleeds, fatigue, arthralgias, low-grade fevers, and night sweats. Two new complaints have surfaced: she has a cough productive of white sputum and she occasionally expectorates quarter-sized clots of blood. She has pleuritic chest pain, but denies dyspnea, tobacco use, and cardiac or pulmonary disease.

She is afebrile with a respiratory rate of 16, blood pressure 120/74, and pulse rate 92. Her oxygen saturation is 98% on room air. There is dried blood in the nares, but the oropharynx is clear. Cardiac and pulmonary exams are unremarkable.

Which initial test is most appropriate?

A) Chest x-ray.
B) Sputum cytologic analysis.
C) Bronchoscopy.
D) Chest CT.
E) CBC.

Discussion

The correct answer is "A." Hemoptysis is alarming to the patient and the physician—we hope. A stepwise approach is warranted with chest x-ray as the first step. Sputum for cytology might help if the suspicion for lung cancer was substantial, but the yield is likely to be low here. She may eventually require bronchoscopy as initial studies indicate. Chest CT is likely to be part of the evaluation, but a chest x-ray should be performed first. Obtaining blood for a CBC is also important, although likely to be normal in the setting of minor hemoptysis.

* *

You obtain the chest x-ray pictured in Figure 3–5. You get the following laboratory results back:

CBC: Leukocytosis, thrombocytosis and normochromic, normocytic anemia.
ESR: 70 mm/hr.
Urine dipstick: Positive for protein, heme, and red cells.

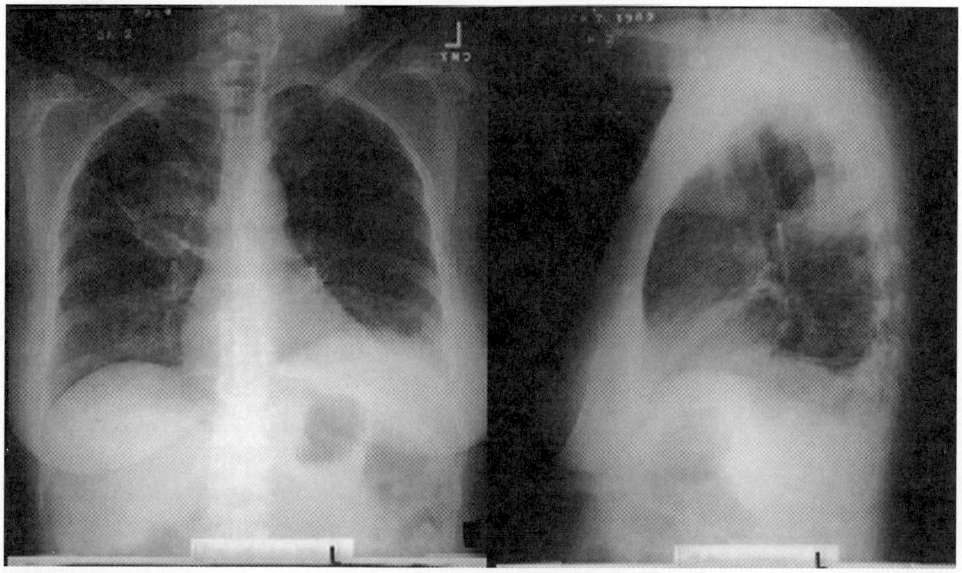

Figure 3–5

Which of the following tests will best assist you in the diagnosis of this patient?

A) Antineutrophil cytoplasmic antibody (ANCA).
B) Antiglomerular basement membrane antibody.
C) Antinuclear antibody (ANA).
D) A and B.
E) A and C.

Discussion

The correct answer is "D." This patient is presenting with the classic triad of Wegener granulomatosis: disease of the upper respiratory tract, lower respiratory tract, and kidneys. She has some of the additional signs and symptoms associated with Wegener granulomatosis as well. Common findings include pleuritic chest pain, myalgias, arthralgias, ptosis, fever, weight loss, and purpuric skin lesions, among others.

The ANCA, and especially c-ANCA which is more specific for Wegener granulomatosis, is present in up to 90% of patients with Wegener granulomatosis. An ANA is not helpful in diagnosing Wegener granulomatosis. An antiglomerular basement membrane antibody may be helpful in diagnosing Goodpasture syndrome, which can be clinically easily confused with Wegener granulomatosis; they both present with respiratory and renal involvement. Thus, anti-GBM antibody will be helpful in differentiating these two (but about 10% of patients with Goodpasture syndrome will also have Wegener granulomatosis—just to add to the confusion). For a partial list of causes of hemoptysis, see Table 3–4.

Table 3–4 CAUSES OF HEMOPTYSIS

Vascular	PE, vasculitides (Goodpasture syndrome, Wegener granulomatosis), arteriovenous malformation
Neoplastic	Bronchogenic carcinoma, metastatic disease
Connective tissue	Lupus, rheumatoid arthritis
Cardiac	CHF, mitral stenosis
Infectious	TB, bronchitis, pneumonia, abscess
Drugs	Anticoagulants, cocaine, solvents
Miscellaneous	Trauma, foreign body, epistaxis, hematemesis

CHF, congestive heart failure.

Which of the following is NOT a radiographic finding of Wegener granulomatosis?

A) Nodules that may be cavitary.
B) Alveolar opacification.
C) Pleural opacities.
D) Widened mediastinum.

Discussion

The correct answer is "D." A widened mediastinum is not one of the classic findings in Wegener granulomatosis. However, one may, on occasion, see hilar adenopathy. All of the other choices can be found in Wegener granulomatosis. In the patient's x-ray (Figure 3–5), a right upper-lobe mass is easily distinguished. In a young, nonsmoking female presenting with these symptoms, such a lung mass should lead to the consideration of Wegener granulomatosis or possibly an infectious process. She is less likely to have a malignant process.

> HELPFUL TIP: A major, and probably the most common cause of hemoptysis is bronchitis. This is especially true in smokers and the elderly.

* *

The diagnostic evaluation is in progress. Laboratory tests are pending, and a chest CT is scheduled. You have arranged for a pulmonologist to see her. When you are on call, the physician covering the ED calls you to admit her for "massive hemoptysis." When you arrive, the patient looks comfortable and has normal vital signs. She begins a fit of coughing, expectorating several ounces of bright red blood. Her systolic blood pressure falls to 80 mm Hg. Her respiratory rate is 40. Her work of breathing has increased considerably. The situation does not improve after 5 minutes of observation, and her O_2 saturation is now 83%.

Remembering the movie "Moulin Rouge" (which has nothing to do with this case except for hemoptysis), what is your first action in this situation?

A) Arrange emergent bronchoscopy.
B) Transfuse 2 units of blood.
C) Perform endotracheal intubation.
D) Provide bolus IV normal saline.
E) Call for emergent surgical evaluation.

Discussion

The correct answer is "C." Massive hemoptysis is variably defined as 100–600 mL of blood expectorated per day, and it can result in hemodynamic compromise and asphyxiation. Quantification of the blood loss by the patient is usually unreliable. The main cause of mortality with hemoptysis is not hypovolemia but rather asphyxiation from blood in the lungs. As with any patient in acute respiratory distress, the airway must be controlled first. The best choice here is to perform intubation. Since this patient is known to have a potential source for bleeding in the right lung, intubation of the left mainstem bronchus may protect the left lung from the blood. Also, placing this patient on her right side (so that the bleeding source is dependent) may protect the left lung. If available, emergent bronchoscopy may allow identification of the bleeding site. However, bronchoscopy is not well suited for stopping the hemorrhage. The most that a bronchoscopist can do is place an endobronchial blocker and seal off the bleeding lobe. Interventional radiology should usually be the first treatment of choice once the bleeding site has been localized. Emergent surgery is indicated if the bleeding remains brisk and not responsive to other interventions. Fluid resuscitation is important. However, before any of these other measures is undertaken, the airway must be protected.

HELPFUL TIP: It is important to understand that patients with hemoptysis do not die of exsanguination but rather drown in their own blood. The volume of blood needed to cause asphyxiation is surprisingly low and nowhere near the volumes that GI bleeders lose. Also, a low oxygen saturation will occur way before you notice any change in the hemoglobin. Therefore, serial hemoglobins make little sense in hemoptysis patients.

* *

The patient stabilizes in the ICU. You plan to start treatment for her Wegener granulomatosis. She does better and is discharged in 2 days.

HELPFUL TIP: The 5-year mortality of untreated Wegener granulomatosis is 90%. These patients need aggressive treatment.

Cyclophosphamide + steroids seem to be the best combination.

Objectives: Did you learn to . . .

- Perform an appropriate evaluation on a patient with hemoptysis?
- Recognize the major causes of hemoptysis?
- Diagnose Wegener granulomatosis?
- Identify and treat massive hemoptysis?

CASE 9

A 35-year-old African American female presents with dyspnea worsening over the last 2 months. She also complains of cough, generalized fatigue, and intermittent low-grade fevers. She does not smoke. Chest x-ray shows hilar adenopathy and small bilateral pleural effusions. Spirometry is consistent with a restrictive pattern.

Of the following, which is the most likely diagnosis?

A) Wegener granulomatosis.
B) Sarcoidosis.
C) Bronchogenic carcinoma.
D) Pneumonia.
E) Microscopic polyangiitis.

Discussion

The correct answer is "B." The findings of hilar lymphadenopathy and a restrictive pattern on spirometry are most consistent with sarcoidosis. The chest x-ray findings do not support the diagnosis of Wegener granulomatosis. Besides, it can't be "A"—we just did that case (and when would you see two Wegener's cases in a row—let alone in your career?). "E" is incorrect. Microscopic polyangiitis is a systemic vasculitis related to Wegener granulomatosis, presenting with similar features as Wegener granulomatosis but without granulomatous disease. Bronchogenic carcinoma is unlikely in this relatively young nonsmoker. The clinical history is not typical of pneumonia, and chest x-ray shows no infiltrate. Tuberculosis, although not an answer option, should also be considered, and the appropriate history and testing should be completed. In fact, TB and sarcoidosis often present in a similar fashion.

Which of the following is NOT commonly associated with sarcoidosis?

A) Hypercalcemia.
B) Elevated ACE levels.
C) Reduced diffusion capacity.
D) Hypothyroidism.
E) Facial or peripheral nerve palsy.

Discussion
The correct answer is "D." Sarcoidosis is marked by the presence of noncaseating granulomas. While sarcoid can infiltrate the thyroid, it rarely, if ever, causes hypothyroidism. Pulmonary sarcoidosis includes a decreased diffusion capacity and decreased vital capacity. Other laboratory findings include hypercalcemia, hypercalciuria, elevated liver and pancreatic enzymes, and elevated ACE levels. Neurologic involvement occurs in up to 5% of patients and frequently presents as facial paralysis but may present as any CNS lesion. Peripheral nerves may also be involved.

Which of the following is NOT found as a part of sarcoidosis?

A) Erythema nodosum.
B) Myocardial infarction.
C) Cardiac arrhythmias.
D) Elevated liver enzymes.
E) Vision loss.

Discussion
The correct answer is "B." Sarcoidosis does not cause myocardial infarctions. While there is cardiac involvement with sarcoidosis, the manifestations are bundle branch block, cardiac arrhythmias, and sudden death. Many organs can be affected by sarcoidosis, including the skin, eye (iritis), heart, lung, liver, nervous system—essentially anywhere granulomas form.

Which of the following is true about ACE levels in sarcoidosis?

A) An elevated ACE level is specific for sarcoidosis.
B) ACE levels often correlates with disease severity in sarcoidosis.
C) ACE inhibitors are effective in the treatment of sarcoidosis.
D) All of the above.

Discussion
The correct answer is "B." One can follow ACE levels to track the progress of the disease. However, since treatment is based on symptoms, following ACE levels is not recommended. "A" is incorrect. ACE levels may be elevated in silicosis, miliary TB, and asbestosis, among others. "C" is incorrect. ACE inhibitors are not used to treat sarcoidosis.

* *

This patient is found to have only pulmonary sarcoidosis with some mild systemic symptoms.

Which of the following is the best initial choice for management?

A) Observation.
B) Oral corticosteroids.
C) Oral antibiotics.
D) Inhaled corticosteroids.
E) Methotrexate.

Discussion
The correct answer is "A." This patient has apparent pulmonary-limited disease and has minimal systemic symptoms. Nearly 50% of patients with sarcoidosis may have spontaneous resolution of their symptoms without treatment. *In fact, treatment may actually prolong the disease process.* If her pulmonary or systemic symptoms worsen or are causing major life problems, she should be started on oral steroids. Systemic corticosteroid therapy is the mainstay of treatment for sarcoidosis. Methotrexate and other immune-modulating drugs may be employed as well and offer a steroid-sparing effect, but these are not first-line agents. Evidence for the use of inhaled corticosteroids is lacking. Antibiotics are not effective.

Objectives: Did you learn to . . .

- Recognize the clinical manifestations of sarcoidosis?
- Manage a patient with mild sarcoidosis?

CASE 10

A 57-year-old male with no prior medical history comes in to clinic with a 1-week history of right rib pain and low back pain. The rib pain is worse with deep breaths and especially bothers him at night. There has been no trauma. He has lost 20 pounds in the last 3 months. He has a cough productive of white sputum. He denies any other symptoms. He smokes one to two packs of cigarettes per day but does not drink alcohol.

* *

Vital signs: temperature 36.5°C, pulse rate 95, blood pressure 110/70, respiratory rate 16. On room air, his oxygen saturation is 96%. There is no adenopathy. His lung sounds are clear on the left and decreased on the right. There is dullness to percussion and decreased tactile fremitus over the right lower lung field.

Based on this patient's history and physical exam, what do you expect to find on chest x-ray?

A) Normal chest x-ray.
B) Cavitary lung lesion.
C) Pleural effusion.
D) Expanded lung fields.
E) Pneumothorax.

Discussion

The correct answer is "C." This patient's findings suggest pleural effusion. Everything is diminished in pleural effusion: there is dullness to percussion, decreased breath sounds, decreased tactile fremitus, and decreased voice transmission. A cavitary lung lesion presents with either a normal exam or findings similar to an infiltrate (e.g., crackles, increased fremitus, and dullness to percussion). Expanded lung fields on chest x-ray are often seen in patients with COPD or asthma, and exam findings include prolonged expiratory phase, wheezing, and resonance to percussion. Pneumothorax presents with hyperresonance to percussion, decreased breath sounds, and decreased fremitus.

HELPFUL TIP: Chest radiographs have a low sensitivity for rib fractures. However, this is really not a problem. The presence or absence of a rib fracture is generally immaterial. What we are interested in is whether or not there is anything underlying the rib fracture, such as a pulmonary contusion or hemothorax.

* *

Your suspicions are confirmed. The chest x-ray shows obliteration of the right hemidiaphragm, and the posterior costophrenic angle is obscured on the lateral view, consistent with pleural effusion. There is also a right upper-lobe lung mass.

Which of the following will provide most information and guidance for your thoracentesis?

A) Supine chest x-ray.
B) Chest CT.
C) Lateral decubitus chest x-ray.
D) Chest ultrasound.
E) Apical view chest radiograph.

Discussion

The correct answer is "D." Prior to performing a thoracentesis, you must know whether the effusion is loculated or freely flowing. Portable ultrasound has become a validated and widely accepted modality to diagnose and access a pleural effusion. Also, ultrasonography has been found to be more sensitive for detection of pleural fluid than a chest radiograph. Chest CT is somewhat more sensitive but far more cumbersome and does not allow a bedside diagnosis and treatment. A decubitus film, with the affected side down, would allow you see the effusion "layer out" unless it is loculated but again is less sensitive. A supine chest x-ray may cause the effusion to "layer out" too, but you will not be able to see it as well, which is why effusions may be missed when a patient is unable to stand or sit upright for his x-ray.

Relative and absolute contraindications to thoracentesis include all of the following EXCEPT:

A) Herpes zoster in the area of needle placement.
B) Coagulopathy.
C) Diaphragmatic rupture.
D) Positive pressure ventilation.
E) History of recurrent laryngeal nerve injury or compromise.

Discussion

The correct answer is "E." Absolute contraindications include chest wall compromise (e.g., burn, cellulitis, herpes zoster, ruptured diaphragm) and cases where chest tube thoracostomy would be more appropriate. Relative contraindications are poor patient cooperation, coagulopathy, anticoagulation therapy, very small effusions (<10 mm on decubitus film view), positive pressure ventilation, and pleural adhesions.

* *

On ultrasound, the effusion appears free floating and not loculated.

What is the next most appropriate step?

A) Referral for surgical drainage.
B) Place a chest tube to drain the effusion.
C) Perform an ultrasound-guided diagnostic thoracentesis at the bedside.
D) Order two pizzas, one for you and one for the patient (you have both had a long day and are hungry).

Discussion

The correct answer is "C." The patient has a relatively large pleural effusion. Ultrasound-guided thoracentesis is a good first step in evaluating this effusion. Referral to a thoracic surgeon may eventually be necessary, but this would not be the first step. Placing a chest tube into an effusion is not recommended at this point, and the diagnostic study should be obtained first. Note that with large effusions, ultrasound guidance is unnecessary.

* *

Ultrasound-guided thoracentesis is successful in obtaining fluid. The fluid is amber and cloudy, with a pH 7.3, LDH 800 IU/L, glucose 65 mg/dL, total protein 5.5 g/dL, WBC 1300/mm^3, RBC 50,000/mm^3. *Serum* studies done the same day include LDH 155 IU/L, glucose 99 mg/dL, and total protein 7.0 g/dL. Cytology, Gram stain, and culture of the pleural fluid are pending.

Which of the following is the most accurate statement regarding the pleural fluid analysis?

A) The fluid is due to infection.
B) The fluid is due to cancer.
C) The fluid is a transudate.
D) The fluid is an exudate.
E) The fluid is orange juice.

Discussion

The correct answer is "D." Pleural effusions are broadly categorized as exudates and transudates (see Tables 3–5 and 3–6). Such a categorization helps to narrow the differential diagnosis. In this case, several elements of the pleural fluid are consistent with an exudate.

LDH and protein can be used to determine whether the pleural fluid is transudative or exudative. A pleural fluid LDH >2/3, the upper limit of normal serum LDH, a pleural LDH:serum LDH ratio >0.6, and a pleural protein:serum protein ratio >0.5 are all suggestive of an exudate. All three of these indicators point to an exudate in this case. Also, exudative effusions tend to have a higher degree of cellularity than transudative effusions. With the information given, it is difficult to determine if the effusion is related to infection, cancer, or some other process.

Table 3–5 CATEGORIZATION OF PLEURAL FLUID AS AN EXUDATE OR TRANSUDATE

Exudate characterized by
- Pleural fluid to serum protein ratio >0.5
- Pleural fluid to serum LDH ratio >0.6
- Pleural fluid LDH greater than 150 mg/dL (two-thirds the upper limit of normal serum LDH)

Table 3–6 CATEGORIZATION OF PLEURAL EFFUSIONS BY CLASS (TRANSUDATIVE VS. EXUDATIVE)

Type of Effusion	Potential Causes
Transudative effusions	Heart failure, cirrhosis, nephritic syndrome, atelectasis, myxedema, pulmonary embolism, urinothorax
Exudative effusions	Bronchogenic carcinoma, metastatic neoplasm, mesothelioma, pneumonia, TB, chylothorax, pancreatitis, esophageal rupture, collagen vascular diseases (rheumatoid arthritis, Sjogren syndrome), trauma, drugs (nitrofurantoin, amiodarone, methotrexate), heart failure with diuretic therapy, pulmonary embolism

Note: CHF and PE can cause exudative and transudative effusions.

* *

The pleural fluid cytology comes back negative. The patient's symptoms and exam have not changed. Repeat radiograph still shows an upper lobe mass.

What is the most appropriate next step in approaching this pleural effusion?

A) Await pleural fluid culture results.
B) Perform bedside chest tube drainage of the effusion.
C) Refer for surgical evacuation of the effusion.
D) Refer for bronchoscopy.
E) Place a chest tube for chemical pleurodesis.

Discussion

The correct answer is "D." The effusion is clearly exudative, and the patient appears to have a lung mass. Biopsy of the lung mass via bronchoscopy is indicated. A negative pleural fluid cytology does not rule out lung cancer. Positive cytology indicates advanced stage lung cancer. Chest tube drainage of a pleural effusion is not recommended except under extraordinary circumstances. Intermittent thoracentesis is preferred and has lower morbidity. Surgical evacuation of the fluid would be indicated if the patient were symptomatic, the effusion was loculated and/or related to infection. If the effusion grows, or is drained and recurs, it may respond to pleurodesis. Otherwise, pleurodesis is not indicated at this time.

> HELPFUL TIP: Patients with malignant pleural effusions are not likely to benefit from surgery since the tumor is not localized and is not resectable by this point. Long-term outcomes with a malignant pleural effusion are bleak.

* *

Now that you have gained expertise with ultrasound of a pleural effusion, your colleague sends you a patient that has a pleural effusion on chest x-ray. Your colleague asks you whether you could "tap" the fluid for him as he does not feel comfortable with the portable ultrasound... Also, he has a tee time in 30 minutes.

On ultrasound, you quickly visualize the chest and see a septated and loculated pleural effusion. What is the next best step?

A) Return the patient back to his doctor--the effusion is too small to access.
B) Perform ultrasound-guided needle thoracentesis.
C) Refer to a thoracic surgeon.
D) Place a small-bore chest tube.
E) Head to the golf course with your colleague. Nothing you can do here.

Discussion

The correct answer is "C." A loculated and septated pleural effusion can very often be seen in empyema and evacuation usually requires surgical intervention. Thoracentesis would unlikely be successful and would expose the patient to an unnecessary procedure after which he would still need to see a surgeon. Placing a chest tube blindly into a loculated pleural effusion is unsafe. That procedure should be done under visualization; most commonly, video-assisted thoracic surgery (VATS) would be utilized.

Objectives: Did you learn to . . .

- Recognize the historical and physical exam findings of pleural effusion?
- List potential etiologies of pleural effusion?
- Narrow the differential diagnosis based on pleural fluid findings?
- Decide when to perform diagnostic and therapeutic thoracentesis?
- Decide when to perform chest tube drainage?

CASE 11

A 60-year-old male presents to the ED for a cough. His symptoms began with a cold 2 weeks ago, and the other symptoms have improved, but the cough has persisted. He has mild production of white sputum with no hemoptysis. The patient denies fevers, night sweats, chills, and weight loss. He's had no chest pain or dyspnea. He smokes one pack of cigarettes per day, works in construction, and does not have a regular doctor. In fact, with some pride, he says, "I haven't seen a doctor in over 30 years." On physical examination, you find a fit-appearing male in no acute distress. His vital signs are normal. His lung sounds are diminished bilaterally, but the remainder of the exam is unremarkable. While breathing ambient air, the patient's oxygen saturation is 94%. You obtain a chest x-ray, which is shown in Figure 3–6.

Your next step is to:

A) Prescribe a 5-day course of azithromycin.
B) Refer the patient to a pulmonologist.
C) Order a high-resolution CT scan of the chest.
D) Have the patient return to you in 3 months to repeat a chest x-ray.
E) Reassure the patient and have him return as needed.

Discussion

The correct answer is "C." The chest x-ray in Figure 3–6 shows a single nodule in the right lower lobe. The nodule is round, less dense than bone, and appears to be >1 cm in diameter. These are sometimes called "coin lesions." There are no other abnormalities. The

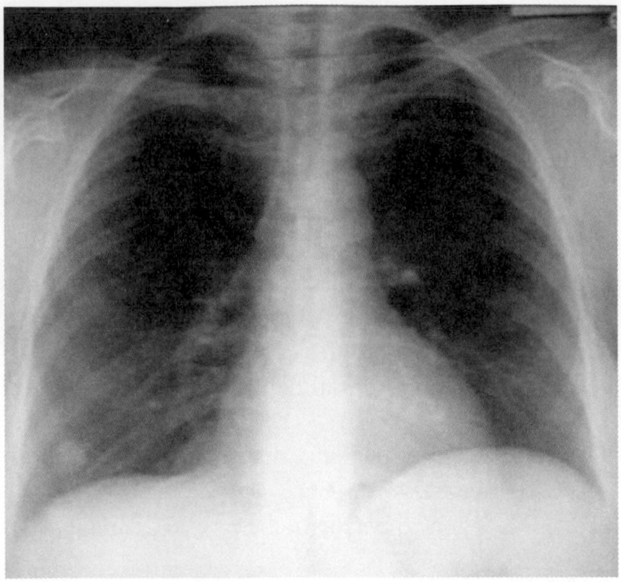

Figure 3–6

most appropriate next step in the evaluation is to order a high-resolution CT scan of the chest. Treatment with azithromycin is inappropriate in this setting, as this patient has no signs of pulmonary infection on exam or chest x-ray. Referral to a pulmonologist is premature without first investigating the nodule by CT scan. Delaying further imaging and evaluation is also inappropriate since 15–75% of solitary pulmonary nodules (SPNs) ≥8 mm are ultimately diagnosed as cancer.

Which of the following is NOT considered a benign pattern of calcification on CT scan?

A) Diffuse, homogeneous calcification.
B) Central calcification.
C) Laminar calcification.
D) Spiculated, irregular calcification.
E) "Popcorn" calcification.

Discussion
The correct answer is "D." We are accustomed to thinking of calcified nodules as being benign, but that is not always the case. Irregular, spiculated calcification is not reassuring. The other answer choices are considered indicative of a benign lesion. Two patterns on CT are relatively specific for cancer: a scalloped border and the corona radiata sign, which is composed of fine linear strands extending out from the nodule.

All of the following are useful to help assess the risk of cancer in a patient with an SPN EXCEPT:

A) Smoking status.
B) Age.
C) Diameter of the nodule.
D) Gender.

Discussion
The correct answer is "D." Determining the probability of cancer in patients with an SPN is an inexact science. The risk of cancer is generally assessed as low, intermediate, or high based on patient and radiograph characteristics. Although men are slightly overrepresented in lung cancer diagnoses, this is generally thought to be due to greater smoking rates in men and to occupational hazards. Gender itself does not help to risk-stratify patients with an SPN. Smoking increases the risk of an SPN being cancer, with greater use increasing the risk of cancer. As with most cancers, increasing age is associated with a higher risk. The diameter of the nodule is also important. If the diameter is <8 mm, the risk of cancer is low. When the diameter is ≥3 cm, the SPN is now referred to as a "pulmonary mass" and is highly likely to be cancerous. SPN >3 cm in diameter should be considered cancer until proven otherwise.

The Fleischner Society has published a set of widely accepted recommendations regarding follow-up of single pulmonary nodules *noted on CT* chest that are <8 mm in diameter. Please see Table 3–7.

* *

Later that week, your patient returns with his CT scan in hand. His cough is somewhat better (therapeutic CT scan radiation therapy . . . you know, like those CT scans in California that were cooking people's brains accidentally?). You review the CT scan with him. It shows a round, smooth nodule measuring 2 cm in diameter and located in the periphery of the right lower lobe. There are no calcifications in the nodule and no other abnormalities.

Which of the following is the most appropriate next step?

A) Referral for bronchoscopy.
B) High-resolution CT scan every 3 months.
C) Chest x-ray every 3 months.
D) Bone scan.
E) Referral to a thoracic surgeon.

Discussion
The correct answer is "E." This patient needs a biopsy. There are several factors that put your patient

Table 3–7 RECOMMENDATIONS FOR FOLLOW-UP AND MANAGEMENT OF NODULES SMALLER THAN 8 MM DETECTED INCIDENTALLY AT NONSCREENING CT

Nodule Size (mm)	Low-Risk Patients	High-Risk Patients
≤4	No follow-up needed	Follow-up at 12 months. If no change, no further imaging needed
>4–6	Follow-up at 12 months. If no change, no further imaging needed	Initial follow-up CT at 6–12 months and then at 18–24 months if no change
>6–8	Initial follow-up CT at 6–12 months and then at 18–24 months if no change	Initial follow-up CT at 3–6 months and then at 9–12 and 24 months if no change
>8	Follow-up CTs at around 3, 9, and 24 months. Dynamic contrast enhanced CT, PET, and/or biopsy	Same as for low-risk patients

Notes: These guidelines apply to newly detected indeterminate nodules in persons 35 years of age or older. Low-risk patients have minimal or absent history of smoking and no other known risk factors. High-risk patients have a history of smoking or of other known risk factors.

at higher risk of having a malignant cause for the SPN, including his age and tobacco use. These put him into an intermediate- to high-risk category for cancer. Although the nodule is smooth on CT, its size is >8 mm and there are no calcifications. This patient should be referred for transthoracic fine-needle biopsy or open biopsy. "A" is tempting but incorrect. Bronchoscopy is insensitive in the peripheral lung, especially when the lesion is relatively small. "B" and "C" are also wrong here but are appropriate in other settings. In this case, repeat imaging over time may delay a diagnosis of malignancy. Without symptoms of bone pain or confirmation that the SPN is a cancer that might metastasize to bone, a bone scan will have a very low yield.

* *

Your patient returns from the surgeon much relieved. Fine-needle biopsy proved the SPN to be a hamartoma. Now your patient wants to quit smoking for good, and he thinks that he will need some assistance. You recommend nicotine replacement products and bupropion, but your patient claims to have had an allergic reaction to bupropion. Fortunately, you know of an effective alternative (unless he is a homicidal maniac . . . it happens you know).

To assist with tobacco cessation, you prescribe which of the following?

A) Varenicline.
B) Fluoxetine.
C) Olanzapine.
D) Metoprolol.
E) Clonidine.

Discussion

The correct answer is "A." Randomized trials have demonstrated the effectiveness of the nicotine partial agonist, varenicline (Chantix™). This FDA-approved medication appears to be at least as effective as bupropion as an aid to smoking cessation. Fluoxetine and other selective serotonin reuptake inhibitors have not demonstrated a benefit. In schizophrenic patients, the use of atypical antipsychotic medications may aid in smoking cessation when compared with typical antipsychotics. Clonidine is sometimes used to help patients who are withdrawing from narcotics, and it may have some limited role in smoking cessation but is not very effective. Depression, very vivid dreams or nightmares, aggressive behavior, etc., are a common side effect of varenicline and your patients should be informed of that prior to prescribing the drug.

HELPFUL TIP (REALLY): Cytisine, an "alternative" medicine, has actually been shown to have benefit in smoking cessation. It is a partial nicotine agonist and is much less expensive than alternatives (*N Engl J Med* 2011;365:1193-1200).

Objectives: Did you learn to . . .

- Weigh risk factors when evaluating an SPN?
- Develop a plan for evaluating a solitary pulmonary nodule?
- Assist a patient with smoking cessation?

CASE 12

A 74-year-old male presents to your ED for weakness, cough, and fatigue. His wife relates an incomplete recovery since his myocardial infarction last year. He continues to have poor appetite and listlessness, and she thinks that he may be depressed. He is short of breath and confused. His wife says that yesterday he developed a fever, chills, and a new cough productive of white sputum. His past medical history is otherwise remarkable for a cholecystectomy. He is taking aspirin, metoprolol, and simvastatin.

Vitals: temperature 39°C, respiratory rate 30, pulse rate 90, blood pressure 140/80. Oxygen saturation on room air is 90%. He is thin, pale, and oriented to person only. The lung examination is remarkable for rales in the left lower field, with dullness to percussion and increased tactile fremitus. The remainder of the exam is normal.

The chest x-ray shows a left lower lobe infiltrate. Other laboratory data currently available: hemoglobin 12.4 g/dL, WBC 14,100/mm^3, platelets 340,000/mm^3, creatinine 1.9 mg/dL, BUN 50 mg/dL, and normal electrolytes, troponin, and CK. An ECG shows normal sinus rhythm.

What is your next step in managing this patient's medical condition?

A) Place a chest tube on the left.
B) Perform chest CT.
C) Administer inhaled bronchodilators.
D) Administer parenteral antibiotics.
E) Perform intubation and mechanical ventilation.

Discussion

The correct answer is "D." Given the clinical picture and chest x-ray findings, the patient most likely has community-acquired pneumonia. Therefore, the administration of parenteral antibiotics is the best choice. "A" is incorrect. Since there is no effusion, a chest tube would be useless. "B" is incorrect. CT is not required in this straightforward case of pneumonia. "C" is incorrect. The patient is not wheezing and there is no indication for bronchodilators at this time. As for "E," since your patient's respiratory status is stable, he does not require intubation.

HELPFUL TIP: Remember that it is impossible to tell a "typical" versus an "atypical" pneumonia by radiograph. Do not base your therapy for community-acquired pneumonia on the radiographic appearance. Atypical organisms can cause lobar consolidation and typical pneumonias can appear diffuse. Note that treatment guidelines make no mention of radiographic appearance.

HELPFUL TIP: The pneumonia severity index is a popular guideline used for deciding whether or not to admit a patient with pneumonia. However, it is so cumbersome that nobody can remember it. Look it up (http://pda.ahrq.gov/clinic/psi/psicalc.asp or http://internalmedicine.osu.edu/pulmonary/cap/10675.cfm, and there is always Wikipedia!).

HELPFUL TIP: A simpler but less well-validated tool exists for determining disposition in a patient with pneumonia—the "CURB-65." Catchy name, too, eh? Here are the variables:

*C*onfusion (based on a specific mental test or disorientation to person, place, or time).

*U*rea (BUN) $>$20 mg/dL.

*R*espiratory rate $>$30 breaths/min.

*B*lood pressure $<$90/60.

*A*ge $>$65 years.

Patients with a score of 0 or 1 have a low risk of death.

Based on patient-specific characteristics and your knowledge of causative factors involved in pneumonia, which of the following is LEAST likely to be the agent causing this patient's infection?

A) *Mycoplasma pneumoniae.*
B) *S. pneumoniae.*
C) *Haemophilus influenzae.*
D) *Pseudomonas aeruginosa.*

Discussion

The correct answer is "D." When a pathogen is identified in adult community-acquired pneumonia, it is usually *S. pneumoniae*. In fact, *S. pneumonia* makes up 40–60% of all cases of community-acquired pneumonia in the elderly. Nontypeable *H. influenzae* composes about 5–10% of cases. Mycoplasma is implicated in 5% of all cases of pneumonia in adults, and it is more common in young adults. *P. aeruginosa* pneumonia is uncommon in healthy elders and more likely to occur in patients with serious underlying lung disease or immunodeficiency. Approximately 5% of patients or more are infected with multiple agents.

On the basis of your assessment of his risk, you decide to admit this patient to the hospital. An IV is in place. Which of the following IV antibiotic regimens do you choose?

A) Penicillin.
B) Azithromycin.
C) Penicillin and gentamicin.
D) Azithromycin and ceftriaxone.
E) Piperacillin/tazobactam and ciprofloxacin.

Discussion

The correct answer is "D." The updated 2007 IDSA/ATS guidelines for pneumonia did not call for significant changes in the approach to treatment. For community-acquired pneumonia treated in the hospital setting, the optimal antibiotic regimen must offer good coverage of *S. pneumoniae*, *H. influenzae*, and atypical organisms such as *Mycoplasma* and *Chlamydia* species. Most *S. pneumoniae* bacteria are resistant to penicillin and about 20–30% are resistant to macrolides such as azithromycin. Therefore, these agents should not be used alone in the treatment of pneumonia in hospitalized patients. Gentamicin has no activity against *S. pneumoniae* but has a role in *P. aeruginosa* infections. Ceftriaxone offers good gram-negative coverage and activity against *S. pneumoniae*. Azithromycin covers atypical organisms. For these reasons, "D" is the best choice. An alternative regimen would be monotherapy with a respiratory fluoroquinolone such as moxifloxacin or levofloxacin. The combination of piperacillin/tazobactam with ciprofloxacin is reserved for patients with more severe pneumonia, requiring ventilation and ICU care.

* *

Initial blood cultures grow *S. pneumoniae*. Sputum Gram stain and culture are negative. The patient initially does well and defervesces after 2 days of IV antibiotics. However, on day 3, he again spikes a fever. He looks moderately ill. Your exam reveals increased dullness to percussion on the left. There is no jugular venous distention (JVD) or peripheral edema. The radiograph is shown in Figure 3–7.

The most likely diagnosis at this point is:

A) Anaerobic abscess.
B) Development of resistant *S. pneumoniae*.
C) Parapneumonic effusion.
D) Transudate secondary to heart failure.
E) Drug-induced transudate.

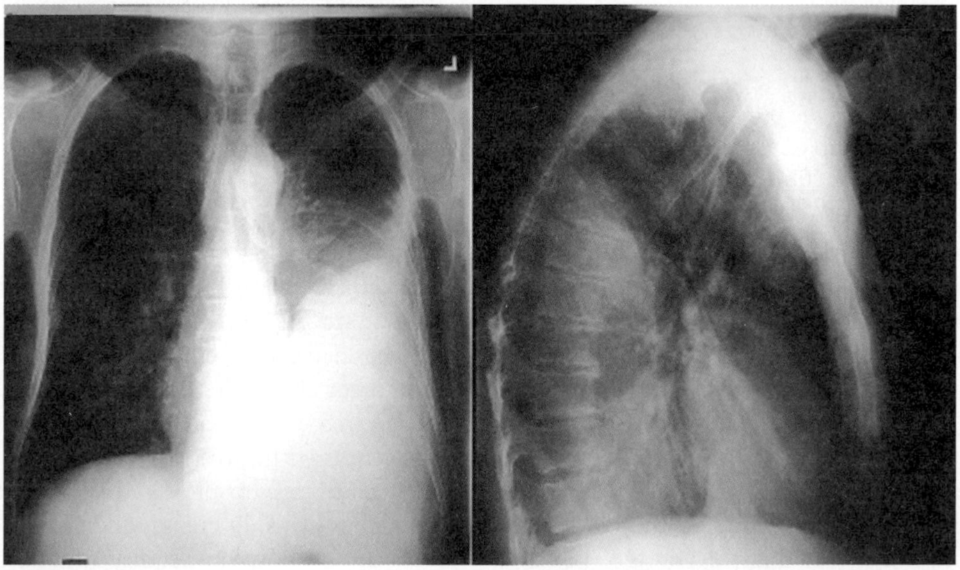

Figure 3–7

Discussion

The correct answer is "C." The most likely problem in this patient is a parapneumonic effusion. "A," an anaerobic abscess, is unlikely given that there are no air/fluid levels and the fact that the fluid appears to be in the pleura. "B" is unlikely. Development of resistance should take more than 3 days, especially since this patient is on two drugs. "D" is unlikely given that this patient does not have a history of CHF, is febrile, and has no JVD, etc. "E" is unlikely. None of the drugs that he is on is known to cause pleural effusions.

* *

You place a chest tube to drain the (nonloculated on ultrasound) pleural effusion and continue the current antibiotic regimen. The patient does well and is discharged 1 week later on clarithromycin after sensitivities conclude that his organism is sensitive.

Six weeks after the onset of illness, he returns for follow-up to ensure clearing of the chest x-ray. He is feeling well. He is alert and oriented, and his lung exam is now normal. There is no lymphadenopathy in the neck or supraclavicular areas. The x-ray still shows left lower lobe infiltrate, unchanged in size from the initial x-ray. The pleural effusion has resolved.

Which of the following is the most appropriate next step in the evaluation and management of this patient?

A) Chest CT.
B) Chest x-ray in 2 weeks.
C) Chest x-ray in 6 weeks.
D) Prescribe amoxicillin/clavulanate.

Discussion

The correct answer is "C." There are no clear guidelines regarding follow-up chest x-ray in patients who had pneumonia. British Thoracic Society published recommendations in 2007 where it advised repeating chest x-ray in 6 weeks in patients with a smoking history. The reason for that recommendation is a chance that the infiltrate would obscure an underlying malignancy. Also, age 50 is the recommended threshold for a follow-up repeat x-ray. Bacteremic pneumococcal pneumonia has been associated with very slowly clearing x-rays, up to 3–5 months in some cases. Thus, repeating the chest x-ray in 2 weeks is unlikely to show resolution. In elderly patients, the chest x-ray takes longer to normalize than in younger patients. The patient is clinically doing well, and does not require treatment for a persistent pulmonary infection. Chest CT would give more information, but in the absence of systemic symptoms, such as weight loss, persistent cough, hemoptysis, or fever, it is unlikely to change the management at this point. It is important to consider the fact that this "infiltrate" may represent a neoplastic process if it does not resolve within several months.

HELPFUL TIP: Even with extensive evaluation (blood culture, sputum culture, etc.), an infectious agent is only identified in 50% of cases of pneumonia. Thus, treatment is usually empiric. Sputum cultures do not alter antibiotic therapy or disease outcome in most patients with pneumonia, and 30% of patients with pneumonia are not able to produce sputum. Blood cultures are of little or no value in pneumonia but are still recommended in most guidelines for hospitalized patients. If possible, do blood cultures before initiating therapy.

* *

Your patient returns a week later looking ill. He has dyspnea, fever, and worsening cough. His temperature in the office is 39°C, and he has a new infiltrate on chest x-ray.

This situation is best described as:

A) Community-acquired pneumonia.
B) Double pneumonia.
C) Hospital-acquired pneumonia.
D) Healthcare-associated pneumonia.
E) Triple pneumonia.

Discussion

The correct answer is "D." The 2005 IDSA/ATS guidelines define high-risk pneumonia based on setting. Healthcare-associated pneumonia is defined as pneumonia occurring in a nonhospitalized patient who has had extensive healthcare contact (meaning IV therapy or chemotherapy within the last 30 days, residence in a nursing home, attendance at a hemodialysis center within the last 30 days, or 2 or more days in an acute care hospital in the last 90 days). Your patient meets this definition due to his recent hospitalization. "C," hospital-acquired pneumonia, is one that develops 48 hours or more after admission to a hospital and did *not* appear to be brewing at the time of admission. The guidelines also distinguish ventilator-associated pneumonia, which occurs in patients 48 hours or more after endotracheal intubation. "B" and "E" are fake foils. Sorry!

Now that he has healthcare-associated pneumonia, you order the appropriate antibiotic regimen consisting of:

A) Linezolid and amphotericin B.
B) Cefepime.
C) Gentamicin and vancomycin.
D) Ciprofloxacin.

Discussion

The correct answer is "B." Since he has received antibiotics in the last 90 days, an antipseudomonal cephalosporin is indicated. Depending on circumstances, other antibiotics may be added to broaden empiric coverage. For example, if there are high levels of resistance to gram-negative bacilli in the area, add an aminoglycoside. If MRSA is suspected, add linezolid or vancomycin. If legionella is likely, add a fluoroquinolone. In this scenario, "A" is incorrect because it doesn't cover pseudomonas and a fungal infection is not likely in this unimmunosuppressed patient. The same is true of "C." "D" may be arguable but is not the preferred empiric choice according to the 2005 IDSA/ATS guidelines. Most important: know your local resistance patterns and your patient's specific characteristics.

HELPFUL TIP: Although infrequently a cause of routine community-acquired pneumonia, *Staphylococcus aureus* is a common cause of bacterial pneumonia during influenza epidemics.

HELPFUL TIP: Proton pump inhibitors and H_2-blockers are associated with an increased risk of pneumonia. Stop them when you can.

* *

In one of life's funny little coincidences, the next day you diagnose this patient's 36-year-old healthy son with a community-acquired pneumonia. Besides a fever, cough, and left lower lobe infiltrate on chest x-ray, he's feeling fine.

Which of the following drug regimens is appropriate for the treatment of this patient in the outpatient setting?

A) Cephalexin 250–500 mg PO QID for 10 days.
B) Penicillin V 250 mg TID for 10 days.
C) Clarithromycin 500 mg BID for 10 days.
D) Doxycycline 100 mg BID for 10 days.
E) C or D.

Discussion

The correct answer is "E." The treatment of community-acquired pneumonia requires coverage of "typical" and "atypical" organisms. Neither "A" nor "B" covers atypical organisms. Guideline-recommended choices for the outpatient treatment of community-acquired pneumonia include doxycycline and macrolides such as clarithromycin. Additional options include the respiratory fluoroquinolones such as moxifloxacin, gemifloxacin, or levofloxacin. However, respiratory fluoroquinolones should not be used in all cases. The IDSA/ATS consensus guidelines recommend that respiratory fluoroquinolones be reserved for patients with serious underlying disease (e.g., COPD, diabetes, immunocompromised states). Of the appropriate regimens, doxycycline and erythromycin are the least expensive, but erythromycin is associated with a high rate of gastrointestinal intolerance.

HELPFUL TIP: 2007 IDSA/ATS guidelines recommend treating patients with CAP for the minimum duration of 5 days. However, prior to discontinuation of treatment, they should also be afebrile for 48–72 hours and should have no more than one of the following criteria of instability: heart rate >100, respiratory rate >24, systolic blood pressure <90, O_2 saturation $<90\%$ on room air, PaO_2 <60 mm Hg on room air, inability to maintain oral intake, confusion. Should the patient have more than one of these criteria, longer antimicrobial therapy is indicated (and hopefully you don't still have them in the community!).

Objectives: Did you learn to . . .

- Recognize the clinical presentation of community-acquired pneumonia in different patient populations?
- Determine the appropriate disposition for a patient with community-acquired pneumonia?
- Initiate outpatient and inpatient treatment for community-acquired pneumonia?

CASE 13

While you are covering the ED, a 60-year-old female comes in by ambulance. She is unresponsive, and her husband states that he found her 30 minutes ago surrounded by bottles of pills and an empty bottle of vodka. She has a history of COPD, hypertension, osteoarthritis, and depression. The EMTs brought in her pill bottles, which include lorazepam, acetaminophen/hydrocodone, hydrochlorothiazide, aspirin, and nortriptyline. Only a few tablets are left in the bottle of hydrochlorothiazide. She is wearing a non-rebreather face mask with 50% oxygen. Her respirations are shallow with a rate of 8. The remainder of her vitals: temperature 36°C, blood pressure 90/50, and pulse rate 90. Oxygen saturation is 88% and increases to 94% with some assisted breaths. One nurse is obtaining a blood gas while another gives naloxone. You decide that this patient cannot protect her airway and choose to intubate her.

The blood gas drawn just before intubation shows pH 7.16, $PaCO_2$ 60 mm Hg, PaO_2 40 mm Hg.

These findings imply which of the following processes?

A) Metabolic acidosis.
B) Metabolic alkalosis.
C) Respiratory alkalosis.
D) Mixed metabolic/respiratory acidosis.
E) Mixed metabolic/respiratory alkalosis.

Discussion

The correct answer is "D." The pH is acidotic (<7.4). In a patient whose baseline $PaCO_2$ is not known to you, you might assume her $PaCO_2$ is usually 40 mm Hg, which is the accepted normal for most patients.

If this is true and the acidosis is purely due to acute respiratory changes, a rise in $PaCO_2$ should be accompanied by a fall in pH equal to $0.08 \times$ (change in $PaCO_2$ from baseline) $= 0.08 \times 20 = 0.16$, resulting in a pH of 7.24.

However, this patient's pH is measured at 7.16, lower than expected for a pure respiratory acidosis presenting acutely. Thus, you can determine that the acidosis is both metabolic (perhaps from lactic acidosis from hypoperfusion) and respiratory.

> HELPFUL TIP: It is clear that low tidal volumes are protective in patients with ARDS/ALI (acute lung injury) and prevent VILI (ventilator-induced lung injury). It is unclear whether the same strategy should be employed for all the patients. There is data that shows that even slightly injured lung is more prone to VILI so it is reasonable to aim at Vt of 6–8 mL/kg of predicted body weight in all patients. Additionally, patients with asthma or COPD can quickly develop dynamic hyperinflation with higher tidal volumes. Ventilated patients with obstructive disease generally need more time for exhalation.

* *

Your patient is on assist-control mode of ventilation. A nasogastric tube, 2 IVs, and a bladder catheter are in place. Gastric lavage yielded no pill fragments, and she has received activated charcoal. She was given IV *N*-acetylcysteine. Her blood pressure has improved to 112/67, and her oxygen saturation is 99%. Her chest x-ray shows an endotracheal tube terminating 3 cm above the carina and no infiltrates. Thirty minutes after you intubated her, with the ventilator rate at 14 breaths/min, FiO_2 100%, and tidal volume at 400 mL, you obtain another ABG: pH 7.35, $PaCO_2$ 45, PaO_2 130. She takes 6–8 spontaneous, assisted breaths, while the ventilator provides the remaining breaths. She appears to be perfusing her periphery well.

It turns out that the patient did not take a tricyclic overdose. Her main problems are alcohol, acetaminophen, and narcotics.

Your next action is to:

A) Decrease the tidal volume to allow for permissive hypercapnia.
B) Increase the tidal volume to achieve a pH of 7.45–7.50.
C) Reduce FiO_2 while maintaining oxygen saturations at or above 90%.
D) Change to pressure support ventilation.

Discussion

The correct answer is "C." Your patient is perfusing well, and her PaO_2 and measured oxygen saturation are much improved. You should now decrease the FiO_2, with the goal being to achieve an FiO_2 of less than 60% while maintaining adequate perfusion and oxygen saturation. An FiO_2 of 100% is somewhat toxic and can lead to airway injury. "A" is incorrect. However, permissive hypercapnia (the CO_2 may be allowed to rise to >80 mm Hg as long as the patient tolerates it) may be useful in ventilated patients with COPD, ARDS, or asthma. But remember that you still need to maintain oxygenation. "B" is incorrect. Your patient is doing reasonably well with her slightly acidotic pH, which has corrected very quickly. It may be inadvisable to attempt to increase her pH beyond 7.40, as she may develop respiratory alkalosis that can then lead to cardiac arrhythmias. Because of her low respiratory rate, she should remain on some type of assisted volume-cycled ventilation. Pressure support ventilation, as its name implies, only augments patient-triggered breaths with increased airway pressure.

> HELPFUL TIP: Permissive hypercapnia is an approach to the ventilated patient where the physician allows CO_2 build up and decrease in pH (even down to levels of 7.1) in order to provide long expiratory times and low minute ventilation to prevent hyperinflation due to airflow obstruction.

In this patient, which of the following ventilator management techniques will unequivocally decrease her FiO_2 requirement?

A) Increase the respiratory rate.
B) Increase the positive end-expiratory pressure (PEEP).
C) Decrease the tidal volume.
D) Addition of inhaled nitric oxide (NO).

Discussion

The correct answer is "B." Two standard techniques are usually employed to improve a patient's oxygenation: increasing FiO_2 and PEEP. PEEP maintains positive pressure in the airways at the end of expiration. Its use increases lung compliance and decreases ventilation/perfusion mismatching, resulting in better oxygenation. Since FiO_2 >60% over periods longer than 48 hours may result in oxygen toxicity, PEEP may be employed to reduce the need for high levels of FiO_2. "A" and "C" are incorrect. Increasing respiratory rate or tidal volume will cause increases in minute ventilation, which reduces $PaCO_2$, but has little effect on PaO_2. Decreasing minute ventilation, through decreased respiratory rate or tidal volume, causes CO_2 retention and increased $PaCO_2$. "D" is incorrect. Nitric oxide has been shown to improve oxygenation in select patients with severe pulmonary hypertension and ARDS, but its use is not appropriate in this patient.

* *

You follow the patient during her hospitalization. The next day she is more alert and is able to follow commands. Her ventilator requirements have decreased. You consider extubation.

All of the following parameters predict a poor outcome for attempted weaning from ventilation EXCEPT:

A) Minute ventilation supplied by ventilator is <10 L/min.
B) PaO_2 <55 mm Hg while on FiO_2 >35%.
C) RSBI (rapid shallow breathing index) of 140.
D) Physical exam findings of increased respiratory effort.

Discussion

The correct answer is "A." Preparing to withdraw a patient from mechanical ventilation—typically called weaning or liberation—relies considerably on physician judgment, but a few objective parameters can be helpful. In general, the patient to be liberated must be awake, alert, and cooperative. She should have reasonably good oxygenation on a lower FiO_2, have PEEP <8 cm H_2O, and be able to generate adequate inspiratory pressures. Minute ventilation from the ventilator of less than 10 L/min is associated with greater success with weaning.

Poor prognostic indicators include a minute ventilation from the ventilator >10 L/min, PaO_2 <55 with FiO_2 >35%, and RSBI (see Helpful Tip) >105. Patients with poor cardiopulmonary reserve or who have significant underlying disease may also have difficulty weaning. Allow patients a period of breathing on their own (e.g., a T-piece) before extubating. This way, if the patient fails, you can simply hook her back up to the ventilator.

> HELPFUL TIP: RSBI is one of the predictors of successful extubation. It is calculated by dividing respiratory rate by tidal volume in liters while patient is maintained on pressure support with minimal settings (pressure of 5–10, PEEP 5–8). For example, patient breathing 20 times per minute with 500 mL Vt has RSBI of 20/0.5 = 40. Patient breathing 34 times per minute with Vt = 210 mL has RSBI of 34/0.21 = 161 and is obviously not ready to be extubated.

> HELPFUL TIP: ICU setting is much different than OR; extubations in the ICU carry higher risk of failure. Do not feel bad if your patient needs to be reintubated. There is no perfect predictor of successful ICU extubation and data shows that up to 15% of ICU patients will require reintubation despite good predictors of successful extubation.

> HELPFUL TIP: Minute ventilation (for the patient) is calculated by multiplying respiratory rate by tidal volume. Thus, a person getting 20 breaths/min from the ventilator at 400 mL/breath generates a minute ventilation = 20 × 400 = 8 L/min.

Objectives: Did you learn to . . .

- Identify patients in need of intubation and mechanical ventilation?
- Recognize a mixed respiratory/metabolic acidosis?
- Calculate expected pH changes in acute respiratory acidosis?
- Institute ventilation with appropriate initial ventilator settings?
- Identify potential complications of ventilation?
- Wean a patient from the ventilator?

CASE 14

A 52-year-old male smoker presents for a 3-month history of productive cough. He reports multiple episodes of pneumonia, but he appears healthy now. Chest x-ray is unremarkable. Chest CT shows enlarged peripheral airways with thickened airway walls in the lower lobes bilaterally. Sputum culture grows several types of bacteria, including *P. aeruginosa*.

Which of the following do you recommend as initial therapy?

A) Corticosteroids.
B) Antibiotics.
C) Chemotherapy.
D) Supplemental oxygen.
E) Wedge resection of the affected lung tissue.

Discussion

The correct answer is "B." This patient's findings are consistent with the diagnosis of bronchiectasis, a chronic inflammatory disease of the medium-sized bronchi. Appropriate initial therapy consists of prolonged courses of antibiotics, usually 2 weeks of a narrow-spectrum antibiotic followed by reassessment. Doxycycline, amoxicillin, clarithromycin, amoxicillin/clavulanate, and trimethoprim/sulfamethoxazole are often used. Respiratory quinolones demonstrate some limited use in patients with *Pseudomonas*. Patients should be directed to discontinue tobacco use and take inhaled bronchodilators. Resection of the affected lung tissue may be necessary, but should not be the initial therapy. Supplemental oxygen therapy is used if oxygenation is poor. Chemotherapy and prolonged oral corticosteroids are not used to treat bronchiectasis.

> HELPFUL TIP: Patients with bronchiectasis are often treated with intermittent or daily antibiotics to prevent acute exacerbations. One regimen is to alternate between trimethoprim/sulfamethoxazole and doxycycline, taking one of these antibiotics for the first 10–14 days of the month. The effectiveness of this intervention is not well studied.

In most adults with bronchiectasis, its cause is:

A) Genetic.
B) Pseudomonas infection.
C) Tobacco smoking.
D) Allergic bronchopulmonary aspergillosis (ABPA).
E) Unknown.

Discussion

The correct answer is "E." There are limited data regarding the etiology of bronchiectasis, but many conditions and environmental exposures seem to have an association. In most patients, no cause is identified. Children are more likely than adults to have an identified etiology of their bronchiectasis, and the most common causes in kids are foreign body aspiration, cystic fibrosis, and gastroesophageal reflux. Identified etiologies in adults include those mentioned for children and pulmonary infections, ABPA, COPD, rheumatic diseases, and cigarette smoking.

Objectives: Did you learn to . . .

- Identify findings consistent with bronchiectasis?
- Treat a patient with bronchiectasis?

QUICK QUIZ: DYSPNEA

A 75-year-old gentleman presents to your office with emphysema diagnosed elsewhere. He reports dyspnea on exertion after 1–2 blocks. He smokes 10 cigarettes per day and does not have underlying cardiac disease. Physical examination is remarkable for fine crackles in both lung bases. Chest x-ray shows increased interstitial markings in the lower lobes. He has no pulmonary function testing on record.

Of the following tests, which is the most likely to confirm or alter the diagnosis?

A) Spirometry, diffusing capacity, lung volumes.
B) Spirometry, ABG, diffusing capacity.
C) ABG, diffusing capacity, lung volumes.
D) ABG, lung volumes, chest CT.

Discussion

The correct answer is "A." This case demonstrates a commonly seen phenomenon: patients who smoke and have dyspnea are assumed to have obstructive lung disease, particularly emphysema. However, pulmonary function tests are required to make the diagnosis of obstructive disease. Furthermore, this patient's chest x-ray shows increased interstitial markings in the lower lung fields suggesting interstitial lung disease. This disease process is associated with a restrictive pattern on pulmonary spirometry. However, lung volumes and diffusing capacity will provide a more complete picture. Thus, spirometry, diffusing capacity, and lung volumes would allow you to make the diagnosis. In interstitial lung disease, spirometry shows a FEV_1/FVC ratio >0.7, a decreased diffusing capacity, and decreased TLC (the hallmark of restrictive lung disease). ABG is unlikely to help diagnose restrictive lung disease, so options "B" through "D" are not correct.

HELPFUL TIP: The diffusing capacity, as measured by DLCO, is low in the following disease states: emphysema, interstitial lung disease (e.g., sarcoid, alveolitis, pulmonary radiation, pulmonary toxicity from drugs such as amiodarone, pulmonary fibrosis), Pneumocystis pneumonia, and pulmonary vascular disease. Anemia will also cause a low DLCO—so a hemoglobin or hematocrit should always be ordered with DLCO.

HELPFUL TIP: DLCO can be *increased* by pulmonary hemorrhage, polycythemia, massive obesity, left-to-right intracardiac shunting, asthma, and left heart failure (increase capillary volume in the lungs).

QUICK QUIZ: PULMONARY INFECTIONS

A 72-year-old woman you admitted to the hospital for pneumonia is having worsening dyspnea and hypoxemia. She is decompensating despite 3 days of antibiotic therapy with intravenous levofloxacin. According to her husband, the couple had been working on their Iowa farm, and made a trip to an old barn to collect manure *a week before the patient developed a cough and fever* (so this is not hypersensitivity pneumonitis nor organic toxic dust syndrome). The barn was noted to be the home of numerous birds. Her respiratory rate is 32, and her oxygen saturation is 89% on 5 L/min of oxygen by nasal cannula. Chest x-ray reveals a diffuse interstitial infiltrate, enlarged mediastinal nodes, and normal heart size.

Which of the following is the most likely culprit for the cause of her current illness?

A) *S. pneumoniae.*
B) *H. influenzae.*

C) *Coxiella burnetii.*
D) *Histoplasma capsulatum.*
E) *Blastomyces dermatitidis.*

Discussion

The correct answer is "D." The case described here is classic for an environmental exposure to a large dose of *Histoplasma* organisms. *Histoplasma* occurs most commonly in the Mississippi and Ohio River valleys, causing a self-limited disease in most persons. Patients who have *Histoplasma* infection frequently develop calcified mediastinal lymph nodes after resolution of the infection. Diagnosis can be made by urinary antigen or bronchoscopic biopsy. The bacterial causes are unlikely to be important factors here, as she was on a broad-spectrum antibiotic for 3 days with no improvement. *C. burnetii*, the agent causing Q fever, is rare and tends to affect workers exposed to fresh animal material, such as placentas. *Blastomyces* is found in the same regions as *Histoplasma*, but the site of exposure tends to be more moist, unlike the dry environment inside a barn. We all have histoplasmosis on x-ray in Iowa.

CASE 15

A 42-year-old female comes to your office with a history of asthma that has been difficult to control. She relates symptoms that have been worsening over the last 4–6 weeks. She received two courses of oral corticosteroids during that time. Her symptoms improved with this therapy but quickly returned after completing the steroids. She denies fever, chills, and night sweats, but complains of a *chronic cough productive of brownish-colored sputum*. She is a homemaker in a suburban area and has no pets. Physical examination reveals wheezing throughout all lung fields but is otherwise normal. Laboratory evaluation includes CBC with increased eosinophils, normal C-reactive protein, and an elevated IgE level of 1250 ng/mL. A high-resolution CT scan of the chest reveals central bronchiectasis.

What is the most likely diagnosis?

A) Hypersensitivity pneumonitis.
B) Acute eosinophilic pneumonia.
C) ABPA.
D) Bacterial pneumonia.
E) Churg–Strauss vasculitis.

Discussion

The correct answer is "C." This patient's history points to the diagnosis of ABPA, which is characterized by the presence of severe asthma, brownish mucus plugs, peripheral eosinophilia above 10%, elevated serum IgE, and central bronchiectasis. IgE elevation is required to be greater than 1000 ng/mL. "A" is unlikely but a bit tricky. First, there is no history of exposure to a causative agent. Second, let's focus on symptoms. Constitutional symptoms—often fever—are present in the acute form of hypersensitivity pneumonitis. However, they need not be present in the subacute and chronic forms of the disease. So, based on symptoms, this could be hypersensitivity pneumonitis. However, the radiologic findings of hypersensitivity pneumonitis would include interstitial lung disease, rather than central bronchiectasis. Thus, this is not likely hypersensitivity pneumonitis.

"B" and "D" are incorrect. Note that she has no significant constitutional symptoms that might be more typical of acute eosinophilic pneumonia or bacterial infection. You would also expect an infiltrate on the chest CT. "E" is incorrect. Churg–Strauss vasculitis is characterized by transient patchy interstitial infiltrates, fever, weight loss, elevated sedimentation rate, abnormal liver enzymes, and a peripheral blood eosinophilia >1000/μL. This is often related to using an oral steroid and a leukotriene inhibitor simultaneously. It *seems* to be related to inhaled steroids because once the patient is on a steroid inhaler, the oral steroid is usually tapered unmasking the vasculitis. Remember that this patient has a normal CBC. Extrapulmonary manifestations distinguish this entity from other eosinophilic conditions.

Which of the following would be the next best step in confirming the diagnosis?

A) Sputum cultures.
B) Transbronchial biopsy.
C) Methacholine challenge.
D) Allergy skin testing for *Aspergillus* species.
E) p-ANCA.

Discussion

The correct answer is "D." Most but not all of the following criteria (see Table 3–8) need to be present in order to make the diagnosis of ABPA. Transbronchial biopsy is unnecessarily invasive, and the other tests will not help to confirm the diagnosis.

Table 3-8 CRITERIA FOR THE DIAGNOSIS OF ALLERGIC BRONCHOPULMONARY ASPERGILLOSIS (ABPA)

• Asthma
• Central bronchiectasis
• Elevated total serum IgE >1000 ng/mL
• Immediate skin test reactivity to *Aspergillus*
• Elevated serum-specific IgE and/or IgG to *Aspergillus fumigatus*
• Peripheral blood eosinophilia >10%
• Pulmonary infiltrates

The most appropriate treatment for this patient with ABPA would include which of the following?

A) Antibiotics.
B) Oral corticosteroids.
C) Leukotriene receptor antagonist.
D) Itraconazole.
E) Inhaled ipratropium bromide.

Discussion

The correct answer is "B." Oral corticosteroids are the treatment of choice for ABPA. Patients are typically treated for several months with tapering doses rather than short courses of steroids. Serum IgE levels and chest x-rays are used to monitor response to treatment. Please note that "D" is incorrect, and azoles are *not* the mainstay therapy in ABPA. The goal of treatment is suppression of the immune system responding to the fungal antigen. There are studies that show benefit of adding an antifungal agent as a steroid-sparing agent. However, there are risks associated with concomitant use of steroids and azoles, namely, marked adrenal suppression. Hence, oral corticosteroids should be your first choice.

Objectives: Did you learn to . . .

- Identify the clinical presentation of ABPA?
- Diagnose and treat a patient with ABPA?

CASE 16

A 16-year-old female comes to your office with complaints of sneezing spells, itchy watery eyes, and nasal congestion for the past 2 years. These symptoms are worse during the spring and fall and when she plays with her cat. She denies any other constitutional symptoms and has no other past medical history. She has tried over-the-counter loratadine without relief. She has lived in the same residence for the past 6 years and denies any other environmental exposures. Her examination reveals pale nasal mucosa and swollen nasal turbinates bilaterally. Her lungs and skin are clear.

You are not clear if this is allergic or vasomotor rhinitis. The most effective way to determine if this is allergic is to:

A) Do a methacholine challenge test.
B) Do a Hansel stain of nasal mucus.
C) Check overall IgE levels.
D) Perform a nasal mucus electrophoresis to visualize allergic bands.

Discussion

The correct answer is "B." The best way to tell if this is allergic is to do a Hansel stain of the nasal mucous. This will show eosinophils if it is allergic. If this is vasomotor rhinitis, eosinophils will be absent. If it is infectious, there will likely be a predominance of neutrophils. "A" is incorrect. A methacholine challenge test is helpful in diagnosing asthma, not allergic rhinitis. Neither "C," IgE levels, nor nasal mucus electrophoresis have any use here (and nasal mucus electrophoresis has no use anywhere that we know of... and it is disgusting). IgE is only elevated in 40% of patients with allergic rhinitis.

A Hansel stain shows eosinophils. Which of the following would be the *most appropriate* next step in managing her symptoms?

A) Recommend allergen-impermeable encasements for mattress and pillow.
B) Use topical decongestant sprays.
C) Change classes of antihistamines.
D) Refer for allergy evaluation, including percutaneous aeroallergen skin testing.
E) Recommend a high efficiency particulate air filter for the home.

Discussion

The correct answer is "C." Although all of the above choices may provide relief for allergic symptoms, the best answer first step would be to try changing the class of antihistamines. Antihistamines (and NSAIDs for that matter) are grouped into classes based on chemical structure. One class may be helpful for a patient when another class does not work.

The other choices are suboptimal. Without skin testing, avoidance measures may be needless, costly, and ineffective. Allergen-impermeable encasements are currently recommended for patients with dust mite allergy. Although filters are often recommended for pet allergies, the data regarding their effectiveness in reducing allergic symptoms is contradictory. Topical decongestant sprays are an inappropriate choice secondary to the addictive nature of these medications and the risk of causing rebound symptoms. Removing a pet from the bedroom may reduce—but not eliminate—allergen exposure. Further evaluation should be performed prior to recommending any such lifestyle modifications. Another reasonable option would be a trial of intranasal corticosteroid.

* *

Your patient's 17-year-old brother is in the next exam room. He is a Boy Scout who just returned from a backpacking trip in the four corners area of New Mexico, Arizona, and (name the other two yourself... this is a quiz book, after all). He has noted myalgias, fever, and chills. He knows that you are reviewing pulmonary medicine for your upcoming board exam, so he presents to your office complaining of dyspnea that has been getting markedly worse over the past several days. He has no URI symptoms such as coryza, rhinorrhea, ear pain, etc. He has noticed nausea, vomiting, and diarrhea with severe abdominal pain. His respiratory rate is 40 with an oxygen saturation of 88%. ("See," he says, "I told you I'm sick.") You place him on nasal oxygen and order a chest x-ray, which shows bilateral pulmonary edema.

Based on the epidemiology and chest x-ray appearance, your best guess at this point in the disease is:

A) Plague.
B) Coccidiomycosis.
C) Hantavirus from Sin Nombre (No Name) strain.
D) Noncardiogenic pulmonary edema from smoking paraquat (you never know what is going on at those Boy Scout camps...).

Discussion

The correct answer is "C." This is a typical history and physical exam for hantavirus. The absence of URI symptoms, the presence of GI symptoms, and the noncardiogenic pulmonary edema are all symptoms/signs of hantavirus. In fact, it may present as an acute abdomen. It is spread by aerosolization of mouse excrement or urine. "B" is incorrect. Although coccidiomycosis, "Valley Fever," is found in the same geographical region, it is present with lower respiratory symptoms, a thin walled cavitary lesion, erythema nodosum (10%), and eosinophilia. It is generally a low grade, subacute process that lasts weeks to months. It does not cause noncardiogenic pulmonary edema. "A," pneumonic plague, while also found in the same area, causes high fever, bloody sputum, pleuritic chest pain, and develops over hours to days. It can be rapidly fatal if not recognized and treated within the first day. As to marijuana and paraquat, "D," it does cause pulmonary edema. And you never *do* know what is going on at those Boy Scout camps.

Laboratory findings suggestive of hantavirus include all of the following EXCEPT:

A) Thrombocytopenia.
B) Leukocytosis with a left shift.
C) A lymphocytic predominance.
D) An immunoblast count <10%.

Discussion

The correct answer is "D." In fact, thrombocytopenia, a 10% immunoblast count, and a left shift constitute the so-called diagnostic triad in a patient with appropriate clinical findings. Immunoblasts are the most immature cell in the lymphocyte line (they still enjoy scribbling on walls and drink irresponsibly). Overall, case fatality rate of hantavirus is up to 50%. Care is supportive. Extra-corporeal membrane oxygenation may be used in seriously ill patients. There is often an oliguric phase that needs careful management to prevent fluid overload. This can be problematic because patients are often hypotensive and there is a proclivity toward giving them fluids.

Objectives: Did you learn to...

- Assess and treat allergic rhinitis?
- Diagnose and manage a hantavirus infection?

BIBLIOGRAPHY

Annema JT, et al. Endoscopic ultrasound added to mediastinoscopy for preoperative staging of patients with lung cancer. *JAMA*. 2005;294:931-936.

Cahill K, et al. Nicotine receptor partial agonists for smoking cessation. *Cochrane Database Syst Rev*. 2007;24(1): CD006103.

Celli BR. The body-mass index, airflow obstruction, dyspnea, and exercise capacity index in chronic obstructive pulmonary disease. *N Engl J Med.* 2004;350:1005-1012.

Centers for Disease Control and Prevention. Antiviral agents for seasonal influenza: Information for health professionals. Available at: http://www.cdc.gov/flu/professionals/antivirals/index.htm, Accessed October 31, 2007.

Daniels JM, et al. Antibiotics in addtion to corticosteroids for acute exacerbations of chronic obstructive pulmonary disease. *Am J Respir Crit Care Med.* 2010;181: 150-157.

Daniels JMA, et al. Antibiotics in addition to systemic corticosteroids for acute exacerbations of chronic obstructive pulmonary disease. *Am J Respir Crit Care Med.* 2010;181(2):150-157.

Ege MJ, et al. Exposure to environmental microorganisms and childhood asthma. *N Engl J Med.* 2011;364:701-709

Gibson PG, et al. Allergic bronchopulmonary aspergillosis. *Semin Respir Crit Care Med.* 2006;27:185-191.

Gravenstein S, Davidson HE. Current strategies for management of influenza in the elderly population. *Clin Infect Dis.* 2002;35:729-737.

Irwin RS, Madison MJ. The diagnosis and treatment of cough. *N Engl J Med.* 2000;343(23):1715-1721.

Jodang W, et al. Outpatient patient treatment in patients with acute pulmonary embolism. *J Thromb Haemost.* 2011;9:1500-1507. Doi: 10.1111/j.1538-7836.2011.04388.x.

Lacasse Y, et al. Clinical diagnosis of hypersensitivity pneumonitis. *Am J Respir Crit Care Med.* 2003;168:952-958.

Laszlo G. Standardisation of lung function testing: Helpful guidance from the ATS/ERS Task Force. *Thorax.* 2006;61:744-746.

Mandell LA, et al. Infectious Diseases Society of America/American Thoracic Society consensus guidelines on the management of community-acquired pneumonia in adults. *Clin Infect Dis.* 2007;1(44, Suppl 2):S27-S72.

National Asthma Education and Prevention Program, Expert Panel Report 3. Guidelines for the diagnosis and management of asthma. 2007. Available at: http://www.nhlbi.nih.gov/guidelines/asthma/asthsumm.pdf, Accessed October 31, 2007.

Naureckas ET, Solway J. Mild asthma. *N Engl J Med.* 2001;345(17):1257-1262.

Ost D, et al. The solitary pulmonary nodule. *N Eng J Med.* 2003;348(25):2535-2542.

Palareti G, et al. d-Dimer testing to determine the duration of anticoagulation therapy. *N Engl J Med.* 2006;355:1780-1789

Pasteur MC, et al. British Thoracic Society guideline for non-CF bronchiectasis. *Thorax.* 2010;65:i1-i58.

Rabe KF, et al. Global strategies for the diagnosis, management, and prevention of chronic obstructive pulmonary disease: GOLD executive summary. *Am J Respir Crit Care Med.* 2007;176(6):532-555.

Shanthi P, Jones P. Corticosteroid therapy in pulmonary sarcoidosis: A systematic review. *JAMA.* 2002; 287(10):1301-1307.

Steinberg KP, Kacmarek RM. Respiratory controversies in the critical care setting. Should tidal volume be 6 mL/kg predicted body weight in virtually all patients with acute respiratory failure? *Respir Care.* 2007;52:556-564

Swenson SJ, et al. CT screening for lung cancer: Five-year prospective experience. *Radiology.* 2005;235:259-265.

Tillie-Leblond I, et al. Pulmonary embolism in patients with unexplained exacerbation of chronic obstructive pulmonary disease: Prevalence and risk factors. *Ann Int Med.* 2006;144:390-396

Van Belle, et al. (writing group for the Christopher Study Investigators). Effectiveness of managing suspected pulmonary embolism using an algorithm combining clinical probability, D-dimer testing, and computed tomography. *JAMA.* 2006;295(2):172-179.

Von Essen SG, et al. Organic dust toxic syndrome: A noninfectious febrile illness. *J Toxicol Clin Toxicol.* 1990;28(4):398-420.

Von Essen SG, et al. After exposure to the hog barn environment. *J Swine Health Prod.* 2005;13:273-276.

Yasufuku K, et al. Comparison of endobronchial ultrasound, positron emission tomography, and CT for lymph node staging of lung cancer. *Chest.* 2006;130: 710-718.

Yu CJ, et al. Ultrasound study in unilateral hemithorax opacification. Image comparison with computed tomography. *Am Rev Respir Dis.* 1993;147:430-434.

4 Allergy and Immunology

Mark A. Graber and Jason K. Wilbur

CASE 1

A 15-year-old girl has a history of acute difficulty breathing when playing basketball. Her symptoms include **inspiratory** wheezing/stridor, increased respiratory rate, throat tightness, and chest discomfort. Premedication with adequate doses of albuterol has no effect.

What is the most likely diagnosis?

A) Exercise-induced asthma.
B) Gastroesophageal reflux disease.
C) Musculoskeletal chest pain.
D) Hyperventilation.
E) Vocal cord dysfunction.

Discussion

The correct answer is "E." Vocal cord dysfunction (VCD) is one of the most common asthma mimics. Patients with VCD present with hoarseness, coughing, dyspnea, and loud **inspiratory wheezing/stridor**, along with other symptoms mentioned above. Pulmonary function testing indicates airway obstruction due to an extrathoracic component. It appears that paradoxical inspiratory vocal cord adduction causes airflow restriction at the level of the larynx, thereby resulting in a flattened inspiratory loop on flow-volume diagram. VCD presents a diagnostic challenge, and often leads to unnecessary treatment of asthma. In this patient, a β_2-agonist was ineffective, even though she displays symptoms with exertion. This argues against answer "A." The distinction between VCD and asthma may be less clear in other patients, since the two disorders sometimes coexist. The clinical history does not support the diagnoses of gastroesophageal reflux disease, musculoskeletal chest pain, or hyperventilation.

* *

You make the diagnosis of VCD. However, the patient also complains of rhinorrhea, itchy eyes, sneezing, and itchy nose. Because you realize that we need to discuss it in this book, you kindly refer her for allergy testing (thank you!).

With regard to radioallergosorbent testing (RAST) for allergic rhinitis, which of the following is true?

A) RAST is less expensive than traditional skin testing.
B) RAST is more sensitive than traditional skin testing.
C) RAST has a limited role in testing those with allergic rhinitis
D) Antihistamine use is a contraindication to the use of RAST.

Discussion

The correct answer is "C." RAST will be negative in up to 25% of those with a positive skin test, has poorly reproducible results, and is more expensive. Thus, skin testing remains the procedure of choice for identifying allergens. RAST can be used if skin testing is unavailable.

Which of the following medications does NOT need to be discontinued prior to aeroallergen skin testing?

A) Intranasal steroid spray.
B) Atenolol.
C) Amitriptyline.
D) Cyproheptadine.
E) Azelastine nasal spray.

Discussion

The correct answer is "A." Intranasal steroid sprays do not need to be discontinued prior to skin testing as they do not interfere with immediate-type hypersensitivity reactions. They are not antihistaminic in nature, as opposed to amitriptyline, cyproheptadine, or azelastine, which may all blunt dermal reactivity. Although azelastine is administered as a nasal spray, its administration may interfere with skin test reactivity within 2 days of usage. Beta-blockers, such as atenolol, have been shown to affect skin test reactivity and should be avoided in patients undergoing skin testing.

* *

Aeroallergen skin prick and intradermal testing reveals positive reactions to dust mites, cat, ragweed, and tree pollens. The patient relates that she gets considerable nasal congestion and has tried over-the-counter decongestants with no relief.

Which of the following interventions would provide the most relief for her nasal symptoms?

A) Diphenhydramine 25 mg PO BID.
B) Montelukast 10 mg PO QHS.
C) Intranasal steroid spray daily.
D) Ipratropium bromide nasal spray BID.
E) Getting rid of the cat. No one should have a cat. They are evil.

Discussion

The correct answer is "C." Intranasal corticosteroids would provide the most relief in this patient by addressing nasal congestion in addition to the other nasal symptoms mentioned. Although antihistamines are very helpful in relieving nasal symptoms such as rhinorrhea, nasal itching, and sneezing, they are generally not as effective for nasal congestion. Likewise, montelukast is a leukotriene modifier, which is approved for treatment of allergic rhinitis, but studies suggest that intranasal steroids are superior. Additionally, nasal steroids are nonsystemic (although a bit may be absorbed). Ipratropium is mainly effective for rhinorrhea only, while nasal saline irrigations promote thinning of nasal secretions and drainage, but neither predictably improves nasal congestion. As to "E," yes, cats are evil and shed. But as family doctors we are supposed to be accepting of our patient's quirks...

> HELPFUL (AND REALLY COOL) TIP: Nasal steroids also seem to improve ocular symptoms. Whether some of the drug gets up the nasolacrimal ducts or is otherwise aerosolized into the eye is unclear. But it works equally for all nasal steroids. Obviously, do not put nasal steroids directly in the eye.

* *

She returns to you a year later, having tried intranasal steroid sprays and high-dose antihistamines, without gaining significant relief. She has instituted appropriate avoidance measures during the interim (there goes the cat), also without improvement in symptoms. You recommend allergen immunotherapy.

All of the following statements are true regarding allergen immunotherapy EXCEPT:

A) Patients should carry emergency epinephrine to all immunotherapy shot appointments.
B) It is unnecessary to stop beta-blocker therapy prior to starting immunotherapy.
C) Patients should be observed in the office for at least 30 minutes after immunotherapy injections.
D) At least 3 years of immunotherapy should be given to avoid recurrence of symptoms.

Discussion

The correct answer is "B." It has been shown that patients taking beta-blockers may be at increased risk of having more severe systemic reactions to immunotherapy, because these medications attenuate the response to epinephrine. Patients should be treated with an alternative antihypertensive during immunotherapy. The current practice parameters for allergen immunotherapy recommend that emergency epinephrine should be readily available for treatment of systemic allergic reactions associated with immunotherapy. To monitor for these immediate reactions, patients should be observed in the office setting for at least 30 minutes after immunotherapy shots are administered. Based on studies of seasonal symptom scores, it is generally recommended that allergen immunotherapy be continued for 3–5 years.

HELPFUL TIP: Beta-blockers should be stopped in patients with a history of anaphylaxis if possible. Beta-blockers amplify anaphylaxis and make it more difficult to treat.

Objectives: Did you learn to . . .

- Recognize symptoms of vocal cord disfunction?
- Recognize symptoms of allergic rhinitis?
- Provide appropriate management for allergic rhinitis?
- Describe the role of immunotherapy in treating allergic rhinitis?

QUICK QUIZ: ALLERGIC REACTIONS

A 52-year-old man with common variable immunodeficiency (CVID) receives his first infusion of intravenous immunoglobulin (IVIG) therapy. Ten minutes into the infusion, he complains of difficulty breathing and generalized pruritus.

Based on the traditional classification of hypersensitivity reactions, which of the following best categorizes this patient's reaction?

A) Type I—Immediate hypersensitivity reaction.
B) Type II—Cytotoxic reaction.
C) Type III—Immune complex reaction.
D) Type IV—Delayed-type reaction.

Discussion

The correct answer is "A." Based on the clinical history and timing of the above event, you should suspect an immediate hypersensitivity reaction (Type I). Type I reactions typically occur within seconds to minutes after exposure to the offending agent and are due to cross-linkage of IgE antibodies that are bound to surfaces of mast cells or basophils, with subsequent release of mediators such as histamine. Pruritus, urticaria, angioedema, laryngeal edema, and possible generalized anaphylaxis can occur. To see why Types II–IV are incorrect, refer to Table 4–1 for definitions of the immunologic reaction types.

QUICK QUIZ: CAN I HAVE THAT BANANA OR NOT?

A slightly deranged patient of yours has a serious latex allergy and wants to play "fruit roulette."

You tell her that all of the following may be associated with cross-reactivity in latex-allergic patients EXCEPT:

A) Celery.
B) Banana.
C) Avocado.
D) Kiwi.
E) Chestnut.

Table 4–1 CLASSIFICATION OF IMMUNOLOGIC REACTIONS

Reaction Type	Mechanism	Clinical Features	Timing
Type I—Immediate	Antigen exposure causes cross-linkage of IgE antibodies that are bound to surfaces of mast cells and basophils, with subsequent release of mediators such as histamine	Anaphylaxis Angioedema Bronchospasm Urticaria	Less than an hour after exposure
Type II—Cytotoxic	IgG or IgM antibodies are directed against antigens on the individual's own tissues, and subsequent complement activation leads to cell destruction	Graft rejection Hemolytic anemia Neutropenia Thrombocytopenia	At least 5 days but sometimes many weeks after exposure
Type III—Immune complex	IgG or IgM antigen–antibody complexes form and deposit within blood vessels and tissues, causing complement activation and neutrophil recruitment, ultimately resulting in tissue damage	Localized Arthus reaction Serum sickness	1 week or more after exposure
Type IV—Delayed	Antigen exposure to sensitized T-cells causes a reaction	Contact dermatitis Stevens–Johnson syndrome	24–72 hours after exposure

Discussion

The correct answer is "A." Celery is so boring; it can't even cause an allergic reaction in those with latex allergy! Symptoms of oral allergy syndrome can include oral pruritus with or without angioedema of the lips, tongue, palate, and posterior oropharynx. Cross-reactivity has been reported between:

- Ragweed antigens and the gourd family and banana.
- Birch pollen allergy may result in sensitivity to apple, carrots, parsnips, celery, hazelnuts, and potatoes.
- Latex-fruit cross-reactivity may occur with banana, avocado, passion fruit, kiwi, and chestnut, but not celery. Your patient should be warned about these potential reactions.

HELPFUL TIP: The vast majority of patients who report penicillin (and other) allergies are not truly allergic. In the case of penicillin, 0.5% of those with reported penicillin allergy had skin reactions and less than 10% had **any** reaction to a full dose of penicillin. Many patients misinterpret an adverse reaction (such as nausea) as an allergy.

HELPFUL TIP: There is essentially no cross-reactivity between penicillin and third-generation cephalosporins. As long as the patient did not have true anaphylaxis, feel comfortable using these drugs in penicillin-allergic patients.

QUICK QUIZ: CONTRAST ALLERGY

A 57-year-old man with chest pain is scheduled for an elective cardiac catheterization. You remember that the patient has a history of generalized urticaria with lip and tongue angioedema shortly after receiving contrast dye for a CT scan several years back.

Which of the following interventions should be recommended for this patient prior to undergoing the planned procedure?

A) Use of higher-osmolality radiocontrast media if possible.
B) Give a test dose of radiocontrast media and proceed as usual if testing is negative.
C) Administration of prednisone and diphenhydramine as premedications.
D) Percutaneous and intradermal skin testing with radiocontrast media.
E) Desensitization procedure for radiocontrast media.

Discussion

The correct answer is "C." Anaphylactoid reactions to radiocontrast material are typically non-IgE-mediated; however, they look very similar to a Type I immunologic reaction and can be severe and life threatening. This patient will require the premedication for this elective procedure. The appropriate premedication regimen for contrast dye allergy includes (1) diphenhydramine 50 mg IM/PO 1 hour before procedure and (2) prednisone 50 mg PO 13 hours, 7 hours, and 1 hour before procedure. "A" is incorrect. Use of **lower-osmolality** radiocontrast media is associated with fewer adverse reactions and is appropriate for contrast-allergic patients. "B" is incorrect. Test dosing for radiocontrast media should not be done; patients with no reaction to test doses have had severe reactions to full doses. Additionally, tests doses themselves have been reported to result in fatalities. Skin testing ("D") **can** be done, but it is of very limited predictive value and **should not** be done. There is no desensitization procedure available.

HELPFUL TIP: **There is no cross-reaction between shellfish and iodine-based contrast material.** The allergy to seafood is an allergy to the protein (tropomyosins) in the seafood not the iodine. Think about it for a second. How many people have you seen dropping dead from an anaphylactic reaction to iodized salt?

CASE 2

An 18-month-old boy comes to clinic with a history of eczematous rash covering his extremities and face. His parents state that it worsens after the ingestion of certain foods. He has had increased fussiness over the last several months, as well as some difficulty gaining weight. Food allergy is suspected.

Which of the following foods is NOT commonly implicated in food allergy?

A) Milk.
B) Corn.
C) Wheat.
D) Soy.
E) Egg.

Discussion

The correct answer is "B." Corn is not often implicated in food allergies (a good thing too, since we are writing this in Iowa, surrounded by corn). Although many foods are potentially antigenic, the great majority of food allergies involve only a few foods. Studies have shown that eight foods account for 93% of reactions, and these foods are, in order of frequency, egg, peanuts, milk, soy, tree nuts, fish, crustacean, and wheat. Although these food allergies may be outgrown, sensitivity to peanut, tree nuts, fish, and crustacean tend to be lifelong.

HELPFUL TIP: Peak incidence of food allergies occurs around age 1 year, with most allergies identified by age 2. Cow's milk and egg allergies tend to resolve by adulthood.

* *

Two months later, this patient required an emergency room visit after developing increased work of breathing, wheezing, and an urticarial rash after eating. He is tested by both percutaneous skin testing and RAST and is found to have egg allergy.

Which of the following vaccinations should NOT be given to this patient in light of his egg allergy?

A) MMR vaccine.
B) Inactivated polio vaccine.
C) *Hemophilus influenzae* B vaccine.
D) Conjugated pneumococcal vaccine (Prevnar).
E) Influenza vaccine.

Discussion

The correct answer is "E." Influenza vaccine should not be given to individuals with egg allergy. Of particular note is "A." "A" is incorrect. It had been common practice to withhold measles vaccination from children with a history of anaphylactic reaction to egg; the measles vaccine is prepared in chick-embryo fibroblast cultures. However, the MMR is safe to use in these children. Options "B," "C," and "D" do not contain egg-related products and can therefore be given safely to this patient.

HELPFUL TIP: As of 2012 the CDC suggests vaccinating egg allergic patients as long their reaction was hives only. See http://www.cdc.gov/mmwr/preview/mmwrhtml/mm6132a3.htm#fig2

Objectives: Did you learn to . . .

- Identify common food allergens?
- Recognize important associations between food allergy and selected vaccines?

CASE 3

A 34-year-old female establishes care in your clinic. Her medical history consists of intermittent abdominal pain and episodes of angioedema in the past with unclear etiology. She has received multiple laparoscopic procedures that were unrevealing. During the initial interview, she relates several past episodes of lip and tongue swelling, for which she has not sought medical assistance. She has tried diphenhydramine without significant improvement. The swelling episodes resolve without intervention after 3–4 days.

Which of the following laboratory tests would be most helpful in establishing the diagnosis in this patient?

A) ANA.
B) C3 complement level.
C) C4 complement level.
D) Complete blood count (CBC).
E) SS-A and SS-B.

Discussion

The correct answer is "C." This patient's presentation should raise concern for hereditary angioedema (HAE), or C1-esterase inhibitor deficiency. This entity is clinically characterized by recurrent episodes of angioedema involving any part of the body. Thus, it can present with laryngeal angioedema (the major cause of death) or recurrent abdominal pain (generally with a normal white count and "always" without peritoneal signs). Urticaria is **not** a feature of this disorder. HAE is caused by a C1-esterase inhibitor deficiency, which allows an overexuberant activation of the complement cascade. For this reason, patients with C1-esterase inhibitor deficiency have chronically low levels of C2 and C4. They may have normal levels of C1-esterase inhibitor but have a nonfunctional allele. Thus, "C" is the right answer and C4 levels should be low if the patient has C1-esterase inhibitor deficiency. Of course, you will also check a C1-esterase inhibitor level keeping in mind that the nonfunctional allele may give a false negative test (e.g., the presence of a nonfunctional C1-esterase inhibitor).

* *

While awaiting the test results, you discuss HAE with your patient.

In order to minimize future attacks of angioedema, you recommend which of the following?

A) Avoidance of estrogen containing medications.
B) Avoidance of ACE inhibitors.
C) Testing and treatment of *Helicobacter pylori.*
D) All of the above.

Discussion

The correct answer is "D." Education is the cornerstone of treatment of HAE. Patients need to know what triggers to avoid and how to identify symptoms early. Most attacks are precipitated by trauma (often head and upper airway trauma), medical procedures (dental and oral surgery in particular), emotional stress, infections, menstruation, or the use of medications, especially oral contraceptives and ACE inhibitors. Interestingly, *H. pylori* infection has been associated with HAE, and *H. pylori* eradication reduces the frequency of angioedema attacks.

* *

Your patient is ultimately diagnosed with HAE.

In this particular patient, which medication would be most helpful in preventing future episodes?

A) Emergency epinephrine.
B) Oral diphenhydramine.
C) Fresh frozen plasma (FFP).
D) Androgens (e.g., danazol)
E) No prophylactic treatment is available.

Discussion

The correct answer is "D." Emergency epinephrine and antihistamines have not generally been effective, as HAE is not allergic in nature. Prophylactic treatment in the form of attenuated androgens (danazol) is available. Attenuated androgens appear to work by up-regulating the synthetic capability of hepatic cells that make C1-esterase inhibitor, thus raising the C4 level and reducing the number and severity of acute exacerbations. Two purified C1-esterase inhibitor replacement protein products (Cinryze and Berinert) were approved by the FDA in 2010 for treatment and prevention of HAE exacerbations. However, they are costly and lack strong efficacy data. Treatment of acute episodes of HAE includes FFP that contains C1-esterase inhibitor, the C1-esterase inhibitor replacement protein products, and bradykinin/kallikrein inhibitors (ecallantide and icatibant). Additionally, these three options could be used as prophylactic treatment in short-term situations, such as prior to surgery in a high-risk patient. However, FFP would not be a long-term preventive measure, so "C" is incorrect.

> HELPFUL TIP: Make sure patients with HAE receive the hepatitis B vaccination series as they may require blood products for acute treatment of angioedema.

Objectives: Did you learn to . . .

- Identify a patient presenting with hereditary angioedema?
- Manage a patient with hereditary angioedema?

CASE 4

Your patient's sister (her biologic sister, not her stepsister or BFF) presents to clinic the next day with a similar history of angioedema symptoms, only less frequent and less severe.

What is the likelihood that she has HAE as well?

A) Infinitesimally small because HAE is a rare disorder.
B) About 25% because HAE is autosomal recessive.
C) About 50% because HAE is autosomal dominant.
D) Almost 100% because you can tell that she's got bad luck.
E) Unknown because multiple gene involvement renders a simple calculation impossible.

Discussion

The correct answer is "C." HAE is transmitted in an autosomal-dominant fashion with incomplete penetrance, which may be why the patient's sister is less symptomatic. New mutations do arise and cause a minority of cases.

* *

Later that same night, you are called to the ED to see a patient with facial swelling. "Really?" you ask. "Yeah, really. Get in here," replies Happy Nurse. This patient is a 35-year-old female friend of your patient with HAE (so, her BFF not her biologic sister). She is worried she has HAE, too. This is the first ever episode of lip and face swelling, associated with itching in her mouth and a few hives on her arm and torso. She had shrimp gumbo for dinner, but has never had a reaction to shrimp before. She denies any recent trauma, surgery, or medication use. She is in no respiratory distress. Her O_2 sat is 99% on room air, and BP is 118/76. On lung exam, there is no stridor or wheezing.

The most appropriate next step in the treatment of this patient is:

A) Supportive care and monitoring overnight in the intensive care unit (ICU).
B) Administration of FFP.
C) Administration of epinephrine IM × 1.
D) Administration of diphenhydramine, cimetidine, and prednisone PO.
E) Prophylactic intubation.

Discussion

The correct answer is "D." This patient is different from your HAE patient. It is unlikely that she has HAE for several reasons: she's never had this reaction before, she has urticaria associated with the angioedema, and she did not experience an inciting event. This episode of angioedema and urticaria is more likely to have been caused by a typical allergic reaction and mast-cell release. For these types of reactions, antihistamines and steroids are the mainstay of therapy. "A" is incorrect because it is overkill to admit her to the ICU, and you should be treating her rather than just monitoring her. "B" is incorrect because FFP treats HAE not allergic angioedema. "C" is incorrect because this patient is not having a full anaphylactic reaction. Epinephrine would be appropriate if she had wheezing, airway compromise, or hypotension. If you chose "E" for a walking, talking patient with no airway compromise, well... that just makes us sad.

Objectives: did you learn to...

- Differentiate HAE from allergic angioedema?
- Manage an anaphylactoid reaction?

Warning: The next section is about immunodeficiency syndromes. As Dante would say: "Abandon hope all ye who enter here." (One of the editors has a dog named Dante and she (the dog) says this all the time... to squirrels). See Table 4–2 for a quick review. The main points and **the most important cases** are mentioned below. For those of you who are gluttons for punishment (gluttony is only Dante's 3rd circle), look at the table.

The main points:

- Rule out the obvious: Does the patient have HIV, cancer, diabetes, lupus, or other chronic disease or is he/she on immunosuppressing drugs that predispose to recurrent infections?
- 1–3% of patients are heterozygous for an IgG subtype deficiency, the most common type of immunoglobulin deficiency. These patients may be asymptomatic or may present with recurrent sinusitis, otitis, skin infections, etc. IgG deficiency can be diagnosed by immunoglobulin electrophoresis. These patients often do not have an appropriate response to vaccinations.
- 1 in 700 patients are IgA deficient. Most are hereditary, but it can also be caused by several drugs (including captopril and thyroxine). Usually this resolves upon stopping the drug. Most patients with IgA deficiency are asymptomatic, although some have recurrent sinus and GI infections. Also, these patients frequently develop autoimmune disease and may have anaphylaxis to blood products.
- Symptomatic immunoglobulin deficiencies can be treated with IVIG. The most common side effects of IVIG administration include renal failure, anaphylaxis, and thromboembolic disease.

CASE 5

A 35-year-old male is seen by you in the hospital setting, after being admitted for pneumonia. Blood cultures reveal *Streptococcus pneumoniae*. The patient was well until age 25 when he began having recurrent infections and developed an autoimmune hemolytic anemia. He also relates frequent sinus infections (real ones... not the kind we so often see) requiring antibiotics 8–10 times a year. His last bout of pneumonia required a stay in the ICU.

You suspect immune deficiency in this individual. What is the most useful test in making the diagnosis in this patient?

A) Complement levels.
B) Immunoglobulin levels.
C) CBC and differential.
D) Bone marrow biopsy.
E) Nitroblue tetrazolium test.

Table 4–2 IMMUNODEFICIENCY SYNDROMES

Syndrome	Age of Onset	Defect/Laboratory Findings	Manifestations	Organisms Likely to Cause Infection
Humoral				
X-linked agammaglobulinemia	Late 1st year of life but up to age 50 (in very mild disease)	Low IgG, almost undetectable IgM, IgD, IgE, and IgA. No B cells	Multiple, recurrent infections (generally start 6–18 months) especially lung, sinuses, ears, CSF. Eventually bronchiectasis and pulmonary insufficiency	*Streptococcus*, *Haemophilus*, *Giardia*
Common variable immunodeficiency	Variable but >2 years of age and mostly by age 30. May be older	Low levels of serum immunoglobulins	Sinus and respiratory infections. GI infections especially Giardia. Enhanced chance of lymphoma as adult. Autoimmune disorders	*Pneumococcus*, *Haemophilus*, *Mycoplasma*, *Giardia*
Hyper IgM syndrome	First 2 years of life	Elevated IgM, no IgG, IgA, IgE (although few may have very low level IgA, IgE)	Recurrent severe sinopulmonary infections. Autoimmune disorders	Encapsulated bacteria, *Giardia*, *Pneumocystis*, *Cryptosporidium*, Histoplasmosis
IgA deficiency	Not before age of 6 months; more severe disease presents by age 5 years	Low IgA levels, normal immunoglobulins otherwise	Most asymptomatic. May have respiratory tract infections. Watch for anaphylaxis with blood products	*Haemophilus*, *pneumococcus*
Cellular				
Myeloperoxidase deficiency	Variable	Poor phagocytic killing	None except in presence of other defects (e.g., diabetes)	Candidiasis
Chronic granulomatous disease	Infant, toddler but occasionally in late life	Neutrophil dysfunction measured by nitroblue tetrazolium testing (and other tests)	Recurrent life-threatening illnesses especially pulmonary, hepatic, skin, and lymphatic abscesses	*Staphylococcus*, *Aspergillus*
Leukocyte adhesion deficiency	Early (poor separation of umbilical stump) or later if mild disease. Those with mild disease rarely have life-threatening illnesses	Poor adhesion of leukocytes to endothelium, etc.	Periodontal and dental infections, recurrent infections of skin, upper and lower airways, bowel, perirectal area	Pseudomonas and other gram-negative rods, *Staphylococcus*

(*Continued*)

Table 4–2 IMMUNODEFICIENCY SYNDROMES (Continued)

Syndrome	Age of Onset	Defect/Laboratory Findings	Manifestations	Organisms Likely to Cause Infection
Hyper IgE (Job syndrome)	First weeks to month of life	Elevated IgE levels, poor leukocyte chemotaxis	Facial abnormalities (hypertelorism; prominent, protruding triangular mandible; broad, somewhat bulbous nose). Eczema, mucocutaneous candidiasis, sinus, pulmonary, and skin infections. Recurrent "cold abscesses" in skin secondary to lack of inflammation	Multiple organisms, but especially *Staphylococcus*, *Haemophilus*, *Candida*
Wiskott–Aldrich	Early. Fatal by age 10 without bone marrow transplant	Low IgM, diminution of cellular immunity ability to respond to polysaccharide capsules	Eczema, thrombocytopenia with purpura, recurrent infections	Encapsulated organisms
Severe combined immunodeficiency syndrome	Early, by 6 months. Death by 2 years	Leukopenia, no mature T-cells, low serum immunoglobulin levels	Colon and lung infections including diarrhea, abscesses	Multiple organisms, including viral
DiGeorge syndrome	Early—in infancy	Absent thymus, Reduced T3 + cells	Recurrent infections but variable in penetrance. Some have normal or near normal immune function. Craniofacial abnormalities, congenital heart disease, chromosomal abnormalities, hypocalcemia	*Pneumococcus*, *Haemophilus*

Discussion

The correct answer is "B." The clinical picture for this patient is most consistent with CVID. CVID, or acquired agammaglobulinemia, is similar to X-linked agammaglobulinemia, but generally has a later age of onset. In addition, it is associated with various gastrointestinal disorders, autoimmune disorders, and malignancy. Immunoglobulin levels are decreased secondary to inadequate B cell differentiation. Therefore, the most useful laboratory for diagnosis of CVID would be serum immunoglobulin levels. With regard to the other options and other tests you might do to evaluate otherwise unexplained immunodeficiency:

- Complement levels will be low in patients with immunodeficiency secondary to complement disorders.
- Nitroblue tetrazolium test will be abnormal in patients with phagocytic disorders.
- Response to vaccines will be muted or absent in humoral immunodeficiency (e.g., immunoglobulin deficiency).
- Delayed hypersensitivity skin testing (e.g., candida and mumps) may indicate a T-cell defect.

Which of the following is the most appropriate treatment plan for this patient?

A) Prophylactic antibiotics.
B) Bone marrow transplantation.
C) Gene therapy.
D) IVIG replacement.
E) No treatment needed.

Discussion

The correct answer is "D." The treatment of choice for CVID includes replacement IVIG, especially in this patient who has a history of life-threatening infections. Prophylactic antibiotics may be required in addition to IVIG in some patients. Gene therapy is not currently possible because the genetic defect has not been identified. Although bone marrow transplantation is useful in other immune-deficient states, it is not indicated in CVID.

> HELPFUL TIP: Patients with CVID develop lymphoproliferative disorders (e.g., non-Hodgkin lymphoma). New adenopathy should be taken seriously.

Objectives: did you learn to . . .

- Describe presenting symptoms of common variable immunodeficiency?
- Recognize treatment options for CVID?

QUICK QUIZ: IgA DEFICIENCY

A 37-year-old female is incidentally found to have an IgA level of 3 mg/dL (below the normal range).

What is the most likely clinical picture in this patient?

A) Pyogenic infections.
B) Thrush.
C) Cold abscesses.
D) Aphthous ulcers.
E) No clinical abnormalities.

Discussion

The correct answer is "E." IgA deficiency is present in approximately 1 in 700 Caucasians in the United States and is the second most common immunodeficiency described. Most of these patients are asymptomatic, but some IgA-deficient patients may present with an increased rate of respiratory tract infections.

> HELPFUL TIP: The evaluation of immunodeficiency should NOT stop when IgA deficiency is discovered since IgA deficiency is often asymptomatic and may be accompanied by a more serious form of immunodeficiency.

QUICK QUIZ: IVIG

Which of the following patients is most likely to develop an anaphylactic reaction in response to the administration of IVIG?

A) A patient with IgA deficiency.
B) A patient with IgG deficiency.
C) A patient with sickle cell anemia.
D) A patient with graft versus host disease.
E) A pregnant patient.

Discussion

The correct answer is "A." Patients with IgA deficiency have preformed IgG or IgE antibodies against IgA, and thus may develop an anaphylactic reaction in response to IVIG (and blood and FFP, for that matter). Patients with IgG deficiency may have a similar problem but it is much less common. Not all patients with IgA deficiency will develop anaphylaxis, but the risk is high enough to be prepared and to reduce the risk by using IgA-depleted IVIG and giving the IVIG slowly.

BIBLIOGRAPHY

Azar AE. Evaluation of the adult with suspected immunodeficiency. *Am J Med.* 2007;120(9):764.

Bowen T, et al. 2010 International consensus algorithm for the diagnosis, therapy and management of hereditary angioedema. *Allergy Asthma Clin Immunol.* 2010;6(1):24.

Calderon MA, et al. Allergen injection immunotherapy for seasonal allergic rhinitis. *Cochrane Database Syst Rev.* 2007, Issue 1. Art. No.: CD001936. DOI: 10.1002/14651858.CD001936.pub2.

Cooper MA. Primary immunodeficiencies. *Am Fam Physician.* 2003;68(10):2001-2008.

Quillen DM. Diagnosing rhinitis: Allergic versus nonallergic. *Am Fam Physician.* 2006;73(9):1583-1590.

Scurlock AM. Food allergy in children. *Immunol Allergy Clin North Am.* 2005;25(2):369-388, vii-viii.

5

Nephrology

Jason K. Wilbur and Mark A. Graber

CASE 1

A 49-year-old female with a 5-year history of diabetes mellitus type 2 presents for an initial visit. She has no known complications of diabetes. She takes metformin, glyburide, and aspirin. On examination, you find a pleasant, obese female in no distress. Her blood pressure is 136/86 mm Hg, pulse 86, respirations 14, and temperature 37°C. As you discuss monitoring her diabetes, you recommend screening for early kidney disease.

Which of the following approaches is the recommended way to screen for diabetic kidney disease?

A) Obtain a 24-hour urine collection for albumin now and again in 3 years.
B) Obtain a spot urine microalbumin every year.
C) Obtain a spot urine microalbumin/creatinine ratio every year.
D) Obtain a urinalysis every year.
E) Obtain a serum creatinine every year.

Discussion

The correct answer is "C." Microalbuminuria is a marker for possible future kidney disease in diabetic patients. The best test to evaluate for microalbuminuria is the urine microalbumin/creatinine ratio. Its advantages include ease of use, relatively low cost, and good correlation with 24-hour urine collections. Some of you may have chosen "B." Microalbumin is the classic way to screen. As a practical matter, many physicians use microalbumin alone as a method of screening for urine protein, but this is not the preferred method. A random spot urine microalbumin/creatinine ratio is normally less than 30 mg/g. Values above 30 mg/g are consistent with 24-hour measures showing abnormal amounts of albumin. Answers "D" and "E" offer measures of kidney function that simply are not sensitive enough to use for screening purposes.

Her microalbumin/creatinine ratio is 42 mg/g. The next step to confirm microalbuminuria is:

A) Repeat urine microalbumin/creatinine ratio.
B) Urine dipstick for protein.
C) 24-hour urine collection for total protein excretion.
D) Serum creatinine.

Discussion

The correct answer is "A." Verification by repeat urine microalbumin/creatinine ratio is sufficient for a diagnosis of microalbuminuria, so 24-hour urine collections need not be performed for confirmation. Since protein excretion must exceed 300–500 mg/day for a urine dipstick to detect proteinuria, urinalysis ("B") is not sensitive enough to detect microalbuminuria and cannot be used for confirmation. Serum creatinine elevation may be a marker for diabetic kidney disease, but it would develop late in the process.

Which of the following can cause a false-negative microalbumin/creatinine ratio?

A) Vigorous exercise.
B) Fever.
C) Cachexia.
D) Poor glycemic control.
E) Large muscle mass.

Discussion

The correct answer is "E." Patients with a large muscle mass have a high rate of creatinine excretion, which may result in a falsely negative microalbumin/creatinine ratio (as the urine creatinine goes up, the ratio obviously goes down). Cachectic patients have the opposite problem, with low amounts of creatinine excretion, resulting in false-positive microalbumin/creatinine ratio. **Fever, vigorous exercise, heart failure, and poor glycemic control can cause transient microalbuminuria, potentially resulting in false-positive microalbumin/creatinine ratios.**

* *

Your patient's other laboratory studies reveal the following: hemoglobin A_{1c} 6.4%, serum creatinine 1.4 mg/dL, and normal electrolytes. A month later, your patient returns. Her blood pressure is 138/84 mm Hg. Her urine microalbumin/creatinine remains elevated on a second measurement. According to an eye exam yesterday, she has nonproliferative diabetic retinopathy.

Because your patient has type 2 diabetes mellitus and microalbuminuria, you realize that her likelihood of progressing to overt nephropathy is:

A) Almost zero.
B) About half that of a similar patient with type 1 diabetes.
C) Nearly equal to that of a similar patient with type 1 diabetes.
D) More than twice that of a similar patient with type 1 diabetes.
E) Absolutely certain (100% chance).

Discussion

The correct answer is "C." Although earlier studies showed a greater progression to overt nephropathy in type 1 diabetics, more recent studies demonstrate a nearly equal rate of progression in types 1 and 2. About 20–40% of Caucasian patients with diabetes type 2 and microalbuminuria will progress to diabetic nephropathy. The rate of progression to nephropathy in non-Caucasian populations is even higher.

What is the most appropriate next step in the evaluation and management of this patient's microalbuminuria?

A) Start an angiotensin-converting enzyme (ACE) inhibitor.
B) Start an angiotensin receptor blocker (ARB).
C) Order renal ultrasound with Doppler of the renal arteries.
D) Start insulin.
E) Refer to a nephrologist.

Discussion

The correct answer is "A." ACE inhibitors should be the first-choice drugs unless there is a contraindication to their use. "B," an ARB, should be second-line choice in the event that the patient cannot tolerate an ACE inhibitor. "C," a renal ultrasound, is not indicated at this point in time. "D" is also incorrect. Your patient already has good glucose control (HbA_{1c} of 6.4%). Consultation with a nephrologist is premature.

HELPFUL (AND VERY IMPORTANT) TIP: ARBs *are not* just an ACE without the cough. A large, recent, meta-analysis showed that ARBs, while lowering blood pressure, have no appreciable effect on MI or cardiovascular mortality ***versus placebo*** (*BMJ* 2011;342:d2234; doi: 10.1136/bmj.d2234). It is sad, really.

* *

The patient has a full urinalysis to rule out renal inflammation (e.g., nephritis) and overt proteinuria (nephrotic syndrome). The urinalysis is entirely negative.

What further investigations must your patient undergo to eliminate other potential causes of proteinuria?

A) Renal biopsy.
B) Renal ultrasound with Doppler of the renal arteries.
C) ANA, ESR, CRP.
D) All of the above.
E) None of the above.

Discussion

The correct answer is "E." No further evaluation is necessary in this patient with microalbuminuria. The combination of diabetic retinopathy (a marker for diabetic renal disease), hypertension (BP >130/80 mm Hg in a diabetic patient), and abnormal protein in the urine as measured by the urine microalbumin/creatinine ratio is sufficient to make the diagnosis of early diabetic nephropathy. Renal biopsy is quite invasive and unlikely to change management. ANA, ESR, CRP, and ultrasound are unlikely to offer new information. If things change (e.g., nephritic urine and gross proteinuria), further evaluation may be indicated.

* *

You continue to follow this patient for several years. She ultimately is admitted for chest pain, rules out for myocardial infarction, but has a positive stress test. She will need to have a cardiac catheterization.

In addition to holding her metformin, which of the following interventions would be most likely to reduce her risk of developing contrast-induced nephropathy?

A) *N*-acetylcysteine and IV saline.
B) *N*-acetylcysteine and mannitol.
C) IV saline.
D) Sodium bicarbonate and mannitol.
E) Mannitol and IV saline.

Discussion

The correct answer is "C." For patients at risk of contrast-induced nephropathy, contrast studies should be avoided if possible. If a contrast study must be done, stop aggravating medications like nonsteroidal anti-inflammatory drugs (NSAIDs). Hydration, usually with IV saline, should be given if there are no contraindications (e.g., heart failure). Nonionic lower osmolality (or even iso-osmolar) contrast agents should be used.

Sodium bicarbonate and *N*-acetylcysteine do not have good evidence for effectiveness. Sodium bicarbonate (isotonic sodium bicarbonate solution at 3 mL/kg for 1 hour before the procedure and continue at 1 mL/kg for 6 hours after the procedure) can be used but it is unclear if bicarbonate improves outcomes over saline alone. *N*-acetylcysteine needs to be started the day before the procedure and the evidence is scant: we don't use it. The diuretics, mannitol, and furosemide may be associated with an *increased* risk of nephropathy, and mannitol in particular has an undesirable side effect profile.

HELPFUL TIP: There is a move to dialyze patients who are already on dialysis within 24 hours of a CT contrast study. There is no good data, however, and studies show potential harm. Their kidneys are already shot... they are on dialysis. What additional harm can you do to their kidneys?

HELPFUL (AND VERY IMPORTANT) TIP: The use of MRI contrast (gadolinium) in patients with renal disease has been associated with a scleroderma-like syndrome (nephrogenic systemic fibrosis). Gadolinium should be avoided in those with a CrCl of <30 mL/min. The data are less compelling in those with a CrCl of 30–60 mL/min. Since nephrogenic systemic fibrosis can affect more than just the kidneys, early dialysis may help prevent this disease by reducing the half-life of the gadolinium.

* *

Upon cardiac catheterization, she is found to have several lesions. She undergoes coronary artery bypass grafting and is discharged. Her creatinine remains stable at 1.4 mg/dL.

A few months later, she presents with gradually increasing dyspnea and cough. Her vitals show temperature 37°C, pulse 76, respiratory rate 24, and blood pressure 92/46 mm Hg. You note crackles at both lung bases. Her heart rhythm is regular and an S4 is audible. She has JVD of 9 cm and 2+ pitting pretibial edema.

The ECG shows sinus tachycardia but **no evidence of potassium toxicity.** Lab results: Troponin-T and CK normal, BUN 70 mg/dL, Cr 2.0 mg/dL, Na 128 mEq/L, K 5.3 mEq/L, HCO_3 19 mEq/L, WBC 14,500 per mm^3, remainder of CBC normal. Urinalysis shows protein and glucose and a specific gravity >1.030, but there are few cells and no casts. Cultures and a chest x-ray are pending.

You suspect that her elevated creatinine is primarily due to which of the following processes?

A) Adverse toxic effects of drugs on the kidney.
B) Heart failure or other prerenal cause of renal failure such as dehydration.
C) Sudden progression of diabetic nephropathy.
D) Urinary obstruction.
E) Urinary tract infection.

Discussion

The correct answer is "B." Your patient has clinical evidence of congestive heart failure (CHF), including edema and rales. With a BUN/Cr ratio greater than 20 and an elevated urine-specific gravity, she appears to have a prerenal azotemia, likely secondary to insufficient cardiac output. Drugs may play a role in her dehydration, but the BUN/Cr ratio of >20 argues against a renal cause of her elevated creatinine. Therefore, the most likely culprit is CHF. Diabetes should not cause a sudden worsening of renal disease. Although it has not been eliminated as a cause, urinary obstruction is not likely since she has good urine output. Answer "E" is incorrect since the urinalysis does not support diagnosis of infection, and CHF explains the overall clinical picture much better.

> HELPFUL TIP: Remember that a BUN/Cr ratio >20 generally indicates a prerenal cause of azotemia. These causes include dehydration and poor renal perfusion (shock such as sepsis, CHF, and hypotension). A BUN/Cr ratio <20 is suggestive of intrinsic renal disease or urinary outlet obstruction. These broad generalizations apply to adults only—use clinical judgment.

Given her diabetes and renal disease, which of the following is the most likely cause of her hyperkalemia?

A) Renal tubular acidosis (RTA) type 1.
B) RTA type 2.
C) RTA type 3.
D) RTA type 4.
E) RTA type 5.

Discussion

The correct answer is "D." RTA type 4 is due to aldosterone deficiency or resistance to the activity of aldosterone. The most common cause of RTA type 4 is hyporeninemic hypoaldosteronism, which is often seen in diabetic nephropathy. The disorder is recognized by hyperkalemia and mild acidosis. RTA types 1 and 2 usually are hypokalemic and these forms of RTA are not associated with diabetes. RTA type 3 is a rare autosomal-recessive disorder. RTA type 5 does not exist.

In an effort to *reduce* her serum potassium level (not temporize), you should do which of the following?

A) Temporarily hold her furosemide and ACE inhibitor.
B) Increase her furosemide and temporarily hold her ACE inhibitor.
C) Administer IV calcium gluconate.
D) Bolus IV normal saline 1–2 L.
E) Give albuterol by nebulizer.

Discussion

The correct answer is "B." Because ACE inhibitors can increase serum potassium, you should stop her ACE inhibitor. "A" is incorrect; stopping the furosemide may lead to worsening CHF symptoms and worsening hyperkalemia. In hyperkalemia, calcium gluconate is used to protect cardiac conduction, but it is not effective for reducing potassium concentrations. A bolus of normal saline is contraindicated in a patient with an acute exacerbation of CHF. Albuterol temporarily reduces serum potassium by forcing potassium into the intracellular space.

> HELPFUL TIP: Note that this is a patient who is asymptomatic with a normal ECG and relatively low potassium of 5.3 mg/dL. If she had ECG changes (or a potassium of 7.5 mg/dL), it would be time for a full court press: calcium, insulin, glucose, sodium polystyrene sulfonate (Kayexalate), nebulized albuterol, etc. Note the absence of bicarbonate. It likely doesn't work and its use has fallen out of favor.

Because her creatinine clearance is low (and she is in CHF) you should also discontinue:

A) Insulin.
B) Metoprolol.
C) Metformin.
D) Aspirin.
E) Simvastatin.

Discussion

The correct answer is "C." Your patient's creatinine increased from 1.4 to 2.0 mg/dL, corresponding to a nearly 50% reduction in creatinine clearance—a rough measurement of glomerular filtration rate

(GFR). When creatinine clearance decreases, patients on metformin are at higher risk of developing the rare adverse effect of lactic acidosis. There is some evidence that patients with mild CHF or slight elevations in creatinine can safely take the drug, but stopping metformin in renal failure continues to be the standard of care.

HELPFUL TIP: A rough estimate of the creatinine clearance can be calculated using the Cockcroft–Gault formula:

Estimated creatinine clearance = (140 − age [year])(body weight [kg])/(72 × (serum creatinine [mg/dL]))

For women, multiply this figure by 0.85. One caveat is that this formula may not reflect early renal injury because of compensatory hypertrophy of the remaining glomeruli. **Normal** for healthy adult is 94–140 mL/min for men and 72–110 mL/min for women.

HELPFUL TIP: There is no perfect equation for calculating the GFR. The abbreviated modified diet in renal disease (MDRD) calculation is increasingly used because it seems to be an accurate representation of kidney function in adults with renal disease. Unlike the Cockcroft–Gault equation, the MDRD makes an adjustment for African American race but does not take weight into account. Both equations adjust for gender. Although the equation is a little complicated, many labs now calculate the MDRD GFR. If you want to calculate it yourself, use the National Kidney Foundation Web site at http://www.kidney.org/professionals/KLS/gfr_calculator.cfm.

From the authors' perspective, any of these are OK. We don't need 2 mL/min accuracy in the CrCl. Just make sure you use one of them.

* *

You administer intravenous furosemide. The night after admission she starts vomiting, and your partner inserts a nasogastric tube, which is left to continuous suction overnight (Don't do this . . . there is almost no indication for an NG tube—especially on continuous suction). The next morning, your patient's lab results are as follows: BUN 49 mg/dL, Cr 2.0 mg/dL, Na 132 mEq/L, K 3.5 mEq/L, and HCO_3 35 mEq/L.

On the basis of history and laboratory data provided, you strongly suspect:

A) Metabolic acidosis.
B) Respiratory acidosis.
C) Metabolic alkalosis.
D) Respiratory alkalosis.

Discussion

The correct answer is "C." Loss of gastric acid, through emesis or gastric suction, can result in a metabolic alkalosis. Although no pH is available to confirm alkalosis, you are able to infer the diagnosis based on the elevation in serum HCO_3.

HELPFUL TIP: Diuretics will often cause a hypochloremic "contraction" alkalosis from volume contraction. Watch for this in your patients on a diuretic.

* *

Your patient recovers surprisingly well from her heart failure. Her creatinine returns to near baseline (1.5 mg/dL). You try to rechallenge the patient with an ACE inhibitor followed by an ARB. However, her hyperkalemia recurs and she is unable to tolerate either of these drugs. With beta-blocker and loop diuretic therapy, her average blood pressure is 130/80 mm Hg. At a follow-up visit, you find no signs or symptoms of CHF.

You want to lower your patient's risk of progressing to end-stage renal disease. To reduce proteinuria, which of the following strategies is best?

A) Add isosorbide dinitrate.
B) Add a nondihydropyridine calcium channel blocker (e.g., diltiazem, verapamil).
C) Add a dihydropyridine calcium channel blocker (e.g., amlodipine, nifedipine).
D) Restrict protein in the diet.

Discussion

The correct answer is "B." Nondihydropyridine calcium channel blockers reduce protein excretion in diabetic patients with nephropathy and slow down the progression of renal disease. Answer "A," nitrates, would be effective for angina and will lower blood pressure but do not demonstrate an effect on diabetic nephropathy. The dihydropyridine calcium channel blockers do not slow down progression to nephropathy to the same degree as some other antihypertensive drugs. The effect of protein restriction on nephropathy has been well studied and it doesn't likely reduce progression of the disease. This is still controversial, however.

HELPFUL TIP: For diabetic nephropathy, always start with an ACE inhibitor and try to maximize the dose. Full dose ACE inhibitor treatment is associated with improved survival in diabetic nephropathy compared with low-dose ACE inhibitor. The dose of ACE inhibitor may be limited by serum potassium level or patient blood pressure. **Sodium restriction added to an ACE inhibitor is actually more effective than adding an ARB for proteinuria and blood pressure control.** (BMJ 2011;343:d4366; http://dx.doi.org/10.1136/bmj.d4366). In this study, the actual sodium in the diet was 2500 mg (although the goal was 1200 mg).

* *

Over the next year, your patient experiences increasing difficulties with glycemic control. Despite your efforts, her proteinuria and serum creatinine increase. As you discuss referral to a nephrologist, she asks about dialysis.

Which of the following is NOT an indication for dialysis?

A) Severe hyperkalemia due to renal failure.
B) Accelerated hypertension.
C) Malnutrition.
D) Persistent nausea and vomiting despite treatment.
E) Bleeding secondary to uremia.

Discussion

The correct answer is "C." In chronic renal failure due to any cause, **absolute clinical indications for initiating dialysis include** persistent nausea and vomiting, pericarditis, fluid overload, uremic encephalopathy, accelerated hypertension, bleeding due to uremia, serum creatinine greater than 12 mg/dL, and severe electrolyte abnormalities that cannot be otherwise handled. These are potentially life-threatening situations that must be dealt with acutely. Malnutrition is a relative indication that occurs more indolently.

HELPFUL (AND VERY IMPORTANT) TIP: **Counter to what you might expect, early dialysis increases mortality.** Do not initiate dialysis until the GFR is 5–7 mL/min/1.73 m^2 **or** the patient is having clinical problems that cannot be otherwise managed (Arch Intern Med 2011;171:39 and N Engl J Med 2010; June 27). Patients on early dialysis die from infection, complications from dialysis (hypotension), problems with their grafts (again leading to infection), etc.

Objectives: Did you learn to . . .

- Screen for microalbuminuria in diabetic patients?
- Evaluate and treat microalbuminuria and proteinuria in diabetic patients?
- Identify prerenal renal failure?
- Describe the features of RTA type 4?
- Identify gastric suctioning as a common cause of metabolic alkalosis in the hospital?
- Discuss when to initiate dialysis in a patient with chronic renal failure?

CASE 2

A 49-year-old African American female with diabetes type 2, hypertension, and hyperlipidemia returns for a follow-up visit. She's had diabetes for 15 years, and her control has been variable over that time. Now, her glycosylated hemoglobin is 8%. She has developed microalbuminuria and diabetic retinopathy. You point out that her renal function has progressively declined, which alarms her since her mother is on hemodialysis. Her creatinine was 1.2 mg/dL 3 years ago, and now it is 1.9 mg/dL. Her GFR is 36 mL/min/1.73 m^2. She weighs 100 kg, and her blood pressure is 120/76 mm Hg.

Which of the following is the most appropriate description of her renal function?

A) Stage 1 chronic kidney disease (CKD).
B) Stage 2 CKD.
C) Stage 3 CKD.
D) Stage 4 CKD.
E) Stage 5 CKD.

Table 5–1 STAGES OF CHRONIC KIDNEY DISEASE

Stage	GFR (mL/min/1.73 m^2)	Comments
1	≥90	Stage 1 defined by evidence of kidney damage (e.g., structural damage, albuminuria) with normal GFR
2	60–89	Mild decline in renal function; about 5.4% of US population
3	30–59	Moderate decline in renal function; about 5.4% of US population (yes, same percent as stage 2)
4	15–29	Severe decline in renal function; approaching need for dialysis
5	<15	End-stage disease

GFR, glomerular filtration rate.

Discussion

The correct answer is "C." She has stage 3 CKD. Table 5–1 defines the various stages of CKD. Not all patients will progress through all of the stages of CKD. On the basis of age alone, many elderly patients may be classified as having stage 1 or 2 CKD, and they may never progress. Knowledge of a patient's CKD stage is useful in determining how to treat, what drugs to avoid, etc.

HELPFUL TIP: Patients with CKD, with or without diabetes, are at increased risk of coronary artery disease, so other risk factors for heart disease should be treated aggressively. In fact, many experts believe that CKD should be treated as a "coronary artery disease equivalent."

* *

You increase the patient's insulin and lisinopril doses, confirm that she is taking aspirin, and convince her to quit smoking (you are very persuasive—not to mention good-looking!). One month later, your patient returns with typical symptoms of a urinary tract infection. Her urine culture grows *Escherichia coli* resistant to trimethoprim/sulfamethoxazole but susceptible to all other antibiotics tested.

The most appropriate antibiotic regimen for this patient's UTI is:

A) Ciprofloxacin 250 mg PO every other day for two doses.
B) Ciprofloxacin 250 mg PO once.
C) Ciprofloxacin 250 mg PO BID for 3 days.
D) Levofloxacin 750 mg PO daily for 7 days.

Discussion

The correct answer is "C." This patient's GFR is 36 mL/min/1.73 m^2 and her creatinine clearance is 56 mL/min (using the Cockcroft–Gault equation given earlier). Therefore, the usual ciprofloxacin dose of 250 mg PO BID for UTI is safe and appropriate. Less frequent dosing may be required for lesser GFR or creatinine clearance. The important thing here is to recall that CKD may require dosage adjustments for many medications. Numerous drugs are renally cleared, so it's always prudent to know the GFR or creatinine clearance and check for dosage adjustments before prescribing.

* *

You assume the UTI cleared because you do not hear from her for a few months. Then her sister brings her in for an acute illness including nausea, emesis, confusion and generalized weakness. These symptoms began yesterday. The only other thing new with her health is heartburn which she has been self-treating with increasingly larger amounts of Tums® (calcium carbonate), taking "handfuls" over the last few days. Her lab results now include creatinine 2.5 mg/dL, calcium 14 mg/dL, and HCO_3 37 mEq/L.

The most appropriate treatment for her now includes:

A) Hydrochlorothiazide (HCTZ).
B) Furosemide.
C) Normal saline IV.
D) A and C.
E) B and C.

Discussion

The correct answer is "C." Your patient is now presenting with a classic case of milk-alkali syndrome. The diagnosis should be recognized by the triad of hypercalcemia, metabolic alkalosis, and renal insufficiency in combination with the history of typical symptoms (described in the case) and excessive calcium carbonate ingestion. Treatment includes removal of the offending agent and treatment of the hypercalcemia with IV saline (to improve renal perfusion and metabolic alkalosis). "A," thiazide diuretics, results in reabsorption of calcium—the opposite of what you want to achieve in a patient with hypercalcemia. "B," furosemide, has fallen out of favor and requires the establishment of euvolemia first. Even then you need 10 L of saline per day with 100 mg of IV furosemide every 1–2 hours. This is usually impractical and hasn't been shown to add anything.

> HELPFUL TIP: Compared with loop diuretics, thiazide diuretics are generally better at lowering blood pressure. However, at a GFR <30 mL/min/1.73 m^2, thiazides are less effective as antihypertensive agents. For stage 4 and stage 5 CKD patients, especially those with hypervolemia, consider using a loop diuretic or metolazone instead of a thiazide.

* *

You get the patient through her episode of hypercalcemia. As your patient's renal disease progresses over the years, you find that she has become anemic with a hemoglobin of 10.1 g/dL. She takes a multiple vitamin. Her iron studies are normal, and her screening colonoscopy last year was normal. The anemia is normocytic and normochromic.

If you were to treat her with an erythropoietic agent (e.g., erythropoietin or darbepoetin), her target hemoglobin would be:

A) 9–10 g/dL.
B) 10–11 g/dL.
C) 13–14 g/dL.
D) >15 g/dL.

Discussion

The correct answer is "B." For patients with CKD and anemia of chronic disease (when other causes of anemia have been ruled out and/or treated), erythropoietic agents should **NOT** be used to achieve "near normal" hemoglobin levels. Target levels should be about 10–11 g/dL. Higher hemoglobin levels are associated with a greater risk of adverse events, including increased risk of mortality, need for dialysis, CHF, graft thrombosis, uncontrolled hypertension, etc. This finding is consistent with a similar finding in cancer patients (JAMA 2010;303(9):857–864; N Engl J Med 2009;361:2019–2032). The **FDA suggests withholding erythropoietin if the Hb >12 g/dL or if the Hb increases by >1 g/dL in any 2-week period.**

Objectives: Did you learn to . . .

- Stage CKD?
- Adjust medication doses based on renal function?
- Recognize and treat milk-alkali syndrome?
- Recognize appropriate targets for treatment with erythropoietic agents?

CASE 3

A 55-year-old male presents to your office for evaluation of blood in his urine. It turns out that he had a life insurance physical and the urinalysis showed 2+ blood on urine dipstick and 2 RBC/hpf. The remainder of the urinalysis and microscopic exam was normal.

After an appropriate history and physical exam, your first step in the evaluation of this urine abnormality is to:

A) Repeat the urinalysis and microscopic exam.
B) Obtain urine for culture.
C) Order a renal ultrasound.
D) Order a CT scan of the abdomen.
E) Order an intravenous pyelogram (IVP).

Discussion

The correct answer is "A." According to the urinalysis, there is a small amount of blood in your patient's urine, but the number of RBCs is actually normal (<3 RBC/hpf). Your first step should be to repeat the urinalysis and urine microscopic exam to determine if this patient actually meets the criteria for microscopic hematuria (≥3 RBC/hpf on two of three properly collected urine specimens, according to the American Urological Association).

A urine culture may prove useful later in the evaluation process but is not necessary now. Likewise, ordering ultrasound, CT, or IVP studies is premature because the diagnosis of microscopic hematuria has not been made.

> HELPFUL TIP: Kidney stones are a very common cause of gross and microscopic hematuria. However, recall that 20% of patients with kidney stones will have no blood in their urine and a normal urinalysis. IgA nephropathy is one of the most common intrinsic renal diseases to cause microscopic hematuria; kidney cysts, including polycystic kidney disease, are common causes as well. Neoplastic diseases, in particular bladder cancer and renal cell carcinoma, may also be discovered during the investigation of microscopic hematuria.

* *

Further history reveals that he smokes one to two packs of cigarettes per day. He has a normal blood pressure and the remainder of the physical exam is unrevealing. On two urine samples, you find microscopic hematuria, with a positive dipstick and 5 RBC/hpf. The rest of the urinalysis is normal, and there are no red cell casts.

In your evaluation of this patient, you include all of the following tests EXCEPT:

A) Urine cytology.
B) CBC.
C) Serum creatinine.
D) CT scan of the abdomen and pelvis with particular note of the kidneys.
E) Renal biopsy.

Discussion

The correct answer is "E." In most cases of microscopic hematuria, renal biopsy is not indicated. However, if an intrinsic renal cause of hematuria is suspected, renal biopsy may prove necessary. Intrinsic renal disease is more likely if there is proteinuria, hypertension, elevated serum creatinine, or an active urinary sediment (e.g., nephritic, dysmorphic red cells, red cell casts).

There is no completely standardized evaluation of microscopic hematuria, and recommendations vary depending on the author. However, the recommendations always include serum creatinine and usually include CBC, coagulation studies, and serum chemistries. Depending on the patient's age, further studies may be indicated. For patients older than 40 years, you should consider studies to evaluate for urinary tract cancers. Urine cytology has low sensitivity but high specificity for bladder cancer and may be quite useful in conjunction with cystoscopy. Imaging of the urinary system is an absolute requirement in the workup of microscopic hematuria in older patients. CT scan appears to have the greatest sensitivity for detecting masses, but ultrasound, IVP, or the combination of the two may also be employed. Cystoscopy should be considered if the CT scan is normal since CT is poor at visualizing bladder abnormalities. See Table 5–2 for a suggested workup for microscopic hematuria.

The US Preventive Services Task Force recommends which of the following screening strategies for detecting microscopic hematuria?

A) Annual urinalysis after age 50.
B) Urinalysis every 2 years after age 50.
C) Annual urinalysis after age 65.
D) Annual urinalysis in all high-risk patients older than 65 years.
E) No screening at any age.

Table 5–2 EVALUATION OF MICROSCOPIC HEMATURIA

After microscopic hematuria has been identified (2 of 3 urine samples with 3 or more RBC/hpf), the AUA recommends the following evaluation:

- Infection identified → treat with antibiotics and repeat urinalysis
- RBC casts, proteinuria, or elevated creatinine → begin evaluation for glomerulonephritis and consider referral to a nephrologist
- No infection or primary renal disease identified in first 2 steps → urine cytology, bladder cystoscopy (if at risk for bladder cancer based on environmental exposures and/or age >40), and CT scan (helical CT if stones suspected, contrast-enhanced CT if stones not suspected)
- If entire thorough diagnostic evaluation negative → follow-up urinalysis, urine cytology, blood pressure, and serum creatinine every 6–12 months.

Discussion

The correct answer is "E." The USPSTF recommends against routine screening for microscopic hematuria to detect urinary tract cancers. In one-time urine specimens in healthy adults, the presence of abnormal numbers of RBCs (≥3 RBCs/hpf) can be as high as 39%. In up to 70% of patients, even after imaging of the upper and lower urinary tract, the source of microscopic hematuria cannot be found. In a low-risk population, the false-positive rate of microscopic hematuria found on urinalysis would be unacceptably high. Also, there is no evidence that early detection of bladder cancer through screening urinalysis improves prognosis.

* *

Your patient returns to discuss his lab and radiology results. His serum creatinine is 1.1 mg/dL, and his CBC, chemistries, and coagulation studies are normal. His urine cytology was negative, as was cystoscopy performed by a urologist. CT scan of the abdomen and pelvis reveals normal size kidneys and no masses, but three stones, measuring 2–3 mm in diameter, are noted in the left renal pelvis. There does not appear to be any obstruction. Your patient denies any history of renal colic.

Regarding the finding of stones in the left renal pelvis, which of the following interventions is warranted at this time?

A) Observation.
B) Lithotripsy.
C) Ureteral stent placement.
D) Ketorolac and fluids by IV.

Discussion

The correct answer is "A." The incidental finding of stones during the evaluation of microscopic hematuria is common. The stones may be the reason for your patient's hematuria. Since the stones are small, they may pass without intervention. Most stones less than 5 mm in diameter will pass spontaneously. No further intervention is warranted in asymptomatic patients. "D" is of particular note. Ketorolac and other NSAIDs are effective in treating the pain of urolithiasis. However, fluid is not helpful in treating acute ureteral colic (unless the patient is dehydrated). Fluid does nothing to "push" the stone out and increases pain. For those of you old enough to remember routine IVPs, remember the 1- and 2-hour delayed films? The body simply shifts the excess fluid to the nonobstructed kidney. This is why there is delayed visualization of the kidney on IVP. So, forgo the fluids during renal colic if the patient is euvolemic.

> HELPFUL TIP: Desmopressin (DDAVP), which decreases urine volumes, can be used to control pain in those with urolithiasis (although we don't recommend it for routine use—there are plenty of good analgesics out there).

* *

Your patient does well for a year. When you see him next, he presents to your office as a late afternoon add-on and complains of severe abdominal pain that woke him from sleep at 3 AM. He describes the pain as "sharp" or "crampy," occurring in his left lower quadrant and radiating to the left testicle. Although the pain has waxed and waned, it has never resolved completely. He is also nauseated and has been vomiting. On exam, he is afebrile and tachycardic and has a blood pressure of 110/56 mm Hg. He appears uncomfortable and is writhing in pain. There is left lower quadrant, flank and costovertebral angle tenderness.

Your next action is to:

A) Prescribe oral ibuprofen and morphine and arrange follow-up tomorrow.
B) Give IM ketorolac and arrange follow-up tomorrow.
C) Bolus 1 L IV saline, administer IV ceftriaxone, and arrange follow-up tomorrow.
D) Send him to the emergency department (ED) for pain management, fluids, and possible admission.

Discussion

The correct answer is "D." In a patient with known kidney stones presenting with classic findings of urolithiasis, the most likely diagnosis is renal colic due to stones. This patient is nauseated and vomiting frequently and may not do well at home overnight. He may not be able to tolerate oral medications and could become dehydrated. Additionally, we don't have a UA; a postobstructive UTI is an indication for admission and possibly stenting. For these reasons, the most appropriate action is aggressive pain management, which can be accomplished in the ED. If the patient is unable to keep down oral pain medications after treatment in the ED, admission to the hospital is warranted.

Narcotic analgesics, IV NSAIDs (e.g., ketorolac), and IV fluids to maintain euvolemia are all appropriate. The role of antibiotics will depend on urinalysis findings, but most cases of acute renal colic do not require antibiotics.

HELPFUL (AND VERY IMPORTANT) TIP: Urolithiasis and abdominal aortic aneurysm can have the same presenting symptoms and signs (including hematuria). For that reason, imaging is mandatory in the older individual in whom an abdominal aortic aneurysm is a consideration. Also, keep testicular torsion on the differential for younger male patients presenting with renal colic symptoms.

* *

You admit the patient to the ED; start IV saline to maintain hydration; and administer narcotics, NSAIDs (ketorolac), and antiemetics. CT scan shows a 5-mm stone in the proximal ureter. There is no hydronephrosis. Serum electrolytes, BUN, creatinine, and CBC are all normal. Urinalysis reveals 2+ blood, 1+ leukocyte esterase, trace protein, pH 6, specific gravity 1.025, 20 RBC/hpf, few calcium oxalate crystals, and otherwise normal.

Which of the following is the most appropriate management at this point in time?

A) Add antibiotics to the current therapy.
B) Continue the current therapy and observe.
C) Refer for extracorporeal shock wave lithotripsy.
D) Refer for endoscopic lithotripsy.

Discussion

The correct answer is "B." There is no reason to change management at this point in time. Many 5-mm stones will pass spontaneously. Although leukocyte esterase is detected on the urine dipstick, there is no compelling evidence of infection (e.g., fever, elevated WBC count, and WBCs on microscopic exam), so antibiotics are not appropriate.

HELPFUL TIP: Stones of 6 mm or greater will pass spontaneously only 10% of the time and those 4–6 mm 50% of the time. Those less than 4 mm pass the great majority of the time. If pain persists or the stone does not pass within 72 hours, consider urologic intervention such as nephrostomy, stent placement, and lithotripsy. Renal injury from obstruction generally does not occur for at least 72 hours (and, amazingly enough, there is only a 20% chance of complications if a nonobstructing stone remains for 4 weeks!).

HELPFUL TIP: Patients discharged from the ED with urolithiasis should be placed on an NSAID in addition to a narcotic. This reduces pain and "bounce back" visits.

Your patient asks how he can avoid kidney stones in the future. Which of the following tests will be most useful in determining the treatments that may prevent future stone formation?

A) Urine culture.
B) Stone recovery and analysis.
C) Urinary calcium excretion.
D) Urinary oxalate excretion.
E) Serum uric acid.

Discussion

The correct answer is "B." The prevention of further stone formation is aided considerably by knowledge of the stone type. You should always attempt to recover the stone and send it for analysis—unless the patient is a well-known stone former and the composition of his or her stones is already known. The other studies listed have value, mostly depending on the stone type. Struvite stones form during bacterial infections of the urinary tract and a urine culture ("A") will help direct therapy when these stones are identified. Calcium oxalate stones are the most common and 24-hour urine collection to determine calcium and oxalate excretion can lead to diagnoses of metabolic disturbances (hyperoxaluria and hypercalciuria). Patients with uric acid stones should be evaluated for symptoms of gout and undergo serum uric acid measurements.

* *

Your patient passes the stone, his pain completely resolves, and he is discharged from the hospital within 24 hours of his admission. The stone is pure calcium oxalate. Studies of his 24-hour urine collection are pending.

In order to reduce his risk of forming more stones, you tell him to incorporate all of the following lifestyle changes EXCEPT:

A) Restrict calcium intake.
B) Restrict oxalate intake (e.g., leafy green vegetables, chocolate).
C) Increase daily water intake.
D) Reduce meat and fish consumption.

Discussion

The correct answer is "A." To prevent recurrent urolithiasis, restricted calcium intake was encouraged in the past. Now, moderate calcium intake (1 g/day) is recognized as beneficial and should be encouraged. Patients should take calcium with meals, which will bind oxylate and prevent its absorption. A low-calcium diet actually leads to an *increased* risk of urolithiasis. Increases in urine oxalate greatly increase the risk of stone formation. Restriction of oxalate in the diet may help to reduce the risk of recurrent urolithiasis. Unfortunately, oxalate is also the end product of numerous metabolic pathways, and significant reduction in urinary oxalate levels often proves difficult (good news for you rhubarb fans).

Increased fluid intake to achieve a urine volume >2 L/day reduces stone formation. Water and citrus juices are traditionally recommended, but most fluids consumed are associated with a positive effect, including drinks with caffeine.

Meat, fish, and poultry are sources of purine, which is metabolized to uric acid. A uric acid crystal can form a pure uric acid stone or serve as a nidus for calcium stone formation. Therefore, a general recommendation to avoid recurrent urolithiasis is to reduce purines in the diet through reduced meat, fish, and poultry consumption.

* *

Urinary citrate inhibits calcium stone formation. Hypocitraturia is a common cause of recurrent urolithiasis. A nonspecific measure to decrease calcium stone formation is to increase citrus fruits in the diet. Lemonade and orange juice are excellent sources of citrate and can also be used to increase urine volume. However, the best studies suggest that lemon juice ***does not*** reduce stones from hypocitraturia and grapefruit juice **increases** stone formation.

Your patient is wondering if he should have his urolithiasis worked up to determine an etiology. All of the following are reasons to pursue a further evaluation in this patient EXCEPT:

A) A strong family history of stones.
B) Black ancestry.
C) Chronic diarrhea.
D) Hypertension.
E) Bariatric surgery.

Discussion

The correct answer is "D." Simply having hypertension is not a reason to work up a patient for renal stones. All of the other choices are correct. Of note is "B." Patients of African ancestry are less likely to have stones. Therefore, the workup is more likely to be positive in these patients. "C" and "D" are also of note. Anything that can cause malabsorption including bowel surgery, history of inflammatory bowel disease, etc., can increase the risk of stones. Thus, evaluation is indicated in these patients.

* *

Because of his strong family history, you decide to proceed with evaluation. Results of your patient's 24-hour urine have returned and are as follows (normal values):

Volume 1.6 L.
pH 6.5.
Creatinine clearance normal.
Calcium 410 mg (100–300 mg).
Uric acid 410 mEq (250–750 mEq).
Oxalate 42 mg (7–44 mg).
Citrate 560 mg (100–800 mg).
Magnesium 3.1 mEq (3–5 mEq).

Which of the following medications is most likely to reduce his risk of developing kidney stones in the future?

A) Allopurinol.
B) Potassium citrate.
C) HCTZ.
D) Sodium bicarbonate.
E) Furosemide.

Discussion

The correct answer is "C." According to the 24-hour urine studies, your patient has hypercalciuria, suboptimal urine volumes (the goal for urine output in urolithiasis should be 2 L/day or more), and no other abnormalities. Patients with urolithiasis and hypercalciuria benefit from long-term treatment with thiazide diuretics, such as HCTZ, which decrease calcium excretion and therefore stone formation. Furosemide increases calcium excretion and has the potential to increase stone formation.

Even though it seems counterintuitive, patients with **calcium** stones and **hyperuricosuria** may benefit from allopurinol. It is thought that hyperuricosuria predisposes to calcium stones. Also, allopurinol is useful in treatment of patients with uric acid stones. Patients with uric acid stones and hyperuricosuria may benefit from alkalinization of the urine with sodium bicarbonate or potassium citrate. In general, dietary citrate should be maximized. Oral potassium citrate is indicated for patients with hypocitraturia.

* *

The patient is wondering whether he can expect to get another stone.

All of the following are true EXCEPT:

A) The peak incidence of kidney stones is age 30.
B) Kidney stones are more common in men than in women.
C) The rate of a second kidney stone is 60–80%.
D) Only people who become dehydrated can expect to have a second stone.
E) Living in a hot climate can predispose to a second stone.

Discussion

The correct answer is "D." While dehydration may predispose to a second stone (and thus "E"), maintaining optimal hydration is not necessarily protective. Kidney stones are more common in men and have a peak incidence at age 30. About 60–80% of patients with a kidney stone will suffer a recurrence.

HELPFUL TIP: Compared with microscopic hematuria, **gross hematuria** is more commonly associated with malignancy and, once confirmed, should prompt a thorough evaluation.

Benign causes of **microscopic hematuria** in adults include vigorous exercise, menstruation, sexual activity, viral illness, and trauma.

Which of these kidney or ureteral stone patients requires hospitalization?

A) Those with high-grade obstruction.
B) Those with intractable pain or vomiting.
C) Those with an associated urinary tract infection.
D) Those with a solitary kidney, transplanted kidney, or in whom the diagnosis is uncertain.
E) All of the above.

Discussion

The correct answer is "E." All of the patients listed above should be admitted. Obviously, patients having uncontrollable pain or vomiting will do poorly as outpatients. Urolithiasis with a coexistent UTI is a significant problem due to the risk of abscess formation, bacteremia, and renal parenchymal destruction. These patients require IV antibiotics and immediate urologic consultation for admission, particularly in the presence of comorbidity. Patients with solitary or transplanted kidneys or in whom the diagnosis of renal colic is unclear should be admitted for monitoring of renal function and further evaluation.

HELPFUL TIP: The use of an alpha-blocker (e.g., tamsulosin) may help speed up stone passage. However, this is true only in proximal stones (near the kidney) that are larger than 4 mm. Distal stones 4 mm or less will pass on their own anyway.

Objectives: Did you learn to . . .

- Define microscopic hematuria?
- Evaluate a patient with microscopic hematuria based on risk and differential diagnosis?
- Describe the difficulties inherent in employing urine studies to screen for urinary tract cancers?
- Evaluate and manage a patient with urolithiasis?
- Identify causes of urolithiasis based on the characteristics of the stone?
- Decide when a patient with urolithiasis should be referred for lithotripsy?
- Use strategies to prevent stone formation based on the characteristics of the stone?

CASE 4

A 29-year-old female presents to your office concerned about protein in her urine. On a routine physical examination for employment, a urinalysis showed 2+ protein. She has no urinary symptoms and denies fever, weight changes, and edema. She is afebrile with a blood pressure of 118/68 mm Hg. Examination is otherwise unremarkable. Repeat urinalysis in the office shows 1+ protein, specific gravity 1.020, pH 6.5, and no blood. The urine microscopic exam is normal.

Which of the following is the most appropriate next action in evaluating this patient?

A) Repeat urinalysis and urine culture.
B) Ultrasound of the kidneys.
C) 24-hour urine collection for protein and creatinine.
D) Random urine protein/creatinine ratio.
E) C or D.

Discussion

The correct answer is "E." You should ask the patient to collect urine for 24 hours for protein and creatinine measurements. Alternatively, random urine protein/creatinine ratios correlate well with 24-hour collections and are much easier to obtain. Besides, who wants to lug around a vat of their own urine all day?

Your patient already has protein on urinalysis twice. Another urinalysis will not help to determine if this is truly a worrisome finding or not. There is no evidence of a UTI (no leukocyte esterase, nitrites, etc., and no symptoms); thus, culture would be very low yield. There is no indication for renal ultrasound at this point.

> HELPFUL TIP: Concentrated or alkaline urine can result in overestimation of urine protein on dipstick.

Which type(s) of protein are detected on a urine dipstick?

A) Albumin.
B) Amino acids.
C) Immunoglobulin light chains.
D) A and B.
E) A and C.

Discussion

The correct answer is "A." The urine dipstick only detects large-molecular-weight proteins—generally this means albumin. Amino acids are not detected. Immunoglobulin light chains, such as Bence Jones proteins, are also not detected on urine dipstick.

* *

After analysis of her 24-hour urine collection, your patient returns. She has 1 g of protein in the 24-hour collection. Creatinine clearance is normal. Serum creatinine, BUN, albumin, glucose, and electrolytes are normal.

Which of the following is the next step in your evaluation and management?

A) Reassure the patient and schedule follow-up urinalysis in 6 months.
B) CT scan of abdomen and pelvis.
C) Measure recumbent urine protein level.
D) Refer for renal biopsy.

Discussion

The correct answer is "C." Proteinuria may be either transient or persistent. Transient proteinuria is often due to fever, exercise, or other causes and is not associated with significant kidney disease. Transient proteinuria is found in 7% of women and 4% of men. It often resolves spontaneously, and subsequent urine tests will probably be negative. However, at this point you don't know if this case will be transient or persistent proteinuria.

Orthostatic proteinuria is a common type of transient proteinuria seen in young, healthy persons. Up to 5% of adolescents have orthostatic proteinuria, and young adults may present with it as well. Protein is spilled in the urine when the patient is upright, but not when recumbent. There are two ways to determine recumbent urine protein: an easy way and a hard way. The easy way is to have the patient void before going to bed, stay supine all night (~8 hours), and collect urine immediately upon waking. This urine is checked for protein/creatinine ratio. Another urine sample must be checked for protein/creatinine after the patient has been upright. If the upright is abnormal and the recumbent is normal, you have diagnosed orthostatic proteinuria. The "hard way" involves splitting a 24-hour urine collection. Orthostatic proteinuria is a benign condition that usually resolves as the patient ages, and it require no additional evaluation.

A finding of 1 g of protein in a 24-hour urine collection is abnormal (normal <0.15 g/day), but it does not yet reach the nephrotic range (>3 g/day). Reassuring the patient at this stage is not appropriate. CT scan of the abdomen and pelvis is unlikely to add any knew information. Referring for renal biopsy is premature.

* *

The patient collects urine in upright and recumbent positions, and both have abnormal amounts of protein. You refer the patient to a nephrologist who recommends follow-up rather than biopsy. Annual follow-up will include blood pressure, serum creatinine, and spot urine protein/creatinine ratio.

In order to prevent worsening proteinuria, the nephrologist also recommends which of the following medications?

A) Amlodipine.
B) Diltiazem.
C) Furosemide.
D) Benazepril.
E) Aspirin.

Discussion

The correct answer is "D." Patients with proteinuria tend to respond well to ACE inhibitors. ACE inhibitors have been shown to reduce proteinuria by 35–40%. This effect is true in nondiabetic patients with proteinuria as well as in diabetic patients. ACE inhibitors appear to be superior to other antihypertensives, including calcium channel blockers. Furosemide would be indicated if your patient develops edema, but loop diuretics should not be used primarily for treatment of hypertension or proteinuria. Aspirin may be indicated for protection against coronary artery disease in patients with risk factors, including CKD, but it is not a primary treatment of proteinuria or hypertension. Remember that NSAIDs can adversely affect renal function.

* *

Unfortunately, over the next few years, your patient develops hypertension. You maximize the dose of benazepril and need to add another drug to control her pressure. Her proteinuria increases to 3.5 g/day, and her plasma creatinine increases to 2.0 mg/dL. She develops edema, and her serum albumin is 2.8 g/dL. The urine shows only protein **and no inflammatory components.**

This patient's current clinical condition is most appropriately described as:

A) Hypertensive nephropathy.
B) Acute renal failure.
C) Focal nephritic glomerulonephritis.
D) Nephrotic syndrome.
E) Floating kidney.

Discussion

The correct answer is "D." While identifying no specific disease state, the term nephrotic syndrome refers to a constellation of signs and laboratory abnormalities. A number of diseases may lead to nephrotic syndrome (keep reading for more on this). When urine protein exceeds 3 g/day, it is often referred to as "nephrotic range" proteinuria. Complete nephrotic syndrome is characterized by nephrotic range proteinuria, edema, hypertension, hypoalbuminemia, and hyperlipidemia (Table 5–3).

Which of the following findings in urine sediment is associated with nephrotic syndrome?

A) Red cell casts.
B) White cell casts.
C) Oval fat bodies.
D) Uric acid crystals.
E) Granular casts.

Discussion

The correct answer is "C." Urine sediment in nephrotic syndrome is typically bland. There is little cellular matter. Oval fat bodies and fatty casts occur in the urine of patients with heavy proteinuria and hyperlipidemia. Fat bodies reflect the increased permeability of the glomeruli and suggest some type

Table 5–3 CRITERIA FOR NEPHROTIC SYNDROME

Required for the diagnosis of nephrotic syndrome
• Albuminuria >3 g/day
• Hypoalbuminemia (serum albumin of <3 g/dL)
• Peripheral edema
Other (nonnecessary) findings:
• Hyperlipidemia
• Thrombotic events

Table 5–4 URINE SEDIMENT FINDINGS AND ASSOCIATED CONDITIONS

Sediment Finding	Associated Condition
Epithelial cell casts	ATN, acute glomerulonephritis
Fat bodies, fatty casts	Massive proteinuria (nephrotic syndrome), fat emboli, polycystic kidney disease, glomerular disease (may not be active as in nephrotic syndrome)
Granular casts	Nonspecific—many renal disorders
Hyaline casts	Concentrated urine, diuretic use, normal finding
Red cell casts	Glomerulonephritis, vasculitis (very specific to these)
Waxy casts	Advanced renal failure
White cell casts	Pyelonephritis, acute interstitial nephritis, various glomerular diseases

ATN, acute tubular necrosis.

of glomerular disease (including nephrotic syndrome) albeit not necessarily active disease. However, fat can also be seen in patients with polycystic kidney disease and fat embolism syndrome.

Red cell casts, the hallmark of glomerulonephritis, are absent in nephrotic urine. White cell casts are associated with interstitial nephritis and pyelonephritis. Uric acid crystals are sometimes seen in gout, hyperuricemia, and urate stone disease. Granular casts are not specific to any particular pathologic process and may be found in acute tubular necrosis, glomerulonephritis, and other renal diseases. See Table 5–4 for more details on urine sediment.

Nephrotic syndrome is not a specific disease entity but can be the end result of a number of processes. Which of the following cause nephrotic syndrome?

A) Diabetes.
B) Minimal change disease.
C) Amyloidosis.
D) Systemic lupus erythematosus.
E) All of the above.

Table 5–5 CAUSES OF NEPHROTIC SYNDROME

- Diabetes
- Amyloidosis
- Systemic lupus erythematosus
- Minimal change disease ("Nil" disease)
- Diffuse glomerulonephritis
- Membranous nephropathy
- IgA nephropathy
- Postinfectious glomerulonephritis (e.g., poststreptococcal GN)
- Membranoproliferative glomerulonephritis
- Various neoplastic diseases (lymphoma, multiple myeloma, lung cancer, etc.)
- Preeclampsia
- Familial kidney disease (Alport disease, Fabry disease)
- Focal and segmental glomerulosclerosis
- Medications (NSAIDs)
- Miscellaneous

Discussion

The correct answer is "E." All of the above can be a cause of **nephrotic** syndrome. Remember that many causes of nephrotic syndrome can present initially with **nephritic** urine. Causes of nephrotic syndrome are summarized in Table 5–5.

Which of the following tests is NOT indicated in most patients with nephrotic syndrome?

A) Hepatitis B and C serology.
B) ANA.
C) Serum and urine protein electrophoresis.
D) Antistreptococcal antibodies (e.g., ASO titer).
E) CA-125 antigen.

Discussion

The correct answer is "E." Evaluation for cancer should be done if there is a specific reason to believe the patient has a malignancy (weight loss, mass on exam, etc.). CA-125 is a marker for ovarian cancer (among others . . . colon, pancreatic, etc.) and need not be done routinely. Plus, it's not a useful screening test for ovarian cancer. In addition to a thorough history and physical, routine evaluation of patients with nephrotic syndrome (and nephritis and glomerulonephritis) include the following:

- Hepatitis B and C serology.
- ANA.
- Serum and urine protein electrophoresis.

- ASO titer.
- Cryoglobulins.
- Serum complement levels.
- ANCA.
- Serum calcium (to rule out sarcoid).
- Antiglomerular basement membrane antibodies.

Use clinical judgment to guide your workup. However, this testing will find the cause of most cases of nephritis/nephrotic syndrome.

* *

The diagnosis in your patient is unclear despite the workup noted above. It is time to consider a renal biopsy.

Absolute contraindications to renal biopsy include which of the following?

A) Hypertension.
B) Use of warfarin for atrial fibrillation.
C) Pyelonephritis.
D) Solitary renal cyst.
E) All of the above.

Discussion

The correct answer is "C." The presence of renal or perirenal infection is a contraindication to renal biopsy. None of the others are absolute contraindications. However, **uncontrollable** hypertension, **irreversible coagulopathy, multiple bilateral cysts**, hydronephrosis, small kidneys (indicative of chronic, irreversible disease), known renal tumor, and lack of consent are all contraindications to renal biopsy. Simply being on warfarin, which can be reversed, is not a contraindication to biopsy.

Which of the following is an indication for renal biopsy?

A) **Persistent** hematuria in a patient with normal renal function and an otherwise negative workup.
B) **Persistent** low-grade proteinuria (1–2 g/day range) with normal blood pressure and creatinine.
C) Suspected case of IgA nephropathy.
D) Nephrotic syndrome likely from diabetes mellitus.
E) **Persistent** low-grade proteinuria with elevated blood pressure and/or elevated creatinine.

Discussion

The correct answer is "E." Patients with low-grade proteinuria and increasing creatinine and blood pressure should have a renal biopsy in order to determine the etiology of their disease. Indications for biopsy are listed in Table 5–6.

Table 5–6 INDICATIONS FOR RENAL BIOPSY

- Nephrotic syndrome **without** a systemic etiology found on other testing
- Hematuria from a glomerular source **with** hypertension or increasing creatinine
- Nephritis **without** a systemic explanation (e.g., no lupus, drug exposure)
- Suspicion of Wegener granulomatosis or polyarteritis nodosum where other tissue is not available
- Acute or subacute renal failure without another explanation (although history will usually result in a presumptive diagnosis)

Objectives: Did you learn to . . .

- Evaluate and follow a healthy-appearing patient with proteinuria?
- Define and diagnose orthostatic proteinuria and understand its significance?
- Manage a patient with progressive proteinuria?
- Recognize nephrotic syndrome?
- Identify causes of nephrotic syndrome?

CASE 5

While covering the ED, a 62-year-old female you have known for several years presents with her husband. Your patient appears very lethargic and is unable to give a coherent history. Her husband tells you that she began having stomach pain, nausea, and diarrhea 2 days ago. Although she has not been vomiting, she has been unable to drink or eat much due to nausea. She takes furosemide for edema and albuterol/ipratropium (Combivent) for COPD. She smokes a pack of cigarettes per day.

On physical examination, her respiratory rate is 30, pulse 104, blood pressure 112/64, and temperature 37.9°C. She is lethargic and disoriented. Oral mucosa is dry. Her lungs show diminished air movement bilaterally. Her abdomen is diffusely tender, but there is no rebound. Rectal exam is negative for occult blood.

The first laboratory test you have available is a room air arterial blood gas (although venous would have been fine, right?): pH 7.12, $PaCO_2$ 33 mm Hg, PaO_2 80 mm Hg, HCO_3 10 mEq/L, and oxygen saturation 92%. Her baseline blood gas is in her medical record, which has been ordered.

This blood gas is most consistent with which of the following processes?

A) Compensated metabolic acidosis.
B) Compensated respiratory acidosis.
C) Poorly compensated metabolic acidosis.
D) Poorly compensated respiratory acidosis.

Discussion

The correct answer is "C." This patient is clearly acidotic, as her pH is well below the normal range of 7.35–7.45. So, obviously, whatever she has, it will be poorly compensated, ruling out "A" and "B." Based on the bicarbonate (HCO_3) level and the history of gastrointestinal losses due to diarrhea, you would suspect a metabolic acidosis. In order to have appropriate respiratory compensation, the $PaCO_2$ should fall 12 points for every 10 point drop in the HCO_3 below the normal level (around 24 mEq/L).

In this case, the HCO_3 is 10 mEq/L (14 points below normal); therefore, the $PaCO_2$ is expected to drop by about ($1.2 \times 14 = 16.8$) or approximately 17.

However, the $PaCO_2$ is not 23 mm Hg; it is 33 mm Hg (close to the normal range of 35–45). The patient's $PaCO_2$ is too high to appropriately compensate for her metabolic acidosis, and she thus has a poorly compensated metabolic acidosis.

There is another way to do this:

The pH should change by 0.8 for every 10 change in CO_2. So, if a patient's CO_2 is 50, the pH should be 7.32 if it is an uncompensated respiratory acidosis. If they are more acidotic (e.g., 7.24), they have a mixed respiratory and metabolic acidosis. If they are less acidotic (e.g., 7.39), they have a compensated respiratory acidosis.

* *

While you are providing supportive care, the patient's lab results are completed: Na 134 mEq/L, K 2.1 mEq/L, Cl 112 mEq/L, HCO_3 10 mEq/L, BUN 29 mg/dL, Cr 1.1 mg/dL, Ca 9.1 mg/dL; CBC: WBC 16,100 cells/mm^3, Hgb 13.9 g/dL, platelets 167,000 cells/mm^3; urinalysis: specific gravity 1.030, remainder normal. Troponin-T, CK, and liver enzymes are normal.

All of the following may be contributing to hypokalemia in this patient EXCEPT:

A) Hypomagnesemia.
B) Furosemide.
C) Acidosis.
D) Beta-agonists such as albuterol.
E) Diarrhea.

Discussion

The correct answer is "C." Acidosis should cause a spuriously elevated potassium and not a low potassium. Magnesium ("A") depletion promotes potassium loss. Thus, hypomagnesemia can contribute to hypokalemia. "B," furosemide and other loop diuretics, causes renal potassium wasting. "D," beta-agonists, such as albuterol, shifts potassium into cells thereby lowering the plasma potassium. Diarrhea ("E") results in direct gastrointestinal losses of potassium.

Other causes of hypokalemia include thiazide diuretics, metabolic alkalosis (often from protracted emesis—although this represents a shift of potassium intracellularly and not a true hypokalemia), hyperaldosteronism, and RTA types 1 and 2.

INTERESTING (BUT USELESS) TIP: Until 1970, "light salt" contained lithium chloride. You could help grandma's hypertension and mania at the same time! Areas in Japan with higher lithium content in the soil have lower rates of depression and suicide.

HELPFUL TIP: Acidosis will spuriously elevate a patient's potassium. The serum potassium goes up by about 1 mEq/L for every decrease in pH of 0.1. Alkalosis will cause an equivalent hypokalemia. So, if the pH is 7.3, 1 mEq/L of the elevated potassium is due to the acidosis.

You do not have any monitored beds available for this patient. The most appropriate initial therapy to correct her hypokalemia (2.1 mEq/L) is to give your patient:

A) KCl 40 mEq PO.
B) KCl 80 mEq PO.
C) KCL 20 mEq/hr IV.
D) KCl 20 mEq IV push.
E) KCl 60 mEq/hr IV.

Discussion

The correct answer is "C." Remember that this patient is vomiting and lethargic. Thus, oral potassium replacement is not going to work. Couple this with the fact that she is profoundly hypokalemic, and IV replacement becomes the treatment of choice. One should not give more than 20 mEq KCl IV per hour without a monitor. It should be given through a large bore peripheral IV or a central line. If you chose "D," you just failed your test. IV push KCl is fatal.

Most commonly, the chloride salt (KCl) is administered to replete potassium stores. In an awake patient with a functional gastrointestinal tract, oral KCl should be administered. Oral and intravenous bioavailability is very similar, but oral doses greater than 40 mEq may not be well tolerated.

HELPFUL TIP: There are no reliably reproducible ways to gauge potassium depletion and amount needed to make a patient eukalemic. The best thing to do is start replacing with KCl and monitor serum potassium levels, adjusting the KCl dose as you go. Be careful when ordering potassium replacement: *hyper*kalemia is most commonly iatrogenic.

In addition to KCl repletion, which of the following interventions do you initiate now in an attempt to correct the acidosis?

A) Bolus normal saline.
B) Sodium bicarbonate.
C) Bolus 5% dextrose.
D) Intubation and mechanical ventilation.

Discussion

The correct answer is "A." On the basis of history, physical exam, and BUN/creatinine ratio, your patient is dehydrated. The first step is to correct the dehydration with intravenous fluids. Normal saline is preferred over dextrose, which might lead to further hyponatremia and hypokalemia. Additionally, **dextrose will not stay intravascular and will actually precipitate a diuresis by making the serum hypotonic.** "B" is incorrect. **There is no evidence that bicarbonate improves outcomes in metabolic acidosis;** correct the underlying problem. In most cases, volume replacement will lead to improvement in acidosis without needing to resort to bicarbonate. Although she is oxygenating well now, if your patient's respiratory condition deteriorates, she may require intubation and ventilator settings could be adjusted to aid in correcting the acid/base disorder.

Objectives: Did you learn to . . .

- Distinguish simple metabolic or respiratory acidosis from mixed acidosis?
- Discuss causes of hypokalemia?
- Manage a patient with metabolic acidosis and hypokalemia?

QUICK QUIZ: RHABDOMYOLYSIS

The primary mechanism by which renal failure occurs in rhabdomyolysis is:

A) Glomerular destruction.
B) Acute tubular necrosis (ATN).
C) Interstitial nephritis.
D) None of the above.

Discussion

The correct answer is "B." Myoglobin deposits in the renal tubules, causing local damage and ischemia, which results in acute tubular necrosis. Findings in the urinary sediment that support acute tubular necrosis include renal tubular epithelial cells and dark brown casts of granular material ("muddy" brown casts).

HELPFUL TIP: Patients with rhabdomyolysis with CK <5000 U/L and clear urine are unlikely to develop acute tubular necrosis but should be monitored to assure dropping CK and adequate renal function.

QUICK QUIZ: NEPHROLOGY

Which of the following is/are associated with polycystic kidney disease?

A) Liver cysts.
B) Cerebral aneurysms.
C) Colonic diverticula.
D) Cardiac valvular disease.
E) All of the above.

Discussion

The correct answer is "E." All of the above are associated with polycystic kidney disease. Of particular importance is the possibility of cerebral aneurysms (5–20%) leading to subarachnoid hemorrhage. However, aneurysm rupture remains fairly rare (but does seem to run in families—and seems to result in a really bad day for your patient). Currently, screening for subarachnoid aneurysms in asymptomatic patients with ADPKD is not recommended.

ADPKD occurs in 1 in every 400–2000 live births and is autosomal dominant. Common extrarenal manifestations of ADPKD include cerebral aneurysms, hepatic cysts, cardiac valve disease, colonic diverticula, and abdominal and inguinal hernias.

QUICK QUIZ: TOO SALTY

A 79-year-old female nursing home resident with moderate dementia presents for worsening confusion over the last 2 days. She just finished antibiotics for a urinary tract infection. Her temperature is 38.1°C, pulse 110, respiratory rate 18, and blood pressure 118/60 mm Hg. She is disoriented and lethargic. Examination of the heart, lungs, and abdomen is unremarkable.

Laboratory studies are as follows: Na 165 mEq/L, K 4.6 mEq/L, Cl 118 mEq/L, HCO_3 28 mEq/L, BUN 31 mg/dL, Cr 1.1 mg/dL. Urine specific gravity is >1.030 and urine osmolality is 700 mmol/kg (elevated reflecting reabsorption of free water). Her CBC is normal.

Initial treatment for this patient should be:

A) Normal saline IV bolus.
B) Dextrose 5% IV bolus.
C) Sterile water IV bolus.
D) Loop diuretics.
E) DDAVP.

Discussion

The correct answer is "A." Demented or delirious patients with an acute febrile illness may not be able to consume enough free water to avoid hypernatremia. Several mechanisms may be at work: free water loss due to illness, impaired thirst, and inability to respond to thirst due to cognitive or physical impairments.

Table 5–7 CAUSES OF HYPERNATREMIA

- GI loss of water
- Osmotic diuresis
- Excess exercise and sweating
- Diabetes insipidus

Note: Generally, regulatory mechanisms will maintain a normal serum sodium. However, this requires access for free water. Immobile patients (especially the elderly) are particularly prone to problems because of their limited mobility and inability to independently access water.

Just as with hyponatremia, the hypernatremic patient should not be corrected too quickly. Sudden changes in plasma sodium may result in cerebral edema. Although there are no standardized guidelines to direct the correction of hypernatremia, most authorities recommend a maximal correction of 0.5–1 mEq/L/hr. In this patient who appears hypovolemic, the primary concern is to give volume. The administration of normal saline will allow you to administer volume while lowering her plasma sodium. Dextrose 5% solution may lower the sodium too quickly. Sterile water should never be administered IV because it will cause massive local hemolysis.

"E" is incorrect. This patient's kidney function is appropriate for her hypernatremia. She is concentrating her urine, as evidenced by her high urine specific gravity and urine osmolality. Therefore, she does not have diabetes insipidus, which is characterized by large volumes of dilute urine. DDAVP is an appropriate treatment for central diabetes insipidus. See Table 5–7 for more on causes of hypernatremia.

HELPFUL TIP: To calculate the free water deficit in a hypovolemic hypernatremic patient, use the following equation:

$$\text{Water deficit} = 0.6 \times \text{weight (kg)} \times [(\text{plasma Na}/140) - 1].$$

In this patient, assuming a weight of 60 kg:

$$\text{Water deficit} = 0.6 \times 60 \times [(165/140) - 1] = 6.4 \text{ L}.$$

CASE 6

A surgical colleague asks you to consult on a patient because of increasing creatinine (We know... this will never happen... just pretend). A 63-year-old woman was admitted for an elective cholecystectomy. She is on postoperative day 3 and has fevers and delirium. Her current medications are morphine, cefotetan, and acetaminophen as needed. She takes nothing by mouth, but has intravenous fluids (5% dextrose/0.45% saline) running at 100 cc/hr. Plasma studies from the day of surgery and this morning are available:

Lab Test	Before Surgery	Day of Consultation
Sodium mEq/L	138	130
Potassium mEq/L	4.5	5.8
Chloride mEq/L	103	105
HCO_3 mEq/L	24	18
BUN mg/dL	15	30
Creatinine mg/dL	1.1	2.0

The BUN/Cr ratio on the day of consultation suggests that:

A) She is dehydrated.
B) She has a prerenal cause of her increased creatinine, such as hypoperfusion.
C) Intrinsic kidney disease is more likely than a prerenal cause.
D) None of the above.

Discussion

The correct answer is "C." A BUN/Cr ratio <20 generally indicates an intrinsic renal cause of renal failure (increasing Cr) while a BUN/Cr ratio >20 indicates a prerenal cause such as hypoperfusion (e.g., CHF, dehydration). In this patient, the BUN/Cr ratio is 15, suggesting intrinsic renal disease.

Which of the following is the most appropriate first step in determining the nature of this patient's elevated creatinine?

A) Give a trial bolus of normal saline.
B) CT scan of the abdomen.
C) Determine volume of urine output.
D) Obtain urine for culture.
E) Give a trial dose of furosemide.

Discussion

The correct answer is "C." Currently, all you know about this patient's kidney function is that it has declined since her admission and that it is not likely from a prerenal cause. It is important to know if this patient is oliguric or has adequate urine output. This is important because it can affect treatment. For example, oliguric or anuric patients may become volume overloaded easily in response to IV fluids. Although hospital measurements of intake and output are often plagued by errors, you should start this evaluation by analyzing the patient's urine output, as well as fluid intake, over the last few days. Urine culture and CT scan may eventually play a role in your evaluation. The decision to give fluids or diuretics cannot be made until more information is gathered.

> **HELPFUL TIP:** Relatively small changes in serum creatinine may reflect renal failure. A patient with a baseline creatinine of 0.7 mg/dL has lost **half** her renal function when her creatinine increases to 1.4 mg/dL, even though this number may still be in the normal range—thus, the need to calculate a creatinine clearance.

* *

Vital signs, intake, and output have been recorded by the nurses for each shift since admission and are provided in Table 5–8.

You have now determined that your patient has become oliguric. Which of the following is most likely to help you narrow the differential diagnosis of renal failure?

A) Calculation of creatinine clearance.
B) Arterial blood gases.
C) CT scan of the abdomen.
D) Fractional excretion of sodium (FENa).
E) Furosemide challenge.

Discussion

The correct answer is "D." In this patient, you know that her BUN/Cr ratio is <20, pointing you toward intrinsic renal disease. But this ratio is not specific enough to rely upon. In oliguric renal failure, the FENa is a useful tool to help differentiate prerenal causes of renal failure from intrinsic renal causes. If the FENa is less than 1%, the kidney is functioning appropriately to conserve sodium and water, and a prerenal cause of failure is more likely. If the FENa is greater than 1%, salt and water losses are excessive, suggesting intrinsic kidney dysfunction. This

Table 5–8 VITAL SIGNS, INTAKE, AND OUTPUT

	Day 1 Shift 1	Day 1 Shift 2	Day 1 Shift 3	Day 2 Shift 1	Day 2 Shift 2	Day 2 Shift 3	Day 3 Shift 1	Day 3 Shift 2	Day 3 Shift 3
BP	118/60	117/63	102/57	80/42	92/48	102/67	105/60	102/56	120/79
Pulse	84	82	92	124	117	106	100	102	93
Temp	37.3	37.0	37.7	40.0	39.1	37.1	38.0	36.9	36.8
RR	12	14	13	15	20	18	20	12	12
IV in (cc)	1800	800	800	800	800	800	800	800	800
Urine out (cc)	1650	1000	750	850	600	400	180	100	80

calculation is only useful in oliguric renal failure (urine output <400 cc/day). Also, FENa may be inaccurate in the elderly, patients receiving diuretics, and in chronic renal failure. The equation used to calculate FENa is:

$$\text{FENa (\%)} = [(\text{urine Na/plasma Na})/(\text{urine Cr/plasma Cr})] \times 100.$$

HELPFUL TIP: This is easy to remember teleologically. If the FENa is <1%, the kidney is working: it is conserving sodium to try to increase serum volume to better perfuse the kidney. This is what a normal kidney should do and the cause of the increased creatinine isn't with the kidney... it could be hypoperfusion from shock, dehydration, etc. If the FENa is >1%, the kidney is unable to hold on to sodium and is therefore not working. Same with urinary sodium. If it is high, the kidney is not able to hold onto sodium and water to increase volume.

HELPFUL TIP: What if the patient is on a diuretic and you cannot make use of the FENa? Use the FEUrea, as urea excretion is not affected by diuretics. Here's the equation:

$$\text{FEUrea (\%)} = (\text{urine urea/plasma urea})/(\text{urine Cr/plasma Cr}).$$

If the FEUrea is <35%, a prerenal cause is more likely. If FEUrea is >50%, acute tubular necrosis is more likely. Caveat: hyperglycemic diuresis increases excretion of urea even in hypovolemic states (e.g., 3+ glucose in the urine can give you a falsely high FEUrea).

* *

On examination, you find a mildly disoriented female in no acute distress. She has lower extremity and sacral edema. You obtain urine studies, showing a specific gravity of 1.020, pH 6, 3 RBCs/hpf, 2 WBCs/hpf, and muddy brown granular casts. The urine creatinine is 6.5 mg/dL and the urine sodium is 45 mEq/L. You calculate the FENa that turns out to be >1%.

Given the clinical course and urine findings, which of the following is the best diagnosis?

A) ATN.
B) Acute interstitial nephritis.
C) Vasculitis.
D) CHF.
E) Lactic acidosis.

Discussion

The correct answer is "A." ATN is a major cause of acute renal failure in hospitalized patients. ATN is the result of toxic and/or ischemic effects on the kidney tubules. Metabolic derangements in ATN include progressive hyponatremia, hyperkalemia, and metabolic acidosis with a high anion gap, all of which are present in this case. Typically patients with ATN have a FENa >1% (or FEUrea >50%) and a urine sodium >40 mEq/L. (Remember, the kidney should be retaining sodium to increase its perfusion. This is not happening here. So it is an intrinsic renal problem.) In this case, FENa is 9.9%. Additionally, "muddy" brown casts (renal tubular cell casts) are often found in the urinary sediment of patients with ATN. All of these findings point to ATN as the cause of renal failure in this patient.

Based on the available data (including the vital signs and urine values), you suspect that ATN in this patient is the result of:

A) Acetaminophen.
B) Hypotension.
C) Intrinsic renal infection.
D) Cefotetan.
E) Any of the above is equally likely.

Discussion

The correct answer is "B." As you review the vital signs, intake, and output, you will notice that the patient had a hypotensive period associated with tachycardia and fever (day 2, shifts 1 and 2). She then developed progressively lower urine output despite stable IV intake. It is likely that she has had an ischemic insult to her kidneys as a result of hypotension and decreased perfusion. While many medications can cause ATN, cefotetan and acetaminophen are relatively safe. More often, cephalosporins cause acute interstitial nephritis (fever, +/− rash, white cell casts, and eosinophils in the urine and perhaps in the peripheral blood).

HELPFUL TIP: In addition to hypoxic insult (shock, hypoperfusion, CHF, etc.), common causes of ATN include medications such as tacrolimus, various ACE inhibitors, some of the penicillin derivatives, gentamicin, tobramycin, cyclophosphamide, several antirejection drugs, and more.

* *

When you go to check on the patient later in the afternoon, she has become more tachypneic and has rales on exam.

Which of the following recommendations do you make for this patient's continuing care?

A) Administer dopamine.
B) Increase IV fluids to 200 cc/hr, using 5% dextrose/0.45% saline.
C) Dialysis.
D) Administer HCTZ.
E) Administer furosemide.

Discussion

The correct answer is "E." The treatment of acute renal failure due to ATN is largely supportive. In this oliguric patient with signs of volume overload, a trial of a loop diuretic is appropriate. Intravenous furosemide dosed at 20–100 mg every 6–12 hours is a reasonable way to start. "A," dopamine, is not effective in the treatment of ATN (it is not "renal sparing" and does not increase GFR). "B," more fluid, is clearly not indicated in this patient who is already fluid overloaded. Why not dialysis you ask ("C")? Early dialysis in ATN is associated with greater mortality and increased kidney damage from hypotension, infection, and complement activation in the kidney. "D," HCTZ, is less likely than furosemide to achieve a good diuretic effect in the setting of a low GFR.

HELPFUL TIP: While traditionally taught, trying to "convert" oliguric to nonoliguric renal failure (by flogging the kidneys with diuretics) is not helpful and is possibly harmful. There is a trend toward greater mortality in patients who are treated this way. There's more: it can cause deafness (eh?), vertigo, and tinnitus. Remember, it doesn't help to flog a dead horse or ailing kidneys.

* *

Your patient has very little response to furosemide, but you match her input and output and she has enough insensible loss to resolve her rales. She begins to eat, and you monitor her fluid intake carefully. You match her fluid intake with output, giving normal saline to match her urine output and suspected insensible losses. You treat her hyperkalemia with sodium polystyrene sulfonate (Kayexalate), which is effective. Her BUN and creatinine continue to rise over the next few days and reach 60 and 4 mg/dL, respectively. The plasma HCO_3 is 18 mEq/L.

You now recommend:

A) Hemodialysis.
B) Sodium bicarbonate.
C) Strict protein restriction.
D) Continuing to match intake and output.
E) All of the above.

Discussion

The correct answer is "D." At this point, there is no reason to change your therapeutic approach. In particular, hemodialysis is not necessary. Indications for hemodialysis in this patient might include symptomatic uremia (e.g., coma, pericarditis), severe hyperkalemia or acidosis unresponsive to other therapies, and complications of volume overload (e.g., pulmonary edema). Sodium bicarbonate is used orally in patients with significant acidosis, but many patients can tolerate mild acidosis associated with renal failure. Dramatic protein restriction will probably help to control uremia, but lower BUN should not be your primary goal. Your patient is recovering from surgery and was probably septic. She requires good nutrition to continue to heal.

HELPFUL TIP: Renal failure due to ATN typically lasts 7–21 days, with renal function returning as the tubular cells regenerate. However, the course is highly variable and depends on the patient's general health and the length and degree of the initial injury.

The most common cause of death from acute tubular necrosis is:

A) Hemorrhage.
B) Dialysis.
C) Infection.
D) Transfusion reaction.
E) CHF secondary to fluid overload.

Discussion

The correct answer is "C." In patients with ATN who die, infection is the usual culprit. It is critical to avoid sepsis in these patients. Also, serious infection resulting in sepsis is a common cause of ATN.

* *

Ten days after her surgery, your patient's urine output increases markedly. Her BUN and creatinine return to their premorbid levels. The National Kidney Foundation makes you an honorary nephrologist and awards you the Bronze Nephron.

Objectives: Did you learn to . . .

- Evaluate a hospitalized patient for renal failure?
- Use urine studies, including urine sodium and FENa, to assist in the diagnosis of acute renal failure?
- Identify acute tubular necrosis?
- Describe common causes of acute tubular necrosis, its treatment, and its prognosis?

CASE 7

While on call, you admit a 75-year-old female for confusion. One month ago, she started HCTZ for hypertension. Her medications include HCTZ 25 mg daily, levothyroxine 0.125 mg daily, aspirin 81 mg daily, sertraline (Zoloft) 50 mg daily, and atorvastatin (Lipitor) 40 mg daily. She has a 50-pack-year history of tobacco use and continues to smoke.

On examination, you find an irritable, confused female in no acute distress. Her admission vitals: BP 100/60, P 120, RR 12, T 36.1°C, weight 50 kg. Her oral mucosa is dry and she has poor skin turgor. She has clear lungs, an S4 on heart exam, and no edema. Her neurological exam is nonfocal.

Laboratory results: Na 110 mEq/L, K 3.0 mEq/L, Cl 70 mEq/L, HCO_3 33 mEq/L, BUN 30 mg/dL, Cr 1.0 mg/dL, glucose 110 mg/dL. Plasma osmolality 220 mOsm/L (normal 270–299 mOsm/L).

Which of the following statements is true regarding the etiology of her hyponatremia?

A) She has pseudohyponatremia.
B) She has isovolemic hyponatremia.
C) She has hypovolemic hyponatremia.
D) She has hypervolemic hyponatremia.

Discussion

The correct answer is "C." The definition of hyponatremia is a plasma sodium concentration below 135 mEq/L. The evaluation of hyponatremia begins with the determination of the validity of the plasma sodium measurement. You must distinguish "true" hyponatremia from pseudohyponatremia, which can be the result of hyperlipidemia, hyperglycemia, or hyperproteinemia. If pseudohyponatremia is present, the calculated osmolality will be significantly lower than measured osmolality. Your patient's calculated osmolality is determined by the formula Osm = 2 (sodium) + glucose/18 + (BUN/2.7), which for her is about 236 Osm. Her measured osmolarity is 220 mmol/kg, and the fact that measured osmolality is higher than calculated rules out pseudohyponatremia.

* *

The next step in the evaluation of hyponatremia is to determine the patient's volume status. This patient has no signs of volume overload, such as edema or crackles, making hypervolemia unlikely. She is tachycardic with a low blood pressure, dry mucous membranes, and a BUN/Cr ratio greater than 20, suggesting she is hypovolemic. Most likely, she has a hypovolemic hyponatremia.

> **HELPFUL TIP**: Always consider "beer potomania" (one of our favorite disease names . . . not to mention one of our favorite food groups). Here's what happens: too much beer (or any alcohol) plus too little solute equals poor free water excretion and hyponatremia.

What further information will help you narrow the differential diagnosis of hyponatremia in this patient?

A) FENa.
B) Urine osmolality and urine sodium concentration.
C) Urine creatinine concentration.
D) Urine potassium and calcium concentration.

Discussion

The correct answer is "B." Urine osmolality can be used to distinguish between impaired water excretion, SIADH, and pathologic water intake (polydipsia). In SIADH, the urine will be inappropriately concentrated with urine osmoles of >100 mOsm/L/kg (the patient is unable to retain sodium). FENa is discussed earlier; it's not helpful for discovering the etiology of hyponatremia. Concentration of potassium and calcium is not likely to add any useful information.

* *

You order urine studies. Urinalysis: specific gravity 1.020, pH 5.0, trace protein, 0–1 RBC/hpf, 0–1 WBC/hpf, otherwise negative. Spot urine Na 70 mEq/L (elevated) and urine osmolality = 700 mmol/kg (elevated).

Given the patient's history, urine studies, and hypovolemic status, what is the most likely diagnosis?

A) SIADH.
B) CHF.
C) Diuretic-induced hyponatremia.
D) Hyponatremia due to reset osmostat.
E) Potato chip deficiency.

Discussion

The correct answer is "C." In order to be useful in the diagnosis of hyponatremia, urine studies must be viewed in the context of volume status, plasma osmolality, and electrolyte levels. This patient's lab results are consistent with SIADH. However, patients with SIADH should be euvolemic or slightly hypervolemic. Thus, her labs and clinical picture are most consistent with diuretic-induced hyponatremia.

The appropriate response of the kidney to hypo-osmolality is to make maximally dilute urine (retain sodium to correct the hypo-osmolality). Thus, the urine should have a specific gravity less than 1.005 and osmolality less than 100 mmol/kg.

Inappropriately concentrated urine (osmolality >100 mmol/kg) occurs when there is limited excretion of fluid and may be observed in SIADH, CHF, cirrhosis, and renal failure. This is also reflected in the urine sodium. If the kidneys respond to hyponatremia as expected, urine sodium concentration should be low, typically less than 20 mmol/L and often less than 10 mmol/L (the kidneys are attempting to retain sodium to increase the serum osmolarity). In the setting of hypovolemia, if the urine sodium concentration is inappropriately high, something is inappropriately spurring the kidney on to excrete sodium (e.g., diuretic use, hypoaldosteronism). In this patient, the elevated urine sodium is likely due to the diuretic.

Diuretic use is the most common cause of hypovolemic hypoosmolality, and thiazides are more commonly associated with hyponatremia than are loop diuretics (furosemide, etc.). Your patient is hypovolemic and hyponatremic, with a high urine sodium concentration and the history of diuretic use: most likely, her hyponatremia is diuretic induced.

"D," a reset osmostat, requires special mention. A reset osmostat, which is responsible for 20–30% of hyponatremia, occurs when the patient's body "adapts" to hyponatremia and gives up trying to correct the problem: the kidneys just throw in the towel. Patients with a reset osmostat will present like SIADH (hyponatremia, euvolemia or slight hypervolemia, and inappropriately concentrated urine) but will be resistant to treatment. If a patient with apparent SIADH does not respond to usual treatment, consider a reset osmostat. Since patients with a reset osmostat generally have mild hyponatremia (125–130 mg/dL) and are generally asymptomatic, trying to correct the sodium by limiting water intake is unnecessary and futile.

HELPFUL TIP: When you encounter a patient with hyponatremic hypo-osmolality, also look at the plasma potassium concentration. Diuretic use is a common cause of hyponatremia, hypokalemia, hypochloremia, and hypo-osmolality occurring simultaneously.

In addition to discontinuing her diuretic, which of the following approaches is the best initial therapy for her hyponatremia?

A) Saline 0.9% 1 L bolus followed by 150 cc/hr.
B) Fluid restriction to 1500 cc/day.
C) Saline 3% 100 cc/hr for 24 hours.
D) Saline 0.45% 100 cc/hr for 24 hours.
E) Saline 3% at 60 cc/hr and furosemide 40 mg IV.

Discussion

The correct answer is "A." This patient is hypotensive and tachycardic and thus needs volume somewhat quickly to address her abnormal vital signs. If this patient was not hemodynamically compromised, you could forgo the fluid bolus. Excessively rapid correction of hyponatremia may lead to pontine myelinolysis.

Sodium concentrations less than 120 mEq/L are considered severe hyponatremia. Patients with acute, severe hyponatremia are almost always symptomatic as a result of the low sodium. By definition, acute hyponatremia has been present for 48 hours or less and chronic hyponatremia for more than 48 hours. As previously discussed, your patient's hyponatremia is due to a diuretic, which she started 1 month ago. Therefore, her hyponatremia is more likely to be chronic.

As a general rule, hypovolemic hyponatremia should be corrected by volume infusion, usually with 0.9% (normal) saline. Fluid restriction ("C"), while good treatment for SIADH, is not appropriate in this patient who is already volume depleted nor is loop diuretic use ("E") appropriate. Both "C" and "E" will exacerbate the problem. Hypo-osmolar solutions, like 0.45% saline ("D"), will lead to more severe hyponatremia.

Your patient has chronic hyponatremia, which needs to be corrected more slowly than acute hyponatremia. Chronic hyponatremia should be corrected no faster than 0.5 mEq/hr or 12 mEq/day. For significantly symptomatic patients with acute hyponatremia, sodium can be corrected more quickly with maximum increases in plasma sodium concentration of 1 mEq/hr or 20 mEq/day.

In order to determine how quickly sodium concentrations will rise, you must know the concentrations of the solution being infused and the patient's plasma sodium. A liter of saline will affect the serum sodium by the following calculation:

$$
\begin{aligned}
\text{Na increase} &= (\text{solution Na} - \text{plasma Na})/(\text{total body water} + 1).\\
\text{Patient's Na} &= 110 \text{ mEq/L}.\\
\text{Na in 3\% saline} &= 513 \text{ mEq/L}.\\
\text{Na in 0.9\% saline} &= 154 \text{ mEq/L}.\\
\text{Total body water} &= \text{weight (kg)} \times 0.5 \text{ (females) or } 0.6 \text{ (males)}.
\end{aligned}
$$

When using 3% saline solution, 1 L will increase the plasma sodium as follows:

$$
\text{Na increase} = (513 - 110)/[(50 \times 0.5) + 1] = 15.5 \text{ mEq/L}.
$$

At 100 cc/hr, the plasma sodium will increase at a rate of 1.55 mEq/hr. This correction is too rapid for chronic hyponatremia.

When using normal saline, 1 L will increase the plasma sodium as follows:

$$
\text{Na increase} = (154 - 110)/[(50 \times 0.5) + 1] = 1.7 \text{ mEq/L}.
$$

Therefore, 1 L of normal saline will increase the plasma sodium by 1.7 mEq initially, and 150 cc/hr will increase the plasma sodium by 0.25 mEq/hr, well within the safe range.

In addition to HCTZ, which medication should you discontinue because of its potential role in hyponatremia in this patient?

A) Aspirin.
B) Atorvastatin.
C) Levothyroxine.
D) Sertraline.

Discussion

The correct answer is "D." Serotonin reuptake inhibitors (SSRIs) and tricyclic antidepressants, among other medications, can stimulate the release of ADH from the pituitary gland, ultimately causing hyponatremia with an SIADH-type presentation. The association between SSRIs and hyponatremia is strong enough to consider measuring plasma sodium levels in elderly patients before and after starting an SSRI. The other medications are not associated with hyponatremia to any significant degree.

* *

Your patient does well, recovers from her hyponatremia, and is discharged. In place of HCTZ, you start an ACE inhibitor for hypertension. You next see her a few months later when she starts to have problems with mild confusion. Her family reports that she is definitely not taking any diuretics. Her vitals are normal. Clinically, she appears **euvolemic** with normal vitals, and her exam is nonfocal. Her plasma sodium is 120 mEq/L, creatinine 1.1 mg/dL, plasma osmolality 240 mmol/kg, and urine osmolality 320 mmol/kg. Urinalysis shows specific gravity of 1.030 but is normal otherwise.

In addition to the lab tests already available to you, which of the following laboratory tests should be done in patients with hyponatremia?

A) CBC.
B) ESR.
C) TSH.
D) Liver enzymes.
E) ADH.

Discussion

The correct answer is "C." Hyponatremia with hypo-osmolality and a normal volume status is often the result of SIADH. However, SIADH is a diagnosis of exclusion. Both hypothyroidism and glucocorticoid deficiency present with similar features and should be ruled out. Hypothyroidism is more common, and at a minimum you must check TSH. Of special note is option "E." Most of the time, ADH levels are not helpful in the diagnosis of SIADH because up to 20% of patients with diagnosable SIADH do not have elevated plasma ADH levels. SIADH is diagnosed on clinical grounds, with characteristic lab data, and lack of a better explanation.

> HELPFUL TIP: In any given patient with hyponatremia, what makes SIADH likely? All of the following data are used to support the diagnosis of SIADH: decreased plasma osmolality; inappropriately concentrated urine (e.g., a urine osmolality of >100 mmol/kg); clinical euvolemia or mild hypervolemia; elevated urine sodium excretion (urine sodium >20 mEq/L); and the absence of diuretic use, hypothyroidism, and adrenal dysfunction.

* *

You order a number of laboratory tests, including TSH, CBC, and electrolytes. In addition to the lab tests mentioned above, abnormal tests include plasma Cl 90 mEq/L, urine Na 50 mEq/L (and urine osmoles, as noted above, are 320 mmol/kg). Thyroid function tests are normal. You diagnose SIADH.

As initial treatment, you prescribe:

A) Demeclocycline.
B) Lithium.
C) Saline 0.9% bolus.
D) Furosemide.
E) Water restriction.

Discussion

The correct answer is "E." The labs and clinical picture are consistent with SIADH (euvolemia, elevated urine sodium excretion, elevated urine osmolarity). Water restriction is the mainstay of therapy in SIADH. Free water should be restricted to 1–2 L/day. Demeclocycline and lithium interfere with the activity of ADH at the collecting tubules, but these drugs are reserved for SIADH patients with severe hyponatremia unresponsive to water restriction. Saline infusion corrects hypovolemic hyponatremia, and furosemide is used in hypervolemic hyponatremia (e.g., CHF, renal insufficiency). Neither of these conditions is present in this patient.

The patient fails water restriction. The *next* step in the treatment of this patient is:

A) Demeclocycline.
B) Lithium.
C) Sodium chloride tablets.
D) IV urea.
E) None of the above.

Discussion

The correct answer is "C." Increasing salt intake and adding a loop diuretic are other ways to treat SIADH in patients who cannot or will not maintain fluid restriction. IV urea, which causes an osmotic diuresis, is the next step to use after the sodium chloride tablets. Demeclocycline and lithium should be reserved for patients who fail the other treatments.

HELPFUL TIP: Conivaptan (Vaprisol®) and tolvaptan (Samsca) both are ADH antagonists that can be used for SIADH. They are third-line agents. Potential problems include exacerbations of heart failure, orthostatic hypotension, and hypokalemia. They must be started in the hospital because of the potential side effects.

Objectives: Did you learn to . . .

- Generate a differential diagnosis for hyponatremia?
- Identify medications that are commonly associated with hyponatremia?
- Use urine osmolality to identify impaired renal water handling?
- Calculate sodium correction using different concentrations of saline?
- Diagnose, evaluate, and treat a patient with SIADH?

CASE 8

A 65-year-old male with a new diagnosis of heart failure returns to your office after starting several new medications within the last month. A cardiologist at an academic health center 100 miles away started these medications but never sent a note, and neither you nor your patient knows what the drugs are (typical of us academic types). Over that same time period, he states that he has felt "worse than I did after my heart attack." At first he was just fatigued, but in the last few days, he has developed **nausea, vomiting, and body aches.**

On examination, his vitals are T 37.1°C, P 70, RR 8, BP 100/58 mm Hg. He has trace pedal edema. His lungs are clear, and his abdomen is diffusely tender. When you stand him up to check his blood pressure, he loses consciousness but quickly recovers when placed supine.

Your nurse draws blood, starts an IV, and obtains an arterial blood gas on room air. ABG: pH 7.52, $PaCO_2$ 49 mm Hg, PaO_2 90 mm Hg, and HCO_3 39 mEq/L.

The blood gas is consistent with the diagnosis of:

A) Metabolic alkalosis with respiratory compensation.
B) Respiratory alkalosis with metabolic compensation.
C) Mixed metabolic/respiratory alkalosis.
D) Mixed metabolic alkalosis and respiratory acidosis.

Discussion

The correct answer is "A." Your patient appears to have a pure metabolic alkalosis with respiratory compensation. His pH is above the upper limit of normal (7.45), and his plasma bicarbonate is elevated as well. In metabolic alkalosis, you can expect the $PaCO_2$ to rise in proportion to the rise in HCO_3. $PaCO_2$ should increase by 0.5–0.75 times the increase in HCO_3 from baseline (usually 24 mEq/L). In this case, the HCO_3 has increased by 15, and the $PaCO_2$ has appropriately increased by 9. And remember, you cannot overcorrect your pH. Thus, the primary process has to be an alkalosis.

Which of the following urine tests will aid in determining the cause of this patient's metabolic *alkalosis*?

A) Urine sodium.
B) Urine potassium.
C) Urine chloride.
D) Urine bicarbonate.
E) Urine creatinine.

Discussion

The correct answer is "C." You can approach the differential diagnosis of metabolic alkalosis by measuring the urine chloride (see next question). The other urine studies are less useful in metabolic alkalosis. Of course, an appropriate history and physical as well as plasma tests are required to determine the correct diagnosis and treatment.

You have admitted the patient and are on your way to the hospital to see him when the lab tests return (you aren't driving and talking on the phone at the same time are you?). **Plasma studies:** Na 140 mEq/L, K 2.5 mEq/L, Cl 94 mEq/L, BUN 18 mg/dL, creatinine 0.9 mg/dL, Ca 8.4 mg/dL, Mg 1.9 mg/dL.

* *

Urine studies: specific gravity 1.025, chloride 45 mEq/L (high).

Of the following choices, which is NOT likely to contribute to metabolic alkalosis in this patient?

A) Corticosteroids.
B) Diuretics.
C) Hypokalemia.
D) Vomiting or NG suction.

Discussion

The correct answer is "D." This makes intuitive sense. If there is NG suction or vomiting, the patient will be low on chloride and thus will have little in the urine (where it is being reabsorbed.) All of the rest of the answers will cause an **elevated** urine chloride and thus are consistent with this patient's picture. With mineralocorticoid excess (aldosterone or extrinsic corticosteroids, "A"), one excretes potassium causing hypokalemia. Hypokalemia prevents the kidneys from optimally reabsorbing chloride ("C"). See Table 5–9 for more on causes of metabolic alkalosis.

* *

You are able to obtain the cardiologist's records and your patient's medications. He started taking captopril, furosemide, and metoprolol in the last month. He also takes aspirin and isosorbide dinitrate.

All of the following are appropriate interventions in this patient EXCEPT:

A) Discontinue furosemide.
B) Administer potassium chloride.
C) Administer hydrochloric acid through an NG tube.
D) Infuse normal (0.9%) saline.
E) Administer ranitidine.

Table 5–9 CAUSES OF METABOLIC ALKALOSIS DIVIDED BY URINE CHLORIDE LEVELS

Low Urine Chloride (<25 mEq/L)	High Urine Chloride (>40 mEq/L)
Vomiting	Hypokalemia (severe)
Nasogastric suctioning	Diuretics (loop or thiazide; early effect)
Factitious diarrhea (laxative abuse)	Alkali load
Cystic fibrosis	Bartter/Gitelman syndromes
Low chloride intake	Primary mineralocorticoid excess (hyperaldosteronism, corticosteroids)
Posthypercapnia	
Diuretics (loop or thiazide; late effect)	

Discussion

The correct answer is "C." Chloride-responsive metabolic alkalosis is usually secondary to volume contraction. Your patient has renal salt and water losses due to a diuretic and has gastrointestinal volume losses due to emesis. Physical exam (except trace edema—but remember that he has heart failure) and laboratory findings support hypovolemia. The diuretic should be discontinued and volume should be replaced. An isotonic solution, such as normal saline, is an appropriate choice. However, you must monitor your patient's volume status closely due to his CHF. Because his potassium is low, he requires KCl. An H2-blocker, like ranitidine, is a good choice for a patient with alkalosis and gastrointestinal illness: it will reduce acid secretion in the stomach (and thus further acid loss) and may offer some symptomatic relief as well.

Hydrochloric acid is an option in severe metabolic alkalosis unresponsive to other therapies. However, it is not given by NG tube. HCl is very corrosive and should only be infused centrally.

Your patient is not responding to the KCl you are administering. You give which of the following electrolytes to aid in repleting his potassium stores?

A) Sodium.
B) Bicarbonate.
C) Calcium.
D) Phosphate.
E) Magnesium.

Discussion

The correct answer is "E." Give magnesium before giving more potassium. Although your patient's magnesium is only slightly low and may in fact be normal by some laboratory reference values, continued hypokalemia in the face of KCl repletion may indicate whole-body magnesium depletion. Serum magnesium levels may not accurately reflect whole-body magnesium stores, especially in patients with CHF. Furosemide causes further magnesium wasting. None of the other electrolytes listed earlier is as important to potassium repletion.

* *

With correction of fluid and electrolyte status, your patient recovers quickly. You try to convey to the cardiologist the importance of good communication. However, as noted by Machiavelli (ca. 1520): "There is nothing more difficult to take in hand, more perilous to conduct, or more uncertain in its success than to take the lead in the introduction of a new order of things."

Objectives: Did you learn to . . .

- Identify metabolic alkalosis?
- Utilize urine chloride in the evaluation of metabolic alkalosis?
- Recognize various causes of metabolic alkalosis?
- Recognize the role of hypomagnesemia in treating hypokalemia?

QUICK QUIZ: HEMATURIA

A 25-year-old **male** medical student presents with blood in his urine. When asked further about this finding, he admits that he was using urine dipsticks at home to check his urine (did you know that 20% of medical students meet the criteria for somatization disorder at some time during medical school? It's true.). He has no gross hematuria, just 1+ blood on his urine self-test. He has no symptoms otherwise. His major concern is that his father had a renal transplant at age 30 for Alport syndrome.

Given that his father had Alport syndrome, what is the probability that this student has it?

A) Certain (100% chance).
B) One in two.
C) One in four.
D) One in eight.
E) Less than 1 in 20.

Discussion

The correct answer is "E." Alport syndrome, also known as hereditary nephritis, typically presents with microscopic hematuria and progresses to complete renal failure. Alport syndrome has a heterogeneous inheritance pattern: 80% of cases are due to X-linked disease, about 15% are autosomal recessive, and about 5% are autosomal dominant. Since most cases are X-linked, males are affected more severely and earlier than females. If your medical student's father had Alport syndrome, it was most likely X-linked, and the patient could not possibly have inherited it. However, there is a 5% chance that the father had autosomal-dominant disease and then a 50% chance that the trait was passed on to the patient; therefore, "E" is correct.

CASE 9

A 33-year-old male presents to the ED complaining of shortness of breath and cough of 10 days duration. He must sleep in a chair due to orthopnea. He has severe fatigue and a mild, diffuse headache. Four days ago, he was seen in an urgent care clinic and diagnosed with bronchitis. He reports no medical problems or surgeries. He quit smoking 1 year ago and denies alcohol and drug use. He has a strong family history of hypertension. The review of systems is otherwise negative.

On physical examination, his vitals are T 36.8°C, P 104, RR 16, and BP 200/118. There are bibasilar crackles with dullness to percussion at the lung bases. The heart, abdomen, and extremities are unremarkable.

His chest x-ray shows cardiomegaly, mild CHF, and bilateral small pleural effusions. An ECG shows sinus tachycardia with left atrial enlargement and left ventricular hypertrophy. Lab results: troponin-T negative, hemoglobin 9.1 g/dL, WBC count and platelets normal, Na 136 mEq/L, K 4.4 mEq/L, Cl 96 mEq/L, HCO_3 19 mEq/L, BUN 108 mg/dL, Cr 11.9 mg/dL, glucose 104 mg/dL, calcium 7.8 mg/dL, albumin 4.0 g/dL.

Which of the following is the most appropriate next step?

A) Prescribe levofloxacin and discharge patient with follow-up the next day.
B) Prescribe furosemide and discharge patient with follow-up the next day.
C) Administer a bolus of normal saline intravenously and admit the patient.
D) Administer furosemide intravenously and admit the patient.
E) Perform thoracentesis for diagnostic purposes.

Discussion

The correct answer is "D." The proper disposition of this patient is the hospital. His uremia is quite severe, and he is symptomatic from his renal failure. He needs further diagnostic tests and requires further monitoring. He has signs and symptoms of volume overload, and he may yet respond to loop diuretics. A trial of IV furosemide is reasonable. Even if it doesn't cause a diuresis, furosemide can decrease pulmonary capillary wedge pressure. The initial diagnosis of bronchitis was most likely erroneous and switching to another antibiotic will only perpetuate that error. As he is volume overloaded, you certainly do not want to administer more volume. If you are willing to attribute his pleural effusions to volume overload due to kidney failure, a thoracentesis is not necessary.

How should the low calcium be approached in the ED?

A) Administer calcium gluconate intravenously.
B) Obtain a serum parathyroid hormone level.
C) Monitor for signs and symptoms of hypocalcemia.
D) Obtain an ionized calcium level.

Discussion

The correct answer is "C." Currently, your patient does not have signs and symptoms of hypocalcemia; therefore, he does not need calcium replacement in the ED. He should be observed for the development of signs and symptoms. Symptoms are mostly neurological—generalized seizures, perioral paresthesias, and carpopedal spasms. The two best-known signs of hypocalcemia are Chvostek and Trousseau sign. Chvostek sign is present if a grimace occurs in response to tapping the facial nerve. Trousseau sign is evoked by inflating a blood pressure cuff above the systolic pressure for 3 minutes and observing for hand spasms.

* *

Since you expect that the patient's hypocalcemia is secondary to renal disease and hyperphosphatemia and you will treat him symptomatically, serum PTH level is not required. As you have access to both the total serum calcium level and the serum albumin, you can calculate the corrected calcium. Thus, it is not necessary to measure ionized calcium. To correct total calcium for decreased albumin, use the following formula: corrected calcium = measured calcium + [0.8 × (normal albumin − measured albumin)].

HELPFUL TIP: If the patient does not respond to furosemide, IV nitroglycerin will likely be successful at reducing this patient's pulmonary edema by decreasing preload and afterload.

Your patient is admitted. Initially, his urine output increases slightly with loop diuretics, but then he becomes oliguric. You ask for a nephrology consult to assist in management of this case. The nephrologist plans to place an IV catheter for dialysis and is considering a renal biopsy. If the patient develops bleeding with these procedures, he may have difficulty achieving hemostasis because of his uremia.

Which of the following treatments is LEAST likely to reduce the risk of bleeding in this patient?

A) Hemodialysis.
B) DDAVP.
C) Cryoprecipitate.
D) Platelet transfusion.

Discussion

The correct answer is "D." The cause of bleeding dysfunction in uremia appears to be the effect of uremic toxins on platelet function. Giving a uremic patient more platelets—especially when there is no thrombocytopenia—will not improve the situation, as the platelet dysfunction due to uremia will occur with the new platelets as well. "A," hemodialysis, will remove toxins related to uremia, improving platelet function. "B," DDAVP, is often the first-line treatment in a bleeding patient with uremia. DDAVP is not generally toxic and quickly reduces bleeding time. It acts by causing the release of factor VIII:vWF multimers from endothelial storage sites. Unfortunately, patients rapidly develop tachyphylaxis to DDAVP; once the multimers are depleted from the endothelial cells, DDAVP will not work until these multimers are replaced (usually a process of several days). "C," cryoprecipitate, will reduce bleeding time. Estrogen is another option for renal failure–related bleeding.

In order to reduce the risk of renal osteodystrophy (elevated serum parathyroid hormone with mobilization of calcium from bone), which of the following medications will you prescribe initially?

A) Calcium carbonate.
B) Aluminum hydroxide.

C) Magnesium hydroxide.
D) Sevelamer (Renagel®).
E) Vitamin D.

Discussion

The correct answer is "A." Renal osteodystrophy occurs when parathyroid hormone levels are elevated and bone is mobilized. This occurs because patients with renal failure cannot clear phosphate. The body tries to compensate by increasing parathyroid hormone secretion, which reduces phosphate and increases serum calcium. However, it also is detrimental to bone and leads to demineralization.

Gastrointestinal binding of phosphate requires large doses of a cation such as calcium (2 g/day). Calcium carbonate is associated with the least potential toxicity; therefore, it is the initial choice for treating hyperphosphatemia to reduce the risk of renal osteodystrophy. Also, you may consider calcium acetate, which is as safe as calcium carbonate and is a more potent phosphate binder but more expensive. Avoid aluminum and magnesium products in renal failure as these ions accumulate and can cause toxicity.

Sevelamer is a cationic polymer that binds phosphate in the gastrointestinal tract and avoids the problems that can occur with the calcium, magnesium, and aluminum compounds. It is expensive and does not seem to be superior to calcium, so calcium products should be tried first.

* *

Patients with chronic renal failure or end-stage renal disease on dialysis should also receive vitamin D. However, vitamin D causes increased gastrointestinal absorption of phosphate, so it should be given only after hyperphosphatemia has been controlled.

HELPFUL TIP: Whenever prescribing calcium for renal osteodystrophy, have patients take it with meals—otherwise it will not bind phosphate. Also, calcium is absorbed better when taken with food.

HELPFUL TIP: Cinacalcet (Sensipar) is another option for treating renal osteodystrophy. By mimicking calcium in the parathyroid, it fools the parathyroid into thinking that the serum calcium is normal and thus reduces the output of parathyroid hormone.

Objective: Did you learn to . . .

- Anticipate complications of renal failure, including hypervolemia, hypocalcemia, platelet dysfunction, and renal osteodystrophy?

CASE 10

A 10-year-old male presents with his mother, who appears very anxious. She reports several episodes of red-brown urine this morning. The patient reports feeling a bit tired, but otherwise has no complaints. His past medical history is unremarkable and he takes no medications. On review of systems, he reports a sore throat that completely resolved a few days ago.

On exam, you find a pleasant young male in no acute distress. He is afebrile. His blood pressure is 140/94 mm Hg, and he has trace pretibial edema. The remainder of the exam is unrevealing.

All of the following tests are likely to be helpful in the workup of this patient EXCEPT:

A) Urinalysis.
B) Abdominal x-ray.
C) CBC.
D) Plasma electrolytes.
E) BUN and creatinine.

Discussion

The correct answer is "B." Abdominal plain films are not useful in almost any situation unless looking for constipation or bowel obstruction. (What did you say? Free air? An upright chest is the most sensitive film for free air—save for CT.) If this patient had a presentation consistent with urolithiasis, an abdominal CT scan may be indicated. All of the other laboratory tests should be ordered.

* *

Urinalysis shows 2+ blood, 2+ protein, specific gravity 1.015, and numerous red blood cells with red cell casts. BUN is 35 mg/dL and creatinine is 1.8 mg/dL. CBC, coagulation studies, and electrolytes are pending.

At this point, all of the following should be considered in the differential diagnosis EXCEPT:

A) Minimal change disease.
B) Henoch–Schönlein purpura.
C) Poststreptococcal glomerulonephritis.
D) IgA nephropathy.
E) Membranoproliferative glomerulonephritis.

Discussion

The correct answer is "A." Minimal change disease usually presents with clinical signs and symptoms of nephrotic syndrome and not gross hematuria. All of the other diseases are associated with hematuria, either microscopic or gross. Henoch–Schönlein purpura, poststreptococcal glomerulonephritis, IgA nephropathy, and membranoproliferative glomerulonephritis all have more "nephritic" features with "active" urinary sediments (dysmorphic red cells, red cell casts, granular casts, white cells, and protein in the urine). Also, these diseases have a similar pathologic process in which immune complexes deposit in the glomeruli, resulting in glomerulonephritis.

* *

CBC, coagulation studies, and electrolytes are all normal. You are suspicious that he may have had streptococcal pharyngitis that was unrecognized.

Which of the following statements best describes the usual course of poststreptococcal glomerulonephritis?

A) Most patients progress to renal failure.
B) After resolution of the initial episode, recurrent episodes of gross hematuria are common.
C) In most cases, hypertension and uremia subside within 1–2 weeks.
D) In most cases, hypertension is persistent and requires treatment.
E) Adults tend to recover more quickly than children.

Discussion

The correct answer is "C." Poststreptococcal glomerulonephritis, characterized by immune complex deposition in the glomeruli, is a self-limited disease in most patients. There is a latent period, averaging 10 days, between pharyngitis and the development of hematuria. Recovery is expected in 1–2 weeks. Unlike IgA nephropathy, recurrent episodes of gross hematuria are rare in poststreptococcal glomerulonephritis. Poststreptococcal glomerulonephritis is more common in children and tends to be more severe when it affects adults. Hypertension and uremia resolve relatively quickly, but microscopic hematuria may persist for 6 months.

Table 5–10 CAUSES OF GROSS HEMATURIA IN CHILDREN

Idiopathic (usually benign with resolution over time)
Urinary tract infection
Trauma
Congenital anomaly
Urethral irritation or trauma
Nephrolithiasis
Sickle cell disease/trait
Coagulopathy
Glomerular disease (e.g., poststreptococcal glomerulonephritis)
Malignancy (e.g., Wilm tumor)
Medications (e.g., hemorrhagic cystitis from cyclophosphamide)

HELPFUL TIP: Renal biopsy is rarely indicated in children with nephritic urine and mild renal failure because the differential diagnosis can be narrowed by the clinical presentation and because many of the diseases are self-limited. In more severe cases, renal biopsy may be necessary to diagnose and treat appropriately. See Table 5–10 for a partial list of causes of hematuria in children.

Objectives: Did you learn to . . .

- Evaluate a child with gross hematuria?
- Generate a differential diagnosis for hematuria and proteinuria in a child?
- Describe the usual course of poststreptococcal glomerulonephritis?

(NOT SO QUICK) QUIZ: I'VE GOT TO PEE . . . AGAIN

A 45-year-old female presents to your clinic complaining of urinary frequency, bladder pain, and urgency. There is no dysuria, however. This has been going on for several months and other practitioners (less skilled than yourself) have treated with a number of antibiotics without any relief. On questioning, she also notes bladder pain during intercourse and some chronic, vague, lower pelvic pain distinct from the bladder pain. A urinalysis and pelvic exam are unremarkable except for bladder tenderness.

The MOST IMPORTANT next step is:

A) Urine culture.
B) Trial of 4 weeks of antichlamydial therapy.
C) Pelvic ultrasound.
D) Psychiatry consult and/or SSRI therapy for somatization disorder.

Discussion
The correct answer is "C." This patient is describing typical symptoms of interstitial cystitis. However, it is critical to rule out other pelvic pathology such as an enlarged uterus sitting on the bladder or ovarian cancer. Other causes of similar symptoms could be bladder irritants (caffeine, alcohol).

All of the following are mandatory at this point EXCEPT:

A) Urine cytology in a high-risk patient (smoker, etc.).
B) Postvoid residual.
C) Cystoscopy and hyperdistention of the bladder.
D) Ruling out a bladder stone.

Discussion
The correct answer is "C." Cystoscopy and hyperdistention are NOT required in order to make the diagnosis of interstitial cystitis. It is a clinical diagnosis of exclusion: Is there anything else causing the symptoms? If not, as Sherlock Holmes said, "Once you eliminate the impossible, whatever remains, no matter how improbable, must be the truth." It is important to rule out tumor (if indicated), stones, neurogenic bladder (thus the postvoid residual). There are biomarkers in the works for this disease, but they have not yet entered the clinical arena.

HELPFUL TIP: Treatment of interstitial cystitis includes possible referral to a pain clinic, support groups, treatment of any other underlying problems (inflammatory bowel disease, etc.), tricyclics, gabapentin, intravesicular DMSO, recurrent hydrodistention of the bladder, etc. What about pentosan polysulfate sodium (Elmiron)? It is way expensive, may take up to 6 months to work, and the benefit is modest at best.

HELPFUL TIP: Why not chronic phenazopyridine (e.g., Pyridium)? Well, you can consider it. But there is a danger of significant methemoglobinemia.

CASE 11

The parents of a 2-year-old female bring her in to your office for a weeklong history of diarrhea. Initially, her stools were loose and watery, but over the last few days, they have become bloody. The patient has appeared to have abdominal pain on occasions, and her appetite is depressed. Despite bloody diarrhea, her parents attempted to care for her at home until she became more lethargic (well, that didn't work... probably the same parents who refused vaccines). They are also worried about some bruising on her extremities.

The nurse takes her vital signs: T 37.2°C, P 145, BP 88/47, RR 40. The patient appears pale, with slight scleral icterus. You note petechiae and purpura on the extremities. Her abdomen is diffusely tender. She responds to commands but appears very lethargic.

While you are arranging her admission to the hospital, some laboratory tests return: Hgb 8 g/dL, Hct 24%, WBC 14,000/mm^3, platelets 50,000/mm^3, Na 128 mEq/L, K 3.9 mEq/L, HCO_3 14 mEq/L, BUN 38 mg/dL, creatinine 2.1 mg/dL. The peripheral blood smear shows schistocytes, "Burr" cells, and grossly reduced number of platelets.

Which of the following is the most appropriate initial management of this patient?

A) Intravenous fluids.
B) Dialysis.
C) Platelet transfusion.
D) Corticosteroids.
E) Antibiotics.

Discussion
The correct answer is "A." The proper initial management consists of supportive therapy. This patient

has signs of dehydration, which would be expected from the history of prolonged diarrhea. She is hyponatremic, and isotonic (0.9%) saline is the IV fluid of choice. Use 20 cc/kg boluses until her blood pressure stabilizes. This patient may also require an RBC transfusion given her anemia. Although she has had diarrhea, her potassium is currently in the normal range, probably due to decreased glomerular filtration. Given her renal failure, potassium should not be in her IV fluids.

Consideration of dialysis is premature. A platelet count of 50,000 is adequate for hemostasis, so answer "C" is incorrect. The schistocytes suggest a microangiopathic hemolytic anemia. Steroids are not generally helpful for this, so "D" is incorrect. Finally, antibiotics may (or may not) be beneficial if the patient has bacterial enteritis, but IV fluids should be administered first.

Based on the available information, which of the following is the most likely diagnosis?

A) Thrombotic thrombocytopenic purpura.
B) Hemolytic uremic syndrome.
C) Postinfectious glomerulonephritis.
D) Henoch–Schönlein purpura.
E) Autosomal-recessive polycystic kidney disease.

Discussion

The correct answer is "B." Hemolytic uremic syndrome (HUS) is the most likely diagnosis. This patient presents with a classic history of uremia and hemolysis preceded by 5–7 days of diarrhea. Patients tend to become oliguric and sometimes anuric.

"A," thrombotic thrombocytopenic purpura (TTP), is a related disorder which is rare in children. TTP tends to occur in young adults, with women making up about 70% of all cases. In contrast to HUS, patients with TTP may present with the classic pentad: thrombocytopenia, fever, mental status changes, renal insufficiency, and hemolytic anemia. Usually, there is a prodrome viral illness with TTP but diarrhea occurs only rarely.

"C," postinfectious glomerulonephritis, usually occurs after pharyngitis or skin infection with group A beta-hemolytic streptococci. Common symptoms include edema and hematuria but not thrombocytopenia or diarrhea. "D," Henoch–Schönlein purpura, is a (usually) transient IgA vasculitis following upper respiratory infections in children and adolescents. Autosomal-recessive polycystic kidney disease is a rare disorder that presents early in childhood with abdominal masses, hypertension, urinary tract infections, and renal failure.

HELPFUL TIP: HUS may occur without diarrhea. This subtype of HUS occurs less frequently, is associated with *Streptococcus* infections, and carries a worse prognosis.

From the blood culture, you expect to find:

A) *Shigella* species.
B) *E. coli*.
C) *Streptococcus pneumoniae*.
D) *Haemophilus influenzae*.
E) None of the above.

Discussion

The correct answer is "E." Although HUS is the result of bacterial enteritis, patients are not bacteremic. Instead, the endothelial damage and hemolysis are caused by Shiga toxin, released from *E. coli* and *Shigella dysenteriae*.

All of the following are true regarding Shiga toxin HUS in children EXCEPT:

A) If dialysis is needed, renal function rarely returns.
B) Half or more of the cases occur in the summer months.
C) Ingestion of contaminated meat is a common source of *E. coli* O157:H7 infection.
D) Cattle are the main vectors of *E. coli* O157:H7.
E) Antibiotics do not reduce the risk of HUS in patients with confirmed *E. coli* O157:H7 infections.

Discussion

The correct answer is "A." All the other statements are true. The prognosis of Shiga toxin HUS in children is generally quite favorable, even if renal failure requires dialysis. HUS is more common in rural areas and in the summer. Cows are the culprits. (In general, that is the answer you should put on the test. Cows are always the culprits except in English dramas where it is the butler.) "E" is of special note. There is controversy over whether or not antibiotics may **increase** the risk of HUS developing in patients with *E. coli* O157:H7 infections; however, it is fairly clear that antibiotics do not reduce the risk. The idea is that bacterial death from antibiotics releases more Shiga toxin leading to HUS. Remember that most cases of bacterial gastroenteritis—*E. coli* O157:H7 included—will clear without antibiotic therapy.

HELPFUL TIP: Other subtypes of *E. coli* as well as *Shigella* can be responsible for HUS. The absence of the O157:H7 subtype of *E. coli* does not rule out HUS.

Objectives: Did you learn to . . .

- Evaluate and manage a child with hypovolemia and renal failure?
- Recognize a clinical history and laboratory findings suggestive of hemolytic-uremic syndrome?
- Identify causes of hemolytic-uremic syndrome?

QUICK QUIZ: ACID–BASE DISORDER

While covering your local ED, a 15-year-old female presents with her father. He reports that he came home from work, found her asleep on the couch, and had difficulty waking her. She is lethargic and complains of nausea, dizziness, and abdominal pain. Apparently, she had muscle aches after gymnastics practice and then took "handfuls" of aspirin to relieve her pain. She was taking three to four tablets every hour or two today but is not sure about her total ingestion. She denies other ingestions.

On physical examination, her vitals are T 39°C, P 110, RR 18, BP 104/68. She is diaphoretic. The neurological exam is nonfocal, but she becomes progressively more lethargic during the exam. An arterial blood gas on room air shows pH 7.38, $PaCO_2$ 23 mm Hg, PaO_2 98 mm Hg, and HCO_3 15 mEq/L. Other lab data: Na 140 mEq/L, K 3.1 mEq/L, Cl 101 mEq/L, HCO_3 15 mEq/L, BUN 19 mg/dL, creatinine 1.1 mg/dL.

The arterial blood gas results are best described as:

A) Metabolic acidosis.
B) Metabolic acidosis and metabolic alkalosis.
C) Metabolic acidosis and respiratory alkalosis.
D) Metabolic alkalosis and respiratory acidosis.
E) Just dandy! Look at the pH, professor.

Discussion

The correct answer is "C." Although the pH is in the normal range, there is an acid–base disorder present. First, there appears to be a metabolic acidosis with an elevated anion gap. The measured HCO_3 is 15 mEq/L, consistent with an acidosis, and the anion gap is 24 (based on the calculation of Na − (Cl + HCO_3), in this case: 140 − (101 + 15) = 24). This patient has taken an inadvertent overdose of aspirin. In salicylate overdoses, a high anion gap metabolic acidosis is often observed. Since salicylates directly stimulate the CNS respiratory center, there is usually a concurrent respiratory alkalosis.

In metabolic acidosis, the $PaCO_2$ should drop by 1.25 mm Hg for every 1 mEq/L drop in HCO_3. In this case, the serum HCO_3 is 9 mEq/L below normal (if the normal is counted as 24), so $PaCO_2$ should be about 29 mm Hg (40 − (9 × 1.25)). However, the measured $PaCO_2$ is 23 mm Hg, indicating the presence of a respiratory alkalosis. Also, the pH is nearly normal despite the presence of a disturbance in measured HCO_3, **which only occurs when a mixed disorder is present.**

* *

Proper treatment of salicylate overdoses includes supportive therapy, urine alkalinization with sodium bicarbonate. Dialysis may also be necessary.

HELPFUL TIP: It is impossible to overcorrect a metabolic abnormality. Thus, a patient with a metabolic acidosis will not become alkalotic or normal unless there is another primary process present (e.g., respiratory alkalosis). Likewise, a patient with a respiratory acidosis from the retention of CO_2 will not become alkalotic or normal unless there is a secondary primary process going on (e.g., metabolic alkalosis).

QUICK QUIZ: DYSURIA

Your nurse comes to you with a patient request. A 25-year-old female called in complaining of 2 days of burning with urination, urgency to urinate, and increased frequency. She has no fever, nausea, abdominal pain, flank pain, or vaginal discharge. The patient wants to know, "Can't I just get some antibiotics?"

She's sure this is a bladder infection, just like the one she had last year. Oh, by the way, she's leaving for Europe tomorrow for her honeymoon.

Your response is to:

A) Prescribe ciprofloxacin 250 mg BID for 3 days.
B) Prescribe trimethoprim/sulfamethoxazole BID for 14 days.
C) Ask her to come in for a urinalysis.
D) Ask her to come in for a urine culture.
E) Recommend cranberry juice.

Discussion

The correct answer is "A." Although you could argue that the diagnosis of UTI should be confirmed by urinalysis, there is plenty of evidence that history alone is sufficiently accurate. If a woman complains of dysuria and increased frequency without vaginal discharge, the likelihood ratio of UTI is about 25 and "posttest" probability is greater than 90% that she has a urinary tract infection (JAMA 2002;287(20):2701). If her urinalysis were completely normal, she may still have an infection and have a false-negative dipstick urine. **Using urine dipstick alone in a woman with urinary symptoms only increases the posttest probability to 81%.** Thus, certain symptoms and historical elements are more useful than urinalysis. For this patient, empiric antibiotic therapy with an appropriate antibiotic (nonrespiratory fluoroquinolone, trimethoprim/sulfamethoxazole, or other) for 3 days is reasonable. Fourteen days of trimethoprim/sulfamethoxazole is overkill. Of course, urine culture is the gold standard for diagnosing UTI, but she will be in Europe by the time you get the results. There is some evidence that cranberry products may reduce the frequency of recurrent UTI (maybe), but cranberry juice does not seem to work for treatment. Trials of cranberry products for UTI suffer from high dropout rates and variability in products and measurements.

HELPFUL TIP: With typical UTI symptoms (e.g., dysuria, frequency) and a negative urine culture or no response to antibiotics, consider other causes: interstitial cystitis, chlamydia urethritis, prostatitis (in men), pelvic inflammatory disease (in women), pelvic mass, herpes genitalis, and drugs (e.g., diuretics, caffeine, and theophylline).

CASE 12

You are asked to consult on a patient who is hospitalized by an orthopedic surgeon. The patient is a 25-year-old female who has a history of osteomyelitis from an open fracture sustained in a skiing accident. She has recently begun to spike a fever to 38.5 and have a rapid increase in her creatinine.

Medications: methicillin, ibuprofen, morphine, lactated Ringer solution IV 100 cc/hr.

Labs: Cr 3.5 mg/dL, BUN 25 mg/dL.

CBC shows mild eosinophilia.

All things being equal, what would you expect to find?

A) FENa >2%, urine sodium <20.
B) FENa <1%, urine sodium <20.
C) FENa >2%, urine sodium >40.
D) FENa <1%, urine sodium >40.

Discussion

The correct answer is "C." Remember... her BUN/Cr <20; therefore, it is likely **not** pre-renal disease (and she's receiving volume and has no history of heart failure). Thus, the patient likely has intrinsic kidney disease. This means that the FENa should be >2% and the urine sodium >40 mg/dL. In this scenario, the kidney is not trying to hold on to sodium in an attempt to correct a prerenal cause of increasing creatinine.

* *

The patient's exam shows a diffuse rash and the urine contains white cell casts. There are no red cells in the urine.

The most likely diagnosis is:

A) ATN.
B) Interstitial nephritis.
C) Renal infarction.
D) Glomerulonephritis.
E) Nephrotic syndrome.

Discussion

The correct answer is "B." The combination of fever, rash, mild eosinophilia, exposure to a new drug (methicillin) and white cell casts in the urine essentially makes the diagnosis of interstitial nephritis. "A" is incorrect. **The patient with ATN may have the same FENa and urine sodium as this patient but should have renal tubular cells and/or granular**

Table 5–11 COMMON DRUGS ASSOCIATED WITH INTERSTITIAL NEPHRITIS

- Penicillins
- Aspirin
- Ciprofloxacin (and likely other fluoroquinolones)
- Allopurinol
- NSAIDs
- Some ACE inhibitors
- Erythromycin

NSAIDs, nonsteroidal anti-inflammatory drugs; ACE, angiotensin-converting enzyme.

casts in the urine. Also, ATN does not cause fever, eosinophilia, or rash. "C," renal infarction, is unlikely in a young patient and the rest of the clinical picture does not fit. "D," glomerulonephritis, is a possibility (e.g., lupus could cause a rash and fever). However, glomerulonephritis is associated with **red cell casts** and not white cell casts. Finally, as you already learned above, nephrotic syndrome presents with a bland urinary sediment. See Tables 5–11 and 5–12 for more details.

How long after drug exposure does interstitial nephritis generally begin?

A) 2–3 days.
B) 10–14 days.
C) Several months.
D) A and B.
E) All of the above.

Discussion

The correct answer is "E." Patients can develop interstitial nephritis anywhere from 1 day to several months after beginning a drug. Rifampin can often cause interstitial nephritis on day 1. Interstitial nephritis can begin within 2–5 days if there has been a prior exposure to the drug, will typically begin within 10–14 days on **first** exposure to a drug, and may delayed for months in the case of NSAID exposure.

Table 5–12 SYMPTOMS/SIGNS/ LABORATORY FINDINGS IN ACUTE INTERSTITIAL NEPHRITIS

- Fever
- Rash (variable, may not be seen in all)
- Acute rise in plasma creatinine
- Active urine sediment that includes white cell casts
- Peripheral eosinophilia and urine eosinophils (in most cases)
- Renal tubular acidosis

Note: Interstitial nephritis secondary to NSAIDs may occur without fever, rash, or eosinophilia.

HELPFUL TIP: Patients with interstitial nephritis will often have eosinophils in the urine and peripheral smear, but eosinophils may be absent especially in those with NSAID-induced interstitial nephritis. Treatment is to stop the offending drug. If this doesn't work, steroids or cytotoxic drugs may be needed.

Objectives: Did you learn to . . .

- Recognize the presenting symptoms of acute interstitial nephritis?
- Describe causes and prognosis of interstitial nephritis?

QUICK QUIZ: SAVE THOSE NEPHRONS!

A 45-year-old male comes to your office to establish care. He reports a history of hypertension treated with verapamil and chlorthalidone. His blood pressure today is 130/78. You order some lab tests and find that his creatinine is 2.5 mg/dL.

You recommend which strategy to preserve his renal function?

A) Start a low-dose ACE inhibitor.
B) Start a high-dose ACE inhibitor.
C) Start furosemide.
D) Start amlodipine.

Discussion

The correct answer is "A." Even in patients with renal dysfunction as evidenced by elevated creatinine, ACE inhibitors can reduce the rate of progression of renal disease. More importantly, ACE inhibitors can be used safely in patients with stage 4 CKD. Due to the risk of rising creatinine and potassium, ACE inhibitors should be started at a low dose and increased slowly, checking creatinine and potassium levels within a week or 2 after making a dose adjustment. Furosemide and amlodipine have not been shown to preserve renal function.

HELPFUL TIP: ACE inhibitors have been shown to be useful in reducing progression of renal disease even when the patient's creatinine is 5.0 mg/dL. But, be very careful in this group.

BIBLIOGRAPHY

Azadi R, et al. Hemolytic uremic syndrome caused by Shiga toxin-producing *Escherichia coli* 0111. *J Am Osteopath Assoc.* 2010;110(9):538-544.

Gill N, et al. Renal failure secondary to acute tubular necrosis: epidemiology, diagnosis, and management. *Chest.* 2005;128(4):2847-2863. Review.

Hou FF, et al. Efficacy and safety of benazepril for advanced chronic renal insufficiency. *N Engl J Med.* 2006;354:131-140.

Kellum J, et al. Acute renal failure. *Am Fam Physician.* 2007;763:418-422.

Kohlstadt I, Frassetto L. Treatment and prevention of kidney stones: An update. *Am Fam Physician.* 2011;84:11.

Levey AS, et al. *K/DOQI Clinical Practice Guidelines for Chronic Kidney Disease: Evaluation, Classification, and Stratification.* Available at: http://www.kidney.org/professionals/kdoqi/guidelines_ckd/toc.htm, Accessed October 20, 2007.

Martinez-Bianchi V, Halstater BH. Urologic chronic pelvic pain syndrome. Prim Care. 2010;37:527-546.

Miller NL, Lingeman JE. Management of kidney stones. *BMJ.* 2007;334(7591):468-472.

Phrommintikul A, et al. Mortality and target haemoglobin concentrations in anaemic patients with chronic kidney disease treated with erythropoietin: a meta-analysis. *Lancet.* 2007;369:381-388.

Schena FP. Management of patients with chronic kidney disease. *Intern Emerg Med.* 2011;6(Suppl 1):77-83.

Simerville JA, et al. Urinalysis: a comprehensive review. *Am Fam Physician.* 2005;71(6):1153-1162.

Strippoli GF, et al. Angiotensin converting enzyme inhibitors and angiotensin II receptor antagonists for preventing the progression of diabetic kidney disease. Cochrane Database Syst Rev. 2006;(4):CD006257.

Tarr PI, et al. Shiga-toxin-producing *Escherichia coli* and haemolytic uraemic syndrome. *Lancet.* 2005;365:1073.

Vincendeau S, et al. Tamsulosin hydrochloride vs placebo for management of distal ureteral stones: a multicentric, randomized, double-blind trial. *Arch Intern Med.* 2010;170(22):2021-2027.

Whitmore KE, Theoharides TC. When to suspect interstitial cystitis. *J Fam Pract.* 2011;60(6):340-348. Review.

6

Hematology and Oncology

Mark A. Graber and Jason K. Wilbur

CASE 1

A 6-month-old boy presents to your office after his mother notices swelling and ecchymosis over his anterior right thigh. She does not recall any trauma to the area. The mother denies any history of bleeding problems, including during his circumcision. On physical exam the child has a large hematoma over his thigh. There are no obvious bony deformities and the child otherwise looks well. You suspect the child may have an inherited coagulation disorder.

Which of the following statements is NOT correct?

A) Child abuse should be included in the differential diagnosis.
B) The child did not bleed during circumcision, so the possibility of hemophilia need not be considered.
C) A careful family history is important in the workup.
D) Coagulation studies (PT, PTT) and CBC should be obtained.

Discussion

The correct answer is "B." The absence of bleeding during circumcision in no way rules out hemophilia. Up to half of hemophiliac patients do not bleed after circumcision. Depending on the severity of factor deficiency, the diagnosis may not be made until the child is very active or even in adulthood, after surgery, etc.

Which of the following statements is true about the patient with a bleeding disorder?

A) Factor deficiencies generally present with mucosal bleeding/petechiae.
B) Hemarthrosis generally reflects a platelet deficiency.
C) Hematomas are usually the result of a factor deficiency.
D) All of the above are true.

Discussion

The correct answer is "C." Generally, petechiae and mucosal bleeding are the result of platelet problems (e.g., mild von Willebrand disease and thrombocytopenia) while hemarthrosis and hematomas are the result of a factor deficiency. Severe von Willebrand disease may present with hemarthrosis and hematomas.

Which of the following is NOT TRUE about hemophilia A?

A) It is an X-linked disorder.
B) It is the result of factor Xa deficiency.
C) It generally leads to mucosal bleeding.
D) It occurs most often in males.

Discussion

The correct answer is "B." Hemophilia A is an X-lined deficiency of factor VIII, which presents with hematomas, bleeding, and hemarthrosis (and not generally mucosal bleeding or petechiae). Deficiency of factor IX, or hemophilia B, also known as "Christmas Disease," is also X-linked but is much less common.

"D" deserves special mention. Hemophilia rarely occurs in females but can occur in two situations: (1) the female patient is a heterozygote who has early inactivation of the second X chromosome during embryogenesis or (2) if both parents are carriers—in which case the father would have the disease overtly.

HELPFUL TIP: von Willebrand disease may be autosomal dominant (Type I), variable (Type II), or autosomal recessive (Type III). There is often a family history of factor deficiency or bleeding, but a percentage of cases occur spontaneously.

Which of the following is indicated when evaluating for a suspected inherited coagulopathy?

A) CBC.
B) PT and PTT.
C) Platelet count.
D) PFA-100.
E) All of the above.

Discussion
The correct answer is "E." The PTT is actually the most sensitive test for hemophilia. "D" deserves special mention. The PFA-100 (**P**latelet **F**unction **A**ssay) tests for (appropriately enough) platelet functioning and will be abnormal in von Willebrand disease. Other qualitative platelet defects are rare, however.

HELPFUL TIP: The PFA-100 can help you make a diagnosis but it doesn't necessarily correlate with the risk of clinical bleeding.

* *

This patient grows up under your excellent tutelage. As a junior high school student, he attends summer camp for hemophiliacs in Transylvania. For some bizarre reason, the councilors decide to have the kids play tackle football (just in case you think we made this up, it did happen to one of your authors while working in the emergency department (ED)—but not at the University of Iowa). The patient presents to the ED with bleeding into two of his joints.

What percent of activity factor will you shoot for when treating this patient?

A) 25–29%.
B) 30–40%.
C) 75–80%.
D) 100%.
E) I don't know how to take tests so I am convinced all of the above are wrong.

Discussion
The correct answer is "B." For a hemarthrosis or other "minor" bleeding, you should maintain a factor level of 30–40% for 72 hours. For more serious bleeding (intracranial, for example), maintain a level of 80–100% for 10 days.

* *

It turns out that this patient has very mild hemophilia and your hospital does not have factor for replacement (or fresh frozen plasma (FFP) or cryoprecipitate—you know, budget cuts).

Which of the following may be useful in this patient?

A) IV desmopressin.
B) Tranexamic acid or aminocaproic acid.
C) IV vitamin K.
D) A and B.
E) All of the above.

Discussion
The correct answer is "D." Patients with mild hemophilia (and some types of von Willebrand disease) will respond to desmopressin with a transient increase in serum von Willebrand factor (vWF) and factor VIII.

HELPFUL TIP: von Willebrand disease Type 1 will respond to desmopressin (as noted above). Types II and III von Willebrand require infusion of factor VIII and vWF (such as Humate-P).

In 2011 (as opposed to 1981) which of the following is likely to be the case in a patient with hemophilia?

A) Hemarthrosis with significant arthritis and joint dysfunction.
B) An extremely low risk of HIV/AIDS from multiple transfusions of FFP.

C) Maturational delay if antifactor antibodies are present.
D) Reduced risk of coronary artery disease (CAD).
E) All of the above are found with hemophilia.

Discussion
The correct answer is "E." "A" is true. Patients still get recurrent hemarthrosis leading to arthritis and joint dysfunction. "B" is true. Screening and use of recombinant factor VIII have led to a marked reduction in HIV in hemophiliacs from a high of 50%. Patients with hemophilia do have delayed maturation, especially if antifactor antibodies are present. And finally, they do have a **reduced risk** of CAD. This is also seen in carriers of hemophilia.
Note: In this chapter, objectives are listed after several short cases, so keep reading.

CASE 2

A 3-year-old girl is brought to you after she is noted to have small pink spots on her lower extremities and bleeding from her gums. She had a URI a couple of weeks ago. You note petechiae on her lower extremities and purpura in her oropharynx. The mother and patient deny any other bleeding. You obtain a CBC, which is normal except for a platelet count of 15,000/mm^3. You suspect idiopathic thrombocytopenic purpura (ITP).

Which of the following may have led to this patient's ITP?

A) MMR vaccine.
B) Infection.
C) Food allergy.
D) Autoimmune hemolytic anemia.
E) A and B.

Discussion
The correct answer is "E." Both infections and the MMR vaccine have been linked to ITP (not autism... got that?... **not autism**). The others are incorrect. Food allergy does not cause ITP and if you chose "D," time to study some more. An autoimmune hemolytic anemia is just that an autoimmune hemolytic anemia. It is a different disease process entirely.

Which of the following is not likely to lead to a sustained (lets say 2 day) increase in the patient's platelet count?

A) IVIG.
B) Steroids (e.g., prednisone).
C) Platelet transfusion.
D) Splenectomy.

Discussion
The correct answer (and what will not yield a sustained increase in platelet count) is "C." Transfused platelets will just be chomped up by Mr. Spleen. However, platelets can be used to temporize if a patient must go to the OR, etc. **Most children can simply be observed. The only indication for treatment is bleeding.** All of the treatments have a downside. **Splenectomy** is associated with a risk of sepsis. If possible, delay splenectomy until after the child is over 5 years old. **Steroids** may cause behavioral problems and long-term problems such as avascular necrosis. IVIG leads to a temporary increase in platelets that may last several weeks but can be associated with renal injury and anaphylaxis among other adverse effect.

HELPFUL TIP: If a child suspected of having ITP looks sick, you need to expand your differential diagnosis. Sepsis with disseminated intravascular coagulopathy (DIC) and thrombotic thrombocytopenic purpura—hemolytic uremic syndrome (TTP–HUS) are also in the differential. ITP is most common in children between the ages of 2 and 4 years. The condition often resolves without specific therapy: 80–90% of pediatric patients are back to normal within a few months, and fewer than 20% of children will remain thrombocytopenic for greater than 12 months. Only 0.1–0.5% develop intracranial bleeding.

HELPFUL TIP: Do not bother checking for antiplatelet antibodies in those with ITP. Patients **without** ITP may have antiplatelet antibodies and the presence of these antibodies is not predictive of outcome.

HELPFUL TIP: For adults with ITP, treatment is generally indicated. Treatment incudes (in order) steroids, Rho(D) immunoglobulin **for Rh-positive patients,** IVIG (which causes a transient rise in platelet numbers), and splenectomy. Other treatment options for refractory cases include rituximab or various immunosuppressive agents. The thrombopoietin-receptor agonists, romiplostim and eltrombopag, stimulate platelet production and can also be used in ITP.

HELPFUL TIP: Failure of ITP to respond to splenectomy may be due to the presence of an accessory spleen, which can often be identified by a liver–spleen radionuclide study.

CASE 3

A 24-year-old female G1 P0 at 39 weeks of gestation presents to your office with a bruise on her anterior tibia, which she noticed after bumping into a coffee table. She has been well during her pregnancy and takes only prenatal vitamins. Her physical exam is unremarkable with the exception of an 8-cm bruise over her right anterior tibia. She has a normal blood pressure (BP), normal reflexes, and no peripheral edema. You obtain the following lab tests: CBC, which demonstrates white blood cell (WBC) 9000/mm^3, hemoglobin (Hb) 11.8 g/dL, and platelet count 95,000/mm^3; negative urinalysis, normal liver enzymes.

What is your next step?

A) Recommend immediate delivery by cesarean section as the infant likely has thrombocytopenia as well and is at high risk for intracranial hemorrhage.
B) Recommend immediate delivery by cesarean section as this disorder will likely progress to eclampsia.
C) Recommend close observation, and reassure the patient that this is typically a self-limited condition.
D) Start prednisone, 1 mg/kg daily, and taper slowly over the next 6 weeks.
E) Recommend splenectomy as soon as possible after delivery.

Discussion

The correct answer is "C." This patient likely has gestational thrombocytopenia, a condition that occurs in up to 5% of pregnant women. It is characterized by mild thrombocytopenia occurring in late gestation; the platelet count is usually >70,000/mm^3 (two-thirds are between 130,000/mm^3 and 150,000/mm^3). The condition resolves after delivery and is not associated with severe neonatal thrombocytopenia. No specific change in routine obstetrical care is warranted, although the anesthesiologist placing an epidural may want a follow-up platelet count closer to the time of delivery.

HELPFUL TIP: A platelet count of >20,000–50,000/mm^3 is generally considered adequate for appropriate clotting.

Objectives: Did you learn to . . .

- Obtain a thorough bleeding history?
- Use laboratory testing to assist in the diagnosis of a bleeding disorder?
- Identify common congenital bleeding disorders?
- Identify and treat common acquired bleeding disorders?

QUICK QUIZ: COAGULATION STUDIES

Which of the following conditions should be considered if both the PT and PTT are prolonged in a patient noted to be oozing from a surgical incision?

A) Severe liver disease, DIC, factor X deficiency.
B) Heparin effect, von Willebrand disease, factor XII deficiency.
C) Warfarin effect, factor VII deficiency, vitamin K deficiency.
D) All of the above.

Discussion

The correct answer is "A." The three factor deficiencies that may prolong both PT and PTT are II, V, and X. Both PTT and PT may be prolonged due to **severe liver disease** and DIC as well. Mild vitamin K deficiency or **mild liver disease** generally affects the PT only. Generally, heparin affects PTT, and warfarin affects PT.

CASE 4

A 42-year-old gentleman presents to the ED with a gastrointestinal (GI) bleeding due to ibuprofen use; his Hb is 6.8 g/dL. He is hemodynamically unstable at this point. You remember that blood actually increases mortality if used incorrectly.

Table 6–1 BLOOD TRANSFUSION INDICATIONS

Indication	Transfuse to Maintain
Transfuse any symptomatic patient (e.g., tachycardia, hypotension, CHF, and angina)	Until no longer symptomatic
Asymptomatic, presurgical, stable patient	Hb 7–8g/dL
Hemodynamically stable postsurgical stable patient	Hb 8 g/dL
Postsurgical patient at risk for ischemic disease (e.g., cardiac and bowel)	Hb 10 g/dL
Hemodynamically stable, nonpregnant, ICU patients >16 years old without ongoing blood loss	Transfuse at 7 g/dL to maintain Hb at 7–9 g/dL
Elderly patients following MI	Transfuse to maintain Hct of >33%

What are the general indications for a transfusion?

A) Hemodynamic instability due to bleeding unresponsive to 2 L of saline.
B) Preoperative Hb of 7–8 gm/dL.
C) Elderly patient after a myocardial infarction (MI) with a hematocrit <33%.
D) Angina with a Hb of 8.5 gm/dL.
E) All of the above.

Discussion

The correct answer is "E." All of the above are indications for transfusion. Additional indications include postoperative Hb of less than 10 gm/dL in patients at risk for ischemic disease (ischemic bowel, CAD, etc.) and an Hb of <7 gm/dL in postoperative patients who are hemodynamically stable. **Transfusion for indications other than this are not beneficial and have been proven harmful.** See Table 6–1 for a list of transfusion indications.

* *

You decide to transfuse 2 units of packed red blood cells (PRBCs). After 30 minutes, the patient complains of dyspnea and back pain. Repeat examination of this patient reveals a diaphoretic man with a pulse of 130 and BP of 88/50. His lung fields are clear (initial vitals before the transfusion were a pulse of 110 and BP of 94/52.

What is your next step?

A) Stop the blood transfusion and begin normal saline through the IV.
B) Increase the rate of transfusion.
C) Administer acetaminophen 650 mg PO.
D) Administer furosemide 40 mg IV.
E) Place a nasogastric tube for lavage.

Discussion

The correct answer is "A." The transfusion must be stopped. The patient is exhibiting signs and symptoms of a hemolytic transfusion reaction, which is generally the result of an ABO incompatibility. Patients may exhibit nausea, flushing, dyspnea, oliguria, back pain, and hypotension. Other findings include markers of hemolysis: hemoglobinuria, elevated serum-free Hb, reduced haptoglobin, and elevated bilirubin. Patients are positive for direct antiglobulin (Coombs) test. Therapy includes IV saline at a high enough rate to initiate a brisk diuresis and prevent Hb from precipitating in the kidneys causing acute tubular necrosis.

> HELPFUL TIP: Additional transfusion reactions include anaphylaxis (especially in those with IgA deficiency), "febrile, non-hemolytic reactions" (which respond to meperidine and acetaminophen), acute pulmonary syndrome, which includes dyspnea and hypoxia.

> HELPFUL TIP: Why do we always order "2 units of packed red cells?" In a nonbleeding patient, the transfusion of one unit of PRBCs can be expected to raise the hematocrit by 3–4% (1 g/dL for Hb). If one unit should be sufficient, give one unit and reassess the patient. Every unit of blood has its own risk of mismatch, contagion, etc.

CASE 5

A 56-year-old male presents to the ED with an acute abdomen, likely from a perforated diverticulum. He is taking warfarin for a DVT that occurred after a total knee arthroplasty. He weighs 65 kg. You are evaluating him for surgery and find the following labs: Hb 14.3 g/dL, platelets 478,000/mm^3, INR 3.5, and PTT 28 seconds.

Which of the following statements about his preoperative management is correct?

A) Platelet transfusion perioperatively will produce the most immediate reduction in risk of bleeding from warfarin.
B) FFP transfusion will produce the most immediate reduction in risk of bleeding from warfarin.
C) Vitamin K administration orally will produce the most immediate reduction in risk of bleeding from warfarin.
D) Vitamin K administration subcutaneously will produce the most immediate reduction in risk of bleeding from warfarin.
E) Cryoprecipitate transfusion will produce the most immediate reduction in risk of bleeding from warfarin.

Discussion

The correct answer is "B." The patient above would benefit most immediately from the administration of FFP. FFP contains all the soluble plasma proteins found in whole blood, including the vitamin K-dependent factors that are depleted by warfarin. If more sustained reversal is desired, the simultaneous administration of vitamin K is effective. **The preferred route of administration of vitamin K is oral.** Giving vitamin K IV is second best—it is associated with a risk of anaphylaxis and lowers INR the same degree as oral vitamin K at 24 hours. Avoid vitamin K SQ or IM, which are less effective than PO and IV routes. The effects of FFP rarely last 24 hours; the effects of vitamin K are usually not apparent for 12–24 hours. The use of cryoprecipitate will not provide the appropriate factors depleted by warfarin. Cryoprecipitate contains vWF, factor VIII, factor XIII, and fibrinogen. Platelet transfusion would not benefit this patient since warfarin does not affect platelet function.

HELPFUL TIP: The INR of FFP is 1.5. No matter how hard you try, you cannot reduce the INR to less than 1.5 with FFP.

Objectives: Did you learn to . . .

- Decide when blood transfusion is appropriate?
- Recognize hemolytic transfusion reactions?
- Treat warfarin-induced hypocoagulability?

CASE 6

A 20-year-old female with acute myeloid leukemia completed her second cycle of consolidation chemotherapy 5 days ago. She presents to the ED complaining of fatigue and fever. She denies cough, dysuria, abdominal pain, sinus drainage, or redness around her Hickman catheter. Her physical exam reveals a temperature of 38.4°C, pulse 100, BP 120/58, and respirations 14. Her exam is otherwise unremarkable, including no redness or tenderness at the Hickman site. **Your magic crystal ball tells you she does not have a line infection.** Her labs reveal the following: WBC 200/mm^3, Hb 9 g/dL, hematocrit 27%, and platelet count 47,000/mm^3. Blood cultures have been drawn.

What is your next step, and what is your rationale?

A) Administer IV amphotericin B; a Candida urinary tract infection is most likely.
B) Administer IV cefepime; she requires empiric coverage for both gram-negative and gram-positive organisms.
C) Administer IV nafcillin; a gram-positive bacterial infection is most likely and broader antibiotic coverage will encourage growth of resistant bacteria.
D) Administer IV vancomycin; she most likely has an MRSA sinus infection.
E) Close observation; there is no evidence of infection and she looks well.

Discussion

The correct answer is "B." This patient has a neutropenic fever, which is a medical emergency. Prompt treatment with broad-spectrum antibiotics has drastically improved the survival of patients with neutropenic fever. Neutropenia is usually defined as neutrophils plus bands (absolute neutrophil count, ANC) $<500/\text{mm}^3$ or $<1000/\text{mm}^3$ when the nadir has not been reached. Most myelosuppressive chemotherapeutic agents produce a reduction in WBCs 4–10 days after completion and nadir at 10–14 days. Fever is defined as a single oral temperature >101°F (38.3°C) or a temperature >100.4°F (38°C) persisting for 1 hour or more. **This** patient does not need vancomycin since the absence of a line infection was stipulated in the history (via crystal ball that always works in our experience).

* *

Broad-spectrum coverage of gram-positive and gram-negative organisms, including pseudomonas, is the

Table 6–2 SUGGESTED ANTIBIOTIC REGIMENS FOR NEUTROPENIC FEVER

High-Risk Patients (ANC $\leq 100/\text{mm}^3$ or expected duration of neutropenia >7 days or significant comorbidity)	
Single Agents	**Combinations**
Cephalosporins • Cefepime • Ceftazidime (some concerns about emerging resistance) Carbapenem • Imipenem • Meropenem	Aminoglycoside + one of the following: • Cefepime • Antipseudomonal penicillin (ticarcillin, piperacillin) • Carbapenem • Extended spectrum quinolone (levofloxacin) if penicillin-allergic • Ceftazidime (some concerns about emerging resistance)
• Add vancomycin if a line infection is suspected, MRSA is likely, patient is clinically more ill (hypotension, etc.), or if no improvement after 3–5 days of empiric therapy. • Add metronidazole for suspected intra-abdominal infections. • Add antifungal (voriconazole, amphotericin B) if still febrile 4–7 days after starting antibiotics. The risk of fungal infection is increased by this point.	
Low-Risk Patients (anticipated neutropenia <7 days, able to take PO, hemodynamically stable, no comorbid conditions, able to comply with daily follow-up) • PO ciprofloxacin and amoxicillin-clavulanate OR • Hospital admission and any of the above regimens for high-risk patients	

Data from Infectious Diseases Society of America. (Freifeld AG et al. Clinical practice guideline for the use of antimicrobial agents in neutropenic patients with cancer: 2010 update by the Infectious Diseases Society of America. *Clin Infect Dis.* 2011;52(4):e56.)

cornerstone of therapy with specific therapy for any localizing symptoms or risk signs. See Table 6–2 for common antibiotic regimens.

> HELPFUL TIP: Patients with a neutropenic fever can have any infection seen in normal hosts, but you should also consider IV catheter infections, perirectal infections and abscesses, and necrotizing enteritis (aka "typhlitis"). Remember that they may not have an inflammatory reaction around a catheter site, abscess formation, infiltrate on chest x-ray, or WBCs in the urine because of the neutropenia. The absence of signs or symptoms should not dissuade the physician from starting empiric antibiotic therapy. Similarly, **the absence of fever in a neutropenic patient with focal infection should be approached as a high-risk situation**.

CASE 7

A 63-year-old male with a diagnosis of non-small-cell lung cancer, undergoing weekly chemotherapy and radiation to a left upper lobe mass, presents to your office. He complains of dull, nonradiating back pain in the lower thoracic/upper lumbar area. He denies trauma or any new activities. He has no associated weakness or paresthesias. He denies difficulties with bowel or bladder function.

What is you initial diagnostic and/or therapeutic approach to this patient?

A) MRI of thoracic and lumbar spine and NSAIDs.
B) Plain films of the thoracic and lumbar spine a COX-2 inhibitor with a 2-week follow-up.
C) Plain films of the thoracic spine and NSAIDs.
D) Prescription for physical therapy and NSAIDs.
E) Urinalysis with culture and antibiotics.

Discussion

The correct answer is "A." This is not your average back pain. Any patient with active malignancy complaining of back pain should be investigated for metastasis. While a plain film of the spine may be useful, the gold standard is MRI. The real emergency is spinal cord impingement. Spinal cord compression may occur from direct extension of metastatic disease from the vertebrae or extension from retroperitoneal or paravertebral disease. Frequently, the pain predates neurological symptoms, and because of the potential for severe, adverse outcomes, you want to catch the disease early to prevent chronic impairment.

* *

The patient undergoes MRI of the spine, which demonstrates a lesion compressing the cord at L1.

Which of the following is NOT an appropriate therapeutic modality?

A) Decompression surgery.
B) Dexamethasone 10 mg bolus IV, followed by 6 mg every 6 hours.
C) Observation with pain control (e.g., with morphine PCA).
D) Radiation therapy to the affected area.

Discussion

The correct answer is "C." Patients with spinal cord compression who have aggressive interventions are more likely to retain function, including ambulation and bowel and bladder control. Steroids will help reduce edema surrounding the tumor and hopefully will relieve pressure on the cord. Radiation can often provide symptomatic relief and reduce the likelihood that the tumor will spread locally to impinge on the cord. Surgical decompression is another option. Of course, if this patient opted for a palliative care approach and had decided upon hospice, "C" might be appropriate, but he is still getting active therapy, and his remaining time could be spent with less pain and better function if one of the other options were chosen.

CASE 8

A 32-year-old woman presents to your office with complaints of dyspnea, constipation, menorrhagia, and fatigue that are new over the last few weeks. She has a distant history of Hodgkin disease treated with chemotherapy and radiation to the chest. Her physical exam reveals a well-developed woman, who appears comfortable at rest with normal vital signs. She has no adenopathy and the remainder of her exam is unremarkable. Her CBC with WBC differential is normal.

Which of these diagnoses can be absolutely ruled out based on this patient's history?

A) Coronary ischemia.
B) Hypothyroidism.
C) Lung cancer.
D) Relapse of the Hodgkin disease.
E) None of the above.

Discussion

The correct answer is "E." The point here is that patients with a history of Hodgkin disease and chest radiation are at risk for a wide range of complications—even years after the disease has been successfully treated. Even though 80% of Hodgkin patients have long-term disease-free survival, one in six patients can be expected to die from late effects of therapy. Although CAD ("A") would be extremely unusual in a normal 32-year-old, a patient with a history of chest radiation has a relative risk of coronary disease of 5–10 times that of age-matched controls. "B," thyroid disease, is highly likely, with over 50% of patients treated with chest radiation requiring thyroid hormone replacement. A TSH would be adequate screening. There is a high risk for secondary malignancy, including breast cancer, lung cancer ("C"), leukemia, sarcoma, and non-Hodgkin lymphoma (NHL). Finally, you should always be concerned about recurrence ("D").

* *

The patient has a normal chest radiograph and ECG. However, her TSH is markedly elevated, and you start her on levothyroxine. You plan to see her back in 8 weeks for reevaluation and will provide additional counseling at that time.

Which of the following preventive health issues is/are necessary to address at follow-up?

A) Early intervention by a fertility specialist if the patient desires pregnancy.
B) Smoking cessation.
C) Yearly mammograms.
D) All of the above.
E) None of the above.

Discussion

The correct answer is "D." Female patients who were treated for Hodgkin disease with chemotherapy and radiation prior to age 20 have up to a 35% incidence of breast cancer by age 40. The typical latency period is 15 years. National guidelines recommend that annual mammography of Hodgkin survivors treated with chest irradiation should begin 5–8 years post-treatment, or age 40, which ever comes first. Smokers with a history of Hodgkin disease have a 20-fold increased chance of developing lung cancer when compared to nonsmokers with a history of Hodgkin disease. Also, female patients with Hodgkin disease have a 69% incidence of premature ovarian failure if treated for their cancer before age 29 and up to 96% if treated after age 30. While these statistics are improving with newer chemotherapy regimens, a patient should seek early referral to a fertility specialist if she desires pregnancy but is unable to conceive.

CASE 9

A 40-year-old male who has just received his **first course of chemotherapy** for Non-Hodgkin Lymphoma (NHL) presents to your ED complaining of weakness, cramps, and decreased urine output. He has no other medical problems and takes no medications except for prochlorperazine as needed for nausea. He has been eating and drinking well. His physical examination reveals a tired-appearing male, with normal vital signs. His head and neck exam reveals bilateral palpable cervical lymph nodes (2 cm). His lungs are clear in the upper lung fields with crackles bilaterally at the bases. Muscle strength is normal, and reflexes are 3+ and symmetric. He exhibits 6 beats of clonus at the ankles. Chest radiograph shows evidence of early pulmonary edema.

What is the most likely set of laboratory values you will find for this patient (reference ranges: potassium 3.5–5 mg/dL, phosphate 2.4–4.1 mg/dL, uric acid 3.5–7.2 mg/dL, calcium 8.5–10.2 mg/dL).

A) Potassium 2.3 mEq/L, phosphorus 3.1 mg/dL, uric acid 4 mg/dL, calcium 9 mg/dL.
B) Potassium 2.6 mEq/L, phosphorus 6 mg/dL, uric acid 5 mg/dL, calcium 12 mg/dL.
C) Potassium 6.5 mEq/L, phosphorus 7 mg/dL, uric acid 18 mg/dL, calcium 6 mg/dL.
D) Potassium 6 mEq/L, phosphorus 6.8 mg/dL, uric acid 5 mg/dL, calcium 6.7 mg/dL.
E) Potassium 4.5 mEq/L, phosphorus 3.2 mg/dL, uric acid 9 mg/dL, calcium 8 mg/dL.

Discussion

The correct answer is "C." This patient most likely has tumor lysis syndrome, which can occur in a patient with a highly responsive leukemia or a bulky lymphoma being treated with chemotherapy (it rarely occurs without treatment). Tumor lysis syndrome occurs when there is rapid release of intracellular contents into the bloodstream. It is characterized by high potassium, high phosphorus, high uric acid, and low calcium. Patients may experience renal failure, arrhythmias, fatigue, muscle cramps, and tetany.

* *

The patient is found to have a creatinine of 8 mg/dL.

What is the most likely cause of this patient's renal failure?

A) Dehydration.
B) Heart failure.
C) Hemoglobinuria.
D) Rhabdomyolysis related to chemotherapy.
E) Uric acid nephropathy.

Discussion

The correct answer is "E." Patients with tumor lysis syndrome have renal failure secondary to uric acid nephropathy. This is caused by the precipitation of uric acid in the kidney, and it can be prevented by the use of allopurinol prior to the administration of chemotherapy. Although dehydration ("A") is not the cause of renal failure, it certainly will exacerbate the situation.

Which of the following is MOST LIKELY to help this patient's current condition?

A) Allopurinol 300 mg orally.
B) Calcium carbonate 500 mg orally.
C) Emergent hemodialysis.
D) IV D5W with 2 amps bicarbonate.
E) IV normal saline 200 mL/hr.

Discussion

The correct answer is "C." The horses are already out of the barn, and in fact they're probably over the hills and through the woods. Allopurinol and oral calcium will not help this situation. The patient already has renal failure from his tumor lysis syndrome. While he may benefit from preventive measures, including aggressive hydration and allopurinol **prior to undergoing chemotherapy**, none of these measures are going to help his current renal failure. Additionally, the patient may develop worsening pulmonary edema if given too much volume with IV fluids.

* *

While awaiting hemodialysis, you should treat the patient's hyperkalemia. Treatment may include IV calcium gluconate, insulin and dextrose, and oral sodium polystyrene sulfonate (Kayexalate). Note that sodium bicarbonate for hyperkalemia has fallen out of favor.

> HELPFUL TIP: Rasburicase has also been approved for the prevention of tumor lysis syndrome. It converts uric acid into a nontoxic, excretable metabolite allantoin. It can also be used after tumor lysis syndrome has started. It has several black box warnings, including anaphylaxis, hemolysis, and methemoglobinemia. Its use is considered high risk in pregnancy.

Objectives: Did you learn to . . .

- Recognize and initiate treatment of some oncologic emergencies, including spinal cord compression, tumor lysis syndrome, and neutropenic fever?
- Recognize late complications of cancer and cancer therapy, including distant radiation and chemotherapy?

QUICK QUIZ: TOO MUCH OF A GOOD THING

A 60-year-old gentleman presents to your office with complaints of fatigue. He has a history of alcoholic cirrhosis, diet-controlled diabetes, and hypertension and currently takes hydrochlorothiazide, enalapril, and monthly testosterone injections. He smokes two packs of cigarettes daily and consumes 6–8 beers nightly. His physical exam reveals an obese, ruddy-faced man with a temperature of 37°C, pulse 90, BP 164/80, and respirations 14. He is found to have a hematocrit of 54%.

Which of the following items in his history is LEAST likely to explain the elevated hematocrit?

A) Alcoholic cirrhosis.
B) Diabetes.
C) Antihypertensive medications.
D) Testosterone injections.
E) Smoking.

Discussion

The correct answer is "B." Diabetes should not cause an elevated hematocrit and often causes anemia secondary to renal disease and reduced production of erythropoietin. Approach an elevated hematocrit with two questions: (1) Is it due to increased RBC mass or decreased plasma volume? (2) Is it primary erythrocytosis or secondary?

This patient has many potential secondary causes of an elevated hematocrit. "A," alcoholic cirrhosis can lead to hepatocellular carcinoma which, along with other malignancies, can result in overproduction of erythropoietin, causing an elevated hematocrit. Diuretics ("C") decrease plasma volume, causing an apparent elevation of hematocrit. Testosterone injections ("D") may cause polycythemia. Finally, he has a significant smoking history ("E") that may produce a secondary polycythemia due to hypoxia and cor pulmonale.

CASE 10

A 30-year-old female presents to your office for a routine visit. She was hospitalized for an appendectomy and at the time of surgery, her platelet count was found to be 1,400,000/mm^3, which her surgeon felt was most likely reactive. She has no other past medical history, is asymptomatic, and exercises three times per week. You repeat the CBC, showing WBC 5000/mm^3, Hb 13 g/dL, and platelet count 800,000/mm^3.

What is your next step in managing this patient?

A) Anticoagulation with warfarin to a goal INR 2–3.
B) Counseling against becoming pregnant.
C) Initiation of hydroxyurea 500 mg BID.
D) No further evaluation or follow-up necessary.
E) Observation and periodic evaluation of her CBC.

Discussion

The correct answer is "E." This patient likely has essential thrombocythemia (ET), which is the most common myeloproliferative disorder in the United States. ET is more common in females. Although patients are typically older when diagnosed, it is not uncommon in younger patients. Patients with ET have a higher rate of mortality than matched controls due to risk of thrombosis (arterial > venous) and bleeding events. In order to diagnose ET, other causes of thrombocytosis (e.g., inflammation, iron deficiency, recent surgery, infection, bleeding, and malignancy) must be excluded. A bone marrow biopsy may be helpful in establishing the diagnosis by demonstrating adequate iron stores and ruling out chronic myelogenous leukemia (CML) or myelodysplasia.

"A" is incorrect. Warfarin would not be appropriate prophylactic therapy and would not be used unless the patient had a thromboembolic event. "B" is incorrect. Although patients with ET have a high rate of spontaneous abortion, the patient can be counseled regarding this risk and aspirin can be considered if the patient has had a prior pregnancy loss. "C" is also incorrect. The patient is at low risk for thromboembolic events (platelet count <1.5 million/mm^3, young age, no comorbid illness or prior events). Hydroxyurea could be considered if the patient was at high risk or symptomatic.

HELPFUL TIP: The most common cause of an abnormally high platelet count is reactive thrombocytosis, which can result from iron deficiency, infection, inflammation, or malignancy. There is no increase in bleeding or clotting risk in patients with reactive thrombocytosis.

CASE 11

A 15-year-old female presents to your office complaining of fatigue. She reports menarche at age 13 and complains of heavy menses. Her physical examination reveals a well-developed, well-nourished, pale female. You find no hepatosplenomegaly. Her labs reveal a WBC of 6000/mm^3, Hb of 8.9 g/dL, hematocrit of 27%, platelet count 400,000/mm^3, MCV 72 fL, red blood cell distribution width (RDW) 16. You order more laboratory tests.

What are the expected findings in this patient?

A) Increased iron, decreased ferritin, increased total iron binding capacity.
B) Decreased iron, decreased ferritin, decreased total iron binding capacity.
C) Increased iron, increased ferritin, increased total iron binding capacity.
D) Decreased iron, increased ferritin, decreased total iron binding capacity.
E) Decreased iron, decreased ferritin, increased total iron binding capacity.

Discussion

The correct answer is "E." This patient likely has iron deficiency anemia related to her heavy menses. Iron-deficiency anemia is characterized by anemia along with a decreased serum iron, decreased ferritin, increased TIBC, and decreased transferrin saturation. The decrease in serum ferritin is proportional to the decrease in total body iron stores. Hypochromic microcytic RBCs are found on peripheral smear. See Table 6–3 for a general guide to the causes of anemia based on red cell indices.

HELPFUL TIP: The prevalence of von Willebrand disease in women with menorrhagia ranges from 5% to 20%. Always make sure to take a good personal and family bleeding history.

HELPFUL TIP: Even if it looks like iron deficiency anemia, always consider other causes of anemia such as B12 deficiency, folate deficiency, and thalassemia. Often patients will have more than one cause for their anemia.

Table 6–3 CAUSES OF ANEMIA BY RED CELL VOLUME

Low MCV (usually <80 fL)	Normal MCV (usually 80–100 fL)	High MCV (usually >100 fL)
Thalassemias	Acute blood loss	B12 deficiency
Iron-deficiency anemia	Early iron-deficiency	Folate deficiency
Sideroblastic anemias	Endocrine (e.g., hypothyroidism)	Alcohol effects
Anemia of chronic disease	Anemia of chronic disease	Hypothyroidism
Lead poisoning	Chronic renal insufficiency	Primary bone marrow disease
	Primary bone marrow disorders	Drug effect
		Liver disease
		Hemolytic anemia

* *

You start iron supplementation therapy in this patient.

Which of the following tests will be the first to indicate that you have instituted appropriate therapy and that the patient is responding?

A) Increase in hematocrit.
B) Increase in reticulocyte count.
C) Increase in serum-free Hb.
D) Decrease in ferritin.
E) Decrease in transferrin saturation.

Discussion

The correct answer is "B." The patient's reticulocyte count will increase first—before the hematocrit ("A"). This should start soon after treatment and maximize at 7–10 days. Pica (if present) should also resolve fairly early. "C" is incorrect. Only in exceptional circumstances (intravascular hemolysis) will there be free Hb in the blood. "D" is incorrect because the ferritin is low in iron deficiency anemia and should increase with therapy. Finally, transferrin saturation ("E") should increase in patients once you start to treat their anemia, but the reticulocyte count increases first.

HELPFUL TIP: Ferritin is not a useful test for iron deficiency in hospitalized patients or in those who are chronically ill. Ferritin is an acute-phase reactant and thus may be elevated in these patients even when the patient has iron-deficiency anemia (where the ferritin should be low).

HELPFUL TIP: There may be no reticulocytosis with treatment of iron deficiency if the patient is simply iron deficient without anemia.

How long should you continue iron supplementation once the patient's labs have normalized?

A) Stop immediately once anemia has resolved.
B) Continue 3–6 months after the anemia has resolved.
C) Continue for 1 year after the anemia has resolved.
D) Indefinite iron supplementation is indicated.

Discussion

The correct answer is "B." Continue iron for 3–6 months once the anemia has resolved. Also address the underlying problem, in this patient her heavy periods, which may respond to hormonal contraception or NSAIDS.

* *

The patient returns in 2 months but her labs, if anything, are worse than at first presentation. The patient swears that she has been taking the iron faithfully.

Which of the following can lead to a failure of iron therapy for iron deficiency anemia?

A) Proton pump inhibitors (PPIs).
B) Incorrect diagnosis.
C) Oral antacids (e.g., calcium carbonate).
D) Atrophic gastritis, celiac disease, or *Helicobacter pylori* infection.
E) All of the above.

Discussion

The correct answer is "E." Anything that neutralizes the stomach pH will interfere with absorption including PPIs, antacids, and loss of acid producing cells (e.g., pernicious anemia). Other GI diseases (celiac disease, *H. pylori*) can also interfere with iron absorption. Tea and some green leafy vegetables can also reduce iron absorption.

HELPFUL TIP: Vitamin C (supplements or orange juice) enhances iron absorption and should be considered if a patient is not responding to iron therapy. Meat can also increase iron absorption (which we hate to say because one of us is a vegetarian... however, the truth hurts).

HELPFUL TIP: A widened RDW and an elevated platelet count are typical of iron deficiency anemia. Conversely, the RDW will be normal in thalassemias.

* *

The patient returns to your office and finally admits she has not been able to take the iron because of side effects. Her Hb is now down to 7.2 gm/dL. She still feels fatigued. The patient will not agree to take any further iron orally. However, she is willing to consider other suggestions.

What is your next step?

A) Encourage the patient to take the iron preparation along with calcium carbonate (Tums) to reduce the GI side effects.
B) Continue her prenatal vitamin only and encourage her to eat more red meat.
C) Give iron sucrose 200 mg IV weekly for 4 weeks.
D) Transfuse 2 units of PRBCs immediately.

Discussion

The correct answer is "C." If oral iron preparations are not tolerated, IV iron preparations are available. Intramuscular preparations are best avoided due to pain at the injection site, skin discoloration, and risk for infection. Options for IV replacement include iron dextran and iron sucrose. Iron dextran carries a risk of anaphylaxis in 0.6–2.3% of patients and other side effects in up to 25% of patients, including bronchospasm, flushing, headache, fever, urticaria, nausea, vomiting, hypotension, seizures, myalgia, arthralgia, and increased thromboembolic events. Iron sucrose has a lower incidence of side effects—typically nausea, constipation, diarrhea, or a transient minty taste—and may be given to patients who have had a previous reaction to iron dextran. "A" is incorrect because calcium will interfere with iron absorption. Not only that but also she has already said she would not take additional oral iron. "B" is incorrect because she needs more iron than can be provided through prenatal vitamins and her diet. Finally, "D" is incorrect as transfusion carries potential risks that could be avoided if she responds to IV iron replacement.

HELPFUL TIP: Any adult patient with microcytic anemia should be evaluated further to clarify the etiology. In adults, GI blood loss is a common cause of microcytic anemia. Colitis, malignancy, or malabsorption from inflammatory disease should be considered in the differential diagnosis. Tailor your workup to the patient's symptoms. If he has symptoms referable to the upper GI tract (e.g., dyspepsia), consider an upper GI endoscopy in addition to colonoscopy.

CASE 12

A 52-year-old woman with a history of rheumatoid arthritis is in your clinic for a 1-month follow-up after having a knee prosthesis removed secondary to a joint infection and osteomyelitis (*Staphlococcal aureus*). You obtain a CBC, revealing a WBC 8000/mm^3, Hb 9.5 g/dL, hematocrit 28%, platelet count 450,000/mm^3, and MCV 83 fL. Serum iron levels are low; serum transferrin receptor is normal, while ferritin is increased.

What is the most likely diagnosis?

A) Iron deficiency anemia due to rheumatoid arthritis.
B) Anemia of chronic disease due to rheumatoid arthritis and osteomyelitis.
C) Hemolytic anemia induced by antibiotics.
D) Acute blood loss during surgery.
E) Myelodysplastic syndrome (MDS) associated with rheumatoid arthritis.

Discussion

The correct answer is "B." Anemia of chronic disease (previously known as anemia of inflammation) is a hypoproliferative anemia that occurs in the setting of chronic infection, inflammation, malignancy, heart failure, diabetes, and other serious health conditions. The anemia is usually mild and characterized by low serum iron, increased ferritin (remember that ferritin is an acute-phase reactant and these patients often have inflammation), decreased serum transferrin, normal (or low) serum soluble transferrin receptor level, and decreased transferrin saturation (see below for more on the soluble transferrin receptor). In addition, the reticulocyte count is typically low, the erythropoietin may be mildly elevated, and the peripheral smear may show hypochromic, microcytic RBCs or normochromic, normocytic RBCs. If differentiation between iron deficiency anemia and anemia of chronic disease is not apparent, a bone marrow biopsy can be obtained to assess iron stores.

HELPFUL TIP: What is that transferrin receptor anyhow? The transferrin receptor can help to differentiate between iron deficiency anemia and anemia of chronic disease. The serum transferrin receptor level is inversely correlated to iron storage levels. **When the iron is low, the soluble transferrin receptor level is high. Thus, high serum transferrin receptor levels are associated with iron deficiency but not with anemia of chronic disease in which iron**

stores are adequate. One caveat: the serum transferrin receptor level will also be elevated in states in which there is rapid cell turnover (hemolytic anemia, for example). However, it should not be checked in this situation so you shouldn't get confused.

CASE 13

A previously healthy 3-year-old female with a history of anorexia and irritability for 3 days is brought to your ED by her mother. On the day of admission, the child is difficult to arouse. You learn that her 6-year-old brother has had some difficulty reaching appropriate developmental milestones, and is a "fussy eater."

Physical examination reveals a slightly pale-appearing child, who responds to tactile stimuli but not to voice. Vitals are normal and her exam is unremarkable except for her decreased level of consciousness. Laboratories include a WBC 8000/mm^3, Hb 10 g/dL, platelets 300,000/mm^3, and MCV 75 fL (microcytic). Her urine dipstick is normal, except for 1 + glucose; there are no ketones in the urine. Her blood chemistries are within normal limits, with the exception of a phosphorous of 2.0 mg/dL. Her peripheral blood smear shows red cells with coarse basophilic stippling.

What is the best working diagnosis at this time?

A) Acute lead poisoning.
B) Anemia of chronic disease.
C) Early diabetic ketoacidosis (DKA).
D) Severe iron deficiency anemia.
E) Unrecognized bacteremia secondary to pyelonephritis.

Discussion

The correct answer is "A." Lead poisoning should be considered in a child presenting with symptoms of encephalopathy and anemia with basophilic stippling on RBCs. Basophilic stippling occurs when ribosome precipitates litter the RBCs and can be seen in alcohol abuse, thalassemias, and heavy metal poisoning. "B," anemia of chronic disease, is unlikely because this illness is acute. "C," DKA, is unlikely because urine ketones are 99% sensitive for DKA. "D" is unlikely because there should be no neurologic symptoms associated with iron-deficiency anemia. "E," pyelonephritis, is unlikely because the patient is afebrile and has a normal white count and negative urine.

HELPFUL TIP: Lead levels >10 μg/dL may cause developmental delay, loss of milestones (especially language), encephalopathy, seizures, cerebral edema, and cognitive impairment. CNS effects are especially problematic in children <6 years old who have an incomplete blood–brain barrier. Lead paint in houses built before the 1970s and use of imported products such as pottery, solder, cosmetics, and crayons (and some toys made in China) still provide sources of lead ingestion.

HELPFUL TIP: **Other symptoms of lead intoxication** include anorexia, decreased activity, irritability, insomnia, hearing loss, peripheral neuropathy, SIADH, decreased renal function, and anemia. **Laboratory findings may include** anemia, signs of hemolysis, coarse basophilic stippling on RBCs, glycosuria, hypophosphatemia, positive qualitative urine coproporphyrin, and moderate increases in free erythrocyte protoporphyrin.

* *

The patient's lead level is 70 μg/dL. Because of your concern about acute lead intoxication and resulting encephalopathy, you decide to admit the child and treat her with dimercaprol.

All of the following are true EXCEPT:

A) Dimercaprol should not be given if the child has a peanut allergy.
B) The child's diet should be monitored for adequate intake of calories, iron, and calcium.
C) The child's sibling should be tested, and arrangements should be made for close follow-up for both children.
D) The dose of dimercaprol should be tripled for patients with glucose-6-phosphate dehydrogenase (G6PD) deficiency.

Discussion

The correct answer is "D." Dimercaprol is a lead chelator used to treat elevated lead levels. It is administered intramuscularly, is water-insoluble, and must be given in a peanut oil vehicle. **It may cause hemolysis in individuals with G6PD deficiency**, so these patients should be monitored closely and not receive larger doses of dimercaprol. It is important to test siblings of an affected child, because the source of lead is often in the house. Close follow-up of affected children is essential to monitor for increasing blood lead levels after treatment, which may indicate the source of lead has not been removed. The absorption of lead can be made worse by malnutrition, iron deficiency, and poor intake of calcium. Iron deficiency frequently occurs in affected patients and may worsen anemia.

> HELPFUL TIP: A large percentage of lead is absorbed into bone with a half-life of greater than 25 years. In periods of physiologic stress, the inert pool of lead can be mobilized and released into the bloodstream, producing signs and symptoms of lead intoxication years after the initial exposure.

CASE 14

A 6-month-old male infant is brought to you for a well-baby checkup. His mother reports that the child has had difficulty with feeding, has frequent colds, and is often irritable. She has noted recurrent episodes of jaundice, especially when he is sick. His physical exam reveals a small child, faintly jaundiced. His temperature is 37.5°C, pulse 160, BP 85/50, and respirations 30. His abdomen is soft with palpable splenomegaly. The remainder of the exam is unremarkable. Laboratories reveal a WBC of 13,000/mm^3, Hb 9 g/dL, platelets 260,000/mm^3, and MCV 60 fL. He is noted to have target cells on peripheral blood smear.

Which one of the following is the most appropriate next step?

A) Order PT/PTT.
B) Order Hb electrophoresis.
C) Transfuse with 1 unit of PRBCs.
D) Test for G6PD deficiency.
E) Test for sickle-cell anemia.

Discussion

The correct answer is "B." The clinical and laboratory presentation is consistent with a hereditary hemoglobinopathy, most likely a thalassemia. The splenomegaly, significant anemia, target cells, and the profoundly low MCV are all suggestive of thalassemia. He has no history of abnormal bleeding, so "A" would not be indicated. Also, as the child does not appear to be in distress, "C" would be an incorrect answer. G6PD-deficient patients experience episodes of hemolytic anemia. Peripheral smear review at that time may reveal bite or blister cells, rather than target cells, so "D" is not the right answer. "E" is incorrect since the peripheral smear would reveal sickle cells if the patient had sickle disease.

* *

Beta thalassemia major is confirmed by Hb electrophoresis.

Which of the following regarding his management is NOT true?

A) Untreated, mortality may approach 80% by 5 years of age.
B) Frequent blood transfusions may be required.
C) The condition will improve with age.
D) The child is likely to have growth retardation and delayed sexual maturation.
E) Without iron chelation therapy, there is a high incidence of mortality with this disease.

Discussion

The correct answer is "C." Beta thalassemia refers to the disease state in which there are mutations in both genes that code for beta globin. Without treatment, mortality from thalassemia major approaches 80% by 5 years of age. Judicious use of transfusions and concurrent chelation therapy with deferoxamine has reduced long-term complications related to the disease. Deferasirox (Exjade), an oral chelating agent, is available. Bone marrow transplant can be curative. Beta thalassemia minor (or beta trait) is much less severe and occurs when only one of the genes is defective.

> HELPFUL TIP: The FDA recently approved deferiprone as an alternative chelating agent in transfusion-acquired iron overload. It is second line but can be administered orally.

> HELPFUL TIP: Alpha thalassemia has a more variable course. There are 4 alpha globin genes. If all 4 genes are defective, intrauterine fetal demise is the rule. When 1 gene is

defective, there is a silent carrier state. When 2 genes are defective, there is a mild microcytic anemia. Here's a memory aid: there are 4 alpha globin genes and "4" looks kind of like the "A" in "Alpha"; beta is the second letter in the Greek alphabet and beta globin has 2 genes.

HELPFUL TIP: Because of the persistence of fetal hemoglobin (HbF) up to 6 months of age, hemoglobinopathies might not be apparent until that time.

HELPFUL TIP: Thalassemias may be erroneously diagnosed as iron deficiency anemia due to a low MCV. Consider testing for thalassemia in a patient with microcytic anemia, normal or increased iron levels, a normal RDW (less reliable), and appropriate ethnic background (e.g., Mediterranean or African descent).

HELPFUL TIP: In other Hb synthesis related news . . . when you see that middle-aged female with abdominal pain and psychiatric symptoms for the tenth (or twentieth or thirtieth) time, think of acute intermittent porphyria before you make the diagnosis of somatization disorder.

CASE 15

A woman brings her 10-week-old infant for evaluation. The child is colicky and irritable after feeding. She was born full term but has not been gaining weight appropriately. The patient's sister has sickle-cell trait, so you obtain a Hb electrophoresis, which ultimately demonstrates SS genotype.

Which of the following is INCORRECT regarding the child's care?

A) The patient should remain on prophylactic antibiotics until the age of 5 years due to a high risk of pneumococcal sepsis.
B) The child may develop splenomegaly and lymphadenopathy related to her disease.
C) The disease provides protection against infection with parvovirus.
D) The child may not develop pain crisis until she is older due to protection from HbF.
E) The child is likely to have a delay in puberty.

Discussion

The correct answer is "C." The patient has homozygous SS sickle-cell disease. This child's mother should be counseled regarding the importance of continuing antibiotic prophylaxis until the age of 5 years because her child is at high risk for pneumococcal sepsis. Sickle-cell disease is protective against malaria, not parvovirus ("C"). In fact, the development of a parvovirus infection can be life threatening due the development of aplastic anemia.

During infancy, children may be noted to have reticulocytosis, hemolytic anemia, and sickling by 10–12 weeks. At 5–6 months, splenomegaly may be noted, and lymphadenopathy may be prominent between 6 months and 5 years. The earliest pain crisis often involves hands and feet (dactylitis), and occurs after the HbF decreases to adult values. This usually does not occur until after age 4. The spleen involutes by 5–8 years. Puberty is delayed by an average of 2.5 years.

HELPFUL TIP: Sickle trait, the condition in which a patient is heterozygous for Hb S, is associated with a normal life expectancy and no symptoms other than occasional hematuria and inability to concentrate urine. Pain crises are extremely rare, and occur only in the settings of low-oxygen atmosphere (e.g., very high altitude) or extreme physical activity (e.g., running a marathon).

* *

The child follows regularly with you for years, and she begins to develop more frequent pain crises in college. She is found to have an elevated C-reactive protein, increased LDH, and decreasing Hb. You explain to her that some measures can be taken to reduce the frequency of pain crises.

These measures include all of the following EXCEPT:

A) Initiation of hydroxyurea therapy.
B) Avoidance of hot showers.
C) Prompt treatment of infections.
D) Adequate hydration and nutrition.
E) Avoidance of emotional stress.

Discussion

The correct answer is "B." Two main features of sickle-cell disease are shortened RBC survival and vaso-occlusion due to poorly deformable RBC membranes. Pain episodes occur due to acute episodes of tissue hypoxemia and microinfarction. Crises can be precipitated by stress, fatigue, cold weather (not hot showers, which cause problems in multiple sclerosis patients), infection, dehydration, acidosis, and poor nutrition. The use of hydroxyurea promotes increased levels of HbF, and HbF is associated with decreased frequency and severity of pain crises.

HELPFUL TIP: Acute chest syndrome (ACS) should be suspected when a sickle-cell patient presents with fever, cough, chest pain, and pulmonary infiltrates on chest x-ray. ACS may be due to infection or pulmonary infarction. Treatment involves aggressive pain management, antibiotics for respiratory pathogens, supplemental oxygen, cautious hydration, and blood transfusion if the patient is significantly anemic. Exchange transfusion may also be required in more severe cases.

Since you first met that little baby girl, 22 years have elapsed, and she is getting married—and you are getting old (the alternative is worse, of course). She is concerned about significant illness related to her disease. You counsel her regarding the most common causes of morbidity and mortality.

All of the following statements are true EXCEPT:

A) ACS and pain crises are the most common causes for hospital admission for patients with sickle-cell disease.
B) Eighty percent of patients develop cholelithiasis by age 35.
C) Strokes may occur in 8% of patients by age 14, may be either symptomatic or clinically silent, and tend to be recurrent.
D) Heart failure, pulmonary fibrosis, pulmonary hypertension, and renal failure complicate fluid management, transfusions, and maintenance of adequate oxygenation.
E) Pregnancy should be avoided under any circumstance.

Discussion

The correct answer is "E." The average life expectancy in patients with Hb SS is 42 years for men and 48 years for women. Maternal mortality occurs in about 1% of pregnancies. All of the rest are true including cerebrovascular events causing seizures and possible cognitive difficulty early in life. Of particular note, renal failure may be the cause of death in up to 10% of cases. Avascular necrosis and osteomyelitis (classically as a result of *Salmonella* infection), chronic skin ulcers, and priapism are also common.

Objectives: Did you learn to . . .

- Recognize the presentation and implication of essential thrombocytosis?
- Evaluate a patient with an elevated Hb or platelet count?
- Obtain a thorough history in an anemic patient?
- Use laboratory parameters to identify the etiology of anemia?
- Initiate treatment of various causes of anemia?
- Identify certain anemias, especially iron deficiency, thalassemias, and sickle-cell disease, based on clinical and laboratory manifestations?

QUICK QUIZ: THE CURIOUS CASE OF THE MISSING VITAMIN

A 72-year-old gentleman is brought to your office because a home health nurse noted he was becoming progressively weaker and more fatigued. He has a history of celiac disease for which he follows a strict gluten-free diet, but he has not been eating well. He also has a history of a seizure disorder and takes phenytoin. His review of systems is positive for dyspnea on exertion and mild anorexia. He has no other symptoms.

Physical exam reveals a thin, pale-appearing man with normal vital signs. His conjunctivae are pale and his tongue is smooth, with moist mucosa and no oropharyngeal lesions. The remainder of the exam is unremarkable. A CBC reveals a WBC of 4500/mm^3, Hb 9 g/dL, hematocrit 28%, platelet count 140,000/mm^3, MCV 102 fL, RDW 14, and B12 level 900 ng/L (normal).

Which of the following statements is most likely FALSE?

A) The patient may have a high homocysteine level.
B) The patient's condition could be made better with a trial of folate replacement.
C) The patient may have a low RBC folate level.
D) The patient's condition will likely require chronic blood transfusions.
E) The patient may have a normal **serum** folate level.

Discussion

The correct answer is "D." This patient likely has folate deficiency, given a normal B12, macrocytic anemia, and risk factors for folate deficiency—old age, poor diet, avoidance of gluten (flour is normally fortified with folate), use of phenytoin, and possible malabsorption due to GI disease (celiac disease in this case, but also any other infiltrating or inflammatory process of the bowel). Dietary deficiency is uncommon in the United States due to supplementation of grain products with folate. Foods naturally high in folate include melons, bananas, leaf vegetables, asparagus, and broccoli. The recommended intake is 400 μg/day, and the body stores approximately a 4-month supply. If he has had recent adequate folate intake, the serum folate level may be normal, but the RBC folate will still be low, reflecting the deficiency (think of it as the HbA1C of folate).

To differentiate folate from B-12 deficiency, check serum homocysteine and methylmalonate levels. Both will be elevated with B-12 deficiency, while only homocysteine will be elevated in folate deficiency. Remember, you must exclude B12 deficiency before replacing folate, because folate replacement can reverse the anemia but will permit progression of neurologic effects of B12 deficiency, so "B" is true.

HELPFUL TIP: Folate replacement is dosed as 1–5 mg daily. If macrocytic anemia persists, other causes must be considered.

QUICK QUIZ: REMEMBER THAT TAPEWORM FROM MEDICAL SCHOOL? HERE IT IS AGAIN

A 47-year-old woman presents to your office complaining of tongue soreness, fatigue, and dyspnea with exertion. She denies unusual bleeding, weight loss, fevers, and night sweats. Her past medical history includes hypothyroidism, for which she takes levothyroxine, and she does not drink alcohol or smoke. Physical exam reveals a tired-appearing woman with lemon-yellow-colored skin, temperature 37°C, pulse 110, BP 120/74, and respirations 12. The exam is otherwise unremarkable. A CBC demonstrates a WBC count 4000/mm^3, Hb 9 g/dL, platelet count 140,000/mm^3, and a MCV of 105 fL. Her B12 level is 100 pg/mL (normal >300 pg/mL) and folate 40 ng/mL.

Which of the following historical elements is LEAST likely to contribute to her condition?

A) History of working as a park ranger in Canada.
B) History of Zollinger–Ellison syndrome.
C) History of hypothyroidism.
D) History of new vegetarian diet started last month.
E) History of GI surgery.

Discussion

The correct answer is "D." Most likely, this woman has pernicious anemia caused by B12 deficiency. Pernicious anemia is caused by immune destruction of parietal cells in the stomach, resulting in decreased absorption of B12. It typically develops in people over the age of 40 and is more common in people of northern European descent or in African Americans, as well as people with type A blood. Laboratory findings include antiparietal cell antibodies in 90% of affected patients (5% of normal individuals) and antibodies to intrinsic factor in 70% of patients. Individuals commonly have other autoimmune diseases such as thyroid disease, diabetes, and vitiligo. Individuals may complain of paresthesias, GI symptoms, sore tongue, or weight loss. The lemon-yellow appearance of the skin is due to anemia and mild jaundice.

Other causes of cobalamin (B12) deficiency include gastrectomy, Zollinger–Ellison syndrome (inability to alkalinize the small intestine), blind loop syndrome, bacterial overgrowth from previous surgery, and ingestion of undercooked fish infested with the tapeworm *Diphyllobothrium latum* (found in

Canada, Alaska, and the Baltics—hence, the history of working as a park ranger). Although a strict vegetarian diet can cause B12 deficiency, there are sufficient stores to last 3–5 years (in other words, more than 1 month).

QUICK QUIZ: SAY, DID HE SWALLOW A PENNY?

A 21-year-old college student is brought to the ED by his friends because of bizarre behavior. His friends state that he has been acting "a little odd" lately, but they are unaware of any drug abuse. He does drink alcohol but is not known as a binge drinker—at least not by modern NCAA Division I Drinking standards. His friends do not know his medical history but state he was taking a prescription drug for a "metabolic disorder," which he stopped several months ago. He is uncooperative, paranoid, and disoriented. You note brownish pigmentation of his corneas on physical exam. This may be the first case of Wilson disease you have ever seen.

Regarding this patient, which of the following is INCORRECT?

A) The patient has likely had episodes of hemolytic anemia in the past.
B) The patient has likely discontinued penicillamine.
C) The patient likely has an elevated ceruloplasmin level on blood test.
D) The patient likely has hepatolenticular degeneration.
E) The patient is at risk for hepatic failure.

Discussion

The correct answer is "C." This patient likely has Wilson disease (an autosomal-recessive defect in cellular copper export), which presents with **decreased** levels of ceruloplasmin, increased liver enzymes, and signs of hemolysis (from the direct toxic effect of copper on the cell). Symptoms typically present in the teens and early twenties. Presenting symptoms may include Kayser–Fleisher rings (golden-brown pigmentation of the cornea), hemolytic anemia, or neurologic symptoms, often mimicking psychiatric illness. Treatment of the disease includes lifelong therapy with penicillamine or trientine (chelating agents), and should be considered even for asymptomatic individuals known to have the disease.

QUICK QUIZ: "HOLE-Y BONES"

A 50-year-old man presents to your office with low back pain of 8 weeks duration. He denies any history of trauma or overexertion. He notes the pain is constant and does not improve with positioning. Also, he has noticed some fatigue. He has no other complaints.

Physical exam reveals a well-nourished male with normal vital signs. His neurologic exam is normal. On musculoskeletal exam, he has midline point tenderness over T12. Plain films reveal a compression fracture at T12. A serum total protein level is 9 mg/dL (elevated), but the remainder of an evaluation for endocrine causes of osteoporosis is normal.

All of the following are necessary for the diagnosis of this patient EXCEPT:

A) Bone scan.
B) Serum and urine protein electrophoresis with immunofixation.
C) Bone marrow aspirate and biopsy.
D) Quantitative immunoglobulins.
E) Skeletal survey.

Discussion

The correct answer is "A." A spontaneous vertebral fracture in a 50-year-old male is definitely not normal. Multiple myeloma should be considered in patients with this presentation.

Multiple myeloma is a clonal disorder of plasma cells. Risk factors include African American race, male sex, and advancing age (median age of 60–65 at presentation). Workup for the diagnosis of multiple myeloma requires a serum and urine protein electrophoresis with immunofixation ("B"). This will help to identify a monoclonal protein. Quantitative immunoglobulins ("D") will help to assess whether this patient has an elevation of immunoglobulins in the range required for the diagnosis of multiple myeloma. A skeletal survey ("E") and bone marrow biopsy ("C") complete the diagnostic workup. A bone scan is not useful because the lytic lesions characteristic of multiple myeloma do not take up radioisotope.

CASE 16

On a routine insurance physical exam, a 55-year-old man was found to have a total protein of 9 g/dL. The remainder of his serum chemistries and his CBC were normal. He is active, feels well, and is not taking any medications. His physical examination is unremarkable. You order a serum and urine electrophoresis with immunofixation and quantitative immunoglobulins. He has a monoclonal spike with 1400 g/dL of IgG kappa. His other immunoglobulins are within normal limits. A skeletal survey demonstrates no lytic lesions, and his bone marrow aspirate and biopsy demonstrate 6% plasma cells (normal is 1–4%). After the bone marrow biopsy, the hematologist sends him back to you for follow-up.

What is your next step in the management of this patient?

A) Monitor blood, including serum immunoglobulins, every 3–6 months and, if stable after 1 year, annually thereafter.
B) Monitor blood, including serum immunoglobulins, every 4 weeks indefinitely.
C) Start on chemotherapy for multiple myeloma.
D) Obtain yearly bone marrow biopsy and skeletal survey.
E) No follow-up is necessary.

Discussion

The correct answer is "A." This patient has monoclonal gammopathy of undetermined significance, or MGUS, which is found in up to 3% of asymptomatic older individuals. A bone marrow biopsy indicating 10% plasma cells is required to make the diagnosis of multiple myeloma; this patient only has 6%. Additionally, this patient has a normal CBC and is asymptomatic (no fatigue, bone pain suggestive of lesions, etc.). Thus, this patient has MGUS. Patients with MGUS typically do well, with only 1% per year progressing to multiple myeloma.

While patients should be reassured of the typically benign nature of this condition, up to 30% will have complications (multiple myeloma, amyloidosis, other myeloproliferative disorders). After several unchanged immunoglobulin levels and normal CBCs, yearly evaluation should be adequate. Any changes in the patient's condition, such as unexplained anemia, increased immunoglobulin levels, renal insufficiency, or bony pain, should prompt further evaluation. An increase in immunoglobulin does not necessarily mean the monoclonal protein is increasing, and a serum protein electrophoresis and immunofixation should be obtained. Repeat bone marrow biopsy is indicated only if the clinical picture is confusing.

CASE 17

A 63-year-old woman presents to your office with complaint of fatigue. She states she felt like she spent the winter taking antibiotics because she developed "one infection after the other." Prior to this past winter, she had been well and did not take any prescription drugs regularly. Physical examination demonstrates a slightly pale, thin woman. Her temperature is 37.5°C, pulse 90, BP 120/58, and respirations 12. Her oropharynx demonstrates purpuric lesions. Her abdominal exam shows no organomegaly, and the remainder of the physical exam is unremarkable.

You obtain blood tests: WBC 2100/mm^3, Hb 8.4 g/dL, and platelet count 20,000/mm^3. A bone marrow aspirate and biopsy are obtained, which demonstrate a hypercellular marrow with 4% blasts, 4% ringed sideroblasts, and megakaryocytes. You talk to the hematologist, who suspects that your patient has a myelodysplastic syndrome (MDS).

Which of the following statements is INCORRECT?

A) The small number of blasts in the bone marrow indicates a better prognosis.
B) The patient cannot have MDS because she has pancytopenia.
C) The patient may benefit from administration of erythropoietin.
D) The patient may develop acute myeloid leukemia.
E) The patient's gender may result in a better prognosis.

Discussion

The correct answer is "B." Patients with MDS can be pancytopenic. MDS includes a number of clonal stem cell disorders characterized by dysplasia and ineffective hematopoiesis of one or more cell lines. The disease is typically one of older adults, with a median age of 65–70 years at onset; however, a better prognosis is associated with age <60 and female gender. There is an increased risk of MDS in smokers, those exposed to benzene or alkylating agents, and with some hereditary disorders. Prognosis depends on the number of blasts, the number of lineages affected, and cytogenetic abnormalities. Median survival ranges from 10 to 66 months, and progression to acute leukemia ranges from 6% to 33% of patients, depending on the subtype of MDS.

Depending on the age and overall performance status of the individual MDS patient, treatment can range from supportive care with blood or platelet transfusions, to treatment with granulocyte colony stimulating factor (GCSF), to chemotherapeutics such as azacytidine, or even to bone marrow transplantation.

Objectives: Did you learn to . . .

- Identify pancytopenia as a presentation of MDS?
- Recognize the presentation of multiple myeloma?
- Identify MGUS?

QUICK QUIZ: IT'S JUST KIDS' STUFF

All of the following are accurate statements about neutrophil counts in children EXCEPT:

A) African American children may have a normal ANC of $1000/mm^3$.
B) Children over the age of 6 should be expected to have a normal ANC of $1500–8000/mm^3$.
C) Neonates typically have a normal ANC of $<500/mm^3$ at birth.
D) Infants typically have 20–30% neutrophils on WBC differential.
E) Five-year-old children have 50% neutrophils on WBC differential.

Discussion

The correct answer is "C." In the pediatric population, neutropenia is typically described as an ANC of $<1500/mm^3$. Up to 30% of African American children have an asymptomatic ANC of $<1000/mm^3$ (e.g., no increased risk of infection). At birth, neutrophils make up the majority of the WBC differential, and this decreases to 20–30% after the first few days of life. At 5 years of age, neutrophils comprise approximately 50% of the differential, and this reaches 70% by puberty.

CASE 18

A 49-year-old male presents to your office complaining of joint pain, fatigue, and increased urination. There is a family history of cirrhosis of the liver, apparently not related to alcohol. He does not take any medications and does not smoke but drinks two glasses of wine each night. Physical examination reveals a thin male with tanned skin (in the dead of winter in Iowa, so he is either rich or sick, take your choice) and normal vital signs. His heart and lung exams are unremarkable. The abdomen is soft, nontender, and nondistended, and his liver edge is palpable 2 cm below the costal margin. He has pain with range of motion in his hips, knees, and MTP joints. The remainder of the exam is unrevealing. Serum electrolytes are normal, but his glucose is 282 g/dL. His transaminases are elevated.

Of the following, what is the most likely diagnosis?

A) Alcoholic hepatitis.
B) Colon cancer.
C) Hemochromatosis.
D) Vitamin B12 deficiency.

Discussion

The correct answer is "C." This patient presents with a "classic" history of hemochromatosis. Symptoms start during or after the fifth decade of life, are initially mild, and progress slowly. "Bronze diabetes" (bronze or tan skin color due to iron deposition accompanied by hyperglycemia) is sometimes noted. Most organs can eventually be involved, but most commonly symptoms are due to liver, cardiac, joint, and testicular involvement.

* *

"A," alcoholic hepatitis, is a consideration, but his reported use is unlikely to result in disease. You also would not expect to see some of the other symptoms (e.g., diabetes and arthritis) in relation to alcoholic hepatitis. "B," colon cancer, is unlikely to present in this way. "D," vitamin B12 deficiency, typically presents with anemia and neurologic symptoms.

Which of the following laboratory values are most consistent with this patient's presentation?

A) Decreased iron, decreased ferritin, decreased transferrin saturation.
B) Decreased iron, decreased ferritin, increased transferrin saturation.
C) Increased iron, decreased ferritin, increased transferrin saturation.
D) Increased iron, increased ferritin, decreased transferrin saturation.
E) Increased iron, increased ferritin, increased transferrin saturation.

Discussion

The correct answer is "E." All of these iron studies are elevated in patients with hereditary hemochromatosis. A normal person maintains approximately 3–4 g of iron in the body. Normal individuals absorb about 1 mg/day of iron (10% of what is ingested), which is precisely balanced with loss through sweat, sloughing of cells, and GI losses. In hereditary hemochromatosis, 2–4 mg of iron is absorbed daily, resulting in the accumulation of iron.

* *

The patient's diagnosis is confirmed, and you counsel him regarding his disease.

All of the following statements are true EXCEPT:

A) This is an autosomal-dominant disease.
B) Affected females typically present later in life due to increased iron losses.
C) Patients may benefit from phlebotomy even after development of symptomatic disease.
D) Patients are susceptible to unusual infections.
E) Patients are at high risk for hepatocellular carcinoma.

Discussion

The correct answer is "A." Hereditary hemochromatosis is an autosomal-recessive disorder. Approximately 10% of Caucasians are heterozygous, and 5/1000 are homozygous for the gene mutation. Patients are at increased risk for infections due to *Listeria*, *Vibrio vulnificus* (sorry, no sushi!), and *Yersinia enterocolitica*. Affected females may present later in life due to increased iron losses from menstruation, pregnancy, and lactation.

Treatment includes phlebotomy or chelation therapy if phlebotomy is contraindicated. Patients should be monitored closely for development of hepatoma, since therapy does not reduce the risk of hepatocellular carcinoma once cirrhosis is present. Family members should be screened for the disease so they can be started on therapy early, in order to prevent the development of cirrhosis.

HELPFUL TIP: Other causes of iron overload include thalassemia, sideroblastic anemia, and frequent blood transfusions.

CASE 19

A 56-year-old man undergoes a laryngoscopy. In an outdated move that is generally not recommended now, his doctor used extra doses of benzocaine spray (like gallons of the stuff) to overcome a strong gag reflex. The patient tolerated the procedure well, but afterward he started to have cyanosis around the lips. You are now seeing him in the ED, and he has a bluish discoloration of his lips and fingertips and is complaining of a headache. You administer oxygen by nasal canula with no improvement in his cyanosis. You draw venous blood for labs, and find that it has an unusual chocolate color.

All of the following statements are likely to be true about this patient EXCEPT:

A) A measured arterial blood gas will demonstrate a normal PaO_2.
B) The pulse-oximeter will show a high-normal oxygen saturation.
C) The patient may require therapy with methylene blue.
D) The patient should not be treated with methylene blue if he has a history of G6PD deficiency.
E) Additional doses of benzocaine can be lethal.

Discussion

The correct answer is "B." This patient has methemoglobinemia, which in his case was likely a result of the benzocaine spray. Methemoglobinemia results when iron in Hb is oxidized from the ferrous to the ferric state and the Hb becomes incapable of binding and transporting oxygen. The blood gas oxygen may look normal because the RBCs cannot release oxygen (and thus remain oxygenated). However, the pulse- oximeter will show a low O_2 saturation. **So, there is often a gap between what you see on the blood gas and what the pulse- oximeter suggests.**

In a normal patient, less than 1% of Hb is found in the methemoglobin form. Depending on the percentage of methemoglobin, presentations will vary. At 10–20%, patients present with cyanosis refractory to oxygen. The arterial blood gas may show a normal PaO_2 with low oxygen saturations. When methemoglobin levels are >30%, patients present with headache, dizziness, dyspnea, and tachypnea. At >50%, patients develop stupor and obtundation, and >70% may be lethal.

Certain drugs such as nitroprusside, sulfonamides, some local anesthetics, and acetaminophen have been found to cause methemoglobinemia.

Treatment of methemoglobinemia is methylene blue. However, patients with G6PD deficiency should not be given methylene blue, and hyperbaric oxygen therapy should be considered instead. Remember, when patients have been exposed to cyanide, you want to **cause** methemoglobinemia. The exact mechanism by which this protects against cyanide is unknown, since patients begin to improve prior to the presence of methemoglobinemia.

HELPFUL TIP: Children with diarrhea may develop methemoglobinemia, although it is rarely clinically significant.

HELPFUL (AND SOMEWHAT USEFUL) TIP: Methylene blue can also cause a serotonin syndrome if used in those on SSRIs, etc.

CASE 20

A 16-year-old sub-Saharan African male presents to your office for progressive fatigue and dyspnea over the last few days. He also has some mild upper respiratory symptoms that are being "treated" with sulfamethoxazole—trimethoprim. (Dr. Feelgood down the street is known to treat all respiratory infections with antibiotics.) On examination, you find a well-nourished male in no distress. He is afebrile but slightly tachycardic. You note mild scleral icterus and pallor of the palmar creases, but the remainder of the exam is unremarkable. A CBC shows normal WBC count and platelets, with Hb 10.2 g/dL. On peripheral smear, "bite cells" and rare Heinz bodies are reported. The LDH and bilirubin are elevated and the serum haptoglobin is low, but the other serum chemistries are normal.

Which of the following is the most likely diagnosis?

A) Hereditary spherocytosis.
B) G6PD deficiency.
C) Sickle-cell disease (homozygous).
D) Sickle-cell trait (heterozygous).
E) Iron-deficiency anemia.

Discussion

The correct answer is "B." The most likely cause of this patient's anemia is G6PD deficiency. He appears to have a hemolytic anemia, as evidenced by the elevated LDH, bite cells, elevated bilirubin, low haptoglobin, and the acute onset of symptoms. Heinz bodies are inclusions in red cells seen on peripheral smear within the first few days of an oxidative stress in patients with G6PD deficiency. Bite cells are formed as the red cells pass through the spleen and the Heinz bodies are removed. The other diagnoses are less likely. Hereditary spherocytosis ("A") is caused by an inherited defect in the red cell membrane, and episodes of hemolytic anemia may be brought on by environmental stress. However, patients generally have a baseline anemia, and spherocytes should be seen on peripheral smear. Sickle-cell disease and trait are discussed in more detail elsewhere. "E," iron-deficiency anemia, does not generally present acutely and is not associated with findings of hemolysis.

HELPFUL TIP: G6PD deficiency is the most common inherited RBC enzyme defect, affecting 10% of the black male population. It occurs more commonly in African and Mediterranean populations.

* *

Hemolytic anemia in G6PD deficiency is caused by oxidative stress on red cells, most commonly as the result of infection or administration of certain drugs.

Which of the following can precipitate a hemolytic crisis in G6PD deficiency?

A) Sulfa antibiotics.
B) Fava beans.
C) Nitrofurantoin.
D) Some antimalarial drugs.
E) All of the above.

Discussion

The correct answer is "E." All of the above can cause a hemolytic crisis in G6PD deficiency. Multiple other drugs can be involved as well including vitamin C, salicylates, isoniazid, and phenytoin.

HELPFUL TIP: Fresh fava beans aren't worth the bother. First you have to shell them and then ***peel each and every bean.*** After all that work, you just end up with a hemolytic crisis if you have G6PD deficiency. Get the canned ones.

Which of the following is the most appropriate intervention for this patient with G6PD deficiency at this point?

A) Admit to the hospital and observe.
B) Admit to the hospital and transfuse 2 units of packed red cells.
C) Recommend supportive care and follow-up in a few days.
D) Recommend splenectomy and refer to a general surgeon.

Discussion

The correct answer is "C." The hemolytic anemia of G6PD deficiency is self-limited and will resolve. This is because in most cases of G6PD deficiency, only about 25% of the RBCs (the older cells) are susceptible to oxidative stress. Severe episodes should be treated in the hospital setting, but most episodes can be managed as an outpatient. Patients should be educated on the drugs and stressors that may precipitate an episode of hemolytic anemia. Splenectomy may limit hemolysis in patients with more severe disease.

Objectives: Did you learn to . . .

- Recognize disorders of iron metabolism?
- Describe symptoms and signs of hemochromatosis?
- Recognize complications related to iron overload?
- Describe findings and treatment of methemoglobinemia?
- Identify clinical and laboratory manifestations of G6PD deficiency and describe its management?

QUICK QUIZ: TOO MANY LYMPHOCYTES

A 72-year-old man presents to your office for follow-up after a recent hospitalization for pneumonia. While he was in the hospital, he had an increased WBC with lymphocytosis. You repeat his CBC and find a WBC of 18,000/mm^3, with 80% lymphocytes, Hb of 14 g/dL, and a platelet count of 200,000/mm^3. You review office records from a visit 1 year ago and find a WBC of 14,000/mm^3 with 76% lymphocytes. You send his peripheral blood for flow cytometry, which is consistent with a diagnosis of chronic lymphocytic leukemia (CLL).

Which of the following statements about this patient is INCORRECT?

A) This patient is at risk for the development of hemolytic anemia.
B) This patient is at risk for serious infection.
C) This patient is likely to experience a relatively benign disease course.
D) This patient should be started on chemotherapy.
E) This patient may develop "B symptoms" (fever, night sweats, weight loss).

Discussion

The correct answer is "D." CLL is characterized by progressive accumulation of long-lived lymphocytes. It is more common in men and tends to be a disease of older adults (median age at diagnosis 65); however, up to 20% of cases occur in patients <60 years of age. Diagnosis is made if a patient has >5000/mm^3 mature-appearing lymphocytes in the blood representing a clonal line (the details are complex . . .). With the use of immunophenotyping, bone marrow biopsy is not necessary for diagnosis, but may be useful for prognosis.

* *

This patient has a low-stage CLL and does not require immediate treatment with chemotherapy. He should be monitored every 6–12 months or sooner if he develops symptoms, such as infections, fatigue, bulky lymphadenopathy, or bleeding. Patients with CLL are at risk for developing autoimmune diseases, including hemolytic anemia, autoimmune thrombocytopenia, pure red cell aplasia, and autoimmune neutropenia.

QUICK QUIZ: TOO MANY NEUTROPHILS

A 46-year-old woman presents to your office for a preoperative evaluation. She is planning an elective hysterectomy for uterine fibroids. She has no significant past medical history. Her review of systems is positive only for sweats. Her physical examination is unremarkable except for a palpable spleen tip. You obtain a CBC, showing WBC count of 50,000/mm^3, Hb 11 g/dL, and a platelet count 350,000/mm^3. On her peripheral blood smear, she has mostly neutrophils and bands, with some metamyelocytes, myelocytes, and basophils as well.

All of the following are likely to be true EXCEPT:

A) The patient has an underlying infection with leukemoid reaction.
B) The patient has a balanced translocation between chromosome 9 and 22.
C) The patient will likely develop progressive leukocytosis, fevers, anemia, and thrombocytopenia if untreated.
D) This condition may be treated with oral tyrosine kinase inhibitors.

Discussion

The correct answer is "A." Although a leukemoid reaction is a possibility, it would be unusual to see a full range of maturation of myeloid cells (e.g., metamyelocytes and myelocytes) in the peripheral blood along with increased basophils and a palpable spleen. Rather, this patient likely has CML, which is a clonal myeloproliferative disorder, characterized by the "Philadelphia chromosome" (translocation between chromosomes 9 and 22), which encodes for an abnormal tyrosine kinase protein. This is the target for the tyrosine kinase inhibitors, such as imatinib (Gleevec), which have resulted in significant improvement in survival. Patients with CML typically present between the ages of 40 and 60. Up to 40% of patients are asymptomatic at presentation. Others complain of weight loss, fatigue, abdominal pain, night sweats, and fever.

QUICK QUIZ: ACUTE LEUKEMIA

You have a febrile 37-year-old male with a very high WBC count, most of which are blasts. Most likely, he has an acute leukemia. A bone marrow has not yet been done, and it is unknown if this is an acute myeloid leukemia or an acute lymphoblastic leukemia.

Which of the following statements is INCORRECT?

A) The patient's fever is likely due to the leukemic cells, and antibiotics should be started only if you identify a specific infection.
B) The patient is at risk for tumor lysis syndrome and should be started on allopurinol.
C) Aggressive inpatient chemotherapy is required for both the treatment of acute myeloid leukemia and acute lymphoblastic leukemia.
D) You should consult a hematologist/oncologist as soon as possible.

Discussion

The correct answer is "A." Patients with acute leukemia and fever should be cultured, and antibiotics should be started as soon as possible since a fever is often the result of a concurrent infection. These patients should be kept well hydrated and given allopurinol to prevent tumor lysis syndrome, as this can occur even without chemotherapy if the tumor burden is high enough. Treatment of acute leukemias requires intensive chemotherapy and should be started as soon as possible, so prompt evaluation by a hematologist/oncologist is imperative.

CASE 21

A 65-year-old male who is on quinine for leg cramps (a non-FDA-approved indication) is brought into the ED. Last night he was complaining of a headache, fever, and numbness on the right side of his face. This morning, he was acting erratically.

His physical examination demonstrates a confused male, with a temperature of 39°C, pulse 110, BP 180/94, and respirations 14. He has a few petechiae on his palate. He is tachycardic and lungs are clear to auscultation bilaterally. His abdomen is soft, without organomegaly. His neurologic examination is difficult to complete due to his inability to cooperate.

Laboratories include WBC 6000/mm^3, Hb 8.4 g/dL, and platelets 50,000/mm^3. Schistocytes are noted on a peripheral blood smear.

All of the following may be expected in this patient EXCEPT:

A) Creatinine of 3.2 mg/dL.
B) LDH of 640 IU/L.
C) Elevated haptoglobin.
D) Elevated indirect bilirubin.
E) Negative direct antiglobulin test (direct Coombs).

Discussion

The correct answer is "C." An elevated haptoglobin would suggest the absence of active hemolysis. The presence of schistocytes suggests ongoing microangiopathic hemolysis, in this case due to TTP. TTP is classically described by a pentad of findings: microangiopathic hemolytic anemia (suggested by schistocytes on peripheral smear), thrombocytopenia, fever, renal insufficiency, and mental status changes. Not all five features need to be present for diagnosis, but your patient seems to have the pentad. The negative direct antiglobulin test (direct Coombs), "E," suggests that the hemolytic anemia is not due to an autoimmune process. Note that the patient is on quinine, one of the drugs that can cause TTP. Clopidogrel and ticlopidine can also cause TTP although it is less common with clopidogrel.

> HELPFUL TIP: Schistocytes are the result of intravascular trauma to RBCs. Any microangiopathic hemolytic anemia can result in schistocytes as can other intravascular trauma such as that secondary to artificial heart valves, HELLP syndrome, malignant hypertension, some malignancies, transjugular intrahepatic portosystemic shunts (TIPS), eclampsia, etc.

Therapy with plasma exchange has reduced the mortality rate from 90% to less than 25%. Other treatments may include glucocorticoids and splenectomy in refractory cases. Platelet transfusion should be avoided as it can worsen the patient's condition.

Which of the following laboratory findings would you expect to see in this patient with TTP?

A) Normal PT/INR.
B) Elevated PTT.
C) Elevated fibrin degradation products.
D) Low level of fibrinogen.

Discussion

The correct answer is "A." Patients with TTP should have a normal PT/INR. This is important because TTP can be confused with DIC, in which the PT/INR should be elevated and fibrinogen should be low.

* *

Your patient is started on plasma exchange. You note that he has not had any change in his Hb or platelet count, and his renal function is worsening.

Which of the following may mimic TTP and should be considered in a poorly responsive patient?

A) Rocky Mountain spotted fever.
B) Disseminated aspergillosis.
C) Disseminated malignancy.
D) Malignant hypertension.
E) All of the above.

Discussion

The correct answer is "E." When patients are poorly responsive to therapy, an alternative diagnosis should be sought. In pregnant patients, preeclampsia or HELLP syndrome can mimic TTP. Autoimmune disease (e.g., systemic lupus erythematosus and scleroderma), malignant hypertension, and disseminated malignancy may also mimic TTP. Infections that can be confused with TTP include Rocky Mountain spotted fever, disseminated aspergillosis, as well as any other disease that can cause mental status changes and a low platelet count such as as Ehrlichiosis, Anaplasmosis, West Nile virus, etc.

CASE 22

A 23-year-old G1 P0 term female goes to emergency cesarean section after she is noted to have placental abruption. She has no other significant medical history. After the delivery, you note that she is having brisk vaginal bleeding and oozing from her venipuncture sites. You obtain laboratories: WBC 9000/mm^3, Hb 8.2 g/dL, platelet count 80,000/mm^3, INR 2.4, PTT 22 seconds, and fibrinogen 80 mg/dL (normal 190–420 mg/dL). Fibrin degradation products are elevated. A CBC at admission was normal.

Which of the following statements is INCORRECT?

A) The patient may benefit from platelet transfusion.
B) The patient may benefit from cryoprecipitate transfusion.
C) The patient may benefit from FFP transfusion.
D) The patient may benefit from crystalloid infusion.

Discussion

The correct answer is "A." This patient is exhibiting signs of DIC, which is characterized by the disordered regulation of normal coagulation. It can be precipitated by a number of conditions resulting in excess thrombin generation and secondary activation of the fibrinolytic system. Thrombin also activates platelets, causing platelet aggregation and consumption. Antithrombin, previously known as antithrombin III, is consumed in this process as well.

Treatment is directed at correcting the underlying cause of DIC whenever possible. Patients may benefit from platelet transfusion to maintain a platelet count above 20,000/mm^3, but transfusion at higher levels can worsen platelet aggregation. Transfusion of FFP will replace consumed factors. Patients with low fibrinogen levels will benefit from transfusion of cryoprecipitate. The use of heparin is generally limited to those with low grade, chronic DIC with thrombotic complications. It may also be considered acutely if there are prominent thrombotic complications.

HELPFUL TIP: Lab findings in DIC include low platelets, prolonged PT/INR, normal or prolonged PTT, low fibrinogen, and increased fibrin degradation products. Further, D-dimer and thrombin time are also increased, antithrombin may be low, and peripheral blood smear will reveal schistocytes. An elevated D-dimer in isolation is not helpful since D-dimer is elevated in many states, including DVT/PE.

HELPFUL TIP: Causes of DIC include sepsis, surgery, malignancy, obstetric complications (amniotic fluid embolism, abruptio placenta, intrauterine fetal death), extensive burns, heat stroke, snake bites, etc.

Objectives: Did you learn to . . .

- Recognize the clinical presentation of TTP?
- Treat a patient with TTP?
- Develop a differential diagnosis for a patient with microangiopathic anemia?
- Distinguish DIC from TTP?

CASE 23

A 22-year-old female college student presents to your office with complaints of an enlarged cervical lymph node and sore throat. She has felt feverish on and off for several weeks but never measured her temperature. She is afebrile today, a rapid strep test is negative, and you treat her symptomatically. You ask her to return if her symptoms do not resolve within 2–4 weeks.

She returns 4 weeks later. The sore throat has resolved; however, she now complains of intense pruritus and sweats at night. The cervical lymph node now measures 3 cm. The remainder of her physical examination is negative.

What is the most appropriate next step?

A) Direct laryngoscopy.
B) Empiric antibiotic trial.
C) Lymph node biopsy.
D) MRI of the neck.
E) Observation for another 4 weeks.

Discussion

The correct answer is "C." The prolonged (>1 month) presence of a large (>1 cm) lymph node deserves a biopsy. MRI of the neck and laryngoscopy may be indicated depending on the biopsy results. Empiric antibiotic therapy ("B") is inappropriate and unlikely to be helpful, as you have no source of primary infection. At this point in time, observation ("E") will just delay the diagnosis.

* *

You obtain a lymph node biopsy that is consistent with nodular sclerosing Hodgkin disease.

Which of the following statements is INCORRECT?

A) The patient has B symptoms.
B) Further staging is necessary.
C) Chemotherapy is palliative only in this patient.
D) Treatment includes both radiation and chemotherapy.

Discussion

The correct answer is "C." Chemotherapy regimens for Hodgkin disease have resulted in response rates of more than 90%, with fewer long-term complications than prior regimens. Despite the fact that it is well known, Hodgkin's is an uncommon disease, with about 8000 cases occurring each year in the United States. It is a disease of young people, occurring typically in patients in their 20s. Patients often present with lymphadenopathy. Symptoms, known as "B symptoms," include weight loss, fever, and drenching night sweats. Other symptoms may include pruritus, diffuse pain after consuming alcoholic beverages (sigh . . . .), and symptoms related to the development of a mediastinal mass. After a diagnostic lymph node biopsy, further staging ("C") includes CT scans, bone marrow biopsy, and routine labs.

> HELPFUL TIP: Non-hodgkin lymphoma is increasing in incidence and is more common than Hodgkin lymphoma. Risk factors for NHL include HIV infection and advancing age.

CASE 24

A 34-year-old woman presents to your office with calf pain and swelling. She denies trauma to the leg. She has no other significant medical history and takes only oral contraceptives. She smokes half a pack of cigarettes daily but does not drink alcohol. Her physical examination is also unremarkable, with the exception of swelling and tenderness of the left calf. A lower extremity Doppler study demonstrates a new thrombus occluding the common femoral vein.

Which of the following would NOT be appropriate in this patient?

A) Start the patient on warfarin to maintain an INR of 2–3.
B) Have the patient scheduled for placement of an inferior vena cava filter.
C) Discontinue hormonal contraceptives.
D) Encourage the patient to stop smoking.
E) Obtain further history regarding her family.

Discussion

The correct answer is "B." This patient has an acute DVT and risk factors for developing a DVT, including smoking, and hormonal contraceptive use. You should start her on heparin (or low-molecular-weight heparin) and warfarin with a goal INR of 2–3. Heparin should be used for at least 5 days and overlapped with therapeutic doses of warfarin that have reached the target INR for at least 48 hours. She should be anticoagulated for at least 3 months. Encourage her to stop smoking and to find an alternative form of birth control.

> HELPFUL TIP: Workup of an inherited or acquired hypercoagulable state is controversial because the treatment of the patient is often not going to change whatever the outcome. When a thromboembolic event is unprovoked, it is probably prudent to screen the patient for hypercoagulable state. When there is a provoked event (e.g., surgery, prolonged immobilization, pregnancy, and oral estrogen), the role of such a workup is less well defined.

The patient returns 3 months later. She has been relatively easy to anticoagulate (somebody has to be, right?), maintaining a stable INR. She stopped smoking and knows to avoid hormonal contraception. She has learned that her mother had a DVT and her maternal aunt died of a pulmonary embolus. Now, the patient wants to know how this new information will affect her long-term care. You decide to screen her for thrombophilia.

Which of the following sets of tests may be performed while she remains on warfarin?

A) Factor V Leiden mutation, antithrombin (previously known as antithrombin III), prothrombin gene mutation.
B) Factor V Leiden mutation, prothrombin gene mutation, antiphospholipid antibodies.
C) Homocysteine, protein C, antithrombin III.
D) Protein C, protein S, antithrombin III.
E) All of them can be done while the patient is on warfarin.

Discussion

The correct answer is "B." There are essentially seven types of thrombophilia for which you might initially test: factor V Leiden mutation, antithrombin III deficiency, prothrombin gene mutation, protein C deficiency, protein S deficiency, antiphospholipid antibody syndrome, and hyperhomocysteinemia. Not all causes of thrombophilia can be tested while on anticoagulant therapy. Factor V Leiden gene mutation, prothrombin gene mutation, homocysteine, and antiphospholipid antibodies are not affected by warfarin. However, warfarin can reduce protein C and S levels (giving false-positive test results) and increase antithrombin levels (giving a false-negative result).

Factor V Leiden mutation is the most common cause of inherited thrombophilia, being found in 3–6% of nonblack blood donors. Antithrombin deficiency (previously known as antithrombin III) is less common, occurring in 1/1000–1/5000 individuals. The homozygous condition is fatal in utero.

Heterozygotes have a 30% chance of developing a thromboembolic event by age 30. Protein C deficiency occurs in 1/200–1/300 people; however, fewer than 1/1000 heterozygotes develop venous thromboses. Protein S deficiency is estimated to occur in 0.03–0.13% of persons and has a clinical presentation similar to protein C deficiency. The prevalence of prothrombin gene mutation varies widely and occurs most commonly in persons of southern European descent. Unlike the other thrombophilias discussed thus far, antiphospholipid antibody syndrome is an acquired disorder that is associated with arterial as well as venous thromboembolic events. Finally, hyperhomocysteinemia is associated with the development of venous thrombosis and atherosclerotic heart disease.

> **HELPFUL TIP:** These tests are not really going to help your patient. The biggest risk factor for having another DVT is having the first DVT. This trumps all of the thrombophilias in determining your patient's subsequent risk.

CASE 25

A 19-year-old gravid female presents during her second trimester and complains of left calf swelling. With the help of Doppler studies, you diagnose her with a DVT.

Which of the following statements is correct?

A) DVT occurs most commonly in the right lower extremity in pregnant women.
B) DVT is common in pregnancy due to increased venous stasis and increased levels of fibrinogen, factor VIII, and vWF.
C) Anticoagulation with heparin introduces no risk to the fetus or mother.
D) DVT is most common in the third trimester.

Discussion

The correct answer is "B." DVT, and the broader category of venous thromboembolism (VTE), occurs two to four times more often in pregnant women compared to nonpregnant controls. Increased risk is found with cesarean delivery versus vaginal delivery. The majority of DVTs occur in the **left** lower extremity of pregnant women, likely due to the compression of the left iliac vein by the right iliac artery as they cross. The increased incidence of VTE is multifactorial, including increased levels of fibrinogen, factor VIII, and vWF; increased venous stasis; increased venous distension secondary to increased estrogen; and anatomic distortion related to the gravid uterus.

VTE occurs **equally during all three trimesters**, but increased lower extremity swelling is frequently seen in normal patients during the third trimester, making the diagnosis less obvious. Treatment of VTE with anticoagulation is more difficult in a pregnant woman. Warfarin crosses the placenta and has teratogenic effects in addition to increased risk of fetal bleeding. Heparin and danaparoid do not cross the placenta, but are associated with a 2% risk of maternal bleeding. Heparin also carries the risks of heparin-induced thrombocytopenia with thrombosis, osteoporosis, and bleeding at the uteroplacental junction. Dosing of unfractionated heparin is difficult during pregnancy, and low-molecular-weight heparin is probably the best choice for anticoagulation. Heparin and warfarin are safe for lactating mothers.

CASE 26

A 52-year-old woman presents to the ED with shortness of breath and respirophasic chest pain. She has been on warfarin for atrial fibrillation. Despite her anticoagulation, you suspect pulmonary embolism (PE) and obtain a spiral CT scan, which shows a thrombus in the right pulmonary artery. Prior to the initiation of any therapy, her coagulation studies return and show INR 2.8 (normal = 1) and PTT 49 seconds (prolonged).

Which of the following is the most appropriate next step?

A) Test the patient for antiphospholipid antibodies.
B) Place an inferior vena cava filter.
C) Repeat the INR and PTT since the patient's sample was probably contaminated with heparin.
D) Confront the patient about her noncompliance with warfarin.
E) Throw up your hands in disgust. Aren't they done with the hematology chapter yet?

Discussion

The correct answer is "A." Patients who have a new VTE while on appropriate anticoagulant therapy should be evaluated for antiphospholipid antibody syndrome. This patient has a prolonged PTT, which is also suspicious for an antiphospholipid antibody. She was an outpatient prior to having her blood drawn and was not taking heparin, so contamination with heparin is unlikely (although heparin definitely causes an increase in the PTT). The increased INR suggests that the patient has been compliant with her warfarin. Caval filters are rarely useful unless the patient is at high risk from anticoagulation. Development of VTE is increased with long-term use of caval filters, and there is no long-term benefit seen with the use of vena caval filters.

> HELPFUL TIP: Previously, retrospective studies resulted in the recommendation that patients with an antiphospholipid antibody and VTE be maintained at an INR of 3–4. This recommendation has changed with newly available prospective data, and these patients should have a target INR of 2.5.

> HELPFUL TIP: Genetic testing is now available for warfarin sensitivity that can help predict which patients will need higher (or lower) doses of warfarin to maintain adequate anticoagulation. However, these tests are very expensive and contribute little to patient care.

CASE 27

A 50-year-old male is admitted to the hospital with a fractured tibia after a motor vehicle collision. You are asked to assist in his perioperative management. The patient is generally healthy but is taking warfarin for a DVT that he developed after a total knee arthroplasty 3 weeks ago. His INR is 1.8, and he is scheduled for open reduction/internal fixation tomorrow.

Which of the following statements is INCORRECT?

A) The patient has an approximate 50% risk of recurrent VTE without appropriate therapy.
B) Heparin should be started preoperatively.
C) Heparin should be continued postoperatively.
D) Resumption of warfarin alone postoperatively is adequate anticoagulation.

Discussion

The correct answer is "D." Perioperative management of a patient with recent VTE is complicated. While there are established guidelines for VTE prophylaxis depending on the type of surgery planned, this patient already has an active thrombotic event. Discontinuing warfarin may result in a rebound hypercoagulable state, and surgery creates a prothrombotic state.

Patients who have a VTE within 1 month of surgery have a 50% risk of a second VTE if not treated aggressively with anticoagulation. These recurrent events carry a mortality rate of approximately 6%. Such patients should be placed on heparin before and after surgery. Starting warfarin after surgery decreases the risk of bleeding compared to restarting full dose heparin but is less effective at preventing VTE immediately postoperatively, so heparin should be employed as well. Patients with a VTE within 1–3 months before a scheduled surgery should be considered for postoperative heparin therapy, while a VTE >3 months before the scheduled surgery should not pose significant additional risk, and established prophylaxis guidelines should be followed.

Objectives: Did you learn to . . .

- Recognize presentation of a patient with Hodgkin disease?
- Describe "B symptoms?"
- Obtain an appropriate history in a patient with clotting problems?
- Recognize common inherited and acquired hypercoagulable risk factors?
- Recognize the risks of VTE in the pregnant patient?
- Identify a patient presenting with antiphospholipid antibodies and understand the management of such patients?
- Describe anticoagulation approaches in perioperative care?

* *

OK, you knew this was coming. A quick primer on the new anticoagulants.

Pradaxa (dabigatran)—A direct thrombin inhibitor. Approved for nonvalvular atrial fibrillation for CVA prevention. May be less bleeding overall than warfarin but prevents fewer MIs and causes more GI bleeds. The dose must be decreased in those with renal disease. There is no way to turn it off: FFP and vitamin K don't work. Forty to sixty percent can be dialyzed off. However, this is difficult to arrange acutely. So you have to watch as they slowly bleed into their brain . . . .

Xarelto (rivaroxaban)—An oral factor Xa inhibitor (similar to enoxaparin). As of late 2011, approved to prevent DVT postoperatively after hip or knee replacement and for stroke prevention in atrial fibrillation. There are multiple drug interactions (though fewer than with warfarin). Not indicated in those with severe renal disease and those with moderate liver disease. A small, recent study looked at reversing rivaroxaban with prothrombin concentrate and it seems to work. (*Circulation* 2011 Oct 4; 124:1573). More study is still needed, of course.

So why can't dabigatran be reversed? Because it is an inhibitor of thrombin. Any new thrombin you infuse will be inhibited. Warfarin, on the other hand, depletes factors. Simply replace the factors depleted by warfarin and you are good to go.

BIBLIOGRAPHY

Abramson N, et al. Leukocytosis: Basics of clinical assessment. *Am Fam Physician.* 2000;62(9):2053-2060.

Allen GA, et al. Approach to the bleeding child. *Pediatr Clin North Am.* 2002;49(6):1239.

American College of Chest Physicians. The Seventh ACCP Conference on Antithrombotic and Thrombolytic Therapy. *Chest.* 2004;126(suppl).

Bain BJ. Diagnosis from the blood smear. *N Engl J Med.* 2005;353:498-507.

Booth KK, et al. Systemic infections mimicking thrombotic thrombocytopenic purpura. *Am J Hematol.* 2011; 86(9):743-751. doi: 10.1002/ajh.22091.

Brandhagen DJ, et al. Recognition and management of hereditary hemochromatosis. *Am Fam Physician.* 2002; 65(5):853.

Freifeld AG, et al. Clinical practice guideline for the use of antimicrobial agents in neutropenic patients with cancer: 2010 update by the Infectious Diseases Society of America. *Clin Infect Dis.* 2011;52(4):e56.

Ganetsky M, et al. Dabigatran: Review of pharmacology and management of bleeding complications of this novel oral anticoagulant. *J Med Toxicol.* 2011;7(4):281-287.

Kearon C, et al. Antithrombotic therapy for venous thromboembolic disease: American College of Chest Physicians Evidence-Based Clinical Practice Guidelines. *Chest* 2008;133(6):454s-545s.

Killip S, et al. Iron deficiency anemia. *Am Fam Physician.* 2007;75(5):671-678.

Landgren O. Monoclonal gammopathy of undetermined significance and smoldering myeloma: New insights into pathophysiology and epidemiology. Hematology Am Soc Hematol Educ Program. 2010;:295-302.

Moake J. Thrombotic thrombocytopenia purpura (TTP) and other thrombotic microangiopathies. Best Pract Res Clin Haematol. 2009;22(4):567-576. Review.

O'Connell TX, et al. Understanding and interpreting serum protein electrophoresis. *Am Fam Physician.* 2005; 7(1):105-112.

Sunga AY, et al. Care of cancer survivors. *Am Fam Physician.* 2005;71(4):699-706.

w3.ouhsc.edu/platelets/index.html (Everything you want to know about platelets.)

www.asco.org (Sponsored by the American Society of Clinical Oncology for physicians.)

www.hematology.org (Sponsored by the American Society of Hematology, with links to many blood disease Web sites.)

www.labtestsonline.org (Information on general hematology/oncology subjects and laboratory testing, also general medicine.)

www.multiplemyeloma.org (Everything about myeloma; sponsored by the Multiple Myeloma Research Foundation.)

www.plwc.org (Web site for patients living with cancer; sponsored by American Society of Clinical Oncology.)

7

Gastroenterology

Mark A. Graber and Jason K. Wilbur

CASE 1

A 43-year-old woman complains of a burning pain in the retrosternal area. Her symptoms started about 2 years ago and initially responded to self-medication with antacids or histamine-2 receptor antagonists (H_2 blockers). However, within the last 4 months, she has had nearly daily problems. She frequently wakes up in the middle of the night with retrosternal, burning pain, radiating to her neck. She also frequently notices an acidic taste in her mouth. While antacids help somewhat, they only provide transient relief. She has otherwise been healthy. She currently takes up to four tablets of cimetidine (200 mg) per day plus the antacids. She denies tobacco or alcohol use. Her physical examination is normal.

Which of the following is NOT considered a "red flag" when it comes to patients with acid reflux/dyspepsia?

A) Weight loss.
B) Trouble swallowing liquids.
C) Trouble swallowing solids.
D) A craving for doughnuts.

Discussion

The correct answer is "D." OK, we will give you this one. One of the most critical parts of patient assessment is to make sure there are no "red flag" symptoms that may indicate more than simple gastroesophageal reflux disease (GERD). Red flag symptoms include dysphagia, weight loss, anemia, aspiration, early satiety or vomiting, and cough. A craving for doughnuts is benign (although eating them is not) and may be seen among the police, college students, book editors, Vash the Stampede, and others.

Which of the following statements is true?

A) All patients with GERD need endoscopy.
B) Routine endoscopy in patients with GERD markedly reduces the risk of esophageal cancer.
C) The sensitivity and specificity of typical symptoms is >90%.
D) Patients over age 45 with new onset symptoms are considered high risk.
E) C and D.

Discussion

The correct answer is "E." Because of the high sensitivity and specificity of symptoms (>90%), most patients do not need endoscopy or any other diagnostic intervention. Patients with refractory GERD or those with new symptoms over age 45 years (50 by some sources) warrant endoscopy. "B" is incorrect. Screening for the presence of Barrett esophagus in patients with GERD is low yield. Targeted, not routine, endoscopy may be beneficial. Even then, the benefit is limited (*J Natl Cancer Inst* 2011;103:1049). This is still a matter of active debate and recommendations may change.

> HELPFUL TIP: The link between *Helicobacter pylori* and GERD is poorly defined. There is no good evidence to support eradication of *H. pylori* for the treatment of GERD. The same is true for nonulcer dyspepsia.

* *

The patient denies any "red flags." Based on this information, you assume that this patient has GERD.

You recommend:

A) Barium swallow study.
B) Esophageal manometry.
C) Endoscopy.
D) Ambulatory pH study of the esophagus.
E) Trial of omeprazole and lifestyle modifications.

Discussion

The correct answer is "E." As noted above, the sensitivity and specificity of classical symptoms (around 90%) allows for the diagnosis of GERD without additional studies. Testing is actually less sensitive than symptoms for GERD with the sensitivity of tests varying between 50% and 70%. Many patients have a false-negative EGD. **While H_2 blockers should still be first-line treatment in patients with GERD,** this patient has already failed cimetidine. Starting a proton pump inhibitor (PPI), like omeprazole, is the next step and is preferred as first-line therapy in patients with severe symptoms. Lifestyle modifications should be made including weight loss (if overweight... maybe it is that doughnut craving); avoidance of carbonated beverages, caffeine, excessive alcohol, and large or late evening meals; avoidance of anticholinergics, calcium channel blockers, NSAIDs, and sedative drugs; smoking cessation; and elevation of the head of the bed using 6-inch blocks.

HELPFUL TIP: Most patients with GERD will have negative endoscopic findings (termed nonerosive reflux disease[NERD]—really, we didn't make this one up). Symptoms do not correlate well with the presence or degree of esophageal inflammation or erosion.

* *

Your patient is willing to try the PPI you prescribe, but she also wants to know about surgery that a friend had.

Regarding surgery for GERD, you can tell her:

A) Bloating and inability to belch do not occur with antireflux surgery.
B) Antireflux surgery should be thought of as first-line because it is vastly superior to medical therapy.
C) Years after antireflux surgery, many patients will require medication for GERD symptoms.
D) Laparoscopic fundoplication will ruin her fabulous bikini body by leaving a large midline scar.

Discussion

The correct answer is "C." Surgery may be an option in select patients with reflux disease. The usual indications for antireflux surgery include failure of medical therapy to control symptoms and failure of medical therapy to prevent complications (e.g., stricture and pneumonia). The most commonly performed surgery is fundoplication, in which the lower esophageal sphincter is "wrapped" to enhance its competency. While fundoplication will alleviate symptoms in 80–95% of patients, there is progressive loss of effectiveness over time (only 40% are without medication after 10 years). Adverse effects of surgery include persistent dysphagia (requiring additional interventions in 3–7%), gas, bloating, and inability to belch. "D" is incorrect because a laparoscopic procedure should result in just a few small scars.

* *

After a trial of your favorite PPI (that her insurance will cover after you play "Guess What's on Our Formulary"), your patient continues to have symptoms. You review lifestyle modifications with her, and she assures you that she has made these changes. You refer her for upper endoscopy (esophagogastroduodenoscopy or EGD). The esophageal biopsy is consistent with the visual report, which shows Barrett esophagus.

All of the following are true regarding Barrett esophagus EXCEPT:

A) Males are more likely to have Barrett esophagus than females.
B) Barrett esophagus is due to a change in the esophageal mucosa from columnar to squamous.
C) Barrett esophagus occurs in 10–15% of patients with erosive esophagitis.
D) Barrett esophagus increases the risk of adenocarcinoma by up to 30-fold.
E) Patients with Barrett esophagus should undergo periodic screening EGD.

Discussion

The correct answer is "B." Barrett esophagus is diagnosed histologically when esophageal mucosal metaplasia has occurred **and the usual squamous epithelial cells have changed to columnar epithelium.** Risk factors for Barrett include long-standing reflux, male gender (6:1 male:female preponderance), middle age, tobacco use, and white race. Barrett esophagus occurs in 10–15% of patients with erosive esophagitis, and it dramatically increases the risk of esophageal adenocarcinoma (30-fold). However, the absolute risk of adenocarcinoma is still small, about 0.12–2% annually. Surveillance for Barrett depends on the level of dysplasia found on initial exam, and guidelines exist that dictate the frequency with which repeat EGD should be performed. Of note, a recent study has called into question the degree to which Barrett esophagus raises the risk of esophageal cancer (N Engl J Med 2011;365:1375), although this study still found the relative risk to be over 11.

HELPFUL TIP: Prokinetic agents, like metoclopramide (Reglan), can be useful in the treatment of GERD. In addition to promoting stomach emptying, metoclopramide increases gastroesophageal sphincter tone.

HELPFUL TIP: Complications of chronic GERD include erosive esophagitis, peptic stricture, and adenocarcinoma of the esophagus. However, the absence of heartburn symptoms does not rule out reflux-related complications since approximately one-fourth of patients with peptic stricture and one-third of those with adenocarcinoma of the esophagus had no heartburn prior to diagnosis. Barrett esophagus can regress with adequate treatment of GERD.

Objectives: Did you learn to . . .

- Describe the diagnosis and management of GERD?
- Use H_2 blockers and PPIs in the management of GERD?
- Recognize complications of GERD and risk factors for Barrett esophagus?

CASE 2

A 53-year-old woman comes to your office complaining of chest pain and problems swallowing. She says food seems to hang up in the retrosternal area. This started several years ago and has gradually progressed and now occurs at least twice per week. Generally, only solid foods cause problems. She has become very careful, only taking small bites and chewing them well before swallowing. Should she experience problems, she has found that drinking additional liquids alleviates her symptoms within minutes. She does not regurgitate food and has not lost weight.

What is the symptom this patient is complaining of?

A) Dysphagia.
B) Globus sensation.
C) Odynophagia.
D) Aerophagia.
E) Phagophobia.

Discussion

The correct answer is "A." Dysphagia, from the Greek *dys* (with difficulty . . . as opposed to "*Dis*" which is a city in Dantes's Hell . . . in addition to being a neologism) and *phagia* (to eat), refers to the sensation that food is being hindered in its passage from the mouth to the stomach. Odynophagia refers to pain upon swallowing, aerophagia to swallowing of air, and globus sensation to a perception of a lump or fullness in the throat that is temporarily relieved by swallowing. Phagophobia is just what you think it is: fear of eating or swallowing.

HELPFUL TIP: Aerophagia is a common and underdiagnosed cause of abdominal symptoms. Generally, patients will complain of belching associated with abdominal bloating, especially after meals. It is not uncommon for patient's to mention that they have to loosen their belt after meals. Aerophagia is exacerbated by gum chewing (which causes frequent swallowing of air), eating quickly, and smoking. Aerophagia can be mitigated by eating more slowly, avoiding carbonated beverages, etc.

What information is important when evaluating this patient with dysphagia?

A) When the sensation first occurs in relation to swallowing.
B) What medications the patient is taking.
C) Whether solids or liquids are affected.
D) The patient's HIV status.
E) All of the above.

Discussion

The correct answer is "E." Taking a careful history is key to evaluating the patient who presents with dysphagia.

Given the above patient's description of symptoms and the location of her discomfort (food sticking in the retrosternal esophagus), what type of dysphagia is she most likely to suffer from?

A) Oropharyngeal dysphagia.
B) Esophageal dysphagia.
C) Functional dysphagia.
D) Aberrant dysphagia.
E) Wandering chestal dysphagia.

Discussion

The correct answer is "B." Dysphagia can be differentiated by where the symptoms seem to occur. Oropharyngeal dysphagia, also known as "transfer dysphagia," arises from difficulty in the upper esophagus and pharynx. Patients complain of food getting stuck immediately upon swallowing, and when asked to point to the location, patients frequently identify the cervical region. Patients with oropharyngeal dysphagia often have more problems with liquids than solids **and may complain that liquid comes out of their nose when they try to swallow** (my brother had this happen with Oreo cookies and milk while laughing when we were kids). Esophageal dysphagia is usually described as beginning several seconds after swallowing, and patients frequently point to the suprasternal notch or retrosternally when trying to localize the area causing symptoms. Patients in whom no cause can be found after detailed investigation are often categorized as having functional dysphagia. There is no such thing as aberrant dysphagia or wandering chestal dysphagia—come on, "chestal" isn't even a real word.

* *

A complete review of systems and physical examination are unrevealing.

Which of the following is the single best test to arrive at a diagnosis in this patient?

A) Barium swallow.
B) Esophageal manometry.
C) EGD.
D) Ambulatory pH study of the esophagus.
E) Diagnostic trial of a high-dose PPI.

Discussion

The correct answer is "C." Visualization of the esophagus is critical in patients with dysphagia. This can either be done by endoscopy or barium swallow. Our patient presents with esophageal dysphagia for solids, which is most consistent with a structural problem, such as a stricture, web, or neoplasm. Endoscopy is the best diagnostic study to evaluate the esophageal mucosa as it allows one to obtain biopsies and perform endoscopic interventions such as dilations, if indicated. While many authorities may recommend a barium swallow first, it does not let one obtain a biopsy or perform an intervention if warranted. Should the endoscopy come back negative, esophageal manometry ("B") may be useful as it will help determine if a motility disorder is the cause of symptoms. While a "diagnostic" trial with PPIs ("E") is an appropriate strategy in patients with noncardiac chest pain, the presence of an alarm symptom, such as dysphagia, requires further testing. "D," an ambulatory pH study, does not help in defining the etiology of the dysphagia.

HELPFUL TIP: Many patients have breakthrough pain at night even when on a PPI. The reason for this is that PPIs only act on cells that have been activated (such as by a meal). PPIs should be taken 30 minutes before eating. Try adding an H_2 blocker at nighttime for patients having breakthrough pain.

HELPFUL TIP: Rebound acid hypersecretion can lead to symptom recurrence if potent antisecretory agents, such as PPIs, are stopped abruptly. Many experts recommend stepping down to H_2 blockers prior to cessation. However, even H_2 blockers can also cause a lesser degree of rebound acid hypersecretion. So, consider tapering these drugs as well.

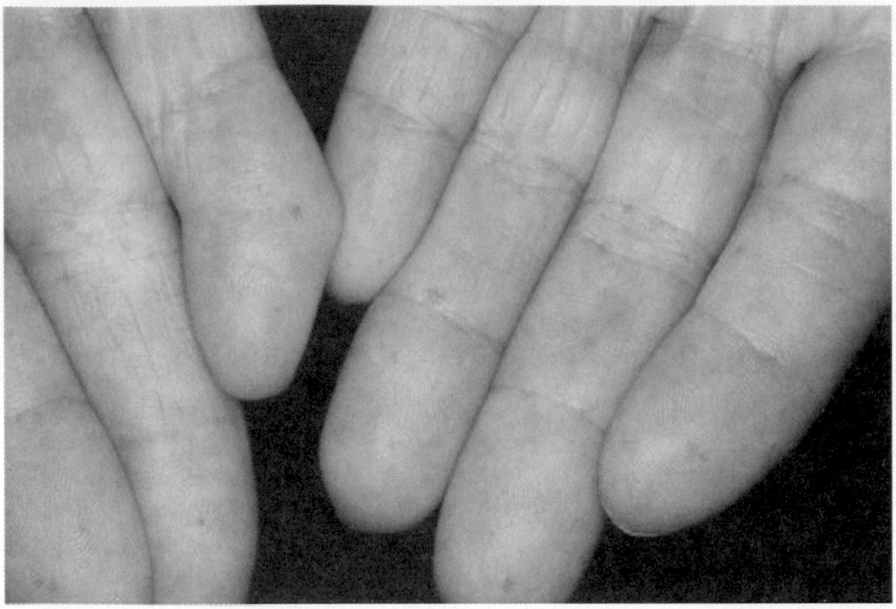

Figure 7–1

* *

The patient returns from her endoscopy. According to the report, she had severe esophagitis with confluent erosions in the distal esophagus. During your physical examination, you find the skin changes shown in Figure 7–1, see also color section. When you ask about these, the patient reports a history of bluish fingertip discoloration with cold temperatures. She also complains that her fingers feel "tight" at times.

With this new information, which of the following diagnoses are you considering?

A) CREST syndrome.
B) Esophageal adenocarcinoma.
C) Metastatic colonic adenocarcinoma.
D) Sicca syndrome.
E) Peptic ulcer disease (PUD).

Discussion

The correct answer is "A." CREST is an acronym for a syndrome that includes **C**alcinosis cutis, **R**aynaud phenomenon, **E**sophageal dysmotility, **S**clerodactyly, and **T**elangiectasias. Figure 7–1 shows telangiectasias on the palmar digital pad. Up to 60% of patients with CREST have erosive esophagitis. Dysphagia is common and is due to esophageal stricture and/or dysmotility.

Given her endoscopic findings and the fact that she likely has CREST syndrome, what treatment do you suggest?

A) H_2 blocker.
B) PPI.
C) High-dose corticosteroids.
D) *H. pylori* eradication.
E) Laparoscopic fundoplication.

Discussion

The correct answer is "B." Severe reflux and dysphagia are hallmarks of CREST syndrome. The esophagus may be amotile with impaired function of the lower esophageal sphincter. The barrier to acid reflux and the motor clearance of refluxing material are affected, requiring chronic and potent acid suppressive medications, such as PPIs. Surgery is **relatively contraindicated**, as the poor contractile function of the esophagus may not generate enough force to overcome a barrier created by fundoplication or other interventions (and thus food will not move into the stomach). *H. pylori* treatment has no role in the management of this illness. Steroids could certainly worsen the GI symptoms by irritating the gastric mucosa. Other causes of esophageal dysphagia are listed in Table 7–1.

HELPFUL (AND IMPORTANT) TIP: It would not surprise us to see this on the board exam. An increasingly recognized cause of dysphagia is **eosinophilic esophagitis.** The classic adult patient presents with dysphagia to solids to the extent that it may cause food impaction. Children often present with feeding problems (age 2), recurrent vomiting (age 8), and chronic abdominal pain (age 12) or food impaction (teenage years). Association with childhood asthma is strong and dietary elimination therapy may be helpful in children. Treatment in adults (and often children) involves swallowing inhaled corticosteroids (fluticasone), montelukast, and, in severe cases, systemic steroids. Systemic eosinophilia is rare.

HELPFUL TIP: Dysphagia that progresses from solids and then to liquids is a classic symptom of esophageal cancer and cannot be ignored.

Objectives: Did you learn to . . .

- Differentiate dysphagia from other gastrointestinal (GI) symptoms?
- Take an adequate history to evaluate the etiology of dysphagia?
- Describe different types of dysphagia and identify various causes of dysphagia?
- Recognize that CREST syndrome as a cause of dysphagia?

Table 7–1 CAUSES OF ESOPHAGEAL DYSPHAGIA

Mechanical Lesions	
Intrinsic	**Extrinsic**
Benign tumors	Aberrant subclavian artery
Caustic esophagitis/stricture	Cervical osteophytes
Radiation esophagitis/stricture	Enlarged aorta
Peptic esophagitis/stricture	Enlarged left atrium
Eosinophilic esophagitis	Mediastinal mass
Diverticula	Postspinal surgery
Malignancy	
Post-GI surgery	
Rings and webs	
Foreign bodies	
Motility Disorders	
Achalasia	
Chagas disease (*Trypanosoma cruzi*)	
Diffuse esophageal spasm	
Hypertensive lower esophageal sphincter	
Nonspecific esophageal motility disorder	
Nutcracker esophagus	
Scleroderma	

QUICK QUIZ: REGURGITATION

You see a 61-year-old woman in your office complaining of halitosis, regurgitation of undigested food 4 hours after eating, and heartburn. She also feels that the food is sticking in her throat.

What is the MOST LIKELY cause of her symptoms?

A) Schatzki ring.
B) Zenker diverticulum.
C) Achalasia.
D) Foreign body.
E) Esophageal web.

Discussion

The correct answer is "B." Late regurgitation of undigested food is pathognomonic for Zenker diverticulum. A Zenker diverticulum is an outpouching of esophageal mucosa that is acquired and typically becomes symptomatic in middle age or later in life. The diagnosis is confirmed by lateral view of a barium swallow. The other diagnoses listed can cause dysphagia and regurgitation but are less likely. "A," Schatzki ring, is a lower esophageal mucosal ring that can "catch" food and cause dysphagia. "C," achalasia, results from a loss of innervation of the lower esophagus and generally occurs in young and middle-aged adults. Patients with achalasia typically have dysphagia with solids and liquids. "D," foreign body, should be diagnosable by history. Elderly adults, children, and patients with psychiatric disease are most at risk for foreign body in the esophagus. "E," esophageal web, is caused by a thin layer of mucosa across the esophageal lumen and presents much like a Schatzki ring.

CASE 3

A 32-year-old woman presents with 3 years of intermittent GI complaints after eating. She describes epigastric pressure and bloating after food intake. Her weight is stable. She denies heartburn, vomiting, diarrhea, constipation, or blood in her stools. She only takes a multivitamin and she has not tried any specific remedies. The physical examination is normal.

What is the MOST LIKELY diagnosis given the information above?

A) Pyrosis.
B) Peptic ulcer disease (PUD).
C) Nonulcer dyspepsia.
D) Stomach cancer.

Discussion

The correct answer is "C." Nonulcer dyspepsia is an ill-defined condition characterized by the presence of recurring intermittent symptoms of epigastric discomfort and fullness with other associated symptoms in the absence of mucosal lesions or other structural abnormalities of the GI tract. Nonulcer dyspepsia is also known as "functional dyspepsia," as there are no identifiable structural or anatomic abnormalities of the GI tract. While about 20% of the general population has nonulcer dyspepsia, only about 20% of these seek medical attention. Pyrosis ("A") means the same thing as heartburn; this patient has no complaints of heartburn. PUD or stomach cancer of 3 years duration would usually be accompanied by other systemic symptoms (such as fatigue, weight loss, or death—is that a systemic symptom?), which the patient denies. In general, the history and physical exam does not allow you to rule out PUD, but young patients without alarm symptoms can be treated empirically without extensive investigation, as the risk of underlying serious pathology is low.

Which of the following symptoms WOULD NOT be a normal symptom of nonulcer dyspepsia?

A) Fullness.
B) Early satiety.
C) Belching.
D) Intolerance to eggs.

Discussion

The correct answer is "D." Nonulcer dyspepsia is characterized by all the other symptoms and also includes such symptoms as abdominal distention, borborygmi (i.e., grandpa's tummy gurgling heard across the room at Thanksgiving), epigastric or substernal pain, anorexia, nausea, vomiting, and abdominal tenderness. "D," intolerance to eggs, is not part of nonulcer dyspepsia. What have you got against eggs? The editors like eggs, poached if possible (which is why we got *Salmonella*). While there are several proposed pathophysiologic mechanisms by which nonulcer dyspepsia may occur, food intolerance is not one of them.

What is the most appropriate next step in this patient?

A) Obtain *H. pylori* serum antibodies.
B) Obtain an abdominal ultrasound examination of liver, biliary tree, and pancreas.
C) Obtain a detailed dietary history.
D) Obtain an upper GI x-ray series.
E) Refer for gastroscopy.

Discussion

The correct answer is "C." Does this seem to be a contradiction to the previous question? Well, we don't mean it to be so. Although food intolerance does not cause nonulcer dyspepsia, the symptoms of the two types of disorders overlap to some degree. Considering the prevalence of selective carbohydrate malabsorption syndromes, high intake of lactose and fructose-containing food and beverages may contribute to GI symptoms in a significant number of patients. Therefore, the history should always contain a detailed assessment of dietary habits. A more extensive workup is not necessary at this point in time as the patient is younger than 45 years of age and has no alarm symptoms. While infection with *H. pylori* causes gastritis and peptic ulcers, **several controlled studies demonstrated no consistent benefit of *H. pylori* eradication in patients with dyspepsia without ulcers.**

> HELPFUL TIP: If you choose to test and treat for *H. pylori*, the preferred testing strategy is 13C urea breath test or stool antigen test (see case 4 later in this chapter).

* *

You obtain a detailed dietary history, suggesting a potential contribution of fructose intolerance and excessive carbonated beverage intake (it's those 5 Giant Gulp soft drinks a day). Her symptoms persist despite appropriate adjustment of food intake. You choose to start the patient on a PPI. One week later, your nurse receives a call from your patient about severe abdominal pain and diarrhea. She has **not** noticed blood in her stool.

What is the best next step?

A) She is having withdrawal from the 5 Giant Gulp pops. Add back the fructose and the 2000 kcal.
B) Check fasting gastrin level.
C) Antibiotic therapy for bacterial overgrowth.
D) Discontinuation of the PPI.
E) Therapeutic trial of an antidiarrheal.

Discussion

The correct answer is "D." Diarrhea is a common adverse effect of PPIs that occurs in at least 5–7% of patients. Discontinuation leads to a rapid resolution in the majority of cases. While reduced stomach acidity from PPIs or H_2 blockers may result in bacterial colonization of the proximal GI tract, the early onset and severity of symptoms described argue against bacterial overgrowth as the etiology of this patient's symptoms. While PPIs can elevate gastrin levels, the hypergastrinemia seen is not comparable to levels seen in Zollinger–Ellison syndrome, which can also cause diarrhea. Stool studies and empiric therapy with antidiarrheals may be considered if discontinuing the PPI does not improve symptoms.

HELPFUL TIP: There are no drugs that have great evidence to support their use in nonulcer dyspepsia. PPIs and H_2 blockers are often used. Prokinetic agents may be helpful, and in the United States this means metoclopramide or erythromycin. Cisapride has been removed from the market secondary to cardiac arrhythmias (QT prolongation with torsades de pointes). Metoclopramide, of course, is associated with tardive dyskinesia and extrapyramidal reactions. Erythromycin causes GI side effects and prolonged QT.

Which of the following IS TRUE of the natural history of nonulcer dyspepsia?

A) Most patients will not have symptom-free periods, instead having constant dyspepsia.
B) Most patients improve with placebo treatment.
C) Most patients will go on to develop ulcers.
D) Spontaneous resolution of symptoms is rare.

Discussion

The correct answer is "B." Up to 60% of patients in placebo-controlled trials respond to placebo, making it difficult to prove efficacy of medications. As the above number suggests, spontaneous resolution of symptoms is common, while many patients will have a chronic, intermittent course characterized by symptom-free periods. Most patients will not develop serious pathology.

HELPFUL TIP: For nonulcer dyspepsia, general management principles call for reassurance by the physician and the avoidance of repeated diagnostic testing. Patients should make appropriate lifestyle modifications (avoid tobacco, caffeine products, and alcohol) and limit or avoid aggravating medications (NSAIDs). Patients should chew their foods slowly and eat more frequent, small meals. Finally, if there is underlying psychiatric morbidity, relaxation training or treatment of specific diseases can be helpful.

HELPFUL TIP: PPIs are not benign drugs and have been associated with (1) increased risk of hip fracture in the elderly, (2) increased risk of pneumonia, (3) increased risk of *Clostridium difficile* colitis, and (4) diarrhea as noted above. Stop them as soon as possible.

Objectives: Did you learn to . . .

- Diagnose and manage nonulcer dyspepsia?
- Appreciate the natural history of nonulcer dyspepsia?
- Recognize important side effects of PPIs?

CASE 4

A 56-year-old woman comes to the emergency department after a sudden episode of hematemesis. Yesterday, she had two bowel movements that were dark, sticky, and foul smelling (like stools should smell like roses). She woke up nauseated and has since twice vomited a small amount of bright red blood. She also feels dizzy. Because of knee pain related to skydiving 1 week ago, she started taking five tablets of naproxen twice a day. She takes no other medicines and denies any significant past medical history.

On physical exam, you find a pale, uncomfortable, but alert patient. She has tachycardia (108 beats/min) and a drop in blood pressure from 116/72 mm Hg supine to 93/65 mm Hg standing. Her abdomen is flat with hyperactive bowel sounds. You note epigastric tenderness but no rebound or guarding. There is melena on rectal examination.

Which of the following steps will be LEAST helpful at this point in time?

A) Admission to the hospital.
B) Immediate treatment with an intravenous (IV) H_2 blocker.
C) Referral for emergent endoscopy.
D) IV access and fluid resuscitation.
E) Laboratory tests including hemoglobin, coagulation studies, and blood type and cross-match.

Discussion
The correct answer is "B." The patient has symptoms and clinical findings of a hemodynamically significant upper GI tract bleed. Although she's "walking and talking" just fine, fluid administration and hospital admission with close monitoring in an intensive care environment are indicated. A baseline hemoglobin and hematocrit (HCT) should be obtained. **However, a normal hemoglobin does not exclude a significant acute bleed, as hemodilution (in the absence of IV fluids) requires several hours.** Given the presentation, a blood transfusion may become necessary in the future; therefore, blood should be sent for to type and cross-match. Early endoscopy should be performed to identify the cause of her bleeding, and endoscopic therapy should be undertaken if appropriate. Treatment with H_2 blockers does not affect the rate of bleeding; these medications do not increase the gastric pH enough to enhance coagulation. Recent studies have demonstrated that IV PPIs do decrease the risk of rebleeding in high-risk patients by increasing gastric pH to enhance coagulation. **However, these studies combined a PPI with endoscopy.**

> **HELPFUL TIP:** Orthostatic vital signs are not that useful in determining a patient's volume status. Many hypovolemic patients are **not** orthostatic and many patients who are euvolemic **have** orthostatic changes (e.g., patients on antihypertensives and the elderly). So, use orthostatic vital signs to confirm your clinical suspicion, but do not use them as an absolute guide to the patient's volume status (*JAMA* 1999;281:1022–1029).

What is the risk of suffering a clinically significant GI event on NSAIDs?

A) 1–4% per year.
B) 5–10% per year.
C) 15–20% per year.
D) 25–30% per year.
E) 45–50% per year.

Discussion
The correct answer is "A." The risk of a clinically significant NSAID-related GI event, including GI bleeding, perforation, or obstruction, is about 1–4% per year.

* *

The patient undergoes endoscopy, which shows a small duodenal ulcer in the bulb with a visible vessel in the ulcer base. Gastric biopsies show chemical gastropathy and no evidence of *H. pylori*. After endoscopic treatment, the patient recovers nicely. Then, 3 months later, she returns to your office for a follow-up evaluation. She is asymptomatic and continues taking a PPI. Her physical examination is normal. Laboratory tests show normal hemoglobin.

What is the best next step?

A) Repeat endoscopy to document healing and rule out malignancy.
B) Upper GI x-ray series to document healing.
C) Switch to a H_2 blocker.
D) Discontinue acid-suppressive medication.
E) *H. pylori* antibody test.

Discussion
The correct answer is "D." While nonhealing ulcers may be due to a neoplasm, the vast majority of **duodenal** ulcers are benign. Therefore, neither endoscopic nor radiologic documentation of healing is necessary. See Table 7–2 for more on risk factors for malignancy in gastric ulcers. "C" is incorrect. Patients with uncomplicated and small (<1 cm) duodenal or gastric ulcers who have received adequate treatment of *H. pylori* or NSAID-induced ulcer do not need long-term therapy directed at ulcer healing as long as they are asymptomatic following therapy. Antisecretory

Table 7–2 RISK FACTORS FOR MALIGNANCY IN GASTRIC ULCERS

- Occurrence in ethnic groups raised in endemic areas (Asians, Latinos, etc.)
- *Helicobacter pylori* infection
- Absence of recent NSAID use
- Absence of concomitant duodenal ulcer or a prior history of duodenal ulcer (duodenal ulcers require higher acid secretion, which is incompatible with the pangastritis typical of most gastric cancers)
- Giant ulcers (>2–3 cm)
- Absence of a protracted ulcer history—in general, the longer the ulcer history, the lower the risk that a gastric ulcer is cancer. Gastric ulcers require acid and gastric cancer usually develops in the setting of atrophic pangastritis

drugs can be discontinued after 4–6 weeks in these patients. "E" is incorrect. Serology for *H. pylori* will not be helpful in this patient. First, histology is as sensitive as other tests for *H. pylori* infection and the patient's biopsies were negative for *H. pylori.* Second, **serologic testing does not tell us if the patient is currently infected;** many patients have antibody positivity even a year after treatment.

> HELPFUL TIP: Sensitivity of serologic testing for *H. pylori* is 90–100%. But this does not indicate current infection and may reflect prior infection. Breath testing is 88–95% sensitive with most false negatives the result of the use of antibiotics and antacids, including H_2 blockers and PPIs. Thus, make sure that the patient has been off antibiotics for at least a month prior to testing and has not taken acid suppressors for 2 weeks prior to testing. This also holds true for CLO testing. Stool antigen testing (94% sensitive, 92% specific) is also available to help with the noninvasive documentation of *H. pylori* infection or eradication.

If your patient had come back *H. pylori* positive, which of the following combinations IS NOT indicated in the treatment of *H. pylori?*

A) Omeprazole, clarithromycin, metronidazole.
B) Cephalexin, omeprazole, amoxicillin.
C) Metronidazole, amoxicillin, omeprazole.
D) Bismuth subsalicylate, metronidazole, tetracycline, lansoprazole.
E) Omeprazole, clarithromycin, amoxicillin.

Discussion

The correct answer (and the regimen you would not want to use) is "B." All of the other regimens can be used to treat *H. pylori* infection. Of note are regimens "A" and "D." There is resistance to metronidazole, so it should only be used when the patient is penicillin allergic OR taking quadruple therapy.

Which of the following IS NOT useful for testing for *H. pylori* eradication after treatment?

A) Serum IgG antibody titers.
B) CLO test.
C) Breath urea test.
D) Radioactive CO_2 blood test.
E) Stool antigen test.

Discussion

The correct answer is "A." Remember the helpful tip above? Only 57% of patients are antibody negative to *H. pylori* a year after successful treatment. Thus, antibody titers cannot document eradication. All of the other tests mentioned are functional tests for the presence of *H. pylori*. The CLO test is done on biopsy specimens and documents the presence of urea splitting. The same is true for the breath urea test and the radioactive CO_2 blood test. In both of these tests, urea is ingested. If *H. pylori* is present, radioactive CO_2 is generated that can be measured in the blood or breath.

> HELPFUL TIP: NSAID-induced ulcers can occur in the stomach, duodenum, and occasionally in the small bowel and colon. However, NSAIDs are more frequently found to be the cause of gastric ulcers (up to 30%) compared to duodenal ulcers (up to 20%).

Objectives: Did you learn to . . .

- Appreciate the role of NSAID use in PUD?
- Manage an acute GI bleed?
- Identify patients at high risk for NSAID-induced GI toxicity?
- Learn about the treatment and diagnosis of *H. pylori?*

QUICK QUIZ: PILL PROBLEMS

Which of these medications would be the LEAST likely cause of esophagitis if stuck in the esophagus?

A) Potassium chloride.
B) Ferrous sulfate.
C) Alendronate.
D) Loratadine.
E) Tetracycline.

Discussion

The correct answer is "D." Many medications can cause "pill esophagitis," including potassium chloride, ferrous sulfate, alendronate, tetracycline antibiotics, and ascorbic acid. Aspirin and other NSAIDs can also cause esophagitis. Smaller pills are less likely to cause problems. In addition to not being irritating, loratadine is tiny.

QUICK QUIZ: THE CASE OF THE HOLY STOMACH

One of your patients presents complaining of diarrhea and epigastric pain unresponsive to H_2 blockers or PPIs. He denies smoking tobacco, taking NSAIDs, or drinking alcohol. Endoscopy reveals several ulcers. Biopsy for *H. pylori* is negative and there is no malignancy.

Which of the following would be the most appropriate laboratory test to obtain in order to discover an etiology for the *multiple* ulcers (and diarrhea)?

A) Vasoactive intestinal peptide (VIP).
B) Gastrin.
C) Glucagon.
D) Somatostatin.
E) None of the above.

Discussion

The correct answer is "B." Some sort of screening test for gastrinoma is warranted in a patient who has recurrent or refractory ulcers. Zollinger–Ellison syndrome is the name given to the state in which there is acid hypersecretion secondary to increased gastrin production, usually from a gastrin-producing tumor (gastrinoma). Up to 1% of patients with PUD have a gastrinoma. Serum gastrin levels should be obtained with the patient fasting **and off PPIs, as PPIs will increase gastrin levels.** If the serum gastrin is elevated, further investigations will need to be performed. Other reasons to consider obtaining a serum gastrin level include ulcers in unusual locations, family history of ulcers, and ulcers associated with reflux esophagitis. "A" is incorrect. VIP actually works to suppress acid secretion. VIPomas do occur (they're actually tumors and not related to VIP patients calling you at all hours), but VIPomas are associated with watery diarrhea and hypokalemia—not ulcers. "C," glucagon, will not be of much help here. Glucagon over secretion results in hyperglycemia and anemia. "D," somatostatin, is a hormone that inhibits the secretion of gastrin and thus would be protective vis-à-vis ulcers. Somatostatin-secreting tumors are very rare.

QUICK QUIZ: GI BLEEDING

Isolated bright red hematemesis (e.g., no tachycardia and no fever), which occurs after several bouts of vomiting or dry heaves, is referred to as:

A) Boerhaave tear.
B) Mallory–Weiss tear.
C) Cameron lesion.
D) None of the above.

Discussion

The correct answer is "B." A Mallory–Weiss tear occurs after repeated trauma to the lower esophageal and gastric mucosa from forceful retching. This can be differentiated from a Boerhaave tear by the (generally) self-limited nature of the bleeding and the absence of other symptoms. A Boerhaave tear is of a similar etiology but occurs higher in the esophagus and is associated with mediastinitis, fever, shock, and death if intervention is not forthcoming. Cameron lesions are small ulcers in patients with a hiatal hernia and are usually an incidental finding, and are thought to be caused by rubbing of the stomach against the diaphragm as the hernia slides. They can bleed, but the history given above is classic for a Mallory–Weiss tear.

QUICK QUIZ: ABDOMINAL PAIN

A 35-year-old female presents to your clinic complaining of onset of severe midepigastric pain, weight loss, and vomiting following meals. Between meals she is asymptomatic. This has been going on for the past 2 years ever since she purposefully lost 25 pounds to attain a healthy weight for her height. Unfortunately, she has continued to lose weight because of the postprandial pain and vomiting. On her exam you notice a midepigastric bruit.

The most likely diagnosis is:

A) Aortic aneurysm.
B) Atherosclerotic disease of the celiac trunk.
C) Superior mesenteric artery (SMA) syndrome.
D) Chronic pancreatitis.
E) None of the above.

Discussion

The correct answer is "C." This is a typical history and physical exam for SMA syndrome. SMA syndrome is more likely to occur in a patient who has lost significant weight, resulting in thinning of the mesenteric fat pad. Here's the pathophysiology: the SMA runs above the duodenum and becomes stretched and partially occluded in response to meals (as the stomach and duodenum expand), leading to mesenteric ischemia and food aversion. SMA syndrome can be diagnosed using Doppler ultrasound to demonstrate increased velocity of blood in the SMA. "A" and "B" are unlikely in a young patient, and "D" should not be associated with a bruit. Celiac artery syndrome may have a similar presentation to SMA syndrome but, obviously, involves the celiac trunk.

CASE 5

A 54-year-old man comes to your office for his annual physical. He is taking naproxen for a recent ankle injury. Based on your recommendation last year, he started taking one aspirin (81 mg) daily. He does not take any other medications. He exercises regularly, does not smoke, and drinks one glass of wine every day. Your examination is completely normal, except that a test for occult fecal blood is positive.

What is the next best step?

A) Upper endoscopy.
B) CBC.
C) Colonoscopy.
D) A and B.
E) B and C.

Discussion

The correct answer is "E." Current recommendations suggest screening for colorectal cancer in all patients over the age of 50 years. Testing for fecal occult blood is one of the accepted methods. However, it should only be performed as screening test in asymptomatic individuals. Moreover, the use of aspirin and/or NSAIDs and foods such as undercooked meat may increase the number of false-positive tests and should thus be avoided. However, once you have a guaiac-positive stool, you must proceed to colonoscopy in a patient over age 50. A CBC is also important to determine if the patient is anemic. Since the patient currently has no symptoms referable to upper GI pathology, evaluation of the upper GI tract should only be considered if the colonoscopy is negative.

> HELPFUL TIP: Iron causes stool to darken. So do iron supplements cause false-positive guaiac tests? No. Guaiac tests rely on the presence of hemoglobin in the stool, not iron. Don't blame a positive guaiac on an iron supplement.

* *

Review of his records shows that he underwent a colonoscopy 3 years ago. Three small adenomatous polyps were found. He also had scattered diverticula in the sigmoid.

Based on this new information, which strategy do you recommend?

A) Colonoscopy now.
B) Colonoscopy in 5 years.
C) Yearly tests for fecal occult blood.
D) Yearly tests for fecal occult blood and colonoscopy in 7 years.
E) Colonoscopy in 7 years.

Discussion

The correct answer is "A." Adenomatous polyps, such as this patient had, are considered precancerous. Recommended follow-up of an adenomatous polyp is by colonoscopy every 3–5 years. So, he did not truly have a "negative" colonoscopy 3 years ago. Plus, we are not doing the colonoscopy in this case for screening; it is diagnostic. We may find another source of his bleeding. If his previous colonoscopy were completely normal (no adenomatous polyps), you could argue for stopping the aspirin and NSAIDs and following up with serial fecal occult blood tests. In this alternative scenario, persistently positive guaiac tests would lead to colonoscopy as well.

> HELPFUL TIP: Adenomatous colon polyps, either pedunculated or sessile, are associated with transformation to cancer. Hyperplastic polyps are considered benign.

> HELPFUL TIP: US Preventive Services Task Force recommends routine screening for colorectal cancer, starting at age 50 years for average-risk patients (this does NOT apply to high-risk patients—positive family history, known adenomatous polyps, etc.). Any of the following modalities is acceptable: annual fecal occult blood testing (FOBT) alone, annual FOBT with sigmoidoscopy every 5 years +/− dual contrast barium enema every 5 years, and colonoscopy every 10 years (without annual FOBT).

* *

The patient underwent colonoscopy. The report from the endoscopist shows 1 small tubular adenomatous polyp in the sigmoid colon that was completely removed. The patient wants to know when he needs another colonoscopy.

Your answer is:

A) In 3 months.
B) In 1 year.
C) In 3 years.
D) In 5 years.
E) In 10 years.

Discussion

The correct answer is "D." The current **postpolypectomy** surveillance guidelines recommend the following:

1. No polyps or only rectal hyperplastic polyps, repeat in 10 years.
2. 1–2 tubular adenomas less than 1 cm in size with only low-grade dysplasia should have repeat colonoscopy in 5 years.
3. 3–10 tubular adenomas, or villous features or high-grade dysplasia should have surveillance in 3 years.
4. Patients with >10 adenomas should be screened more frequently and familial colon cancer syndromes should be considered.
5. If a sessile polyp is removed in piecemeal fashion, then a repeat exam in 3 months is appropriate to assure complete removal.
6. If prep is not good, repeat colonoscopy at earliest convenience is indicated.

Patients presenting with hereditary nonpolyposis colorectal cancer (HNPCC) or "Lynch syndrome" are more likely than patients with sporadic colon cancer to have which of the following findings?

A) Left-sided colon cancers.
B) Late age onset of colon cancer.
C) Multiple colon cancers diagnosed simultaneously.
D) An unusual desire to visit Lynchburg, Tennessee, and a dedication to all things Jack Daniels.

Discussion

The correct answer is "C." Patients with HNPCC (Lynch syndrome) are at increased risk of developing colon cancer. About 2–3% of colon cancers occur in patients with Lynch syndrome. Transformation from an adenoma to cancer is faster in patients with Lynch syndrome. In addition, many of the neoplasms are located in the right colon, so "A" is incorrect. Compared to sporadic colon cancer patients, those with Lynch syndrome are younger at the time of diagnosis, more frequently present with multiple colon tumors, and are more likely to have extracolonic tumors—especially endometrial cancer. This is a genetic disorder, and the occurrence of colorectal and/or **endometrial** cancer in three relatives before the age of 50 should suggest HNPCC. The current recommendation is to perform surveillance colonoscopies at least every 3 years in these patients.

> HELPFUL TIP: Current guidelines recommend earlier screening colonoscopy for asymptomatic patients with a family history of colon cancer, although the recommendations vary by organization. For example, the American Cancer Society (ACS) recommends screening colonoscopy at age 40 or 10 years before the age of diagnosis for any patients with a first-degree relative with colon cancer diagnosed under age 60 (e.g., if mom had colon cancer at 48, start your screening at 38). The ACS

recommends screening colonoscopy at age 40 for patients with a first-degree relative with colon cancer over the age of 60.

Objectives: Did you learn to . . .

- Describe the limitations of FOBT?
- Choose the appropriate tests and screening and surveillance intervals for colorectal neoplasias?
- Learn how family and personal history of colorectal neoplasia affects screening and surveillance strategy?

CASE 6

A 28-year-old graduate student comes to your office complaining of diarrhea. About 6 months ago, she noted a sudden onset of loose stools. While she initially attributed these symptoms to "stomach flu," her problem has persisted. She currently has about four to six loose bowel movements per day with nighttime defecations. She has not seen blood in her stool. In addition, she complains of cramps located in the left and occasionally right lower abdomen. The cramps are made worse with food intake and often are associated with a need to defecate. She has lost about 8 kg unintentionally within the last 3–4 months. She denies any travel or antibiotic use. On physical examination, you notice some tenderness in the right lower quadrant. You see a painless anal fissure in the anterior commissure, and by the appearance, you judge that the fissure is probably chronic in nature.

What do you recommend as the next step in the evaluation and management of this patient?

A) Loperamide.
B) Referral to a holistic clinic for a coffee colonic cleansing regimen (using fair trade, shade grown organic coffee only)
C) Check titers of atypical antineutrophil cytoplasmic antibodies (ANCA).
D) Colonoscopy.
E) Botulinum toxin injection into the area of the anal fissure.

Discussion

The correct answer is "D." The patient's history and physical findings with a painless, anteriorly located anal fissure and diarrhea are consistent with Crohn disease. The best next step in her evaluation is colonoscopy with inspection of the terminal ileum. You may want to do some stool testing before colonoscopy; and testing for *Giardia*, *C. difficile* toxin, and other pathogens would be reasonable. But of the choices presented, colonoscopy is the best option. "A" is inappropriate since this is long-standing with weight loss; symptomatic control is fine but we need to figure out what is going on with this patient. "B" is incorrect. She has diarrhea . . . her colon is already clean. "C," serologic testing, is a reasonable choice but not the best. Here is why. Crohn disease is associated with antibodies against saccharomyces (ASCA), while ulcerative colitis (UC) patients are more often positive for ANCA. However, the sensitivity of these tests is only about 60%. Moreover, there is about a 20% overlap (e.g., ANCA positive in Crohn disease), raising further questions about the overall usefulness of these tests. ASCA can also be positive in celiac disease. "E" is also incorrect. Fissures are one of the anal manifestations of Crohn disease and should be approached by treating the underlying disease rather than using surgical techniques, botulinum injection, etc. Botulinum injections, nitroglycerin ointment, and nifedipine have all been used for anal fissures with success, but we need to diagnose this patient and address the underlying disease.

HELPFUL TIP: In Crohn disease, about 25% of patients have disease confined to the colon. Another 40% have disease in the ileum and cecum, and 30% have disease confined to the small bowel. The remainder has more diffuse disease and/or disease in the proximal GI tract.

Which of the following is *true* regarding the pathophysiology and natural history of Crohn disease?

A) Crohn disease is a genetic disorder, transmitted in an autosomal-dominant fashion.
B) Crohn disease is a relapsing/remitting disease, and 30% of patients will improve spontaneously.
C) Patients with Crohn disease rarely progress to disease requiring surgery.
D) Maintenance therapy with glucocorticoids will reduce the rate of recurrence of Crohn disease.
E) GI fistulae and abscesses are rare complications of Crohn disease.

Discussion

The correct answer is "B." Crohn disease and UC are both relapsing/remitting diseases. Up to 30% of initial exacerbations of Crohn disease will remit without any intervention. While there is a genetic component to inflammatory bowel disease (IBD) (up to a 100-fold increase in risk among first-degree relatives with IBD), no single, autosomal-dominant gene has been identified. "C" is incorrect because half or more of patients with Crohn disease will ultimately require some sort of surgery. "D" is incorrect. Unfortunately, chronic glucocorticoid administration does not lower the rate of relapse. There are many complications of IBD (see next question), and GI abscesses and fistulae occur with a relatively high frequency (20–40%) in Crohn disease.

> HELPFUL TIP: Although considered a disease of young adults, there is a bimodal distribution of IBD with a second peak in the 70s.

Extraintestinal features of IBD include all of the following EXCEPT:

A) Alopecia.
B) Arthritis.
C) Sclerosing cholangitis.
D) Uveitis.
E) Cholelithiasis.

Discussion

The correct answer is "A." Alopecia is not an extraintestinal manifestation of IBD. Arthritis related to IBD (enteropathic arthritis) is fairly common and usually migratory in nature, involving the large joints. Spondyloarthropathy may also be seen. Sclerosing cholangitis and autoimmune hepatitis can occur and may be fatal. Eye disease may include uveitis and episcleritis. Importantly, the main treatment of extraintestinal manifestations is to treat the IBD. IBD spondyloarthropathy and pyoderma gangrenosum are important exceptions, as these do not always improve with treatment of the underlying IBD.

> HELPFUL TIP: Toxic megacolon is a potentially deadly complication of IBD that should be suspected in a patient with IBD who presents with fever, abdominal pain, and shock. Also consider other causes of intestinal obstruction.

* *

Returning to your patient, you next see her in the emergency department, where she presents with fever, abdominal pain, and bloody diarrhea. She is tachycardic and slightly hypotensive but alert and oriented. You suspect a relapse of her Crohn disease.

All of the following are important aspects of her management at this time EXCEPT:

A) Surgical consultation.
B) IV access and fluid administration.
C) Glucocorticoids.
D) Thalidomide.
E) Metronidazole.

Discussion

The correct answer is "D." Thalidomide has been used as chronic therapy for IBD, but it is not indicated in the acute setting. The patient should be stabilized, and this includes IV access and fluid resuscitation. An exacerbation (or relapse) of IBD can be treated with glucocorticoids in the acute setting, and antibiotics are often helpful. It appears that metronidazole has beneficial effects that are not solely due to its antimicrobial properties. In this patient, who may have an abscess or obstruction, further evaluation (e.g., labs and abdominal CT) and surgical consultation are necessary.

Which of the following is indicated in the long-term treatment of IBD?

A) Azathioprine.
B) Methotrexate.
C) 5-ASA moieties.
D) Loperamide.
E) All of the above.

Discussion

The correct answer is "E." All the options are indicated for the treatment of IBD. Of special note are the 5-ASA drugs (e.g., Pentasa and Asacol). These have fewer side effects than sulfasalazine and are the initial drugs of choice for maintenance, once control of symptoms has been obtained. Systemic steroids (e.g., prednisone) are useful acutely to induce remission but should be tapered and stopped as soon as possible.

Additional drugs for treatment of IBD include cyclosporine, 6-mercaptopurine (6-MP), infliximab, and adalimumab (just say Humira®, it's much easier), among others. Antidiarrheal drugs such as loperamide are useful to control symptoms. However, be sure to avoid antidiarrheal drugs in patients who may have impending toxic megacolon. Probiotics and lactose avoidance may also be useful (although there is less good evidence for these).

* *

Because of cost considerations, your patient will be discharged on sulfasalazine.

Which of the following is an absolute contraindication to the use of sulfasalazine?

A) Sulfa allergy.
B) Aspirin allergy.
C) Anemia.
D) A and B.
E) B and C.

Discussion

The correct answer is "D." Sulfasalazine contains both sulfa and salicylate moieties and thus is contraindicated in patients with sulfa or aspirin allergy.

Which of the following is LEAST likely to be a complication of infliximab (Remicade®, an anti-tumor necrosis factor (TNF)-alpha antibody) therapy for IBD?

A) Sepsis.
B) Headache.
C) Abdominal pain.
D) Diarrhea.
E) Anemia.

Discussion

The correct answer is "E." Anemia will generally improve with the treatment of IBD. Anemia in IBD is often due to a combination of iron deficiency and anemia of chronic disease, but IBD can cause an autoimmune hemolytic anemia as well. All of the rest are common—or particularly severe in the case of sepsis—complications of infliximab. In fact, ongoing infection is an absolute contraindication to the use of infliximab.

All of the following characteristics differentiate UC from Crohn disease EXCEPT:

A) The risk of colon cancer is greater in UC than in Crohn disease.
B) Histologically, UC appears as transmural disease, whereas Crohn disease involves only the mucosal and submucosal layers.
C) UC almost always involves the rectum, whereas Crohn disease may or may not.
D) In UC, the diseased segments are continuous, while "skip" areas of healthy bowel are seen in Crohn disease.

Discussion

The correct answer is "B." Histologically, UC involves only the mucosa and submucosal tissue, while Crohn disease is transmural. All of the other statements are true. UC involves the rectum in 95% of cases and advances proximally.

> HELPFUL TIP: Medical and surgical treatments of UC and Crohn disease are similar. Patients with long-standing UC with frequent relapses are candidates for colectomy.

> HELPFUL TIP: IBD increases the risk of colon cancer, so more frequent and earlier colonoscopies are recommended. Recommendations vary, but most recommend colonoscopy every 1–2 years in patients with UC after 8 years with disease. Screening parameters in those with Crohn disease is less well established.

> HELPFUL TIP: Indications for surgery in those with IBD include perforation, obstruction, massive hemorrhage, toxic megacolon, and severe and persistent disease that impair function or quality of life. Surgical resection should be considered for intolerable extracolonic disease including arthritis and skin lesions. However, ankylosing spondylitis (secondary to Crohn disease) and liver dysfunction do not respond to colectomy.

Objectives: Did you learn to . . .

- Diagnose IBD?
- Differentiate Crohn disease from UC?
- Manage a patient with IBD?
- Recognize extraintestinal manifestations and complications of IBD?

CASE 7

A 52-year-old woman complains of abdominal pain, bloating, and constipation. Her symptoms started about 5 years ago and became more bothersome within the last 6 months. She describes a dull pain in the left lower abdomen. This pain is alleviated by passing gas or having a bowel movement. The pain is generally related to eating, and she has had intermittent diarrhea and constipation with constipation predominating. Two years ago, she underwent a screening colonoscopy, which was completely normal. Her review of systems is notable for a weight gain of about 5 pounds within the last 3 years. She is taking only a multivitamin daily. Her physical examination is normal.

Which is the best next step?

A) Defecogram.
B) Barium enema.
C) Anorectal manometry.
D) TSH level.
E) Colonoscopy.

Discussion

The correct answer is "D." The patient's presentation with pain and constipation meets criteria for constipation-predominant irritable bowel syndrome (IBS) (see Table 7–3). This patient underwent colonoscopy for screening 2 years prior to presentation; so further evaluation for colon cancer ("B" and "E") can be delayed unless there is another indication. Secondary causes of constipation, such as hypothyroidism, medication side effects or hypercalcemia, should be ruled out as appropriate. Therefore, a TSH level should be obtained prior to deciding on additional diagnostic or therapeutic steps. At this point in time, anorectal manometry and defecogram are unnecessarily invasive procedures, and neither will help you to determine if this patient has IBS.

Table 7–3 ROME III CRITERIA FOR IRRITABLE BOWEL SYNDROME

Continuous or recurrent abdominal pain or discomfort, at least 3 days per month in the last 3 months, with symptoms starting at least 6 months prior to diagnosis, *and* associated with at least 2 of the following:

- Relief with defecation
- Change in stool frequency
- Change in stool form

Adapted from Longstreth GF, et al. Functional bowel disorders. *Gastroenterology*. 2006;130:1480. Copyright 2006, with permission from Elsevier.

* *

The patient is euthyroid. Hypercalcemia and other electrolyte abnormalities have been ruled out. Since she does not use medications other than the multivitamin, you decide to initiate treatment of IBS. Based on available evidence, you suggest using fiber supplements.

What do you tell your patient to expect?

A) Complete resolution of her symptoms.
B) Increase in stool frequency and stool volume with less need for straining.
C) Increase in stool frequency but worsened abdominal pain.
D) Decrease in abdominal pain and bloating.
E) Enlightenment and absolute bliss.

Discussion

The correct answer is "B." Although there is not much evidence for its efficacy, the mainstay of therapy for IBS is fiber. Fiber supplements increase stool volume and frequency and soften stools, thereby alleviating symptoms of constipation. While bowel habits can be successfully changed with bulking agents for constipation or loperamide for diarrhea-predominant IBS, pain is generally not affected by these measures. In fact, increased fiber intake may transiently worsen some symptoms due to fermentation and generation of gas, potentially resulting in flatulence or bloating. "E" requires special mention. Bliss and enlightenment can only occur with proper colon purging procedures provided at a very expensive resort!

HELPFUL TIP: IBS has a relatively good prognosis, and up to 60% of patients improve on placebos in trials, making it hard to show benefit of any treatment. There is no increase in mortality, and symptoms usually improve over time.

HELPFUL TIP: Regardless of the advertising, and even though the authors spin their results as positive, don't start all of your IBS patients on rifaximin (41% improved on rifaximin vs. 32% on placebo!). The NNT is 11 (which means 10 patients are paying up to $1200/month for no benefit), there are no long-term studies (and IBS is a long-term condition), and the benefit is modest at best (N Engl J Med 2011;364:22–32).

Which of the following has NOT demonstrated efficacy in IBS?

A) Peppermint oil.
B) Hyoscyamine.
C) St. John wort.
D) Psyllium.
E) All of the above are effective.

Discussion

The correct answer (and the one that does not work) is "C," St. John wort. With regard to the others, psyllium has an NNT of 11, hyoscyamine has an NNT of 5, and peppermint oil has an NNT of 2.5 (*BMJ* 2008; 337:a2313). Amazingly, St John wort is actually less effective than placebo! SSRIs and tricyclic antidepressants (TCAs) are also effective.

In terms of other drugs, Tegaserod (Zelnorm®) has been removed from the market because of cardiovascular side effects but is available on a "compassionate use" protocol for women with constipation-predominant IBS that have failed other treatments. Alosetron (Lotronex®) was approved for diarrhea-predominant IBS, removed from the market due to ischemic colitis, and re-released under a protocol similar to Zelnorm.

HELPFUL TIP: Some patients with constipation-predominant IBS will respond to oral SSRI medications such as fluoxetine or paroxetine that seem to increase bowel transit times.

Objectives: Did you learn to . . .

- Evaluate a patient with constipation?
- Diagnose and manage IBS?

CASE 8

A 32-year-old male complains about fatigue and episodic abdominal pain. His pain is located in the periumbilical region and the left lower quadrant. It is cramp-like in nature and is associated with flatulence and diarrhea. Passing gas alleviates his symptoms. He notes that milk and other dairy products worsen his symptoms. His weight has remained stable. His prior medical history, family and social history, and physical examination are unremarkable. Laboratory tests reveal hemoglobin of 11.5 g/dL and a normal blood glucose and TSH.

What is the most appropriate next step in your evaluation?

A) Lactose breath test.
B) Dietary trial of strict lactose avoidance.
C) Enteroclysis.
D) Colonoscopy.
E) Tissue transglutaminase antibody titer.

Discussion

The correct answer is "B." The patient's symptoms are consistent with lactose intolerance. He may have malabsorption secondary to lactose intolerance, which may be partially responsible for his anemia. If his symptoms resolve with a trial of a lactose-free diet, you have your diagnosis. Further follow-up should include rechecking his CBC and perhaps other studies, such as stool for occult blood. If these symptoms are new, he could have a secondary form of lactase deficiency (e.g., Crohn disease or bacterial overgrowth) or a coincidental problem with the absorption of this carbohydrate.

* *

The patient tries a lactose-free diet, but this is of no benefit and his abdominal cramping and diarrhea continue. At this point, you are considering additional diagnoses.

Which of the following is LEAST likely in this patient?

A) Bacterial overgrowth syndrome.
B) Gluten-sensitive enteropathy.
C) *Giardia lamblia*.
D) *C. difficile*.
E) Whipple disease.

Discussion

The correct answer is "E." It is unlikely that this patient has Whipple disease, which is a result of an infection with *Tropheryma whippelii*. Whipple disease is associated with nondeforming arthritis, weight loss, fever, diarrhea, etc. All of the others are possibilities in this patient. "A," bacterial overgrowth syndrome, presents with bloating, diarrhea, dyspepsia, and possible malabsorption and weight loss. It can occur as a result of bowel dysmotility, bowel redundancy or diverticula, chronic pancreatitis, etc. "B," gluten-sensitive enteropathy (nontropical or celiac sprue), presents with similar symptoms including malabsorption. "C," *Giardia* infection, can be chronic and presents with gas, diarrhea, and occasionally constipation. Finally, *C. difficile* infection (pseudomembranous colitis) can also be chronic in nature with chronic diarrhea and blood loss.

* *

You continue to work up this patient's diarrhea with stool cultures, stool for *C. difficile* toxin, direct immunofluorescence analysis for *Giardia* and *Cryptosporidium*, and three stools for ova and parasites. All of the studies are negative. You now turn your attention to possible bacterial overgrowth syndrome.

The best test(s) for bacterial overgrowth syndrome is (are):

A) Quantitative stool culture.
B) Stool leukocytes.
C) 72-hour fecal fat.
D) [14-C] d-xylose breath test.
E) B and D.

Discussion

The correct answer is "D." The d-xylose breath test takes advantage of the fact that the bacteria responsible for bacterial overgrowth syndrome (gram-negative aerobes) catabolize d-xylose. The breath test measures radioactive CO_2 that is formed as a result of bacterial breakdown of radioactive d-xylose. The glucose breath test, in which glucose is administered to the patient and breath hydrogen is measured, is also helpful and commonly used. However, it is less sensitive and specific than the d-xylose test and has a 30–40% false-negative rate. Workup of bacterial overgrowth syndrome should also include an upper GI endoscopy and possible small bowel biopsy. GI hypomotility, small bowel dilatation, or small bowel diverticula support the diagnosis of bacterial overgrowth syndrome. Of the others, "B," stool leukocytes are pretty useless in general and do not have a good correlation with infectious causes of diarrhea (high false-positive and false-negative rates). "C," fecal fat collection, is useful in documenting fat malabsorption syndromes, including those secondary to severe pancreatic insufficiency (e.g., cystic fibrosis with >90% pancreatic dysfunction) and short bowel syndrome.

HELPFUL TIP: Another option to diagnose bacterial overgrowth is empiric treatment for 7–10 days with medications to cover aerobes and anaerobes (cephalexin plus metronidazole, TMP/SMX plus metronidazole, amoxicillin/clavulanate). Definitive treatment may require surgical intervention to shorten the bowel, resect diverticula, etc.

* *

This patient's d-xylose test is negative and you consider the possibility of gluten-sensitive enteropathy (celiac disease).

Of the following, the BEST test for the diagnosis of gluten-sensitive enteropathy is:

A) Antiendomysial antibodies.
B) Tissue transglutaminase antibodies.
C) Antigliadin antibodies.
D) Radiolabeled wheat flour absorption test.
E) None of the above.

Discussion

The correct answer is "B." Tissue transglutaminase antibodies are sensitive and specific for severe gluten-sensitive enteropathy but may be falsely negative in mild-to-moderate cases. Antiendomysial IgA antibodies are also relatively sensitive and very specific for gluten-sensitive enteropathy. Antigliadin antibodies are less sensitive and specific and have fallen out of favor. The definitive test ("gold standard") is a small bowel biopsy and should be considered if your clinical suspicion is high and the patient has negative antibodies. Patients with positive antibodies should also have and endoscopy; the diagnosis should be confirmed by endoscopy and biopsy before committing the patient to a gluten-free diet for life.

HELPFUL TIP: Up to 1:200 Caucasians living in the United States may be affected with gluten-sensitive enteropathy (while 1:20 grocery store aisles appear to be devoted to gluten-free products).

* *

The results of his tissue transglutaminase test are positive. You educate him about gluten-sensitive enteropathy (celiac disease) and have an endoscopy performed. A small bowel biopsy demonstrated blunted villi with a significant increase in intraepithelial lymphocytes, consistent with gluten-sensitive enteropathy. With a gluten-free diet, the patient experiences a significant increase in his energy level. Two years later he comes for a routine visit. He has gradually reintroduced some wheat products into his diet and tolerates this very well.

What do you recommend?

A) Resume gluten-free diet.
B) Continue dietary challenge and repeat examination in 6 months.
C) Repeat small bowel biopsy.
D) Check tissue transglutaminase antibody titer.
E) Avoid wheat, but try barley or rye products.

Discussion

The correct answer is "A." While there is no good data on the benefit of a long-term gluten-free diet in patients who can tolerate small amounts of gluten, several factors argue for continuing a gluten-free diet. The first is that many patients will have subclinical nutrient deficiencies if they reintroduce gluten. For this reason, patients with gluten-sensitive enteropathy should be screened for osteoporosis and take a multivitamin. This is especially true in pediatric patients where deficiencies may lead to stunted growth. The second is that there is some data that patients who reintroduce gluten may have increased mortality from GI lymphoma despite the fact that they are tolerating the gluten well.

HELPFUL TIP: With a gluten-free diet, antibodies (tissue transglutaminase, antigliadin, antiendomysial) often return to normal levels.

HELPFUL TIP: Patients with gluten-sensitive enteropathy must be compulsive about their diet. Rice, corn, and soybean-based flours are safe to consume. Oats are often contaminated with wheat.

Objectives: Did you learn to . . .

- Evaluate a patient with diarrhea?
- Recognize clinical manifestations of gluten-sensitive enteropathy?
- Manage a patient with gluten-sensitive enteropathy?

CASE 9

A 22-year-old previously healthy male reports a 3-day history of explosive and watery diarrhea. He is having up to 6 bowel movements per day. He recalls eating at a new Mexican restaurant 5 days ago. His head sinks a little low as he recalls drinking a "fish bowl" sized margarita . . . or at least he **thinks** he remembers drinking it! He denies fever, blood in his stool, or recent travel. Multiple people ate the same food but he is the only one who is sick. His vital signs are normal (including supine and standing blood pressures), and the remainder of the physical exam is remarkable only for mild, diffuse abdominal tenderness.

What is the most likely diagnosis?

A) Celiac sprue.
B) Viral gastroenteritis.
C) Lactose intolerance.
D) Small bowel bacterial overgrowth.
E) *C. difficile* colitis.

Discussion

The correct answer is "B." This is always a dilemma. It can be difficult to differentiate acute gastroenteritis from food poisoning. What makes gastroenteritis more likely is that there is no clustering of cases among people who ate the same food. With only 3 days of symptoms, it would be premature to diagnose "A," "C," or "D." Without recent antibiotic exposure, "E" would be unlikely in an otherwise healthy male. See Table 7–4 for a differential diagnosis for diarrhea.

Table 7–4 DIFFERENTIAL DIAGNOSIS FOR DIARRHEA

Acute diarrhea
- Bacteria (e.g., *Campylobacter*, *Salmonella*, and *Clostridium*)
- Viruses (e.g., Norwalk and rotavirus)
- Parasites (e.g., *Giardia*)
- Protozoa (especially in HIV-infected patients)
- Medications
- Anything that causes chronic diarrhea

Chronic diarrhea
- Inflammatory (e.g., IBD and radiation enteritis)
- Osmotic (e.g., gluten-sensitive enteropathy and lactase deficiency)
- Secretory (e.g., Zollinger–Ellison syndrome and villous adenoma)
- Disordered motility (e.g., irritable bowel syndrome and overflow from fecal impaction)

What is the MOST appropriate next step in the care of this patient at this point?

A) Order a CBC.
B) Order electrolytes.
C) Order stool examination for ova and parasites.
D) Recommend hydration and antidiarrheals as needed.
E) Order an abdominal film.

Discussion

The correct answer is "D." No workup is needed for a mild case of acute diarrhea, since such cases are usually self-limited. Generally, the history and physical exam should provide the diagnosis and indicate need for further workup. Further workup and treatment are indicated if the patient has severe or bloody diarrhea, dehydration, systemic toxicity, or severe pain.

HELPFUL TIP: Patients with severe, bloody diarrhea, and fever (T >101 F, >6 stools per day) should be treated with a 3–5-day course of a fluoroquinolone while awaiting stool culture results. **Bloody diarrhea in an afebrile patient should suggest *Escherichia coli* 0157:H7.** These patients should **not** get antibiotics because of an increased risk of hemolytic–uremic syndrome.

* *

You treat the patient with oral rehydration and prochlorperazine for some nausea and he does well. He returns to see you a few weeks later after a trip to Mexico. He liked that fish bowl-sized margarita so much that he decided to go for an original (remember that we live in a college town… this could easily be true!). He has diarrhea that began a couple of days after his arrival in Cancun and has now been present for 5 days. (*Note:* this question was written before all of the beheadings in Mexico. We see no reason to change it now… it is still a good question. If it makes you feel better, just substitute Belize for Mexico.) He has had frequent, watery diarrhea with nausea but no vomiting. He has noticed no blood in the stool. He was very careful to avoid salads and water but did have some ice in a soft drink.

The most likely organism causing illness in this patient is:

A) *Salmonella*.
B) *Shigella*.
C) Enterotoxigenic *E. coli*.
D) Enterohemorrhagic *E. coli*.
E) *Campylobacter*.

Discussion

The correct answer is "C." Entero**toxigenic** *E. coli* is the most common cause of traveler diarrhea in patients traveling to Mexico. Entero**hemorrhagic** *E. coli* is less likely and should be associated with bloody diarrhea. The others are much less likely to be causes of traveler diarrhea.

HELPFUL TIP: Many physicians would not treat a patient with *Shigella* unless that patient is clinically ill (e.g., fever). Treatment with antibiotics is **relatively** contraindicated in *Salmonella* because it prolongs the carrier state. However, use judgment in the patient who is particularly ill.

Which of the following is/are appropriate for the treatment of this patient's traveler diarrhea (remember, he has no vomiting)?

A) Oral rehydration.
B) Antidiarrheals.

C) Eat any food (e.g., no need for a bland diet with slow advancement).
D) All of the above.
E) None of the above.

Discussion

The correct answer is "D." This patient has non-bloody diarrhea and no systemic signs, so it should be safe to treat him with antidiarrheal agents (e.g., loperamide) and avoid antibiotics. Oral rehydration is the rule unless a patient is too nauseated or has some other reason that he cannot take adequate fluids by mouth. Patients (including children) should eat anything they can tolerate. The concept of "gut rest" is passe and actually leads to increased bowel permeability and more persistent diarrhea. **Lactose deserves special mention.** The American Academy of Pediatrics has changed their recommendations about lactose in diarrhea. They recommend withholding lactose **only** in children less than 3 months of age. This seems to be the group in which transient lactase deficiency occurs.

> HELPFUL TIP: *Klebsiella oxytoca* can produce an antibiotic-related diarrhea that is indistinguishable from *C. difficile*. In those with a negative stool for *Clostridium* antigen, consider (1) false-negative test (some of the newer strains of *Clostridium* are not detected by traditional stool antigen) or (2) *K. oxytoca* or (3) the *C. difficile* toxin degenerates rapidly at room temperature (no toxin may be detectable after 2 hours of exposure to room temperatures) or (4) ELISA tests generally only test for Type A antigen. The patient may have an antigen Type B producing strain **or** there may be a mutation of antigen Type A.

Objectives: Did you learn to . . .

- Evaluate a patient with acute diarrhea?
- Treat acute diarrhea?
- Recognize different bacterial causes of diarrhea?

CASE 10

A 49-year-old man comes to your office, requesting testing for hepatitis C. He recently attended his 25-year college reunion where an old friend he had "partied" with during experimentation with injectable drugs related that he has cirrhosis due to hepatitis C. The patient is otherwise healthy and denies any symptoms except for occasional fatigue after a long day at work. Physical examination of the patient is unremarkable. There are no stigmata of chronic liver disease.

Which of the following is the most appropriate course of action?

A) Check a quantitative Hepatitis C virus (HCV) PCR ("viral load").
B) Order a recombinant immunoblot assay (RIBA).
C) Order HCV antibody test (enzyme immunoassay).
D) Order a qualitative HCV PCR.
E) Order ALT and AST.

Discussion

The correct answer is "C." The sensitivity and specificity of the present-day HCV antibody test are excellent; thus, this is the best test to perform in this situation. Rarely, patients with immunologic impairment, such as HIV infection, have HCV viremia without detectable antibody, but this would not be a concern in this otherwise healthy patient. Quantitative HCV PCR is not a reliable means for diagnosing HCV infection because currently used methods are insensitive at low levels of viremia; thus, infection cannot be ruled out if the level of HCV viremia is below the lower limit of detection of the test. RIBA is an old test that is no longer used. **Qualitative** HCV PCR is the most sensitive test for the presence of HCV RNA, with a limit of detection that is lower than that of quantitative PCR. It is useful to establish the presence of viremia, but is more expensive than antibody testing and thus not a first-line test. Many patients with chronic HCV infection have normal liver enzymes and can still have progressive disease; therefore, in a high-risk patient, ALT and AST are not appropriate for screening for HCV.

* *

The patient returns several weeks later to discuss his test results. His HCV antibody test is positive. A liver panel obtained that day shows an ALT of 48 IU/L (normal range, 0–20) and an AST of 39 IU/L (0–31). His albumin and total bilirubin are within normal limits. He is extremely anxious about his liver.

To most accurately assess the degree of liver disease, your next step is to:

A) Obtain a liver–spleen scan to assess for evidence of cirrhosis.
B) Reassure the patient that his mild liver test abnormalities rule out cirrhosis.
C) Refer for percutaneous liver biopsy.
D) Order abdominal ultrasound with Doppler's to assess for evidence of cirrhosis.
E) Obtain abdominal CT to assess for evidence of cirrhosis.

Discussion

The correct answer is "C." Having established that the patient has hepatitis C with elevated liver enzymes, the next step is to determine the severity of his liver disease. Although his liver function tests are reassuring, it does not exclude the possibility of advanced fibrosis or even well-compensated cirrhosis. You would not be incorrect to order ultrasound imaging in addition to the liver biopsy.

* *

The patient agrees to a liver biopsy, which is scheduled for the following week. Nonetheless, he is still very concerned about his situation and asks what you think the chances are that he already has cirrhosis.

Regarding the development of progressive liver disease in hepatitis C, all of the following are true EXCEPT:

A) Approximately 20% of patients with chronic HCV infection will develop serious liver disease.
B) Heavy alcohol use is a risk factor for development of serious liver disease.
C) Acquisition of HCV infection after the age of 40 is associated with increased risk of developing serious liver disease.
D) HCV genotype impacts on the probability of developing end-stage liver disease.
E) Males are more likely than females to develop serious liver disease.

Discussion

The correct answer is "D." While only a minority of persons infected with HCV develop serious liver disease (20%), the likelihood of progression is difficult to predict in an individual patient. Nonetheless, male gender, heavy alcohol use, and acquisition of HCV infection after age 40 are associated with increased risk of progressive liver disease, while genotype is not. Additionally, Japanese ancestry, acquisition of hepatitis C from a blood transfusion, and daily marijuana use have been associated with an increased risk of progression.

HELPFUL TIP: Patients who have a persistently normal ALT, acquired hepatitis C before age 35, are female, do not drink alcohol, and have minimal or no fibrosis on liver biopsy are unlikely to progress to end-stage liver disease.

* *

The patient is concerned that he may transmit the virus to his wife or children. They are tested and are found to be negative for HCV antibody. He is relieved but asks for advice to prevent infecting them.

You tell him all of the following EXCEPT:

A) No change in sexual practices is recommended for couples in a long-term monogamous relationship in which one partner is HCV+ and the other HCV−.
B) The use of condoms is recommended for couples in a long-term monogamous relationship in which one partner is HCV+ and the other HCV−.
C) Hepatitis C is not spread by hugging, sneezing, or sharing a drinking glass.
D) Household members of persons infected with HCV should not share items that might be contaminated with small amounts of blood such as razors or nail clippers.
E) Parenteral exposure to infected blood is a major route of transmission of HCV.

Discussion

The correct answer is "B." HCV is spread by parenteral contact with infected blood. In contrast to hepatitis B, sexual transmission of HCV is inefficient and appears to be a minor route of spread. Additionally, the efficacy of latex condoms in preventing disease is not known. **The NIH and the USPHS do not recommend condom use for patients in a stable, long-term, and monogamous relationship. That**

said, using condoms will likely reduce an already low risk even further.

* *

The patient's liver biopsy shows mild-to-moderate inflammatory activity and portal and periportal fibrosis (stage 2). He is relieved to find out that he does not have cirrhosis, but remains very concerned about his hepatitis and wants to do everything possible to "get rid of" the hepatitis C. He asks about treatment of his HCV.

You tell him which of the following?

A) Combination therapy with interferon and ribavirin results in sustained virologic responses (SVR) in 40–70% of patients treated.
B) Combination therapy with interferon and ribavirin can cause numerous side effects including cytopenias, flu-like symptoms, worsening of autoimmune conditions, depression, and hemolytic anemia.
C) The HCV genotype is a strong predictor of response to treatment.
D) Newer treatment regimens including protease inhibitors (telaprevir and boceprevir) are much more effective than the tradition combination of interferon/ribavirin.
E) All of the above.

Discussion

The correct answer is "E." But, "A," combination therapy with interferon and ribavirin is the old treatment of HCV. The HCV genotype **was** a major factor determining the likelihood of achieving sustained virological response (SVR), although not the likelihood of progression to end-stage liver disease. Genotype 1 (including 1a and 1b) is the most difficult to clear, while genotypes 2 and 3 are the most responsive to treatment. Stage of fibrosis is also a factor, with patients with stages 3 and 4 (bridging fibrosis and cirrhosis) being less likely to achieve SVR. Higher baseline viral levels also tend to predict poorer response to treatment. Combination therapy is expensive and is associated with significant toxicities. The major concerns with ribavirin are hemolytic anemia and teratogenicity, while the interferons (standard or the long-acting pegylated forms) have a long list of potential side effects, of which neuropsychiatric problems, such as depression and irritability, are often the most troublesome.

OK now the game changer: Telaprevir and boceprevir are protease inhibitors that have shown benefit in genotype 1 hepatitis C. For now, they are being used in combination with interferon and ribavirin. However, recent studies suggest they may be just as effective without the use of interferon, the side effects of which are a major limitation to the current regimens. It is not clear if the protease inhibitors are effective against genotypes 3 and 4 but they do have some activity against genotype 2.

Objectives: Did you learn to . . .

- Evaluate a patient at risk for hepatitis C?
- Understand the natural history of the disease process in hepatitis C?
- Describe the transmission of hepatitis C?
- Discuss treatment issues for a patient with hepatitis C?

CASE 11

A 24-year-old female graduate student from China comes to your office complaining of fatigue for the past month. She has also had a poor appetite and has lost about 3 pounds over this period. She reports that she was told that she had "hepatitis" when she was about 10 years old but does not recall what type. She is otherwise healthy and takes no medications. She has no history or percutaneous exposures or blood transfusion. Her grandfather died of "liver cancer."

Physical examination reveals a thin, tired-appearing woman. The liver edge is palpable 2 cm below the right costal margin and is slightly tender. There is no ascites, splenomegaly, or cutaneous stigmata of chronic liver disease.

Laboratory studies are remarkable for mild anemia (hemoglobin 9.1 g/dL). Liver tests reveal elevated aminotransferases (ALT 289 IU/L, AST 158 IU/L), albumin 3.2 g/dL, and total bilirubin 1.5 mg/dL (normal 0.2–1.0 mg/dL).

Diagnostic possibilities at this point include:

A) Hepatitis A.
B) Hepatitis B.
C) Hepatitis C.
D) Autoimmune hepatitis.
E) All of the above.

Discussion

The correct answer is "E." Constitutional symptoms such as fatigue and anorexia can be seen with any form of acute or chronic liver disease; thus, they are not helpful in establishing a differential diagnosis. The first priority is to rule out infectious hepatitis including hepatitis A, B, and acute hepatitis C. Autoimmune hepatitis deserves consideration, particularly in female patients. While HCV infection is a worldwide problem, HBV infection is endemic in Asia and Africa, and the possibility of chronic hepatitis B also warrants special attention in this patient.

Appropriate laboratory studies at this point include which of the following?

A) Quantitative HCV PCR.
B) Hepatitis B surface antigen (HBsAg).
C) Anti-hepatitis A antibodies (IgG and IgM).
D) B and C.
E) All of the above.

Discussion

The correct answer is "D." As discussed previously, the quantitative HCV PCR is not a useful test for diagnosing HCV infection. HCV antibody testing would be a better choice. Both HBsAg and anti-HAV are useful tests in this patient. HBsAg is helpful to assess for HBV infection (acute and chronic) and anti-HAV antibodies will rule out acute hepatitis A infection. A positive total anti-HAV (positive IgG) with a negative IgM would indicate past infection, while a positive IgM would suggest acute HAV infection. Interpreting the HBV antigens (Ag) and antibodies (Ab) can be confusing, and Table 7–5 may help.

* *

The patient's results show a positive HbsAg, indicating ongoing hepatitis B infection. She is immune to hepatitis A and is hepatitis C negative.

After being out of contact for 4 months, she returns for a follow-up visit. She tells you that she took an herbal medicine her mother sent from China and has been feeling much better recently. Her HBsAg remains positive, but her liver enzymes, albumin, and total bilirubin are now completely normal.

Appropriate actions at this time include:

A) Treatment with interferon-alpha 5 million units daily for 16 weeks.
B) Order hepatitis Be antigen, anti-HBe, and HBV DNA level.
C) Begin periodic screening for hepatocellular carcinoma with ultrasound and alpha-fetoprotein (AFP).
D) A and C.
E) B and C.

Discussion

The correct answer is "E." The HBe antigen reflects viral replication. Loss of HBeAg indicates decreased viral replication and less of a risk of progression to cirrhosis. Loss of HBeAg may occur spontaneously; it is also the therapeutic endpoint of antiviral treatments of HBV infection (interferon, lamivudine, adefovir). If she is negative for HBeAg and is anti-HBe antibody positive (anti-HBe +) or has low or undetectable levels of HBV DNA, she has a low level of viral replication and will not benefit further from antiviral treatment.

Her liver panel should be monitored periodically, as should the AFP and ultrasound. Even asymptomatic HBV carriers with minimal liver disease are at risk for hepatocellular carcinoma, and screening is recommended in chronic HBV carriers (men >40 years old, women >50 years old, in those with family a history of HCC, in cirrhotic patients and in those of African ancestry >20 years of age). Our patient had positive family history of HCC.

Table 7–5 HEPATITIS B VIRAL SEROLOGIES FOR DIFFERENT PHASES OF INFECTION

Antigen/Antibody	Acute	Chronic	Recovered	Vaccinated/Immune
HBsAg	+	+	−	−
HBeAg	+	+	−	−
Anti-HBsAb	−	−	+	+
Anti-HBcAb	+ (IgM)	+ (IgG)	+ (IgG)	−
Anti-HBeAb	−	+/−	+	−
HBV DNA	+	+/−	+/−	−

HBs, surface antigen or antibody; HBc, core antigen or antibody; HBe, "e" antigen or antibody; Ag, antigen; Ab, antibody.

* *

The patient returns to discuss the results of her tests. Laboratory results show that she is positive for HBsAg and is anti-HBe positive. Her HBV DNA is undetectable using an unamplified assay, making her a carrier without evidence of viral replication (no chronic, active, hepatitis B). AFP is within limits and abdominal ultrasound is unremarkable. She continues to feel well. She also tells you that she will be getting married in 2 months. She asks you what can be done to prevent her fiancé and future children from becoming infected with HBV.

All of the following are accurate responses to her question EXCEPT:

A) No special precautions need to be taken because she has undetectable HBV and is therefore not infectious.
B) If her fiancé has not been immunized against HBV, he should be tested and vaccinated if not immune.
C) If her fiancé is not immune to HBV, they should use barrier contraceptives (e.g., condoms) until he has completed his HBV vaccination series.
D) She should cover any open cuts or scratches with a bandage and clean up any blood spills with bleach.
E) Administration of hepatitis B immune globulin (HBIG) and HBV vaccination begun immediately after birth is 95% effective in preventing perinatal transmission of HBV.

Discussion

The correct answer is "A." Although patients with higher levels of HBV DNA are more infectious than those with lower levels of viral DNA, the risk of transmission in the latter case is not zero. In the case of this patient, having "undetectable" HBV DNA simply indicates a level of HBV DNA that falls below the limit of detection of an unamplified assay (on the order of 10^5 copies/mL). Also, the positive HbsAg means she is still a carrier. Thus, precautions should be taken to prevent sexual or household transmission to her fiancé (use of condoms, immunization if required, etc.) and to her future children (HBIG and HBV vaccination).

VERY HELPFUL (IF LONG) TIP: **ALT and AST can be elevated secondary to:**

- **Viral agents**: Hepatitis (A, B, C, D, E), CMV, Epstein–Barr virus, and other viruses.
- **Drugs and chemicals**: Acetaminophen overdose, the "glitizones," HMG-CoA reductase inhibitors, INH, griseofulvin, anticonvulsants, NSAIDs, chemicals (carbon tetrachloride, etc.), alcohol, and many other agents.
- **Primary liver diseases**: Primary sclerosing cholangitis, primary biliary cirrhosis (positive antimitochondrial antibody (AMA)).
- **Metabolic diseases**: Wilson disease (decreased ceruloplasmin), hemochromatosis, alpha$_1$-antitrypsin deficiency, and cystic fibrosis.
- **Mechanical difficulties**: Ductal obstruction secondary to common duct stone or carcinoma (especially pancreatic, hepatoma, metastatic), Budd–Chiari syndrome (thrombosis of the hepatic vein).
- **Cholestasis** from central venous nutrition (CVN), pregnancy, or ceftriaxone therapy.
- **Infiltrative processes**: Fatty liver (especially those with diabetes, hypothyroidism, obesity; determine by U/S), amyloid, granulomatous hepatitis, liver abscess (including amebic or echinococcal; diagnosis by U/S or CT; may have eosinophilia), AIDS-related lymphoma, or other neoplasm.
- **Other**. Congestive heart failure (CHF), celiac sprue, muscle diseases (e.g., polymyositis).

Alkaline phosphatase may be elevated secondary to:

- Pregnancy, type O or B blood after a fatty meal.
- **Liver**: Cholestasis, partial obstruction of the biliary ducts, primary sclerosing cholangitis, adult bile ductopenia, primary biliary cirrhosis, sarcoidosis, and other granulomatous disease.
- **Bone diseases** such as Paget disease and metastatic disease.

For elevated liver tests, workup should include (in approximate order, which may vary depending on patient presentation):

- Rule out toxin exposure (alcohol, drugs).
- Hepatitis A, B, and C serology.
- Serum Fe, TIBC, transferrin saturation (hemochromatosis).
- Ultrasound or CT imaging (ultrasound first).

- mANA and antismooth muscle antibody (autoimmune hepatitis but only 28–40% sensitive).
- Serum alpha$_1$-antitrypsin.
- Serum protein electrophoresis (elevated levels in autoimmune hepatitis, 80% sensitive).
- Antiendomysial antibodies or tissue transglutaminase (gluten-sensitive sprue).
- Serum ceruloplasmin (Wilson disease).

Objectives: Did you learn to . . .

- Generate a differential diagnosis for patients with abnormal liver enzymes?
- Identify patients at risk for hepatitis B?
- Use the various hepatitis B antigens and antibodies to determine a patient's infection status?
- Describe the route of transmission of hepatitis B?

QUICK QUIZ: HEPATITIS C

All of the following are significant side effects of interferon therapy for hepatitis C EXCEPT:

A) Depression.
B) Hypoglycemia.
C) Aggression and homicidal behavior.
D) Myalgias.
E) Leukopenia.

Discussion

The correct answer is "B." Interferon therapy is fraught with adverse effects including those listed above. Flu-like symptoms of myalgias, malaise, fever, chills, headache, and weight loss are particularly common.

CASE 12

A 73-year-old man comes to your office, complaining of abdominal and ankle swelling, decreased energy, and poor appetite for the past 2 months. He dates the onset of his symptoms to a "reaction" to penicillin given for dental work. He says that before taking the penicillin, he was in excellent health and walked 3 miles per day. Now he is too weak and tired to even care for his own yard.

His past medical history is remarkable for coronary artery bypass surgery done 6 years ago. He also recalls having "yellow jaundice" (as opposed to the purple kind . . .) when he was stationed in Korea. He has no significant family history. He "drank a bit" on the weekends when he was in the service but has drunk very little alcohol in the past 50 years. He also quit smoking about 50 years ago. His medications are aspirin 81 mg daily and ibuprofen 600 mg as needed for knee pain due to degenerative joint disease.

Diagnostic considerations suggested by the history should include which of the following?

A) Adverse drug reaction to penicillin.
B) Malignancy.
C) Cirrhosis.
D) CHF.
E) All of the above

Discussion

The correct answer is "E." The patient's history of abdominal and lower extremity swelling suggests fluid overload. Penicillin is known to cause interstitial nephritis and secondary nephrotic syndrome, which can lead to fluid retention. Sources of fluid overload besides the kidneys should be considered in this patient, including liver and heart disease. Malignancy, especially with liver involvement, can cause ascites. He is on an NSAID, which can cause fluid retention, although rarely to this degree.

* *

Physical examination reveals a fragile-appearing elderly man with temporal wasting. There is no JVD. The lungs are clear to auscultation. The heart sounds are regular, with no murmurs or gallops. The abdomen is protuberant with bulging flanks. Shifting dullness is present. There is 2+ ankle edema bilaterally and scattered telangiectasias on skin exam. He has no asterixis.

Which of the following findings would you expect on laboratory exam?

A) Elevated hemoglobin and HCT (17.5 gm/dL and 55%).
B) Decreased platelet count of 80,000/mm^3.
C) Elevated serum albumin.
D) BUN/Cr ratio <20.
E) All of the above.

Discussion

The correct answer is "B." This patient likely has portal hypertension given his ascites and stigmata of liver disease (spider angiomata/telangiectasias). Blood is shifted toward the spleen because of the increased portal pressure (the blood, like the rest of us, likes the path of least resistance). Shunting of blood through the spleen results in thrombocytopenia through increased platelet destruction. "A" is wrong since liver patients often have anemia. "C" is incorrect because liver patients frequently have a low albumin. And, "D," a BUN/Cr ratio <20 is associated with intrinsic kidney disease (see Chapter 5).

* *

Diagnostic paracentesis is performed and approximately 50 mL of clear light yellow fluid are obtained.

Appropriate laboratory studies on the ascitic fluid include which of the following?

A) pH.
B) Albumin.
C) Lactate.
D) Triglycerides.
E) All of the above.

Discussion

The correct answer is "B." The ascitic fluid albumin is needed to calculate the serum-ascites albumin gradient (SAAG), which is helpful to distinguish between ascites resulting from portal hypertension from ascites due to other causes. Lactate and pH have been proposed as markers for spontaneous bacterial peritonitis (SBP) but have proven to be unreliable. Measurement of triglycerides is useful to confirm chylous ascites; however, in the absence of grossly milky-appearing fluid, there is no need to perform this test.

> HELPFUL TIP: In addition to albumin, all ascitic fluid should be sent for cell count and cultures. A cell count showing ≥ 250 polymorphonuclear leukocytes/mm^3 is presumptive evidence of SBP. Gram stain is nearly useless since bacterial counts are low enough that bacteria are rarely seen on Gram stain.

* *

Your patient's lab tests reveal an ascitic fluid total protein is 2.5 g/dL with an albumin of 1.9 g/dL. A liver panel reveals normal aminotransferases, normal bilirubin, serum albumin 3.3 g/dL, and alkaline phosphatase 147 IU/L. Electrolytes, BUN, and creatinine are within normal limits.

Which of the following is the most accurate interpretation of these results?

A) The SAAG is 1.7, which is consistent with portal hypertension as its cause.
B) The SAAG is 1.7, which rules out portal hypertension as its cause.
C) The SAAG is 1.4, which is consistent with portal hypertension as its cause.
D) The SAAG is 1.4, which rules out portal hypertension as its cause.
E) The serum-ascites gradient confuses me, so I don't want to do it.

Discussion

The correct answer is "C." The SAAG can tell us whether the fluid is a transudate or exudate. The SAAG is simply the difference between the serum albumin and the ascitic fluid albumin, or $3.3 - 1.9 = 1.4$, in this case. **A SAAG of $\geq$ 1.1 indicates portal hypertension with 97% accuracy.** Remember this by remembering that a high SAAG means high pressure in the portal system.

> HELPFUL TIP: Ascites from any cause of portal hypertension will have a high SAAG. Aside from cirrhosis, portal hypertension also may result from schistosomiasis, sarcoidosis, portal vein thrombosis (Budd–Chiari syndrome), congenital hepatic fibrosis, CHF, myxedema, etc. **Causes of a low SAAG include** serositis from connective tissue disorders, nephrotic syndrome, pancreatic-related ascites, and peritoneal carcinomatosis among others.

In addition to a complete evaluation to determine the cause of his portal hypertension, which of the following is/are appropriate action(s) at this time?

A) Refer the patient to a nutritionist for instruction on a low-sodium diet.

B) Discontinue ibuprofen and prescribe a COX-2-selective inhibitor for arthritis.
C) Prescribe spironolactone 100 mg daily and furosemide 40 mg daily.
D) A and C.
E) A, B, and C.

Discussion

The correct answer is "D." The initial approach to the management of ascites due to portal hypertension is sodium restriction and diuretics. The goal is a 2-g sodium diet (which is impossible to follow). The majority of patients will **not** have an adequate response to sodium restriction alone, so it is reasonable to begin diuretics at the outset. Spironolactone, which is an aldosterone antagonist, is useful because portal hypertension is a state of hyperaldosteronism. Spironolactone tends to cause hyperkalemia, an effect that can be mitigated by the coadministration of furosemide. Once-daily doses are appropriate for initial therapy; adjustments are made based on the patient's electrolytes, renal function, and response to treatment. NSAIDs should be avoided, due to sodium retention and GI bleeding. **COX-2-selective inhibitors have no advantage over nonselective NSAIDs in this regard.** Other approaches to the patient's knee pain should be considered, including intra-articular injections, acetaminophen (up to 2 g daily is likely safe in cirrhosis), and narcotics, provided encephalopathy is not a problem.

* *

A few months later, your patient comes to the emergency department "feeling sick." He complains of diffuse abdominal pain and swelling, stating that his abdomen feels "tense." On examination, you find a pale, uncomfortable male with a temperature of 38.3°C. His other vital signs are normal. His abdomen is tense, distended, and diffusely tender with hypoactive bowel sounds. You perform a paracentesis that shows 400 polymorphonuclear leukocytes/mm^3.

What is the most appropriate next step in the evaluation and treatment of this patient?

A) Discharge to home with increased doses of spironolactone and furosemide.
B) Discharge to home with amoxicillin and the same doses of diuretics.
C) Perform a large-volume paracentesis for symptomatic relief and discharge to home.
D) Admit to the hospital and start IV ceftriaxone.
E) Admit to the hospital and place a peritoneal tube for drainage.

Discussion

The correct answer is "D." This patient meets criteria for spontaneous bacterial peritonitis (SBP) ($\geq$250 polymorphonuclear leukocytes/mm^3 in the ascites fluid) and has clinical findings to suggest infection. This patient could become unstable quickly, so discharge from the emergency department is not recommended. Increasing doses of diuretics and/or large-volume paracentesis may be required, but these interventions should only be considered in the setting of hospital admission. Broad-spectrum antibiotics are the standard of care for SBP, and IV third-generation cephalosporins (ceftriaxone, cefotaxime) are typically the first-line agents in hospitalized patients. Amoxicillin ("B") is not sufficient.

In addition, albumin in the dose of 1.5 g/kg on day 1 followed by 1 g/kg on day 3 reduces the chance of renal failure and death and therefore should be given to all patients with SBP. Further studies of this are pending. Also, send the ascites fluid for culture. Blood cultures, CBC, and serum chemistries and PT/PTT should be obtained as well. Consider imaging the abdomen with ultrasound or CT. Further tests should be ordered as indicated.

> **HELPFUL TIP:** The most common organisms in SBP include *Streptococcus pneumoniae, E. coli,* and *Klebsiella.*

> **HELPFUL TIP:** Fluoroquinolones and TMP/SMX have been used to decrease the frequency of SBP episodes. Prophylaxis is indicated in anyone with an episode of SBP, an ascitic fluid albumin of <1.5 g/dL especially if the Cr >1.2 mg/dL, the Na is <130 mg/dL or the BUN >25 mg/dL.

Objectives: Did you learn to . . .

- Generate a differential diagnosis for ascites?
- Analyze ascitic fluid to determine potential causes of ascites?

- Initiate treatment of a patient with ascites?
- Diagnose and manage SBP?

CASE 13

A 42-year-old male with known hepatitis C who is also a heavy drinker presents to your office because of increasing confusion. He hasn't noticed much of anything (hey, most of his life has been like this . . .), but his family states that he is somewhat confused and on occasion difficult to wake up. He has a known history of end-stage liver disease. He is supposed to be on a low-protein diet but decided that it was time to start the Atkin low-carbohydrate diet to "lose that gut" (he even found himself a "low carb" beer). So, he has increased his intake of protein.

Which of the following is NOT a common cause of hepatic encephalopathy?

A) GI bleeding.
B) Constipation.
C) High-carbohydrate diet.
D) Up-regulation of GABA receptors.

Discussion

The correct answer is "C." High-carbohydrate diets are not associated with hepatic encephalopathy. Alternatively, high-protein diets are associated with hepatic encephalopathy as is answer "D," up regulation of GABA receptors in the CNS. Similarly, a GI bleed ("A") delivers a large protein load to the GI tract. **Thus, any patient with hepatic encephalopathy should be evaluated for a GI bleed.** Other causes of acute hepatic encephalopathy include constipation, sedative use (e.g., benzodiazepines), and hypokalemic metabolic alkalosis.

HELPFUL TIP: An elevated ammonia level is associated with hepatic encephalopathy, although there is not a direct linear correlation between serum ammonia level and mental status.

* *

You decide to admit the patient to the hospital for treatment of his hepatic encephalopathy.

Which of the following IS NOT part of the treatment of hepatic encephalopathy secondary to alcohol use?

A) Lactulose.
B) Polyethylene glycol (e.g., GoLytely and MiraLax).
C) Oral antibiotics.
D) Fluid and electrolyte management.

Discussion

The correct answer is "B." Polyethylene glycol plays no role in the treatment of hepatic encephalopathy. While it would make intuitive sense that it would work since lactulose works, this is not the case. The mechanism of action of lactulose is dependent on bacterial metabolism of lactulose into lactic and acetic acids. This reduces the pH of the colon leading to precipitation of nonabsorbable ammonia in the colon, which reduces serum ammonia levels. **Enemas (soap suds, etc.), on the other hand, may help acutely** by removing colonic contents. "C" is of particular note. Oral antibiotics (neomycin, metronidazole and others) should be reserved for patients who do not respond to lactulose. Their efficacy is more limited.

* *

The patient does well on a regimen of lactulose and oral metronidazole.

What other problems do you need to worry about in this patient?

A) Elevated bleeding time.
B) Elevated PT/INR.
C) Thrombocytopenia.
D) A and B.
E) All of the above.

Discussion

The correct answer is "E." Patients with end-stage liver disease tend to have a lack of vitamin K-dependent clotting factors (and thus elevated PT/INR) and have thrombocytopenia due to shunting of blood from the liver to the splanchnic bed because of elevated portal pressures. However, 50,000 platelets are generally considered adequate. Additionally, it is likely that there is platelet dysfunction in cirrhosis, although the clinical significance is not clear.

* *

It turns out that this patient has also been drinking again, but he made it through his hospital stay without going through withdrawal. Esophageal varices were noted on EGD. He is ready for discharge.

Which of the options is indicated for this patient at the time of discharge, assuming he is hemodynamically stable?

A) Nadolol.
B) Isosorbide dinitrate.
C) Pentoxifylline.
D) Vitamin K.
E) All of the above.

Discussion

The correct answer is "E." All of the above are indicated in the further treatment of this patient. "A" and "B" will reduce portal pressures and reduce the risk of variceal bleeding. "C," pentoxifylline, has anti-TNF activity and reduces mortality when used acutely (at least in the first 4 weeks after an event of alcoholic hepatitis). "E," vitamin K, is indicated because of liver failure-induced coagulopathy.

HELPFUL TIP: Prednisolone (40 mg/day) and tapered over 2–4 weeks may have some benefit in severe alcoholic hepatitis. The evidence is contradictory, although it will probably be the right answer on the test.

* *

The patient does relatively well and abstains from alcohol. In addition to the medications noted above, you have the patient on spironolactone and furosemide and a low-salt diet to reduce edema and ascites. He seems to be following your instructions well but returns to the clinic because of increasing dyspnea, abdominal distention, and pain. On exam, he has no peritoneal signs but obviously has massive ascites. You are considering a large-volume paracentesis in your office.

Which of the following statements best reflects the current thinking on large-volume paracentesis?

A) A patient who has over 4 L of fluid removed should receive IV albumin.
B) There is no consistent data with regard to the use of albumin in large-volume paracentesis.
C) Under no circumstance should more than 5 L of ascites be removed at one time.
D) Given this patient's dyspnea, large-volume paracentesis is contraindicated.
E) If more than 10 L of ascites fluid is removed, and equal volume of normal saline should be replaced intravenously.

Discussion

The correct answer is "B." It is still unclear who needs albumin replacement. "A" is incorrect. There is clearly no need for albumin in patients who have less than 5 L of fluid removed. However, for patients who have more than 5 L of fluid removed, the standard of care is replacement with albumin although the data are limited. "C" is incorrect. In some studies, up to 10 L of ascitic fluid has been removed (don't try this one at home . . .). "D" is incorrect. In fact, respiratory compromise is one reason to do a large-volume paracentesis. Removal of fluid will help with diaphragmatic excursion and may help with the resolution of pleural effusions. "E" just sounds wrong, don't you agree? That's a lot of fluid shifting.

HELPFUL TIP: A meta-analysis of albumin in paracentesis was published that suggested 6–8 gm of albumin/liter of ascites removed be given those having more than 5l removed (*Heptalogy* 2012 Apr;55:1172).

* *

You remove 4 L of fluid via paracentesis, and the patient feels better. In the meantime, however, he has had a variceal bleed and has been hospitalized yet again. He needs something else done, and you refer him for a transjugular intrahepatic portosystemic shunt (TIPS) procedure to help reduce portal pressures, prevent the reaccumulation of ascites, and hopefully prevent further bleeding.

Which of the following statements best reflects the status of TIPS?

A) TIPS is ineffective in controlling acute variceal bleeding.
B) TIPS unequivocally improves survival from end-stage liver disease.
C) TIPS is associated with an increased risk of hepatic encephalopathy.
D) Once placed, TIPS remains effective for at least 3 years.
E) TIPS is only indicated for waiters, bar tenders, and cab drivers.

Discussion

The correct answer is "C." TIPS is clearly associated with an increased risk of hepatic encephalopathy. "A" is incorrect. TIPS is **effective** in controlling variceal bleeding. "B" is incorrect. In fact there may be some survival **disadvantage** to TIPS. However, the data is still equivocal. "D" is incorrect because TIPS shunts tend to clot and may need to be evaluated for patency by Doppler if ascites reaccumulates or other symptoms occur. Newer devices, however, tend to clot off less often.

HELPFUL TIP: Overdiuresis can lead to hepatorenal syndrome, which is characterized by oliguric renal failure. Sepsis, GI bleeding, etc. can also lead to hepatorenal syndrome. The mechanism has more to do with altered circulation to the kidneys from hepatic disease than with the diuresis itself.

Objectives: Did you learn to . . .

- Recognize causes of hepatic encephalopathy and identify patients at risk?
- Manage a patient with hepatic encephalopathy?
- Discuss risks and benefits of TIPS and large-volume paracentesis?

QUICK QUIZ: AUTOIMMUNE LIVER DISEASE

Which of the following is a marker for primary biliary cirrhosis?

A) Antimitochonrial antibodies (AMA).
B) Antismooth muscle antibodies.
C) $Alpha_1$-antitrypsin.
D) Polyclonal antibodies on serum protein electrophoresis.

Discussion

The correct answer is "A." AMA are found in primary biliary cirrhosis (95% sensitive and 98% specific). "B," antismooth muscle antibodies, are found in autoimmune hepatitis. "C," **reduced levels** of $alpha_1$-antitrypsin, are found in hepatitis from $alpha_1$-antitrypsin deficiency (surprise!). "D," polyclonal antibodies, are found in autoimmune hepatitis.

HELPFUL TIP: The diagnosis of sclerosing cholangitis is made by cholangiography, which demonstrates strictures and dilatation of intrahepatic and/or extrahepatic ducts.

CASE 14

A 31-year-old man comes to your office for evaluation of "abnormal liver tests." He had labs for disability insurance and the following was noted: elevated total bilirubin (2.1 mg/dL) with normal direct bilirubin. The AST, ALT, GGT, albumin, and alkaline phosphatase are normal. A CBC obtained at that time was unremarkable.

The patient feels generally well. When you ask about jaundice, he recalls that once when he was sick with the "flu" while in college, his roommate told him that he "looked a little yellow." He went to the student health service a few days later when he felt better and was told there was nothing to be concerned about. He drinks 6–8 beers/week and takes ibuprofen once or twice a month for knee pain.

Physical examination is unremarkable. A repeat liver panel shows a total bilirubin of 1.7 mg/dL with normal direct bilirubin and normal AST, ALT, and alkaline phosphatase. CBC and reticulocyte count are also normal. A blood smear, LDH, and haptoglobin are normal.

The most likely diagnosis is:

A) Crigler–Najjar syndrome type I.
B) Choledocholithiasis.
C) Gilbert syndrome.
D) Hemolytic anemia.
E) Occult acetaminophen abuse.

Discussion

The correct answer is "C." Gilbert syndrome is the most common inherited disorder of bilirubin metabolism, affecting up to 5% of Caucasians. It is characterized by isolated mild unconjugated hyperbilirubinemia, with serum bilirubin levels usually less than 3 mg/dL. However, bilirubin levels in patients affected with Gilbert syndrome can increase with fasting or during febrile illnesses, though rarely exceeding 6 mg/dL. Crigler–Najjar syndrome type I is a rare disorder leading to severe unconjugated neonatal jaundice and neurologic impairment due to kernicterus. Both choledocholithiasis and acetaminophen hepatotoxicity would be unlikely to cause an isolated increase in unconjugated bilirubin; the LFTs should be elevated with these. The normal blood smear, reticulocyte count, normal LDH, and normal haptoglobin make significant hemolysis unlikely. Thus, this presentation is most consistent with Gilbert syndrome.

* *

Several months later, the patient's older sister comes to see you. She had gone to a local health fair where screening liver tests were found to be abnormal. She recalled her brother mentioning something about a familial problem causing liver test abnormalities and wonders if she has the same thing.

She is 39 years old with good general health, although she wishes she could lose weight. She says she has been 30–40 pounds overweight for at least 10 years and is now at her heaviest weight ever. She is not taking any medications, drinks no alcohol, and is a nonsmoker. She denies any risk factors for viral hepatitis.

Physical examination reveals an obese woman. Blood pressure is 138/88; BMI is 35 kg/m^2. There is no scleral icterus or other cutaneous stigmata of chronic liver disease. The abdomen is protuberant with the liver edge palpable about 3–4 cm below the right costal margin and is slightly tender to palpation. There is no splenomegaly and no evident ascites.

Her liver panel from the health fair 3 months ago shows the following: ALT 87 IU/L (normal range, 0–20), AST 53 IU/L (0–31), alkaline phosphatase 110 IU/L (30–115), total protein 7.8 g/dL (6.0–8.0), albumin 4.2 g/dL (3.3–5.0), total bilirubin 0.9 mg/dL (0.2–1.0), and direct bilirubin 0.1 mg/dL (<0.2).

Appropriate steps at this time include all of the following EXCEPT:

A) Repeat the liver panel.
B) Counsel the patient that her labs suggest Gilbert syndrome.
C) Counsel the patient regarding weight loss.
D) Recommend a serologic evaluation to assess for chronic viral and autoimmune hepatitis if the liver test abnormalities persist.

Discussion

The correct answer is "B." As discussed above, Gilbert syndrome is defined by isolated unconjugated hyperbilirubinemia. This patient's pattern of liver test abnormalities with aminotransferase elevations clearly indicates a different type of problem. If these abnormalities persist, an evaluation for causes of chronic aminotransferase elevations is warranted (see differential earlier in this chapter of elevated liver enzymes). Chronic viral hepatitis and autoimmune hepatitis would be among the diagnostic considerations. Given the apparent hepatomegaly and tenderness on physical examination, an imaging study of the liver is also indicated.

* *

The repeat liver panel is remarkable for ALT 129 IU/L and AST 76 IU/L. The other tests are normal. HBsAg and HCV antibody are negative. Antinuclear and antismooth muscle antibodies are <1:40 (normal). The ultrasound examination shows an enlarged liver with increased echogenicity, suggestive of diffuse fatty infiltration.

Regarding nonalcoholic fatty liver disease (NAFLD), or nonalcoholic steatohepatitis (NASH), all of the following are true EXCEPT:

A) It is frequently associated with one or more features of the metabolic or insulin resistance syndrome.
B) It is more common in men than women.
C) The histologic features can closely mimic those of alcoholic hepatitis.
D) It may cause cirrhosis in a minority of patients.

Discussion

The correct answer is "B." NAFLD is more common in women and is among the most common causes of elevated liver enzymes. NAFLD refers to a spectrum of histologic findings that range from simple steatosis to an aggressive injury pattern. NAFLD often occurs in association with obesity, dyslipidemia, and/or glucose intolerance, hypothyroidism, and occurs more commonly in women than men. While most patients with NAFLD will not develop progressive liver disease, a minority are at risk to develop cirrhosis. Female gender and the presence of diabetes increase the risk of progression to cirrhosis.

HELPFUL TIP: Vitamin E 800 mg/BID has been shown to be helpful in NASH (*N Engl J Med* 2010;362:1675). Some physicians have also been using metformin although the data are sketchy.

In this patient with NAFLD, all of the following are appropriate actions EXCEPT:

A) Obtain a fasting lipid panel.
B) Obtain fasting serum glucose.

C) Recommend weight loss to get her BMI to the normal range.
D) Start a "glitizone."

Discussion

The correct answer is "D." Weight loss, including from gastric surgery, can improve NAFLD. However, too rapid weight loss may be counterproductive in the setting of NAFLD, as mobilization of peripheral fat stores may worsen hepatic steatosis. Also, addressing underlying metabolic illnesses (e.g., diabetes and hypothyroidism) would be important elements in treatment. Treating hyperlipidemia and diabetes can also improve NAFLD. Glitizones have been shown to be ineffective in NAFLD as has ursodeoxycholic acid.

HELPFUL TIP: In France, they force feed geese to produce fatty liver (Foie Gras). In the United States, we do it to ourselves...

Objectives: Did you learn to...

- Evaluate a patient with abnormal liver tests?
- Recognize the clinical and laboratory presentation of Gilbert syndrome?
- Describe findings of nonalcoholic liver disease?
- Manage a patient with "benign" liver disease?

QUICK QUIZ: GI BLEED

Which of the following has shown benefit in reducing mortality from variceal GI bleeding?

A) Vasopressin.
B) Somatostatin/octreotide.
C) Band ligation of varices.
D) TIPS.
E) C and D.

Discussion

The correct answer is "E." Unfortunately, while medical treatment may benefit the patient by reducing bleeding, there is no evidence that vasopressin or somatostatin reduce mortality. In fact, vasopressin may **increase** mortality because of associated GI ischemia. TIPS and ligation of varices via an endoscope have a positive impact on mortality. Somatostatin reduces rebleeding when used with endoscopic therapy but does not affect mortality.

CASE 15

A 70-year-old female presents to the emergency department complaining of midepigastric pain associated with vomiting. This started approximately 12 hours ago and now she notes vomiting, fever, and myalgias. Her vital signs are blood pressure 110/70, pulse 115, and temperature 38.5°C. On exam, the patient is quite tender in the midepigastric region with guarding and some rebound. Her past history is significant only for lone atrial fibrillation and a seizure disorder for which she is taking phenytoin.

Your next steps in the diagnosis of this patient should include all of the following EXCEPT:

A) Chest radiograph.
B) CBC.
C) Liver enzymes.
D) Abdominal CT with contrast.
E) Amylase.

Discussion

The correct answer is "D." An abdominal CT is not indicated in this patient as part of the initial workup. "A," an upright chest radiograph, is the single best plain radiograph for finding free abdominal air and is indicated for this reason. Additionally, the etiology of abdominal pain may also include pneumonia and other thoracic pathology that may be evident on a chest radiograph. Liver enzymes, amylase, and CBC are indicated since midepigastric pain with fever can be related to pancreatitis, acute cholecystitis, etc.

* *

The laboratory results are as follows: elevated AST and ALT (mild), normal amylase, mildly elevated white count (13.5×10^3 cells/mm^3), and elevated GGT.

The correct interpretation of these results is:

A) The patient does not have pancreatitis.
B) The elevated GGT is specific for biliary outlet obstruction.
C) The elevated AST and ALT may indicate biliary outlet obstruction.
D) None of the above.

Discussion

The correct answer is "C." Early in the course of biliary outlet obstruction (e.g., biliary colic and common duct stone), the AST and ALT may be mildly elevated. "A" is incorrect because the amylase is only 80% sensitive for pancreatitis. Twenty percent of patients with pancreatitis have a normal amylase—a false-negative test. "B" is incorrect because GGT is nonspecific. GGT is an inducible enzyme and can be elevated in response to alcohol and various medications including phenytoin.

HELPFUL TIP: In alcohol-related liver disease, the AST is generally 2× the ALT.

* *

The patient has a history of atrial fibrillation and is not on anticoagulation (appropriately since she has "lone atrial fibrillation" as defined by the new criteria; see the cardiology section). You are concerned that there may be bowel ischemia from an embolism.

Which of the following is true of mesenteric thrombosis and bowel ischemia?

A) Patients generally have guarding and rebound early in the course.
B) The pain is out of proportion to the exam and patients may have a normal initial exam.
C) A serum lactate level is helpful and specific for the diagnosis of bowel ischemia.
D) The best study to diagnose this disease entity is CT with contrast.

Discussion

The correct answer is "B." Patients with small bowel ischemia from either embolism or mesenteric thrombosis will generally present with severe abdominal pain and an exam that is unremarkable. Late in the course there will be guarding, rebound, and other peritoneal signs as the bowel perforates. However, early in the course of the illness, severe pain with a relatively benign exam is consistent with the presentation of bowel ischemia. "A" is incorrect for the reasons started above. "C" is incorrect because the serum lactate can be elevated in a number of states, not just bowel ischemia. However, abdominal pain plus lactic acidosis should raise the suspicion that there may be bowel ischemia. "D" is incorrect because radiographic findings on CT scan are present in only about 65% of patients with mesenteric thrombosis/embolism. The **best** study remains angiography.

* *

Since the patient's exam includes guarding and rebound, you put the diagnosis of bowel ischemia lower in your list of possibilities. Based on the elevated white count and elevated ALT and AST, you order an ultrasound of the right upper quadrant, which shows evidence of a common duct stone. There is thickening of the gallbladder wall but no pericolic fluid noted. You decide that there is a mild cholecystitis and want to admit the patient to the hospital. Clearly, this patient needs to be started on antibiotics.

Which antibiotic is the most appropriate choice for this patient?

A) IV clindamycin.
B) IV vancomycin.
C) IV gentamicin.
D) IV ampicillin/sulbactam.

Discussion

The correct answer is "D." The most appropriate antibiotic choice available for this patient is ampicillin/sulbactam (Unasyn). The main organisms that need to be covered are gram-negative organisms and anaerobes (*E. coli*, *Enterococcus*, *Klebsiella*, and *Enterobacter*). Ampicillin/sulbactam will cover all of these organisms. "A" is incorrect because clindamycin, while it covers gram positives and anaerobes, does not cover most gram-negative organisms. Additionally, many enterococci are resistant. "B" is incorrect because vancomycin only covers gram-positive organisms. "C" is incorrect because gentamicin does not cover anaerobic organisms. Other antibiotic options for treating this patient include cefotetan and cefoxitin, among others.

* *

The patient is admitted to the hospital. She is treated with ampicillin/sulbactam and pain medication.

The next step for this patient is:

A) Percutaneous "T" tube placement to drain the gallbladder.
B) 2 weeks of IV antibiotics followed by cholecystectomy.

C) Endoscopic retrograde cholangiopancreatography (ERCP) with sphincterotomy.
D) Lithotripsy.

Discussion

The correct answer is "C." The patient should have an ERCP with sphincterotomy in an attempt to retrieve the stone in her common bile duct. "A" is incorrect because in this healthy patient, percutaneous drainage would certainly be a third-line procedure. "B" is incorrect because the patient essentially has a closed abscess (the gallbladder blocked by a stone), which requires drainage. If the patient had cholecystitis **without** obstruction, prolonged antibiotics followed by cholecystectomy would be an option. However, **in patients with cholecystitis without obstruction outcomes are overall better with an early cholecystectomy.** "D" is also incorrect and would be a less desirable approach than is ERCP with sphincterotomy.

HELPFUL TIP: Studies have shown improved outcome in patients with severe gallstone pancreatitis and/or cholangitis that receive early (within 72 hours after admission) ERCP with biliary sphincterotomy.

* *

The ERCP is successful but the patient develops worsening pain in the midepigastric region.

Which of the following is the most common adverse consequence of ERCP?

A) Pancreatitis.
B) Contrast allergy.
C) Perforation.
D) Bleeding.
E) Sepsis.

Discussion

The correct answer is "A." Of the complications listed, pancreatitis is the most common, with an incidence of about 5% of patients after ERCP. In fact, elevations in pancreatic enzymes (mostly not significant) occur in up to 75% of patients post-ERCP. The others are less common and in order of descending incidence are bleeding, perforation, sepsis, and contrast allergy (rare).

* *

Although you suspect that this patient has pancreatitis secondary to the ERCP, you also consider other potential causes of pancreatitis.

All of the following are causes of pancreatitis EXCEPT:

A) Viral infection.
B) HMG-Co A reductase inhibitors (e.g., atorvastatin).
C) Alcohol.
D) Indinavir.
E) Spider bites.

Discussion

The correct answer is "E." The most common causes of acute pancreatitis are ethanol ingestion, biliary tract disease, and endoscopic procedures with biliary tract disease being the most common cause in the United States. "A" is true. Common viruses that can cause pancreatitis include HIV, hepatitis viruses, EBV, and Coxsackieviruses. "B" and "D" are true. Many other drugs can also cause pancreatitis: of note are didanosine (DDI), some diuretics, some NSAIDs, some antibiotics, etc. See Table 7–6 for more on drugs that cause pancreatitis. The venom of a scorpion bite can result in pancreatitis, but spider bites are not known to do so.

* *

You check laboratory studies and the patient does indeed have worsening pancreatitis from the ERCP. The surgeon on the case recommends against using

Table 7–6 DRUGS ASSOCIATED WITH PANCREATITIS

Drugs with Definitive Association	Drugs with Probable Association
Thiazide diuretics	Acetaminophen
Sulfonamides	Salicylates
Azathioprine/ 6-Mercaptopurine	Metronidazole
	Nitrofurantoin
Furosemide	Erythromycin
Estrogens	NSAIDs
Tetracycline	ACE inhibitors
Valproic acid	Methyldopa
Pentamidine	Steroids
Valproic acid	
Dideoxyinosine	

morphine and would prefer meperidine in this patient, mumbling something about that's the way they always did it in residency.

All of the following are true EXCEPT:

A) There is no evidence that meperidine is superior to morphine even in gallbladder and pancreatic disease.
B) Meperidine is more likely than morphine to cause seizures in this patient.
C) Meperidine is more likely than morphine to cause confusion and agitation in elderly patients.
D) When used in combination with an SSRI, morphine is more likely to cause a serotonin syndrome than is meperidine.

Discussion

The correct answer is "D." Meperidine (and tramadol) may cause a serotonin syndrome when combined with an SSRI. This is not a problem with morphine. The rest are all true. There is no evidence to support the tradition that meperidine is superior to morphine in biliary or pancreatic disease. Meperidine is metabolized into normeperidine that can cause agitation and seizures. Thus, "B" and "C" are correct. In general, then, morphine is a much cleaner drug to use for pain management than is meperidine.

* *

You have the patient's pain well managed with morphine, despite grumbling from your surgical colleague.

Which of the following treatments is *routinely* indicated in pancreatitis?

A) NG tube with intermittent suction.
B) H_2 blockers (e.g., cimetidine) or PPIs (e.g., lansoprazole).
C) IV antibiotics.
D) NPO order.

Discussion

The correct answer is "D." "A" is incorrect because there is no indication for an NG tube in the patient who is not vomiting. "B" is incorrect because H_2 blockers or PPIs do not change the outcome in pancreatitis. "C" is incorrect unless there is evidence of infection (e.g., fever) or necrotizing pancreatitis—and even then there is controversy. The routine treatment of pancreatitis includes avoiding oral intake (NPO status), administering IV fluids, and providing pain management.

* *

Your patient is NPO, receiving appropriate IV fluids. However, over the next couple of days, her condition worsens. She begins to vomit and have increased pain as well as tachycardia and fever. The patient wants to know what her chances of surviving this bout of pancreatitis are, so you break out a chart and your smart phone.

All of the following are part of Ranson criteria EXCEPT:

A) Patient's age.
B) Patient's white count on admission.
C) HCT at 72 hours.
D) Glucose on admission.

Discussion

The correct answer is "C." The HCT at **48 hours** is one of Ranson criteria. The other criteria are outlined in Table 7–7.

HELPFUL TIP: The Ranson criteria are neither particularly sensitive nor specific for severe pancreatic disease and cannot be completed before 48 hours of hospitalization. The Apache score accounts for blood pressure, oxygenation, temperature, respiratory rate, creatinine, GCS, etc., and is a better predictor of survival. Finally, an HCT of 44% or greater at admission and failure to decrease at 24 hours is also an excellent predictor of necrotizing pancreatitis and multiorgan failure.

Table 7–7 RANSON CRITERIA

On admission	• Age >55 years • WBC >16,000 • Glucose >200 • LDH >350 • AST >250
At 48 hours	• Hematocrit reduction by >10% • Bun increase of >5 • Calcium <8 • pO_2 <60 • Base deficit >4 • Fluid sequestration of >6 L

Note: Mild pancreatitis is defined by presence of 1–3 Ranson criteria; mortality increases with the presence of 4 or more.

* *

Because of the patient developed a fever and vomiting, you begin IV antibiotics and place an NG tube. Since the patient is vomiting and it seems as though it will be a protracted course, the patient will need nutrition.

The BEST way of providing nutrition for this patient is:

A) Full enteral feeds via the NG tube.
B) Central venous nutrition (CVN), TPN.
C) Clear liquid diet.
D) Peripheral nutrition with 10% dextrose and lipids.

Discussion
The correct answer is "B." Nutrition is critical for inpatients because of increased metabolic demand. The best choice from this list is CVN. "A" is incorrect because we want to avoid food in the stomach. "C" is incorrect for the same reason. "D" is better than giving enteric feeding but will not provide amino acids, vitamins, or enough calories.

HELPFUL TIP: **Enteral nutrition is preferred over CVN for pancreatitis** as long as the feeding is done below the ligament of Treitz. Jejunal feeding does not stimulate pancreatic enzymes and is associated with fewer complications than is CVN.

Which of the following IS NOT a complication of CVN?

A) Infection.
B) Cholestasis.
C) Hypoglycemia.
D) Ileus.

Discussion
The correct answer is "D." Infection, cholestasis, and hypoglycemia can all be a result of CVN. Hypoglycemia generally occurs when stopping CVN because of increased levels of circulating insulin. This can be mitigated by tapering CVN or administering IV dextrose.

* *

Since the patient has continued to do poorly, you order a CT scan of the abdomen that shows evidence of a pseudocyst.

Which of the following IS NOT true about a pancreatic pseudocyst?

A) Pseudocysts occur in 10% of patients with pancreatitis.
B) Pseudocysts can be drained by forming a fistula with the stomach endoscopically.
C) Pseudocysts can lead to the formation of arterial pseudoaneurysms that can cause severe bleeding.
D) Open drainage is the preferred method of treatment.
E) Not all pseudocysts require drainage.

Discussion
The correct answer is "D." The formation of a fistula with the stomach using an endoscope is actually the preferred method of drainage. The one major contraindication to endoscopic treatment is a pseudoaneurysm. Injury to an artery can cause significant bleeding that is difficult to control.

HELPFUL TIP: CT scan can be used to look for a pseudoaneurysm before endoscopic drainage. An aneurysm should also be suspected in these circumstances: evidence of an upper GI bleed, a drop in the HCT, or a sudden expansion of the pseudocyst.

Objectives: Did you learn to . . .

- Recognize and diagnose mesenteric thrombosis?
- Identify causes of acute pancreatitis?
- Diagnose and manage a patient with acute pancreatitis?
- Manage the complications of pancreatitis?
- Use parenteral nutrition in a hospitalized patient?
- Describe the principles of narcotic choice in parenteral pain management?

QUICK QUIZ: GALLSTONES

A 40-year-old female presents to you with gallstones found on a "full body CT scan" performed at Live4Ever Imaging Technologies, Inc. She is anxious that she will become sick like her sister who had an emergent cholecystectomy for her gallstone pancreatitis. She asks you if she should have her gallbladder removed. She is asymptomatic and her liver enzymes are normal.

Which of the following should you recommend?

A) Laparoscopic cholecystectomy because of family history of severe gallstone pancreatitis.
B) Ultrasound to confirm gallstones and to check for common bile duct stones.
C) No treatment or follow-up is needed unless she develops symptoms.
D) ERCP with sphincterotomy to allow stones to pass without obstructing common bile duct or compressing pancreatic duct.
E) Recheck liver enzymes and if elevated recommend cholecystectomy.

Discussion

The correct answer is "C." Asymptomatic gallstones do not need special attention since 70–80% remain asymptomatic. Only 2–3% of patients will present with acute cholecystitis or other complications and therefore prophylactic cholecystectomy is not indicated. American Indian populations have high risk of stone associated gallbladder cancer and are an exception to this rule. Diabetics or sickle cell disease patients have higher risk of complications from gallstones but still **should not** have their gallbladder removed if asymptomatic. Family history of complication from gallstones is not an indication for prophylactic cholecystectomy.

CASE 16

A 58-year-old woman with type 2 diabetes mellitus comes to your clinic with nausea, vague epigastric abdominal pain, bloating, early satiety, and intermittent vomiting for 3 weeks. Her past medical history is significant for hypertension and hyperlipidemia and her diabetes is complicated by retinopathy and neuropathy. She is on metformin, glyburide, lisinopril, aspirin, and simvastatin.

She is afebrile and not ill appearing on exam. She has gained 5 kg in the last year. She has mild epigastric tenderness without rebound or guarding. Bowel sounds are normal and there is no abdominal distention. Labs show normal CBC and differential with HbA1c of 9.4%. You suspect diabetic gastroparesis.

Which statement is *FALSE* regarding diagnosis of gastroparesis?

A) On scintigraphy (gastric emptying study) >50% of the standard meal present in stomach at 2 hours suggests gastroparesis.
B) On scintigraphy >10% of the standard meal present in the stomach at 4 hours suggests gastroparesis.
C) EGD looking for evidence of food after an uncontrolled restaurant meal is a good test for diagnosing gastroparesis.
D) Gastroparesis can be diagnosed by exhaled radiolabeled CO_2 measurement.

Discussion

The correct answer (the false statement) is "C." Simply looking for retained gastric contents at an unspecified time after an unspecified ingestion is not the way to diagnose gastroparesis. The most widely used test for diagnosing gastroparesis is radionucleotide scan. The patient is given standardized meal containing 99m technetium sulfur colloid in low-fat eggs, and nuclear activity is measured at 2 and 4 hours, respectively. If radioactivity in the stomach is >50% at 2 hours or >10% at 4 hours, the patient is considered to have delayed gastric emptying. You can do a liquid phase gastric emptying study if you suspect dumping syndrome, but it is not necessary to evaluate for gastroparesis. "D," radiolabeled CO_2 breath test, correlates well with nuclear scintigraphy and is easier to perform in the community setting. However, a radiolabeled CO_2 breath test requires normal small bowel, pancreas, liver, and lung function.

* *

You order a radionucleotide gastric emptying study, and it shows that 75% of the meal was present in the stomach at 2 hours and 20% at 4 hours. You diagnose gastroparesis.

The best long-term treatment option for her is:

A) Cisapride.
B) Domperidone.
C) Erythromycin.
D) Metoclopramide.
E) Improved glucose control.

Discussion

The correct answer is "E." The treatment of diabetic gastroparesis is often difficult and frustrating for patients and clinicians. Although not proven in prospective trials, most experts believe improved glucose control with dietary and lifestyle modification is the key to long-term success in diabetic gastroparesis. All of the above medications ("A"–"D") have shown benefit in the short term to reduce symptoms associated with diabetic gastroparesis. Cisapride was removed from the market because of prolongation of the QT interval. Domperidone is not available in the United States but is used in other countries for gastroparesis. Erythromycin and metoclopramide are effective and available. However, both can cause cramps, and erythromycin can cause nausea while metoclopramide may cause tardive dyskinesia or dystonia. Other macrolides are not effective.

* *

You add insulin to the diabetic regimen in an attempt to tighten glucose control and prescribe metoclopramide 5 mg 30 minutes before meals.

In addition to this you recommend all of the following dietary and lifestyle modifications EXCEPT:

A) Increase dietary fiber.
B) Change from four large to six small meals daily.
C) Moderate exercise.
D) Decrease dietary fat.
E) ADA 1800 kcal diet.

Discussion

The correct answer is "A." Fiber and raw vegetables can form gastric bezoars (phytobezoar) in gastroparesis and this is commonly seen on endoscopy. Bezoars cause early satiety and bloating and add to the symptom burden of gastroparesis. If a bezoar is found, it can be dissolved using cellulase (Kanalase®) or *N*-acetylcysteine orally. More frequent, smaller meals help with symptoms; and moderate exercise can be helpful but excessive exercise may slow gastric emptying. Your patient is gaining weight, so it is important to reinforce the ADA diet. Fat slows gastric emptying; therefore, dietary fat should be reduced to less than 40 g/day.

Which of the following medications can exacerbate preexisting gastroparesis?

A) Fluoxetine.
B) Oxycodone.
C) Angiotensin-converting enzyme (ACE) inhibitors.
D) Metformin.
E) Insulin.

Discussion

The correct answer is "B." Oxycodone and all narcotics reduce GI motility and are rarely tolerated by patients with gastroparesis. This can be clinically challenging, and attention to the cause of pain and alternative management options should be explored. Fluoxetine does not have significant effects on gastric motility, but TCAs and other drugs with anticholinergic activity do and are not good options for pain syndromes in gastroparesis. ACE inhibitors do not affect GI motility. Although metformin is associated with GI side effects, it does not affect GI motility. Insulin has no adverse effect on GI motility. Other medications that reduce gastric emptying are dopaminergic agents, antiadrenergic antihypertensives, calcium channel blockers, and anticholinergic agents. All drugs known to affect gastric motility should be stopped prior to obtaining a gastric emptying study.

HELPFUL TIP: The last resort in severe, unremitting gastroparesis with weight loss and brittle diabetic control can be to place percutaneous endoscopic jejunostomy. The patient is then placed on jejunal feedings temporarily while diabetic control and nutritional balance are regained (if possible).

Objectives: Did you learn to . . .

- Diagnose gastroparesis?
- Identify medications that can exacerbate gastroparesis?
- Manage gastroparesis?

QUICK QUIZ: GI BLEED

You admit a 65-year-old woman with end-stage renal disease on hemodialysis. She is being admitted because of recurrent episodes of melena requiring transfusions. She is anemic with low ferritin, iron, and iron saturation. The gastroenterologist performs an upper and lower endoscopy without any bleeding source found. Subsequently, a capsule enteroscopy shows multiple small angiodysplasias throughout the small bowel, without any large, endoscopically treatable, lesions.

Your patient is discharged after a blood transfusion. Her hemoglobin is 11 g/dL. At follow-up 1 month later, her hemoglobin is 9 g/dL. The patient is on maximum doses of erythropoietin with dialysis and is still having guaiac-positive stools. She refuses to take oral iron because of constipation.

Which of the following is the best next step in the management of this case?

A) Prescribe iron dextran or sucrose IV with dialysis to maintain her iron stores.
B) Try to prevail upon the gastroenterologist to repeat endoscopy and treat any angiodysplasia lesions that can be reached.
C) Prescribe octreotide.
D) Order a Meckel scan.
E) Prescribe estrogen–progesterone.

Discussion

The correct answer is "A." This is an appropriate situation for the administration of iron IV. It is safer than blood transfusions and can be given on an outpatient basis during hemodialysis. There are rare occurrences of anaphylaxis with iron dextran, and a test dose should be given. Some reports suggest iron sucrose is safer. "B," repeat endoscopies with treatments of angiodysplasias, may help but should be adjunctive therapy to maintenance of iron stores. The scope only reaches the proximal jejunum and the patient has lesions throughout the small bowel. "C," octreotide, has been reported in case series to have a beneficial effect, but no randomized trials have been performed and it cannot be recommended at this time. "D," a Meckel scan (done to look for Meckel diverticula), would be redundant as another cause has been found and the patient does not fit the age group. "E," hormone replacement therapies, initially seemed effective at reducing bleeding from angiodysplasia but randomized trials failed to show benefit.

HELPFUL TIP: Angiodysplasias are commonly missed and are associated with increasing age, end-stage renal disease, aortic stenosis, hereditary telangiectasias (autosomal dominant), and are more likely to bleed in patients on long-term anticoagulation and antiplatelet therapies. Other commonly missed lesions include Cameron lesions (small ulcers caused by rubbing of hiatal hernia sac against diaphragm) and PUD.

HELPFUL TIP: Capsule endoscopy of the small bowel using a small camera can be helpful if a small bowel follow-through does not show a source of bleeding. Other possibilities include tagged red blood cell (RBC) scan and angiography that are only really useful in overt bleeding. The tagged RBC scan needs 0.1 mL/min bleeding rate and angiography requires 0.5 mL/min bleeding rate to detect bleeding sites.

QUICK QUIZ: GI BLEED

A 30-year-old female comes to your clinic with the complaint of intermittent blood on toilet paper for 3 years. She says she always has been constipated and takes polyethylene glycol (MiraLax) on regular basis. She has no family history of colorectal cancer and is asymptomatic and has no weight loss. On exam, she does not appear anemic and abdominal exam is normal. Rectal exam is normal and nontender. Anoscopy is normal.

What is the most appropriate action?

A) Reassurance.
B) Anusol suppositories three times/week for 6 weeks; follow up as needed.
C) Flexible sigmoidoscopy.
D) Colonoscopy.
E) Anorectal manometry.

Discussion

The correct answer is "C." The message is that everybody reporting persistent blood in stools without lesions seen on anoscopy warrants endoscopic evaluation. Colon cancer is rare in this age group but can happen. The symptom of red blood per rectum suggests that the cause could be found distal to descending colon and likely in the rectum. If there is only a single episode of bleeding, some would argue for a more conservative approach in patients less than 50 years of age without other alarm symptoms (constitutional symptoms or change in bowel habits). In this young patient, a full colonoscopy is not necessary unless there is a strong family history of colorectal cancer or other symptoms suggestive of colitis such as urgency, weight loss, or diarrhea. Anorectal manometry is not useful in the evaluation of rectal bleeding. Anusol suppositories can be helpful to reduce pain associated with hemorrhoids, but if bleeding is the only symptom, fiber supplements and stool softeners are sufficient. If the patient is older than 50 years with rectal bleeding, full colonoscopy is indicated.

CASE 17

A 73-year-old male comes to your office with a 3-day history of left lower quadrant abdominal pain. He has felt cold and clammy at times but has not checked his temperature. He has had no nausea, vomiting, or diarrhea. The pain does not worsen after meals, but his appetite has been poor since this started. On review of systems, he reports increased urinary frequency and urgency for the same amount of time. He has had no surgeries on his abdomen. He has diabetes mellitus type 2 and is on glipizide. He also takes aspirin 81 mg/day. He has always declined screening colonoscopy, stating, "If it ain't broke, don't fix it"—apparently, his family motto. On exam, he is in no distress with blood pressure 125/75 mm Hg, pulse 90, respirations 15, and temperature 38.5°C. His heart sounds are normal, and his chest is clear bilaterally. He has moderate left lower quadrant tenderness without rebound tenderness or guarding. There is no abdominal distention or organomegaly. Bowel sounds are normal, and the rectal exam is normal without stool in ampulla. Urinalysis is normal.

What is the most likely diagnosis?

A) Ischemic colitis.
B) Colon cancer with large bowel obstruction.
C) Irritable bowel syndrome.
D) Pyelonephritis.
E) Diverticulitis.

Discussion

The correct answer is "E." Diverticulitis is the most likely cause of the patient's pain. Fever associated with acute onset abdominal pain located in left lower quadrant makes this pain more likely to be due to diverticulitis. Diverticulitis can, however, occur in any part of the colon. Ischemic colitis ("A") can present with abdominal pain in this location but is usually associated with bloody diarrhea, so it is less likely. IBS ("C") almost never presents in this age group, is not associated with fevers, and is a chronic condition not acute. Pyelonephritis ("D") was a good thought until the urine dipstick returned normal. Urinary symptoms are common in diverticulitis because of bladder irritation. Colon cancer with large bowel obstruction ("B") would present with severe abdominal pain and distention. In obstruction, bowel sounds are typically hyperactive with intermittent rushing.

The most appropriate next step in the workup of the patient is?

A) CT scan of abdomen and pelvis with IV and oral contrast.
B) Surgical consult.
C) Gastroenterology consult.
D) Abdominal ultrasound.
E) Colonoscopy.

Discussion

The correct answer is "A." CT scan is very sensitive and specific for diverticulitis and can simultaneously evaluate for other causes of abdominal pain. In general, CT scan is indicated if the patient has peritoneal signs or mass suggesting diverticular abscess formation. In a patient who has had previously documented attacks and who has none of the above symptoms, empiric treatment is appropriate. Surgical and/or GI consults may be indicated but are premature at this point. Abdominal ultrasound can diagnose diverticulitis and/or abscess, but it is less sensitive than CT scan. Colonoscopy is only indicated in the acute setting if obstruction is present or if colitis is thought to be more likely. In the setting of acute diverticulitis, the risk of perforation during colonoscopy is increased, and colonoscopy is preferably delayed until inflammation has subsided. Note that you do not want to use rectal contrast if there is a question of a perforation (or that you may cause a perforation).

HELPFUL TIP: In the absence of a CT scanner, it is reasonable to admit a patient with a classic history of diverticulitis, give IV antibiotics, and perform serial abdominal exams. If the patient improves rapidly, you can schedule colonoscopy when the attack has resolved. If the patient worsens, he goes immediately to a center that has a CT scan and a surgeon (do not pass go, do not... you get the idea).

* *

You get the CT scan the same day and have the patient return to your office to discuss the results. The CT scan shows inflammation in the sigmoid colon with some outpouching structures suggesting diverticulosis. There is a 1.5 cm fluid collection posterior to the sigmoid colon suggesting pericolonic abscess. No other findings were noted, and the colon above sigmoid appeared normal. No free air was seen.

Which of the following is the most appropriate next step in management?

A) CT guided drainage of the abscess.
B) Surgical consult for immediate diverting colostomy and abscess drainage.
C) Admission with IV antibiotics and serial abdominal exams.
D) Discharge to home on levofloxacin and metronidazole.
E) GI consult for endoscopic ultrasound guided transcolonic drainage of abscess.

Discussion

The correct answer is "C." This patient should be admitted for IV antibiotics. Mild attacks of diverticulitis can be managed on an outpatient basis. Our patient has small abscess that requires inpatient therapy. In addition, he is immunosuppressed by his diabetes, and all immunosuppressed patients with diverticulitis should be admitted for IV antibiotics since they are more likely to develop complications and need surgery. "A" is not the best choice. It is reasonable to ask the radiologist if this abscess can be drained, but the likely answer is no, because it is very small and is posterior to colon. "B" is also incorrect. The patient does not have peritoneal signs, and the abscess likely will respond to IV antibiotics. Thus, immediate surgery is not indicated. As discussed above, colonoscopy (and by extension endoscopic ultrasound) is relatively contraindicated in the setting of acute diverticulitis. "E" is also incorrect. No gastroenterologist has been found crazy enough to try to drain abscesses by a transcolonic approach to our (and Pubmed's) knowledge. However, maybe the emerging Natural Orifice Transluminal Endoscopic Surgeons (NOTES) will attempt this in the future but not on our patient today. (Editor's note: we didn't make this one up either... They have been doing cholecystectomies via a transvaginal approach....don't ask us why...)

> **HELPFUL TIP:** Antibiotic regimens for diverticulitis must include both gram-negative and anaerobic coverage. Some common regimens include ciprofloxacin + metronidazole, ampicillin/sulbactam, amoxicillin/clavulanate, ampicillin + gentamicin + clindamycin, and ceftriaxone + metronidazole.

* *

The patient is admitted and he responds to IV antibiotics and supportive measures. A repeat CT scan 2 weeks later shows resolution of the abscess. The local gastroenterologist performs colonoscopy 2 months after the attack and confirms left-sided diverticulosis with otherwise normal colonoscopy.

Which of the following statements is true about this patient's prognosis?

A) When the patient has his second attack of uncomplicated diverticulitis, a resection of the diseased segment is always indicated (sigmoid colectomy).
B) 50% of patients will have a repeat attack within 5 years.
C) He has 20–30% chance of perforation of diverticulitis in 2 years.
D) He has 30% chance of diverticular bleeding in next 2 years.
E) 33% of patients will have a second attack.

Discussion

The correct answer is "E." Only 33% of patients with an episode of diverticulitis will have a second episode. There is no set rule for the number of attacks needed before partial colectomy is indicated. The commonly used rule of three attacks is not based on prospective evidence. The decision has to be individualized, but the tendency is to operate on healthy young people with frequent attacks while opting for observation of elderly patients with comorbidities (even if they have more than three attacks). Perforation of diverticulitis is rare and occurs in only 5–10% of patients within 2 years of the initial event. Diverticular bleeding happens in 3–5% of patients with diverticulosis and the risk is not increased with diverticulitis; if GI bleeding occurs during an episode of presumed diverticulitis, other diagnoses should be strongly considered.

* *

On a weekend call 6 months later, your patient presents to the emergency department after experiencing sudden onset of bright red blood per rectum mixed within stools. He has passed five stools in last 3 hours and the last one had blood clots. He feels dizzy but has not passed out. He stopped taking his aspirin after his last illness, but otherwise his health and medications are unchanged. His abdomen is nontender and bowel sounds are normoactive. Rectal exam reveals fresh blood on the glove but no masses in rectum. Hemoglobin is 10 g/dL, and you place two large bore IVs and admit him to the hospital. He has no more bowel movements overnight, his hemoglobin is 8.2 g/dL the next morning, and he is feeling well. You assume that the bleeding was diverticular.

Which of the following statements is true?

A) Urgent colonoscopy is needed to localize and treat the lesion.
B) Colonoscopy is needed but can be done on an outpatient basis.
C) Tagged RBC scan followed by angiography is indicated to prevent rebleeding.
D) No further workup is indicated at this point.
E) Sigmoid colon resection is indicated because of the dogmatic diverticular duo (diverticular bleed and diverticulitis).

Discussion

The correct answer is "D." The patient has classic presentation of diverticular bleeding with rapid onset and spontaneous resolution of bleeding (75% stop spontaneously). The patient underwent colonoscopy recently and the only finding was diverticulosis. Since the patient has stopped bleeding, colonoscopy is unlikely to help in the management of his condition. For the same reason, colonoscopy does not need to be done as outpatient. If the patient had continued to bleed, there would be two options for managing this patient and both are acceptable. One approach is to perform rapid colonic lavage by placing an NG tube and giving 6 L (1.5 gallons) of polyethylene glycol (GoLytely) over 4 hours and perform colonoscopy to try to find the bleeding site and treat it. Often multiple blood-filled diverticuli are seen, and the source of the bleed cannot be identified. The second approach is to perform a tagged RBC scan to confirm active bleeding, followed by selective angiography to identify the bleeding vessel and embolize it. The approach taken depends on the local expertise available. Without treatment, 25% of patients eventually rebleed and of those who rebleed, 50% will have a third bleed.

Objectives: Did you learn to . . .

- Identify signs and symptoms of diverticulitis?
- Appreciate the natural history of diverticular disease?
- Manage complications of diverticular disease?

BIBLIOGRAPHY

David D. Diverticulitis. *N Engl J Med.* 2007;357:2057.

Eisenberg JM. Managing chronic gastroesophageal reflux disease. AHRQ Comparative Effectiveness Reviews. Available at: www.effectivehealthcare.ahrq.gov/gerdupdate.cfm, Accessed January 16, 2012.

Heidelbaugh JJ, Bruderly M. Cirrhosis and chronic liver failure: Part I. Diagnosis and evaluation. *Am Fam Physician.* 2006;74(5):756-762.

Heidelbaugh JJ, Sherbondy M. Cirrhosis and chronic liver failure: part II. Complications and treatment. Am Fam Physician. 2006;74(5):767-776.

Jiang D. Care of chronic liver disease. *Prim Care.* 2011; 38:483-498; viii-ix.

Lanza FL, et al; Practice Parameters Committee of the American College of Gastroenterology. Guidelines for prevention of NSAID-related ulcer complications. *Am J Gastroenterol.* 2009;104:728-738.

Longstreth GF, et al. Functional bowel disorders. *Gastroenterology.* 2006;130:1480.

Malfertheiner P, et al. Peptic ulcer disease. *Lancet.* 2009; 374:9699.

Rockey DC. Occult gastrointestinal bleeding; primary care. *N Engl J Med.* 1999;341(1):38-46.

Swaroop VS, et al. Severe acute pancreatitis. *JAMA.* 2004;291:2865-2868.

Tack J, et al. Functional gastroduodenal disorders. *Gastroenterology.* 2006;130:466.

United States Preventive Services Task Force. Screening for Colon Cancer. 2008. Available at: http://www.ahrq.gov/clinic/uspstf/uspscolo.htm, Accessed January 16, 2012.

Whicomb DC. Acute pancreatitis. *N Engl J Med.* 2006; 354:2142.

8

Infectious Diseases

Mark A. Graber

CASE 1

Flu season is right around the corner and you are preparing your clinic for the onslaught. First things first . . . you need to know how much vaccine to order and who will be receiving it. The Centers for Disease Control and Prevention (CDC) annually publishes recommendations for administering influenza vaccine to the American public.

The CDC recommends vaccination for all of the following groups, EXCEPT:

A) Health-care workers.
B) Nursing home residents.
C) Egg-allergic, febrile neonates.
D) Diabetics.
E) The elderly.

Discussion

The correct answer is "C." Those 6 months old or younger (including neonates) should not be vaccinated, nor should children who are febrile. The only other absolute contraindication to influenza vaccination is a known hypersensitivity to eggs or to other components of the influenza vaccine. See note on page 172 for new 2012 allergy information.

> HELPFUL TIP: Vaccinate all persons older than 6 months annually. There are **four types** of vaccine available: trivalent inactivated influenza vaccine (the old-fashioned flu shot), intradermal vaccine (Fluzone) for patients 18–64 years of age, high-dose intramuscular vaccine for the elderly, and the intranasal live attenuated influenza vaccine. Live attenuated influenza vaccine (i.e., FluMist) is indicated only for healthy, nonpregnant persons aged 2–49 years, including health-care workers **except those health-care workers caring for the very immunosuppresed such as bone marrow transplant patients.** Contact with patients with HIV, etc. is not a contraindication to the live attenuated virus.

* *

Oh, no! The virus has struck. Like a zombie apocalypse, it started with just a few cases, but now it's out of control. Every other patient who calls complains of influenza-like illness.

During this outbreak, what intervention(s) is/are most appropriate for all your unvaccinated, frail nursing home patients who have no symptoms of febrile respiratory illness?

A) Antiviral prophylaxis with oseltamivir.
B) Antiviral prophylaxis with amantadine.
C) Influenza immunization.
D) A and C given together.
E) B and C given together.

Discussion

The correct answer is "D." Persons at high risk for complications of influenza can still be vaccinated after an outbreak of influenza has begun in the community, but development of antibodies in adults can take up to 2 weeks. **Thus, chemoprophylaxis should be considered for persons at high risk during the time from vaccination until immunity has developed.** "A" alone might be appropriate for individuals who have a contraindication to vaccination and wish to protect themselves from influenza. "B" is not correct because influenza A is increasingly resistant to M2 drugs (amantadine, rimantadine), and influenza B has never been sensitive: it is no longer recommended. Answer "C," vaccination alone, can be used in individuals **without** known high-risk conditions (chronic disorders including asthma, diabetes, renal dysfunction, immunodeficiency, or cardiovascular disease). But, as noted above, vaccine alone is inadequate for those who are institutionalized and the chronically ill. These higher risk patients also need to be covered by oseltamivir until immunity has developed (2 weeks).

HELPFUL TIP: Sensitivity and specificity of rapid diagnostic tests for influenza (70–75% and 90–95%, respectively) are lower than viral culture. **Resistance of influenza A to oseltamivir has been rising and was 99% in 2009.** Resistance varies by year, however, and the reverse was true in 2010 (99% of H1N1 isolates tested were **susceptible** to oseltamivir).

Which of these patients would qualify for antiviral therapy during an influenza outbreak?

A) A healthy 29-year-old male who presents 72 hours after onset of symptom onset **and** has a positive rapid test for influenza.
B) A 70-year-old patient hospitalized with influenza who presents 72 hours after onset of symptoms.
C) A pregnant women who presents within 48 hours of symptom onset and has a positive rapid test for influenza
D) B and C only
E) All of the above (A, B, and C).

Discussion

The correct answer is "D." **In outpatients**, antiviral drugs are reserved for high-risk groups including pregnancy, age >65 years, significant underlying medical illness (DM, immunosuppression, morbid obesity, asthma, etc.), nursing home residents and children age <2 years. Normal risk outpatients should be prioritized lower on the treatment ladder. However, the CDC does recommend that antiviral drugs be considered for otherwise healthy outpatients with confirmed influenza who can start medication within 48 hours of symptom onset. All hospitalized patients should be treated even if it is >48 hours after onset of symptoms.

* *

The director of nursing at your community nursing home calls about an outbreak of febrile respiratory infections. In the last 24 hours, three patients have become ill on the dementia care unit. All residents of the home were vaccinated with the current year's influenza vaccine in November. Several of the aides have not been vaccinated and two recently left work after complaining of feeling tired, feverish, and achy.

You suspect an influenza outbreak and take the following actions EXCEPT:

A) Quarantine the nursing home and restrict access to visitors, new admissions, and ill staff.
B) Hospitalize all patients suspected of having influenza.
C) Limit the interaction of ill residents with non-ill residents.
D) Administer antiviral prophylaxis to all well residents.
E) Provide influenza vaccine to any unvaccinated residents.

Discussion

The correct answer is "B." Moving sick patients only risks spreading the infection to the hospital. In addition to measures above, employees should be assigned to one work area only to prevent spread via the staff. Activities, visits, and gatherings in central common areas should be curtailed during the outbreak.

HELPFUL TIP: Influenza vaccine is only about 50% effective in nursing home patients. Still, there is some herd immunity and vaccination is recommended as the primary way to prevent an influenza outbreak.

HELPFUL TIP: The most common cause of bacterial pneumonia complicating influenza is *S. pneumoniae*. However, *S. aureus* pneumonia (usually uncommon in the community) is an important entity during influenza outbreaks and generally presents with more severe symptoms.

HELPFUL TIP: **Pneumococcal vaccine:** Indications for **pneumococcal vaccination** include patients with chronic illness at high risk for invasive pneumococcal disease (e.g., diabetes, chronic pulmonary disease, and cardiovascular disease), institutionalization, age 65 or older, immunocompromised state, and **tobacco use**. Note that the tobacco use indication is relatively recent and applies to all patients age 19–64 years old. Patients with an immunosuppressive disorder (e.g., HIV, asplenia, renal failure, and organ transplant) should have a one-time revaccination at least 5 years after initial vaccination.

Objectives: Did you learn to . . .

- Describe who should receive influenza vaccine?
- Identify appropriate interventions to halt the transmission of influenza in community and health-care influenza outbreaks?
- Lead a successful influenza prevention program in a health-care setting?
- Prescribe influenza antivirals appropriately?

CASE 2

An 80-year-old female fell, broke her hip, and underwent intraoperative repair with pinning of the fracture. She developed a local infection at the site of the repair and was treated with a 10-day course of oral clindamycin. She is transferred to the nursing home for rehabilitation and has developed loose, watery stools. Today when you visit her she reports feeling diffuse abdominal discomfort and has had 10 bowel movements. She is very concerned because she cannot work with the therapist and risks losing her Medicare benefit for skilled nursing.

You plan to do the following:

A) Begin loperamide (Imodium) as needed to prevent diarrhea during the therapy sessions.
B) Obtain stool specimens for *Clostridium difficile* toxin.
C) Obtain an abdominal CT scan looking for evidence of obstruction.
D) Ask your favorite gastrointestinal (GI) doctor to perform emergency endoscopy for evaluation of lower GI bleed.
E) Obtain stool specimens for ova and parasites.

Discussion

The correct answer is "B." *C. difficile* is the most common **bacterial** cause of infectious diarrhea in hospitalized patients in the United States (*Campylobacter jejuni* is the most common bacterial cause overall). The antibiotics most commonly associated with *C. difficile* diarrhea are clindamycin, fluoroquinolones, and broad-spectrum cephalosporins. The assay for *C. difficile* cytotoxin is only about 75% sensitivity (enzyme immunoassay). There are several subtypes of toxin, some of which are not detected by this assay. Although symptomatic therapy is important, answer "A" is incorrect because antiperistaltic agents should be avoided in patients with *C. difficile*. Although other causes of diarrhea are possible, the most cost-effective approach in this patient would be stool assay for *C. difficile* repeated on two to three specimens (to improve sensitivity) prior to any other more invasive procedure.

HELPFUL TIP: The gold standard test for detecting *C. difficile* in the stool is the cytotoxin assay, but it is not commonly performed because it takes up to 2 days to perform and is more costly.

* *

A stool specimen reveals the presence of *C. difficile* toxin A. The patient is nontoxic with a normal complete blood count (CBC) and creatinine.

The preferred, first line, treatment of this patient should include:

A) *Dificid* (fidaxomicin)
B) Lactose restriction and acidophilus milk products.
C) Metronidazole 500 mg PO TID for 10 days
D) Vancomycin 250 mg PO QID for 10 days.
E) B and C.

Discussion

The correct answer is "C." Treatment includes supportive care, discontinuation of the offending antimicrobial agent, and initiation of oral metronidazole 250 mg four times daily or 500 mg three times for 10 days. Metronidazole is preferred over vancomycin because of the nearly identical efficacy and relapse/reinfection rates, lower cost, and lower theoretical risk of promotion of vancomycin-resistant *Enterococcus faecalis* (VRE). Consider vancomycin first line if the patient has severe disease (white blood cell (WBC) $>15,000$, creatinine $>1.5\times$ baseline). *Dificid* (fidaxomicin) has recently been approved for *C. difficile* colitis. However, the NNT = 10 to prevent one recurrence. It is certainly NOT first (or even second) line.

Risk factors for *C. difficile* infection in nursing home patients include:

A) Advanced age.
B) Recent acute hospitalization.
C) Proton pump inhibitor (PPI) use.
D) Long-term residence in a chronic care facility.
E) All of the above.

The correct answer is "E." Risk factors for acquisition of *C. difficile* infection in nursing home patients are similar to that of hospitalized patients and include hospitalization, advanced age, GI surgery/procedures and antibiotic exposure and, importantly **PPI use.**

> HELPFUL TIP: *C. difficile* diarrhea and colitis can be caused by **any** antibiotic, including metronidazole and vancomycin. The probability of diarrhea seems highest with clindamycin. Fluoroquinolones are increasingly associated with *C. difficile* infection, including a highly toxigenic strain. Simply stopping the antibiotic can lead to resolution in 25% of the cases.

* *

Failure to resolve *C. difficile*-associated diarrhea after a 10-day course antibiotic therapy is common. Guess what? Your patient's diarrhea has persisted.

The most reasonable treatment approach is to:

A) Repeat a course of oral metronidazole.
B) Treat with a course of oral vancomycin.
C) Treat with a course of intravenous (IV) vancomycin.
D) A or B.
E) B or C.

Discussion

The correct answer is "D." Relapse is very common. Typically about 20% of patients have a recurrence of symptoms within about 1 week of completing therapy. These patients usually respond to retreatment with either metronidazole or vancomycin. IV vancomycin is **ineffective** treatment of *C. difficile* since vancomycin does not enter into the GI tract from the vascular space.

> HELPFUL TIP: *C. difficile* toxin degrades at room temperature. A stool that has been at room temperature for 2 hours will likely be negative for *C. difficile* toxin even the toxin was initially present. A newly identified cause of *C. difficile* negative pseudomembranous colitis is *Klebsiella oxytoca.* Consider this if stool studies are negative for *C. difficile.* Finally, a positive stool culture is not diagnostic of pseudomembranous colitis. *C. difficile* is a normal gut flora. You need a positive toxin to make the diagnosis of *C. difficile*-associated diarrhea or pseudomembranous colitis.

> HELPFUL TIP: The use of probiotics seems to help prevent *C. difficile* colitis and may prevent recurrences. **In particularly recalcitrant cases, stool transplants have been done.** Patients are given "healthy" stool via NG tube to reestablish normal GI flora. Yum. No, we are not making this up. Any volunteers?

Objectives: Did you learn to . . .

- Recognize the presentation of *C. difficile* infection?
- Identify risk factors for the development of *C. difficile* diarrhea and colitis?
- Treat patients with initial and recurrent *C. difficile* infections?

CASE 3

You are called to the emergency department (ED) to examine a 40-year-old man with fever and headache. His past history is remarkable only for a splenectomy secondary to trauma at age 10. He is not allergic to any antibiotics. Upon exam you note that he has meningeal signs. Nondilated fundal exam shows sharp disc margins, and he is neurologically intact with a nonfocal exam.

The most appropriate action is:

A) Obtain a head CT so that you can safely proceed with lumbar puncture.
B) Order IV penicillin as you prepare to perform lumbar puncture.
C) Perform a lumbar puncture (LP) immediately and begin antibiotic therapy empirically.
D) Order IV erythromycin as you prepare to perform lumbar puncture.
E) Order IV vancomycin and IV ceftriaxone as you wait for the CBC. If the CBC is abnormal, you will do the LP.

Discussion

The correct answer is "C." Once you suspect bacterial meningitis, rapid diagnostic evaluation and emergent treatment are imperative, including lumbar puncture and blood cultures. **If lumbar puncture is going to be delayed, then appropriate empiric antimicrobial and adjunctive therapy should be given without delay**. Head CT is necessary only in those who are immunocompromised (HIV/AIDS, those receiving immunosuppressive drugs, transplant recipients), have a history of CNS disease (brain tumor and stroke), develop new onset seizures, display papilledema on exam, or who have an abnormal/focal neurologic deficit or abnormal level of consciousness. Antibiotics for a 40-year-old male should cover *Neisseria meningitidis* and *S. pneumoniae*, and would include vancomycin and ceftriaxone (answer "E"). However, answer "E" is not the best choice. Never wait for a CBC to determine if an adult needs an LP. The decision to do an LP is a clinical one.

HELPFUL TIP: **The standard of care for suspected meningitis is to administer antibiotics within 30 minutes of the patient presenting to the ED. Draw the blood cultures and give the antibiotics.** You won't change the CSF culture results if you give a single dose of antibiotics prior to CT scan. However, it is considered prudent to do the LP within 2 hours of administering IV antibiotics.

* *

Results of the cerebrospinal fluid (CSF) obtained after lumbar puncture are as follows: cloudy, WBC count 5000 cells/mm^3, 95% neutrophils, glucose 20 mg/dL, and gram-positive cocci in pairs.

The most likely pathogen is:

A) *S. pneumoniae.*
B) *Listeria monocytogenes.*
C) *S. aureus.*
D) *N. meningitidis.*
E) *Pseudomonas* species.

Discussion

The correct answer is "A." Gram stain examination of CSF may permit rapid identification of the causative organism in bacterial meningitis with a sensitivity of 60–90%. Prior antibiotic therapy (e.g., a partially treated meningitis... not a single dose of antibiotics in the ED) may reduce the sensitivity by 20%. The likelihood of a positive Gram stain is highest in cases of *S. pneumoniae* (a gram-positive diplococcus). Only about one-third of *L. monocytogenes* meningitis cases demonstrate a positive Gram stain. Answer "D" requires special mention. *N. meningitidis* is a diplococcus but is gram negative.

An adjunctive therapy that has been shown to improve neurologic outcomes in pneumococcal meningitis is:

A) Dexamethasone.
B) Activated protein C.
C) Vasopressors.
D) CSF shunt implantation.
E) Monoclonal antibody directed against the capsule antigen of the bacterium.

Discussion

The correct answer is "A." The Infectious Disease Society of America (IDSA) guideline recommends adjunctive dexamethasone to be administered to all adult patients with pneumococcal meningitis. No other adjunctive therapy has proven benefit. Since the organism is not usually known at the time of initiation of therapy, dexamethasone should be given empirically until the causative organism is identified. If the meningitis is not due to *S. pneumoniae*, dexamethasone should be discontinued.

Patients should receive standard supportive therapies in an intensive care setting. Complications, when they occur, usually develop within the first 2–3 days of therapy. Complications include sepsis, mental status changes, and electrolyte abnormalities.

Highly resistant *S. pneumoniae* infections of the CNS should be treated with:

A) Third-generation cephalosporin.
B) Vancomycin and a third-generation cephalosporin.
C) High-dose penicillin G.
D) Ampicillin.
E) Vancomycin, gentamycin and rifampin.

Discussion

The correct answer is "B." Vancomycin should be combined with a third-generation cephalosporin (e.g., ceftriaxone and cefotaxime) for highly resistant pneumococcus. Do not use vancomycin alone; it does not cover gram-negative organisms. The newer generation fluoroquinolones have enhanced in vitro activity against *S. pneumoniae* and may be used as alternative agents. **However, fluoroquinolones are not recommended unless the patient cannot tolerate or is allergic to standard drugs.**

HELPFUL TIP: Resistance to penicillins (and others) is noted by the minimum inhibitory concentration (MIC). For penicillin, highly resistant pneumococcus has an MIC of >2 μg/mL, intermediate resistance is 0.12–1 μg/mL while sensitive is <0.06 μg/mL.

HELPFUL TIP: The combination of Kernig and Brudzinski signs carries a sensitivity and specificity of 5% and 95%, respectively. Thus, the great majority of patients do not manifest these signs when they have meningitis, and they are useless to rule out meningitis. The sensitivity and specificity of nuchal rigidity (stiff neck) is 30% and 68%, respectively. In adults, the classic triad of fever, nuchal rigidity, and altered mental status was found in only 46%, with 85% having fever, 70% having neck stiffness, and 67% having mental status changes.

Objectives: Did you learn to . . .

- Diagnose meningitis?
- Identify the most likely causative organism based on epidemiology and patient characteristics?
- Describe proper use of empiric antibiotics and steroid therapy for bacterial meningitis?

QUICK QUIZ: BIG MENINGITIS ON CAMPUS

What is the most common bacterial cause of meningitis in college-aged patients who live in dormitories?

A) *N. meningitidis.*
B) *S. pneumococcus.*
C) *L. monocytogenes.*
D) *Haemophilus influenzae.*
E) *Escherichia coli.*

Discussion

The correct answer is "A." Although *S. pneumococcus* is the most common cause of bacterial meningitis in the adult population in the United States, *N. meningitidis* remains the leading cause in adolescents despite vaccination and is particularly prevalent in the setting of dormitory living (e.g., college or military). In addition, the presence of petechial (or purpuric) rash in the lower extremities and pressure points is typical of *N. meningitidis*. The advent of vaccination has made *H. influenzae* a less common cause. *L. monocytogenes* is more prevalent in those over age 50, infants, and immunocompromised. *E. coli* is a common cause for meningitis in neonates and infants but is very uncommon in adolescents and adults.

QUICK QUIZ: SPLEENLESS IN SEATTLE

Patients undergoing elective splenectomy should receive all of the following in EXCEPT:

A) Pneumococcal polysaccharide vaccine (Pneumovax).
B) *H. influenzae* type B conjugate vaccine.
C) Influenza vaccine.
D) Meningococcal vaccine.
E) Oral polio vaccine.

Discussion

The correct answer is "E." Oral polio vaccine is no longer recommended in the United States for anyone. The risk of developing polio from the live vaccine outweighs the benefit of oral administration. All patients undergoing elective splenectomy should receive preoperative vaccination against encapsulated organisms at least 14 days prior to splenectomy; this includes vaccines against *S. pneumoniae*, meningococcus, and *H. influenzae* type B (all encapsulated bacteria). Offer influenza vaccination annually at the appropriate time. Splenectomized individuals should be reimmunized against pneumococcus at 5-year intervals. Patients who have undergone splenectomy need to be educated about seeking prompt medical attention for fever.

CASE 4

A 74-year-old woman is in your office for a complete physical. As part of her routine labs, you obtain a urinalysis (although why is beyond us . . . there is no recommendation for a screening urinalysis for any nonpregnant patients). On further questioning, she has actually had stress urinary incontinence for a number of years, which is unchanged. She reports no fevers, hematuria, dysuria, flank pain, or other symptoms. The urinalysis shows 10–20 WBC/hpf and is nitrite positive on dipstick. A culture of the urine shows 100,000 cfu/mL of *E. coli.*

How should you treat this patient?

A) Trimethoprim-sulfamethoxazole DS 1 tab PO BID for 10 days.
B) Erythromycin 500 mg PO q 6 hours for 14 days.
C) Ampicillin 250 mg PO q 6 hours for 10 days.
D) Ceftriaxone 1 g IM every day for 3 days.
E) With courtesy and respect, but not with antibiotics.

Discussion

The correct answer is "E." A positive urine culture in an asymptomatic patient (e.g., asymptomatic bacteriuria) should not be treated with antibiotics. Asymptomatic bacteriuria is a very common finding, especially in elderly females, persons with indwelling catheters, and institutionalized persons. Treatment does not reduce the incidence of symptomatic infection. Treatment also does not reduce mortality in frail elderly patients, and does not improve **chronic** urinary incontinence symptoms. Persistent asymptomatic bacteriuria does not result in renal insufficiency or the development of hypertension.

Which statement is true of asymptomatic bacteriuria?

A) The finding of pyuria in a urinalysis distinguishes urinary tract infection (UTI) from asymptomatic bacteriuria and guides treatment decisions.
B) The prevalence of asymptomatic bacteriuria in women is unrelated to age, function, or hormonal status.
C) Asymptomatic bacteriuria need not be treated in the pregnant patient.
D) None of the above.

Discussion

The correct answer is "D." None of the statements are true. Answer "A" is incorrect because the finding of pyuria with low numbers of WBCs in a urinalysis specimen is nonspecific, common, and frequently unrelated to infection. Answer "B" is incorrect. The prevalence of asymptomatic bacteriuria in women increases with age, declining functional capabilities, and institutionalization. More than 10% of community-dwelling women over the age of 65 and up to 50% of elderly women in nursing homes will have asymptomatic bacteriuria. Answer "C" is incorrect. Pregnancy is one state in which treating asymptomatic pyuria/bacteriuria is indicated. The risk of infection from asymptomatic bacteriuria is high in pregnant patients.

HELPFUL TIP: Treat asymptomatic bacteriuria in the following patients: those with urinary tract obstruction (functional or anatomic), nephrolithiasis, pregnancy, planned urinary instrumentation, and children with **grade V vesicoureteral reflux only** (it is not helpful in grades I–IV reflux).

HELPFUL TIP: Not all pyuria is from UTI. Other pathologic causes of pyuria include vaginitis (infectious and atrophic), urethritis (*Chlamydia trachomatis, Neisseria gonorrhoeae*), and genital herpes infections.

* *

A few years later, the same patient is now 80 years old (you're still paying off your med school loans and will probably work until you're 80), and she is admitted to a nursing home. Her initial tuberculosis (TB) skin test with 5-tuberculin unit injection of purified protein derivative (PPD) was interpreted as 0 mm diameter of induration after 48 hours.

What is your next step?

A) Repeat the PPD now.
B) Repeat the PPD in 2 weeks.
C) Repeat the PPD in 1 year.
D) Declare the patient free of TB.
E) Obtain a chest x-ray.

Discussion

The correct answer is "B." Because the prevalence of a positive PPD (Mantoux test) doubles between the first and second tests in initial nonresponders, the U.S. Public Health Task Force recommends a two-step PPD by the Mantoux method for screening high-risk populations (e.g., persons living in nursing homes). If the first PPD is negative, a second test should be performed approximately 2 weeks later in order to detect the "booster phenomenon." Individuals admitted to a nursing home with a positive PPD and no symptoms of active TB may be presumed to have a distant history of infection.

HELPFUL TIP: False-positive PPDs can be due to bacillus Calmette–Guérin (BCG) vaccine and infection with other mycobacteria. However, most patients who had the BCG vaccine will experience a decline in immunity (a maximum of 20% will have a positive PPD due to BCG 10 years after the vaccine was given). If there is concern about a potential false positive test, an interferon gamma release assay should be performed. False negatives occur when immunity is impaired. If you suspect impaired immunity, use an interferon gamma release assay.

* *

The PPD is repeated 2 weeks later and is interpreted again as 0 mm diameter of induration after 48 hours. You reassure the patient that her tuberculin test is negative.

What would most accurately represent a positive tuberculin skin test in <u>THIS</u> patient?

A) Erythema 5 mm in diameter.
B) Induration 5–10 mm in diameter.
C) Erythema of 10 mm in diameter.

Table 8-1 INTERPRETATION OF PPD SKIN TESTS

Diameter of Induration	Positive in These Situations
5–10 mm	Chest x-ray consistent with past or current infection; HIV positive; recent close contact of person with active TB.
10–15 mm	Institutionalized persons; IV drug users; immunocompromised states other than HIV; children less than 4; children exposed to high-risk adults, health-care workers.
≥15 mm	Persons without risk factors. These are people who probably should not have been tested in the first place (e.g., the general public without any exposure to TB).

D) Induration 10 mm in diameter.
E) Erythematous induration of any size.

Discussion

The correct answer is "D." Here is the bottom line. Routine screening is not recommended for low-risk patients (e.g., community dwelling individuals from a low-risk country). Screen only the following: contacts of those with TB, HIV infected patients, IV drug users, those with predisposing factors to TB infection (diabetes, immunosuppressive drugs, lung cancer, etc.), foreign-born individuals arriving in the United States within the last 5 years, health-care workers, nursing home and other institutionalized individuals and the homeless. Measure the induration and not the erythema. The definition of a positive PPD changes with the population tested. See Table 8–1.

HELPFUL TIP: Whole blood interferon gamma release assay (e.g., QuantiFERON-TB Gold test) is Food and Drug Administration (FDA)-approved for use in any situation in which the PPD is currently employed. It is more expensive and should not be the front-line screening test but may help in situations in which the PPD result is questionable. QuantiFERON and other such tests are **not 100% sensitive and should not** be used in patients who are symptomatic; they are for asymptomatic screening only and cannot differentiate latent from active infection.

* *

A year later, the nursing home calls about her annual PPD. You examine the patient and find the diameter of induration is 12 mm. The patient denies cough, weight loss, fever, or chills.

The most appropriate next step in this case is to:

A) Obtain a chest radiograph and, if normal, initiate isoniazid 300 mg and pyridoxine for 9 months.
B) Obtain a chest radiograph and, if normal, observe the patient annually for signs of active TB (weight loss, cough, fever, etc.).
C) Obtain a chest radiograph and, if abnormal, initiate isoniazid 300 mg once daily and pyridoxine for 9 months.
D) Obtain sputum specimens for acid-fast bacilli (AFB) stains and mycobacterial culture and sensitivity testing; and initiate therapy with isoniazid, pyridoxine, pyrazinamide, and rifampin for 6 months.
E) Obtain a interferon gamma release assay, and if negative, observe the patient annually for signs of active TB (weight loss, cough, fever, etc.).

Discussion

The correct answer is "A." The patient lives in a high-risk setting (nursing home). The results of her Mantoux test 1 year ago suggest that she was not infected with *Mycobacterium tuberculosis* at that time. She has newly converted—probably due to exposure to an active case of TB in the facility. **The risk of developing active disease following TB infection is greatest in the first 2 years following infection. The risk/benefit ratio favors prophylactic therapy with isoniazid (INH) for the patient who has converted within the last 2 years, as long as there is no sign of active disease and the chest x-ray is negative. Pyridoxine should also be given to prevent peripheral neuropathy.** However, a negative chest x-ray does not mean that you can forego prophylactic therapy, and thus "B" is incorrect. Answer "C" is incorrect because an **abnormal** chest radiograph must be followed with collection of sputum specimens for AFB staining and culture. Answer "D" is incorrect because a chest radiograph is necessary to evaluate all patients with a positive Mantoux skin test. Sputum specimens should be collected and multiple drug regimens initiated only in patients with signs and symptoms of active disease based on clinical history, exam, and radiographic findings. Answer "E" is incorrect. Since this patient has converted from 0 to 12 mm induration in 1 year, her pretest probability is high enough that performing an interferon gamma release assay adds nothing.

HELPFUL TIP: A 3-month course of INH plus rifapentine (note, not rifampin) once weekly has been shown to be superior to a 9-month course of daily INH. As of the writing of this book, the 3-month regimen is not yet the current standard of care.

HELPFUL TIP: If active disease is diagnosed, appropriate therapy should be initiated with a 4-drug regimen for 6–8 weeks followed by a simpler regimen for 4–7 months once sensitivities are known (average 6 months total). A number of regimens are available, and all include isoniazid and rifampin. INH alone is never appropriate for active TB. First-line drugs used for active TB include isoniazid, rifampin, pyrazinamide, and ethambutol. Ethambutol may be dropped if the organism is sensitive to INH, RIF, and PYR. Second-line drugs include levofloxacin, streptomycin, and others. Regimens vary by location and local resistance patterns. Contact your local health department.

* *

The patient's son is somewhat distraught that his mother has TB. He asks if she should have received a vaccine before coming into the nursing home.

Regarding the BCG vaccine, which of the following statements is true?

A) Foreign-born persons who received the BCG vaccine should never have a PPD administered.
B) The BCG vaccine is most efficacious for older adults, and children benefit much less from the vaccine.

C) A PPD in an individual with a remote history of BCG vaccine should be interpreted as if the BCG had not been given.
D) The BCG vaccine is made from killed *M. tuberculosis*.

Discussion

The correct answer is "C." The PPD should be interpreted exactly the same way in those who have and have not had BCG. "D" is incorrect. The BCG vaccine is made from attenuated *Mycobacterium bovis*. "B" is incorrect. BCG is most efficacious in children but protection from the vaccine wanes over a few years. Even in children, it is a poor vaccine, protecting children from TB only about 50% of the time. Persons vaccinated with BCG should still be evaluated by PPD (only if appropriate), and an increase in induration >10 mm (age <35 years) or >15 mm (age ≥ 35 years) from baseline is considered positive.

* *

Prior to starting INH, you measured the patient's aminotransferase levels, which were normal. Now, 3 months into treatment, her alanine aminotransferase (ALT) is 42 IU/L (about twice the upper limit of normal).

Your next step is to:

A) Stop her INH since she has had a few months of treatment.
B) Continue the INH as scheduled and follow up with clinical and laboratory monitoring.
C) Switch to rifampin and pyrazinamide.
D) Refer her to a hepatologist for liver biopsy.
E) Start her on milk thistle.

Discussion

The correct answer is "B." While liver injury is a significant problem with isoniazid, the drug need not be stopped unless the liver enzymes rise to more than three times the upper limit of normal. Others would suggest that even then the drug can be continued and that only signs and symptoms of hepatitis (fatigue, anorexia, nausea, and vomiting) along with further liver enzyme elevations should prompt discontinuation of the drug. Answer "A" is incorrect because she should have 9 months of prophylactic therapy. Answer "C" is incorrect because rifampin and pyrazinamide have potentially more hepatotoxicity than INH! Finally, "D" and "E" are incorrect. Neither liver biopsy nor milk thistle (touted for its benefit in liver disease) is likely to be useful.

HELPFUL TIP: Unfortunately, TB has developed resistance to numerous first-line agents. There is drug-resistant TB, multidrug-resistant TB (MDR-TB), extensively drug-resistant TB (XDR-TB), and now totally drug-resistant TB. The differences:

- Drug-resistant TB is resistant to one of the first-line drugs (INH, rifampin, ethambutol, streptomycin, pyrazinamide).
- MDR-TB is resistant to at least INH and rifampin and possibly more drugs.
- XDR-TB is resistant to at least INH, rifampin, fluoroquinolones, and aminoglycosides or capreomycin or both.
- Totally drug-resistant TB is, as its name implies, resistant to all antibiotics currently used to treat TB. It has been seen in a few cases in Italy, Iran, and India.

Objectives: Did you learn to . . .

- Interpret tuberculin skin test results?
- Describe the BCG vaccine and how patients who receive it should be approached?
- Recommend appropriate treatment of a positive PPD?
- Recognize complications of isoniazid therapy?
- Define and recognize the importance of drug-resistant TB?
- Determine who needs to be treated for asymptomatic bacteriuria?

CASE 5

A 37-year-old woman with a history of mitral valve prolapse and mitral regurgitation presents for evaluation. She reports no symptoms of shortness of breath or exercise intolerance. She plans to undergo health-screening procedures, including dental exams for routine cleaning and filling of several caries, pelvic exam with removal of an intrauterine device (IUD), and colonoscopy in the next year.

According to the American Heart Association (AHA) 2007 guidelines on the prevention of infective endocarditis, what should she receive prior to these procedures?

A) Amoxicillin 2 g PO.
B) Azithromycin 500 mg PO.
C) Clindamycin 600 mg PO.
D) Nothing.

Discussion

The correct answer is "D." In 2007, there were major changes to the AHA guidelines on infective endocarditis prevention. The one change that would seem to affect the greatest number of patients in primary care practices is the "downgrading" of mitral valve prolapse with regurgitation, which is no longer considered a high-risk condition. If the patient had a condition for which prophylaxis was warranted, all of the other regimens (A, B, C) are options depending on the patient's allergies, etc.

According to the AHA 2007 guidelines on the prevention of infective endocarditis, which of the following conditions is NOT a high-risk condition for the adverse outcome of infective endocarditis?

A) Bioprosthetic aortic valve.
B) Mechanical aortic valve.
C) Congenital heart disease completely repaired with prosthetic material.
D) Bicuspid aortic valve.
E) Previous history of infective endocarditis.

The correct answer is "D." The guidelines recommend antibiotic prophylaxis for conditions considered to be high risk for adverse outcomes of infective endocarditis. High-risk conditions include prosthetic valves (bioprosthetic homograft and allograft valves and mechanical valves), previous infective endocarditis, and complex cyanotic congenital heart disease.

HELPFUL TIP: Moderate-risk conditions, **for which prophylaxis is *not* indicated**, include acquired valvular dysfunction, such as rheumatic heart disease, hypertrophic cardiomyopathy, bicuspid aortic valve, and mitral valve prolapse with auscultatory evidence of valvular regurgitation and/or thickened leaflets.

HELPFUL TIP: Infective endocarditis is much more likely to result from transient bacteremia that occurs with routine dental care at home, like brushing and flossing, than from dental, GI, and GU procedures. Accordingly, good oral hygiene to lower the risk of bacteremia is more important than prophylactic antibiotics.

If your patient had a mechanical aortic valve, appropriate endocarditis prophylaxis includes:

A) Ampicillin IV 2 hours prior to **colonoscopy** if biopsy of lesions is anticipated.
B) Ampicillin IV 2 hours prior to **pelvic exam and IUD removal.**
C) Amoxicillin PO 2 hours prior to routine dental **cleaning.**
D) Amoxicillin PO 2 hours prior to any **injection of local anesthesia and filling of caries.**
E) All of the above.

Discussion

The correct answer is "C." For high-risk conditions (e.g., mechanical aortic valve), antibiotic prophylaxis is recommended by the AHA prior to cleaning of teeth and removal of plaque. The risk of endocarditis is highest for dental procedures that might traumatize the oral mucosa, such as tooth extractions, periodontal procedures, and cleaning of teeth with removal of adherent plaque. Answers "A," "B," and "D" are incorrect. Prophylaxis is not recommended prior to these procedures. The risk of endocarditis is low for procedures such as lower GI endoscopy and pelvic exam with IUD removal, because the microorganisms likely to cause transient bacteremia following these interventions are not capable of adhering to cardiac valve tissues. Antibiotic prophylaxis is not recommended for restorative dental procedures (e.g., fillings).

* *

All of the evaluations, including the dental exam, seem to go well. However, 1 month later, she returns to see you for gradually (perhaps even subacutely?) worsening fever, malaise, and night sweats. You are concerned that she may have developed infective endocarditis.

The evaluation of a patient suspected of having subacute bacterial endocarditis (SBE) should include all of the following EXCEPT:

A) Three sets of blood cultures obtained at 1-hour intervals within the first 24 hours of assessment.
B) Auscultation of chest for evidence of new or changing murmur.
C) Transthoracic or transesophageal echocardiogram.
D) Spiral chest CT.
E) Electrocardiogram.

Discussion

The correct answer is "D." Spiral chest CT is not indicated in the diagnosis of SBE. History is important: onset of infection can sometimes be related to a recent dental extraction, IV drug abuse, or invasive medical procedure. Symptoms generally begin insidiously and may include weakness, fatigue, fever, night sweats, arthralgias/myalgias, and hematuria. "C," echocardiography, is indicated. The yield for visualization of vegetations for transthoracic echocardiography is 60–77% and increases to 96% with transesophageal echocardiography. A prolongation of the PR interval on an electrocardiogram may suggest involvement of the cardiac conduction system.

* *

You carefully examine the patient and find that she is febrile and slightly tachycardic.

You look for signs of infective endocarditis, paying particular attention to all of the following EXCEPT:

A) Osler nodes.
B) Painless erythematous macules on the palms and soles.
C) Splinter hemorrhages.
D) Painless nodules over bony prominences.
E) Roth spots.

Discussion

The correct answer is "D." Classical physical exam findings of SBE include intermittent fever; petechiae; conjunctival hemorrhage; splinter hemorrhages under the nails; erythematous painful nodules on the fingers, palms, and soles (Osler nodes); fundic hemorrhages (Roth spots); painless erythematous macules on the palms and soles (Janeway lesions); and new diastolic murmur. Answer "D" is not a physical exam finding in SBE. Painless nodules over bony prominences are observed in rheumatic fever and are one of the Jones' criteria. Remember that in a modern medical practice, most patients with SBE will not present with these findings, and you must maintain a high degree of suspicion for SBE in the appropriate clinical scenario.

> HELPFUL TIP: Laboratory evaluation in endocarditis may be remarkable for anemia, leukocytosis, elevated erythrocyte sedimentation rate (ESR), and microscopic hematuria.

Which of the following is/are included in the major criteria of the modified Duke criteria for endocarditis?

A) Positive blood cultures.
B) Janeway lesions (painless macules on palms and soles).
C) Echocardiographic evidence of valvular vegetation.
D) A and B.
E) A and C.

The correct answer is "E." The modified Duke criteria were developed to provide clinicians with standardized criteria for the diagnosis of endocarditis. They have been validated by pathologic examination and are more sensitive than other endocarditis criteria systems. See Table 8–2.

> HELPFUL TIP: Three words about blood cultures—more is better. The sensitivity of blood cultures for endocarditis and bacteremia is directly related to the amount of blood taken for culture and the number of cultures drawn. Three sets of blood cultures are recommended for suspected endocarditis, and at least 20 mL should be drawn for each culture. Timing of blood cultures is less important, but sick patients should have the cultures drawn in rapid succession (e.g., over an hour or 2).

* *

You draw a CBC, which shows leukocytosis with a "left shift" (e.g., a high percentage of bands and other

Table 8–2 DUKE CRITERIA FOR BACTERIAL ENDOCARDITIS

Definite endocarditis is established by the presence of 2 major criteria and at least 1 minor criterion. Probable endocarditis is established by the presence of 1 major and 1 minor criterion, or 3 minor criteria.	
Major Duke criteria	• New valvular regurgitation • Echocardiographic evidence of vegetations • Two positive blood cultures of an organism known to cause endocarditis • Single blood culture or antibody evidence of *Coxiella burnetii* (Q fever)
Minor Duke criteria (not an exhaustive list but these are the most common manifestations)	• Fever • Vascular phenomena (e.g., Janeway lesions, splinter or conjunctival hemorrhages, and septic emboli) • History of predisposing illness (e.g., IV drug abuse, heart lesion, and artificial valve) • Immunologic phenomena (e.g., glomerulonephritis and Osler nodes)

immature neutrophils). Chest x-ray and urinalysis are unrevealing. You draw blood cultures and admit her to the hospital and start antibiotics. The next morning two blood cultures are reported to grow gram-positive cocci in clusters. You start IV vancomycin and order a transesophageal echocardiogram. Indeed, the echocardiogram shows a small vegetation on her mitral valve. Blood cultures return showing methicillin-sensitive S. *aureus*.

What is the most appropriate treatment of this patient now?

A) Nafcillin 2 g IV q 4 hours for 4–6 weeks.
B) Penicillin G 2 million units IV q 2 hours for 4–6 weeks.
C) Vancomycin 1 g IV q 12 hours for 4–6 weeks.
D) Ceftriaxone 1 g IV q 24 hours for 2 weeks.
E) Levofloxacin 500 mg IV q 24 hours for 4–6 weeks.

Discussion

The correct answer is "A." Nafcillin is the drug of choice for the treatment of methicillin-sensitive *S. aureus* endocarditis. Vancomycin should be reserved for patients with penicillin allergy or patients with methicillin-resistant *S. aureus* (MRSA). Neither ceftriaxone nor levofloxacin would be considered appropriate therapy for staphylococcal endocarditis.

> HELPFUL (AND IMPORTANT) TIP: **Patients who have a sensitive organism actually do better with nafcillin than with vancomycin.** So, save vancomycin for MRSA or other resistant organisms. Other options for hospital-acquired MRSA include linezolid and tigecycline.

* *

While hospitalized, the patient develops symptoms of heart failure and worsening mitral regurgitation by echocardiogram. The heart failure is managed medically, but the regurgitation is now categorized as "severe." She has had 3 days of antibiotics.

Which of the following is the most appropriate course of action?

A) Complete 6 weeks of antibiotics and manage her heart failure medically for the foreseeable future.
B) Complete 6 weeks of antibiotics and manage her heart failure medically, if possible; plan for valve replacement after 6 weeks of antibiotics.
C) Refer her for emergent valve replacement surgery.
D) Refer her for immediate coronary catheterization.
E) Refer her for heart transplant.

Discussion

The correct answer is "B." Progressive heart failure and worsening valvular function are indications for surgery. However, it is generally preferable to complete the course of antibiotics first if the patient's heart failure can be effectively medically managed. Thus, "C" is incorrect. Answers "D" and "E" are incorrect, as there is no indication for coronary catheterization or heart transplant.

> HELPFUL TIP: Other indications for surgery in cases of endocarditis include multiple embolic events, infections that are difficult or impossible to treat adequately with

medications (e.g., fungal infections), cardiac conduction abnormalities due to infection, persistent bacteremia, partially dehisced prosthetic valve, and perivalvular infection (e.g., cardiac abscess and fistula).

Which of the following organisms is most often responsible for causing infective endocarditis?

A) *E. coli.*
B) *Streptococcus viridans.*
C) *Proteus mirabilis.*
D) None of the above.

Discussion

The correct answer is "B." *S. viridans* is the most likely organism to cause endocarditis. Gram-negative organisms, such as *E. coli* and *P. mirabilis*, are infrequent causes of infective endocarditis. Other organisms that cause endocarditis include the HACEK organisms (*Haemophilus* species, *Actinobacillus actinomyces comitantes*, *Cardiobacterium hominis*, *Eikenella* species, and *Kingella kingae*). In summary, organisms typically found causing endocarditis are *S. aureus*, *S. viridans*, enterococci (aerobic, gram-positive organisms in chains that are GI or vaginal flora), *Streptococcus bovis*, and HACEK organisms.

Objectives: Did you learn to . . .

- Determine who is an appropriate candidate for infective endocarditis prophylaxis?
- Recognize signs and symptoms of infective endocarditis?
- Diagnose infective endocarditis?
- Prescribe appropriate treatment for infective endocarditis?

QUICK QUIZ: DRUG INTERACTIONS

Which of the following is/are contraindicated in patients taking linezolid?

A) MAOIs.
B) SSRI.
C) Gentamicin.
D) Vancomycin.
E) A and B.

Discussion

The correct answer is "E." Linezolid can cause serotonin syndrome when combined with SSRIs, lithium, MAOIs, and other serotonergic drugs.

CASE 6

A 10-year-old boy presents with his mother, complaining of intense itching, worse at night, since the first week of school. He has numerous excoriations in the interdigital web spaces, wrists, and anterior axillary folds. His infant sister (10 kg) has recently developed intensely pruritic linear lesions on her palms, soles, face, and scalp. Their mother works in a nursing home and has developed pruritus **and reddish-brown nodular lesions** in her axillae and perineum that have persisted several months after she treated herself with a lotion that was provided at her place of work. As you exam the patient, your skin begins to itch.

The most likely ectoparasite affecting this family is:

A) Head lice (pediculosis).
B) Chiggers (mites).
C) Ticks.
D) Fleas.
E) Scabies.

Discussion

The correct answer is "E." Scabies' mites (*Sarcoptes scabiei*) burrow into the epidermis, lay eggs, and hatch larvae in cycles of 3–4 days. The most notable clinical symptom is intense pruritus that is worse at night. The typical lesion is small, erythematous, and papular and may resemble eczema in quality and distribution. About 7% of individuals develop a nodular variant (like the mother in this case). Transmission is typically by direct contact and infestations may appear as epidemics in institutions like nursing homes. The organism may be spread by fomites as well, although to a lesser extent. Young children and infants often have involvement of palms, soles, face, and scalp. A clinical diagnosis may be made in the setting of pruritic rash, typical distribution, and multiple family members affected.

What is the next best step in this case (remember that one child weighs 10 kg)?

A) Removal of the individual organisms.
B) Tetracycline 10 mg/kg divided TID for all affected family members.

C) Single-dose oral ivermectin 200 μg/kg, repeated in 2 weeks for all affected family members.
D) Symptomatic treatment with topical steroids and oral antihistamines.
E) Single-dose oral ivermectin 200 μg/kg repeated in 2 weeks for the mother; one application of 5% permethrin cream for all other family members for 8–14 hours, followed by showering.

Discussion

The correct answer is "E." Permethrin cream is the topical medication of choice. Ivermectin, an antihelmintic medication, is indicated for adults with nodular disease (like the mother in this case), in epidemic settings, and for treatment of scabies crustosa. Answer "B" is incorrect because tetracycline is not helpful in this situation and should be avoided in children. Answer "C" is incorrect because oral ivermectin should be avoided in infants weighing <15 kg due to concerns about increased penetration of the blood–brain barrier. Finally, "D" is incorrect because scabies should be treated with specific therapy rather than simply symptomatic therapy.

HELPFUL TIP: All family members should be treated, regardless of the presence or lack of symptoms. Microscopic exam of a skin scraping may identify the mite but has poor sensitivity. Other viable treatment alternatives include crotamiton 10% solution precipitated sulfur in petroleum and lindane (but avoid lindane in children <2 years old).

* *

You successfully treated the whole family. They are now comfortable, happy, and totally confident in your abilities. The mother returns with her girl, who is now 3 years old, with a new complaint. Apparently, the patient has complained of her "bottom" hurting, a symptom that her mother has interpreted to mean perineal pain. The pain is worse at night and the child has awoken several nights complaining of vaginal pain. The mother thinks that she may have a bladder infection, but there are no urinary symptoms. In the office, the patient complains only of "itchy butt" and her exam is normal.

What is the next best step in diagnosis of this problem?

A) Reassurance that this is "just a stage."
B) Vaginal speculum exam with cultures.
C) "Scotch tape" test.
D) Stool collection for ova and parasites.
E) Referral to a pediatric behavioral disorders specialist.

Discussion

The correct answer is "C." The presentation is consistent with pinworm (*Enterobius vermicularis*) infection. Clinical manifestations of pinworm infection are related to the life cycle of the parasite, in which the adult worm resides in the colon, exits the anus at night, lays eggs in the perianal skin, and may also infest the female GU tract. Typical symptoms include pruritus ani, vulvitis, vaginal pain, poor sleep, and—rarely—abdominal pain (pinworms can migrate and cause appendicitis, and other intra-abdominal illness). The diagnostic test of choice is the "Scotch tape" test. Clear cellophane tape is wrapped around a tongue depressor, sticky side up, and used to sample the perianal area first thing in the morning before bathing. Multiple specimens should be obtained and stored in a refrigerator (it's a good thing OSHA has no jurisdiction in the home). The tape is then examined microscopically for the characteristic ova.

* *

Your "Scotch tape" test is a success, proving your clinical suspicions.

The best intervention is to:

A) Treat the patient with mebendazole 100 mg PO once, repeat in 2 weeks, and encourage good hand washing for the whole family.
B) Treat the patient and the entire family with mebendazole 100 mg PO daily for 14 days.
C) Treat the patient and the entire family with mebendazole 100 mg PO once, and repeat in 2 weeks.
D) Treat the patient with metronidazole 500 mg PO once, and repeat in 2 weeks.

Discussion

The correct answer is "C." As with scabies, the entire family should be treated. Mebendazole is the agent of choice, although other antiparasitic agents (albendazole, pyrantel pamoate) may also be used. Pyrantel

HELPFUL (AND VERY IMPORTANT) TIP: The CDC no longer recommends fluoroquinolones for traveler diarrhea acquired in Southeast Asia because of resistance. The current recommendation is to use azithromycin for traveler diarrhea in Southeast Asia.

HELPFUL TIP: The CDC maintains a user-friendly and up-to-date travel website at http://wwwnc.cdc.gov/travel. Always check here first to assure you are giving the right vaccines and advice.

* *

Finally, you discuss the medication options for malaria prophylaxis.

Which of the following is TRUE?

A) Mefloquine (Lariam) is relatively contraindicated for Jane due to her history of psychiatric illness.
B) Doxycycline would be a safe and effective option for the whole family.
C) Although malaria is resistant to chloroquine in many parts of the world, it can still be used for prophylaxis in West Africa.
D) Atovaquone/proguanil (Malarone) is contraindicated for Jane and Jack due to their sulfa allergy.
E) A month is too long a time to use malaria prophylaxis safely; recommend against it.

Discussion

The correct answer is "A." Mefloquine is an effective, once-a-week prophylaxis for malaria. However, it carries a significant risk of CNS side effects including vivid or disturbing dreams. There have been case reports of the medication inducing psychosis, so the drug is relatively contraindicated for patients with a history of psychiatric illness (such as Jane Smith). "B," doxycycline, may be a good option for the parents, but is contraindicated in children because of their age and risk of tooth discoloration. "C" is incorrect. Malaria throughout Africa, India, Southeast Asia, and South America is now assumed to be resistant to chloroquine. Finally, "D" atovaquone/proguanil is relatively contraindicated in patients with G6PD deficiency due to a risk of hemolysis, but it does not contain sulfa.

* *

Weeks pass, and you hear nothing more until you are called to the acute care clinic, where Jack Smith has been brought in by his parents for fever and lethargy. Jack had been treated in Lagos, Nigeria, for **malaria** with an unknown medication, and he subsequently recovered. Jack was apparently well until 10 days after returning home, when he developed rapid onset of a fever and shaking chills. He also complained to his parents of generalized abdominal pain and watery, nonbloody diarrhea. The parents treated him at home for a day with ibuprofen and acetaminophen, but he seemed to worsen. He became lethargic, stopped drinking and eating, and the fever continued.

Jack appears drowsy and listless but is arousable. He does not respond to questions about current symptoms, but cooperates with an exam. Findings are temperature 39.1°C, pulse 136, blood pressure 100/50, and respiratory rate 24. His neck is supple with mild lymphadenopathy. He is tachycardic with a mild flow murmur. His abdomen is nontender with a palpable spleen. No rash or petechiae are noted. The rest of the exam is unremarkable. A recurrence of malaria is suspected.

What is the best method for confirming this diagnosis?

A) Blood culture.
B) Malaria serology.
C) Malaria antigen test.
D) Thin and thick blood smears.
E) Stool ova and parasite.

Discussion

The correct answer is "D." Malaria is usually diagnosed by blood smear. The thick blood smear is the more sensitive screening test, and the thin blood smear is used to identify the species of parasite. There are antigen tests that are rapid but have higher false positives and false negatives. Thus, if one suspects malaria and the rapid test is negative, thick and thin smears are still indicated. The blood smear remains the gold standard. Malaria serology and cultures are used only in experiments and are not helpful for diagnosis of an individual patient. Of note, PCR-based testing has excellent sensitivity and specificity but is expensive and not widely available. The malaria parasite cannot be identified in stool.

* *

You begin IV fluids and arrange hospital admission. The relevant laboratory tests are drawn and sent, including CBC, blood cultures, tests for malaria, chemistry profile, blood type and screen, and urinalysis. A lumbar puncture is performed and the CSF is normal. In the meantime, the laboratory calls with the report that *P. falciparum* has been identified.

What antimicrobial should be chosen as initial therapy?

A) PO hydroxychloroquine (Plaquenil), since many hospitals do not stock chloroquine.
B) PO mefloquine (Lariam).
C) PO quinine.
D) IV quinidine, since IV quinine is not generally available in the United States.
E) IV atovaquone/proguanil (Malarone).

Discussion

The correct answer is "D." Clearly, since this patient is ill and not tolerating oral intake, an IV route for malaria treatment is indicated. IV atovaquone/proguanil does not now exist, so the only available option is quinine. But IV quinine is not available in the United States, so its isomer, quinidine (the antiarrhythmic) is used instead. In patients from chloroquine-sensitive zones (currently Central America and the Middle East), treatment with chloroquine is acceptable. Hydroxychloroquine is an option if chloroquine is not available.

> HELPFUL TIP: Artesunate, another antimalarial, clears parasitemia faster than quinidine but is not approved by the FDA. It is available from the CDC on protocol.

* *

Despite a frightening hospital course that included generalized seizures, hypoglycemia, hematuria, renal insufficiency, and an exchange transfusion, Jack eventually recovers completely. The Smith family thanks you for your help and hopes you'll accompany them on their next trip to Africa.

Objectives: Did you learn to . . .

- Identify important elements of a patient's travel plans and unique risks when providing counseling for overseas travel?
- Identify preventative measures for malaria, including chemoprophylaxis and insect bite avoidance?
- Diagnose traveler diarrhea and describe its prevention and treatment?
- Recognize the signs and symptoms of malaria, describe methods of diagnosis, and initiate therapy?

QUICK QUIZ: CRITTERS IN CREIGHTON

A family comes to see you because the two children, ages 7 and 4, have developed itchy scalps. The parents seem unaffected. So far, they have not tried any treatments. On examination of both children, you find erythematous papules on the occiput and small white eggs firmly attached to the hair shaft about 1 cm from the scalp.

The most appropriate treatment is:

A) Application of 1% permethrin cream to all family members for 10 minutes followed by rinsing, combing out all nits with a special louse comb, and decontaminating affected garments and bed linens. Repeat in 7 days.
B) Elimination of animal or fomite sources of infestation and use of insect repellents.
C) Removal of any adherent organisms and oral doxycycline for 14 days.
D) Application of 5% permethrin cream to all family members for 8–14 hours, followed by showering.
E) Shave everyone's head.

Discussion

The correct answer is "A." These are head lice. Pediculosis infestations of the hair and scalp are usually asymptomatic but can present with itching. The diagnosis is made by demonstration of the louse or nits, which fluoresce a pale blue under a Wood's light. Treatment with topical agents such as permethrin cream for two applications and wet combing to remove nits is recommended by the CDC. Ivermectin may be effective in cases of resistant organisms. It is reasonable to recommend washing clothing and bedclothes of an infested person, but head lice do not survive off the scalp longer than 48 hours. Answer "B" is appropriate for chiggers (mites) or fleas. Answer "C" is appropriate for ticks (if also associated with a tick-borne illness). Answer "D" is a treatment of scabies (note the difference in strength of permethrin).

CASE 9

A 19-year-old female college student presents to student health services with "the flu." She has noted a fever of 38.9°C and myalgias. She is treated with symptomatic care and discharged back to her dormitory. Three hours later her roommate finds her lethargic and difficult to arouse, so she calls 911. On exam her blood pressure is 70/30 with a pulse of 145. Her neck is supple, but she is lethargic and complaining of severe muscle aches. She denies headache. There is a fine macular rash over her abdomen.

The most important historical factor(s) in this case is (are):

A) History of splenectomy.
B) Use of tampons.
C) History of acetaminophen overdose.
D) A and B.
E) All of the above.

Discussion

The correct answer is "D." "A" is important since patients with a splenectomy can get sick rather rapidly from pneumococci and other encapsulated bacteria. Answer "B" is important because this patient may have toxic shock syndrome, which is related to the use of tampons. Answer "C" is not important. First, shock is not a prominent feature of acetaminophen overdose (if it occurs at all). Additionally, acetaminophen overdose is not associated with a rash.

* *

The patient is able to give you the additional history that she does not use tampons and has not taken any medication except for occasional acetaminophen and ibuprofen in recommended doses. She has her spleen... in a jar in her dorm room—no, wait, we mean in her left upper quadrant. It's her ex-boyfriend's spleen in the jar.

On the basis of this information you decide that:

A) It is unlikely that this is toxic shock syndrome given that she does not use tampons.
B) The combination of acetaminophen and ibuprofen in this patient with the flu has led to hypotension.
C) Given that she is immunocompetent and has her spleen intact, this cannot be sepsis since it started so quickly.
D) Toxic shock, which was a big problem in the 1980s and early 1990s, no longer occurs since the advent of less absorbent tampons.
E) None of the above.

Discussion

The correct answer is "E." Answer "A" is incorrect because up to 50% of cases of toxic shock occur as the result of staphylococcal infections unrelated to tampons. These may be ingrown toenails, infected abrasions, etc. Answer "B" is incorrect. Acetaminophen and ibuprofen are frequently combined without difficulty. Answer "C" is also incorrect. Splenectomized patients are more prone to sepsis from encapsulated organisms, but the fact that the patient has a spleen does not grant invincibility. Sepsis obviously occurs in the normal host as well. Finally, "D" is incorrect. While absorbent tampons are a major culprit in toxic shock syndrome, as noted above, there are other causes. Thus, toxic shock syndrome is not going away anytime soon.

The organism(s) responsible for toxic shock syndrome is (are):

A) *Staphylococcus.*
B) *H. influenzae.*
C) *Streptococcus.*
D) A and B.
E) A and C.

Discussion

The correct answer is "E." There are two types of toxic shock syndrome, one caused by *Staphylococcus* and the other by *Streptococcus*. There are certain subtypes that make the toxin responsible for toxic shock syndrome and only certain hosts are thought to be susceptible. Of note, most patients with streptococcal toxic shock are bacteremic, whereas those with staphylococcal toxic shock are not.

Which of the following would you NOT expect to find on laboratory testing of this patient with suspected toxic shock syndrome?

A) Creatinine of 2.0 mg/dL (normal 1 mg/dL).
B) Elevated ALT/AST.
C) Platelets of 450,000/mm^3.
D) Elevated CPK.

Discussion

The correct answer is "C." By the definition of toxic shock syndrome, the platelet count should be

<100,00 mm^3 in Staph related toxic shock. All of the other findings are representative of the multisystem dysfunction that categorizes toxic shock syndrome.

* *

Your patient is a little more alert, most likely due to your charming wit. A second set of vitals shows: blood pressure 72/44, pulse 140, respirations 24, temperature 39°C. Labs are pending.

What is the single best next step in the care of this patient?

A) Start IV nafcillin.
B) Place two large-bore IV lines and start aggressive fluid replacement.
C) Start IV norepinephrine.
D) Give a single dose of IV dexamethasone.
E) Transfuse two units of packed red cells.

Discussion

The correct answer is "B." Treatment is mainly supportive. She's in shock. Two large-bore IV lines should be placed with fluids running wide open, and norepinephrine (or other pressor) should be available if her pressure does not improve rapidly. Answer "A" is of special note. Patients with classic toxic shock syndrome (staphylococcal) are not septic. Therefore, while an antistaphylococcal drug is important (as is locally treating the site of infection with incision and drainage, toenail removal, etc.), the antistaphylococcal drug is not to treat bacteremia. However, the patient should receive an antibiotic because we are presuming there is a localized infection somewhere, and we don't know what bacteria is responsible yet. Answer "D" and "E" are incorrect since neither steroids nor blood products are currently indicated.

> HELPFUL TIP: Norepinephrine is the pressor of choice in almost all situations. It has superior survival when compared to dopamine in sepsis and is clearly better in cardiogenic shock. (Although we still hear residents say, "Leave 'em dead with Levophed.")

Objectives: Did you learn to . . .

- Identify signs and symptoms of toxic shock syndrome?
- Describe the pathophysiology of toxic shock syndrome?
- Initiate management for a patient with sepsis and toxic shock syndrome?

CASE 10

One of your patients has recently been in Indonesia for a prolonged period of time. Upon return to the United States, he develops a febrile illness 5 days after landing in Iowa (yes, we have airports). When he presents to the ED, he recalls being bitten by a particularly large and persistent mosquito just before boarding the airplane. On arrival to the ED, he complains of severe, diffuse body pain, headache, and eye pain and eye redness. Vitals show a temperature of 38.5, pulse 145. Labs show a low white count and thrombocytopenia. He does **not** note cyclic fevers. His eosinophil count is normal. A Giemsa stain of the blood show no organisms.

The most likely cause of this illness is:

A) Pneumococcal sepsis.
B) Dengue fever.
C) Malaria.
D) Filariasis.

Discussion

The correct answer is "B." This patient has Dengue fever. Dengue fever is most common in Asia but also occurs in Africa (as well as in Haiti and elsewhere). Patients typically present with fever, conjunctivitis, headache, retro-orbital pain, leukopenia, and thrombocytopenia. The *sine-qua-non* of Dengue fever is severe myalgias and arthralgias, hence the moniker "break bone fever." More mild forms do occur, however. "A" is incorrect since patients with pneumococcal sepsis will *generally* not have thrombocytopenia and a low WBC count (yes, we know there are exceptions). "C" is incorrect because the patient does not have cyclic fevers and a blood smear is negative. Filariasis, "D," presents with eosinophilia and microfilaria in the bloodstream. Again, this should be evident on the blood smear.

* *

With supportive care, the patient recovers. However, not having learned his lesson he returns to Indonesia. When he returns to Iowa, he presents again to the ED, suspecting that he has Dengue fever.

Signs and symptoms of a second occurrence of Dengue fever include all of the following EXCEPT:

A) Capillary leak with hypovolemia and hemoconcentration.
B) Hemorrhagic complications including capillary fragility.
C) Onset >14 days after exposure.
D) Severe thrombocytopenia.

Discussion

The correct answer is "C." If a returning traveller presents more than 14 days after return to home, Dengue fever can be effectively ruled out. In this case, think of other infectious diseases including malaria. The incubation period of Dengue fever is 3–7 days. The rest are correct. Patients with their ***second or subsequent*** episode of Dengue fever can present with capillary leak syndrome, marked thrombocytopenia, and severe hemorrhage. It is usually the second or subsequent infection that leads to mortality.

HELPFUL TIP: The treatment of Dengue fever is supportive care. In many countries, treatment is begun with albumin to replace the circulating volume (given the capillary leak syndrome). However, saline is just as good and a lot less expensive.

Objectives: Did you learn . . .

- The presentation of Dengue fever?
- The difference between the first and subsequent episodes of Dengue fever?

BIBLIOGRAPHY

Annane D, et al. Septic shock. *Lancet.* 2005;365:63.
Bratton RL, Corey R. Tick-borne disease. *Am Fam Physician.* 2005;71(12):2323-2330.
Centers for Disease Control and Prevention. Section on traveler's health. Available at: http://wwwnc.cdc.gov/travel/, Accessed January 12, 2012.
Centers for Disease Control and Prevention. Section on influenza. Available at: http://www.cdc.gov/flu/professionals/index.htm, Accessed January 12, 2012.
Frieden TR, et al. Tuberculosis. *Lancet.* 2003;362:887-899.
Hirschmann JV. Fever of unknown origin in adults. *Clin Infect Dis.* 1997;24:291-300.
Lew DP, Waldvogel FA. Osteomyelitis. *N Engl J Med.* 1997;336:999-1007.
Mylonakis E, Calderwood SB. Infective endocarditis in adults. *N Engl J Med.* 2001;345:1318.
Nichol KL, et al. Effectiveness of influenza vaccine in community-dwelling elderly. *N Engl J Med.* 2007;357:1373-1381.
Schroeder MS. Clostridium difficile-associated diarrhea. *Am Fam Physician.* 2005;71(5):921-928.
Sterling TS, et al. Three months of rifapentine and isoniazid for latent tuberculosis infection. *N Engl J Med.* 2011;365:2155.
Tal S, et al. Fever of unknown origin in older adults. *Clin Geriatr Med.* 2007;23:649-668, viii.
Tolan RW Jr. Fever of unknown origin: A diagnostic approach to this vexing problem. *Clin Pediatr.* 2010;49:207-213.
Wendel K, Rompalo A. Scabies and pediculosis pubis: An update of treatment regimens and general review. *Clin Infect Dis.* 2002;35:S146-S151.
Wilson W, et al. Prevention of infective endocarditis: Guideline from the American Heart Association. *Circulation.* 2007;116(15):1736-1754.

9

HIV/AIDS

Regina Won and Jack T. Stapleton

Note: The antiretroviral treatment of HIV/AIDS (HAART) has become increasingly complex. Thus, this chapter focuses on the primary care aspects of HIV/AIDS including initial evaluation, drug side effects, and infectious disease prophylaxis.

CASE 1

A 23-year-old female presents to your clinic complaining of sore throat, fever, and body aches. She reports that the illness began about a week ago and has persisted despite therapy with NSAIDs, acetaminophen, and sore throat lozenges. She denies cough, abdominal pain, nausea, or vomiting, but reports a persistent headache. Her past medical and surgical history is unremarkable. The patient smokes about one pack of cigarettes a week, drinks occasional alcohol, and denies other drugs, including intravenous (IV) use. She is heterosexual, and has had eight sexual contacts in the past year. She takes oral contraceptives, and her partners usually do not use condoms.

On exam her vital signs are T 38.9°C; P 112; BP 115/68; R 20.

The patient has pharyngitis and enlarged tonsils with exudates. There is diffuse cervical lymphadenopathy, but the neck is supple. There are enlarged nodes in her axilla and inguinal areas as well. The spleen is palpable and nontender. The rest of the exam is unremarkable. You obtain a throat culture, blood count, and heterophile antibody (Monospot), and consider testing for HIV.

An appropriate laboratory test to rule out the acute retroviral syndrome would be:

A) HIV-1 antibody by ELISA and Western blot.
B) HIV-1 antibody by rapid detection method.
C) HIV **DNA** by PCR.
D) CD4 T lymphocyte count.
E) Combined HIV-1 **antibody and antigen** ELISA test.

Discussion

The correct answer is "E." This presentation is consistent with an acute retroviral syndrome, which occurs very early in the infection and is characterized by a mononucleosis-like illness that can last several weeks. Current HIV diagnostic ELISA methods include the option for both antibody and antigen detection. Since the antibody to HIV will not develop for at least 2–8 weeks after infection and the retroviral syndrome typically occurs before seroconversion, HIV antibody tests, including rapid detection methods, may well be negative. During the acute HIV infection, HIV viral loads are very high, and patients are more infectious compared to other times during their HIV infection. Consequently, the HIV antigen assay, which measures HIV p24 protein, is typically positive during this period. Not all laboratories have adopted the HIV antibody–antigen ELISA, so the alternative approach would be to measure the HIV RNA by PCR. However, since this test is much more expensive, the antibody–antigen ELISA is preferred in this setting. The HIV **DNA** PCR assay is not standardized and should not be used in this setting. The CD4 count is not a reliable way of diagnosing HIV infection; it can become depressed with any acute illness or may be normal in early HIV disease.

* *

The ELISA returns positive for HIV antigen and negative for antibody. After appropriate treatment and counseling, blood was sent for CD4 count, HIV RNA testing and, drug-resistance (genotype) testing. Follow-up is arranged for the patient, and she returns in 4 weeks with no complaints or symptoms. A complete history and physical are performed. The patient has mild cervical lymphadenopathy and no other findings.

Laboratory studies are ordered and show:

WBC 3200 cells/mm^3

Chemistry panel (normal)

Hct 42%

Liver enzymes (normal)

Platelets 185,000 cells/mm^3

CD-4 lymphocytes 645 cells/mm^3

HIV viral load 5000 copies/mL

HIV genotype has K103N mutation.

At her next visit, what baseline studies should be ordered?

A) PPD.
B) RPR.
C) Repeat HIV ELISA.
D) Hepatitis B and C antibody.
E) All of the above.

Discussion

The correct answer is "E." During the initial assessment of an HIV-infected person, all of these studies are important. A positive PPD (>5 mm induration in a person infected with HIV) warrants isoniazid and pyridoxine therapy for 9 months if the patient is found to have latent disease (no active disease). Since patients with any sexually transmitted infection (STI) are at risk for another STI, screening for syphilis with an RPR is recommended. The same rationale applies for hepatitis B and C, which can be acquired via the same routes as HIV. The patient has documented HIV by virtue of the positive HIV antigen–antibody ELISA and positive HIV RNA; however, documentation of seroconversion is important, and a repeat HIV antibody ELISA should be sent at 12 weeks and positives confirmed by HIV Western blot. Genotype testing for resistance against certain medications should be performed at baseline regardless of whether antiretroviral (ARV) therapy will be initiated or deferred.

* *

The patient is counseled appropriately about all the results.

What is the most important factor in determining when to start highly active antiretroviral therapy (HAART)?

A) A rising viral load.
B) A decrease in CD4 count.
C) The development of an opportunistic infection.
D) The patient's willingness and ability to comply with the difficult regimens involved.
E) An undetectable viral load (<50 copies/mL).

Discussion

The correct answer is "D." The decision to start HAART is a difficult one that must be done on an individual basis. There is much controversy about when is the best time to start therapy. The most important consideration by far, however, is the willingness of the patient to strictly adhere to complicated medical regimens. **Poor compliance virtually guarantees the development of resistance, hampers treatment of the patient in later stages, and risks the spread of resistant strains to other patients.** If a patient is ready to start therapy, the CD4 count is used to guide the optimum time for initiating therapy. At CD4 counts <200 cells/mm^3, the risk of death rises considerably. Current guidelines (as of 2011 Department of Health and Human Services [HHS] panel) state that therapy should be started at CD4 counts <350 cells/mm^3 or if there is a history of AIDS defining illness. For CD4 counts between 350 and 500 cells/mm^3, the HHS panel was divided and no consensus regarding therapy was reached. At CD4 counts >500 cells/mm^3, the risk for disease progression may be outweighed by the risk of toxicity of the drugs, and the HHS panel was evenly divided on HAART for HIV-infected people with >500 CD4 cells/mm^3. These numbers represent general rules in treatment, and other compelling indications may dictate variations in the approach to treating a specific individual. Evidence does not support using the viral load as an independent determinant of initiating therapy.

HELPFUL TIP: Starting HAART with a CD4 count of >500 cells/mm^3 is advocated by some. It is clear that early treatment reduces partner-to-partner transmission by 96% (Nat Inst of Allergy and Inf Diseases; http://www.niaid.nih.gov/news/newsreleases/2011/Pages/HPTN052.aspx).

HELPFUL TIP: Current guidelines recommend treatment **immediately** for pregnant women at any stage of HIV infection, including during the acute retroviral syndrome. Treatment of others during the acute retroviral syndrome is considered optional, and there is no proven long-term benefit. HIV medications suitable for use during pregnancy must be used.

HELPFUL (BUT CONFUSING) TIP: *Pneumocystis carinii* is no longer *P. carinii.* It is now *Pneumocystis jiroveci.* We didn't do it, honest. It was some microbiologist-taxonomist who wanted to confuse us all. Just to add to the confusion, *P. jiroveci* pneumonia is still often abbreviated "PCP" for in **P**neumo**C**ystis jiroveci **P**neumonia.

Aside from considering HAART and stressing the importance of partner notification, what other intervention should be offered at this stage?

A) Pneumococcal and hepatitis B vaccines.
B) Trimethoprim/sulfamethoxazole (TMP/SMX) DS one tablet per day for the prevention of *P. jiroveci* pneumonia
C) Azithromycin 1250 mg per week for the prevention of *Mycobacterium avium* complex (MAC).
D) Fluconazole 100 mg per day for the prevention of cryptococcal meningitis.

Discussion

The correct answer is "A." Adequate immunizations at a clinical stage when the patient is likely to benefit from the vaccines (i.e., CD4 >500 cells/mm^3) are important. **Live vaccines, such as the MMR, should be avoided in immunocompromised persons, generally considered those HIV-infected persons with a CD4 count <200 cells/mm^3.**

Table 9–1 RECOMMENDED PROPHYLAXIS IN HIV+ PATIENTS

CD4± Count	Organism	Recommended Prophylaxis
<200	*Pneumocystis*	TMP/SMX or dapsone (should make sure patient is not G6PD deficient)
<100	Toxoplasmosis	TMP/SMX
<50	Mycobacterium avium complex (MAC)	Azithromycin or rifabutin

TMP/SMX for PCP prevention is indicated when the CD4 drops below 200 cells/mm^3. Azithromycin is indicated for MAC prophylaxis when the CD4 count drops below 50 cells/mm^3. Fluconazole is used for chronic suppression after the treatment of cryptococcal meningitis or for the treatment of esophageal candidiasis; but it is not currently used as prophylaxis. There is no survival benefit to prophylaxis for cryptococcal meningitis. See Table 9–1 for recommended prophylaxis in patients with HIV.

HELPFUL TIP: Partner notification is very important. State laws vary considerably regarding partner notification, and state health departments are usually very helpful in facilitating this. Some states have criminal transmission statutes for having sex without telling the partner of one's HIV status. Prosecution may not require actual transmission.

* *

After consultation with an HIV specialist, the patient elects not to start therapy at this time and is scheduled for follow-up with regular checks of her viral load and CD4 count. After 1 year, the patient's lab values have changed: CD-4 lymphocytes 280 cells/mm^3; viral load 75,000 copies/mL

In the past year, she has been treated three times for lobar pneumonia and once for oral candidiasis (without esophageal disease).

Does this patient meet the CDC case definition for the acquired immune deficiency syndrome (AIDS)?

A) No, because she has not had an AIDS-defining illness.
B) No, because her CD4 count is >200 cells/mm^3.
C) No, because she has only been diagnosed with HIV infection for 1 year.
D) Yes, because she has had recurrent (two or more episodes) of lobar pneumonia.
E) Yes, because her viral load is >10,000 copies/mL.

Discussion

The correct answer is "D." The 1993 revised CDC HIV classification system requires a case of HIV infection be reported as AIDS if the CD4 count is less than 200 cells/mm^3 OR the patient develops an AIDS defining illness. These AIDS defining illnesses include *esophageal* (not oral) candidiasis, cryptococcal infection, disseminated histoplasmosis, invasive cervical cancer, tuberculosis, HIV wasting disease, and *recurrent pneumonia* (more than one episode per year). Other infections, Kaposi sarcoma, and certain lymphomas may also define AIDS in an HIV-infected person. Duration of infection and viral load are not currently criteria.

* *

The patient is started on tenofovir/emtricitabine (Truvada) and ritonavir-boosted atazanavir once daily. Efavirenz (Sustiva) was not used due to the original resistance testing, and because the patient is of childbearing age and Sustiva is contraindicated during pregnancy. She does well with the treatment, and tolerates the medications. On a later routine follow-up, she reports mild fatigue, but is otherwise well.

Her lab results over several visits are listed in Table 9–2.

Current labs also include WBC 4500 cells/mm^3, Hb 12.1 g/dL, platelets 128,000 cells/mm^3, total bilirubin 2.1.

Table 9–2 CASE 1, LAB RESULTS

	January	March	May
CD4 count	204 cells/mm^3	178 cells/mm^3	244 cells/mm^3
Viral load	5500 copies/mL	<50 copies/mL	<50 copies/mL

At this point, what changes, if any, should be made to the patient's regimen?

A) The patient has failed HAART treatment, and the drug regimen should be changed.
B) The patient has suffered a severe adverse effect (hyperbilirubinemia) from the drug regimen and all three drugs should be changed.
C) The patient has failed to reconstitute her immune system (CD4 count still less than 200 cells/mm^3), so one of her drugs should be changed.
D) The patient is doing well and her regimen should be continued. The hyperbilirubinemia is a side effect associated with atazanavir.

Discussion

The correct answer is "D." The patient's viral load is suppressed, which is the primary goal of HAART. The patient has not suffered any major adverse reactions. Indirect hyperbilirubinemia is commonly seen with atazanavir, and other hepatic enzymes should be followed regularly to ensure that the change in laboratory studies is only due to the atazanavir. It can be mild, but can become severe on occasion. **Criteria for changing drug regimens include** <1 $\log_{10}$ reduction in viral RNA by 8 weeks (e.g., 100,000 to 10,000 is a 1 $\log_{10}$ reduction), failure to depress viral RNA to undetectable levels by 6 months, repetitive detection of viral RNA after initially achieving undetectable levels, persistent decline in CD4 counts (on at least two measurements), or significant clinical deterioration. The expected rise in CD4 counts is much slower than the fall in HIV RNA, and little or no change may be seen in the first 6 months of therapy.

> HELPFUL TIP: When changing drug regimens for virologic failure, it is important to repeat genotype testing while on their current regimen to determine whether the patient's virus has now developed resistance to their current ARV regimen.

* *

The patient's HAART regimen is maintained. However, she misses her next two appointments, and returns to clinic 6 months later. She reports taking all of her medications but complains of a 10 pound unintended weight loss. She also notes increased frequency of night sweats but no fevers. A physical exam is unremarkable except for a gaunt appearance and temporal muscle wasting.

Her lab results show:

CD4 count: 78 cells/mm^3
Viral load: 6400 copies/mL
CBC: WBC 2400 cells/mm^3
Hb: 11.3 g/dL
Platelets: 145,000 cells/mm^3
Total bilirubin: 1.8.

Repeat CD4 count and viral load 2 weeks later shows:

CD4 count: 32 cells/mm^3
Viral load: 7100 copies/mL.

At this point, what changes, if any, should be made to the patient's regimen?

A) The patient has failed HAART treatment and her ARV regimen should be adjusted.
B) Since her hyperbilirubinemia has persisted, the patient is assumed to have suffered a severe adverse affect from her atazanavir, so it alone should be changed.
C) The viral load is not over 50,000 copies/mL, so the current regimen should be continued.
D) The patient is doing well and her regimen should be continued. The hyperbilirubinemia is a side effect associated with atazanavir.

Discussion

The correct answer is "A." The patient has failed HAART based on several criteria, including the reemergence of detectable viral RNA after it had been completely suppressed and a falling CD4 count (see explanation of previous question, above). Her ARV therapy should be changed once the results of the repeat genotype testing are known.

* *

A new ARV therapy regimen is recommended based on the genotype results along with PCP and MAC prophylaxis. Two weeks later, the patient's CD4 count rises to 175 cells/mm^3 and she had more energy. However, she returns to clinic 3 weeks later (5 weeks after starting her new HIV regimen) and is complaining of severe shortness of breath. She says that she had been taking her HIV medications and the azithromycin, but that she lost her PCP prophylaxis prescription (TMP/SMX), and had forgotten to get a new one. Her current illness began 6 days ago as a fever and mild cough. She developed significant dyspnea with minimal exertion, and now is even short of breath at rest. Her chest hurts bilaterally, worse with inspiration. She has drenching night sweats. She denies hemoptysis, sputum production, nausea, vomiting, or abdominal pain.

Physical exam reveals the following vital signs:

T 39°C
BP 90/60
P 135
RR 38
Oxygen saturation 78% (RA).

The patient is in severe respiratory distress and in the tripod position. Neck exam reveals bilaterally enlarged lymphadenopathy. She has no cardiac murmurs. The lung exam shows diffuse rales and tachypnea. The abdomen is nontender, and the remainder of the exam is unremarkable. She does not respond to oxygen and becomes unresponsive.

Aside from respiratory isolation, what should be done next?

A) Sputum culture.
B) Bronchoalveolar lavage (BAL) for direct immunofluorescence (DFA).
C) IV fluids and rapid sequence intubation.
D) Oxygen, furosemide, and nitroglycerin.
E) Chest x-ray, blood count, CD4 count, and viral load.

Discussion

The correct answer is "C." The patient is in extremis—in severe distress and impending respiratory failure. She is also hypotensive and tachycardic and must be stabilized before any further workup is done. "D," Oxygen, furosemide, and nitrates are useful treatments of congestive heart failure, but this is unlikely in such a young person. *P. jiroveci* pneumonia (PCP) is a more likely diagnosis that explains all the findings. Given the timing of the onset of symptoms in the setting of a rapid CD4 response to ARV therapy, this is likely related to immune reconstitution inflammatory syndrome (IRIS).

> HELPFUL TIP: IRIS is well named. It is identified by a paradoxical **symptomatic** worsening of a preexisting infectious process as the immune system reconstitutes with ARV therapy. Basically, the body's immune response is wrecking havoc at the sites of infection (including CMV retinitis, TB causing increased fever, malaise and weight loss, and increased signs of cryptococcal meningitis and obviously, PCP). The infection may be under treatment or subclinical yet becomes symptomatically worse when IRIS develops.

* *

After appropriate resuscitation, laboratories and a chest x-ray are obtained. The x-ray is shown in Figure 9–1.

Laboratory results are:

WBC 3,400 cells/mm^3
Hb 11 g/dL
Platelets 180,000 cells/mm^3
Creatinine 2.4 mg/dL
LDH 1,280 IU/L
PT 12.4 sec, PTT 27 sec
Liver enzymes normal
ABG: pH 7.56, $PaCO_2$ 23 mm Hg, PaO_2 72 mm Hg (on 100% FiO_2)
Sputum and blood cultures are pending.

What should be the initial antibiotic therapy?

A) Four drug antituberculosis regimen.
B) Azithromycin or levofloxacin IV.
C) TMP-SMX IV.

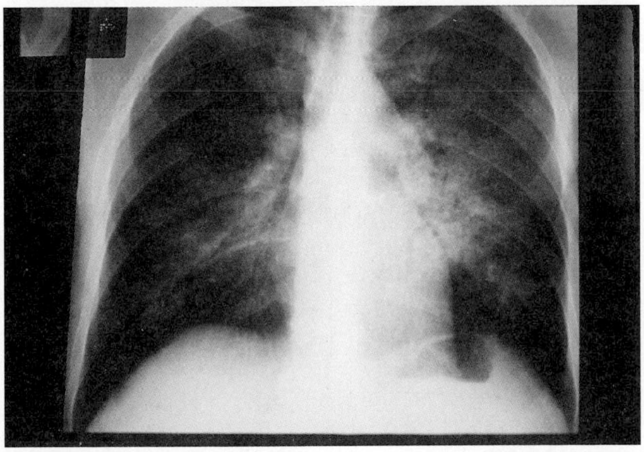

Figure 9–1 **Chest radiograph**

D) TMP-SMX IV, preceded by corticosteroids.
E) No antibiotics initially—just wait for the culture results.

Discussion

The correct answer is "D." The patient is acutely ill, and likely has PCP. Steroids decrease the mortality in patients with severe PCP (PaO_2 <70 on room air or arterial–alveolar O_2 gradient >35 mm Hg). The best antibiotic for PCP is TMP-SMX. Pentamidine IV may be used in cases of sulfa allergy, but it has been associated with hypotension and hypoglycemia. Although the classic chest x-ray appearance for PCP is bilateral interstitial infiltrates, it can present differently (as in this case). Initially normal x-ray exams are not uncommon. **Since the infecting organism is not known with certainty, it would prudent to add empiric therapy for bacterial pneumonia with ceftriaxone and azithromycin pending bronchoscopy results.** PCP does not grow in standard cultures; but it can be visualized with silver stain on BAL or with direct fluorescent assay. It can still be isolated within 48 hours after starting therapy.

* *

The patient is admitted to the ICU and given antibiotics. Her condition stabilizes until 4 hours into her ICU stay. At that time, her respiratory rate on assist-control ventilation dramatically increases from 18 to 42. Peak airway pressures according to the ventilator are greater than 60 cm of water, when they were less than 30 cm water previously. **Breath sounds are absent on the right side of her chest, and her trachea is deviated to the left.** Heart sounds are audible, but tachycardic. Neck veins are distended bilaterally.

What is the next appropriate step, BEFORE a repeat chest x-ray is taken?

A) Give Versed 2 mg IV for sedation, the patient must be very anxious.
B) Pull the ET tube back 1–2 cm, as it is likely in the right mainstem bronchus.
C) Perform a blind pericardiocentesis, as the patient is developing tamponade.
D) Insert a large Angiocath into the left second intercostal space to relieve the tension pneumothorax on the left.
E) Insert a large Angiocath into the right second intercostal space to relieve the tension pneumothorax on the right.

Discussion

The correct answer is "E." The patient has developed a dreaded complication of PCP, a pneumothorax. The organism, *Pneumocystis*, has a propensity to cause blebs (cysts) in the lung tissue. Since the patient was receiving positive pressure ventilation, a tension pneumothorax developed and requires immediate needle decompression. This should be done without waiting for a portable chest x-ray. When the pneumothorax is later confirmed, a tube thoracostomy may be performed under controlled conditions.

* *

Following a protracted ICU admission, the patient improves, and is restarted on the HIV medication regimen that was selected based on her drug resistance testing (zidovudine, raltegravir, ritonavir, and darunavir). She is discharged, and in response to this life-threatening complication, she is highly motivated and becomes very adherent with her medications. Two years later her CD4 is 385 cells/mm^3, her HIV RNA concentration is <50 copies/mL (nondetectable), and she recently started a job that she enjoys.

Objectives: Did you learn to . . .

- Identify the signs and symptoms of the acute retroviral syndrome?
- Use appropriate tests for diagnosis of HIV infection?
- Evaluate a patient with HIV and monitor that patient's progress?
- Review the preventative health measures important in patients with HIV infection?
- Understand the guidelines for initiating and changing HAART?
- Recognize some of the more common medications used to treat HIV and their side effects?
- Recognize some of the more common opportunistic infections in patients with HIV?
- Recognize IRIS?

CASE 2

A 32-year-old female presents to the office seeking prenatal care. Her last normal menstrual period was 2½ months before her visit. She believes that she is pregnant and has tested positive with a home pregnancy test. She has been pregnant twice before, with one living child and one spontaneous abortion (G_3P_1). She is married to the father of the children. She has no health problems but does smoke ½ pack of cigarettes per day. She also admits to occasional alcohol use (one drink every 2 weeks). She denies illicit drug use, including IV drug use.

Besides prenatal vitamins with iron and folate, you recommend:

A) Smoking cessation.
B) Confirming the home pregnancy test with a **serum** HCG in your lab.
C) HIV testing and counseling.
D) A and C.
E) All of the above.

Discussion

The correct answer is "D." Smoking during pregnancy is associated with lower birth weight and preeclampsia, and smoking in the house with a young child is associated with respiratory diseases, especially asthma. Although confirming pregnancy by examination (uterine size or fetal heart tones) and/or urine HCG is appropriate, serum HCG is unnecessary and expensive. Additionally, when used correctly, home pregnancy tests are highly sensitive and specific. But really, this is the HIV chapter, and we want you to know that HIV screening should be included in the routine panel of prenatal tests for **all women** seeking prenatal care. Routine testing for HIV in expectant females has dramatically reduced the HIV prevalence in children in developed countries. Vertical transmission of HIV is still a tremendous problem in Africa and other developing regions of the world.

> HELPFUL TIP: The CDC now recommends universal HIV testing for all individuals between age 13 and 64 "in all health care settings." If the prevalence of HIV is <1/1000 in your region, routine screening is not warranted (Branson et al, 2006). Special consent is **not** necessary prior to testing for HIV and a patient's general consent for medical care is enough. The CDC recommends that testing of all pregnant women be routine and offered as an "opt out" test.

* *

You explain that HIV testing is routine, but that the patient can "opt-out," and the patient agrees to HIV testing. Her pregnancy is confirmed. She is found to be ELISA positive for HIV and subsequently Western blot positive for HIV.

What does this mean?

A) She has been infected with HIV in the last month.
B) She has a false positive test for HIV.
C) She has antibodies to HIV and must be immune.
D) She is infected with HIV and infection occurred a minimum of 2–4 weeks ago.
E) Not enough information to judge: order a HIV DNA PCR.

Discussion

The correct answer is "D." The ELISA is the highly sensitive "screening" HIV antibody test, and the Western blot is the highly specific "confirmatory" test. A positive result for both is a reliable indication for the presence of HIV antibody and indicates infection at some point in the past. Since seroconversion (development of antibodies) is not detected before 2–4 weeks after infection, and may not occur for up to 3 months, recent infections may not test positive. HIV RNA PCR and the HIV antigen ELISA can detect HIV infection before seroconversion. Natural resistance to HIV is uncommon, but may occur due to a homozygous deletion within the gene for one of the HIV entry coreceptors (CCR5). The rate of disease progression in HIV-infected people varies widely. Some genetic traits that lead to slower disease progression include heterozygous deletion of the CCR5 gene and certain HLA genotypes.

* *

Your patient is understandably shaken by the news of this test result. She is most concerned about her unborn child.

What should you tell her?

A) Her child is almost certainly also infected.
B) A therapeutic abortion at this point is the only humane thing to do.
C) With effective therapy, the risk of transmission to the child can be lowered to less than 2%.
D) With effective therapy, the risk of transmission to the child can be lowered to 15%.
E) Despite effective therapy, the risk of transmission remains at 25%.

Discussion

The correct answer is "C." Although it is possible for HIV to infect the unborn fetus, the large majority of transmission from mother to child occurs due to exposure to maternal genital-tract virus. The most important variable for transmission is the HIV viral load (HIV RNA concentration in plasma) in the mother. ARV drugs reduce perinatal transmission by several mechanisms, including lowering maternal antepartum viral load and providing infant pre- and postexposure prophylaxis (PEP). Therefore, combined antepartum, intrapartum, and infant ARV prophylaxis is recommended to prevent perinatal transmission of HIV.

Ideally, the mother should have her HIV suppressed (undetectable viral load) on combination antiretroviral therapy (HAART) prior to delivery. Waiting to start therapy until the second trimester is recommended by some; however, if a patient is on HAART and becomes pregnant, continuing therapy during the first trimester is recommended. If the HIV viral load (HIV RNA concentration in plasma) is nondetectable at 36 weeks, the transmission risk is <2%.

Current guidelines recommend also adding continuous infusion of zidovudine to the mother during labor, and postpartum prophylactic medications for the newborn. Women who present in labor without HIV testing during pregnancy, or with undocumented HIV infection, should be tested by rapid HIV ELISA. If this is positive, continuous infusion zidovudine should be started. Current guidelines do not recommend additional intrapartum drugs in this setting, including nevirapine, which has been shown to cause rapid resistance when used in this setting.

* *

Your patient is somewhat relieved that her baby can be protected, and wants to know what can be done to treat her. She feels fine, is now in the second trimester, and would rather not take medications unless she had to.

Some additional laboratory tests are ordered:

CD4 count: 756/mm^3
HIV viral load: 80,000 copies/mL
Hb: 11.2 g/dL
BUN/Cr: 11 mg/dL / 0.7 mg/dL.

What should you tell her about HAART in pregnancy?

A) To minimize the risk of transmission to her child, she should start triple ARV therapy as soon as possible.
B) ARV medications are teratogenic and should be avoided at all costs during pregnancy, except just before delivery.

C) Since her CD4 count is normal and she feels well with no sign of opportunistic infections, starting HAART is not indicated.
D) Her renal function makes HAART relatively contraindicated.
E) Her hemoglobin level makes HAART relatively contraindicated.

Discussion
The correct answer is "A." ARV therapy is recommended for all pregnant women regardless of their viral load to prevent transmission to the child. Factors that increase risk of transmission of HIV include high maternal viral load, low maternal CD4 count, advanced clinical stage of her HIV, and lack of maternal use of ARV therapy. Vaginal delivery is also a risk factor—but only if the mother did not receive antepartum ARV therapy. Although the patient's hemoglobin is low, it does not preclude her from taking therapy. Her renal function is normal, so it should not be an issue.

* *

The patient is started on HAART (Combivir plus Kaletra) and tolerates her regimen well. Repeat laboratory results at a return visit 4 weeks later are as follows:

CD4 count: 692/mm^3
HIV viral load: 5500 copies/mL
Hb: 10.9 g/dL

Her HAART seems to be effective. Her viral load has decreased by one $\log_{10}$.

What do you recommend regarding *P. jiroveci* pneumonia (PCP) prophylaxis?

A) She should start prophylaxis with TMP-SMX immediately, because PCP in pregnancy can be particularly severe.
B) She should start PCP prophylaxis with inhaled pentamidine, because TMP-SMX is contraindicated in pregnancy.
C) PCP prophylaxis is not indicated, since her CD4 count is greater than 200/mm^3
D) PCP prophylaxis is not a major concern for pregnant patients.

Discussion
The correct answer is "C." PCP is particularly severe in pregnant patients, but prophylaxis is not generally indicated for CD4 counts >200 cells/mm^3. TMP-SMX is associated with hyperbilirubinemia in newborns, but is still indicated for PCP prophylaxis. Oral dapsone is another option, as is inhaled pentamidine.

* *

She continues her ARV therapy, but at 36 weeks, her viral load is still detectable (2500 copies/mL). You recommend changing the ARV, but at the next appointment (37.5 weeks), the patient tells you that she did not fill the new prescriptions, and admits that she has not been adherent with her medications. As this visit, you renew discussions about adherence, and about delivery plans with the patient.

Which of the following is/are true regarding the delivery?

A) A cesarean section (C-section) is likely to reduce the risk of transmission to her infant.
B) A C-section section is indicated, because this patient's viral load remains greater than 1000 copies/ mL despite HAART.
C) A C-section should be performed at 38 weeks gestation, prior to the onset of labor.
D) Peripartum ZDV should be given to the mother and infant.
E) All of the above.

Discussion
The correct answer is "E." If a patient achieves effective suppression with ARV therapy (undetectable viral load), the risk of transmission is minimal, and the mode of delivery should depend on the preferences of the mother and the other usual obstetric factors. Vaginal delivery is not contraindicated if the mother's viral load is suppressed. If, as in this patient's case, the viral load is >1000 copies/mL, current guidelines recommend delivery by C-section at 38 weeks. When performed at 38 weeks, prior to the onset of labor, the relative risk of transmission is reduced by 50%. Perinatal ZDV, as discussed above, may also help reduce the risk of transmission. Also, the premature rupture of membranes (PROM) should be addressed promptly in HIV-infected mothers. Children born to mothers more than 4 hours after rupture are **twice** as likely to acquire HIV.

* *

The patient delivers a healthy, 3-kg male infant via C-section. The postpartum course is uneventful. Blood taken from the infant at day 1 and at 2 weeks both test positive for HIV antibodies.

What does this mean?

A) The infant is infected with HIV.
B) Although technically HIV positive, the infant's infection status is unclear from the information given.
C) Maternal HIV antibodies are expected to be circulating in the infant, but it can be assumed that no transmission of infection took place.
D) A positive test at day 1 is expected due to maternal antibodies, but a repeat positive at 2 weeks indicates infant antibody production and is evidence of infection.
E) None of the above.

Discussion

The correct answer is "B." Children born to HIV-positive mothers will test positive for HIV antibodies as maternal antibodies are acquired across the placenta for at least the first 6 months. Maternal HIV antibodies may persist and interfere with interpretation of a positive HIV antibody test; therefore, HIV antibody testing is not recommended to diagnose an HIV infection in infants.

How should the HIV status of the infant be determined?

A) Serial HIV antibody tests: a fourfold drop in titer can be considered negative.
B) p24 antigen testing in the first 48 hours of life.
C) Viral load by PCR in the first 48 hours of life.
D) Viral load by PCR at 1–2 weeks, 14–21 days and 4–6 months.
E) p24 antigen and PCR viral load on cord blood samples.

Discussion

The correct answer is "D." The best test to assist with diagnosis of HIV infection is viral load by PCR, and a positive test (by DNA PCR or RNA assays) indicates likely HIV infection. Confirmation of HIV infection is provided by two positive virologic tests obtained from separate blood samples. The sensitivity of virologic testing increases rapidly by 2 weeks. One can consider obtaining virologic testing within the first 48 hours in newborns who are at high risk for HIV infection, such as infants born to HIV-infected mothers who did not receive prenatal ARV therapy or who had HIV viral loads >1000 copies/mL close to the time of delivery. If this returns positive, this would indicative of an intrauterine infection rather than intrapartum infection, which is normally acquired during delivery. "A" is incorrect. HIV antibody testing is useless in infants, and quantified titers are not typically generated. "B" is incorrect because the p24 antigen is less sensitive and specific than the viral load in this setting. "E" is incorrect. Tests done on the cord blood may be contaminated with maternal blood and do not give an accurate assessment of the infant's status.

What should you advise your patient about breast-feeding her son?

A) HIV is not transmitted by breast milk.
B) HIV is transmitted by breast milk, but the benefits of breast-feeding outweigh the risk of transmission in this setting.
C) HIV is transmitted by breast milk, but her son will be protected from serious infection due to maternal antibodies in the breast milk.
D) HIV is transmitted by breast milk, and breast-feeding should be avoided if possible.

Discussion

The correct answer is "D." Postpartum transmission of HIV from mother to child occurs in 10–14% of breast-feeding mothers. This is not a major problem in developed nations, where there is reliable access to formula. HIV-positive mothers should be discouraged from breast-feeding in the developed world. The recommendations may be different in developing areas of the world, where mother's milk may the only clean source of nutrition available to the infant. In fact, in many developing nations, the benefit of breast-feeding outweighs the risk of HIV transmission due to inadequate access to good nutrition and risk of diarrheal illnesses. The World Health Organization (WHO) suggests that "when replacement feeding is acceptable, feasible, affordable, sustainable and safe" bottle feeding is the best option (http://www.who.int/child-adolescent-health/NUTRITION/HIV_infant.htm).

* *

Despite the best efforts of your patient and all the physicians and nurses participating in her care, her child tests positive by PCR for HIV at 4 weeks and 4 months. Now, you need to think about how to treat this child with HIV.

Which of the following is true about the use of HAART in children?

A) Treatment should be initiated immediately for all children as soon as HIV infection is diagnosed.
B) Since they are just little adults with relatively big heads compared to their torsos, treatment indications for children and adults are the same.
C) HAART is highly toxic in children and treatment should be reserved until the child's life is in immediate danger from HIV-related complications.
D) No one really knows the best approach, but treatment is recommended in most children and should be given to all infants <1 year.
E) Treatment indications for children are similar to those for adults, but monotherapy is preferred over combination therapy.

Discussion

The correct answer is "D." Recommendations for when to start therapy differ by the age of the child. CD4 counts and HIV RNA viral loads vary by age in children and both markers are poor predictors of disease progression and mortality in children <12 months of age. The risk of rapid progression of the disease and mortality is high in infants, and current guidelines recommend initiating therapy for all infants <12 months regardless of their clinical status, CD4 percentage, or viral load. For children older than 1 year of age, treatment is recommended for AIDS or significant symptoms referable to HIV, regardless of CD4 count. For asymptomatic children >1 and <5 years old, the CD4 percentage is more accurate than the absolute numbers of CD4 cells. HIV therapy is recommended for all children who have a CD4 percent value of <25%. Therapy is also recommended for children 5 years of age or older with an absolute CD4 count <500 cells/mm^3. HAART regimens are more difficult to choose and adjust in children because of a limited number of pediatric (nonpill) formulations and a lack of data about long-term efficacy and safety. However, combination therapy can effectively and safely suppress viral load and stimulate immunologic reconstitution. Monotherapy is NOT recommended.

Which of the following statements regarding the natural history of HIV complications in children is true?

A) Hepatobiliary complications, such as AIDS cholangiopathy, are more common in children.
B) Kaposi sarcoma frequently occurs in young children.
C) Focal brain lesions in children are almost always due to toxoplasmosis.
D) Many children show cognitive and motor deficits, but frank AIDS dementia is uncommon.
E) Lymphocytic interstitial pneumonitis (LIP) is more common in adults than in children.

Discussion

The correct answer is "D." Twenty-five percent of children with HIV infection demonstrate some cognitive and motor deficits. They face problems with verbal expression, attention deficits, hyperactivity, and hyperreflexia. LIP is characterized by diffuse reticulonodular infiltrates and hilar lymphadenopathy and occurs in up to 40% of children with perinatally acquired HIV. LIP is very rare in adults. Kaposi sarcoma is associated with a herpes virus infection and is very rare in children. Toxoplasmosis, usually presenting as focal mass brain lesions, is a reactivation of previous infection, and is therefore also very rare in children. Hepatobiliary complications are more common in adults than in children, but the reason for this is unclear.

What should you recommend for this infant regarding PCP prophylaxis?

A) Prophylaxis is unnecessary because children do not get PCP.
B) Prophylaxis is unnecessary if the child's CD4 count is >200 cells/mm^3.
C) Prophylaxis is unnecessary until the child reaches 1 year of age.
D) Prophylaxis with TMP-SMX is contraindicated in infants less than 6 months of age due to the risk of hyperbilirubinemia.
E) Prophylaxis with TMP-SMX as the first-line agent should be initiated at 4 weeks of age because the highest risk for PCP in children is at 3–6 months of age.

Discussion

The correct answer is "E." The highest incidence of PCP occurs in the first year of life with peak onset at 3–6 months of age. TMP/SMX is still considered first-line therapy for prophylaxis and should be started at 4–6 weeks of age. CD4 counts are naturally higher in children and decrease to adult levels by age 6 years. PCP prophylaxis is recommended for all HIV-infected infants <12 months regardless of CD4 count or percentage. It should be continued until 1 year of age and be reassessed for continued need based on age-specific CD4 count or percentage thresholds. If this drug is not tolerated, dapsone or aerosolized pentamidine are acceptable alternatives.

* *

The child tolerates his HAART very well and demonstrates a consistently suppressed viral load. He gets further follow-up by a pediatric infectious disease specialist. The mother returns to you for further care. She had been taking the previously prescribed HAART, but quit all her medications 3 months ago because she had forgotten to take a couple of doses and did not want to "screw things up."

Her latest laboratory results show the following:

CD4 count: 254 cells/mm^3

HIV viral load: 50,000 copies/mL

(Previously CD4 count: 692/mm^3; HIV viral load: 5000 copies/mL).

What do you tell her now?

A) She should have continued to take the medications because now the HIV has a "foothold" and it will be much harder to treat.

B) It would not have mattered if she took the medications or not. Her disease is progressing as expected.

C) With the degree of drop seen in her CD4 count, the virus must be resistant, and further HAART is futile.

D) She should have continued the medications, even if she was missing doses. A little of ARV activity is better than nothing.

E) She did the right thing by stopping the medications. If a patient is not able to comply fully, it is better to not take any HAART at all.

Discussion

The correct answer is "E." Starting HAART is a very difficult and serious decision and should be made after careful and complete counseling. If taken intermittently, HAART can easily become ineffective. Patients missing frequent doses of HAART are likely to have a more precipitous course to their HIV infection. Once multidrug resistance develops, it can be difficult to find an effective regimen to slow disease progression.

* *

After the drug resistance genotype testing did not identify any mutations associated with drug resistance, she agrees to try Atripla (efavirenz, emtricitabine, tenofovir) one tablet PO QHS. She does not want any more children and is using effective contraception as the efavirenz component in Atripla is teratogenic.

She is slightly drowsy from the Atripla, and repeat labs show an improvement in her viral load:

CD4 count: 261 cells/mm^3

HIV viral load: 7000 copies/mL.

You explain that if her viral load continues to fall and becomes undetectable, she can expect an improvement in her CD4 count over the next 1–2 years, and that the drowsiness from the Atripla should improve over the next few weeks. You take this office visit as an opportunity to catch up on preventative medicine. On one prior occasion 6 years ago, she had an abnormal Pap smear result that returned to normal after a repeat exam and colposcopy. Prior to her diagnosis of HIV, she had never been diagnosed with a STI. A pelvic exam today reveals a normal appearing cervix. A sample for Pap smear is collected and sent to pathology.

How often should this patient get screened for cervical cancer with Pap smear?

A) Cervical cancer is inevitable, so you should recommend prophylactic radical resection.

B) She must be tested every 6 months, regardless of results of this Pap smear.

C) If she has two negative Pap smears 6 months apart and a normal CD4 count, she may be screened per the usual guidelines for HIV-negative women.

D) She may be screened per the usual guidelines for HIV-negative women.

E) She has almost no chance of developing cervical cancer and screening may be discontinued.

Discussion

The correct answer is "C." Human papilloma virus (HPV), implicated as a cause of cervical cancer, has a higher prevalence and demonstrates a more aggressive course in women with HIV infection. If the patient has a relatively normal CD4 count and has had two normal smears at 6-month intervals, Pap smears can be done at 1-year intervals. **However, if the patient has a CD4 count less than 200 cells/mm^3, screening every 6 months is recommended.** Any detection of cervical intraepithelial neoplasia is treated the same as with HIV-negative women. Remember that it is not unusual for multiple STIs to be transmitted together, so consider testing for other STIs when obtaining a Pap smear.

HELPFUL TIP: Any STI causing genital ulcers (e.g., herpes) increases the risk of transmission of HIV.

Aside from an increased risk of aggressive HPV and a high rate of menstrual disorders, how does the natural history of HIV infection in women differ from that in men?

A) Women have a lower rate of progressive multifocal leukoencephalopathy (PML) and bacterial pneumonia.
B) Women are more likely to present with oral thrush and recurrent genital candidiasis.
C) Women with the same level of medical care as men have significantly shortened survival.
D) HAART is more effective and better tolerated in women.
E) Most women in the United States acquire HIV from same-sex partners.

Discussion
The correct answer is "B." The natural history of HIV infection in women and men is very similar. Women with the same level of access to medical care have similar survival rates to men, and HAART is equally effective (and hazardous) in both sexes. Women are more likely to present with recurrent, refractory vaginal candidiasis, oral thrush, PML, and bacterial pneumonias. The majority of women in the United States with HIV have acquired it from heterosexual contact. The second largest route of exposure for U.S. women is IV drug use. Female who have sex with other women are at low risk of contracting HIV; the opposite is true for men who have sex with other men. Worldwide, heterosexual contact is by far the most common means of transmission.

Objectives: Did you learn to . . .

- Interpret HIV antibody and viral load tests?
- Evaluate the risk of vertical transmission of HIV?
- Reduce the risk of vertical transmission of HIV?
- Interpret HIV tests in the neonatal period?
- Use HAART in children?
- Identify some difference in the clinical manifestations of HIV in women and children?

CASE 3

A 39-year-old female working as a nursing assistant in your hospital comes into the emergency department looking quite upset. About 30 minutes earlier, she was helping to move a patient with known HIV when his IV was pulled out and he bled. Several drops of blood got on her hands, but she washed them immediately and thoroughly. On exam, she has intact skin on the hands, no signs of trauma, and no residual blood on her.

The most appropriate action to take is:

A) Reassure her that her risk of contracting HIV for this event is almost zero.
B) Obtain HIV antibody testing.
C) Start her on HAART for prophylaxis.
D) Have her return in 6 weeks for HIV antibody testing.
E) B and D.

Discussion
The correct answer is "A." Fortunately, HIV is not the most efficient virus when it comes to spreading itself. Health-care workers are at risk of contracting HIV when working with HIV-infected patients, but exposure to infected bodily fluid must occur through a percutaneous route or contact with a mucous membrane or nonintact skin. Even percutaneous exposure (e.g., open bore needle) with HIV-infected blood carries a transmission rate of only about 0.3%, and the mucous membrane exposure to HIV-infected blood carries a 0.09% risk. Therefore, contacting an infected patient's blood with intact skin is very low risk.

* *

The patient is reassured that her risk of contracting HIV is negligible. She looks a little sheepish when she tells you, "In all the commotion I knocked over the urinal and spilled the patient's urine on my leg." She changed clothes and washed her leg. You inspect her and find some eczema in the area where the urine was spilled.

Now, you recommend that she:

A) Not worry, as the risk of transmission from this event is negligible also.
B) Start zidovudine for 4 weeks for prophylaxis.

C) Be tested for HIV by viral load.
D) Start HAART.

Discussion

The correct answer is "A." Your patient now has an area of nonintact skin, which is a concern. However, urine is not considered infectious unless it is grossly bloody. Other bodily fluids not considered infectious: feces, vomitus, sputum, tears, sweat, nasal secretions, and saliva. Any visibly bloody fluids, blood, semen, and vaginal secretions are all considered infectious. Other bodily fluids not already mentioned (e.g., CSF and amniotic fluid) should be considered potentially infectious.

HELPFUL TIP: HIV PEP should be considered for contact of nonintact skin or oral or genital mucosa with potentially infected body fluid (see above) from a source that is HIV positive or has an unknown HIV status. PEP should be started with a two- or three- drug regimen as soon as possible and continued for 4 weeks. There are many options for prophylaxis with various advantages and disadvantages; one of the most commonly used is zidovudine/lamivudine (Combivir).

Objective: Did you learn to . . .

- Identify when a health-care worker is at risk for contracting HIV?

BIBLIOGRAPHY

Branson BM, et al. Revised recommendations for HIV testing of adults, adolescents, and pregnant women in health-care settings. *MMWR Recomm Rep.* 2006;55(RR-14):1-17.

Centers for Disease Control and Prevention. Guidelines for the prevention and treatment of opportunistic infections among HIV-exposed and HIV-infected children. Recommendations from CDC, the National Institutes of Health, the HIV Medicine Association of the Infectious Diseases Society of America, the Pediatric Infectious Diseases Society, and the American Academy of Pediatrics. *MMWR.* 2009;58(RR-11):45-47.

Centers for Disease Control and Prevention. Updated U.S. Public Health Service guidelines for the management of occupational exposures to HIV and recommendations for postexposure prophylaxis. *MMWR.* 2005;54(RR-9):1-11.

Khalsa AM. Preventive counseling, screening, and therapy in the patient with newly diagnosed HIV infection. *Am Fam Physician.* 2006;73:271-280.

Panel on Antiretroviral Therapy and Medical Management of HIV-Infected Children. Guidelines for the use of antiretroviral agents in pediatric HIV infection. 2011; pp. 1-268. Available at: http://aidsinfo.nih.gov/ContentFiles/PediatricGuidelines.pdf, Accessed September 30, 2011.

Panel on Treatment of HIV-Infected Pregnant Women and Prevention of Perinatal Transmission. Recommendations for use of antiretroviral drugs in pregnant HIV-1-infected women for maternal health and interventions to reduce perinatal HIV transmission in the United States. 2011;14:1-207. Available at: http://aidsinfo.nih.gov/contentfiles/PerinatalGL.pdf, Accessed September 30, 2011.

10

Endocrinology

Mark A. Graber

CASE 1

A 27-year-old female presents to the office with the chief complaint of chronic fatigue for 4 months. She has gained 17 pounds in 3 months, despite a decreased appetite. She also complains of depression, increased sleep, a disturbing lack of energy, hair loss, and cold intolerance. Her past medical history is unremarkable, and she takes no medications. She has never had any surgeries.

Which of the following physical exam findings would be expected?

A) Tachycardia.
B) Exophthalmos.
C) Fine tremor.
D) Peripheral sensory loss.
E) Delayed relaxation in reflexes.

Discussion

The correct answer is "E." The history given is consistent with a hypothyroid state. Symptoms of hypothyroidism include thinning hair, dry skin, a hoarse, deep voice, bradycardia, and a prolonged relaxation in the reflexes. Tachycardia and a fine tremor are more typical of hyperthyroidism, and exophthalmos is characteristic of Graves disease (one specific cause of hyperthyroidism). Proximal muscle weakness may occur in hypothyroidism, but sensory loss is not typical (although hypothyroidism can contribute to carpal tunnel syndrome and may be the initial presenting symptoms).

How can the diagnosis of hypothyroidism best be confirmed?

A) Elevated thyroid-stimulating hormone (TSH) level.
B) Low TSH level.
C) Thyroid biopsy.
D) Radionucleotide scan.
E) Serum thyroglobulin.

Discussion

The correct answer is "A." The TSH is the most sensitive test for both hypo- and hyperthyroidism, and changes in the TSH can precede abnormalities in serum thyroxine (best measured as free T4) level. An elevated TSH occurs when the pituitary detects insufficient thyroid hormone production, and TSH production is shut off when an excess of thyroid hormone is circulating. If the pituitary produces insufficient TSH, a low TSH will result despite inadequate T4. Therefore, adding serum-free T4 to a TSH assay is required to demonstrate hypothalamic or pituitary hypothyroidism (as in the case of a pituitary adenoma, for example). Since these disorders are rare, and often suggested by other clues in the history and physical, TSH alone is usually sufficient for initial screening for thyroid disease. "C," a biopsy, is used to evaluate thyroid masses and nodules. "D," radionucleotide scan, is also used in the evaluation of thyroid masses and can (mostly) differentiate functioning adenomas from carcinomas and benign cysts. "E," the serum thyroglobulin measurement, is used to **monitor** thyroid carcinoma (and is *not* the initial screening).

* *

Her laboratory results are normal except for glucose 115 mg/dL, TSH 22.3 uIU/mL (reference range 0.27–4.20), free T4 0.56 ng/dL (reference range 0.93–1.70)

Based on prevalence, labs, and presentation, what is the MOST likely cause of this patient's disease?

A) Autoimmune hypothyroidism.
B) Iatrogenic hypothyroidism.
C) Tuberculosis infiltration of the thyroid gland.
D) Nonfunctioning pituitary adenoma.
E) Congenital hypothyroidism.

Discussion

The correct answer is "A." Autoimmune hypothyroidism (Hashimoto thyroiditis) is the most common cause of hypothyroidism in areas where these is adequate iodine. If this patient had a pituitary adenoma causing hypothyroidism, the TSH (as well as the free T4) would be low, since the pituitary is the source of TSH. Congenital hypothyroidism causes a severe mental retardation and constellation of other signs and is tested for at birth as part of routine neonatal screening. Tuberculosis is a rare cause of hypothyroidism, but is the most common cause of **adrenal** failure worldwide.

> HELPFUL TIP: Outside the United States, iodine deficiency is the most common cause of hypothyroidism in the world, with an estimated 2 billion persons being iodine deficient although not all being hypothyroid.

How should this patient be managed?

A) I^{131} administration.
B) Surgical excision of thyroid gland.
C) Start synthetic thyroxine hormone at 25 micrograms (µg) PO QD, and recheck symptoms and TSH in 2 months.
D) Start synthetic thyroxine hormone at 200 µg PO QD, and recheck symptoms and TSH in 2 months.
E) Start synthetic thyroxine hormone at 25 µg PO QD, and double every week until the patient experiences weight loss, tremor, and poor sleep (and the desire to find a new doctor).

QD - quaque die (every day).

Discussion

The correct answer is "C." The patient is deficient in thyroid hormone and needs supplementation. Two strategies may be used (1) start with 25 µg daily and titrate up every 1–2 months until the TSH is in the normal range or (2) start with full-dose therapy based on weight (1.6 µg/kg daily) and adjust based on TSH in 1–2 months. Either option is appropriate in young, otherwise healthy adults. **But older patients (>65 years old) or those with multiple comorbidities should be started at a low dose (25 µg daily).** If the patient is titrated up to 200 µg of levothyroxine and does not seem to be responding, the diagnosis needs to be reconsidered or the patient's compliance needs to be carefully assessed. **Iron and food will decrease the absorption of levothyroxine by as much as 40%.** It usually takes 6–8 weeks for the body's endocrine response and TSH to reach a steady state. The goal of therapy is a euthyroid state with the patient experiencing neither hyper- or hypothyroid symptoms. "A" and "B" are treatments of **hyper**thyroidism. Surgical excision and radioablation with I^{131} are approaches to the treatment of Graves disease. Both can result in iatrogenic hypothyroidism that requires lifelong thyroid hormone therapy.

> HELPFUL TIP: We generally recommend starting levothyroxine at a low dose for a couple of reasons. First, titrating the dose up will assure that you do not overshoot. Second, if patients are started at 100 µg, for example, (a common final dose), it can cause metabolic stress, especially in the elderly, resulting in angina, atrial fibrillation, etc.

* *

You start the patient on 25 µg l-thyroxine (Synthroid) and schedule a return appointment in 2 months. At follow-up, she reports a general improvement in symptoms but is not "back to normal." She reports continued constipation, a lack of energy, and feeling depressed. She has not lost any further weight and reports a thickening of her hair. Laboratory results are as follows: TSH 11.8 uIU/mL (0.27–4.20) and free T4 0.75 ng/dL (0.93–1.70).

What adjustments, if any, should be made to her regimen?

A) None, she will continue to improve at the current dose.
B) Increase the dose to 50 μg/day, and recheck in 2 months.
C) Increase the dose to 200 μg/day, and recheck in 2 months.
D) She is becoming hyperthyroid, so cut the dose to 12.5 μg/day, and recheck in 2 months.
E) L-thyroxine is ineffective in this patient. Change her to desiccated thyroid tissue (e.g., Armour Thyroid).

Discussion

The correct answer is "B." This patient has improved from her initial presentation, but she is clinically and chemically (elevated TSH) still hypothyroid. The half-life of thyroxine is about 1 week, so she has had plenty of time to reach steady state. It is doubtful that her thyroid levels will change much after 2 months on this dose, so it is now time to increase her dose. Since you started with a low dose, doubling of the dose is a reasonable increase that is unlikely to make her hyperthyroid. "E" deserves special mention. Desiccated thyroid is generally avoided due to variability in concentration of thyroid hormone content.

> HELPFUL TIP: Poor compliance is the most common reason for failure of medical therapy. Other causes include malabsorption, drug interactions (e.g., rifampin and amiodarone), drug–food interactions, or drugs that reduce absorption (e.g., iron and sucralfate).

* *

Your patient worries about taking too much thyroid hormone.

Which of the following can result from oversuppression of the TSH (iatrogenic hyperthyroidism)?

A) Renal failure.
B) Pulmonary fibrosis.
C) Hirsutism.
D) Osteoporosis.
E) Loss of secondary sex characteristics.

Discussion

The correct answer is "D." Hyperthyroidism, either iatrogenic or endogenous, causes osteoporosis. For this reason, it is important to monitor the TSH and assure that the patient is not overreplaced.

Objectives: Did you learn to . . .

- Recognize the presentation of hypothyroidism and its most common causes?
- Identify common physical exam findings consistent with hypothyroidism?
- Describe the basic medical and laboratory management of patients with hypothyroidism?

CASE 2

A 32-year-old male presents complaining of severe anxiety. For the last 4 months, he has had difficulty sleeping, progressively worsening nervousness, a 25-pound weight loss, and constantly feels "too warm." He feels "shaky" and has difficulty concentrating. He denies diarrhea, but reports having normally shaped stools four to five times per day, more than usual for him. The patient denies neck or eye discomfort, and has not noticed any neck swelling. He has no other significant medical history. His mother, who died 3 years ago from coronary artery disease (CAD), had a "thyroid problem," but he doesn't know any more details.

Physical exam reveals an anxious young adult male. He has a noticeable resting tremor. You note mild exophthalmos, conjunctival injection, and lid lag. His thyroid is diffusely, mildly enlarged and a bruit is audible over the gland. The cardiac exam reveals tachycardia with a flow murmur. The rest of the exam is unremarkable.

What is the most likely diagnosis?

A) Viral thyroiditis.
B) Graves disease.
C) Anaplastic thyroid carcinoma.
D) Hyperactive thyroid adenoma.
E) Surreptitious thyroid hormone ingestion.

Discussion

The correct answer is "B." This is a classic presentation of Graves disease. The family history, the symptoms and signs of hyperthyroidism (especially the diffusely enlarged goiter with a bruit), and the exophthalmos are all typical. Conjunctival injection is also frequently noted. "A" is unlikely. Viral thyroiditis can cause hyperthyroidism and a goiter, but the thyroid gland is usually tender. Also, viral thyroiditis will likely not last 4 months, but is usually self-limited to <6 weeks. Anaplastic carcinoma is a devastating disease with a dismal prognosis: the thyroid gets very large very quickly, but the disease does not present with hyperthyroidism. A hyperactive adenoma and surreptitious ingestion of thyroid hormone would not cause a goiter or exophthalmos.

HELPFUL TIP: 75% of patients with viral thyroiditis will progress from 2 weeks of self-limited hyperthyroidism to 3–6 months of hypothyroidism that is also self-limited. The hyperthyroid phase is best treated with NSAIDs, beta-blockers, and prednisone if needed.

Which of the following tests is most SPECIFIC for Graves disease?

A) Antithyrotropin receptor (aka anti-TSH receptor) antibody.
B) Antithyroglobulin antibody.
C) Antithyroid peroxidase antibody.
D) Markedly suppressed TSH.
E) A and C.

Discussion

The correct answer is "A." Graves disease is an autoimmune process, and lymphocytes in the thyroid gland itself are responsible for a large amount of the thyroid autoantibodies produced. Although several types of antibodies can be tested for, antithyrotropin receptor antibody is the most specific.

- **Antithyrotropin receptor antibody (anti-TSH receptor antibody)** is found in 80–95% of patient's with Graves disease but also in 10–20% of those with other forms of autoimmune thyroiditis.
- **Antithyroglobulin antibodies** are found in Graves disease, autoimmune thyroiditis, some patients with type 1 diabetes and in up to 20% of the general population.
- **Antithyroid peroxidase antibody** is elevated in Graves disease, autoimmune thyroiditis, type 1 diabetes, and some pregnant patients, etc.

* *

Your patient's laboratory results are as follows: complete blood count (CBC) is normal and TSH is undetectable.

How should the patient be treated acutely?

A) Propranolol and methimazole started immediately.
B) Control the patient's symptoms with propranolol now, then start propylthiouracil (PTU) when the patient feels better.
C) Iodine (Lugol solution).
D) Radioablation with I^{131}.
E) Thyroidectomy.

Discussion

The correct answer is "A." There is no need to wait before starting methimazole (Tapazole), which blocks production of thyroid hormone. PTU can also be used but methimazole is preferred because (1) it affords better control and (2) PTU is associated with more liver toxicity and bone marrow suppression (although these adverse effects can occur with both drugs). PTU is still preferred during pregnancy. Propranolol is helpful for controlling the symptoms of hyperthyroidism (tachycardia, tremor, etc) and prevents the conversion of T4 to active T3. "C" is incorrect, as iodine will provide further substrate for the body in the production of thyroid hormone and should not be given unless a thyroid-blocking agent has been started. Iodine is useful during thyroid storm to prevent the release of stored thyroid hormone, but it is given 1 hour after PTU or methimazole. Radioablation is used for patients who prove refractory to medicine or have poor compliance. Thyroidectomy is rarely used for Graves disease in current medical practice because of the ease and efficacy of radioactive iodine administration (except in the case of pregnancy and few other unusual cases).

Which of the following is/are possible side effects of PTU and methimazole therapy?

A) Granulocytopenia.
B) Aplastic anemia.
C) Elevated liver transaminases.
D) Inhibition of fetal thyroid gland.
E) All of the above.

Discussion

The correct answer is "E." All of the above are known side effects of antithyroid drugs (thioamides).

Granulocytopenia occurs in about 0.5% of patients and is a sudden, idiosyncratic reaction. **Classically, patients present with a severe sore throat. If you have a patient on PTU or methimazole with a sore throat or fever, check a CBC.** Aplastic anemia may occur but is rare. For these reasons, patients starting these medications should have a baseline CBC. Mild, transient elevation of the liver transaminases is common, and the drug should be discontinued if the level is greater than three times normal. Both PTU and methimazole cross the placenta and will inhibit the fetal thyroid, increasing the risk for congential hypothyroidism. The risk to a fetus posed by the drugs is less than the danger posed by a mother with accelerating hyperthyroidism, so the medications should be used even during pregnancy if indicated. PTU is generally regarded as slightly safer in pregnancy. Nonetheless, you should use the smallest dose possible. If a pregnant patient is not controlled with PTU, consider surgical thyroidectomy.

HELPFUL TIP: Avoid radioactive iodine treatment during pregnancy since it will affect the fetus as well.

* *

The patient is interested in treating the ophthalmopathy.

What method has been used successfully to treat Graves disease-related exophthalmos?

A) Orbital radiation.
B) Glucocorticoids.
C) Octreotide.
D) Hydroxyurea.

Discussion

The correct answer is "B." Glucocorticoids have been shown to be effective in treating Graves ophthalmopathy. Intravenous (IV) steroids are more effective than oral but either can be used. Orbital radiation and octreotide have both been used but with little success. Hydroxyurea works for sickle cell and thrombocytosis but not, to our knowledge, for Graves ophthalmopathy.

* *

Your patient complies with the recommended regimen and improves. He is not symptomatic at a return visit in 2 months, and his eye pathology has not progressed. After 6 months of good control, the patient elects to have cosmetic eye surgery to repair his exophthalmos, having not responded well to glucocorticoids. A preoperation physical is unremarkable. Laboratory studies prior to surgery are normal except TSH 0.21 uIU/mL (0.27–4.20) and free T4 3.01 ng/dL (0.93–1.70).

After an uneventful surgery, you are called to the postanesthesia room by the oculoplastic surgeon. She reports that the patient has become very anxious and has a sinus tachycardia of 165 bpm. A quick review of the chart reveals no known allergies, no personal or family history of reactions to anesthesia, and the only medication is methimazole (propranolol had been discontinued 2 months earlier due to lack of symptoms).

Physical exam shows T 39.8°C, BP 98/25, RR 34, and P 166. The patient is agitated but alert and in acute distress. He is tachypneic, tremulous, and is unable to carry on a conversation. He seems confused and distracted. The skin is diaphoretic and flushed. His mucous membranes are dry, and his surface veins are flat; there is no JVD. Pulmonary exam reveals diffuse rales. Reflexes are brisk, his mental status is as noted above, but the rest of the neurological exam is unremarkable.

What is the cause of this patient's symptoms and signs?

A) The patient became fluid overloaded during the surgery due to excessive hydration.
B) The patient has neuroleptic malignant syndrome (NMS).
C) The patient has thyroid storm induced by the stress of surgery.
D) The patient has endocarditis and suffered a valve rupture.

Discussion

The correct answer is "C." The syndrome of thyroid storm is characterized by fever, tachyarrhythmias, altered mental status, and high output cardiac failure. It is induced by a major stress (infection, surgery, myocardial infarction, etc.) in a patient with underlying hyperthyroidism (usually undiagnosed). This patient, although **clinically** well controlled, had a **low TSH and high free T4 prior to surgery**, suggesting he may have suffered a recurrence of disease or had stopped taking his medications. The patient is not fluid overloaded, as evidenced by his clinically dry status (intravascular depleted → dry mucus membranes, flat neck veins); thus "A" is incorrect. The pulmonary edema (rales) is due to high output failure. NMS presents with altered mental status and hyperthermia (due to increased metabolic activity). But, the patient is not currently taking neuroleptics. A ruptured valve due to endocarditis would fit the patient's clinical picture, but he had no fever preceding the surgery. For endocarditis to progress to valve rupture, it must be long-standing, and there is nothing in the presurgical evaluation or history to suggest this.

Which of the following IS NOT a sign/symptom of thyroid storm?

A) Hypothermia.
B) Right upper quadrant pain.
C) Diffuse muscle weakness.
D) Atrial fibrillation.
E) Hypomania, confusion, other central nervous system (CNS) signs and symptoms.

Discussion

The correct answer is "A." Patients with thyroid storm generally will be **hyper**thermic. The rest are correct and are symptoms of thyroid storm. "B," right upper quadrant pain, is from liver congestion secondary to high output congestive heart failure (CHF) and is a bad sign.

HELPFUL TIP: Thyroid storm is a clinical diagnosis consisting of hyperthermia, tachycardia, CNS dysfunction, and signs and symptoms of peripheral hyperthyroidism. While most patients will have an elevated T3 and free T4, there is no laboratory level of these hormones that defines thyroid storm.

HELPFUL TIP: A pheochromocytoma can be confused with hyperthyroidism. Both include tachycardia and possible hypertension. Interestingly, serum catecholamines **are normal** (certainly high normal—but normal) in thyroid storm. Catecholamines will be elevated in patients with a pheochromocytoma.

How should this patient now be treated?

A) Administer aggressive fluid hydration, cooling measures, benzodiazepines, and dantrolene.
B) Administer fluid hydration, cooling measures, beta-blockade (IV propranolol), methimazole, corticosteroids, then iodine 1 hour later.
C) Administer fluid hydration, dopamine drip for his hypotension, and antibiotics; consult cardiovascular surgery immediately.
D) Hold fluids; administer nitroglycerin drip and furosemide for his heart failure; consider an intra-aortic balloon pump.
E) Administer fluid hydration and antibiotics; consider norepinephrine drip if patient becomes more hypotensive.

Discussion

The correct answer is "B." This is the appropriate management for thyroid storm in the correct sequence of therapies. This patient is in extremis (hypotensive and tachycardic) and needs fluid hydration, despite his pulmonary edema. Cooling measures address his hyperthermia, and beta-blockade (propranolol) will improve his high output failure (and reduce the pulmonary edema). Corticosteroids help block release of thyroid hormone and decreases peripheral conversion of T4 to T3. Additionally, corticosteroids will treat any underlying adrenal insufficiency. Methimazole prevents thyroxine synthesis. This must be given before iodine. The iodine blocks any further release of thyroid hormone. "A" is the appropriate management of NMS. "C" is an appropriate approach for valve rupture from endocarditis. "D" describes the management of severe heart failure. "E" describes essential steps in the treatment of sepsis.

HELPFUL TIP: In patients with hyperthyroidism, diarrhea is a sign that can presage thyroid storm.

* *

Your patient is treated appropriately and eventually recovers. He continues on methimazole and propranolol and remains in good control. You can try tapering the medications in 6 months to see how he does. Graves disease will often burn out in 6–18 months.

Objectives: Did you learn to . . .

- Identify the more common causes of hyperthyroidism?
- Recognize the presentation of Graves disease?
- Manage hyperthyroidism and describe the indications and risks of each treatment option?
- Recognize and treat thyroid storm?

CASE 3

You are seeing a 45-year-old female in your office. As part of a routine blood panel, the patient's TSH is noted to be elevated at 7.2 uIU/mL (0.27–4.20 uIU/mL). She has a normal free T4 and is asymptomatic.

The best option is to:

A) Start levothyroxine at a low dose to normalize the TSH.
B) Begin T3 at a low dose.
C) Reassure the patient and have her follow-up for repeat thyroid studies.
D) Begin a workup for central hypothyroidism.
E) Begin methimazole.

Discussion

The correct answer is "C." There is convincing evidence that **asymptomatic** patients with a mildly elevated TSH (generally <10 uIU/mL) and normal free T4 do not benefit from treatment in terms of quality of life, etc. In fact, treated patients tend to have more symptomatic anxiety. The term for this condition (asymptomatic, TSH between 5 and 10, and normal free T4) is subclinical hypothyroidism. Follow-up thyroid studies are indicated, although the interval may differ depending on the clinician's judgment. Of note, many patients will have transient changes in their thyroid hormone levels due to comorbid illness, viral thyroiditis, etc. The thing to do is recheck rather than start treatment. (see http://www.liebertpub.com/thy for new thyroid clinical guidelines.)

* *

The patient returns in a year and has developed overt hypothyroidism, and you start her on levothyroxine. Her TSH and free T4 normalize within 2 months. But a few months later, she storms into the office demanding a prescription for T3 because she still feels tired and is gaining weight. TSH remains normal at this time.

Your response is:

A) Write a prescription for T3 (Cytomel).
B) Tell her that no well-done study shows that T3 is of any help.
C) Intramuscular haloperidol and lorazepam . . . darned if you are going to sit around and take this kind of abuse in your own office.
D) Refer to a specialist . . . in Siberia.

Discussion

The correct answer is "B." Although patients may cite anecdotal evidence, no well-done study has shown an advantage to T3, even after thyroidectomy (much of $T4 \rightarrow T3$ conversion is done peripherally). Her symptoms are likely due to depression, excess calorie intake, deconditioning, insomnia—something other than low T3. (Next she will come in with chronic Lyme disease and want IV doxycycline for a year.)

> HELPFUL TIP: T3 preparations tend to have rapid gastrointestinal (GI) absorption and relatively short half-lives, leading to erratic T3 serum levels. It is best to avoid T3 in the vast majority of patients with hypothyroidism.

Objectives: Did you learn to . . .

- Describe subclinical hypothyroidism?
- Negotiate your way out of prescribing T3?

QUICK QUIZ: THYROID TESTS

A 52-year-old male is being seen in your clinic for weight loss, tachycardia, and anxiety. You suspect hyperthyroidism and decide to check blood work. The patient has a low TSH suggestive of hyperthyroidism but has a normal free T4.

The most likely explanation of this patient's symptoms and laboratory findings is:

A) He has pituitary dysfunction with a pending central hypothyroidism.
B) He has an isolated T3 hyperthyroidism.
C) He likely has Addison disease.
D) He is taking aspirin that interferes with the assay for free T4.

E) He it taking aspirin that interferes with the assay for TSH.

Discussion

The correct answer is "B." Five percent of patients with hyperthyroidism have an isolated T3 hyperthyroidism. Thus, if you suspect hyperthyroidism and the patient has a low TSH but a normal free T4, check a T3-RIA. It is also worth noting that TSH is more sensitive than free T4 for thyroid dysfunction. Of note, "D" and "E" are incorrect. However, many drugs can interfere with thyroid-binding globulin and cause changes in the measurable amounts of **total** T4 and T3 in the serum. In most cases, the free T4 and free T3 (unbound thyroid hormones) are not affected by the changes in thyroid-binding globulin levels.

QUICK QUIZ: HYPERTHYROIDISM

Which of the following cause(s) hyperthyroidism?

A) Lithium.
B) Amiodarone.
C) Peginterferon alfa-2A.
D) Phenytoin.
E) B and C.

Discussion

The correct answer is "E." Amiodarone (see Helpful Tip) and Peginterferon Alfa-2a can cause hyperthyroidism. "A" and "D," lithium and phenytoin respectively, cause hypothyroidism. Phenytoin reduces TSH secretion so patients may have a low TSH and a low T4.

> HELPFUL TIP: Amiodarone is interesting because it can cause **hyper**thyroidism or **hypo**thyroidism. It has multiple effects on the thyroid gland and on metabolism of T4 and T3, which can result in **hypo**thyroidism. It carries a huge iodine load, which can result in **hyper**thyroidism. Somewhere between 2% and 30% of patients taking amiodarone will have thyroid dysfunction. Amiodarone is highly lipophilic and may have a half-life as long as 100 days, resulting in toxicity long after the drug is stopped.

CASE 4

A 45-year-old female presents to the office complaining of a "ball in my neck." She noticed a lump in her anterior neck approximately 1 month ago. She is not sure if it has increased in size. She has not noticed any other lumps or masses. She denies dysphagia, odynophagia, neck pain, cough, weight loss, fever, chills, sweats, or a change in bowel habits. She also denies any hyperthyroid or hypothyroid symptoms. In 1993, she immigrated to the United States from Kiev, Ukraine, where she had lived for most of her life—including all of the 80s (you remember—Madonna, leg warmers, Chernobyl). She has no family history of thyroid or other endocrine disorders, but several relatives in Kiev have been diagnosed with various cancers.

Which of the following factors from history INCREASES the likelihood that the nodule is malignant?

A) Nodule not increasing in size.
B) No regional adenopathy.
C) Age >40 years.
D) Male gender.
E) History of possible radiation exposure.

Discussion

The correct answer is "E." This patient lived in Kiev, near the Chernobyl nuclear power plant during and after the reactor accident in 1986. She was exposed to radiation and, like her family members, is at significantly increased risk for cancer, especially thyroid malignancies. Other clinical factors that suggest a malignant etiology include (in general, not necessarily in this patient) a nodule >2 cm or increasing in size, dysphagia, hoarseness, regional lymphadenopathy, a fixation to the surrounding tissues, female gender, age <40, and family history.

> HELPFUL TIP: There are a lot of cancer survivors walking around who received radiation to the neck (e.g., mantle radiation for Hodgkin lymphoma). These patients are at increased risk of developing thyroid cancers.

* *

Physical exam reveals an obese female in no acute distress. Her head, eye, nose, and oral exam are normal. She has a 2 cm firm nodule on the right pole of the thyroid. The nodule moves along with the other subcutaneous structures upon swallowing. She has no lymphadenopathy. The rest of the exam is normal.

Which of the following next steps would be most likely to yield a definitive diagnosis?

A) Thyroid ultrasound.
B) Fine needle aspiration (FNA).
C) Thyroid scan (Tc^{99}).
D) Serum thyroglobulin level.
E) Serum calcitonin level and CEA level.

Discussion

The correct answer is "B." FNA can conclusively prove or disprove the presence of neoplasm and should be considered for all thyroid nodules and cysts. That is the bottom line; the rest is interesting, but do the FNA.

A thyroid scan will identify if a nodule is actively processing thyroid hormone ("functional" or "hot") or is not metabolically active ("nonfunctional" or "cold"). A "hot" nodule may cause hyperthyroidism, is **usually** nonmalignant ("hot is not") and can be treated with I^{131}. A cold nodule is either an adenoma or a malignancy and a biopsy is mandated. A serum thyroglobulin is the tumor marker for thyroid carcinoma and should be drawn before thyroidectomy. **It has no value as a diagnostic test in the initial evaluation before malignancy is determined but can be followed as a marker. Antithyroglobulin antibodies may interfere with the assay, however.** Serum calcitonin and CEA levels are elevated in the case of medullary carcinoma, but would have low yield in the initial evaluation. An ultrasound may be useful in evaluating a nodule that has low malignant potential or in assisting FNA.

* *

Fine needle aspirate reveals probable papillary carcinoma. A serum thyroglobulin level, TSH, basic chemistries, a blood count, and a blood type are ordered.

What should be done next?

A) Observe the nodule for 1 month.
B) Computerized tomography (CT) of the head and neck with contrast.
C) Radiation therapy with I^{131}.
D) Radiation therapy with external beam radiation.
E) Suppression of TSH levels with thyroxine.

Discussion

The correct answer is "B." Surgery for removal of the tumor is the most appropriate next step, but a CT scan is indicated to delineate the extent of the neoplasm. Radiotherapy with I^{131} is used after surgery for metastatic disease, but external beam radiation is not used for thyroid cancers except for the palliative therapy of anaplastic carcinoma. Because these tumors are TSH responsive, suppression of TSH level **following surgery** for papillary carcinoma is achieved with thyroxine (usually 2.2–2.5 μg/kg—fairly high dose to completely suppress TSH production).

> **HELPFUL TIP:** The most common thyroid cancer is papillary carcinoma. Medullary carcinoma may be associated with an elevated calcitonin and other endocrine malignancies (e.g., multiple endocrine neoplasia II [MEN II]).

Objectives: Did you learn to . . .

- Recognize the major risk factors influencing the development and prognosis of thyroid carcinomas?
- Evaluate a thyroid nodule?
- Describe the management of papillary carcinoma, the most common of the thyroid cancers?

CASE 5

A 78-year-old female is brought to the emergency department (ED) for strange behavior. According to her family, she has been more sleepy and weak throughout the last week. She is acting more withdrawn and depressed and seems to respond to nonexistent external stimuli (similar to our small children's imaginary play friends). When asked about her depression, she reports she is sad because a man in a clown suit who trains poodles keeps telling her she is going to die. She complains of abdominal cramps and blames it on "being plugged up," and her family reports no bowel movement for 2 days. She also notes chronic bone pain in her hips and back. That's about all you can get before the bad news clown returns . . .

A physical exam is notable only for a 3 cm irregular mass in her right breast (we're very impressed that you did a breast exam in the ED). The family thinks it is new. Her neurological exam is normal, except for her apparent confusion.

What finding would you expect from an ECG?

A) Peaked T-waves.
B) Diffuse ST-segment elevations.
C) Long QT interval.
D) Short QT interval.
E) B and D.

Discussion
The correct answer is "E." This patient is likely to have hypercalcemia, probably from an undiagnosed metastatic breast cancer. The ECG in a patient with significant hypercalcemia will show a short QT interval; rarely there is diffuse ST elevation. **Hypo**calcemia is associated with a long QT interval, which can occasionally lead to arrhythmias due to an R on T phenomenon (an R-wave of a PVC fuses with the previous T-wave predisposing to torsades de pointes). Hypercalcemia produces symptoms in the CNS (confusion, psychosis, depression), GI system (abdominal pain, cramps, constipation), kidneys (nephrolithiasis, polyuria, renal insufficiency), and musculoskeletal system (weakness, myopathy, osteoporosis). To help you remember the symptoms of hypercalcemia, use the phrase "stones, bones, moans, groans, and psychiatric overtones." Peaked T-waves are associated with hyperkalemia, and diffuse ST-segment elevations is a finding in pericarditis (and rarely hypercalcemia).

Which of the following tests should now be done?

A) Electrolytes, including a calcium level.
B) CBC.
C) TSH.
D) Chest x-ray.
E) All of the above.

Discussion
The correct answer is "E." The differential diagnosis for altered mental status in an elderly person is relatively large, and many more tests might be appropriate. In addition to hypercalcemia, hyponatremia or hypernatremia are possibilities in this case. This patient has several symptoms of hypothyroidism, so a TSH is critical. Rarely, hyperthyroidism may present in the elderly with lethargy rather than hyperkinetic activity—a presentation known as apathetic hyperthyroidism. Infections are common causes of altered mental status in the elderly. A CBC may reveal an elevated white blood cell count, a left shift, or anemia. The chest x-ray may detect a subclinical pneumonia or, more likely in this case, a mass from metastatic cancer.

* *

Your patient's total serum calcium level is reported as 15.3 mg/dL (upper limit 10.4 mg/dL).

What is the NEXT step in her treatment?

A) Moderately aggressive normal saline hydration.
B) IV chlorthalidone administration.
C) IV calcitonin administration.
D) IV bisphosphonate infusion.
E) Gallium nitrate infusion.

Discussion
The correct answer is "A." Although "C" and "D" may be indicated, adequate hydration and establishing urine output is critical to the treatment of hypercalcemia and should be the next step. A normal saline infusion will increase urinary calcium excretion by inhibiting proximal tubular sodium and calcium reabsorption. **Note that IV furosemide (and diuretics in general) are falling out of favor and should not be used. Hydration is the most important goal.** An IV bisphosphonate infusion should then be started and will lower the calcium level over 2–4 days. Calcitonin has a limited duration of action and can be used in emergencies where saline is ineffective. Gallium nitrate is an older treatment that has fallen out of favor with the advent of the reliable and safe bisphosphonates. It can still be used in refractory cases. "B" is of special note. Chlorthalidone and other thiazide diuretics **increase** calcium levels and are contraindicated.

* *

The patient is treated appropriately for her hypercalcemia and her mental status improves. A biopsy of her breast mass is done and reveals an infiltrating ductal carcinoma. A bone scan reveals diffuse metastatic disease.

Which of the following statements about the mechanism for malignancy associated hypercalcemia is/are TRUE?

A) Decreased bone reabsorption increases the serum calcium.
B) Secretion of osteoclast-inhibiting factors increases the serum calcium.

C) Secretion of parathyroid hormone (PTH)-like substances increases the serum calcium.
D) Direct erosion of bone by tumor cells never plays a role.
E) All of the above.

Discussion

The correct answer is "C." Malignancy increases the serum calcium level by secreting osteoclast-**activating** (not inhibiting as in answer "B") factors leading to increased bone resorption (thus "A" and "B" are false). Secretion of PTH-like substances causes retention of calcium by the kidneys, which elevates the serum calcium. Direct erosion of bone by tumor cells also contributes to the release of calcium from the bones (and predisposes the patient to fractures). The neoplasms most commonly associated with hypercalcemia are cancers of the breast, lung, prostate, and kidney as well as multiple myeloma and a few other hematologic cancers.

Your patient's cancer cannot be cured. How can her chronically elevated calcium level be managed?

A) Oral glucocorticoids 20–40 mg/day.
B) Oral phosphates.
C) Oral bisphosphonates.
D) All of the above.

Discussion

The correct answer is "D." Glucocorticoids decrease intestinal calcium absorption, but in and of themselves can lead to bone density loss and an increased risk for fractures. Oral phosphates can decrease intestinal calcium absorption and bone reabsorption of calcium. Bisphosphonates, as previously discussed, decrease the serum calcium and increase bone density.

Objectives: Did you learn to . . .

- Recognize neoplastic causes of hypercalcemia?
- Identify presenting symptoms of hypercalcemia?
- Understand the mechanisms underlying hypercalcemia in malignancy?
- Initiate emergency treatment for symptomatic hypercalcemia?

CASE 6

A 42-year-old male presents to the office for routine follow-up of his hypertension. He denies any complaints. He has primary hypertension, for which he takes benazepril 20 mg PO daily and hydrochlorothiazide 25 mg PO daily. The patient takes no other medications. His vital signs are as follows: BP 135/70, P 72, R 18, and T 98.6°F. The physical exam is completely normal. His calcium is elevated at 12.8 mg/dL (upper limit normal 10.4). The rest of his electrolytes, BUN, and creatinine are normal as is a CBC and ECG.

You consider what you know about hypercalcemia.

Which of the following is/are responsible for spuriously elevated serum calcium?

A) Pseudopotassium transport.
B) Fever and active metabolic state.
C) Use of alendronate or risedronate.
D) Prolonged application of the tourniquet while drawing blood.
E) All of the above.

Discussion

The correct answer is "D." Prolonged application of the tourniquet or a high calcium meal before a blood draw can both cause a spuriously elevated serum calcium. In fact, 50% or so of patients have a normal calcium when it is checked a second time. So, the next step after finding an elevated calcium is to repeat the test. "C" will cause a low calcium level. "A" doesn't exist that we know of . . . sorry.

Assuming you repeat the lab value and the calcium remains elevated, your next step is:

A) A bone scan for occult cancer.
B) Immediate dialysis.
C) Nothing, since the patient is asymptomatic.
D) Discontinue the hydrochlorothiazide and recheck calcium in 2 weeks.
E) Discontinue the benazepril and recheck potassium in 2 weeks.

Discussion

The correct answer is "D." This patient has hypercalcemia. Asymptomatic hypercalcemia is not uncommon on routine screening examinations. It should be addressed because it is always abnormal and can be treated early before any symptoms develop. In this patient, the most likely cause is hydrochlorothiazide. Thiazide drugs increase the renal reabsorption of calcium (remember the case above?). Angiotensin-converting enzyme (ACE) inhibitors may cause hyperkalemia but are usually not associated with hypercalcemia. An investigation for occult cancer may be indicated in this patient's future, but it is reasonable to address the potential adverse drug effect first. Dialysis is not indicated.

* *

The patient stops taking the hydrochlorothiazide and returns for a laboratory draw in 2 weeks. The calcium level is now 12.9 mg/dL. "Rats," you say. "Where's my thinking cap—I mean iPad?"

What should you do next?

A) Wait another month and recheck before taking any other action.
B) Order a 24-hour bisphosphonate infusion.
C) Perform prostate and testicular exam for masses, chest x-ray, and intact PTH (iPTH).
D) Perform prostate and testicular exam for masses, CT of the chest, abdomen, and pelvis, and bone scan.
E) Perform prostate and testicular exam for masses, chest x-ray, then reassure patient if normal.

Discussion

The correct answer is "C." In this patient, it is reasonable to rule out primary hyperparathyroidism while also checking for other obvious causes. A chest x-ray will rule out significant lung masses and sarcoidosis. A testicular and prostate exam for masses is important so that **large** tumors in these organs do not go unnoticed (remembering that a digital rectal exam is neither sensitive nor specific as a screening/diagnostic test for prostate cancer). An elevated iPTH in the presence of a calcium level >12 mg/dL confirms the diagnosis of hyperparathyroidism. The test for iPTH will not significantly cross-react with the PTH-like hormone produced by neoplasms. Unless the history or physical is suspicious for lymphoma, or some other occult neoplasm, a pan-body scan is a waste of money and exposes the patient to unnecessary radiation. At this point, it is not necessary to acutely lower the calcium level because the cause has not been identified and the patient is asymptomatic. See Table 10–1 for more causes of hypercalcemia.

Table 10–1 CAUSES OF HYPERCALCEMIA

Pseudohypercalcemia
Excessive calcium intake
Hypervitaminosis D
Hyperparathyroidism (primary and secondary)
Hyperthyroidism
Malignancy
Hypervitaminosis A
Adrenal insufficiency
Pheochromocytoma
Rhabdomyolysis
Familial hypocalciuria
Immobilization
Medications
Lithium
Megestrol
Methyltestosterone
Mycophenolate
Tacrolimus
Tamoxifen
Theophylline (toxicity)
Thiazides

* *

The patient's complete exam is normal as is the chest x-ray. The iPTH level is twice the upper limit of normal.

How should this patient be treated?

A) Immediate CT of the chest, abdomen, and pelvis.
B) IV bisphosphonate infusion.
C) Daily dialysis until the calcium level is normal.
D) Referral for parathyroidectomy.
E) Referral for thyroidectomy.

Discussion

The correct answer is "D." This patient has primary hyperparathyroidism. He has an elevated parathyroid hormone in the presence of hypercalcemia. This is usually caused by a functional parathyroid adenoma and is best treated in otherwise healthy patients with a parathyroidectomy. This can be done without significant loss of thyroid tissue. In elderly patients with mild hyperparathyroidism and asymptomatic hypercalcemia, medical management is an option. If the patient had a low or normal PTH level, occult cancer should be considered (check for

PTH-like hormone in the serum), and a bone scan or body CT may be warranted. Although bisphosphonates will lower the serum calcium and may be used in an emergency, a parathyroidectomy is curative. Dialysis is not indicated in this patient.

* *

Your patient undergoes a parathyroidectomy and is discharged from the hospital. The pathology report on the removed tissue confirms the presence of a parathyroid adenoma and no malignancy. He returns for his first postoperative appointment 1 week later, and he is complaining of weakness. He says that the day after the surgery he felt fine, but has progressively gotten weaker "all over" since that time. Last night, he was kept awake by recurrent muscle spasms in his legs and arms. He denies fever, chills, nausea, or vomiting. He says he is eating, drinking, and passing urine normally. He has had no hematuria or dysuria. His vital signs are normal.

On physical exam, he appears anxious. Just after taking the patient's vital signs, his left arm develops a muscle spasm and an involuntary flexion of the wrist that lasts for about 20–30 seconds. Tapping the cheek just anterior to the tragus causes the ipsilateral face to twitch. The rest of cranial nerve exam is normal. His neck wound is healing well, with minimal erythema and no tenderness. The rest of the physical exam is unremarkable.

What is causing this patient's symptoms?

A) He suffers from vitamin D deficiency.
B) This patient has MEN II and also has a pheochromocytoma.
C) Too much parathyroid tissue was removed during the surgery.
D) The stress of the surgery precipitated thyrotoxicosis.
E) The stress of the surgery precipitated the onset of multiple sclerosis.

Discussion

The correct answer is "C." This patient likely has hypocalcemia due to excessive removal of parathyroid gland tissue. This is a rare, but unfortunate, complication of parathyroid gland removal and is usually detected in the immediate postoperative course. The patient's physical exam demonstrates Chvostek sign (tapping over the facial nerve elicits a twitch) and Trousseau signs (carpopedal spasm after placement of a blood pressure cuff). Vitamin D deficiency, although a cause of hypocalcemia, is unlikely to develop so quickly. The usual causes of vitamin D deficiency are malabsorption or inadequate intake, but there is nothing in the patient's history to suggest this. There is nothing to suggest MEN II (hyperparathyroidism, medullary thyroid carcinoma, and pheochromocytoma). There is also nothing here to suggest pheochromocytoma (episodic diaphoresis, labile blood pressure, recurrent palpitations and near-syncope). There is no clinical evidence of thyrotoxicosis (tachycardia, tremor, etc.).

* *

A calcium and albumin level is sent, as well as a CBC and routine chemistry panel. Everything is normal except: calcium 5.1 mg/dL (8.8–10.4 mg/dL) and albumin 3.0 g/dL (3.4–5.0 g/dL). His phosphate level is 4.2 mg/dL (2.5–4.5 mg/dL).

Does this patient have hypocalcemia?

A) No, the serum calcium level is normal.
B) No, the serum calcium level when corrected for the albumin is normal.
C) Yes, because the serum (calcium × phosphate) product is >20.
D) Yes, because the serum calcium level is still low when corrected for albumin.
E) Not enough information given to determine.

Discussion

The correct answer is "D." The patient's calcium level is low, even after correcting the hypoalbuminemia. To correct for albumin, add 0.8 mg/dL to the serum calcium level for each 1 g/dL the albumin is <4 g/dL. In other words, corrected serum calcium = [(4–albumin) × 0.8] + measured serum calcium, or in this case the equation is $[(4-3) \times 0.8] + 5.1 = 5.9$ mg/dL. When evaluating hypocalcemia, it is prudent to check a BUN and creatinine to rule out renal failure as a cause (from renal osteodystrophy . . . see Chapter 5 for more information).

HELPFUL TIP: If you don't want to correct for albumin, check an ionized calcium. An ionized calcium will also be useful in patients with monoclonal gammopathy or multiple myeloma. Occasionally, these proteins can also bind calcium.

How should this patient now be treated?

A) Calcium gluconate 1 g by rapid IV push.
B) Correct his hypomagnesemia with IV MgSO4.
C) Administer IV normal saline 1 L bolus.
D) Calcium carbonate 1–4 g with vitamin D PO daily.
E) No therapy, as the calcium level will correct itself.

Discussion

The correct answer is "D." The patient now requires oral calcium supplementation, usually with vitamin D to stimulate absorption. He will likely require it lifelong. This patient has neither hypomagnesia nor hyperphosphatemia, nor any other electrolyte abnormalities. If he had, correcting either would also raise the serum calcium. "A" deserves special mention. IV calcium gluconate or calcium chloride can be used in severe hypocalcemia. But they should not be given by rapid IV push but rather by slow push over a couple of minutes.

Objectives: Did you learn to . . .

- Describe the evaluation and treatment of primary hyperparathyroidism?
- Recognize the signs and symptoms of hypocalcemia and hypercalcemia?
- Recognize the causes of hypercalcemia and hypocalcemia?
- Evaluate and treat hypocalcemia?

CASE 7

A 36-year-old female presents to the office complaining of difficulty losing weight for 2 years. She seeks a prescription drug to aid in these efforts. She has tried every fad diet she comes across, but nothing seems to help. She tries to exercise regularly, but manages only walking a couple of miles each week. A nutritional history reveals that she is eating a sensible low-fat diet. Her past medical history includes hypertension treated with medications for the last 3 years and noninsulin-dependent diabetes mellitus (DM) for the last year. She also has been seeing a psychiatrist over the last 6 months for emotional lability, which she blames on anxiety over her inability to get pregnant. The patient takes glyburide 5 mg PO daily and benazepril (Lotensin) 40 mg PO daily. A review of systems reveals thinning hair, irregular menses, delayed wound healing and infertility (she's been trying to get pregnant for over 1 year).

What advice do you offer this patient now?

A) She is eating right; she just needs to exercise more.
B) Low-fat diets are ineffective; she needs to reduce her carbohydrate intake.
C) She has failed lifestyle modifications, and appetite suppressant medications are indicated.
D) She is likely depressed, and needs to continue psychiatric therapy and probably should start treatment with a selective serotonin-reuptake inhibitor (SSRI).
E) Reserve any dietary advice at this time, as she first needs a medical workup.

Discussion

The correct answer is "E." The patient's symptoms of weight gain and associated findings on review of systems (emotionally labile, thinning hair, infertility, irregular menses, and delayed wound healing) suggest a secondary cause, most likely an endocrine abnormality. (What else would you expect? This is the endocrine chapter after all . . .)

HELPFUL TIP: Did you notice that she is trying to get pregnant and is on an ACE inhibitor . . . for shame. Her doctor should talk to her about that.

* *

Her vitals in the office: P 88, BP 155/94, R 20, and T 37.7°C. On physical exam, you note an obese female with truncal obesity and thin extremities. She has thinning hair, round facies, hirsutism, and a buffalo hump at her upper back. Her skin is hyperpigmented with abdominal striae. The rest of the exam is unremarkable.

Based on this patient's history and physical exam, what diagnosis is most likely?

A) Hypothyroidism.
B) Hyperthyroidism.
C) Cortisol excess secondary to chronic steroid therapy.
D) Cortisol excess secondary to an endogenous process (Cushing disease).

E) Cortisol deficiency secondary to autoimmune adrenal insufficiency.

Discussion

The correct answer is "D." This patient has the classic symptoms and signs of Cushing *syndrome*, or cortisol excess. This may be due to corticosteroid therapy (the most common cause), ectopic ACTH production from neoplasms of the lung, pancreas, kidney, etc, adrenal neoplasms producing cortisol, or ACTH production from a pituitary neoplasm (termed Cushing *disease*). Her condition is unlikely due to steroid therapy, as this should have been revealed in her medical history. At this point in the evaluation, it is not clear what the source of ACTH is, just that there is excess ATCH being produced.

* *

Labs are sent, most of which are normal except for an elevated glucose of 210 mg/dL and an elevated 24-hour urinary free cortisol of 115 μg (normal <100 μg). Based on these findings, a dexamethasone suppression test is ordered. The patient is given huge, supratherapeutic dexamethasone for 2 days, and then serum ACTH is drawn, and another 24-hour urine collection is done. The repeat values are serum ACTH is slightly elevated and 24-hour urinary free cortisol is 78 μg (normal).

What is the source of this patient's cortisol excess?

A) An ACTH-producing tumor.
B) A cortisol-producing adrenal tumor.
C) Surreptitious use of oral steroids.
D) Not enough information to determine.

Discussion

The correct answer is "A." When the patient was given exogenous steroids during the test, there was a partial suppression of cortisol production (mild decrease in 24-hour urinary free cortisol). But more importantly, the serum ACTH level remained normal despite the high steroid load. It should have been low in the presence of dexamethasone, or any exogenous steroid, which would act to shut off ACTH production in the normal patient.

Normal mechanisms provide negative feedback on the pituitary gland (the source of ACTH) when cortisol levels are high. If ACTH is still being produced despite a high steroid load, then there must be an ACTH-producing neoplasm somewhere in the body (either ectopic production from a lung, renal, or pancreatic cancer, or an ACTH-producing pituitary tumor that has escaped normal regulatory feedback mechanisms).

HELPFUL TIP: In the case of a **cortisol-producing adrenal neoplasm,** the high exogenous steroid doses should effectively suppress ACTH production because the pituitary functioning is appropriate. The urinary free cortisol remains high (the tumor produces cortisol independent of ACTH control). However, since the pituitary is functioning, the baseline ACTH would have been low to begin with.

* *

On physical exam, the patient has a visual field cut.

What is the best next step in this patient's evaluation?

A) Ultrasound of kidneys to assess for masses and adrenal flow.
B) CT scan of the brain to rule out metastatic lesions and assess pituitary size.
C) CT scan of the adrenals to evaluate for adrenal neoplasms.
D) MRI of the pancreas to evaluate for neoplasms.
E) MRI of the pituitary gland to evaluate for a neoplasm.

Discussion

The correct answer is "E." The previous studies strongly suggest Cushing syndrome and the visual filed cut suggests a pituitary source of excess ACTH (e.g., ACTH-producing tumor of the pituitary gland). An MRI of the pituitary is the best means to confirm this. CT scan may suggest enlargement of the sella turcica (where the pituitary gland sits), but it is insensitive for detecting abnormalities in the pituitary, especially microadenomas.

HELPFUL TIP: If the MRI is negative, then the more rare case of ectopic ACTH production from occult cancer must be considered, and a body CT scan is indicated.

Objectives: Did you learn to . . .

- Recognize the common presenting signs and symptoms of Cushing syndrome?
- Identify the causes of cortisol excess and how they are best evaluated?

CASE 8

JFK, a 38-year-old male, presents to the office with the chief complaint of weakness. He reports that he lacks the energy to complete his previously busy work schedule (such as invading Cuba) and has cut his hours back the last 2–3 weeks, which has recently become a financial hardship. JFK also reports poor appetite and a 20-pound weight loss over the last month. He has had alternating periods of diarrhea and constipation. He also reports often feeling faint and has come near to passing out after standing up quickly a few times. This is different for him from baseline. He has no previous medical or surgical history. He denies medications or allergies. He reports that several of his relatives on his mother's side have had thyroid problems. "I caaan't go on like this," he complains in an accent that betrays his Boston roots.

On physical exam, his vitals reveal BP 85/38, P 85, R 20, and T 37°C. The rest of the exam is normal except for hyperpigmentation of buccal mucosa and weakness in the proximal musculature (5−/5 strength in both upper and lower extremities). Skin: Hyperpigmentation of the elbows, knuckles, knees, and the palmar creases. No edema.

What is the most likely cause of this patient's symptoms?

A) Hyperthyroidism
B) Hypothyroidism
C) Adrenal gland hyperactivity
D) Adrenal insufficiency
E) Depression

Discussion

The correct answer is "D." Several clues point you in this direction. First, the hyperpigmentation found at stress/crease points on the peripheral skin suggests the diagnosis of adrenal insufficiency. The low blood pressure and orthostasis is also more likely to be seen in adrenal insufficiency.

This patient has a number of symptoms consistent with both depression and hypothyroidism, but his physical exam suggests another diagnosis. A patient with depression and no underlying medical cause would have a normal physical exam. A patient with hypothyroidism may have a slightly low blood pressure, but not markedly low as in this patient. The heart rate in symptomatic hypothyroidism is usually low. Hypothyroidism may also cause changes in the hair, skin, and thyroid gland that are not seen here. Finally, the patient's reflexes are normal, rather than delayed. There is nothing in this case to suggest hyperthyroidism or cortisol excess.

* *

Laboratory results show a low sodium (129 mg/dL), low glucose (69 mg/dL), and high potassium (5.4 mg/dL) along with a normal TSH and a mildly low hemoglobin.

Based on the information provided thus far, what is the best test to diagnose this patient's condition?

A) Cosyntropin stimulation test.
B) Random serum cortisol.
C) Bone marrow biopsy.
D) Plasma renin.
E) Ultrasound of kidneys to measure their size.

Discussion

The correct answer is "A." The laboratory chemistry results (hyperkalemia, hyponatremia, and hypoglycemia), combined with the history and physical exam, strongly suggest a mineralocorticoid deficiency. A cosyntropin stimulation test uses synthetic ACTH to try to induce a burst of cortisol secretion. No increase in the serum cortisol in response to the cosyntropin suggests that the adrenal glands are unable to respond to the body's mineralocorticoid and glucocorticoid needs. A positive cosyntropin test makes the diagnosis of adrenal insufficiency. A random serum cortisol is definitely second best, as cortisol levels normally fluctuate widely throughout the diurnal cycle. Plasma renin is used in the evaluation of mineralocorticoid excess (hyperaldosteronism) and should be low in this state. "E" is not likely to be helpful. Even in the case of adrenal insufficiency, the kidneys are unlikely to change in size. Although an ultrasound may show small, shrunken adrenals that have been destroyed by tuberculosis infection, a CT scan is a better tool for assessing the adrenals. "C" is way off base. This patient has no indication for a bone marrow biopsy.

> **HELPFUL TIP:** An early morning serum cortisol level is often low in patients with adrenal insufficiency. However, this test alone is insufficient for screening, as it has a high false negative rate. But a low (<5 μg/dL) early morning serum cortisol is likely to be due to adrenal insufficiency.

* *

Further laboratory results are as follows:

Random serum cortisol: 12 μg/dL (normal ≥ 20 μg/dL).

Serum cortisol 1 hour after 0.25 mg cosyntropin IV: 13.5 μg/dL (the rise in cortisol is expected to be >7 μg/dL).

Based on the prevalence in the United States, what is the most likely underlying cause of this patient's condition?

A) Autoimmune disease.
B) Invasive carcinoma.
C) Meningococcal septicemia.
D) Sarcoidosis.
E) Tuberculosis.

Discussion

The correct answer is "A." All the conditions listed are known causes of primary adrenal insufficiency, and all cause this disorder by destruction of the adrenal glands. This will result in a lack of adrenal hormone secretion and a blunted response of the adrenals to ACTH—hence, the minimal rise of cortisol despite administration of synthetic ACTH (cosyntropin). A cortisol rise of <7 μg/dL (in response to cosyntropin) with a baseline cortisol <20 μg/dL is suggestive of primary adrenal insufficiency. Autoimmune destruction is by far the most common cause in North America, and invasion of the adrenals by tuberculosis is the most common cause worldwide.

Without measuring the serum ACTH or 24-hour urine ACTH level, it is still possible to tell the difference between primary (lack of adrenal response to ACTH) and secondary (lack of ACTH) adrenal insufficiency.

Which of the following suggests primary adrenal insufficiency (e.g., adrenal destruction) rather than secondary?

A) Elevation of cortisol by cosyntropin test of >7 μg/dL.
B) Presence of hyperpigmentation on physical exam.
C) Presence of neuropathy on physical exam.
D) Predominant symptoms of depression.

Discussion

The correct answer is "B." Hyperpigmentation at skin creases occurs in primary adrenal insufficiency (but not secondary adrenal insufficiency). This is because in primary adrenal insufficiency, the **pituitary** is intact. As a result, the ACTH level is high, as is the level of melanocyte-stimulating hormone. It is this melanocyte-stimulating hormone that causes hyperpigmentation. An elevation of cortisol by >7 μg/dL during the cosyntropin test would suggest an intact adrenal system with a pituitary problem. Hypoglycemia and depression are symptoms common to all causes of adrenal insufficiency. Neuropathy is not a common finding in adrenal insufficiency.

> **HELPFUL TIP:** Patients with primary adrenal insufficiency **may** present with low serum sodium and high serum potassium (although many will have normal electrolytes). This is primarily because of loss of the aldosterone system. Patients with secondary adrenal insufficiency (e.g., pituitary cause) have intact adrenal glands and therefore intact aldosterone. Thus, they will generally have normal electrolytes and less dehydration, hypotension, etc.

How should this patient now be treated?

A) Prednisone 60 mg PO for 5 days, then slowly tapered over 2 weeks.
B) Cosyntropin 0.5 mg SC daily indefinitely.
C) Corticosteroids (prednisone 5 mg or hydrocortisone 15 mg) daily indefinitely.
D) Corticosteroids (prednisone 5 mg or hydrocortisone 15 mg) daily plus mineralocorticoid (fludrocortisone 0.1 mg) daily indefinitely.
E) Adrenal transplant.

Discussion

The correct answer is "D." This patient requires chronic corticosteroid supplementation, and, because he has primary adrenal insufficiency, he also requires mineralocorticoid supplementation. Cosyntropin treatment would have no effect since the adrenals are not functioning. A short burst of prednisone is important if this patient experiences a sudden stressor, such as an infection, but it is not the primary therapy. Medical therapy is fairly effective, so adrenal (or renal) transplant is not a usual treatment option.

* *

JFK is treated appropriately and, after 4 weeks, is feeling much better, has regained most of his lost weight and in fact feels well enough to take on both Castro *and* Khrushchev (local competitors to his dry-cleaning business). He no longer suffers spells of lightheadedness or depression. To celebrate his new good health, he and a blond starlet go out for a lavish seafood dinner, including fresh oysters. Within 8 hours of the meal, JFK develops severe cramping abdominal pain and profuse watery diarrhea (so much for the date . . .). He tries to treat himself at home with Pepto-Bismol and oral fluids, but gets progressively weaker. After 12 hours of intestinal symptoms, he calls for an ambulance because he is too weak to stand.

Upon presentation in the ED: Vital signs: P 130, BP 70/20, R 30, and T 38°C.

General: Diaphoretic, ill-appearing male in severe distress.

After establishing adequate IV access, what should be done next?

A) Order a chest x-ray.
B) Start "renal-dose" dopamine through a peripheral line.
C) Give 2 L normal saline by bolus.
D) Start normal saline at 125 cc/hr.
E) Give levofloxacin 500 mg IV.

Discussion

The correct answer is "C." This patient is severely volume depleted and needs crystalloid immediately. All other treatment concerns, although may eventually be done, are secondary.

* *

Fluid is run in quickly, yet he remains hypotensive. Did you forget something?

What should have been done simultaneously for this patient when the fluids were started?

A) Intubation by rapid sequence and mechanical ventilation.
B) Administration of a phenylephrine drip.
C) Administration of 4 mg dexamethasone IV.
D) Administration of 100 mg hydrocortisone IV.
E) C or D.

Discussion

The correct answer is "E." This patient has adrenal insufficiency and requires additional "stress doses" of steroids in times of severe physical stress (e.g., infection, trauma, and chest pain). The steroids he regularly takes for his disease may not be sufficient during these periods, precipitating Addisonian crisis. Without this additional treatment, the patient may experience intractable hypotension and possibly death.

HELPFUL TIP: If you suspect adrenal insufficiency crisis, start steroids immediately even if you do not have laboratory confirmation. Dexamethasone is an option for treatment, and it will not interfere with the cortisol assay when doing a cosyntropin stimulation test. **But note that dexamethasone does not have mineralocorticoid activity and should be replaced by hydrocortisone succinate just as soon as the cosyntropin stimulation test is done.**

Objectives: Did you learn to . . .

- Recognize the presentation of adrenal insufficiency?
- Evaluate a patient with adrenal insufficiency?
- Treat a patient chronically for adrenal insufficiency and when in adrenal crisis?

QUICK QUIZ: DIABETES DIAGNOSIS

Which of the following can be used to diagnose diabetes mellitus (DM)?

A) Fasting blood glucose on one occasion.
B) Glycosylated hemoglobin (HbA_{1c}) on one occasion.
C) A random blood sugar of >160 mg/dL.
D) None of the above.

Discussion

The correct answer is "D." Here is why. The diagnosis of DM requires **two** elevated fasting blood sugars or ***two*** **HbA_{1c} levels** of >6.5%. It can also be diagnosed if the patient has a random blood sugar of >200 mg/dL with signs and symptoms of DM (polyuria, polydipsia, weight loss, blurred vision).

QUICK QUIZ: DIABETES DIAGNOSIS

Which of the following statements is FALSE?

A) The diagnosis of diabetes can be made if a fasting blood sugar is 126 mg/dL or higher twice, confirmed on a different day **or** a random blood sugar is over 200 mg/dL in a patient with symptoms (polyuria, polydipsia).
B) Impaired fasting blood glucose is defined as a fasting level of 100–125 mg/dL.
C) Patients with adult onset type 1 diabetes (also known as latent autoimmune diabetes in adults or slowly progressing type 1) are generally thin.
D) Patients with adult onset type 1 diabetes comprise about 10% of patients diagnosed with diabetes type 2.
E) Patients with adult onset type 1 diabetes manifest significant insulin resistance.

Discussion

The correct answer is "E" (which is a false statement). Patients with adult onset type 1 diabetes **do not** have insulin resistance. Adult onset type 1 diabetes (also known as latent autoimmune diabetes in adults or slowly progressing type 1) is a relatively new concept. Patients with adult onset type 1 diabetes develop diabetes as an adult, which is similar to those with DM2. However, they are generally thin, not hypertensive and do not have the rest of the constellation of disease in DM2 (low HDL, high triglycerides). Generally, they need insulin relatively early in the course of their treatment, although they will initially respond to oral hypoglycemic agents. The rest of the statements are all correct. Note especially the criteria for making the diagnosis of DM in answer "A."

HELPFUL TIP: The American Diabetes Association (ADA) suggests that a blood sugar of 100 mg/dL is now "prediabetes" and represents "impaired fasting glucose." The authors think calling a normal blood sugar prediabetes is absurd. So does the European Diabetes Epidemiology Group that advocates using the original 110 mg/dL as impaired fasting glucose. Take it for what it is worth . . .

CASE 9

You are called to the ED to see a 17-year-old young man brought in by his parents who found him in his room at home. He is lethargic, but not unconscious or comatose. He is unable to give a coherent history. His parents state that they have been concerned because the patient has been losing weight in the last 2 months, and acting more tired than usual. They are worried that he might be abusing drugs, but have not found any drugs or drug paraphernalia in the home. They have observed no other signs of illness. The family history is positive for hypertension in multiple family members, and the patient's mother has hyperlipidemia. There is no family history of kidney or liver disease, heart attacks or strokes, diabetes, or cancer. Your exam discloses the following:

Vital signs: T 36.9°C, P 125, BP 98/54, respirations are deep with a rate of 28.

Mental status: Lethargic, arouses to pain. Nonverbal.

HEENT: Mucous membranes dry, tongue fissured. Fruity aroma on breath.

Lungs: Clear to auscultation throughout, no wheezes or stridor.

Heart: Regular rapid rate, no murmur or gallop.

Abdomen: Soft, mild generalized tenderness without guarding or rebound. No masses or organomegaly.

Test results are as follows:

ECG: Sinus tachycardia, otherwise normal.

Hemogram: Hb 17.9 g/dL; WBC 16,200 cells/mm^3, predominantly neutrophils.

Platelets: 650,000 cells/mm^3.

Electrolytes: Sodium 131 mEq/L, potassium 5.7 mEq/L, chloride 97 mEq/L, bicarbonate 10 mEq/L.

Renal: BUN 63 mg/dL, creatinine 1.8 mg/dL, glucose 635 mg/dL.

ABG (room air): pH 7.20; $PaCO_2$ 27 mm Hg; PaO_2 101 mm Hg, bicarbonate 10 mEq/L

Serum ketones: Positive.

You diagnose diabetic ketoacidosis (DKA) with dehydration >10% and admit the patient to the intensive care unit. As the first stage of therapy you wish to replace the lost fluid volume.

Which of the following regimens is the most appropriate initial intervention?

A) 5% dextrose in 0.45% (half-normal) saline to run at 150 cc/hr.
B) 0.45% (half-normal) saline with 20 mEq potassium/L, to run at 150 cc/hr.
C) 0.9% (normal) saline 1 L to infuse as quickly as possible.
D) 0.9% (normal) saline with 20 mEq potassium/L to run at 1000 cc/hr.
E) 5% dextrose in 0.225% (quarter-normal) saline with 20 mEq potassium/L to run at 1000 cc/hr.

Discussion

The correct answer is "C." Initial volume replacement should be with isotonic saline infused at a rapid rate (in the absence of cardiac disease) until the volume deficit is corrected. "D" is of special note. In general, potassium should be added to the **second liter** of fluid unless the patient is already hypokalemic on the first blood gas (getting a potassium, glucose, and sodium on the first blood gas is good policy). Potassium replacement is essential even in the hyperkalemic patient, as correction of the ketoacidosis leads to a rapid shift of potassium into the intracellular compartment. Remember that an acidosis artificially increases the serum potassium by shifting potassium extracellularly. The potassium increases by approximately 1 mEq/L for every pH point of 0.1 below 7.4 (so, a pH of 7.3 will increase the potassium from 4 to 5 mEq/L). See Chapter 5 for more on acidosis, alkalosis, and the effects on potassium. "D" is incorrect because you would like the first liter to infuse as quickly as possible in DKA and not over an hour. Besides, 20 mEq of potassium IV in 1 hour should not be routine and only given if the patient has continuous cardiac monitoring.

> HELPFUL TIP: Urine ketones are >99% sensitive for DKA. Thus, checking serum ketones is superfluous in most cases.

What is the most appropriate initial insulin regimen for this patient?

A) Subcutaneous NPH insulin, 1 unit/kg; repeat as necessary.
B) IV regular insulin, 5 unit IV bolus, followed by constant infusion at 0.05–0.1 U/kg/hr; adjusted as needed.
C) Subcutaneous regular insulin, 0.5–1 unit/kg; adjust dose by fingerstick blood glucose results.
D) Intramuscular regular insulin, 5–10 units hourly; adjust dose by fingerstick blood glucose results.
E) Insulin glargine 10 units daily adjusted based on fasting glucose levels.

Discussion

The correct answer is "B." A bolus of IV regular insulin, followed by a constant infusion, adjusted to reduce the blood glucose level by 50–75 mg/dL/hr, is the appropriate therapy. This may frequently require <0.1 U/kg/hr, but 0.05–0.1 U/kg/hr is a good place to start. Intramuscular insulin administration is an alternative, but absorption is unreliable, especially in hypotensive patients. Long-acting insulins and subcutaneous insulin administration have no place in the initial management of DKA.

> HELPFUL TIP: Although tradition, the bolus of regular insulin is unnecessary and does not change outcomes. Starting a drip of regular insulin is the critical step here.

Which of the following types of insulin can be administered IV?

A) NPH insulin.
B) Lantus insulin.
C) Lente insulin.
D) Ultralente insulin.
E) None of the above.

Discussion

The correct answer is "E." The only insulin that can be administered IV is regular insulin.

* *

The patient's status improves, and you recheck his blood sugar. His glucose is now 200 mg/dL and his insulin drip is still at 5 units per hour. His pH is 7.30 with a bicarbonate level of 14 mEq/L.

Given that his glucose has almost normalized, your reaction at this point is to:

A) Administer bicarbonate in order to finish correcting the pH.
B) Decrease the rate of the insulin infusion to 2 units per hour.
C) Add 10% dextrose to his treatment.
D) Consider the addition of an oral hypoglycemic agent.
E) None of the above.

Discussion

The correct answer is "C." This patient is still acidotic and will need continued insulin to reverse his catabolic state. Thus, the appropriate treatment is to increase the amount of sugar he is getting. Remember, DKA is not primarily a result of too much sugar but rather of too little insulin. "A" is incorrect. **Bicarbonate plays no role in the treatment of DKA no matter what the pH**. In fact, the administration of bicarbonate actually prolongs acidosis and ketosis and produces a paradoxical CNS acidosis. Additionally, it shifts the oxygen disassociation curve to reduce oxygen delivery to the tissue. Finally, **the only predictor of cerebral edema in children treated for DKA is the administration of bicarbonate.** So, there is no need to restrict fluids in children being treated for DKA (although this does NOT mean you should overhydrate them).

The common causes of DKA include all of the following EXCEPT:

A) Missed insulin.
B) Infection.
C) Myocardial infarction.
D) Dietary indiscretion.
E) Metabolic stress.

Discussion

The correct answer is "D." Dietary indiscretion does not generally precipitate DKA. DKA is actually a state caused by a lack of insulin rather than by increased intake of carbohydrates. Certainly dietary indiscretion will complicate glucose control, but it will not precipitate DKA. All of the other options can cause DKA.

Which of the following statements is FALSE:

A) The Somogyi phenomenon occurs when a patient's blood sugar becomes elevated and there is a reactive hypoglycemia.
B) Patients who are being treated appropriately for DKA may have an increase in serum ketones during treatment.
C) There is no correlation between the WBC count and the presence of infection in patients with DKA.
D) Glucagon is an inappropriate treatment of patients with alcoholic **hypo**glycemia.

Discussion

The correct answer (and false statement) is "A." Consensus is that the Somogyi phenomenon **does not exist regardless of what we were taught** (N Engl J Med 1987;317(25):1552). **If you see it on the test though,** it was thought to occur when a patient becomes **hypoglycemic** (often in the middle of the night) and there is a reactive hyperglycemia from adrenergic outpouring. All of the rest are true statements. "B" is correct because beta-hydroxybutyrate is metabolized to acetoacetic acid that will increase serum ketone measurements. "D" is a true statement. Patients with alcoholic hypoglycemia have exhausted their glycogen stores and are also generally NAD deficient and thus have impaired gluconeogenesis. Thus, glucagon will not work. Another group on which glucagon will not work is the infant or child who becomes hypoglycemic overnight and has a seizure in the morning. They have already depleted their stores of glycogen.

HELPFUL TIP: Consider the possibility of a silent myocardial infarction in a diabetic patient who is generally well controlled but suddenly has elevated blood sugars.

HELPFUL TIP: Twenty percent of patients with DKA have "normoglycemic" DKA with a blood sugar under 300 mg/dL.

* *

It is time to transition this patient to a home-going insulin regimen.

Which of the following answers is FALSE regarding the use of insulin in this patient?

A) Insulin detemir and insulin glargine are both long acting, essentially equivalent, and can (almost always) be used once a day as basal insulin.

B) If you use NPH, start with 0.1–0.2 U/kg/day and give 2/3 in the AM and 1/3 HS.
C) Regular insulin should be given in relation to meals to cover blood sugars and generally requires 0.1–0.2U/kg/day as a start.
D) Metformin can markedly reduce the need for insulin in this patient.
E) This patient's insulin need may markedly diminish over the next 2 weeks.

Discussion

The correct answer (which is false) is "D." Metformin is used only in DM2. Our patient has DM1. The rest are true. Insulin detemir and glargine can both be used once a day in most patients (although not always). The starting dose of both regular and NPH insulin is about 0.1–0.2 U/kg/day for a total initial insulin dose of 0.2–0.4 U/kg/day to start. "E" refers to the "honeymoon period." Patients usually present with DM in relation to some metabolic stress. Once this stress resolves, the need for insulin may decrease markedly. Thus, close monitoring is required.

> HELPFUL TIP: There is little outcome advantage to insulin glargine versus NPH. Cost and convenience should be the main considerations in choosing one versus the other.

* *

This patient presents to your clinic 4 months after his hospitalization. He has noted postprandial fullness, reflux and occasional vomiting. You do a gastric emptying study that shows delayed gastric emptying.

Which of the following are appropriate drugs for treating this patient's delayed gastric emptying?

A) Omeprazole.
B) Metoclopramide.
C) Ranitidine.
D) Erythromycin.
E) B and D.

Discussion

The correct answer is "E." Both metoclopramide and erythromycin will speed gastric emptying. A third drug, cisapride, is available on compassionate use protocol. It was removed from the general market secondary to prolonged QT and subsequent torsades de pointes. **It is clear that diabetic gastropathy is at least somewhat reversible with good glucose control.** The higher the sugar, the worse the stomach empties.

> HELPFUL TIP: Remember that erythromycin causes a prolonged QT. Also remember that chronic metoclopramide is associated with extrapyramidal side effects that may be permanent.

Objectives: Did you learn to . . .

- Diagnose a patient with DKA?
- Initiate therapy in DKA?
- Identify causes of DKA?
- Realize that the Somogyi phenomenon is scary but not real (like Godzilla)?
- Prescribe treatment for diabetic gastroparesis?

QUICK QUIZ: DIABETES PREVENTION

Which intervention has been shown to have the *greatest effect* in preventing or delaying the onset of DM2 in patients with impaired fasting glucose or impaired glucose tolerance?

A) Dietary modifications and increased activity.
B) Early glipizide treatment.
C) Early metformin treatment.
D) Intensive fitness training.
E) Weight loss >25% of baseline.

Discussion

The correct answer is "A." Metformin has been shown to have some benefit in delaying progression to diabetes but is less effective than diet and activity modifications. The studies showing benefit from lifestyle modifications used much less aggressive targets for weight loss and activity level than the 25% listed in answer "E." Thus, "E" is incorrect. Other medications that have been used (successfully) to reduce progression to diabetes include the glitazones and acarbose. **However, exercise and diet are superior to drugs. The benefit of drugs is marginal. And the glitazones have significant downsides including edema and increased cardiac events.**

QUICK QUIZ: DIABETIC RETINOPATHY

Which of the following interventions has NOT been shown to prevent loss of vision in patients with retinopathy due to type 2 diabetes?

A) Laser photocoagulation therapy.
B) Aspirin.
C) Tight glycemic control.
D) Tight blood pressure control.

Discussion

The correct answer is "B." Aspirin has not been shown to be of any benefit in the Early Treatment Diabetic Retinopathy Study. All the other options have been shown to be useful in retarding the development of diabetic retinopathy or preventing its progression to visual loss.

CASE 10

You are seeing a new patient in your office. He is a 47-year-old man with a presenting complaint of fatigue for several months. He denies fever, rigors, cough, nausea, or diarrhea. He has lost about 10 pounds. Upon questioning him you discover that he is also having nocturia most nights and is thirsty all the time. He has asthma, for which he uses an albuterol metered dose inhaler occasionally; he has no other chronic medical problems and takes no other medications on a regular basis. He has a family history of diabetes, hypertension, and heart disease. He smokes about one pack per day, and he works as a teacher at the local high school. He is aware of no occupational exposure to toxins.

Physical exam reveals the following: T 37°C, BP 135/83, P 72, BMI 38 kg/m^2. Aside from obesity, the remainder of the exam is normal.

Laboratory test results reveal the following: normal CBC, BUN/creatinine, electrolytes. You ask him to return to the office the next day for fasting lab tests, which reveal the following

Fasting blood glucose: 131 mg/dL.
HbA_{1c}: 7.5%.

Does this patient have diabetes?

A) Yes; he has an elevated fasting glucose.
B) Probably; he needs a second fasting glucose to confirm the diagnosis.
C) No; his fasting glucose is not >mg/dL.
D) Yes; he has the classic symptoms of diabetes: fatigue, weight loss, and thirst.
E) Probably not; his HbA_{1c} is not >8%.

Discussion

The correct answer is "B." The ADA criteria for the diagnosis diabetes require two fasting blood glucose measurements ≥126 mg/dL on different days. As noted above, another option is to recheck the HbA_{1c}: two values above 6.5% will diagnose diabetes. Finally, a random blood sugar of 200 mg/dL with symptoms allows one to make the diagnosis of diabetes.

Assuming another fasting blood glucose level is elevated, what further study must be done to complete the diagnosis of diabetes and determine whether the patient has type 1 or type 2 diabetes?

A) C-peptide level.
B) Antiislet cell antibodies.
C) Serum insulin level.
D) Antiinsulin antibodies.
E) None of the above.

Discussion

The correct answer is "E." This patient's age, history, examination (BMI 38), and laboratory findings are consistent with the diagnosis of DM2. None of the other studies listed needs to be performed. However, if questions remain regarding the type of diabetes (which will then affect therapy, prognosis, follow-up, etc.), you may choose to perform further studies. In DM1, the C-peptide level (a marker of endogenous insulin production) is low. If it is equivocal, give a glucose load (e.g., large meal) and see if it goes up. If it goes up, the diagnosis is likely DM2. Antiislet cell antibodies are present in 80% of type 1 diabetics and, if found, are essentially diagnostic of type 1 diabetes. "C," the serum insulin level, is generally not helpful; and "D" is incorrect because antiinsulin antibodies have a low sensitivity.

HELPFUL TIP: To be complete, antiglutamic acid decarboxylase (anti-GAD) antibodies are present in 70% of patients with DM1 at the time of diagnosis.

The pathologic factors involved in type 2 diabetes in adults include:

A) Pancreatic beta-cell destruction through a yet undetermined infectious process.

B) The production of antiinsulin antibodies that cause precipitation of insulin/antibody complexes.
C) Resistance to the effects of insulin at peripheral tissues and a relative insulin deficiency that is progressive over time.
D) An autosomal-dominant process, with the diabetes gene located on the long arm of chromosome 18.
E) Too much exercise and a complete lack of a "beer gut."

Discussion
The correct answer is "C." DM2 is the result of the development of insulin resistance at the peripheral tissues (e.g., fat and muscle cells) and a relative lack of insulin compared to the increasing amount that the body requires. "A" is incorrect. However, autoimmune destruction of beta-cells in the pancreas is responsible for causing diabetes type 1. "B" is wrong although there are anti-insulin antibodies found in **DM1**. "D" is incorrect as well, but there is a strong genetic component to DM2. The exact genetic factors that cause DM2 in adults have not been completely elucidated, but there does not appear to be a single gene responsible transmitted in an autosomal-dominant fashion. "E" is incorrect because lack of exercise, weight gain, dietary factors, and truncal obesity (the "beer gut") predispose persons to the development of DM2.

* *

You obtain a second fasting blood glucose 2 days later, and it is 145 mg/dL. You meet with the patient and his wife to go over the test results and explain the diagnosis of diabetes. Given his age, habitus, and lack of exercise, you feel certain that this patient has type 2 diabetes. You provide some basic education on the nature of diabetes, its natural history, and what can be done to manage it.

What is the most important next step for this patient?

A) Initiation of insulin therapy.
B) Initiation an ACE inhibitor
C) Referral to an endocrinologist.
D) Diabetic education classes.

Discussion
The correct answer is "D." A general education program that includes information on diet, disease management, and the family's role in successful diabetes care is the most important intervention listed. While specialist consultation may be useful in complex diabetic patients or in those who are not responding to treatment, generalist physicians can, and do, provide care to the majority of patients with diabetes. Insulin therapy is not indicated at this point, and an ACE inhibitor may or may not be helpful depending on the patient's blood pressure and urine protein.

Which of this patient's other conditions does NOT have a direct impact on his diabetes?

A) Asthma.
B) Elevated blood pressure.
C) Smoking.
D) Obesity.
E) Elevated LDL cholesterol.

Discussion
The correct answer is "A." Hypertension and hyperlipidemia have been clearly shown to increase the risk of microvascular complications in patients with DM2. Smoking is an additional risk factor for coronary heart disease (CHD). Obesity is common in type 2 diabetics; even a modest weight loss can lead to significant improvements in blood glucose and lipid profiles. Asthma does not have a direct impact on his diabetes, but taking systemic corticosteroids for an exacerbation certainly will complicate his diabetes management.

* *

You find that the patient's blood pressure is elevated (systolic pressure $\geq$130 or diastolic pressure $\geq$80 mm Hg).

Which class of medications is the best choice for initial therapy of hypertension in diabetics?

A) ACE inhibitors.
B) Calcium-channel blockers.
C) Loop diuretics.
D) Vasodilators.
E) Beta-blockers.

Discussion
The correct answer is "A." ACE inhibitors have been shown to provide renal protection in patients with type 1 and type 2 diabetes. Patients with microalbuminuria and hypertension will certainly benefit from an ACE inhibitor. Loop diuretics (e.g., furosemide) are not indicated for the **primary** treatment of hypertension in diabetics (or, really, anyone else).

Angiotensin receptor blockers (ARBs) are a good alternative in the patient with microalbuminuria if an ACE inhibitor is not tolerated. **However, ARBs, while they decrease proteinuria, likely do nothing to reduce adverse cardiovascular outcomes** or morality in those with diabetic nephropathy. Vasodilators and calcium-channel blockers are not optimal choices in this patient although nondihydropyridine calcium channel blockers are an option for renal protection. "E," beta-blockers, are no longer considered first line for treating hypertension in patients without cardiac disease.

> **HELPFUL (BUT CONFUSING) TIP:** It turns out that tight control of BP (<130/80) in DM2 does little to reduce cardiovascular disease. Some are now arguing for a BP goal of 140/90 with tighter control only if it can be easily achieved with little impact on the patient's life. Whoops, once again everything we thought we knew is wrong (*JAMA* 2010; 304:61). We would still use the 130/80 goal for the test, though.

* *

After 3 months of dietary therapy and lifestyle modifications, the patient returns to see you. While he has been adherent to the recommendations given by you and the diabetes education staff, his HbA_{1c} remains elevated at 8.7%. You decide to begin pharmacologic therapy.

Which medication is the *most* appropriate *first-line* therapy for an obese patient with type 2 diabetes?

A) A "glitazone" (e.g., Actos).
B) A sulfonylurea.
C) Insulin.
D) Metformin.
E) A "gliptin" (e.g., Januvia).

Discussion

The correct answer is "D." Metformin does not cause weight gain (unlike most other treatments for diabetes) and thus is the drug of choice in obese patients. It is effective, inexpensive, well tolerated by most patients, and has very little risk of hypoglycemia. Studies comparing effects on end-organ disease show better outcomes with metformin than with sulfonylureas. "A," the glitazones, are falling out of favor because of the possibility of increased cardiovascular events (rosiglitazone was removed from the market for its cardiovascular risk, and pioglitazone can exacerbate CHF). Sulfonylureas are also effective and well tolerated, but have a significant risk for hypoglycemia and are associated with weight gain. All other oral drugs are best considered second-line agents. "E" is of special note. "Gliptins" block the degradation of the body's endogenous incretin, which helps to lower blood sugar. Gliptins can be used as an "add-on" therapy if traditional hypoglycemic agents are not effective and have the benefit of some weight loss.

> **HELPFUL TIP:** In addition to the gliptins that help prevent the breakdown of endogenous incretins, incretin mimetics have been developed. The first of these is called excnatide (Byetta). It is given by subcutaneous injection and is weight neutral or may even cause weight loss. The second is liraglutide (Victoza) and more are on the way.

Which of the following is a notable side effect of incretin mimetics (e.g., exenatide)?

A) Bone marrow suppression.
B) Pancreatitis.
C) Elevated triglycerides.
D) Elevated blood pressure.
E) Malabsorption of carbohydrates.

Discussion

The correct answer is "B." These drugs can cause pancreatitis although it is rare and the association has recently been questioned. **Victoza use is associated with a greater incidence of pancreatitis as well as some thyroid tumors.**

Metformin should NOT be used in which class of patients?

A) Patients with COPD.
B) Patients with impaired renal function.
C) Patients with leukemias or lymphomas.
D) Postmyocardial infarction patients with normal systolic function.
E) Patients with insufficient fat stores.

Table 10–2 RECOMMENDATIONS FOR MEDICAL TREATMENT DIABETES MELLITUS TYPE 2

First Line	Second Line	Third Line	Fourth Line
Metformin	Sulfonylureas (but not glyburide or chlorpropamide) Insulin	Pioglitazones (likely should avoid this class) Exenatide	Liraglutide Pramlintide Sitagliptin Saxagliptin

Note: Bromocriptine has been used for diabetes as well, but it results in only a 0.5% decrease in HbA_{1c} and has many side effects. Its role in diabetes therapy has not yet been determined.

Data from Nathan DM, et al. Diabetes: A consensus algorithm for the initiation and adjustment of therapy. *Clinical Diabetes.* 2009;27: 4-16.

Discussion

The correct answer is "B." Patients with renal disease are at a higher risk of lactic acidosis, the most severe complication of metformin therapy, although it is exceedingly rare (0 patients of 75,000 in one study). Patients with pulmonary or neoplastic diseases may take metformin unless they also have severe hepatic or renal failure. Postmyocardial infarction patients may use metformin as long as they do not have CHF, but metformin should be held for 48 hours after contrast studies (Table 10–2).

Which one of the following is NOT a risk factor/marker for lower-extremity amputation in patients with diabetes?

A) Diabetic retinopathy.
B) Bony deformity of the feet or ankles.
C) CRP level.
D) Abnormal monofilament testing for sensory function.
E) Severe nail pathology.

Discussion

The correct answer is "C." The risk of ulcers or amputations is increased in patients who have had diabetes for 10 years or more, are male, have a history of poor glucose control, or have evidence of microvascular complications of diabetes. Bony deformities, loss of protective sensation, and severely dystrophic toenails are also risk factors for amputation. An elevated CRP in and of itself is not a known risk factor for amputation, but CRP may be elevated if there is lower extremity infection present.

* *

At the next visit, you review the patient's medical record and try to assure that he is up to date on his preventive health care.

Which of the following is NOT true regarding preventive services in diabetics?

A) Patients diagnosed with diabetes type 2 should have a dilated eye exam at the time of diagnosis.
B) Patients with type 1 diabetes should have a dilated eye exam at the time of diagnosis if they are over age 12, or have had diabetes type 1 for 5 years.
C) Patients with diabetes type 1 should have a urine microalbumin checked every 6–12 months after age 12.
D) A urine microalbumin should be checked at least yearly in all type 2 diabetics.
E) A foot examination using a 10-g nylon microfilament should be done annually for all diabetics.

Discussion

The correct answer is "B." Patients with diabetes type 1 should have an eye exam **5 years** after the diagnosis and then yearly. Age at the time of diagnosis is not a factor in determining when an eye exam should be done. See Table 10–3 for more screening information.

* *

Speaking of prevention, your patient, now 48 years old with his diabetes controlled, asks if he should be taking an aspirin daily to protect his heart.

You respond:

A) "Take aspirin 325 mg daily because it will lower your risk of myocardial infarction."
B) "Diabetes does not automatically qualify you for aspirin therapy. Let's check your Framingham score."
C) "The risks and benefits of aspirin in your case are unknown."
D) "Take it by the truckload. I've got a lot of stock in Bayer."

Table 10–3 SUMMARY OF SCREENING RECOMMENDATIONS

DM type 1:
- Urine microalbumin starting at age 12 and then every 6–12 months.
- Dilated eye exam 5 years after diagnosis and then annually.
- HbA_{1c} every 6 months for stable patients achieving glycemic goals, every 3 months patients changing therapy or not meeting glycemic goals.
- Blood pressure screening at every visit.
- Foot exam and screening for polyneuropathy at diagnosis and annually.

DM type 2: Same as DM1 above, except:
- Eye exam **at time of diagnosis** and then yearly.
- Urine microalbumin at the time of diagnosis and then every 6–12 months.

Data from American Diabetes Association. Standards of medical care in diabetes—2011. *Diabetes Care.* 2011;34:S11-S61.

Discussion

The correct answer is "B." The aspirin-for-prevention debate rages on. As of 2012, the recommendations promote an individual approach to myocardial infarction prevention with aspirin. Previously, diabetes was thought to confer a heart disease risk equivalent to that of a patient with known coronary disease. This is no longer the case, so diabetics should not universally receive aspirin (see chapter 2). However, aspirin appears to be beneficial for patients with a 10-year cardiovascular disease risk >10%. Therefore, using a risk calculator (e.g., Framingham) for appropriate patients (like a 50-year-old male with diabetes and hypertension) will help determine who to treat with aspirin. If you decide to prescribe aspirin for primary CAD prevention in a diabetic, use 81 mg daily.

* *

Unfortunately, this patient follows the "rule" of type 2 diabetes and ends up on multiple medications. When he returns to your clinic a few months later, he is complaining of shortness of breath and lower extremity edema.

Which of the following drugs (by itself—not in combination with other drugs) is the most likely cause of this patient's edema, shortness of breath, and possible heart failure?

A) Metformin.
B) Glyburide.
C) Pioglitazone.
D) Lisinopril.
E) Insulin.

Discussion

The correct answer is "C." The "glitazones" (thiazolidinediones) tend to cause edema as one of their major side effects. Thus, they are contraindicated in patients with a history of heart failure. Some drug combinations can cause edema, including the combination of glimepiride and metformin.

* *

Because of the problem with edema, you decide to change this patient to a sulfonylurea, and you choose to start glyburide. The patient does well on this for several weeks but is then found unconscious in his home with a blood sugar of 20. He is rapidly revived by the paramedics with an amp of D50. You are called to see the patient in the ED. He is currently awake, conversant, and eating ("a great excuse for a couple of cookies, Doc"). He would like to go home since he is back to his baseline.

Which of the following is TRUE about patients with hypoglycemia?

A) Type 1 diabetics on NPH insulin should be admitted for observation after a hypoglycemic episode.
B) Type 2 diabetics controlled with insulin should be admitted for observation after a hypoglycemic episode.
C) Patients on metformin have a higher risk of hypoglycemia than those taking only a sulfonylurea.
D) Patients on oral hypoglycemic agents should be admitted for observation after a hypoglycemic episode.
E) All of the above are true.

Discussion

The correct answer is "D." Patients on an oral hypoglycemic agent should be admitted for observation. This is because of the somewhat erratic absorption of oral hypoglycemic agents and their prolonged effect. The patient may have an additional episode of hypoglycemia for up to 36–48 hours after the initial episode. This is not true of patients on NPH insulin who are using a drug that is relatively short acting. Finally, one of the benefits of metformin is that it rarely (if ever) causes hypoglycemia. Its main action is to reduce gluconeogenesis and release of glucose from the liver (although it also improves skeletal muscle use of glucose).

* *

It turns out that one of your partners has started this patient on a beta-blocker for its cardioprotective and antihypertensive effects while you were on vacation. The patient wants to know if this may have prevented him from noticing the signs and symptoms of hypoglycemia.

Your response is:

A) "Beta-blockers reduce your ability to recognize hypoglycemia and the drug should be stopped."
B) "Beta-blockers reduce your ability to recognize hypoglycemia but the benefits are worth it."
C) "Beta-blockers do not decrease your ability to recognize hypoglycemia to any great degree. Don't worry about it."
D) "ACE inhibitors are better drugs because they do not contribute to hypoglycemia in diabetics."
E) "My partner's smarter than me, so I'm sure it's fine."

Discussion

The correct answer is "C." Beta-blockers do not significantly interfere with patients' ability to recognize hypoglycemia. The main thing that contributes to unawareness of hypoglycemia in diabetics is the rate of glucose drop (a slow drop is less likely to be noticed) and autonomic insufficiency (patients cannot respond with tachycardia, sweating, etc. to the outpouring of adrenergics). "D" is incorrect. ACE inhibitors, like beta-blockers, are actually associated with hypoglycemia in diabetics.

* *

You admit the patient and advise him to carry a source of glucose with him at all times and everybody has a happy outcome until...

The patient has developed persistent hyperglycemia despite being on maximal doses of metformin and glyburide. He is willing to begin insulin therapy, but wants to give himself as few injections as possible.

Which of the following regimens would be best for him?

A) A single injection of insulin glargine (Lantus™) at bedtime.
B) A single injection of 70/30 NPH/regular insulin at bedtime.
C) A baseline bedtime injection of insulin glargine and up to three injections of short-acting insulin with meals.
D) Two-thirds of the total daily insulin dose (divided two-thirds of NPH and one-third of regular) in the morning, and the remainder (divided equally, NPH and regular) in the evening.

Discussion

The correct answer is "A." Because of its slow release, insulin glargine provides a steady-state insulin level throughout 24 hours and is less likely to cause nocturnal hypoglycemia. Other options include insulin detemir and ultralente insulin (off the market in the United States), both of which have prolonged action. A single injection of 70/30 insulin is a reasonable alternative, but should be given at dinnertime, not at bedtime. Multiple daily insulin injections may be necessary for type 1 diabetics, but rarely are so for type 2 patients. Choice "D," the combination of NPH and regular, is a reasonable option and is only second best in this scenario because it involves 2 injections daily and is slightly more complicated. If you are trying to start with the simplest possible regimen, choose something like "A."

HELPFUL TIP: Sulfonylureas and insulin work in the same manner: they both increase circulating insulin levels. For this reason, some choose not to use these two drugs together.

* *

Your patient is hospitalized for acute diverticulitis and requires urgent partial colectomy.

Which of the following statements regarding the management of diabetes in hospitalized patients is TRUE?

A) Hyperglycemia in the hospital has minimal if any effect on outcomes of myocardial infarction.
B) A standardized sliding-scale insulin regimen is adequate to control hyperglycemia in all hospitalized diabetic patients.
C) Insulin requirements will be lower for acutely ill, hospitalized diabetic patients.
D) Metformin should be discontinued in seriously ill, hospitalized patients.

Discussion

The correct answer is "D." In general, one should consider discontinuation of metformin in severely ill, hospitalized patients due to contrast studies, changes in fluid balance, changes in glomerular filtration rate, etc. "A" is incorrect. Hyperglycemia is associated with worse outcomes in hospitalized patient with cardiac disease or who are in the intensive care unit. "B" is also incorrect. Sliding-scale regimens, if used at all, should be individualized to each patient, rather than prescribed as a standardized regimen. It is clear from most recent studies that a sliding scale is not actually the best way to control blood sugars in hospitalized patients. Continuing some type of "normal" insulin regimen is best, using supplemental insulin as needed. The stress of acute illness and surgery will likely increase insulin requirements in most diabetics, not decrease them.

HELPFUL TIP: Chasing the insulin for tight control in the hospital is counterproductive and does not improve outcomes! Even though patients with hyperglycemia may do worse, it is clear that the elevated glucose is a marker for metabolic stress and thus for sicker patients. Shoot for a blood sugar of between 120 and 180 mg/dL. This has been found to be superior to intensive glycemic control.

* *

He does well and is ready for discharge. He asks about self-monitoring of blood glucose.

How often should a type 2 diabetic on oral hypoglycemic agents measure his or her blood glucose?

A) Once or twice a week, at varying times during the day.
B) Four times daily, before meals, and at bedtime.
C) Twice a day, fasting, and 2 hours after a meal.
D) Once or twice a day, fasting, and before a meal.
E) Routine blood sugars are not indicated on a daily basis for type 2 diabetics.

Discussion

The correct answer is "E." Daily measurements of finger stick sugars in patients on oral hypoglycemic agents do nothing to improve glycemic control (BMJ 2012 Feb 27; 344:e486). In these patients, we are not reacting to daily fluctuations in glucose control but rather making changes in response to the HbA$_{1C}$. Occasional random sugars are not unreasonable to get a general idea about glycemic control. **Type 2 diabetics on insulin (and all type 1 diabetics) should measure their blood glucose at least daily, and ideally twice a day, regardless of the presence or absence of symptoms.**

Objectives: Did you learn to . . .

- Recognize diagnostic criteria for diabetes?
- Differentiate diabetes type 1 from type 2?
- Evaluate a patient with new onset DM2?
- Identify risk factors for complications of diabetes?
- Initiate oral therapy in diabetes?
- Manage a patient on insulin?
- Manage diabetes in the hospital setting?

CASE 11

A 32-year-old female presents to your office complaining of "hypoglycemia." She notices that about 2–3 hours after a meal she gets nauseated, shaky, and irritable. When she wakes up in the morning, she generally feels well even though she eats dinner at about 5:00 PM and does not eat any snacks afterward and generally does not have breakfast until 8:00 AM.

You can tell her that:

A) She likely has an insulinoma.
B) She likely will have normal blood sugars when she feels shaky.
C) Hypoglycemia does not exist as an entity in this form and she likely has anxiety.
D) She likely has "fasting" hypoglycemia.
E) None of the above.

Discussion

The correct answer is "E." "A" is incorrect because a patient with an insulinoma should be hypoglycemic after a 15-hour fast (5:00 PM–8:00 AM). "B" is incorrect. This patient may have postprandial hypoglycemia that occurs 2–4 hours after eating. The process leading to postprandial hypoglycemia is as follows: the patient has a large meal with simple carbohydrates, the serum insulin level increases in response but overshoots, and the patient becomes transiently hypoglycemic for 15–20 minutes 2–4 hours after eating. This is associated with adrenergic outpouring in an attempt to correct the problem. It is the adrenergic outpouring that causes the symptoms of tremor, nausea, etc. "C" is incorrect because hypoglycemia does exist. "D" is incorrect. The patient does not have symptoms of fasting hypoglycemia, which occur 4–6 hours (or longer) after the last meal.

All of the following are associated with postprandial hypoglycemia EXCEPT:

A) Early diabetes.
B) Diuretics.
C) Alcohol intake.
D) Postgastrectomy syndrome.
E) Beta-blockers.

Discussion

The correct answer is "B." Diuretics tend to increase the blood sugar a bit. In addition to the list above, aspirin, ACE inhibitors, pentamidine, and renal failure may be associated with postprandial hypoglycemia.

You advise this patient to do all of the following EXCEPT:

A) Increase the amount of simple carbohydrates with her meals.
B) Increase the amount of complex carbohydrates with her meals.
C) Eat smaller, more frequent meals.
D) Initiate diphenhydramine 25 mg QID.
E) A and D.

Discussion

The correct answer (and what you would not want to do) is "E." The problem is caused at least in part by a high intake of simple carbohydrates, leading to a rapid and high peak of the blood sugar followed by an excessive release of insulin. Thus, one would want to decrease the amount of simple carbohydrates in the diet. Of note is "D." Delaying gastric emptying (using an agent like propantheline, an anticholinergic/antispasmodic) doesn't seem to make a difference (but might make the patient sleepy enough that she doesn't notice the symptoms!).

INTERESTING (BUT MAYBE NOT SO HELPFUL) TIP: Gin and tonic and ackee fruit (from Caribbean islands) are two known causes of hypoglycemia. In "gin and tonic hypoglycemia" (the actual name of the syndrome), alcohol prevents effective counterregulatory measures. Ackee fruit, common in the Jamaican diet, contains "hypoglycin" that prevents gluconeogenesis.

HELPFUL TIP: For insulinoma, watch the patient during a **controlled** fast during which the patient is observed and can be treated for hypoglycemia if necessary. If you are considering self-induced hypoglycemia with insulin (e.g., factitious hypoglycemia), measure the c-peptide. This will be **low** if the patient is being administered exogenous insulin because pancreatic insulin production will be shut off in response to hypoglycemia (remember, however, that it will also be low in type 1 diabetics).

Objectives: Did you learn to . . .

- Evaluate a patient with possible hypoglycemia?
- Treat a patient with postprandial hypoglycemia?
- Identify causes of hypoglycemia?

CASE 12

A 24-year-old female presents to the office complaining of amenorrhea. Six months ago, her menses became irregular and light. For the last 4 months, she has not had a period at all. This is causing her great distress, as she constantly worries about being pregnant. She does desire to have children "some day," but not now. She has run multiple home pregnancy tests, all of which have been negative. Last week, she developed clear leakage from her nipples, and the patient is now convinced she is pregnant and that the home pregnancy tests must be faulty. She requests that you perform "a real pregnancy test."

Which of the following may cause her amenorrhea?

A) Emotional stress.
B) Pregnancy, despite multiple negative tests.
C) Thyroid dysfunction.
D) Pituitary tumor.
E) All of the above.

Discussion

The correct answer is "E." The differential diagnosis for amenorrhea is rather broad, but includes all of the above diagnoses. The most common cause in a woman of childbearing age is, of course, pregnancy. Although urine-based pregnancy tests have become very sensitive (able to detect as little as 20 IU/mL of β-hCG), the patient may have been using the tests incorrectly and was getting false negative results. Other causes of amenorrhea include hypothyroidism, strenuous exercise or anorexia, emotional stress, pituitary tumor, certain medications (e.g., phenothiazines, dopaminergic agents, chemotherapy, and estrogens), and end-organ (ovarian) failure or agenesis. See Chapter 15 for a more thorough discussion of amenorrhea.

* *

Further history from the patient reveals menarche at age 12, no previous pregnancies, and no previous history of menstrual irregularities. She participates in low-impact exercise regularly and does not engage in long-distance running or other demanding endurance sports. Review of systems reveals frequent mild headaches, the aforementioned nipple discharge, but no visual disturbances or symptoms of hypothyroidism.

Physical exam demonstrates a well-developed, well-nourished (neither obese nor excessively thin) adult female. She has appropriate secondary sex characteristics, no hirsutism, and a normal thyroid gland to palpation. Galactorrhea is noted on breast examination. The pelvic exam is normal, with appropriately developed external genitalia, vagina, and cervix. The uterus is palpable and small, and the ovaries are neither palpable nor tender.

In addition to a serum β-hCG and a TSH, what other test(s) should be ordered?

A) Karyotype, to evaluate for testicular feminization and Turner syndrome.
B) Adrenal MRI, to evaluate for adrenal hyperplasia.
C) Prolactin level.
D) All of the above.
E) None of the above.

Discussion

The correct answer is "C." A prolactin level is an essential component of this evaluation. A prolactinoma is the most common form of pituitary adenoma, and it can cause secondary amenorrhea, galactorrhea, and infertility (or impotence in men). Expansion of the mass in the sella turcica may cause headaches or visual field defects (bitemporal hemianopsia), but the tumors are more often too small to have any local effects. Adrenal hyperplasia is unlikely in the patient because of a lack of virilizing characteristics from androgen excess (such as hirsutism). Also, adrenal imaging is not usually the first step in the diagnosis of this disorder (24 urine collection for cortisol and 17-OHS is indicated if adrenal hyperfunction is suspected). A karyotype is not indicated in this patient because she has secondary amenorrhea, or amenorrhea that has developed after a period of time of normal menses. Patients who complain of never having a menstrual cycle are considered to have primary amenorrhea, which may be evidence of either Turner syndrome (XO genotype) or complete androgen insensitivity (aka testicular feminization, which has an XY genotype with end-organ resistance to testosterone, resulting in a female phenotype). Both cases result in ovarian agenesis and, therefore, no menstrual cycles.

* *

You obtain laboratory tests, and the results are as follows:

TSH 3.1 IU/mL (0.27–4.20), β-hCG undetectable, prolactin 150 ng/mL (3.4–24.1).

What is the best next step in this patient's evaluation?

A) Reassure patient that stress is causing her lack of periods and she will improve when she learns to deal with her life.
B) No additional tests at this time, but return in 2 weeks for a repeat prolactin level.
C) Admit the patient to the hospital and start bromocriptine therapy STAT.
D) MRI brain to evaluate for pituitary mass.
E) Refer patient for neurosurgical intervention.

Discussion

The correct answer is "D." This patient has a high prolactin level and symptoms of prolactin excess. In the absence of medications causing an elevated prolactin (phenothiazines, narcotics, estrogens, etc.) and a normal TSH, this prolactin result is virtually diagnostic for a prolactinoma. Imaging is indicated regardless of visual symptoms. A visual field exam by confrontation is insensitive for a minor loss of field. If she had a mild elevation in prolactin (up to two times the upper limit of normal), and no other symptoms/signs, then repeating the level over several visits may be appropriate. If the level remains elevated, imaging and medical therapy should then be considered. Neurosurgical intervention is not immediately indicated, since a trial of medical therapy is usually the first step in treatment.

* *

This patient undergoes a brain MRI, which shows a 1.3 cm pituitary mass.

How should this finding be interpreted and managed?

A) This is a microadenoma, and the result can be ignored.
B) This is a microadenoma, and medical therapy with a dopamine agonist is indicated.
C) This is a macroadenoma, so medical therapy is futile, and the patient should be referred for surgery.
D) This is a macroadenoma, but medical therapy with a dopamine agonist should still be attempted.
E) This is a macroadenoma, which tends to be self-limited, so therapy can be held for 6 months when a repeat scan will be done.

Discussion

The correct answer is "D." A pituitary tumor <1 cm in size is considered a microadenoma, and tumors 1 cm or greater in size are considered macroadenomas. The treatment implications are slightly different. In both cases, medical therapy with a dopamine agonist (e.g., bromocriptine and cabergoline) is indicated. Successful shrinkage of even macroadenomas is possible with this therapy. Remember that the secretion of prolactin is under a negative feedback loop. As CNS dopamine levels go up, prolactin levels go down. When dopamine levels go down, prolactin levels go up.

> HELPFUL TIP: Many psychoactive medications inhibit dopamine and can result in hyperprolactinemia. Resist the knee-jerk reaction of stopping a psychoactive medication in a patient found to have hyperprolactinemia. High prolactin levels do not kill patients, but untreated mental illness does. Risks, benefits, and likelihood that the drug is to blame must all be considered.

* *

The patient is started on bromocriptine and is scheduled for follow-up in 3 weeks. She returns earlier than scheduled due to severe nausea and lightheadedness. No other new symptoms have occurred. The patient's vital signs are normal, but the systolic blood pressure decreases by 20 mm Hg and the pulse increases by 20 beats/minute upon standing.

Aside from a bolus of IV fluids, how should you address this problem?

A) This is a common side effect from bromocriptine. Decrease or stop the bromocriptine, and consider another type of dopamine agonist, such as cabergoline.
B) Admit her to the hospital and arrange for a STAT head CT scan to rule out bleeding from the pituitary adenoma.
C) Repeat the pregnancy test.
D) She is having an anaphylactic allergic reaction. Administer epinephrine and diphenhydramine immediately.
E) She has failed medical therapy and must be referred for neurosurgical intervention.

Discussion

The correct answer is "A." The most common side effects of dopamine agonists are nausea, postural hypotension, and difficulty concentrating. These symptoms tend to be lessened when lower doses are used and the dose is increased very slowly. Cabergoline tends to be better tolerated than bromocriptine.

* *

The patient is able to tolerate cabergoline, and continues the medication for 6 months. During this time, the prolactin level decreases slowly. She has had resumption of her menses. A repeat MRI is done after 6 months and shows a marked decrease in size of the adenoma. The patient has reached that magical inflection point in life where she recognizes that her own mortality is inevitable, and she desires to get pregnant "as soon as I can." She wants to know if she should have surgery to remove the adenoma.

What is/are the indication(s) for transsphenoidal pituitary surgery?

A) Failure to respond to dopamine agonists.
B) Failure to tolerate dopamine agonists.
C) Treatment of large adenoma in a patient who desires pregnancy, despite efficacy of medical therapy.
D) A and B.
E) All of the above.

Discussion

The correct answer is "E." Surgery should be reserved for those patients who fail to respond to or cannot tolerate medical therapy. Note that visual field defects are not a specific indication for surgery, since medical therapy can be effective in decreasing the size and related local effects of the tumor. If a patient desires pregnancy and has a large mass (>3 cm), surgery may be considered as an adjunct to medical therapy. During pregnancy, there is a physiological increase in the size of the pituitary gland. If such a patient becomes pregnant (without a prior reduction in tumor size) and discontinues the dopamine agonist for the duration of pregnancy, the adenoma may increase to a clinically important size before delivery.

HELPFUL TIP: Bromocriptine and cabergoline are classified as category B for pregnancy risk (in other words, they are generally considered safe). These medications can be continued during pregnancy, but a careful risk–benefit analysis and discussion between patient and physician must occur before making treatment decisions.

* *

The patient wants to know how long she should be on cabergoline or bromocriptine and when a trial off of the medication is indicated.

You let her know that:

A) Patients with a pituitary adenoma have to be on medication chronically to suppress the tumor.
B) A trial off of a dopamine agonist should be done at 6 months.
C) Dopamine agonists can be stopped at 1 year and tumor shrinkage will be sustained.
D) Prolactin levels can be allowed to rise after menopause without problem unless visual symptoms or other local symptoms develop.
E) None of the above.

Discussion

The correct answer is "D." Dopamine agonists can be stopped at menopause. Follow-up can be done using blood levels of prolactin. If prolactin levels rise, an MRI can be done to see if the adenoma is becoming larger. If not, there is no reason to treat the adenoma in postmenopausal patients. "A" is incorrect. A trial off of medications at 1 year is reasonable. If prolactin levels remain under control, there is no need to continue medication. "B" and "C" are incorrect. A trial off of drugs should be tried at 1 year (not 6 months). Tumors recur in a large number of cases, so patients **may** need chronic treatment.

Objectives: Did you learn to . . .

- Generate a list of potential causes of secondary amenorrhea?
- Evaluate a patient with secondary amenorrhea?
- Diagnose and treat hyperprolactinemia secondary to a pituitary prolactinoma?

CASE 13

A 39-year-old female presents to the office complaining of amenorrhea. She has had normal menses until 8 months ago, when they became infrequent and then stopped. She insists she cannot be pregnant, because she denies sexual activity "in years." She believes she is going through "the change" but wants to know why she is reaching menopause at a much earlier age than other women she knows. On review of systems, she complains of headaches "for years" and recent onset of weakness and fatigue. She also complains of arthritis in the hip and knees, something she attributes to "getting old." She reports that her hands are swollen, and her rings do not fit any more. She denies other complaints.

On physical exam, vitals are normal. The patient is an adult female of average height, with a noticeably large jaw and hands. Her hair is thick and coarse, and hirsutism is present. Her thyroid gland is slightly enlarged, but regular in shape. No bruit or tenderness is present. The point of maximal impulse is displaced laterally, but the heart rhythm is regular with no murmurs. The rest of the exam is normal.

What is the most appropriate next step?

A) Reassure the patient that menopause is a normal process and offer estrogen replacement therapy for symptomatic relief (but warn the patient about risks of long-term use).
B) Tell the patient you suspect depression and offer a regimen of counseling combined with SSRI therapy.

C) Although she is likely depressed, tell the patient she may suffer from growth hormone (GH) excess, and recommend sending a serum insulin-like growth factor (IGF-I) level.
D) Tell the patient to get a life (you know of one for sale cheap on ebay).

Discussion

The correct answer is "C." This patient represents a classic presentation of acromegaly due to GH excess, and the best single test for this is the IGF-I level. Although GH levels will often be elevated, the IGF-I does not vary from hour to hour and is not dependent on food intake, as is the case with GH. An elevated GH after a glucose load is also very suggestive of GH excess. Acromegaly of adult onset (after fusion of the long bones) does NOT result in increased height, but does cause coarsening of facial features, prognathism, and thickening of the feet and hands. These changes can be very subtle, and there is generally a lag of **12 years** before diagnosis. Comparing older photographs of the patient to their current appearance may be a clue (a driver's license photograph may be a convenient source). Patients with acromegaly also develop hypertrophy of certain organs (such as the thyroid and heart) and may present with CHF due to cardiomyopathy. Eighty-five percent of females with acromegaly have at least some menstrual dysfunction and 60% are amenorrheic.

HELPFUL TIP: Premature ovarian failure is defined as menopause at age 40 or younger (two standard deviations below the mean).

* *

The patient's IGF-I is elevated, and her TSH is normal. An MRI is performed that reveals a pituitary mass slightly <1 cm in diameter.

What is the most effective therapy for this condition?

A) Weekly anti-IGF-I antibody infusions.
B) Bromocriptine therapy.
C) Transsphenoidal pituitary resection.
D) Somatostatin analogs (such as octreotide).
E) Pegvisomant (GH receptor antagonist).

Discussion

The correct answer is "C." Acromegaly is caused by a GH-secreting pituitary tumor. Surgery is the treatment of choice for patients with a microadenoma (1 cm or less in diameter) or for patients with a macroadenoma that appears to be fully resectable. Somatostatin analogs and pegvisomant (Somavert®) may be useful adjuncts to surgery, and are an option for patients who are not surgical candidates. Bromocriptine is not very effective, and only about 10% of acromegaly patients will achieve normal IGF-I levels with bromocriptine; however, cabergoline seems to work in about half of patients. Cabergoline has an advantage over somatostatin analogs in that it can be taken orally. Radiation is also an option for therapy, especially for those patients who are not surgical candidates and do not tolerate or do not respond to medical therapy. "E," anti-IGF-I antibody (if it existed as a medication), would not have an effect on a GH-secreting tumor. But it does not exist. It's a made-up answer, so it's wrong. By the way, there's no made-up stuff on the real exam . . . we think.

Objectives: Did you learn to . . .

- Recognize signs and symptoms of GH excess?
- Evaluate and manage a patient with GH excess?

QUICK QUIZ: GROWTH HORMONE

A boy of 6 years is brought into the office by his concerned mother due to "growing too slowly." She has noticed that he is significantly shorter than his classmates at school, and she wants something done about it. She heard a report on the nightly news about a new medication that makes children grow taller and insists on getting it for her son. Both parents want their son to play in the NBA or NFL and believe he will not make it unless he "gets a lot taller really soon." She informs you in no uncertain terms that if you don't prescribe this "growing pill," she will just find someone that will.

You believe this mother is in need of some education about GH deficiency.

What are the *approved* indications in children and adolescents for GH replacement therapy?

A) GH deficiency.
B) Growth failure due to chronic renal insufficiency, intrauterine growth retardation with lack of "catch up" growth by age 2, Turner syndrome, and Prader–Willi syndrome.
C) An adolescent male who wishes to play basketball but is only 5 feet 9 inches on a good day.
D) A and B.
E) All of the above.

Discussion

The correct answer is "D." GH replacement is specifically approved for GH deficiency and growth failure due to chronic renal insufficiency, intrauterine growth retardation and no "catch up" growth by age 2, Turner syndrome, and Prader–Willi syndrome. It has been approved for use in "idiopathic short stature" (more than two standard deviations below the mean height for age). Not all patients with GH deficiency require GH replacement, because not all will suffer the negative end-organ effects, such as marked short stature, growth failure, hypoglycemia in infancy, and central distribution of body fat.

HELPFUL TIP: As with acromegaly, IGF-I should be checked when considering short stature secondary to pituitary failure. It is also important to check IGF-binding protein-3 levels. Low levels of IGF-binding protein-3 may cause problems with binding of IGF to the proper receptors.

HELPFUL TIP: Even when used appropriately, GH only leads to a couple of inches increase in adult height.

QUICK QUIZ: DIABETES

Which of these drugs can be used in patients with either type 1 or type 2 diabetes?

A) Nateglinide (Starlix).
B) Pramlintide (Symlin).
C) Precose (Acarbose).
D) Glimepiride (Amaryl).
E) A and B.

Discussion

The correct answer is "B." Pramlintide is a synthetic analogue of amylin, which is secreted by the body along with insulin. This drug (1) prolongs gastric emptying leading to lower spike in serum glucose, (2) suppresses postprandial glucagon secretion (again lowering blood sugars) and (3) suppresses hunger leading to lower calorie intake. **It should only be used in patients who are already on insulin but can be used for both type 1 and type 2 diabetes.** Nateglinide (Starlix) is a meglitinide that releases glucose from the pancreas similar to sulfonylureas. Precose (Acarbose) is an alpha-glucosidase inhibitor that prevents the conversion of starches to simple sugars in the GI tract and thus slows absorption of glucose from the GI tract. Finally, glimepiride (Amaryl) is a sulfonylurea.

BIBLIOGRAPHY

American Diabetes Association. Standards of medical care in diabetes—2011. *Diabetes Care.* 2011;34:S11-S61.

Betterle C, Morlin L. Autoimmune Addison's disease. *Endocr Dev.* 2011;20:161-172.

Carroll MF. A practical approach to hypercalcemia. *Am Fam Physician.* 2003;67:1959.

Findling JW. Diagnosis and differential diagnosis of Cushing's syndrome. *Endocrinol Metab Clin North Am.* 2001;30:729.

Finklestein BS. Effect of growth hormone therapy on height in children with idiopathic short stature: A meta-analysis. *Arch Pediatr Adolesc Med.* 2002;156:230.

Fraser WD. Hyperthyroidism. *Lancet.* 2009;374:145-158.

Grozinsky-Glasberg S, et al. Thyroxine-triiodothyronine combination therapy versus thyroxine monotherapy for clinical hypothyroidism: Meta-analysis of randomized controlled trials. *J Clin Endocrinol Metab.* 2006;91:2592.

Herrick B. Subclinical hypothyroidism. *Am Fam Physician.* 2008;77:953.

Kearns AE. Medical and surgical management of hyperparathyroidism. *Mayo Clin Proc.* 2002;77:87.

Kim N. Evaluation of a thyroid nodule. *Otolaryngol Clin North Am.* 2003;36:17.

Moghissi ES, et al. American Association of Clinical Endocrinologists and American Diabetes Association consensus statement on inpatient glycemic control. *Diabetes Care.* 2009;32:1119-1136.

Montori VM, Fernández-Balsells M. Glycemic control in type 2 diabetes: Time for an evidence-based about-face? *Ann Intern Med.* 2009;150:803-808.

Nathan DM, et al. Diabetes: A consensus algorithm for the initiation and adjustment of therapy. *Clinical Diabetes.* 2009;27:4-16.

Norris SL, et al. Effectiveness of self-management training in type 2 diabetes: A systematic review of randomized controlled trials. *Diabetes Care.* 2001;24:561-587.

Sherlock M, et al. Medical therapy in acromegaly. *Nat Rev Endocrinol.* 2011;7:291-300.

Tritos NA, et al.; Medscape. Management of Cushing disease. *Nat Rev Endocrinol.* 2011;7:279-289.

Unger J. Latent autoimmune diabetes in adults. *Am Fam Physician.* 2010;81:843.

U.S. Preventive Services Task Force. Screening for gestational diabetes mellitus: U.S. Preventive Services Task Force recommendation statement. *Ann Intern Med.* 2008;148:759-765.

11
Rheumatology

Bogdan Cherascu

A few words on "rheumatology panels." Doing a "rheumatology panel" will never be the right answer. *The diagnosis of rheumatologic disease is clinical with specific clinical criteria for each illness.* While antinuclear antibody (ANA), rheumatoid factor (RF), erythrocyte sedimentation rate (ESR), and C-reactive protein (CRP) may be useful in supporting a clinical diagnosis and assessing disease activity, these tests have **poor specificity** and may be positive in a variety of disease states. A positive ANA without a clinical diagnosis is meaningless. Likewise, RF helps to gauge prognosis (seropositive vs. seronegative) in rheumatoid arthritis, but has very limited value as a diagnostic test. False-positive RF can be found in Wegner granulomatosis, many viral infections, primary lung disease, sarcoid, primary liver disease, and other autoimmune diseases. ESR and CRP may support the clinical impression of inflammatory disease, but are again nonspecific.

CASE 1

A 43-year-old female presents with body aches and stiffness, which are worse in the morning. She further describes a low-grade fever and pain in her hands, feet, and left knee. She feels that her grip strength is diminished. These symptoms started rather abruptly 2 weeks ago and have not responded to acetaminophen.

She frequently camps with her family. She remembers that 1 week they could not go because her 8-year-old daughter had a fever, mild diarrhea, abdominal pain, and a skin rash ("legs, arms, and especially face were red and warm, and she seemed 'flushed' all the time"). Her daughter's symptoms resolved in a few days, she did not see a doctor, and no one else was sick. She has no other illnesses, and review of systems is otherwise negative.

On physical examination, her vitals are normal. She is unable to close her hands completely. Although your exam is somewhat limited by pain, there appears to be swelling of all metacarpophalangeal (MCP) and proximal interphalangeal (PIP) joints. You detect a bulge sign (indicating effusion) upon examining the left knee. Also, you notice mild erythema over the MCPs.

If found on physical exam, which of the following would be LEAST useful in helping you in narrow your diagnosis?

A) Bilateral metatarsophalangeal (MTP) joint swelling and tenderness.
B) Painless oral ulcerations, with clean edges.
C) Firm, slightly tender subcutaneous nodules at the olecranon bursae.
D) A "bull's eye" rash in the right axilla.
E) Icterus and tender hepatomegaly.

Discussion

The correct answer is "A." This patient presents with a picture of a polyarticular inflammatory arthritis of unclear etiology. While important to note, MTP joint swelling would not add much to the picture of subacute, symmetrical, small joint polyarthritis that you have already found on your examination. Your differential diagnosis will include acute viral arthritis, specifically parvovirus B19 (due to the daughter's history of acute illness resembling erythema infectiosum), coxsackievirus, hepatitis B (answer "E"), and HIV. Also on your differential will be Lyme disease ("D") (although small joint symmetrical arthritis would be atypical), rheumatoid arthritis ("C," the presence of rheumatoid nodules would be helpful although these would be unlikely in early disease), and other inflammatory disorders. "B," painless ulcerations, are associated with systemic lupus. Painful ulcers are consistent with Bechet disease.

* *

After you sneak off to do a little reading, you examine her again. She has no rash. You detect bilateral pain and swelling of MTPs 3 and 4. There are no oral ulcerations and no lymphadenopathy. She is not icteric, and her abdomen is diffusely, mildly tender. There is no hepatomegaly. You decide to order some blood tests.

If positive, which of the following serologic tests would be MOST helpful in ruling in a specific diagnosis?

A) Positive ANA.
B) Elevated white count.
C) Positive parvovirus B19 IgG and IgM.
D) Positive urinalysis for white blood cells (WBCs).
E) Elevated ESR and CRP.

Discussion

The correct answer is "C." The presence of IgM antibodies to parvovirus B19—or rising titers of IgG antibodies—indicates acute viral infection, which may present with symptoms and signs seen in this patient. Answer "A," positive ANA, will not help you rule in a diagnosis at this point. While the ANA is a highly sensitive test, it is not specific and has a low positive predictive value. "B," "D," and "E" are all important findings but do not lead you toward a specific diagnosis. Table 11–1 presents a framework for who should be tested for and diagnosed with rheumatoid arthritis.

HELPFUL TIP: Note that the diagnosis of RA no longer requires 6 weeks of symptoms, although longer duration of polyarthritis makes RA more likely. Similarly, it would be unusual for parvovirus B19 to cause symptoms for 6 weeks. However, the virus can cause prolonged joint pain in 10% of affected adults.

Table 11–1 WHO SHOULD BE TESTED FOR RHEUMATOID ARTHRITIS?

Patients who:	
1. Have at least 1 joint with definite clinical synovitis (swelling)	
2. With the synovitis **not better explained by another disease**	
A. Joint involvement	
1 large joint	0
2–10 large joints	1
1–3 small joints (with or without involvement of large joints)	2
4–10 small joints (with or without involvement of large joints)	3
>10 joints (at least 1 small joint)	5
B. Serology (at least 1 test result is needed for classification)	
Negative RF and negative ACPA	0
Low-positive RF or low-positive ACPA	2
High-positive RF or high-positive ACPA	3
C. Acute-phase reactants (at least 1 test result is needed for classification)	
Normal CRP and normal ESR	0
Abnormal CRP or abnormal ESR	1
D. Duration of symptoms	
<6 weeks	0
>6 weeks	1

Diagnose rheumatoid arthritis if: Score of categories A–D is at least 6/10.
Data from Aletaha D. 2010 Rheumatoid arthritis classification criteria: An American College of Rheumatology/European League Against Rheumatism collaborative initiative. *Arthritis Rheum.* 2010;62:2569-2581. (doi: 10.1002/art.27584.)

* *

Her lab results return as follows:

Hepatitis B: Surface antibody positive, surface antigen negative.
CMV: IgG positive, IgM negative.
Parvovirus: IgG positive, IgM negative.
Rheumatoid factor: 1:160 (positive $\geq$1:40)
Anticitrullinated protein antibody (ACPA)*: 64 units (strong positive >60 units)
ANA: Negative.
ESR: 58 mm/hr.

*Anticitrullinated protein antibody (ACPA) is also known as Anti-CCP (Anticyclic citrullinated peptides). This is a fairly specific marker for rheumatoid arthritis. Anti-CCP antibodies are very specific for RA; however, their sensitivity is 70% and therefore may be negative in RA.

Note that based on results so far, she has 7 points (4–10 joints involved, high titers of RF and CCP antibody, and elevated ESR).

Which of the following is the most appropriate next step?

A) Bilateral hand x-rays.
B) CT of the chest.
C) Smith antibody, double-stranded DNA (dsDNA), complement levels.
D) Start methotrexate 15 mg PO weekly with or without low-dose prednisone and follow up in 4–5 weeks.
E) Start prednisone 60 mg PO QD and follow up in 4–5 weeks.

Discussion

The correct answer is "D." This patient most likely has seropositive rheumatoid arthritis (see criteria above, Table 11–1). The patient should be started **on weekly methotrexate, at a moderate dose, along with folic acid 1 mg daily and prednisone 10–20 mg daily. There is a "window of opportunity" when treating early RA; an early remission *may* lead to sustained remission.**

Note that investigating other systemic involvement should be included as part of her initial evaluation. It is appropriate to obtain CBC, liver function tests, electrolytes, BUN, creatinine and, UA (to rule out glomerulonephritis). Answer "A" is incorrect. She is presenting fairly early after the onset of symptoms, so it is unlikely that hand x-rays will provide any significant findings. Answer "B" is also incorrect. Without further symptoms, signs of lung involvement (e.g., pulmonary osteoarthropathy and respiratory symptoms), a CT scan would be inappropriate. As to "C," she has no other symptoms of lupus and also had a negative ANA, so further testing for lupus (Smith antibody, dsDNA [also known as antinative DNA antibodies], complement levels) is not appropriate. Answer "E" is incorrect. The correct dose for prednisone is 10–20 mg/day.

HELPFUL (IF LONG) TIP: In all cases of RA, and especially in those with a poorer prognosis, disease-modifying antirheumatic drugs (DMARDs) should be instituted promptly, and escalated fairly rapidly, with goal being disease remission. Methotrexate is the DMARD of choice, but combination therapy (methotrexate plus hydroxychloroquine or sulfasalazine) or triple therapy (methotrexate, hydroxychloroquine, and sulfasalazine) improves outcomes over methotrexate alone. Low-dose prednisone is indicated for immediate symptomatic relief. Recent data suggests that low-dose prednisone in the first 6 month up to 2 years after diagnosis is associated with better prognosis and more sustained remission. Occupational therapy referral is helpful in identifying and treating functional impairment due to RA. Vitamin D 800 IU/day and calcium 600–800 mg BID should be initiated with prednisone therapy to help prevent steroid-induced osteoporosis. Evaluation of bone density (DEXA scan) and a bisphosphonate (e.g., alendronate and risedronate) should also be initiated if >5 mg of prednisone is to be used for >3 months.

HELPFUL TIP: Rheumatoid arthritis typically has an insidious onset with a fluctuating course; however, a significant minority of patients (perhaps one-third) will experience rapid onset, over days to weeks.

* *

She returns in 4 weeks and is now about 7 weeks into her illness. She reports a moderate response to your intervention (you started methotrexate 15 mg weekly and 1 mg folic acid daily and prednisone 20 mg), but now she has 1–2 hours of morning stiffness. She continues to complain of pain in her hands and feet, with poor grip. In fact, she had to take time off from work during the last week. On exam, she has persistent swelling of MCPs 2–5 bilaterally and MTPs 3 and 4 bilaterally. Also, you note swelling in the left wrist and both knees. However, now she has no erythema and seems less tender.

You take a step back and want to reconsider your diagnosis.

What exam finding is so general that it would NOT help you support/reconsider your diagnosis?

A) Pleural rub auscultated on lung exam.
B) Firm, slightly tender subcutaneous nodules at the olecranon bursae.

C) Faint pink rash over chest, which is not visible 15 minutes later.
D) Reduced passive flexion in left knee.
E) Left foot drop.

Discussion

The correct answer is "D." While important to note, limitation of passive movements of the knees is indicative only of knee effusion (or pain), which you have already observed, and is not specific for any particular etiology. She responded modestly to methotrexate and prednisone but clearly still has arthritis. What can you use to expand or limit your differential diagnosis? "A" is indicative of possible lupus. Diagnostic criteria for lupus include serositis, which may be detectable as a pleural rub on auscultation of the lungs (also, look for malar rash, discoid lesions, alopecia, and oral ulcerations). Although not part of the diagnostic criteria for the disease, rheumatoid arthritis may also present with pleuritis or pericarditis. Rheumatoid nodules (answer "B") are found RA. A salmon-colored, evanescent macular rash ("C") would lead you to consider adult Still disease. Still disease is also known as juvenile idiopathic arthritis (JIA, discussed in Chapter 13), presents with an evanescent rash, intermittent fever, and arthritis. "Adult onset" Still disease is Still disease with onset after age 16. A finding of isolated foot drop ("E") may be the result of mononeuritis multiplex, a feature of vasculitides, and paraneoplastic syndromes.

Since your patient is taking methotrexate, you caution her to avoid which of the following?

A) Aspirin.
B) Sulfonamide antibiotics.
C) Ibuprofen.
D) Folate.
E) Penicillin antibiotics.

Discussion

The correct answer is "B." Methotrexate is a folate antagonist. Antifolate medications, such as sulfonamide antibiotics, must be avoided in patients taking methotrexate; the combination may result in pancytopenia. Supplemental folate, 1 mg daily, reduces the adverse effects of methotrexate. Patients with RA are often treated with aspirin or NSAIDs in combination with methotrexate. Penicillin antibiotics can be administered safely with methotrexate.

HELPFUL TIP: Drug interaction programs often warn about concomitant use of NSAIDs and methotrexate, as well as aspirin and methotrexate. These warnings are most relevant to high-dose methotrexate used to treat cancer, not the lower doses used for inflammatory arthritis.

* *

At her first return visit, she had only mild improvement so you (rightly) added hydroxychloroquine (good job!). Initial hand x-rays demonstrate mild periarticular osteopenia. Liver function tests, urinalysis, CBC, BUN, and creatinine are normal. She returns 6 weeks after starting the hydroxychloroquine and is much improved, having returned to work full-time. She tells you that she still has problems with opening jars and about 45 minutes of morning stiffness, "but nothing like it was."

What is the BEST course of action to follow now?

A) Continue her current therapy and follow up in 6–12 months with transaminases, RF, and hand x-rays.
B) Continue her current therapy and follow up in 3–4 months with transaminases, RF, and hand x-rays.
C) Continue current therapy and follow up in 3–4 months; arrange for monthly BUN, creatinine and CBC; and schedule for an annual ophthalmology exam.
D) Continue her current therapy and arrange for monthly transaminases and CBC; schedule for an annual ophthalmology exam; and schedule follow-up in another 2–3 months.
E) Instruct her to discontinue methotrexate, taper the prednisone dose, and continue hydroxychloroquine; arrange follow-up in 1 year.

Discussion

The correct answer is "D." She seems to be responding to therapy, and a 3-month trial on her current medications (during which the methotrexate dose may be increased) is indicated. A slow prednisone taper should be initiated only after disease remission is achieved. Guidelines for monitoring her DMARD regimen require monthly transaminases and CBC for methotrexate and an annual eye exam to assess for hydroxychloroquine-related retinal toxicity. Hand x-rays are recommended at 2-year intervals. Answer "E" is clearly incorrect: DMARD therapy reduces her risk of joint destruction and disease progression, and it should not be discontinued.

* *

At her next visit 3 months later, she feels better. Although she still has difficulty opening jars, she now has <30 minutes of morning stiffness and almost no pain. On exam she has no rash, and no nodules, no evidence of serositis. She now has swelling over MCPs 2–4 on the right and 2–3 on the left. Her grip is still somewhat weak but improved. Laboratory data shows an ESR of 28 mm/hr, CRP 0.7 mg/dL, and normal transaminases and CBC.

Which of the following is the most appropriate next step?

A) Increase methotrexate to 25 mg a week and refer to rheumatology.
B) Stop methotrexate and switch to leflunomide 20 mg/day.
C) Increase prednisone to 60 mg QD.
D) Discontinue all medications except methotrexate.
E) Discontinue methotrexate, taper prednisone, and continue hydroxychloroquine.

Discussion

The correct answer is "A." Despite her initial response, she has evidence of ongoing inflammatory activity by history and exam. Discontinuing or reducing medication is inappropriate. According to published guidelines, consultation with a rheumatologist is now indicated—if it had not been sought sooner. She has had a fair initial response to methotrexate, prednisone, and hydroxychloroquine. Further benefit may be gained with increasing the methotrexate dose. However, she will likely need addition of a biologic agent. Answer "B" is incorrect. Since she had an initial response to methotrexate, it would be wise to further increase the methotrexate dose, rather than substituting another agent (leflunomide). Answer "C" is incorrect. Doses of prednisone this high are not indicated for rheumatoid arthritis.

This patient wants to get pregnant. You can tell her that:

A) Symptoms remit in 70% of women when they get pregnant.
B) It is inappropriate to get pregnant while on methotrexate.
C) Rheumatoid arthritis is a contraindication to pregnancy.
D) Prednisone cannot be taken during pregnancy.
E) A and B.

Discussion

The correct answer is "E," both "A" and "B" are correct. RA is an autoimmune disease, and it tends to remit during pregnancy when a woman is relatively immunosuppressed. Methotrexate is class X for pregnancy and is actually used in ectopic pregnancy to arrest fetal growth. Women and men on methotrexate should use an effective form of contraception, and continue contraception for 3 months after stopping methotrexate.

"D" is incorrect since prednisone is often used to control RA during pregnancy, when methotrexate is contraindicated.

* *

The patient is also concerned about her future. She enjoys running and other activities.

You can let her know that:

A) RA tends to progress without any remissions to involve almost all joints in all patients.
B) Ninety percent of the joints that will be involved are involved during the first year.
C) Patients with RA have the same life expectancy as the general public.
D) Renal involvement is common with RA and is a major source of morbidity and mortality.
E) She won't need to worry about having a life after she gets pregnant and has a child. All her energy will be absorbed by that little parasite . . . er, child.

Discussion

The correct answer is "B." Ninety percent of the joints that will eventually be involved with RA are involved during the first year. Answer "A" is incorrect. Up to 40% of patients will go into remission with 10% going into a long-term remission. Another 30% have an intermittent course with exacerbations and remissions. Additionally, drugs can induce a remission. Answer "C" is incorrect. RA reduces the life expectancy by up to 10 years. Finally, "D" is incorrect. Renal disease is a rare complication of RA. It can be a result of some of the medications used for RA, however.

HELPFUL TIP: Does joint replacement work in RA? Yes. Remember, however, that the life span of an artificial joint may be 15 years max with current technology. Thus, replacement should not be undertaken lightly in a young (or any) patient.

Objectives: Did you learn to . . .

- Describe an appropriate diagnostic strategy for polyarthritis?
- Recognize the diagnostic criteria for rheumatoid arthritis?
- Develop a management strategy for rheumatoid arthritis?
- Recognize the importance of early DMARD therapy for rheumatoid arthritis?
- Identify the uses and adverse effects of medications used to treat rheumatoid arthritis?

QUICK QUIZ: ARTHRITIS IN CHILDHOOD

A concerned mother brings in her 2-year-old son with a history of fever for 1 week. She had expected the fever to resolve by now and is worried. According to his mother, the patient also has a rash, poor appetite, and lethargy. On exam, he looks ill and his temperature is 39.0°C. There is a diffuse, erythematous, macular rash, and peeling skin on the fingertips. The oropharynx is injected and the tongue is bright red with white papillae. Cervical lymph nodes are enlarged and tender.

Based on the available information, what is your leading diagnosis?

A) Rheumatic fever.
B) Parvovirus B19 infection.
C) Kawasaki syndrome.
D) JIA.
E) Varicella infection.

Discussion

The correct answer is "C." Kawasaki syndrome is an acute vasculitis of unknown etiology which is most often seen in children. Kawasaki syndrome presents with at least 5 days of fever, polymorphous rash, conjunctival injection, mucous membrane involvement (e.g., "strawberry" tongue), cervical lymphadenopathy, and extremity findings of erythema and desquamation. The usual treatment is aspirin and IVIG. Steroid therapy is controversial and does not seem to improve outcomes. There may be cardiac involvement with the formation of coronary artery aneurysms.

"A," rheumatic fever, which is rare in developed countries, is recognized by the Jones criteria. The major Jones criteria consist of polyarthritis, carditis, Sydenham chorea, erythema marginatum, and subcutaneous nodules. (Here's a fun mnemonic: "JONES" with a heart shape in place of the "O," so that J = joints, O = carditis, N = nodules, E = erythema marginatum, and S = Sydenham chorea). "B" is incorrect. Children are generally less ill appearing with parvovirus B19 infection (fifth disease). "D," JIA, would be unusual at such a young age, and is discussed in Chapter 13. "E" is incorrect, as this is obviously not varicella.

CASE 2

A 62-year-old male whom you have followed for hypertension for several years presents with complaints of worsening fatigue and aching in his back, shoulders, and neck. He notes 3 months of symptoms unresponsive to acetaminophen.

Further history reveals that your patient has experienced stiffness of the neck and shoulders each morning for over 30 minutes. He occasionally has difficulty getting out of bed. Vital signs are normal. There is no evidence of synovitis of the hands, wrists, and elbows. Active range of motion in the neck and shoulders is slow but full. There is tenderness to palpation of the shoulders, upper back, and neck, but no apparent muscle atrophy.

Which of the following is the most appropriate next step in the diagnosis of this illness?

A) Obtain an ESR and CRP.
B) Obtain a urinalysis.
C) Prescribe a diagnostic trial of steroids.
D) Order a rheumatology panel, including ANAs, uric acid, ESR, CRP and RF.
E) Perform shoulder radiograph.

Discussion

The correct answer is "A." This patient's presentation is consistent with the diagnosis of polymyalgia rheumatica (PMR). Elevations of ESR and/or CRP contribute further evidence to such a diagnosis and are useful in following the treatment of PMR. While a urinalysis may be important in some rheumatologic illnesses (e.g., lupus, Behçet syndrome, and Wegener granulomatosis), PMR is not likely to be associated with renal disease.

Answer "C," a trial of steroid therapy, may be appropriate, but an ESR should be obtained first to further clinch the diagnosis. At this point all we know is that he has bilateral shoulder and neck pain, which could be mechanical from the cervical spine, etc. As you already know from earlier discussion, "D" is incorrect: a "rheumatology panel" will typically include tests that are not indicated, and positive results can be misleading. In the absence of small joint symptoms or exam findings, an RF is not indicated. Likewise there is no history to suggest an ANA-related disorder. Answer "E" is incorrect. This patient does not need shoulder radiographs. In a patient with bilateral shoulder pain and neck pain, a neck radiograph may be more useful than shoulder imaging. Neck radiographs help to evaluate for cervical canal narrowing and degenerative disc disease, which may result in pain and neurologic findings in the upper extremities. An MRI of the neck might be useful if cervical spine disc disease or a syrinx were suspected. Diagnostic criteria for PMR are given in Table 11–2.

HELPFUL TIP: Physical exam findings of PMR are subtle. Active ROM in the affected areas is often limited by pain, but passive ROM should be full. Strength is intact. In general, PMR affects shoulders to a greater degree than hips, and PMR affects hips more than the neck. The essential pathology is inflammation of the synovia, and muscles are not directly involved.

Table 11–2 GENERALLY ACCEPTED CRITERIA FOR DIAGNOSIS OF PMR

- Age >50 years
- Pain/aching for at least 1 month involving 2 of the following areas: neck, shoulders/proximal arms, and pelvic girdle
- Morning stiffness
- ESR >40 mm/hr
- Exclusion of other potential causes of the symptoms except giant cell arteritis

HELPFUL TIP: Patients with PMR often have a low-grade fever and a normocytic anemia.

The sensitivity of an elevated ESR in the diagnosis of PMR and giant cell arteritis (GCA, AKA, temporal arteritis) is:

A) 100%.
B) 95%.
C) 85%.
D) 75%.
E) 65%.

Discussion

The correct answer is "C." Up to 15% of patients with PMR or GCA (a closely related disorder—keep reading) have a false-negative ESR. Using ESR and CRP together is 97–99% sensitive for GCA. Double false negatives of ESR and CRP are uncommon, but do occur. Thus, in the patient in whom GCA is suspected but in whom there is a normal ESR and/or CRP, biopsy is still recommended. In those suspected of PMR, a trial of steroids is still recommended.

HELPFUL TIP: PMR is uncommon in non-white populations. The mean age of onset is approximately 70 years. Women are affected twice as often as men.

* *

You order radiographs of the neck, which demonstrate mild degenerative disease. A CBC is unremarkable, except for a mild thrombocytosis. The ESR is 80 mm/hr. You relate these findings to the patient and tell him that your presumptive diagnosis is PMR.

Which of the following is the most appropriate initial treatment in this case?

A) Naproxen 500 mg BID.
B) Prednisone 15 mg QD and aspirin 81 mg QD.
C) Aspirin 650 mg BID.
D) Prednisone 50 mg QD.
E) Referral to physical therapy.

Discussion

The correct answer is "B." Steroids are the treatment of choice in PMR. Doses of prednisone ranging from 10 to 20 mg QD usually control the disease. Higher doses (up to 30 mg/day) should be tried if there is no response in 1–2 weeks. If the patient fails to respond to low-dose steroids, the diagnosis of PMR should be reconsidered. Answer "A" is incorrect. NSAIDS may provide some symptomatic relief but are not the treatment for PMR. Answer "C" is incorrect. **When added to prednisone, low-dose aspirin, 81 mg/day decreases the risk of vision loss in temporal arteritis. However, high-dose aspirin therapy without steroids is not recommended.** Answer "E" is incorrect. Since patients usually respond quickly to steroids, physical therapy is not necessary—although you could hardly be faulted for employing physical therapy as part of your overall treatment approach.

HELPFUL TIP: Looking at the long-term outcomes, initial low-dose therapy for PMR works better than high-dose therapy. Patients have fewer relapses and are spared some of the adverse effects of high-dose steroids.

* *

You prescribe prednisone 15 mg QD, aspirin 81 mg daily, and calcium and vitamin D supplementation. Your patient presents for follow-up 4 weeks later, reporting that he is greatly improved. On examination, there is no muscle tenderness with range of motion or joint inflammation. His ESR is 20 mm/hr. You believe that the patient's disease is now in remission.

Which of the following is the most appropriate next step in his management?

A) Discontinue prednisone and initiate naproxen.
B) Continue the current dose of prednisone for the next 12 months.
C) Continue the current dose of prednisone for the next 6 months.
D) Taper prednisone by 1–2 mg every 2 weeks to reach the minimum effective dose.
E) Taper prednisone by 5 mg over 2 weeks and then discontinue the dose.

Discussion

The correct answer is "D." Relapse of PMR occurs more frequently when steroids are abruptly discontinued or tapered too quickly. However, due to complications associated with steroid therapy, the dose should be reduced as soon as possible; therefore, maintaining prednisone 15 mg QD for 6–12 months is inappropriate. The usual recommendation is to reduce the dose of prednisone by 10% every 1–2 weeks until the minimum effective dose is reached. While tapering the steroid dose, the patient should be monitored with an ESR and/or CRP every 2–4 weeks. If symptoms worsen, the steroid dose should be increased slightly to achieve symptomatic control. If the ESR increases to 40 mm/hr or greater and the patient is asymptomatic, consider continuing the same dose of steroid until the ESR normalizes, then continue the taper. However, an isolated elevation in ESR without symptoms is not a reason to **increase** the steroid dose.

Which of the following is true regarding the prognosis of PMR?

A) PMR is associated with an increased risk of mortality.
B) Most patients with PMR will require steroid therapy for life.
C) Up to 50% of patients who initially have a successful remission will experience a relapse while tapering prednisone.
D) A relapse of PMR requires high-dose steroids (prednisone 50 mg QD) for successful treatment.

Discussion

The correct answer is "C." Relapses occur in 30–50% of patients after induction of a remission and should be treated by resuming or increasing prednisone. Usually, successful treatment of a relapse requires increasing the prednisone dose by a few milligrams. Answer "A" is incorrect. Although the pathogenesis of PMR is incompletely understood, it has features in common with vasculitides, including potential vascular complications of GCA. However, PMR is not associated with an increase in mortality. Answer "B" is incorrect because PMR is a self-limited disease, and most patients recover within a few months to a few years. Thus, patients require steroids for 6 months to 2 years, but steroid therapy is typically not life-long. Relapses of PMR after prednisone has been successfully stopped are seen in about 20% of cases, and can occur up to years later.

* *

Your patient does well and is able to taper off steroid therapy over a year. Three months after stopping steroids, he presents to the ED one night. His shoulder and neck pain and stiffness have returned, as well as severe fatigue and feeling feverish. He has lost 5 pounds in 2 weeks. He is now experiencing frequent left-sided headaches. Finally, he is most concerned about a new visual disturbance starting today. He notes that he has a "hole" in his vision. On physical examination, there is ta prominent, tender vessel palpable at the left temporal area. Funduscopic exam of the left eye shows a pale disc with blurred margins. The remainder of the neurologic exam is normal. The ESR is 70 mm/hr.

Which of the following is the most likely diagnosis for the visual symptoms?

A) PMR.
B) Stroke.
C) GCA.
D) Multiple sclerosis.
E) Acute angle-closure glaucoma.

Discussion

The correct answer is "C." Many of the patient's symptoms can be explained by PMR ("A"), but visual symptoms do not occur with this disease. GCA is a related diagnosis that is commonly seen in conjunction with PMR. Most experts now agree that PMR and GCA are different presentations of the same disease process. With the new symptoms of localized headache and tenderness of the temporal artery and the previously known findings consistent with PMR, this patient now meets diagnostic criteria for GCA (see Table 11–3). The visual symptoms described are typical of GCA and can occur acutely or chronically. As to the other answers, vision loss in multiple sclerosis is attributable to optic neuritis, which is associated with pain and presents initially in a younger population. Acute angle-closure glaucoma is associated with eye pain and redness. The lack of other symptoms makes stroke less likely.

Table 11–3 DIAGNOSTIC CRITERIA FOR GIANT CELL ARTERITIS

Three of the following must be present:

- Age ≥50 years at onset of symptoms
- New localized headache
- Temporal artery tenderness or decreased pulsation
- ESR ≥50 mm/hr
- Temporal artery biopsy findings consistent with vasculitis

HELPFUL TIP: The initial visual loss in temporal arteritis is peripheral, while the vision loss in macular degeneration is initially central. If you think about it, this makes sense. GCA basically causes an anterior ischemic optic neuropathy (AION) secondary to involvement of the retinal artery by vasculitis. The further you are from the artery, the poorer the perfusion.

Which of the following is the most appropriate initial management of this patient?

A) Withhold treatment for now and arrange for temporal artery biopsy within 48 hours.
B) Refer to a neurologist as soon as possible.
C) Refer to an ophthalmologist as soon as possible.
D) Initiate prednisone 20 mg QD, and refer for temporal artery biopsy.
E) Admit and administer methylprednisolone 1 g intravenously (IV).

Discussion

The correct answer is "E." When symptoms of vision loss occur, aspirin 81 mg daily and IV methylprednisolone 1 g daily for 3 days, followed by aspirin and prednisone 40–60 mg daily is the standard of care. Compared to PMR, higher doses of steroids are necessary to treat GCA. In the absence of vision loss, prednisone doses of 40–60 mg QD are usually required to relieve symptoms. "A" is incorrect. You do not want to withhold treatment from this patient whose vision is at risk (see "helpful tip" below). Answers "B" and "C" are incorrect for the same reason. However, an ophthalmologist will be absolutely necessary in the care of this patient; so, option "C" would be the very next thing on your list. Answer "D" is incorrect because a dose of 20 mg of prednisone is generally not going to be effective in GCA.

HELPFUL TIP: Temporal artery biopsy is vital to the accurate diagnosis of GCA. Characteristic giant cell inflammation pathology can be seen for up to 4 weeks after initiating high-dose corticosteroids. However, **corticosteroid therapy should never be delayed for fear of reducing the inflammatory findings on the temporal artery biopsy**.

* *

Six years after his diagnosis of GCA, your patient has experienced several remissions and relapses. Although he has been able to discontinue steroids on occasion, he is taking prednisone 5 mg QD with good symptomatic control.

One night, 3 AM in the ED... the weather is cold and the coffee is colder... your patient presents with tearing substernal chest pain radiating to his back. He is alert but anxious and diaphoretic. His left radial pulse is diminished compared to the right. His heart rate is 120 bpm, and his blood pressure is 92/56 mm Hg.

Which of the following studies will confirm the most likely diagnosis?

A) Chest radiograph.
B) Chest CT.
C) ECG.
D) ABG.
E) Troponin-T.

Discussion

The correct answer is "B." Your patient's symptoms are classic for a dissecting thoracic aortic aneurysm, which is often mistaken for a myocardial infarction. Thoracic aortic aneurysm is a late complication of GCA; aortic aneurysms generally occur an average of 6–7 years after the initial diagnosis of GCA. Thoracic aortic aneurysms occur 17 times more often in patients with GCA when compared to the general population. The diagnosis of thoracic aortic aneurysm is confirmed by CT scan of the chest, echocardiogram, or angiogram. While the other studies listed should be done, none of them is going to make the diagnosis of a dissecting aneurysm for you.

HELPFUL TIP: With the initiation of steroids in PMR or GCA, start calcium 1200–1500 mg daily and vitamin D 400–800 IU daily for osteoporosis prevention. If diagnosis is confirmed, a bone density should be done and bisphosphonates instituted based on FRAX calculated risk of fracture (do you see a pattern here of prophylaxis for osteoporosis when starting steroids?). Aspirin 81 mg/day, if not contraindicated, reduces the risk of vision loss and perhaps stroke in patients with GCA.

Objectives: Did you learn to...

- Describe the appropriate evaluation, including physical exam and laboratory test, of diffuse pain in the older patient?
- Recognize the diagnostic criteria for PMR and GCA?
- Describe the appropriate management, including medical therapy, of PMR and GCA?
- Identify complications of PMR and GCA?

QUICK QUIZ: OSTEOARTHRITIS

The preferred initial therapy for elderly patients with arthralgia due to osteoarthritis is which of the following?

A) NSAIDs.
B) COX-2 inhibitors.
C) Acetaminophen.
D) Combination narcotic analgesics.
E) Early joint replacement.

Discussion

The correct answer is "C." Because of greater risk of gastrointestinal (GI) and renal toxicity in the elderly, NSAIDs should be avoided if possible and limited if used in this population. As for COX-2 inhibitors, the advantage in GI side effects is questionable, and the cost is much greater than traditional NSAIDs. The best initial choice for osteoarthritis pain in the elderly (and almost everybody, for that matter) is acetaminophen with doses scheduled three to four times per day. In older patients, do not exceed 3 g of acetaminophen per day. Combination narcotic analgesics are employed when acetaminophen alone does not suffice and NSAIDs are contraindicated. Although elderly patients should be considered candidates for joint replacement, it is not appropriate as the initial therapy.

HELPFUL TIP: Other treatments of osteoarthritis that have some demonstrated benefit for short-term pain control include topical capsaicin cream, topical NSAIDs, intra-articular steroid injection, and intra-articular hyaluronic acid injection. A single, high volume, injection of the latter has been approved by the FDA for treatment of primary osteoarthritis of the knee. Glucosamine, with or without chondroitin, has not shown benefit in rigorous trials. None of these treatments has demonstrated clinically significant, long-term benefit.

CASE 3

A 22-year-old graduate student presents to the ED on a Monday night with an acutely swollen left knee. He admits to "wild partying" over the weekend but only had a couple of beers. His knee was OK then. However, when he woke up this morning, he noticed the knee was swollen and painful (so was his head, but that's another matter). By early afternoon, he had difficulty bearing weight. He denies fever, but feels tired.

He reports a history of JIA (previously termed juvenile rheumatoid arthritis), and has had ankle and knee swelling previously, but not to this degree. He took prednisone intermittently, as well as hydroxychloroquine and methotrexate, for his JIA until age 18. He then continued on hydroxychloroquine until 8 months ago, when he stopped it because he felt fine. He denies any other medical problems. He smokes only when drinking—which happens way too often.

What other information from the history would be most helpful in establishing the diagnosis?

A) Sexual history, including sexual orientation, practices, and last contact.
B) History of gout or pseudogout (calcium pyrophosphate dihydrate disease, CPPD).
C) History of IV drug use.
D) A and B.
E) A and C.

Discussion

The correct answer is "E." While all of these points are important in the history, this patient is too young to have gout or pseudogout (although there are very rare syndromes of familial hyperuricemia and early gout). Although there are several etiologies possible for this patient's presentation, the most critical to identify and treat is septic arthritis. As such, the history and exam should focus on those clues that point toward an infectious etiology and its source. The clinician must also consider noninfectious inflammatory arthropathies.

* *

Your patient is heterosexual and *thinks* he had intercourse Saturday night but admits that his memory is somewhat blurry (maybe he had more than the "couple" of beers he claims). He denies a history of gout and IV drug use. He complains of poor sleep and feeling stiff in the mornings and evenings lately.

What findings on physical exam would be LEAST helpful in determining the diagnosis?

A) A few vesiculopustular lesions on the back, arms, and legs.
B) Swollen, tender, nonerythematous MCP joints.
C) Nontender hepatomegaly.
D) Diastolic murmur at the right sternal border.
E) Whitish discharge from the tip of penis.

Discussion

The correct answer is "C." Although nontender hepatomegaly is important to notice and may indicate presence of liver disease, it is unlikely to help identify the etiology of this patient's arthritis. Hepatitis B arthritis usually presents as a symmetric polyarthritis, although it can be migratory or additive (sequential joints becoming involved without resolution in the initial joints). Answer "A" is helpful: a vesiculopustular rash occurs in disseminated gonococcal infections. Answer "B" is helpful: the presence of other swollen joints should prompt consideration of noninfectious inflammatory arthritis, and the swelling of the MCPs in particular may be a clue for active rheumatoid arthritis. Answer "D" is helpful: a diastolic murmur is always abnormal and may be a clue for endocarditis (which may seed joints causing infectious arthritis). Finally, "E," penile discharge, can result from acute gonorrheal infections.

HELPFUL QUESTION: Here's a Zen meditation: If he did have intercourse but doesn't remember it, did it ever really happen (except for the STIs, of course)? Also, what is the sound of one hand clapping?

* *

On exam, vitals show pulse 112 bpm, temperature 38.2°C, and normal blood pressure. He has no other swollen joints, no skin rash, no penile discharge, and no heart murmur. You palpate a smooth, nontender liver edge 2 cm below the costal margin; it percusses to 15 cm. You note mild cervical lymphadenopathy and whitish pharyngeal exudates.

Which of the following is the most appropriate NEXT step in the management of this patient?

A) Order hepatitis serologies.
B) Order blood cultures, pharyngeal cultures, and abdominal ultrasound.
C) Administer ceftriaxone 1 g IV and inject the knee with triamcinolone.
D) Perform knee aspiration.
E) Prescribe prednisone 20 mg PO QD and arrange consultation with a rheumatologist.

Discussion

The correct answer is "D." Did you get distracted by a big liver? If so, redirect your attention to the knee. The single most important step in evaluating acute monoarthritis is joint aspiration, which will allow differentiation between inflammatory and noninflammatory disease. Although blood and pharyngeal (as well as urethral) cultures should also be sent in this case, obtaining these studies must not delay joint aspiration. Without determining whether the arthritis is infectious, it would be inappropriate—and potentially hazardous to the patient—to start treatment with steroids. Answers "C" and "E" are incorrect because you would **not** want to give steroids—especially intra-articular steroids—to a patient with an infected joint. Analysis of the synovial fluid will aid in determining the appropriateness of treating with antibiotics or anti-inflammatory medications. While you would probably use empiric antibiotics (treat as septic until proven otherwise), you will need to first obtain cultures (knee aspiration, also systemic—blood, pharyngeal, penile, rectal).

HELPFUL TIP: CBC, sedimentation rate, and CRP are not useful in diagnosing a septic joint. While they may be somewhat sensitive, they are hopelessly nonspecific. You have to tap the joint regardless! (Just keep saying, "Yeah... I'd tap that.").

* *

You have obtained blood cultures, pharyngeal cultures, and urethral cultures. A metabolic profile, CBC, and hepatitis B and C serologies are pending. Knee aspiration yields 45 cc of turbid, blood-tinged fluid.

You send the synovial fluid for all of the following studies EXCEPT:

A) Cell count and differential.
B) Crystal analysis.
C) Culture.
D) Glucose and protein.
E) Gram stain.

Discussion

The correct answer is "D." In contrast to analysis of some other bodily fluids (e.g., cerebrospinal fluid [CSF], pleural fluid, and ascitic fluid), chemistry analysis on synovial fluid is of little diagnostic value. Low glucose levels in synovial fluid are associated with the degree of inflammation but not its cause. Likewise, synovial protein levels do not help differentiate between types of arthritis. Cell count with differential, Gram stain, and cultures should be routine when suspecting infection; crystal analysis is also part of the standard examination, but in such a young patient would likely not help much (you would not be able to rule out infectious etiology even with positive crystal analysis: they may occur together.)

* *

The synovial fluid analysis reveals the following findings: 50,000 WBC/mm^3, 95% polymorphonuclear cells, and no crystals. Gram stain shows gram-negative diplococci. The same Gram stain findings are obtained from the urethral, but not the pharyngeal, swab. Cultures are pending.

Which of the following studies will be most important to the OVERALL care of this patient?

A) HIV testing and RPR.
B) Chest x-ray.
C) ANA and RF.
D) Uric acid.
E) ESR and CRP.

Discussion

The correct answer is "A." His presentation is very suggestive of disseminated gonococcal infection with acute arthritis, and the presence of diplococci is virtually diagnostic. Therefore, the clinician must also consider the presence of other sexually transmitted diseases and screen the patient appropriately. Assays for hepatitis B and C have been sent, and tests for chlamydia, HIV, and syphilis should now be performed. Also, the patient must be counseled regarding safe sexual practices (e.g., condom use, abstinence, reduced alcohol use, moving to Antarctica . . . we live in a college town). In this setting, the other studies are less relevant to his overall health.

HELPFUL TIP: Gonococcus is cultured from the joint fluid only about 50% of the time in patients with gonococcal arthritis. Thus, a PCR of the joint fluid and urethral cultures should be done if the Gram stain is negative.

Which of the following is the most appropriate treatment plan for this patient?

A) Ceftriaxone 1 g IV once, followed by cefixime 400 mg PO bid for 14 days. Follow up in 7 days.
B) Admit to hospital, administer ceftriaxone 1 g IV QD, and perform repeat knee aspirations.
C) Admit to the hospital and administer IV and intra-articular ceftriaxone 1 g QD.
D) Ciprofloxacin 500 mg PO BID for 14 days. Follow up in 7 days.
E) Penicillin G 4 MU IV once, followed by amoxicillin 500 mg PO TID for 14 days. Follow up with a rheumatologist.

Discussion

The correct answer is "B." In order to ensure the best outcome, this patient should be admitted for monitoring and repeated joint aspiration. Purulent fluid tends to collect rapidly in the joint spaces in patients with septic arthritis, necessitating frequent drainage until antibiotics work and inflammation begins to subside. Most cases of gonococcal arthritis respond to needle aspiration, but arthroscopic or open debridement is occasionally necessary. Because IV antibiotics have good penetration into synovial fluid, intra-articular antibiotics are not recommended. When culture, PCR, and sensitivity results become available, antibiotic therapy should be tailored to the sensitivities.

HELPFUL TIP: The initial antibiotic of choice in gonococcal arthritis is ceftriaxone, administered IV. In cases in which drug allergies or other contraindications prohibit the use of ceftriaxone, IV spectinomycin is an acceptable alternative. Remember that there is now fluoroquinolone-resistant gonococcus. Because of this, fluoroquinolones are no longer recommended as treatment of gonorrhea.

* *

Within 48 hours, your patient shows signs of improvement. His knee appears much better, there is no recurrent effusion, and he is afebrile. He wants to leave the hospital. By the way, his chlamydia PCR turned up positive.

Which of the following management strategies do you recommend?

A) Continue the hospital admission and ceftriaxone 1 g IV QD.
B) Discharge with ciprofloxacin 500 mg PO BID.
C) Discharge with penicillin V 500 mg PO TID.
D) Discharge with cefixime 400 mg PO BID and doxycycline 100 mg PO BID.
E) Daily emergency center visits for ceftriaxone 1 g IV QD.

Discussion

The correct answer is "D." Since the patient is improving, continued hospitalization and IV antibiotics are not needed. Thus, answer "A" is incorrect. Without knowing the antibiotic sensitivities of the gonococcus, you should assume that it is penicillin-resistant, making "C" a poor choice. Once local and systemic signs are resolving, you can safely discharge the patient with oral antibiotic therapy, using cefixime 400 mg BID (or an acceptable alternative based on culture and susceptibilities) to complete a 7–14 day course. In cases of gonococcal infection, you should presumptively treat for concurrent chlamydia infection. Thus, while "B" is technically correct for the treatment of gonococcus, it is not the best choice for this patient. Answer "D" provides treatment of chlamydia as well.

HELPFUL TIP: Septic arthritis occurs most often in large joints, such as the knee and hip. Factors that predispose a patient to septic arthritis include advancing age (especially >80 years), rheumatoid arthritis, joint prostheses, recent joint surgery, diabetes, and skin infection.

What is the mortality rate of septic arthritis?

A) 0.5%.
B) 5%.
C) 10%.
D) >15%.

Discussion

The correct answer is "C." The mortality rate of septic arthritis is 10%, with up to one-third of survivors having persistent joint problems, such as limited range of motion, pain, and swelling. Note that the mortality is probably not due to the infection alone but rather to a combination of the underlying illness (e.g., immunosuppression) plus the infection.

Objectives: Did you learn to . . .

- Describe the appropriate evaluation of monoarthritis?
- Appropriately manage a patient with septic arthritis?
- Identify risk factors for septic arthritis?
- Recognize the prognosis of septic arthritis?

CASE 4

A 55-year-old male presents to your office complaining of severe left knee pain of 2 days' duration. Although he was also out partying over the weekend (is there a pattern here to the patients in our practice?), he went home early. He denies any previous history of knee pain or arthritis. He has felt feverish over the last 2 days. He recalls a similar episode of pain in his right great toe 2 years before, but the pain resolved in a few days and he did not seek medical attention. He has hypertension treated with chlorthalidone but is otherwise healthy. He drinks about a case of beer per week—unless he's been partying. His family history is remarkable for osteoarthritis.

Physical examination reveals an uncomfortable-appearing obese male in no acute distress. His temperature is 37.9°C, blood pressure 168/98 mm Hg, and pulse 84 bpm. The left knee is red, warm, and diffusely tender with a palpable effusion.

Which of the following is the most appropriate next step to accurately diagnose this condition?

A) Radiograph of the affected knee.
B) CBC.
C) Uric acid level.
D) Knee aspiration and synovial fluid analysis.
E) Diagnostic steroid injection.

Discussion

The correct answer is "D." We don't mean to sound like a broken record, but the diagnostic study of choice in a monoarthritis is synovial fluid analysis. Synovial fluid analysis allows the clinician to determine whether there is an inflammatory, infectious, or crystalline cause of the arthritis. Answer "A" is incorrect. Radiographs are typically not helpful acutely in inflammatory arthritis (but would be indicated if there was trauma or suspicion of tumor). Answers "B" and "C," a CBC and uric acid level, are useful when infection or gout is suspected (and, in fact, the uric acid is often normal during an acute gout attack). However, neither of these lab results will be diagnostic. Finally, steroid injection must be avoided in monoarthritis until the possibility of infection is eliminated.

* *

You successfully aspirate 5 cc of clear yellow synovial fluid from the left knee. While the patient is waiting, the laboratory reports the following findings: 5000 WBC/mm^3, Gram stain negative for bacteria, needle-shaped negatively birefringent crystals are noted.

These synovial fluid findings are most consistent with which of the following diagnoses?

A) Osteoarthritis.
B) Septic arthritis.
C) CPPD ("pseudogout").
D) Gout.

Discussion

The correct answer is "D." Monosodium urate crystals of gout are needle-shaped as seen in this patient's synovial fluid (a good way to remember this is that being stuck with a needle hurts—and so does gout).

Table 11–4 DIAGNOSTIC CRITERIA FOR ACUTE GOUT

Presence of characteristic urate crystals in the joint fluid **or** tophus proved to contain urate crystals by chemical means or polarized light microscopy **or** presence of 6 of the following 12 phenomena:

1. More than 1 attack of acute arthritis
2. Maximal inflammation developed within 1 day
3. Attack of monoarticular arthritis
4. Joint redness observed
5. First MTP joint painful or swollen
6. Unilateral attack involving first MTP joint
7. Unilateral attack involving tarsal joint
8. Suspected tophus
9. Hyperuricemia
10. Asymmetric swelling within a joint (radiograph)
11. Subcortical cysts without erosion (radiograph)
12. Negative joint fluid culture for microorganisms during attack of joint inflammation

Data from Wallace SL, Robinson H, Masi AT, Decker JL, McCarty DJ, Yu TF. Preliminary criteria for the classification of the acute arthritis of primary gout. *Arthritis Rheum.* 1977 Apr; 20(3):895-900.

Calcium pyrophosphate dihydrate crystals are rod-, square-, or rhomboid-shaped and positively birefringent in polarized light. Thus, the synovial fluid findings given above are most consistent with gout. Answer "B" is incorrect. Normally, synovial fluid contains <180 WBC/mm^3, but it is generally considered noninflammatory if the WBC count is <2000/mm^3. Low WBC counts are seen in the synovial fluid of osteoarthritic joints. Synovial fluid containing ≥2000 WBC/mm^3 is consistent with an inflammatory process. When there are >100,000 WBC/mm^3, the monoarthritis is considered septic until proven otherwise. See Table 11–4 for the diagnostic criteria for gout.

HELPFUL TIP: Serum uric acid is often normal during an acute attack of gout (probably because it precipitates in the affected joints); thus, you cannot rely on serum uric acid levels alone to diagnose gout or refute this diagnosis.

HELPFUL TIP: A polarizing microscope is not required to see crystals in synovial fluid! Look under a standard light microscope for either needle-shaped (uric acid) or rhomboid/square (calcium pyrophosphate) crystals.

In general, all of the following are risk factors for gout EXCEPT:

A) Tobacco use.
B) Alcohol use.
C) Obesity.
D) Diuretic use.
E) Family history.

Discussion

The correct answer is "A." Your patient exhibits many of the risk factors for gout, which include male sex, obesity, high-protein diet, high social class (well, we're not so sure about his social class), use of diuretics (either loop or thiazide), alcohol, and family history. However, tobacco use is not associated with gout.

HELPFUL TIP: Many patients with hyperuricemia do **not** develop gout or nephrolithiasis; it is unclear whether asymptomatic hyperuricemia should be treated with uric acid-lowering agents, and research is ongoing to answer this question.

Which of the following is the NEXT step in the management of this patient?

A) Prescribe allopurinol.
B) Prescribe acetaminophen.
C) Discontinue chlorthalidone.
D) Prescribe naproxen.
E) Therapeutic joint aspiration.

Discussion

The correct answer is "D." An acute attack of gout should first be treated with NSAIDs, such as naproxen or indomethacin. The doses prescribed should be at the upper limit for the particular NSAID (e.g., naproxen 500 mg TID). Earlier treatment is associated with greater relief of symptoms and shorter duration of the acute event. Other potential first-line agents are steroids and colchicine. Narcotic pain medication is also appropriate.

"A" is incorrect. Allopurinol is indicated for prophylaxis of gout when hyperuricemia is documented, but its use in the acute setting is **inappropriate**. Initiation of allopurinol may actually cause or worsen exacerbations of gout. "B" is incorrect because acetaminophen lacks the anti-inflammatory properties of NSAIDs and is less effective. Discontinuing chlorthalidone, "C" (a thiazide diuretic), may reduce uric acid levels over time but is not likely to improve symptoms in the acute setting. Joint aspiration is not therapeutic in gout, but may be helpful in pseudogout. Another option for treatment of acute gout is colchicine, given as one dose of 1.2 mg, followed by 0.6 mg twice daily for 1–2 weeks, and then 0.6 mg daily for 2–6 months. **Note that this is a much lower dose than we have been used to giving!**

HELPFUL TIP: Oral or intra-articular steroid administrations are also options for patients who have contraindications to NSAIDs, who have failed NSAID therapy, or who have more severe attacks. Steroids are just as efficacious as NSAIDS and may be more appropriate for patients with CHF, ulcers, or kidney disease. Narcotic pain medication may be needed as an adjunct to your anti-inflammatory. The only currently available colchicine is a brand name drug (Colcrys) and very expensive when compared to generic NSAIDS or steroids.

* *

You start an NSAID. He returns in a few days to discuss his labs and x-rays. A radiograph of the left knee demonstrates an effusion but is otherwise unremarkable. His uric acid level is 10.1 mg/dL (the upper limit of normal for your lab is 7.2 mg/dL). CBC, creatinine, sodium, and potassium are normal. You instruct the patient to reduce his alcohol intake and try to lose weight to decrease his risk of gout attacks and for overall health. You don't see him again for a year (was it something you said?). He has been using naproxen frequently, and he recalls five acute attacks of gout.

Which is the most effective regimen to start now in this patient to reduce the frequency of gout attacks?

A) Twice-daily colchicine.
B) Daily allopurinol.
C) Daily probenecid.
D) Twice-daily colchicine and daily allopurinol.
E) Daily probenecid and allopurinol.

Discussion

The correct answer is "D." Low doses of colchicine administered twice daily have been shown to reduce the frequency of gout attacks 75–85%. This patient also has hyperuricemia and is likely to benefit from lowering his uric acid level. Remember that the initiation of allopurinol may precipitate or worsen an acute attack of gout. Therefore, allopurinol should be initiated only with concurrent use of colchicine or an NSAID.

Probenecid is a uricosuric agent that also reduces the frequency and severity of acute gout attacks but has multiple drug interactions (including allopurinol) and contraindications (e.g., decreased renal function); however, it may well be indicated in the patient who does not achieve his target with allopurinol alone. An attempt should be made to lower uric acid to 6–7 mg/dL with one medication before considering a combination of drugs.

HELPFUL TIP: Febuxostat (Uloric) is an alternative to allopurinol. However, it is rather expensive (10× the cost of allopurinol) and there is postmarketing data suggesting that there is a higher incidence of cardiovascular events in those on febuxostat when compared to allopurinol.

HELPFUL TIP: Although colchicine is recommended as prophylaxis when allopurinol is initiated, it should be discontinued within 6 months (if possible) due to the potential side effects of GI irritation, diarrhea, and myopathy.

All of the following are side affects of allopurinol EXCEPT:

A) Aseptic meningitis.
B) Rash.
C) Leukopenia.
D) Fever.
E) GI disturbance.

Discussion

The correct answer is "A." Additional side effects include elevated liver enzymes, glomerulonephritis, aplastic anemia, and vasculitis. Not a pretty drug, but look on the bright side... it's not associated with meningitis!

HELPFUL TIP: Probenecid should be avoided in patients with a creatinine of clearance <50 ml/min, as it is ineffective and there may be an increased risk of toxicity.

* *

It is 9 years later. America has a system for universal health care. Doctors have jetpacks. WAKE UP! It's all a dream. But your favorite gout patient is real, and he's back. He's had 9 years of acute intermittent gout attacks. ("Of course I took my medication, Doc.") He presents complaining of pain in his knees and feet that has been present for several months. He has also developed swelling and pain in his hands. The pain is less intense than his attacks of gout, but occurs in the same areas and never completely resolves between attacks. He has no morning stiffness, no muscle complaints, and no other systemic complaints. You find diffuse edema of both hands and palpable hard nodules on the knees.

Which of the following is the most likely cause of his current symptoms?

A) Rheumatoid arthritis.
B) Osteoarthritis.
C) Gout.
D) PMR.
E) Lack of universal health care and jetpacks as promised by presidential candidates.

Discussion

The correct answer is "C." This patient has a long history of acute intermittent gout. After years of acute attacks, patients with gout may develop a form of the disease called chronic tophaceous gout (the nodules are deposits of uric acid called tophi; tophus for a single nodule), in which the intercritical periods are no longer free of pain. There are no clinical associations between gout and the other rheumatic conditions mentioned and, therefore, no reason to suspect that another rheumatic disorder is causing the chronic pain.

HELPFUL TIP: Hyperlipidemia occurs in 80% of patients with gout—check lipids.

HELPFUL TIP: In addition to being a fun word, podagra is a useful diagnostic tool. The first MTP joint is affected in 90% of patients with gout, and the initial attack involves the first MTP joint in 50%.

CASE 5

Citing your characteristic compassion and attention to detail, your patient refers a friend he met at Gouty Retirees in Love with Life (GRILL). This friend of his is a 65-year-old female who reports a history of joint swelling, pain, and redness, usually involving her knees, wrists, and hands; she has never had first MTP joint involvement. Although she has never had a joint aspiration performed, she has been treated for gout for 5 years. She faithfully takes her medication but has found allopurinol unhelpful. She is currently asymptomatic, but uses ibuprofen for acute attacks. The joint exam is unremarkable, without joint effusion—but, again, she is currently asymptomatic.

Which of the following studies is most appropriate for this patient?

A) "Diagnostic" knee injection with steroids.
B) CBC.
C) Rheumatoid factor.
D) Radiographs of the knees and wrists.
E) Serum uric acid.

Discussion

The correct answer is "D." The initial evaluation should include radiographs of the affected joints, which may lend clues to the diagnosis. Radiographs may reveal osteophyte formation typical of osteoarthritis, subchondral cysts, and chondrocalcinosis typical of CPPD, or erosions with an overhanging edge typical of gout. Chondrocalcinosis is most often seen in the knees and triangular fibrocartilage of the wrists. Answer "A," an injection of steroids, might help relieve symptoms, but it will not be diagnostic. Answer "B," a CBC, is nonspecific and will not be helpful. Answer "C" is also not going to be helpful given this patient's symptoms, which are not suggestive of RA. Also, RF may be present in inflammatory arthritides other than rheumatoid arthritis, and so will not be helpful. "E," uric acid, is not diagnostic; but if normal during the intercritical period, it might provide evidence against the diagnosis of gout.

> HELPFUL TIP: The crystals of gout (uric acid) and pseudogout (calcium pyrophosphate) can be seen in synovial fluid during intercritical periods. If there is an effusion even in the absence of acute symptoms and you are thinking gout or pseudogout, tap that joint!

* *

Your patient's knee radiographs demonstrate chondrocalcinosis (see Figure 11–1). Examination of synovial fluid from the knee shows positively birefringent, rhomboid crystals consistent with CPPD (pseudogout).

Which of the following do you recommend to decrease her risk of recurrent acute attacks of pseudogout?

A) Serial joint aspiration.
B) Daily allopurinol.
C) Twice-daily colchicine.
D) Serial intra-articular steroid injections.
E) Chondroitin sulfate.

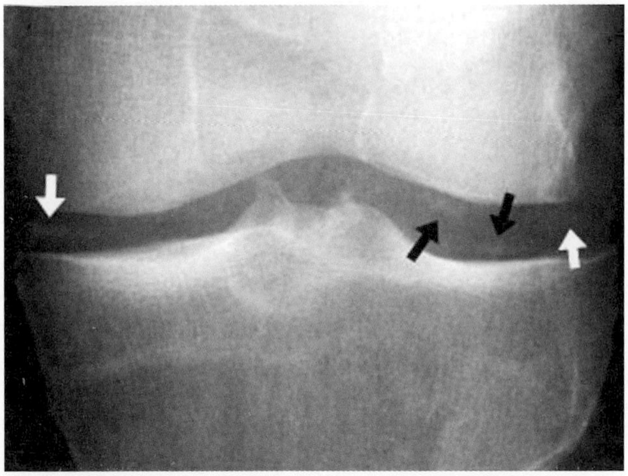

Figure 11–1 **Chondrocalcinosis of the knee joint. (Note arrows highlighting calcification.)**

Discussion

The correct answer is "C." Pseudogout is diagnosed by the presence of CPPD crystals (described above) in synovial fluid and/or typical x-ray findings (basically, chondrocalcinosis). Although prophylaxis is more predictably successful in gout, colchicine 0.6 mg BID has been shown to reduce the frequency of pseudogout attacks in CPPD. NSAIDs or colchicine may be used in acute attacks. Answers "A" and "D" are incorrect. While joint aspiration and steroid injection may be helpful during acute attacks, they have no role in prophylaxis. Answer "B" is also incorrect. Since CPPD is not caused by abnormalities in uric acid metabolism, allopurinol has no role in the management of pseudogout. Finally, chondroitin sulfate does not appear to be useful in osteoarthritis, let alone pseudogout.

> HELPFUL TIP: Gout is more likely to occur during middle age and is more common in men. Pseudogout has a peak incidence later in life and is about equally prevalent in both males and females.

CPPD (pseudogout) is associated with which of the following?

A) Hypothyroidism.
B) Hyperparathyroidism.
C) Amyloidosis.
D) Hemochromatosis.
E) All of the above.

Discussion

The correct answer is "E." All of the above are associated with pseudogout. Additional associated conditions include hypophosphatemia and hypomagnesemia. For this reason, order the following studies in patients newly diagnosed with CPPD: thyroid-stimulating hormone (TSH), calcium, phosphate, magnesium, transferrin saturation, and alkaline phosphatase.

> HELPFUL TIP: Precipitants of gout and pseudogout (CPPD) include trauma, surgery, severe medical illness, and alcohol overindulgence.

Objectives: Did you learn to . . .

- Evaluate recurrent monoarthritis?
- Describe the diagnostic implications of synovial fluid findings?
- Define diagnostic criteria for gout and CPPD?
- Manage a patient with gout and describe adverse effects of the medications used to treat gout?
- Implement appropriate therapy for CPPD?

QUICK QUIZ: CRYOGLOBULINEMIA

Cryoglobulinemia, a vasculitic disease caused by antibodies that precipitate in cold temperatures, is most often caused by which of the following viral infections?

A) HIV.
B) Hepatitis B.
C) Hepatitis C.
D) Parvovirus B19.

Discussion

The correct answer is "C." Hepatitis C is found in 80% of vasculitis cases associated with mixed cryoglobulinemia. Although up to 50% of patients with hepatitis C have cryoglobulins, only a minority of patients have clinical vasculitis. Because of the increasing prevalence of hepatitis C, cases of cryoglobulinemia will most likely increase as well. As to the other answers, hepatitis B and parvovirus B19 infection may cause a symmetric polyarthritis. HIV is less commonly a cause of cryoglobulinemia and is associated with reactive arthritis. The symptoms of mixed cryoglobulinemia associated with HCV infection typically include arthralgias, fever, renal disease, palpable purpura, and neuropathy.

CASE 6

A 13-year-old male presents to your office with his father. The patient complains of pain in his wrists, elbows, and knees bilaterally. He has felt fatigued and has been unable to work his usual summer job as a busboy at his father's restaurant. (Eh? What happened to child labor laws?) He complains of intermittent fevers and an evanescent rash that appears during febrile episodes but is short lived. All of these symptoms have emerged in the last 6 weeks, after a week-long backpacking trip in Minnesota. He has no significant past medical history. His only medication is acetaminophen daily for joint pain. He denies tobacco use, alcohol use, and sexual activity.

The differential diagnosis should include all of the following EXCEPT:

A) Lyme disease.
B) JIA.
C) PMR.
D) Viral illness.

Discussion

The correct answer is "C" of course. From earlier in the chapter, you will recall that the diagnosis of PMR can only be made in persons over the age of 50 years. JIA is a chronic arthritis of childhood that can present in a variety of ways, but must include arthritis of one or more joints, lasting 6 weeks or more, with symptom onset before age 16 years. Likewise, Lyme disease has several presentations, presenting with arthritis early or late in the course. Many viral illnesses can result in arthralgias and/or arthritis. Any of the diseases listed may have associated symptoms of fatigue, malaise, headache, and myalgias. One factor that makes Lyme disease a more likely diagnosis is the history of being outdoors in an endemic area (90% of Lyme disease in the United States occurs in New York, New Jersey, Connecticut, Rhode Island, Massachusetts, Pennsylvania, Wisconsin, and Minnesota).

Which of the following findings on physical examination would be more consistent with Lyme disease than JIA?

A) Bell palsy.
B) Temperature $\geq$38°C.
C) Rash.
D) Lymphadenopathy.
E) A and C.

Discussion

The correct answer is "A." All of the other findings are seen in both Lyme disease and JIA. Neurologic symptoms, including Bell palsy ("A") and even meningitis, may occur with Lyme disease but not JIA. Rash ("C") is present in both diseases but differs substantially. The characteristic rash of Lyme disease is erythema migrans. The rash of JIA is macular, salmon-pink, and brought on by heat. Erythema migrans occurs in about 80% of patients with acute Lyme disease. The lesion is often described as "targetoid," meant to convey a red circular rash with central clearing. However, most patients do not have the classic lesion. Instead, most patients present with a mildly to brightly erythematous patch in the axilla or belt line, where the tick bite occurs. The tick itself is rarely seen. Erythema migrans is usually not painful or pruritic. Both Lyme disease and JIA may have associated systemic findings, including fever and lymphadenopathy, so neither "B" nor "D" is a good discriminator.

* *

Physical examination reveals a thin male in no acute distress. His temperature is 37.3°C, pulse 100 bpm, and blood pressure 120/70 mm Hg. Small, nontender, mobile lymph nodes are palpable in the neck and axillae. There is a large, warm, erythematous patch with central clearing at the patient's left axilla. There is limited range of motion in his right wrist and left elbow. An effusion is palpable at the left knee, which is diffusely tender.

If you were to aspirate the patient's knee—so often the right answer in this chapter—which of the following would you expect to find in the synovial fluid?

A) Greater than 100,000 WBC/mm^3.
B) Predominance of eosinophils.
C) Monosodium urate crystals.
D) Spirochetes.
E) Predominance of polymorphonuclear cells.

Discussion

The correct answer is "E." This patient is presenting now with classic features of Lyme disease. If synovial fluid is obtained in a patient with Lyme arthritis, analysis of the fluid reveals leukocytes, most commonly polymorphonuclear cells. "A" is incorrect. If the synovial fluid has >100,000 WBC/mm^3, you should consider septic arthritis (arthritis in Lyme disease is mostly an immunological phenomenon rather than true septic arthritis). "B" is incorrect because eosinophils are not the predominant cell in synovial fluid of Lyme arthritis. "C" is wrong since monosodium urate crystals are observed in gout—an unlikely cause of this patient's joint complaints. Finally, "D" is wrong. In general, *Borrelia burgdorferi* spirochetes, the causative organism in Lyme disease, are not observed in the synovial fluid.

* *

You strongly suspect Lyme disease and decide not to aspirate the knee effusion.

Which of the following is true regarding laboratory tests for Lyme disease?

A) Serologic tests are reliable within 1 week of the tick bite.
B) Serologic tests are useful in screening for Lyme disease.
C) Blood cultures remain positive for *B. burgdorferi* for months after the tick bite.
D) Serologic tests remain positive for up to 10 years after antibiotic treatment.
E) The diagnosis of Lyme disease is based on serologic tests.

Discussion

The correct answer is "D." Serologic tests for Lyme disease can remain positive for up to 10, and in some cases 20, years after exposure. Thus, serologic tests alone are not diagnostic of active Lyme disease. "E" is incorrect: the diagnosis of Lyme disease is clinical with laboratory tests used to confirm the diagnosis. A positive ELISA test is not adequate to make the diagnosis of Lyme disease. Positive or equivocal ELISA tests should be confirmed with Western blot analysis. "A" is incorrect: serologic assays may be falsely negative early in infection. "B" is incorrect. Because of the high false-positive rate, serologic assays should not be used as a screening tool in the general population. "C" is incorrect: positive blood cultures for *B. burgdorferi* are rarely obtained. When cultures do grow *B. burgdorferi*, it is only early in the disease. Cultures of skin biopsied from the erythema migrans lesion are more likely to be positive.

For this patient, whose weight is 50 kg and who has no known allergies, which course of therapy is safest and most efficacious?

A) Amoxicillin 500 mg PO TID for 1 week.
B) Ceftriaxone 2 g IM, single dose.
C) Doxycycline 100 mg PO BID for 4 weeks.
D) Levofloxacin 250 mg PO QD for 2 weeks.
E) Erythromycin 250 mg PO QID for 4 weeks.

Discussion

The correct answer is "C." Recommended therapy for Lyme arthritis (without neurologic disease) is 4 weeks of either amoxicillin 500 mg TID, doxycycline 100 mg BID, or cefuroxime axetil 500 mg BID. This patient is old enough to take doxycycline, which is generally avoided in children <8 years old due to tooth discoloration. The duration of amoxicillin prescribed here is too short, so "A" is wrong. If this patient was younger and doxycycline was contraindicated, a **4-week** course of amoxicillin or cefuroxime would be the preferred therapy. Ceftriaxone is prescribed when neurologic abnormalities are present (such as Bell palsy or meningitis), and it must be dosed daily for 2–4 weeks. Levofloxacin is not indicated for Lyme disease. Treatment with erythromycin for 4 weeks, while an acceptable alternative, appears to be less efficacious.

HELPFUL TIP: There is no known resistance of *B. burgdorferi* to standard antibiotic regimens.

* *

Several hours after starting antibiotics, your patient's father calls to reports worsening symptoms of fever, shaking, and dizziness.

You recognize this condition as which of the following?

A) An allergic reaction to the antibiotic.
B) *B. burgdorferi* sepsis.
C) Secondary bacterial infection.
D) A cytokine-mediated reaction to the antibiotic-mediated killing of spirochetes (Jarisch–Herxheimer reaction).
E) The expected, natural course of Lyme disease.

Discussion

The correct answer is "D." A Jarisch–Herxheimer reaction occurs in 5–15% of patients treated with antibiotics for Lyme disease. (Remember syphilis? Lyme is also a spirochete disease.) The reaction is mediated by the release of cytokines and occurs within hours of initial administration of antibiotics. In Lyme disease, the reaction is self-limited and usually resolves within a day. Only supportive treatment is necessary, and antibiotics should be continued. "A" is incorrect because this reaction is not typical of a drug allergy. "B" is incorrect because *B. burgdorferi* does not cause sepsis. "C" is incorrect because it is unlikely that a secondary bacterial infection has occurred so quickly. Finally, this does not represent the natural history of Lyme disease ("E"). See Table 11–5 for more on the natural history of Lyme disease.

Table 11–5 STAGES OF LYME DISEASE

Early localized disease (Stage I): Occurs days to a month after the tick bite and includes erythema migrans, fatigue, fever, malaise, myalgias, arthralgia, arthritis, headache, and lymphadenopathy. Except for erythema migrans, it can be confused with a viral illness.

Early disseminated disease (Stage II): Occurs weeks to months after the tick bite; 5–10% have cardiac manifestations (atrioventricular block of any degree, myocarditis/pericarditis, and heart failure) and 10–15% have neurologic manifestations (see below).

Late disease (Stage III): Occurs months to years after the tick bite and includes myalgias, arthralgias, fatigue, polyarthritis, and neurologic symptoms (encephalopathy, cognitive dysfunction, and peripheral neuropathy).

HELPFUL TIP: Lyme disease symptoms typically improve a few days after starting antibiotics.

* *

Since he spends much of his free time hunting deer in Minnesota (loves his gun ... "Everyone should have one," he quips), your patient's father is worried about contracting Lyme disease himself.

What do you recommend for primary prevention of Lyme disease?

A) Weekly tick checks.
B) *N,N*-diethyl-m-toluamide (DEET) application prior to hunting.
C) Daily doxycycline when in endemic areas.
D) Lyme vaccine.
E) Kill as many deer as possible in order to reduce the risk of Lyme disease transmission to humans.

Discussion

The correct answer is "B." Primary prevention is best accomplished with the use of insect repellents when in endemic areas. Also, when in endemic areas, tick checks should be performed daily (not weekly as in answer "A"). A tick that has been attached for <24 hours is not likely to transmit *B. burgdorferi*. Unfortunately, the species that transmits Lyme disease (ticks of the *Ixodes ricinus* complex) are very small and difficult to see. "C" is incorrect. There is no role for routine prophylactic antibiotics. However, if a tick bite from the appropriate species is noticed, a single dose of doxycycline 200 mg administered orally reduces the risk of erythema migrans. The dose should be administered within 72 hours of a known *I. ricinus* tick bite. "D" is not an option for this patient. In 2002, the vaccine was removed from the U.S. market due to low demand. When it was available, antibody titers tended to wane quickly and protection was not complete. After the administration of three vaccinations, the efficacy of the vaccine to prevent Lyme disease was 76% at best. "E" is just plain wrong... what with Bambi and all... And furthermore, the white-footed field mouse, not the white-tailed deer, is the major reservoir of *B. burgdorferi* bacteria.

CASE 7

Your young patient's mother presents with diffuse aching and stiffness worsened by cold weather and stress. She recalls being treated for Lyme disease herself 2 years ago. The physical examination is remarkable for tender points bilaterally at the occiput, trapezius, lateral epicondyle, gluteus, and knee. There is no redness, swelling, or synovial thickening at the knees and elbows. There is no rash.

You suspect that her symptoms are due to which of the following?

A) Chronic Lyme disease.
B) Osteoarthritis.
C) Fibromyalgia.
D) Rheumatoid arthritis.

Discussion

The correct answer is "C." Fibromyalgia is a diagnosis of exclusion, but compared to the other choices, the history and exam findings are most consistent with this diagnosis. If the patient was successfully treated for Lyme disease, she is unlikely to present with late-stage disease. Fibromyalgia may occur coincidentally after treatment of Lyme disease, but it is not due to ongoing infection and does not respond to antibiotics. In fact, a lot of patients who think that they have chronic Lyme disease are actually suffering from depression, fibromyalgia, etc.

> **HELPFUL TIP:** If Lyme meningitis is suspected, confirm by analysis of CSF. Lyme meningitis must be treated with IV ceftriaxone or penicillin G.

Objectives: Did you learn to...

- Describe the appropriate evaluation of polyarthritis?
- Diagnose Lyme disease?
- Describe the stages of Lyme disease?
- Implement appropriate therapy for Lyme disease?
- Discuss preventive strategies for Lyme disease and describe some of the complications of the disease?

CASE 8

A 42-year-old female who was referred by an orthopedic surgeon presents to your office with multiple joint complaints. The orthopedist has seen her for left knee pain, intermittent swelling, occasional "clicking and locking," present for about 10 years. After knee radiograph and exam, the orthopedist diagnosed a chronically damaged meniscus, but he wants the patient evaluated by you for her other joint complaints.

Laboratory data ordered by her orthopedist (apparently, just to confuse you) show an ANA 1:40 (speckled pattern) and an ESR 20 mm/hr. The patient moved to the United States from Guam 4 years ago. She reports poor sleep and feeling quite depressed. She feels that she has no friends, and she has had trouble adjusting to the colder weather. You notice she has a bottle of water with her and upon your specific questioning she states, "I have to sip some water throughout the day. I've done this for the last 15 years because my mouth gets so dry." She denies problems with skin rash, cavities, swallowing, and eye pain. She does not use artificial tears.

Which of the following findings in this patient is the most likely to be a sign of inflammatory arthritis?

A) Spider angiomas (telangiectasia) on the back and abdomen.
B) A positive "bulge sign" on left knee exam.

C) Presence of 16/18 fibromyalgia tender points, with nontender control points.
D) Incomplete left grip.
E) Presence of a holosystolic murmur at the left sternal border, without radiation.

Discussion

The correct answer is "D." Although her symptoms are suggestive of fibromyalgia and depression, it is critical to differentiate between an inflammatory and a noninflammatory condition, especially since many inflammatory disorders (e.g., systemic lupus erythematosus [SLE], RA, and Sjögren syndrome) may masquerade as fibromyalgia. An incomplete grip in an otherwise healthy young woman is suggestive of synovitis, which can be further assessed by careful small joint exam. When synovitis is present, it is always abnormal and suggests an inflammatory arthritis, requiring further evaluation. "A" is incorrect because telangiectasias on the abdomen and trunk are typically related to liver disease, while those found on hands and nail beds are associated with scleroderma and other rheumatic diseases. "B," a positive knee "bulge sign" (swelling of the knee joint that bulges inferiorly when compressed superiorly), indicates fluid in the left knee joint. But from the patient's history and your orthopedic colleague's determination, this finding is chronic and mechanical in nature. "C," the presence of 16/18 tender points, would argue for fibromyalgia but would not help to differentiate between inflammatory and noninflammatory disorders. Finally, a holosystolic murmur ("E"), localized to the left sternal border and present in a healthy young woman, is nonspecific and most likely functional. If there were other signs and symptoms of cardiac disease, the murmur might indicate a more serious disorder.

* *

On physical examination, you find a "bulge sign" on the left knee, but no other joint swelling. She has 16/18 tender points and normal range of motion and strength. The neurological exam is grossly normal, except for poorly defined numbness and pain to touch on the left side of her face. You also notice a **mildly tender, hard, nodular swelling behind the angle of the mandible** on the left in the area of the parotid gland. Her oral mucosa appears dry. Her conjunctiva is mildly, symmetrically injected.

All of the following studies and interventions are appropriate EXCEPT:

A) CBC, transaminases, uric acid, ESR, CRP.
B) Anti-SS-A (Ro), anti-SS-B (La), anti-dsDNA, RF, serum protein electrophoresis.
C) Prescribe trazodone 50 mg PO QHS and recommend aerobic exercises.
D) Prescribe prednisone 20 mg PO QD, with calcium and vitamin D supplement.
E) Maxillofacial MRI.

Discussion

The correct answer (and the thing to avoid right now) is "D." Although prednisone may be used to treat symptoms of autoimmune diseases, at this time the diagnosis is not secure, and initiating steroid therapy exposes the patient to potentially unnecessary risk. She has findings of Sjögren syndrome—red (possibly dry) eyes, dry mouth, and enlarged parotid glands. However, the differential of mass in the parotid gland must include malignancy (e.g., lymphoma), sarcoidosis, and other autoimmune diseases. The laboratory tests offered in answers "A" and "B" may help assess other organ involvement of Sjögren syndrome and also aid in confirming the diagnosis. Other potential manifestations of Sjögren syndrome include generalized vasculitis, interstitial lung disease, cirrhosis, peripheral and cranial neuropathies, possibly thyroid disease, and renal disease leading to proteinuria and renal tubule dysfunction. Although not listed as an option, chest radiograph may also be helpful, assessing for findings associated with the diseases on your differential: Sjögren syndrome (interstitial lung disease), sarcoidosis (adenopathy and interstitial disease), and lymphoma (adenopathy). Answer "E" is also important because although parotid enlargement may be seen in Sjögren syndrome, it is usually symmetrical and nontender. An imaging study is appropriate to rule out a neoplastic process. Finally, "C" is correct. Her symptoms of fibromyalgia may respond to trazodone and exercise, and these low-risk interventions are appropriate at this juncture.

* *

She starts trazodone and exercise and feels better. The tests you order return as follows: negative SSA, SSB, and dsDNA; elevated RF; no monoclonal protein on SPEP but diffusely elevated globulins. A chest x-ray is normal. Her ESR is 35 mm/hr and CRP 0.5. A maxillofacial MRI shows an enlarged left parotid, with an ill-defined 2×3×1.5 cm dense signal in the center without neurovascular compromise.

What is the most appropriate next step in the management of this patient?

A) Continue your current management and adopt a "watchful waiting" approach.
B) Refer for biopsy of the left parotid.
C) Initiate prednisone 20 mg PO QD, with calcium and vitamin D.
D) Refer for lip biopsy.
E) Perform a gallium scan.

Discussion
The correct answer is "B." Even though her presentation is suggestive of Sjögren syndrome, the presence of a mass-like formation on MRI is concerning for lymphoma, and further evaluation (e.g., biopsy) is required. Additionally, the negative SSA and SSB, while not excluding Sjögren syndrome, will make a biopsy necessary for diagnosis. Although a lip biopsy ("D") may be diagnostic of Sjögren syndrome, the parotid biopsy should be done first due to the presence of a mass. The elevated RF and polyclonal gammopathy are consistent with Sjögren syndrome, and the ESR may be elevated due to increased globulins. Gallium scan ("E"), used in the past for diagnosis of lymphoma, has poor sensitivity and specificity.

* *

Results of the parotid gland biopsy report read, "Lymphocytic infiltrate, no malignant cells noted." You then order flow cytometry, and it has no markers for lymphoma. Her biopsy scar has healed nicely, and she has no pain or numbness. You believe that she probably has Sjögren syndrome.

What would you do next?

A) CT chest/abdomen/pelvis.
B) Start prednisone 20 mg PO QD, with calcium and vitamin D.
C) Recommend sugarless lemon drops and artificial tears as needed and continued trazodone and exercise.
D) Wide excision of the parotid gland.
E) Tell her a sad story to assess lacrimation.

Discussion
The correct answer is "C." Lemon drops will stimulate saliva production, helping with her dry mouth. Artificial tears may also be indicated for dry eyes. At this time your working diagnosis is Sjögren syndrome, and definitive diagnosis by lip biopsy is not likely to alter your therapy; and "D" is way too aggressive anyway. If you require a more definitive diagnosis, a lip biopsy would be better. Since she has responded to trazodone and exercise and there is no evidence of systemic involvement, no further anti-inflammatory therapy ("B") is warranted. If she were to develop arthritis or other signs of systemic involvement (e.g., cognitive dysfunction or peripheral neuropathy), prednisone would be an option. Further workup for lymphoma, such as CT scanning ("A"), does not appear warranted. However, she will require active surveillance, since patients with Sjögren syndrome carry an increased risk of developing lymphoma.

> HELPFUL TIP: Sicca symptoms (dry eyes and mouth) are extremely common, especially in the elderly, and should be confirmed by objective physical findings. Definitive diagnosis of Sjögren syndrome relies on the presence of anti-SS-A or anti-SS-B antibodies or histopathologic gland findings on minor salivary gland (lip) biopsy.

CASE 9

Once again, your fabled diagnostic and therapeutic abilities have earned you a well-deserved referral. Your patient is very happy with the way things are going with her Sjögren syndrome. She refers her sister-in-law to you. The sister-in-law is 46 years old and reports having been diagnosed with fibromyalgia several months ago. She takes only acetaminophen and codeine as needed for pain.

Which of the following is the BEST medication option for treating fibromyalgia?

A) Tramadol (Ultram).
B) Hydromorphone (OxyContin).
C) Acetaminophen with codeine.
D) Nortriptyline (Pamelor).
E) Fluoxetine (Prozac) or another SSRI.

Discussion
The correct answer is "D." Of those listed, the tricyclic antidepressant (TCA) nortriptyline is the best

treatment option. Narcotics (answers "A–C") can be used but are third- or fourth line after TCAs. However, patients may develop tolerance so that narcotics become less effective over time. Fluoxetine will treat depression, which can be associated with fibromyalgia, but will not treat the sleep disorder, which is a major problem in fibromyalgia. NSAIDs can be effective, good sleep hygiene is necessary, but low-impact exercises and reconditioning is the most therapeutic intervention for fibromyalgia.

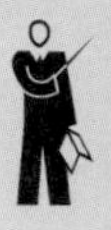

HELPFUL TIP: Fibromyalgia is a common yet poorly understood syndrome characterized by diffuse chronic pain accompanied by other somatic symptoms, accompanied by poor sleep, fatigue, and stiffness, in the absence of identifiable disease. In order to diagnose fibromyalgia, 11 of 18 trigger points must be tender (see Figure 11–2), symptoms must be present for at least 3 months, and other rheumatic conditions must be excluded. There is a female predominance in fibromyalgia, with perhaps 75% of patients being women.

All of the following are associated with fibromyalgia EXCEPT:

A) Irritable bowel syndrome.
B) Subjective fullness/swelling of hands and feet.
C) Paresthesias.
D) Fatigue.
E) Night sweats.

Discussion

The correct answer is "E." All of the others are associated with fibromyalgia. Additional symptoms include headaches, depression, sleep disturbance (which may actually be the etiology), other GI symptoms, and urethral spasm with dysuria and urgency.

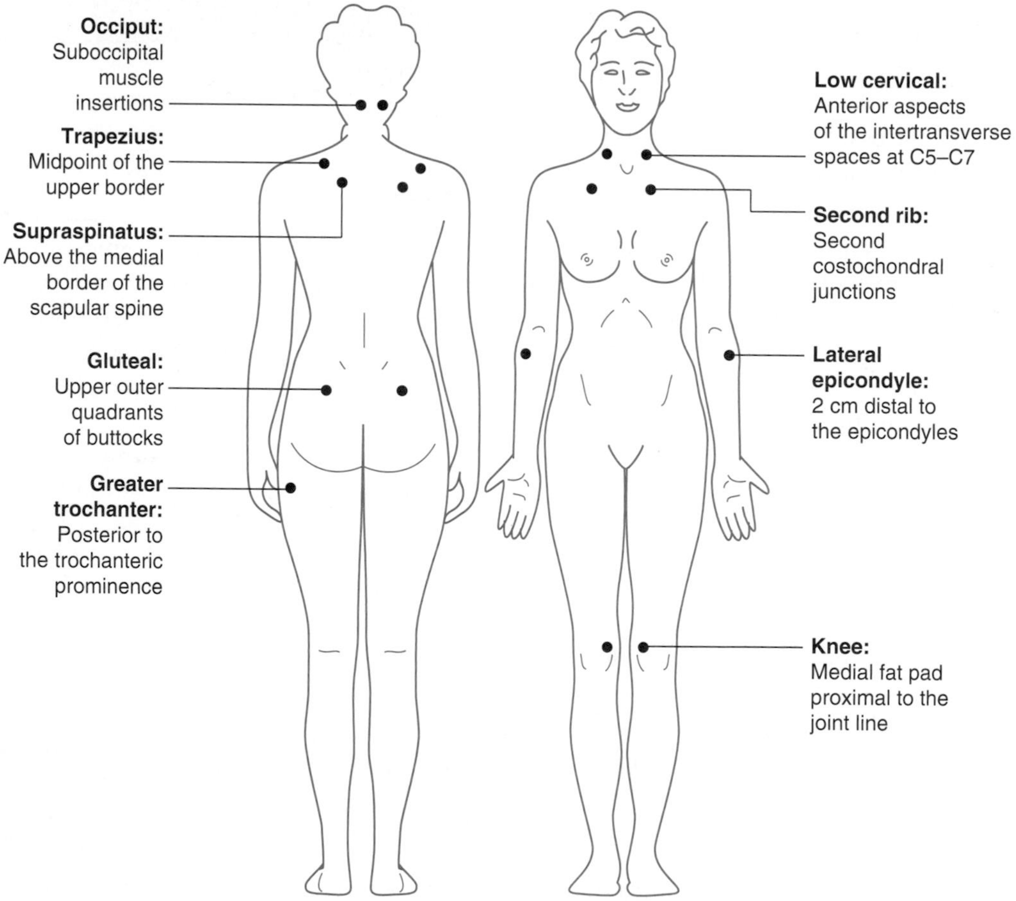

Figure 11–2 **Tender points in fibromyalgia.**

> HELPFUL TIP: Although some SNRIs (Duloxetine, Savella) are FDA approved for fibromyalgia, they are not as effective as the TCAs.

Objectives: Did you learn to . . .

- Describe the appropriate evaluation of polyarthralgia and sicca symptoms?
- Define diagnostic criteria for fibromyalgia and Sjögren syndrome?
- Implement appropriate therapy for fibromyalgia and Sjögren syndrome?

QUICK QUIZ: OSTEOARTHRITIS

All of the following systemic diseases are secondary causes of osteoarthritis EXCEPT:

A) FIbromyalgia.
B) Hemochromatosis.
C) Hyperparathyroidism.
D) Amyloidosis.

Discussion

The correct answer is "A." One of the most common secondary causes of osteoarthritis is previous joint trauma. Systemic diseases that can lead to osteoarthritis include hemochromatosis, hyperparathyroidism, and amyloidosis. FIbromyalgia does not cause osteoarthritis. Any disease, such as diabetes, that leads to a neuropathy can predispose to osteoarthritis (Charcot arthropathy).

CASE 10

A 25-year-old Asian American female presents to your office complaining of bifrontal headaches, occurring intermittently over the last year. Also, she complains of fatigue that seems to be slowly worsening. Over the last 2–3 months, she has developed generalized joint pain and stiffness. The remainder of the history, including a detailed review of systems, is unremarkable.

On physical examination, you find a thin female in no acute distress. She is afebrile with a blood pressure of 110/62 mm Hg and a pulse of 72 bpm. The joint exam shows full range of motion and no swelling. There is mild anterior cervical lymphadenopathy. Close inspection of her skin reveals erythema of the malar eminences and the nose laterally, with involvement of the nasolabial folds. You note flaking and scaling in the eyebrows.

The RASH is most characteristic of which of the following diagnoses?

A) Dermatomyositis.
B) Systemic lupus erythematosus (SLE).
C) Seborrheic dermatitis.
D) Psoriasis.

Discussion

The correct answer is "C." The classic rash of SLE is the malar, or "butterfly," rash with erythema over the malar eminences, bridging over the base of the nose. However, the nasolabial folds are spared. Involvement of the nasolabial fold characteristically occurs in seborrheic dermatitis. In dermatomyositis, facial lesions involve the upper lids and have a light reddish-purple hue (the so called "heliotrope rash"). Flat-topped, violaceous papules over the knuckles (Gottron papules) are classic features of dermatomyositis. The typical lesions of psoriasis include erythematous papules and plaques with silvery scales, noted more commonly on extensor surfaces.

Which of the following diagnoses or descriptions most accurately describes your patient's disease process at this point in time?

A) Fibromyalgia.
B) Somatoform disorder.
C) Polyarthritis.
D) Polyarthralgia.
E) Rheumatoid arthritis.

Discussion

The correct answer is "D." Your patient complains of pain in multiple joints but has no findings of inflammation of the joints; therefore, the designation of "polyarthralgia" fits best at this time. If multiple joints were inflamed, you would use the term polyarthritis. At this time, you do not have enough information to make any of the other diagnoses.

* *

You screen for depression and anxiety and find neither. You recommend acetaminophen for joint pain and headaches and encourage her to exercise regularly. She returns 2 months later feeling worse. She has severe fatigue and joint pain, most commonly involving her hands and knees. She has taken a leave of absence from her job as a high school English teacher. New symptoms include sores in her mouth as well as chest pain, which is worse with inspiration. On exam you note the presence of a cardiac friction rub. There is diffuse tenderness to palpation of both knees and a small effusion apparent in the left knee. Her left hand demonstrates slow, incomplete grip. The facial rash is barely noticeable. There are two nontender ulcerations of the oral mucosa. The remainder of the examination is unchanged from her previous visit.

Her disease process and current findings are most suggestive of which of the following diagnoses?

A) Lymphoma.
B) SLE.
C) Fibromyalgia.
D) Reactive arthritis.
E) CREST syndrome.

Discussion

The correct answer is "B." While she does not meet all the criteria for a diagnosis of SLE, this presentation is more consistent with SLE than any of the other options. Several findings point toward SLE: arthritis, cardiac friction rub (presumably due to pericarditis), and painless oral ulcers. Keep reading for more on the diagnostic criteria for SLE.

* *

You recognize that your patient may be at higher than normal risk for developing SLE.

All of the following groups have a higher incidence of SLE than the general population EXCEPT:

A) Family members of patients with SLE.
B) Females.
C) Asian Americans.
D) African Americans.
E) Caucasians.

Discussion

The correct answer is "E." Compared to other groups, Caucasians have a lower risk of SLE. The peak incidence of SLE occurs in the third to fifth decades of life. Women are 5–10 times more likely than men to be diagnosed with SLE. First-degree relatives of patients with SLE are at higher risk as well. Twin studies have shown a 25–50% concordance rate among monozygotic twins.

* *

You consider that this might represent drug-related lupus, but your patient denies using any medications except for acetaminophen.

In drug-related lupus, you expect to see all of the following EXCEPT:

A) Negative ANA.
B) Rapid resolution of symptoms after discontinuing the drug.
C) Polyarthralgia.
D) Negative anti-dsDNA.
E) Low-grade fever.

Discussion

The correct answer is "A." Patients with drug-induced lupus will generally have a positive ANA. However, it can be differentiated from SLE by a negative anti-dsDNA. Drug-related lupus presents with a lupus-like syndrome, with the most common features being arthralgias, myalgias, fatigue, malaise, and low-grade fever. Pericarditis and pleuritis are occasionally present. Skin, renal, and neurologic involvement are rare.

* *

Your patient returns with a painful, swollen left knee, and she wants to do something about it. You also discuss the following laboratory test results: WBC 5100 cells/mm^3, Hb 11.0 g/dL, platelets 309,000 cells/mm^3; BUN 10 mg/dL, creatinine 1.0 mg/dL; ESR 77 mm/hr; ANA 1:1280 with a nucleolar pattern; urinalysis +1 protein, otherwise negative; chest x-ray shows no cardiomegaly and normal lung fields; ECG shows normal sinus rhythm. You believe that your patient has SLE.

Which of the following management plans do you suggest to the patient?

A) Start ibuprofen 600 mg PO TID and refer to a rheumatologist (3–6 month wait—sheesh, they are busy).
B) Start prednisone 20 mg PO QD and hydroxychloroquine 400 mg PO QD, schedule for follow-up in 1 month, and refer to a rheumatologist (3–6 month wait).
C) Start methotrexate 10 mg PO weekly, prednisone 60 mg PO QD, and hydroxychloroquine 400 mg PO QD, and schedule follow-up in 1 month.
D) Start prednisone 60 mg PO QD and refer to a rheumatologist (3–6 months wait).

E) Start ibuprofen 600 mg PO QD and adopt a "watchful waiting" approach with follow-up in 6 months.

Discussion

The correct answer is "B." Your patient now meets diagnostic criteria for SLE, according to the American College of Rheumatology. See Table 11–6 for the diagnostic criteria for SLE. **Note that a positive ANA is only one of the criteria and is not required for the diagnosis of lupus.** Prompt treatment of her symptoms is important. NSAIDs, such as ibuprofen, are useful in treating arthralgias, mild arthritis, and mild pleurisy and pericarditis. In this case, oral (or perhaps intra-articular) steroids are indicated for immediate symptomatic relief of her arthritis, and a low-to-moderate oral dose should be used (20 mg rather than 60 mg). Vitamin D and calcium supplements should be prescribed with the steroids. Methotrexate can be used in recurrent, persistent arthritis. In the event of more serious renal, hematologic, or neurologic disease, high-dose steroids are employed. Hydroxychloroquine may provide relief of musculoskeletal and constitutional symptoms and may also have a steroid-sparing effect. Ideally, this patient should also be referred to a rheumatologist, but appropriate treatment should be started in a timely fashion.

Table 11–6 DIAGNOSTIC CRITERIA FOR SYSTEMIC LUPUS ERYTHEMATOSUS

SLE requires the presence of 4 of the 11 findings below, not necessarily occurring at the same time.

1. Malar rash
2. Discoid rash
3. Photosensitivity
4. Oral ulcers (usually painless)
5. Arthritis (involving 2 or more peripheral joints)
6. Serositis (pericarditis or pleuritis)
7. Renal disorder (proteinuria >0.5 g/day or cellular casts)
8. Neurologic disorder (seizures or psychosis)
9. Hematologic disorder (hemolytic anemia, leukocyte count <4000/mm^3, lymphocyte count <1500/mm^3, or platelet count <100,000/mm^3)
10. Positive ANA
11. Immunologic disorder (anti-DNA, anti-Smith, or antiphospholipid antibodies, or a false-positive serologic test for syphilis)

Data from Tan EM, Cohen AS, Fries JF, Masi AT, McShane DJ, Rothfield NF, et al. The 1982 revised criteria for the classification of systemic lupus erythematosus. *Arthritis Rheum.* 1982;25:1271-1277.

Close follow-up is necessary due to the potential adverse effects of these medications (e.g., diabetes with prednisone).

* *

Over the next year, your patient does very well. She establishes a relationship with a rheumatologist and is in remission when she sees you next. She is interested in becoming pregnant and wishes to seek your advice prior to trying to conceive. ("Start a college fund early," you say. "Oh, that's not what you meant?") Fortunately, she has been able to discontinue prednisone and continues to tolerate hydroxychloroquine.

With regard to pregnancy and SLE, your patient is at higher risk for all of the following EXCEPT:

A) Premature birth.
B) Infertility.
C) Intrauterine fetal demise.
D) Spontaneous abortion.

Discussion

The correct answer is "B." Women with SLE have a greater risk of premature birth, spontaneous abortion, and intrauterine fetal demise compared with otherwise healthy women. However, these patients appear to have comparable rates of fertility. Pregnancy outcomes are best when the patient is in remission 6–12 months before conception. Pregnancy appears to have a variable affect on SLE, with some patients experiencing exacerbations of the disease.

* *

Your patient does well with her pregnancy but develops recurrent DVTs in the subsequent few years. You wish to evaluate her for antiphospholipid antibody syndrome.

Which of the following results would you expect to find in a patient with antiphospholipid antibody syndrome?

A) Elevated PT/INR.
B) Low PT/INR.
C) Elevated aPTT.
D) Shortened bleeding time.
E) High-fibrin degradation products.

Discussion

The correct answer is "C." Even though they are prone to clotting, patients with antiphospholipid antibody syndrome have a paradoxically elevated aPTT. If this abnormality does not correct in vitro with addition of normal serum, it is presumptive evidence of antiphospholipid antibody syndrome. Besides venous thrombus formation, women with antiphospholipid antibody syndrome are more likely to have late fetal demise and multiple spontaneous abortions.

HELPFUL TIP: Antiphospholipid antibody syndrome is caused by three separate types of antibodies: anticardiolipin antibodies, lupus anticoagulant, and anti-beta-2-glycoprotein I antibodies. These can be detected by direct assay, but there is only an 85% concordance between the presence of antiphospholipid antibody syndrome and laboratory detection of the causative antibodies.

HELPFUL TIP: Only about 10% of patients with lupus have antiphospholipid antibodies.

Which of the following statements is (are) true?

A) Patients with anticardiolipin antibodies should be treated prophylactically even if they have never had a clot, in order to prevent the development of clots.
B) Percent factor II activity is an appropriate way to monitor the response to heparin in patients with antiphospholipid antibody syndrome.
C) Antifactor Xa should be used to monitor the activity of enoxaparin if monitoring is required.
D) A and C
E) B and C.

Discussion

The correct answer is "E." Both "B" and "C" are true statements. Since patients with antiphospholipid antibody syndrome have an elevated aPTT, this value cannot be used to monitor anticoagulation with standard heparin. Percent factor II activity is the most appropriate way to monitor these patients if they are on standard heparin. Antifactor Xa is used to monitor anticoagulation with enoxaparin. "A" is incorrect because there is no evidence that prophylactic treatment reduces complications (although there is significant controversy in this area). Clearly, after a patient has had a thrombotic event, or has another indication, she needs anticoagulation.

HELPFUL TIP: Unfractionated heparin, low-molecular-weight heparin, and aspirin are all used in the treatment of antiphospholipid antibody syndrome in pregnancy. Warfarin is FDA Class X and is teratogenic (remember, it is rat poison!).

Which of the following drugs used to treat lupus is associated with macular damage, corneal opacities, and ciliary muscle dysfunction?

A) Azathioprine.
B) Prednisone.
C) Hydroxychloroquine.
D) Cyclophosphamide.
E) Methotrexate.

The correct answer is "C." Hydroxychloroquine is associated with macular damage, corneal opacities, and ciliary muscle dysfunction, and its use requires yearly eye exams. Other SLE drugs and side effects are noted in Table 11–7.

Objectives: Did you learn to . . .

- Identify clinical manifestations of SLE?
- Define diagnostic criteria for SLE?
- Recognize the waxing and waning course of SLE?
- Implement appropriate treatment of the patient with SLE?
- Recognize adverse effects of medications used in the treatment of SLE?
- Describe some characteristics of antiphospholipid antibody syndrome?

Table 11–7 TOXICITIES ASSOCIATED WITH MEDICATIONS USED TO TREAT SLE

- NSAIDs: gastrointestinal bleeding, renal dysfunction, hypertension
- Steroids: diabetes, hypertension, hyperlipidemia, osteoporosis, cataract formation, weight gain, infections
- Hydroxychloroquine: macular damage, ciliary muscle dysfunction, corneal opacities, myopathy
- Azathioprine: infections, myelosuppression, hepatotoxicity
- Cyclophosphamide: infections, myelosuppression, hemorrhagic cystitis
- Methotrexate: infections, myelosuppression, hepatic fibrosis

CASE 11

A 22-year-old white female presents to your office with the chief complaint of "blue fingers." She reports a history of intermittent bluish discoloration of the fingertips on both hands when they are exposed to cold temperatures. Although she believes the symptoms are worse now, she cannot recall how long they have been present. She has never had ulcers on her fingers or toes.

With no further information, what is the most likely explanation for these digital color changes?

A) Atherosclerotic disease of the extremities.
B) Acrocyanosis.
C) Scleroderma.
D) Physiologic response to cold.

Discussion

The correct answer is "D." At this point all we know is that this patient's fingers turn blue upon exposure to cold. This is a normal physiologic response—vasoconstriction in response to cold. "A" is incorrect. Peripheral vascular disease is the result of atherosclerotic disease of the extremities and typically occurs in older individuals; manifestations include claudication and skin ulceration. "B" is incorrect. Raynaud phenomenon must be distinguished from acrocyanosis, (a rare vasospastic disorder of persistent coldness and bluish discoloration of the hands and feet, not just fingers and toes, which may follow a viral infection). "C" is also incorrect. Scleroderma by itself does not cause blue fingers.

HELPFUL TIP: Over 80% of cases of Raynaud phenomenon that present to a primary care physician's office are due to an exaggerated physiologic response to cold or emotional distress. Although Raynaud phenomenon occurs in most patients with scleroderma (90–95%), the converse is not true. Thus, the presence of Raynaud phenomenon is not synonymous with the presence of scleroderma.

HELPFUL TIP: Buerger disease (thromboangiitis obliterans) is strongly associated with tobacco abuse and presents with distal small vessel ischemia and symptoms that are similar to Raynaud phenomenon. It eventually progresses to infarction of tissue, frequently requiring digit amputation.

* *

Further history reveals that the patient uses no medications. She has been healthy all of her life. Her mother and aunt have had blue fingers in cold temperature, too. She denies tobacco use. The review of systems is unremarkable.

All of the following are expected findings in patients with primary Raynaud phenomenon EXCEPT:

A) Symmetric involvement of the hands.
B) Well-demarcated cyanosis.
C) Digital ulcerations.
D) Normal ESR.

Discussion

The correct answer is "C." Primary Raynaud phenomenon is diagnosed when other causes of Raynaud phenomenon have been eliminated. Primary Raynaud phenomenon is not typically destructive, and digital ulcerations generally occur when the phenomenon is secondary to some other disease process (e.g., scleroderma and SLE). Primary Raynaud phenomenon is almost always symmetric. Raynaud phenomenon can be differentiated from a normal response to cold temperatures by the demarcation between pale or cyanotic fingertips and normal-appearing skin. A normal response to cold may include mottling, with indistinct borders between pale and purple-colored skin, and paresthesias of the involved area. In Raynaud's patients, the distal-most portion of the involved digit is pale or cyanotic, and the transition to normal skin color is abrupt. Since primary Raynaud's is not due to an inflammatory condition, markers of inflammation such as the ESR are usually normal.

HELPFUL TIP: Nail fold capillary microscopy (NCM) can be used to examine the nail fold capillaries of patients with Raynaud phenomenon. NCM involves placing a drop of oil (a drop of surgical lubricant also works well) on the cuticle of one or more digits and visualization of the nail fold capillaries through an ophthalmoscope set at 40 diopters (40 green). Usually the ring fingers (or symptomatic fingers) are examined. Normal capillaries are symmetric, nondilated loops. Distorted, dilated, or absent capillaries suggest secondary Raynaud phenomenon.

* *

You perform a physical examination, including NCM (what's the CPT code for that one, eh?), which is essentially normal. There is currently no discoloration of the fingers.

What is the next most appropriate step in the evaluation and management of this patient?

A) Cold provocation.
B) Doppler ultrasound of the extremities.
C) Blood viscosity testing.
D) ANA.
E) A trial of therapy, nonpharmacologic and/or pharmacologic.

Discussion

The correct answer is "E." Given that she is symptomatic, a trial of drug therapy is warranted. "A," cold provocation, is not recommended, as the diagnosis is based on a convincing history of episodic cyanosis. The results of cold provocation are inconsistent. "B," Doppler ultrasound, might be useful if you were considering large vessel disease from atherosclerosis, etc. However, it is not likely to be helpful in this patient. "C," blood viscosity testing, is not something that is done routinely. "D," an ANA, will be low yield in this case, nonspecific, and would not rule in or rule out disease. However, patients with Raynaud phenomenon and a positive ANA may have a higher risk of developing a systemic autoimmune disease. Based on her age, symmetric involvement, lack of ulcerations, and lack of other symptoms, this patient most likely has primary Raynaud phenomenon unrelated to an underlying disease. A secondary cause (e.g., scleroderma) is more likely with any of the following: patients are 30 years old or older; attacks are asymmetric or associated with skin ulcers; there are symptoms suggestive of systemic involvement (e.g., arthralgias, dyspnea, reflux, and weight loss). If you are concerned about secondary Raynaud phenomenon, an ANA would be indicated.

HELPFUL (FINGER) TIP: Most patients with secondary Raynaud phenomenon will develop symptoms of their underlying autoimmune disease within a few years of onset of Raynaud phenomenon.

* *

After reviewing the diagnosis with your patient, you make several recommendations to help reduce the frequency of attacks: avoid cold temperatures, reduce emotional stress, and avoid tobacco and medications that cause vasoconstriction (e.g., sympathomimetic drugs).

Your patient returns 10 months later with new complaints. Both hands are swollen, stiff, and painful. She complains of multiple joint aches and fatigue despite sleeping well. Her appetite is normal, and she has no GI complaints. Although she has no rash, she complains of itchy hands (surely a sign of cancer, she thinks). On exam, you note that there is diffuse, nonpitting edema of her fingers and hands. She has difficulty making a fist. She has no skin findings. Her CBC is normal. Her ANA is strongly positive with a nucleolar pattern.

Which of the following is the most likely explanation of these findings?

A) Raynaud phenomenon.
B) Rheumatoid arthritis.
C) Scleroderma.
D) CREST syndrome.
E) Iron Fist of Ivan the Terrible syndrome.

Discussion

The correct answer is "C." This patient is now presenting with symptoms of scleroderma, also called systemic sclerosis. Scleroderma encompasses a heterogeneous group of conditions, which are variable in severity but share a common pathophysiologic mechanism—fibrosis of the skin and other organs. The pathology of scleroderma also involves small vessel vasculopathy, a process that leads to Raynaud phenomenon and ischemia of other tissues. Scleroderma may affect the joints, skin, lungs, kidneys, heart, and GI system. Fifty percent of patients with scleroderma have depression.

A positive ANA can be helpful when you suspect scleroderma based on clinical findings. ANA by indirect immunofluorescence will report nuclear staining pattern. Centromere or nucleolar patterns are most highly associated with systemic sclerosis, but other patterns (such as speckled) are also seen. Patients with systemic sclerosis may have a negative ANA.

These findings are now much more than you would expect to see with Raynaud phenomenon; thus, "A" is incorrect. Diffuse swelling and stiffness is present rather than specific synovitis, so "B" (RA) is less likely. CREST syndrome ("D") is a type of systemic sclerosis with the acronym standing for calcinosis cutis, Raynaud phenomenon, esophageal dysmotility, sclerodactyly, and telangiectasia. Your patient does not have all of the findings of CREST syndrome—yet!

HELPFUL TIP: Further diagnosis and categorization of scleroderma can be accomplished with the aid of more specific serologic tests, which are less readily available (e.g., anticentromere—ANA if done by ELISA—or Scl-70 antibodies). Treatment is mainly symptomatic, though immunosuppressive therapies are showing promise in the long-term management of organ-threatening disease, such as interstitial lung disease.

* *

Because of the digital ulcers you observed and the increasing pain of her Raynaud phenomenon attacks, you decide to prescribe medication for Raynaud phenomenon.

Which of the following is the best therapy for reducing the frequency of attacks of Raynaud phenomenon?

A) Amlodipine 5 mg daily.
B) Nifedipine 10 mg as needed.
C) Nitroglycerin 2% ointment daily.
D) Diltiazem 30 mg as needed.
E) Prazosin 1 mg twice daily.

Discussion

The correct answer is "A." All of the medications listed are potentially helpful treatments when Raynaud phenomenon does not respond to conservative measures. However, the most appropriate choice is daily amlodipine. Dihydropyridine calcium-channel blockers, like amlodipine, have been shown to reduce the frequency of attacks by about 50% compared with placebo. They must be scheduled, rather than used as needed (thus "B" is incorrect). Diltiazem is not as effective as the dihydropyridine calcium-channel blockers. In systemic sclerosis, the benefit of calcium-channel blockers is often offset by their exacerbation of GERD. In these patients, ACE inhibitors or angiotensin receptor blockers (ARBs) are also beneficial for Raynaud phenomenon. Topical vasodilators like nitroglycerin have a role if calcium-channel blockers are not effective or the patient cannot tolerate them. There is less evidence that prazosin is effective, but alpha-antagonists have a role if other therapies are unsuccessful. Sildenafil, a phosphodiesterase inhibitor, appears to promote healing of digital ulcers.

Which of the following is NOT indicated for acute ischemic crisis related to Raynaud phenomenon?

A) Aspirin.
B) Beta-blocker.
C) Nifedipine.
D) Digital or wrist nerve block.
E) Topical nitroglycerin.

The correct answer is "B." Beta-blockers are not indicated in the treatment of an ischemic crisis related to Raynaud phenomenon. Beta-blockers actually cause peripheral vasoconstriction and may worsen the problem. Peripherally, **beta-agonists** cause vasodilatation. Thus, when a beta-blocker is used, the patient ends up with an unopposed alpha-adrenergic response, which worsens vasoconstriction. All of the other therapies are useful in acute ischemic crisis. Of particular note is "D." A nerve or wrist block with lidocaine effectively causes a sympathectomy, leading to decreased vascular tone. As mentioned above, sildenafil appears to be beneficial in healing ischemic ulcers and for acute ischemic crisis.

HELPFUL TIP: Raynaud phenomenon may be secondary to connective tissue disease, cancer, some chemotherapeutic agents, exposure to toxins (e.g., polyvinyl chloride), trauma, or entrapment syndromes such as thoracic outlet and carpal tunnel syndromes. History and physical examination must focus on evaluation of these potential causes.

Objectives: Did you learn to . . .

- Identify complications of Raynaud phenomenon and diseases associated with it?
- Develop a strategy for the prevention and treatment of symptoms of Raynaud phenomenon?
- Recognize clinical features of scleroderma?

CASE 12

A 17-year-old male presents to your office with a history of low back pain worsening over the past few months. He recalls having intermittent back pain for at least a year. The pain does not radiate. He runs cross-country and track without exacerbating his back pain. He denies fevers, weight loss, weakness, incontinence, and history of trauma. He is unaware of any family history of back pain. He is otherwise healthy.

What further information will help you differentiate between potential causes of his back pain?

A) Relief with acetaminophen.
B) Morning stiffness.
C) Relief with rest.
D) A and C.
E) B and C.

The correct answer is "E." Determining the pattern of the pain is critical. Inflammatory causes of back pain are characterized by morning stiffness and improvement with activity. In contrast, degenerative back disease causes pain that is exacerbated by activity and relieved with rest. Inflammatory back pain typically presents in younger patients; degenerative back pain typically does not present before age 30 or 40. Acetaminophen and other analgesics may relieve pain from either category of disease and so will not help you narrow the diagnosis.

> HELPFUL TIP: In a young patient with back pain, also consider fractures (e.g., spondylolysis, a bilateral pars defect), infection, disc disease, and osseous malignancies.

* *

On further questioning, your patient reports morning stiffness and pain that improves with stretching. Activity does not seem to aggravate his back but inactivity does. He has had no penile discharge, rash, or conjunctivitis and denies diarrhea or other GI symptoms. On physical examination, your patient is surprised to find it impossible for him to touch his toes, which he had been able to do a few months ago in track practice. Range of motion in the neck, arms, and legs is normal. A focused neurologic exam is normal. There is mild, diffuse tenderness over the lumbosacral spine and with percussion over the sacroiliac joints.

The history and physical exam are most consistent with a diagnosis of:

A) Reactive arthritis (formerly Reiter syndrome).
B) Osteoarthritis of the lumbar spine.
C) Degenerative disc disease.
D) Ankylosing spondylitis.
E) Vertebral body tumor.

The correct answer is "D." The history and exam are most consistent with ankylosing spondylitis, a seronegative (RF negative) spondyloarthropathy. Ankylosing spondylitis is the most common form of spondyloarthropathy and is thought to have a prevalence of 1% in Caucasian populations. Historically, there is a 5:1 male-to-female ratio (but this may also be because ankylosing spondylitis is less recognized in women). Studies based on radiographic appearance and human leukocyte antigen (HLA) B27 typing show a much lower ratio. In addition to the historical features mentioned in the answer to the previous question, there is often a family history of ankylosing spondylitis in patients ultimately diagnosed with the disease.

"A" is incorrect. Reactive arthritis occurs in reaction to an infection (*Chlamydia* urethritis, GI infection, etc.) and presents with mono- or oligoarthritis, usually of the joints in the leg. This patient's age makes osteoarthritis and degenerative disc disease less likely, so "B" and "C" are wrong. Also, he has no neurologic findings that you might expect with disc prolapse. Malignancy is associated with constitutional symptoms (fever and weight loss), neurologic involvement, and steadily worsening pain that is not relieved by activity—none of which are present in this case. Physical examination findings of spondyloarthropathies are listed in Table 11–8.

Table 11–8 PHYSICAL FINDINGS IN THE SPONDYLOARTHROPATHIES

- Limited range of motion in the spine
- Tenderness at the sacroiliac joints
- Tenderness at tendon insertions, particularly the Achilles tendon and plantar fascia synovitis
- Anterior eye symptoms (anterior uveitis in 30–40%)

Time for some tests! Which of the following is the one BEST test that can be used to confirm the diagnosis of ankylosing spondylitis?

A) ANA.
B) Lumbar spine radiographs.
C) HLA-B27.
D) ESR.
E) Sacroiliac joint radiographs.

Discussion

The correct answer is "E." The hallmark of ankylosing spondylitis is sacroiliitis on pelvic radiographs. Although there are no universally accepted criteria for diagnosing spondyloarthropathies, x-ray evidence of sacroiliitis in the setting of a consistent clinical picture is sufficient to diagnose ankylosing spondylitis. Unfortunately, in early ankylosing spondylitis, x-rays are often inconclusive. MRI is more sensitive for detecting early sacroiliitis, but the cost will be prohibitive in many cases. The rest of the answers are incorrect. Ankylosing spondylitis is not associated with a positive ANA. Lumbar spine x-rays may be useful in ruling out other conditions and do show some changes in ankylosing spondylitis but may miss early disease. HLA-B27, a class I HLA gene, is present in about 90% of white patients and 50–80% of nonwhite patients with ankylosing spondylitis and is generally associated with spondyloarthropathies. However, HLA-B27 is not specific. It is present in many normal individuals as well and is of very little diagnostic value (although it does have a good negative predictive value). ESR is slightly elevated in most cases of spondyloarthropathy, but again it is not specific.

* *

Lumbar spine x-rays show squaring of the vertebral bodies. Pelvic x-rays identify mild symmetric sacroiliitis. You are now confident of the diagnosis of ankylosing spondylitis.

Which of the following management plans is best for this patient?

A) Aspirin 650 mg PO QID (or Zorprin or other extended release aspirin BID) and physical therapy referral.
B) Naproxen 500 mg BID and physical therapy referral.
C) Orthopedic referral for early surgical consideration.
D) Prednisone 40 mg QD and fitting for a back brace.
E) Naproxen 500 mg BID and fitting for a back brace.

Discussion

The correct answer is "B." NSAIDs are the mainstay of medical therapy for active phases of spondyloarthropathy. Patients generally experience significant relief from NSAIDs, and any additional benefit from systemic steroids is questionable. Sulfasalazine is a second-line drug. Interestingly, aspirin tends to be less effective in these patients. Thus, "A" is incorrect. The management of ankylosing spondylitis should also include an exercise regimen designed specifically for the patient, and physical therapy may play a key role. The use of braces is not helpful and may actually exacerbate the patient's symptoms. Orthopedic surgery only becomes necessary in cases of advanced ankylosing spondylitis when kyphosis or peripheral joint symptoms become severe.

* *

After 3 months of physical therapy and NSAIDs, your patient returns. He has noticed minimal benefit, and now you find limitation of his neck range of motion.

What is the most appropriate next step in the evaluation and management of this patient?

A) Discontinue naproxen and switch to indomethacin 50 mg TID.
B) Begin methotrexate 15 mg per week and folic acid 1 mg QD
C) Begin prednisone 60 mg QD.
D) MRI of the cervical spine.
E) Continue naproxen and refer to rheumatology.

Discussion

The correct answer is "E." The patient is losing range of motion despite NSAID therapy. Referral to a rheumatologist to consider anti-TNF therapy (e.g., infliximab [Remicade]) is the best next step. Anti-TNF agents can halt disease progression and often improve range of motion in early disease. "A" is incorrect. Switching NSAIDs may provide some minor additional benefit but is unlikely to arrest disease progression. "B" is incorrect: methotrexate may be beneficial for the peripheral arthritis of spondyloarthropathies, but not for the axial skeleton disease. "C" is incorrect since systemic steroids have no value in treating spondyloarthropathies. Local corticosteroid injections are often beneficial for enthesopathy and peripheral arthritis. "D" is incorrect. MRI of the cervical spine will show inflammatory changes of the spine, but will not change your management.

* *

The patient fails to keep his rheumatology appointment and returns to you 1 year later. He is taking over-the-counter naproxen. His neck is very stiff, with even less range of motion. He relates that he has been having crampy abdominal pain, and loose stools with bloody mucous. He is having dyspnea with mild exertion. On exam, his neck range of motion is worse, and back flexion is limited with straightening of his lumbar lordosis.

What is the next most appropriate step in the evaluation and management of this patient?

A) Discontinue naproxen.
B) Check CBC with differential and iron panel.
C) Consult gastroenterology for EGD and colonoscopy.
D) Consult rheumatology and tell patient he must keep his appointment.
E) All of the above.

Discussion

The correct answer is "E." The patient could have enteropathic arthritis in association with inflammatory bowel disease. NSAIDs can exacerbate inflammatory bowel disease, and cause ulcers with chronic use, so discontinue the naproxen ("A"). A CBC and iron panel may reveal iron deficiency anemia, which would explain the patient's dyspnea on exertion. Subspecialty evaluations by a gastroenterologist and rheumatologist are indicated both to confirm the diagnosis and to help with long-term disease management. Anti-TNF agents—like infliximab and adalimumab—but not etanercept—are beneficial for both the spondyloarthropathy and inflammatory bowel disease in enteropathic arthritis.

> HELPFUL TIP: The most common spondyloarthropathies are ankylosing spondylitis, psoriatic arthritis, enteropathic arthritis, and reactive arthritis. These are pathogenically similar diseases that may be difficult to differentiate in early stages, but lack of differentiation does not generally affect therapy.

Enteropathic arthritis occurs frequently in patients with inflammatory bowel disease, and has features in common with ankylosing spondylitis, including inflammatory back pain and sacroiliitis. However, it may also occur after a GI infection such as *Salmonella*, *Yersinia*, *Shigella*, or *Campylobacter*. Finally, other illnesses such as celiac disease may cause a reactive spondyloarthropathy.

Objectives: Did you learn to . . .

- Recognize clinical manifestations of spondyloarthropathies, particularly ankylosing spondylitis?
- Differentiate between types of spondyloarthropathies?
- Develop an appropriate evaluation for the patient presenting with inflammatory back pain?
- Appropriately manage a patient with ankylosing spondylitis?

QUICK QUIZ: SPONDYLOARTHROPATHIES

Which of the following is NOT a characteristic of reactive arthritis?

A) Conjunctivitis.
B) Keratoderma blenorrhagicum.
C) HLA-B8.
D) Urethritis.
E) Arthritis.

Discussion

The correct answer is "C." Reactive arthritis (formerly Reiter syndrome) is associated with HLA-B27 and not HLA-B8 (which is found in sclerosing cholangitis). All of the other choices are seen with reactive arthritis, including keratoderma blenorrhagicum, which is a rash found especially on the soles of patients with reactive arthritis. The urethritis is generally due to *Chlamydia trachomatis*.

> HELPFUL TIP: The onset of reactive arthritis is less insidious than that of ankylosing spondylitis, with some patients presenting with an acute illness that includes fever, acute joint swelling, and rash (keratoderma blenorrhagicum). Generally, reactive arthritis resolves within 12 months. Antibiotics are not effective as treatment of reactive arthritis (although may be indicated for the underlying infection).

CASE 13

A 52-year-old female presents to your office for an initial visit and complains of mild pain and weakness in her hips and thighs. The symptoms have been present for months. About 2 years ago another doctor diagnosed her with psoriasis because of a rash on her hands and elbows, which has since resolved. Otherwise, she reports being relatively healthy and taking no medications. She is a smoker. She has had no recent health screening. On physical exam, her vitals are normal. She has considerable difficulty getting out of her chair. Her strength is symmetrically diminished in the quadriceps and hip flexors. The rest of the exam is unremarkable.

Which of the following diagnostic tests do you order first?

A) Muscle biopsy.
B) Electromyography (EMG).
C) TSH.
D) ANA.
E) Troponin-T.

Discussion

The correct answer is "C." Hypothyroidism (along with many other diseases) can cause a proximal muscle weakness. A muscle biopsy or EMG study is premature without first evaluating for myopathy with serum enzyme levels (CK, aldolase). "D," an ANA, is not likely to be helpful. Autoimmune diseases, such as polymyositis and dermatomyositis, cause myopathy, but ANA is not specific for these diseases. Finally, although CK-MB may be elevated in patients with myopathy, troponin-T (answer "E") is an enzyme relatively specific to cardiac muscle and should be normal.

* *

You order TSH and CBC, which are normal. ESR, CK, and AST are elevated. An EMG demonstrates abnormalities of the paraspinal muscles. Your patient returns to discuss her test results and complains that her psoriasis is back. There are violaceous plaques on her knuckles and elbows and around her eyes.

You recommend the following management plan for the disease:

A) Ultraviolet light therapy.
B) Topical steroids.
C) Oral steroids.
D) Topical emollients.
E) Acetaminophen.

Discussion

The correct answer is "C." This patient now has findings that support a diagnosis of dermatomyositis. To diagnose idiopathic inflammatory myopathy, such as dermatomyositis or polymyositis, certain criteria must be present (see Table 11–9). This patient has three of these criteria plus skin changes consistent with dermatomyositis. Violaceous plaques on the knuckles are commonly called Gottron papules. Similar lesions are often observed over pressure points (e.g., elbows). Because dermatomyositis is a systemic condition, treatment should likewise be systemic. Local topical therapies do not treat the disease, and oral steroids are typically the first-line agents. Hydroxychloroquine is helpful when the rash does not respond to corticosteroids. Addition of immunosuppressive drugs, such as methotrexate or azathioprine, may be indicated.

Table 11–9 DIAGNOSTIC CRITERIA FOR POLYMYOSITIS AND DERMATOMYOSITIS

Three of four are required:
• Elevated muscle enzymes (CPK and aldolase)
• Symmetrical proximal muscle weakness
• Abnormal EMG
• Consistent findings on muscle biopsy
Note: Skin findings must be present in order to diagnose dermatomyositis.

You diagnose dermatomyositis. Which of the following tests and exams should now be ordered?

A) Pap and pelvic exam, CA-125, and pelvic ultrasound.
B) Screening mammogram.
C) Chest radiograph.
D) Fecal occult blood screening.
E) All of the above.

Discussion

The correct answer is "E." Adult onset dermatomyositis has a particularly strong association with malignancy; the risk is up to six times greater than in the general population. Therefore, upon diagnosing dermatomyositis, a thorough history and physical exam must be performed. All patients should undergo age-appropriate cancer screening tests (e.g., Pap smear, fecal occult blood testing, and mammography). Also, other tests generally recommended include CBC,

Quadriceps - R. Femoris, vastus medialis, intermedius and lateralis.
Test- "Kick out", Nerve - L2, L3 L4
Hip flexor- Pulls the knee upward, ↓Hip flexion seen in Thomas test +ve

metabolic profile, liver function tests, urinalysis, and chest x-ray—especially important in smokers. Since the patient is over age 50, colonoscopy is indicated.

HELPFUL TIP: The association of dermatomyositis with GI malignancy, especially colon cancer, is particularly strong. You may consider an alpha-fetoprotein, given this association. Some suggest CA-125 in all women with dermatomyositis, as well as a pelvic ultrasound or CT of the abdomen and pelvis to rule out ovarian cancer.

HELPFUL TIP: Other causes of proximal muscle weakness include alcohol use, muscular dystrophy, medications (e.g., penicillamine and HMG-CoA reductase inhibitors), Cushing syndrome, viral infections, hypothyroidism and diabetes mellitus. The list goes on, including myasthenia gravis and Eaton–Lambert syndrome.

Objectives: Did you learn to . . .

- Recognize symptoms and signs of dermatomyositis and polymyositis?
- Describe how inflammatory myopathies are evaluated and diagnosed?
- Appreciate the relationship between malignancy and inflammatory myopathy?

QUICK QUIZ: OSTEOARTHRITIS

Compared with rheumatoid arthritis, osteoarthritis has a greater predilection for which of the following joints?

A) MCPs.
B) DIPs.
C) Knees.
D) Wrists.

Discussion

The correct answer is "B." Osteoarthritis tends to affect the DIP and PIP joints in the hand, sparing the MCPs, whereas rheumatoid arthritis affects the MCPs and spares the DIPs. Both disease processes may involve the knees and wrists.

BIBLIOGRAPHY

American College of Rheumatology criteria for diagnosing Rheumatoid Arthritis – http://www.rheumatology.org/practice/clinical/classification/index.asp

American College of Rheumatology 2008 Recommendations for the Use of Nonbiologic and Biologic Disease-Modifying Antirheumatic Drugs in Rheumatoid Arthritis – http://www.rheumatology.org/practice/clinical/guidelines/index.asp

Bhate C, Schwartz RA. Lyme disease: Part I. Advances and perspectives. *J Am Acad Dermatol.* 2011;64:619-636.

Bhate C, Schwartz RA. Lyme disease: Part II. Management and prevention. *J Am Acad Dermatol.* 2011;64:639-653.

Botzoris V, Drosos AA. Management of Raynaud's phenomenon and digital ulcers in systemic sclerosis. *Joint Bone Spine.* 2011;78(4):341-346. Epub 2010 Dec 22.

Clauw DJ. Fibromyalgia: An overview. *Am J Med.* 2009;122(12 Suppl):S3-S13.

Dougados M, Baeten D. Spondyloarthritis. *Lancet.* 2011;377:2127-2137.

Firestein GS, et al. eds. *Kelley's Textbook of Rheumatology.* 8th ed. Philadelphia: Elsevier Saunders; 2008.

Haile Z, Khatua S. Beyond osteoarthritis: Recognizing and treating infectious and other inflammatory arthropathies in your practice. *Prim Care.* 2010;37(4):713-727, vi.

Klippel JH, et al., eds. *Primer on the Rheumatic Diseases.* 13th ed. Atlanta: Arthritis Foundation; 2007.

Margaretten ME, et al. Does this adult patient have septic arthritis? *JAMA.* 2007;297:1478.

Nam JL, et al. Current evidence for the management of rheumatoid arthritis with biological disease-modifying antirheumatic drugs: a systematic literature review informing the EULAR recommendations for the management of RA. *Ann Rheum Dis.* 2010;69:976-986.

van Hecke O. Polymyalgia rheumatica – Diagnosis and management. *Aust Fam Physician.* 2011;40:303-306.

Villa-Forte A. Giant cell arteritis: Suspect it, treat it promptly. *Cleve Clin J Med.* 2011;78:265-270.

12

Orthopedics and Sports Medicine

Jon Van Heukelom

General note: If you have a choice between acetaminophen and an NSAID for an acute injury, acetaminophen will always be the right choice. Most acute injuries are not inflammatory and acetaminophen is a lot safer without gastropathy or platelet inhibition (Table 12–1).

CASE 1

A 5-year-old boy presents with acute onset of left anterior thigh and hip pain that began 2 days ago with no known prior trauma. He reports that it initially "loosened-up" after he had been out of bed for a few hours but has become worse again by afternoon. His pain is exacerbated by weight bearing and active or passive range of motion (ROM). His mother notes that he had a cold 7–10 days ago, but has been asymptomatic until he complained of thigh pain two nights ago. She also notes that he has had a low-grade fever. He has no other significant constitutional symptoms and appears to be in some pain, but otherwise he appears well.

Based on the information obtained thus far, which of the following is the most likely diagnosis?

A) Osteomyelitis.
B) Rheumatic fever.
C) Slipped capital femoral epiphysis (SCFE).
D) Legg–Calve–Perthes disease (LCPD).
E) Transient (toxic) synovitis.

Discussion

The correct answer is "E." This presentation is classic for transient (toxic) synovitis (aka transient tenosynovitis), a condition most commonly presenting in the 2–6-year age range and more commonly seen in boys (male:female ratio of 2–3:1). It often is preceded by a viral respiratory infection, although numerous studies have failed to demonstrate a specific viral or bacterial agent. Physical exam reveals a limp or refusal to walk and complaint of pain over the groin and/or proximal thigh. There is pain with ROM testing, especially during abduction. Most children will be afebrile with a temperature of $\leq 38°C$.

Appropriate diagnostic workup might include which of the following?

A) Joint aspiration.
B) Plain film radiographs.
C) Erythrocyte sedimentation rate (ESR).
D) CBC with differential.
E) All of the above.

Discussion

The correct answer is "E." All of the above may be appropriate as transient synovitis is a diagnosis of exclusion. Patients with mild symptoms may be observed without further investigation. However, if the pain is significant, if ROM is significantly impaired, or if the temperature is $>37.5°C$, further diagnostic workup is indicated. Laboratory findings consistent with transient synovitis include clear joint fluid aspirate, normal CBC, and a mildly increased ESR. Blood cultures, ASO titer, bone scan, and MRI may also be of benefit to rule out other possibilities (e.g., septic arthritis, rheumatic fever, and SCFE). **It is of extreme importance to differentiate transient synovitis from**

Table 12–1 TERMINOLOGY FOR DESCRIBING A FRACTURE

Closed fracture. Fracture that does not communicate with the outside.

Open fracture. Fracture that communicates with the external environment.

Comminuted fracture. Consisting of three or more fragments.

Avulsion fracture. Fragment of bone pulled from its normal position by a muscular contraction or resistance of a ligament.

Greenstick fracture. Incomplete, angulated fracture of a long bone, particularly in children.

Torus fracture. Described as a buckle fracture or compression of the bone without cortical disruption. Seen especially in the distal forearms of children.

septic arthritis. Unfortunately, there is no combination of physical findings and laboratory tests short of joint fluid that will tell you absolutely that this is transient synovitis. It requires clinical judgment; decide which patients you are worried enough about that you want to commit them to hip joint aspiration.

HELPFUL TIP: Septic arthritis is an orthopedic emergency and commonly presents with an elevated temperature, general malaise, pronounced pain—often with spasm and guarding. Generally, you will also have an elevated white blood cell (WBC) and ESR, **although neither these nor fever is a good enough indicator to rule out a septic joint by their normality or absence.** Joint fluid will have numerous WBCs. Blood cultures are positive in 30–40% of patients.

What is the most appropriate treatment for this patient with transient synovitis?

A) Open fixation.
B) Immobilization.
C) Antibiotics.
D) Surgical decompression.
E) Ibuprofen and rest.

Discussion

The correct answer is "E." Conservative treatment is warranted: the appropriate initial treatment is rest and observation. Transient synovitis generally responds well to oral NSAIDs. Home care is acceptable; however, admission is indicated if the diagnosis is equivocal or if significant pain management is required. For septic arthritis, prompt administration of an intravenous (IV) antibiotic—directed at the most likely infecting pathogen and altered as necessary based on culture results—is indicated. Surgical irrigation of the joint is often necessary and early orthopedic consultation is needed.

Objectives: Did you learn to . . .

- Recognize the clinical presentation of transient synovitis?
- Differentiate transient synovitis from septic arthritis?
- Treat a patient with transient synovitis?

CASE 2

A 6-year-old white male is brought in by his parents because he is complaining of pain in his hip and anterior thigh. He is walking much less than usual since the pain began about 4 weeks ago. You order a plain radiograph, which shows mild sclerosis with some increased density of the femoral head. An MRI is ordered, which the radiologist interprets as "demonstrating osteonecrosis of the femoral head."

What is the most likely diagnosis in this patient?

A) Osteomyelitis.
B) Septic arthritis.
C) SCFE (Slipped Capital Femoral Epiphysis).
D) LCPD (Legg-Calfe-Perthes Disease).
E) Sickle cell anemia.

Discussion

The correct answer is "D." LCPD is idiopathic osteonecrosis of the femoral head. It is unilateral in 90% of cases, and the typical age range is 4–8 years, but patients may be as young as 2 years and as old as 12 years. "A" is a possibility, although there should be evidence of osteomyelitis on MRI. "B" is discussed in the previous case. "C," SCFE, generally occurs in obese children (usually male) who are in early adolescence. "E," sickle cell anemia, can cause osteonecrosis of the femoral head also, but the disease is rare in white populations. LCPD is less common in blacks.

Which of the following factors most affects the outcome in patients with LCPD?

A) Age at onset of illness.
B) Findings of subchondral fractures or fragmentation.
C) Early appropriate treatment.
D) Severity of pain and ability to bear weight.
E) Bilateral involvement.

Discussion
The correct answer is "A." Compared to older children, younger children generally have a longer time for remodeling to occur via molding of the femoral head within the acetabulum; and therefore, younger children have less flattening of the femoral head.

Which of the following is the best initial treatment for this patient?

A) Joint replacement.
B) Osteotomy.
C) Rest and traction.
D) Opioids.
E) Corticosteroid injection of the hip joint.

Discussion
The correct answer is "C." The initial treatment for a patient with LCPD typically includes rest, traction, and the use of an abduction brace. The objectives are to increase ROM in the hip and to reduce the risk of significant deformity. In general, patients should be seen by a specialist. "A" is incorrect because joint replacement is not an option. "B" is incorrect. While osteotomy may be used, it is typically reserved for older children and patients who are not progressing well with conservative therapy. "D" and "E" are not appropriate interventions in this patient with mild pain and no joint inflammation.

LCPD is difficult to treat largely because of the long duration of treatment and activity restrictions required. Periods of rest with traction, casting or bracing, and surgical intervention may be indicated over 1–2 years of treatment and observation. Even with the best of care, prognosis is fair with need for total hip replacement reaching approximately 50% by middle age due to severe degenerative arthritis.

Objectives: Did you learn to . . .

- Recognize the clinical presentation of LCPD?
- Manage a patient with LCPD?
- Identify when a patient with LCPD should be referred for further evaluation?

CASE 3

A 15-year-old female cross-country runner presents to your clinic with the chief complaint of knee pain. She describes a gradual increase in her symptoms during the first 3 weeks of the season. She wants to run varsity this year and has done extra running and hill training after practice each day. She describes anterior knee pain in the patellar region with little or no swelling, but complains of crepitus and pain exacerbated by stair climbing and running.

The most likely diagnosis for the condition described is:

A) Osgood–Schlatter disease.
B) Chondromalacia patellae.
C) Patellofemoral pain syndrome (PFPS).
D) Femoral stress fracture.

Discussion
The correct answer is "C." PFPS is a common overuse syndrome seen more frequently in runners and female athletes (thus the moniker "runner's knee"). PFPS may involve lateral subluxation or mal-tracking within the femoral groove due to vastus medialis weakness. Mal-tracking may be observed clinically and subluxation may be seen on plain films using a Merchant view. "B," Osgood–Schlatter disease, is also related to overuse but is two to three times more common in males, particularly in athletes engaging in repetitive jumping. The pain of Osgood–Schlatter is generally well localized to the tibial tubercle. Radiographic evidence of fragmentation of the epiphysis or heterotropic ossification anterior to the tubercle may be seen but is not necessary for diagnosis. "C," chondromalacia patella, is softening of the articular cartilage of the patella as seen on arthroscopy and may be a result of long-term patellofemoral dysfunction. This is a surgical diagnosis and the term should be avoided clinically.

What is the preferred treatment for this female runner?

A) Arthroscopic debridement.
B) Decreased activity level and quadriceps strengthening.
C) Evaluation for "Female Athlete Triad."
D) Casting or immobilization.
E) Corticosteroid injection.

Discussion

The correct answer is "B." Quadriceps strengthening is usually initiated by resisted straight leg raises (SLRs) to minimize patellofemoral compressive forces. NSAIDs and cross-training may also be of benefit. Consider physical therapy referral for exercise instruction and trials of therapeutic modalities such as orthotics. Recalcitrant cases and patients with recurrent dislocation/subluxation should be referred to orthopedics for consideration of surgical intervention.

* *

Three months later, the same patient presents complaining of knee pain over the medial knee joint. Again, this pain is exacerbated by knee flexion and she notes popping and snapping when she stands from sitting. Your exam shows tenderness about 1 cm medial to the patella with palpable fullness in the area.

The most likely diagnosis is:

A) Osteosarcoma
B) Medial collateral ligament (MCL) strain
C) Plica syndrome
D) PFPS
E) Meniscal tear

Discussion

The correct answer is "C." This is the typical presentation of plica syndrome. The plica is a synovial remnant that did not resorb properly during development. It can be irritated, usually chronically or subacutely, especially in sports that require repeated flexion of the knee (rowing, cycling, running). Treatment includes rest, ice, quadriceps strengthening, and NSAIDs. If conservative management fails, steroid injection or arthroscopy may alleviate the symptoms.

> HELPFUL TIP: The plica should be palpable. A medial/inferior plica is the most common (between the patella and the medial joint line). It can also occur laterally and either above or below the mid-pole of the patella.

Objectives: Did you learn to . . .

- Identify and manage patellofemoral syndrome?
- Recognize plica syndrome?

CASE 4

A mother brings her 18-month-old son in for well child check. Her only new concern today is that he seems to walk "bow-legged." He has been somewhat pigeon-toed since he could pull himself up and cruise along walls and furniture at home. On exam you find the child's feet to be pointing inward. The foot is flexible and looks normal. The patellae are in a neutral position facing directly forward.

What is the most likely diagnosis in this patient?

A) Cerebral palsy.
B) Excessive femoral retroversion.
C) Forefoot varus.
D) Internal tibial torsion.
E) Bilateral developmental dysplasia of the hip (DDH).

Discussion

The correct answer is "D." This represents a case of intoeing (pigeon-toeing), which is often caused by internal tibial torsion. Internal tibial torsion is characterized by a flexible, normal foot, with the patellae in a neutral position. The condition can be diagnosed by examining the child on his knees. Normally, there should be approximately 30 degrees of external rotation of the feet in this position. With internal tibial torsion, the toes will be pointing inward. Additionally, when the child is sitting with legs dangling over a table, the lateral malleolus will be anterior to the medial malleolus, which is the opposite of what is normally observed. Finally, the hips must be normal in order to confirm this diagnosis. "A" is incorrect because you would expect other findings in a patient with cerebral palsy. "B" is incorrect. In fact, femoral retroversion is synonymous with "outtoeing," which is the opposite of intoeing (of course!). Excessive femoral **anteversion** can be a cause of intoeing. "C" is incorrect because the foot exam does not show varus deformity. Finally, "E" is incorrect, although bilateral

DDH can be quite difficult to diagnose if not caught early in the newborn period. With DDH one would expect external rotation of the leg rather than intoeing.

What is the treatment of choice for this child?

A) Referral for bilateral osteotomy.
B) Shoe modification and bracing.
C) Physical therapy referral.
D) Serial casting.
E) Reassurance and watchful waiting.

Discussion

The correct answer is "E." Spontaneous resolution is the norm for most intoeing and outtoeing deformities. Most will spontaneously correct by age 7 or 8. Children continuing to have difficulty with persistent trips and falls or grossly unsightly gait beyond this time may benefit from a rotational osteotomy. Children with neuromotor disorders and cerebral palsy are more likely to require surgical intervention.

HELPFUL TIP: Another cause of intoeing is femoral torsion that is diagnosed by placing the patient prone with the hips in neutral and knees flexed to 90 degrees. Feet are rotated away from midline to measure internal rotation (anteversion). For external rotation (retroversion), place one hand on the buttocks and move one leg through midline until the pelvis begins to tilt. Typically, normal external rotation is 45 degrees, and normal internal rotation is 35 degrees. Rotation greater than this is considered excessive if it is accompanied by a limited ROM in the opposite direction. Additionally, when a patient with femoral torsion is seated with legs dangling, the patellae will **not** face forward (they face inward for intoeing and outward for outtoeing).

Objective: Did you learn to . . .

- Evaluate and manage intoeing and outtoeing in children?

CASE 5

A 13-year-old male presents to the clinic with his mother for difficulty walking. He is unsure of when the problem first began, but has noticed it getting worse over the last week. It has forced him to stop playing sports. He reports a dull pain in the left hip but denies trauma. On examination, you find an obese male in no distress. There is loss of internal rotation at the left hip joint. When his hip is flexed to 90 degrees, this loss of ROM is more pronounced.

What is the most likely diagnosis in this case?

A) DDH.
B) Septic arthritis.
C) SCFE.
D) LCPD.
E) Juvenile rheumatoid arthritis.

Discussion

The correct answer is "C." SCFE occurs most commonly in active, overweight, adolescent males. Shear forces across the relatively weak physis causes displacement. **Slippage is generally gradual, but may occur acutely.** Mean age at presentation is 12 for females (range 10–14) and 13 for males (range 11–16). Endocrinopathies should be considered in those presenting atypically or outside the typical age range. Watch for development of a similar process in the contralateral hip over time.

Which of the following is the first study you order to confirm the diagnosis?

A) AP and frog-lateral radiographs.
B) CT scan.
C) MRI.
D) ESR.
E) None; physical exam is sufficient.

Discussion

The correct answer is "A." Radiographs of the hip should demonstrate displacement of the femoral head, which can then be classified as mild, moderate, or severe. "B" and "C" are incorrect because the radiograph is diagnostic in most cases. "D" is incorrect since SCFE is not an inflammatory condition. "E" is incorrect. Imaging should be obtained in order to confirm the diagnosis and rate the severity.

The treatment of choice for this patient is:

A) Antibiotics.
B) Immobilization.
C) Physical therapy.
D) Surgical decompression.
E) Surgical fixation.

Discussion

The correct answer is "E." The goals of treatment of SCFE are to prevent further slippage, promote closure of the physis, and to minimize the risk of osteonecrosis or chondrolysis. These aims are best accomplished through referral to an orthopedic surgeon and, ultimately, surgical fixation. "B" and "C" are incorrect because they delay definitive therapy and will not produce the desired result. "A" and "D" are incorrect because SCFE is not an infectious process.

Objectives: Did you learn to . . .

- Recognize the clinical presentation of a child with SCFE?
- Treat a patient with SCFE?

CASE 6

A worried mother presents with her 4-year-old son for evaluation of lower extremity pain. She reports the boy has complained of some vague bilateral leg pains over the past several weeks after vigorous physical activities. She became alarmed after he had awakened the past two nights crying in pain. The boy reports the pain is hardly noticeable during the day. Recently, the pain has been in the bilateral distal thighs; however, his mother notes times of unilateral pain. The boy and his mother both deny constitutional symptoms now or over the past several weeks. Examination reveals an afebrile, well-developed male in no distress. The musculoskeletal exam is normal.

The most likely diagnosis for the condition described above is?

A) Ewing sarcoma.
B) Growing pain.
C) Kohler disease.
D) Leukemia.
E) Osteochondritis desiccans.

Discussion

The correct answer is "B." Growing pain is a diagnosis of exclusion, although history and physical exam usually suffice for excluding more serious diagnoses. It is a condition of unknown etiology, but is thought by some to be a result of overuse/over activity on an immature musculoskeletal system. It is most frequently seen in otherwise healthy, active children aged 2–5, with some older children affected as well. Pain is commonly bilateral or/and localized to the calf, but may be felt at the ankle, knee, or thigh. Pain may be felt during the day after vigorous activities but is more common in the evening or causing awakening at night. Presentation with constitutional symptoms should lead to radiographic and/or metabolic workup.

Which of the following should you entertain when a patient presents with typical growing pain?

A) Osteomyelitis.
B) Tumor.
C) Juvenile rheumatoid arthritis.
D) All of the above.
E) None of the above.

Discussion

The correct answer is "D." It is important to consider other potential causes of what would otherwise appear to be growing pain. Although you may not find it necessary to perform any laboratory or radiologic studies, you should at least keep these and other diagnoses in mind when taking your history and performing your exam. Remember, growing pain is a diagnosis of exclusion.

> HELPFUL TIP: Severe or persistent pain during the day **is not** "growing pain." By definition, "growing pain" occurs primarily at night and is better during the day.

Treatment for growing pain includes:

A) Reassurance, rest, and short-term use of NSAIDs.
B) Amputation.
C) Chemotherapy and radiation.
D) Casting and bracing followed by physical therapy.
E) Staging of the disease is required prior to initiation of therapy.

Discussion

The correct answer is "A." OK, so this was just a fun one. Do not do anything drastic for a benign condition! Those of you who chose "B," amputation, will find themselves in one of Dante's circles (or in court—which is worse?) . . . and clearly need a coffee break.

* *

The same boy returns with his mother years later. He is now 12 years old and requires a physical examination for junior high school sports. You plan to evaluate him for scoliosis.

Which of the following screening methods is the most sensitive for detecting scoliosis?

A) Observe the patient from the front with a loose-fitting shirt on. Measure the difference in shoulder height.
B) Observe the patient from behind, with shirt off, while he bends forward at the waist. Look for elevation of the ribs or paravertebral muscle mass on one side.
C) Observe the patient from the front, with shirt off, while he bends forward at the waist. Look for elevation of the ribs or paravertebral muscle mass on one side.
D) Observe the patient from the side, with shirt off, while he bends forward at the waist. Look for elevation of the ribs or paravertebral muscle mass on one side.

Discussion

The correct answer is "B," which is known as the "forward bending test." This test is more sensitive than the other methods described. The forward bending test is accomplished by having the patient bend at the waist with feet together and hands hanging free. Observe the patient from behind and note any elevation of the ribs or paravertebral muscle mass on one side. The elevation should be measured in degrees (inclinometers are available), and an inclination of 5 degrees or more should be evaluated further. Options "A," "C," and "D" are **not** accepted methods of screening for scoliosis.

HELPFUL TIP: **Routine screening for scoliosis is a recommendation "D" by USPSTF.** Routine scoliosis screening **is not** recommended. It may be appropriate in patients who have noticed pain or some other abnormality. However, we understand that old habits are hard to break.

HELPFUL TIP: Scoliosis is a lateral curvature of the spine, usually accompanied by rotation and generally occurring in the thoracic or lumbar areas. It can occur with excessive kyphosis (posteriorly convex curvature) or lordosis (anteriorly convex curvature).

* *

On forward bending test, you find slight elevation of the left paravertebral muscles mass, which you estimate to be 7 degrees. The remainder of the examination is normal. You decide to obtain radiographs that show 12 degrees of angulation (Cobb angle).

This patient's scoliosis is most likely:

A) Congenital.
B) Idiopathic.
C) Related to a tumor.
D) Secondary to infection.

Discussion

The correct answer is "B." Most scoliosis that develops during adolescence is idiopathic. When there is no pain, fever, weight loss, or other warning signs (e.g., neurologic symptoms), the curvature is unlikely to be due to tumor or infection. "A," congenital scoliosis, typically presents earlier in life.

The most appropriate initial management plan for this patient includes:

A) Bracing.
B) Observation.
C) Physical therapy.
D) Surgery.

Discussion

The correct answer is "B." In an otherwise healthy patient with a curvature measured at <20 degrees, observation is appropriate. "C" is incorrect because physical therapy and exercise regimens do not seem to limit the progression of scoliosis. "A" and "D" are incorrect because bracing and surgery are typically not warranted for this degree of scoliosis. Repeat examination and possibly repeat radiographs are warranted, but if the scoliosis remains stable and mild, the patient is not likely to experience any significant progression of disease with aging.

HELPFUL TIP: Bracing for scoliosis should be limited to those with idiopathic scoliosis and 20–40 degrees of angulation. Bracing is only effective if the child is still growing and <1 year past menarche if female.

Objectives: Did you learn to . . .

- Consider a broader differential diagnosis in a patient presenting with typical "growing pain?"
- Initiate conservative treatment for a patient with growing pain?
- Screen a patient for scoliosis?
- Develop an approach to the adolescent with scoliosis?

QUICK QUIZ: TRAUMATIC INJURIES

A 2-year-old girl is brought in refusing to move her right arm. Earlier today she threw a tantrum at the store when her father refused to buy her the new "Extra Sweet Panda Candy" (advertising hits them young . . .). Dad was holding on to her arm when she flopped to the floor. She immediately began crying and refusing to move her right arm. In the office, she is well but holds her right arm adducted, flexed, and pronated. (The candy's in the other hand. Guilt is a powerful weapon.) Despite every trick you know you can't get her to move that arm. You inspect and palpate the entire extremity and clavicle and find no crepitus, swelling, or tenderness.

What is your next diagnostic step?

A) Obtain an x-ray of the elbow.
B) Actively supinate the forearm and flex the elbow while applying pressure over the radial head.
C) Obtain a blood culture.
D) Consult orthopedics.
E) Perform a skeletal survey.

Discussion

The correct answer is "B." This child has a "nursemaid elbow" that is due to subluxation of the annular ligament rather than subluxation or dislocation of the radial head. It occurs in toddlers due to traction via pulling on a pronated and extended arm. Symptoms are immediate and care is sought due to child's refusal to move the arm. The diagnosis is clinical. Manual reduction may be done via supination/flexion or hyperpronation. Sedation is not needed. A palpable click may be felt. The child usually regains immediate movement of the arm and relief of discomfort. Immobilization is not needed but parents should be told that recurrent subluxations may occur and therefore pulling on the arm should be avoided. "A" would be correct if there was concern for a fracture based on findings of swelling, history of trauma, or focal tenderness. "C" is not needed since this presentation is not consistent with osteomyelitis or septic arthritis. "D" is incorrect as this may be managed by any primary-care provider. "E" is unnecessary as a nursemaid elbow is not a marker of abuse, although traumatic injuries in children should always make one consider abuse.

HELPFUL TIP: The patient with nursemaid's elbow should be using the arm normally within minutes. If the child still refuses to use the extremity after adequate observation, reconsider your diagnosis and whether the reduction was successful. Note that many will spontaneously reduce while radiographs are being done. Both flexion and supination and extension and pronation have been used to reduce nursemaids elbow.

HELPFUL TIP: When dealing with pediatric orthopedics, always remember that child abuse is in the differential diagnosis. Be sure that the reported mechanism of the injury is consistent with the findings on exam and radiograph.

* *

After successful reduction, you see the same 2-year-old child a month later presenting to your clinic with the parents who state that the child has been crying and has refused to walk since tripping over a toy a couple of hours ago. You look at the child and find no signs of abuse. The injured area is represented by the lower leg image in Figure 12–1.

Your approach at this point is to:

A) Consult Child Welfare since this is almost always abuse.

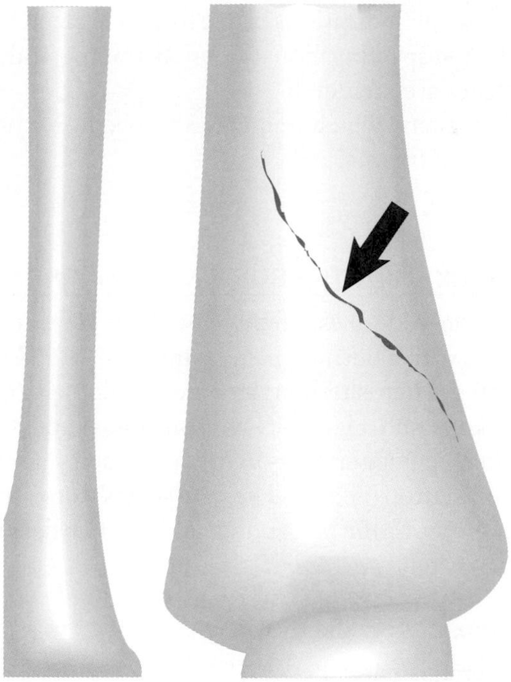

Figure 12–1

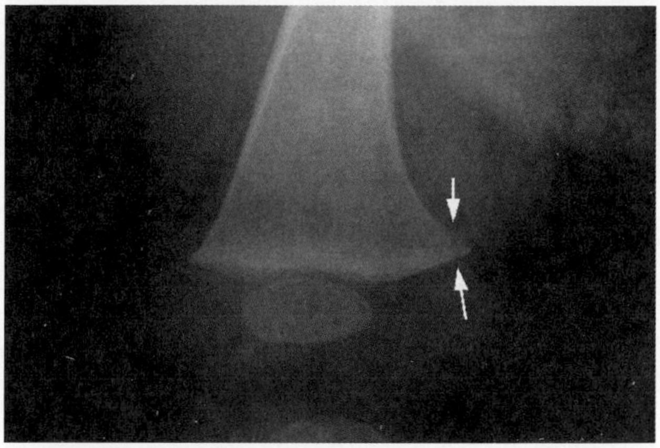

Figure 12–2

B) Consult orthopedics for casting and further treatment.
C) No treatment necessary for this particular fracture in a 2-year-old.
D) A and B.

Discussion

The correct answer is "B." This is a typical "toddler's fracture" that consists of a spiral fracture of the tibia usually from insignificant rotational trauma (e.g., running and falling with a twisting motion). There should not be an associated fibular fracture. "A" is incorrect because this type of fracture is not usually from abuse. A midshaft fracture would more likely be from abuse. "C" is incorrect because this fracture needs to be treated.

Objectives: Did you learn to . . .

- Recognize the clinical presentation and treatment of radial head subluxation?
- Recognize a "toddler's fracture?"

CASE 7

A mother presents to your clinic with her 10-month-old son. She is concerned that he has been very irritable since she arrived home from work, particularly when his legs are touched. She states that he has been crying "nonstop" since she arrived home. He was well when she left for work this morning, leaving the patient under the care of her boyfriend, Tony "the Hustler" Jones. The patient's mother denies any fevers, vomiting, diarrhea, or cough. On exam, he is generally fussy, worsening with palpation of his left leg, particularly around his knee. You also note five bruises on his anterior and posterior chest. The remainder of the exam is unremarkable. You obtain the following radiograph of his left knee (Figure 12–2).

Which of the following mechanisms is most likely responsible for the above fracture (marked with the helpful arrow sign)?

A) A low-energy fall (fall off a low couch).
B) A high-energy fall (fall out of a second story window).
C) A low-energy rotational force (tripping causing the foot to twist inward).
D) A high-energy tension or shearing force (a violent twisting of the leg).
E) Any of the above could result in the injury.

Discussion

The correct answer is "D," a high-energy tension or shearing force. The above radiograph depicts a metaphyseal corner fracture that is highly specific for nonaccidental trauma (child abuse). These fractures are typically caused by shaking of the child with flailing of the extremities or with forceful yanking or twisting or the arm or leg. The incidence of these fractures decreases substantially as children grow beyond 1 year of age.

In which of the following patients is a skeletal survey indicated for concern of nonaccidental trauma?

A) A 1-year-old male with multiple bruises but no other localizing injuries.
B) A 2-year-old female with an intracranial injury on brain CT.
C) A 6-month-old male with a known metaphyseal corner fracture.
D) An 18-month-old female with burns consistent with nonaccidental trauma.
E) A skeletal survey is indicted for all the above patients.

Discussion

The answer is "E," all of the above. The American Academy of Pediatrics consensus guidelines on the radiographic evaluation of child abuse state that a skeletal survey should be obtained for all children younger than 2 years of age who may have experienced maltreatment. Skeletal surveys should also be considered for children between the ages of two and five depending on the clinical scenario. The following images are generally included in a skeletal survey: skull, cervical spine, chest, pelvis, thoracic spine, lumbar spine, humerus, radius, ulna, hands, femur, tibia, fibula, and feet.

Which of the following fractures is considered highly specific for nonaccidental trauma?

A) Posterior rib fractures.
B) Clavicle fractures.
C) Distal radius fractures.
D) Spiral fractures of the tibia.
E) Supracondylar fractures.

Discussion

The correct answer is "A." In addition, the following fractures have moderate to high specificity for nonaccidental trauma: metaphyseal fractures, multiple fractures (especially if bilateral), fractures of different ages, epiphyseal separations, vertebral body fractures, digital fractures, scapular fractures, sternal fractures, and complex skull fractures.

Objectives: Did you learn to . . .

- Recognize a metaphyseal corner fracture and what implications this fracture has?
- Know the indications to perform a skeletal survey when suspecting nonaccidental trauma and what images are included?
- Understand which fractures are specific for nonaccidental trauma?

QUICK QUIZ: THE BURNIN' HIP O' FIRE

A 35-year-old obese female with a large pannus presents with a burning pain in anterior–lateral thigh. It started when she bought a new wide belt (ornate with skulls and Harley-Davidson logos) and started wearing hip hugger pants in order to display her tasteful sacral tattoo (yikes!). The pain seems worse on days when she wears the belt and seems better on days when she hangs out "*au natural*" at home.

The most likely diagnosis is:

A) Meralgia paresthetica.
B) Supratrochanteric bursitis.
C) Tropical pyomyositis.
D) Ruptured plantaris muscle.

Discussion

The correct answer is "A." Meralgia paresthetica is described as a burning pain in the anterior–lateral thigh and is caused by compression of the lateral femoral cutaneous nerve. It is most common in those who wear tight jeans and wide belts and who are obese. Treatment is to relieve the inciting cause. Tricyclic antidepressants or other medication for neuropathy may also be helpful. "B," supratrochanteric bursitis, occurs when there is inflammation of the bursa over the greater trochanter of the femur. Patients complain of pain in the lateral hip and outer thigh. There is point tenderness over the greater trochanter. Treatment is a steroid injection of the bursa. "C," tropical pyomyositis, is a deep infection of the muscle that is often caused by *Staph*. It is increasingly recognized in the United States. Finally, "D," a ruptured plantaris muscle, occurs in the calf and is not related to the thigh. It is often caused by planting of the foot forcefully (such as in tennis or basketball) and patients may report a "pop" followed by calf/gastrocnemius pain.

CASE 8

A concerned father presents to your clinic with a 1-month-old daughter. He is worried that his daughter appears to be pigeon-toed, and his mother-in-law is sure (as most mother-in-laws are) that the child will need immediate surgery for correction. Your exam reveals a pleasant, well-developed 1-month-old female with moderate medial deviation of the forefoot bilaterally. A line bisecting the heel passes through the fourth toe on each foot. The lateral borders of the feet are convex; the heels are in a normal neutral position. The feet are flexible.

The above description is best characterized as?

A) Clubfoot.
B) Internal tibial torsion.
C) Flexible flatfoot.
D) Excessive femoral anteversion.
E) Metatarsus adductus.

Discussion

The correct answer is "E." The above is a classic description of the foot shape of metatarsus adductus. In the normal foot, a line bisecting the heel would pass between the second and third toes. In those with metatarsus adductus, it passes through the fourth toe. In addition to the heels remaining in a neutral position—indicating that the problem is isolated to the shape of the foot and **not** to an internal rotation of the tibia—the forefoot is flexible and easily straightened into normal position. This is as opposed to metatarsus varus in which the forefoot is rigid.

HELPFUL TIP: Clubfoot (talipes equinovarus) is observed at birth. Patients are more often males (2:1 male:female ratio) and present with the following findings: calcaneus seems to be drawn inward and upward, moderate forefoot adduction, and the foot can be placed in a neutral position by passive manipulation. These patients can be treated successfully with early referral for serial casting and manipulation (i.e., the Ponseti method, which we are obligated to promote since Dr. Ignacio Ponseti developed it at the University of Iowa).

The most appropriate treatment for the above case would be?

A) Surgical reconstruction.
B) Serial casting.
C) Physical therapy referral for stretching and exercise.
D) Watchful waiting and reassurance.
E) Orthopedic outflare shoes.

Discussion

The correct answer is "D." Spontaneous correction occurs in most children. Parents can begin a regimen of gentle foot stretching. It gives them something to do but **does not change the outcome.** Care should be taken to avoid keeping the child in the prone position with the feet in an inward position. If the **deformity is severe and inflexible, serial casting and/or surgical intervention may be indicated.** A **rigid** metatarsus adductus in a child >3 months or a residual problem in a child with a flexible metatarsus adductus >6 months is an indication for pediatric orthopedic referral.

Objectives: Did you learn to . . .

- Identify a patient with metatarsus adductus?
- Discuss treatment approaches to metatarsus adductus?

CASE 9

A 5-year-old girl who has recently recovered from chicken pox presents with her mother for evaluation of left leg pain and refusal to walk. The mother reports that she has complained of worsening pain over the last 4–5 days. She started to limp noticeably yesterday and refused to walk this morning. Also, the mother reports general malaise and subjective fever. The patient complains of pain over the distal thigh and knee. The mother has not seen any swelling of the knee, and the patient denies trauma.

Exam reveals a pleasant 5-year-old female who appears uncomfortable, but nontoxic and in no acute distress. Her temperature is 38.5°C. The left **distal thigh** (not the joint) is painful to palpation, and slightly warm. The knee joint has no effusion and the ROM is full with only mild discomfort on knee motion. There is no hip joint involvement.

What is the most common bacterial pathogen associated with this patient's condition?

A) Group A Streptococcus.
B) Group B Streptococcus.

C) *Haemophilus influenzae.*
D) *Staphylococcus aureus.*
E) None of the above. This is not an infection.

Discussion
The correct answer is "D." The acute nature of the symptoms, presence of fever, and minimal involvement of the joint makes osteomyelitis the most likely diagnosis. Additionally, osteomyelitis is associated with chicken pox in children.

> HELPFUL TIP: *Pseudomonas aeruginosa* is commonly associated with osteomyelitis in the setting of a plantar puncture wound through a tennis shoe.

* *

Allow us to digress.

The most common organism causing osteomyelitis in patients with sickle cell disease is:

A) *Neisseria gonorrhoeae* (Gonococcus).
B) Polymicrobial.
C) *Salmonella* species.
D) *S. aureus.*
E) *Streptococcus* species.

Discussion
The correct answer is "C." *Salmonella* species are responsible for up to 85% of bone and joint infections in patients with a history of sickle cell disease. *Staphylococcus*, which is responsible for the majority of bone infections in the general population, is responsible for <25% of infections in patients with sickle cell disease.

> HELPFUL TIP: Most cases of childhood osteomyelitis are the result of hematogenous spread rather than by direct contamination of the bone.

Identification of the pathogen in a case of osteomyelitis is typically made by:

A) ASO titer.
B) Blood culture.
C) Joint aspiration, culture, and Gram stain.
D) Pathology report following open biopsy.

Discussion
The correct answer is "B." A blood culture will reveal the offending organism in 40–50% of cases. Joint aspiration is not typically indicated unless there is strong evidence of joint involvement. After 7–10 days, osseous changes may be seen on plain film radiographs, MRI, and bone scan. If changes are identified and a neoplastic process is ruled out, aspiration at the site of periosteal elevation and bony destruction should be considered if a pathogen has not yet been identified by blood culture. "A," an ASO titer, would not be helpful here since this tests for *Strep pyogenes* infection. An ASO titer would be helpful if looking for rheumatic fever. "D," surgical biopsy, may be required if blood cultures do not reveal a pathogen and the patient is not responding appropriately to empiric antibiotics.

> HELPFUL TIP: Treatment of osteomyelitis requires 4–6 weeks of antibiotics. Surgical debridement is usually (if not always) required as well.

Objectives: Did you learn to . . .

- Diagnose osteomyelitis in a child?
- Identify common pathogens involved in osteomyelitis?

CASE 10

A 45-year-old female with a history of rheumatoid arthritis, on chronic low-dose prednisone, presents to your clinic with 2 days of right knee pain. The patient reports that her knee has been swollen and painful to touch, and she now is having difficulty bearing weight due to the pain. She has had previous knee pain, but nothing this severe. She denies any trauma, fevers, chills, knee surgery, illegal drug use, or risky sexual behavior. On examination, she is well appearing, afebrile, and has a moderate right knee effusion with limited ROM. There is no overlying erythema, but the knee feels warm to touch.

Which of the following diagnostics is the most valuable to rule in or rule out the diagnosis with the highest potential morbidity?

A) Plain films of the affected knee.
B) WBC count.
C) ESR.
D) Arthrocentesis.
E) MRI.

Discussion

The correct answer is "D." The most concerning diagnosis with the highest potential morbidity in this patient is septic arthritis. Her history of rheumatoid arthritis as well as long-term steroid use put her at high risk. In a patient in whom you are concerned about septic arthritis, the most important piece of diagnostic data that you can obtain comes from synovial fluid analysis. While plain radiographs, a WBC count, an ESR, and CRP may be obtained (your friendly neighborhood orthopedic surgeon will surely want to know them), they are neither sensitive nor specific enough to rule in or rule out septic arthritis in a high-risk patient.

Which of the following signs or symptoms has sufficient sensitivity to rule out septic arthritis if absent?

A) Joint edema or effusion.
B) Fever.
C) Sweats.
D) Significantly restricted ROM.
E) **None** of the listed signs or symptoms has sufficient sensitivity to rule out septic arthritis if absent.

Discussion

The correct answer is "E." Unfortunately, there are no clinical signs or symptoms that have sufficient sensitivity to rule out septic arthritis.

* *

You effortlessly obtain 10 ccs of cloudy synovial fluid that is sent to the lab for Gram stain, culture, cell count, and crystal analysis. The Gram stain is negative with cultures pending. The synovial WBC count is 51,000/μL with >90% polymorphonuclear cells. The crystal analysis shows calcium pyrophosphate crystals. You obtain a peripheral WBC count that is 11,000/μL and an ESR is 55mm/hr.

What is the most appropriate next course of action based on these finding?

A) Prescribe high-dose prednisone for a flair of her rheumatoid arthritis
B) Start IV antibiotics and obtain emergent orthopedic consultation.
C) Treat her for pseudogout.
D) Recommend rest, ice, compression, and a prescription for oxycodone.

Discussion

The correct answer is "B." Various cutoffs for synovial WBC counts have been proposed, ranging from >25,000/μL to >100,000/μL with sensitivities ranging from 13% to 88%. A synovial WBC count of 51,000/μL does not rule out septic arthritis in this patient. When the percentage of polymorphonuclear cells is >90%, this significantly increases the likelihood of septic arthritis. Don't let the fact that the crystal analysis showed calcium pyrophosphate crystals dissuade you from suspecting septic arthritis as both gout and pseudogout can coexist with septic arthritis.

Objectives: Did you learn to . . .

- Recognize the clinical presentation of septic arthritis?
- Understand the limitations of using signs and symptoms to rule out septic arthritis?
- Describe the appropriate workup for a patient with suspected septic arthritis?

QUICK QUIZ: MY BIG FAT GREEK KNEE PAIN

A 55-year-old obese female comes to your office complaining of knee pain when she walks. She had an MRI at an urgent care center, which showed some meniscal damage. She is tender inferiorly and medial to the patella on the proximal tibia (but not on the joint line).

Which of the following is true?

A) Washing out her knee by arthroscopy will help to relieve her symptoms.
B) The finding of a meniscal injury on MRI correlates well with symptoms of pain.

C) Based on its location, pes anserinus bursitis is the likely cause of her pain.
D) Baklava is Dr. Wilbur's favorite food.

Discussion

The correct answer is "C." The pes anserinus bursa is located on the medial, proximal aspect of the tibia and is where the tendons of the sartorius, gracilis, and semitendinosus attach. It often becomes inflamed causing significant and chronic knee pain. Steroid injections are the treatment of choice. "A" is incorrect. Several studies have found that washing out the knee and trimming the cartilage is of no benefit. "B" is also incorrect. MRI of the knee is not particularly useful for determining if a meniscal injury is the source of pain. Similar to herniated disks, many asymptomatic patients have meniscal injuries on MRI limiting our ability to assign symptoms to an MRI finding. This is especially true in the elderly with arthritis where >90% will have meniscal damage. As to "D," it obviously does not relate to the case. We call that "test taking skill." If you chose "D," woe is with you...

QUICK QUIZ: ORTHOPEDIC INFECTIONS

The most common organism causing septic arthritis in the teenage years is:

A) *N. gonorrhoeae* (Gonococcus).
B) Polymicrobial.
C) *Salmonella* species.
D) *S. aureus*.
E) *Streptococcus* species.

Discussion

The correct answer is "A." Gonococcus is the most common organism isolated from the joints of sexually active, teenage individuals.

CASE 11

A 28-year-old male presents to your clinic for evaluation of lower back pain (LBP). Yesterday morning he first noticed the discomfort, manifesting as stiffness and soreness in the lower back. The day before had been spent running a floor polisher. He describes his pain as sharp in nature and 8/10 in intensity. He denies radiation of the pain, sensory changes, and constitutional symptoms. He is concerned this may be an injury to a disk and that he may be permanently disabled due to his extreme pain.

Which of the following signs or symptoms would be "red flags" indicating the need for early imaging and/or referral?

A) Pain radiating down one or both legs into the posterior thigh.
B) Severe pain, prompting the patient to request narcotics.
C) Pain greater with active lumbar extension than with forward flexion.
D) New onset erectile dysfunction with back pain.
E) None of the above.

Discussion

The correct answer is "D." The onset of erectile dysfunction is suggestive of neurologic involvement and warrants further investigation. None of the other options are suggestive of significant disease requiring immediate intervention ("A" certainly could represent disk disease; however, this does not require immediate intervention).

Early imaging should be obtained in all of the following presentations of low back pain EXCEPT:

A) Neurologic symptoms such as bowel or bladder dysfunction and impotence.
B) History of fever, night sweats, and weight loss.
C) History of cancer.
D) Trauma.
E) Age >30 years.

Discussion

The correct answer is "E." Patients **over** the age of 50 should have early imaging. See Table 12–2 for other criteria that should prompt early imaging.

> HELPFUL TIP: Several of the indicators listed in Table 12–2 are associated with cauda equina syndrome. Cauda equina syndrome is the result of an acute reduction in the volume of the spinal canal resulting in compression and paralysis of multiple nerve roots distal to the conus medullaris. It is often caused by central disk herniations, epidural abscesses and hematomas, fractures, and other trauma. Cauda equina syndrome is an orthopedic emergency, and MRI and surgical consultation should be sought without delay.

Table 12–2 CRITERIA SUGGESTING THE NEED FOR EARLY IMAGING FOR BACK PAIN

Bowel or bladder dysfunction
New onset of impotence
Fevers or night sweats
Unplanned weight loss
Night pain
Personal history of cancer
Saddle anesthesia
History of recent trauma (e.g., fall or direct blow… NOT twisting or lifting)
Age >50 or <18
Patient with current or recent use of steroids
Any suspicion of an infectious or neoplastic cause for low back pain
Pain for >6 weeks

HELPFUL TIP: Patients who **do not** have films done initially actually have better outcomes than those who do. When we order imaging studies, we "medicalize" the illness, causing the patient to expect a longer recovery and the need for intervention in order to get better.

Upon physical examination, you note the vital signs are normal. Straight leg raise (SLR) testing on the right leg at 55 degrees reproduces the patient's pain in the lower back and a painful "tightness" in the posterior thigh. He complains of the same discomfort on the left at 30 degrees.

Based on these findings, which of the following statements is true?

A) This is a positive SLR test bilaterally and is specific for disk herniation.
B) This is a positive SLR test on the left and is specific for disk herniation.
C) This is a positive SLR test on the right and is specific for disk herniation.
D) This is a negative SLR test bilaterally.

Discussion

The correct answer is "D." The SLR test can be performed in several ways, which are listed here.

- **Seated active:** with the patient seated on the exam table, the examiner asks that he dorsiflex the foot and extend the knee.
- **Seated passive:** with the patient seated on the exam table, the examiner passively extends the knee, and radicular symptoms will be exacerbated with passive ankle dorsiflexion.
- **Lying passive:** with the patient in a supine position, the examiner holds the knee in full extension and passively flexes the hip, and radicular symptoms will be exacerbated with passive ankle dorsiflexion.

In all cases, the test is positive when radicular symptoms occur (e.g., pain and paresthesias down the leg below the level of the knee—not back or thigh pain from muscle stretching) between 25 and 75 degrees of hip flexion while lying or with knee extension while seated. The symptoms will be exacerbated with active or passive ankle dorsiflexion. However, the SLR is neither sensitive nor specific for disk disease. "Crossover" pain with radicular symptoms in the leg not lifted is very specific for disk disease.

* *

Even though SLR is negative, you continue your neurologic exam. You note symmetric patellar reflexes, diminished Achilles reflex on the right, and symmetric strength in the legs except for decreased strength with ankle eversion on the right. You also note decrease in gross sensation to light touch over the right lateral malleolus.

Which of the following nerve roots is most likely compromised?

A) L3.
B) L4.
C) L5.
D) S1.
E) S2–4.

Discussion

The correct answer is "D." A summary of nerve root innervation is given in Table 12–3.

Appropriate initial treatment for this patient's acute back pain should include which of the following?

A) Strict bed rest.
B) Pain control.
C) Corset or lumbar belt.

Table 12–3 EXAM FINDINGS OF LUMBAR AND SACRAL SPINAL NERVE ROOTS

Nerve Root	Reflex	Motor	Sensory	Test
L2 – 3	None	Quadriceps	Anterior thigh	Strength with leg raising
L4	Patella	Tibialis anterior (foot dorsiflexion, inversion)	Medial lower leg and foot	Stand on heels, inside of foot
L5	Medial hamstring (difficult to assess)	Extensor hallucis longus (dorsiflexion of big toe)	Dorsal foot	Hold up toe
S1	Achilles	Peroneus longus and brevis (ankle eversion) and plantar flexion of foot	Lateral foot	Stand on toes, inside of foot
S2–4	Anal wink	Intrinsic foot muscles, anal sphincter tone	Perianal	

D) Referral for epidural steroid injection or endoscopic disk resection.
E) A and B.

Discussion

The correct answer is "B." In acute mechanical back pain (no longer than 6 weeks), regardless of the method of treatment, 40% are better within 1 week, 60–85% in 3 weeks, and 90% in 2 months. Negative prognostic factors include more than three episodes of back pain, gradual onset of symptoms, and prolonged absence from work. **Bedrest does not contribute to a return of function and may worsen outcomes.** Early mobilization of the patient is best for allowing him to continue activities as tolerated. Acetaminophen is a great drug for pain control and has fewer side effects than do the NSAIDs.

Chiropractic care and acupuncture may be useful.

HELPFUL TIP: For low back pain, early mobilization and walking is important. Epidural steroid injections, while intuitively appealing, have been shown to be of no long-term (and little short term) benefit (*Journal of Bone and Joint Surgery*. 2012;94:1353-1358, and others).

* *

You prescribe your pain medication of choice and recommend rehabilitation exercises.

Which of the following has been shown to be effective at reducing the recurrence of back injury in the workplace?

A) Back support belts.
B) "Back School" that teaches proper lifting techniques, stretches, etc.
C) Increasing physical fitness and muscle tone.
D) A and C.
E) B and C.

Discussion

The correct answer is "C." The only thing that has been unequivocally shown to reduce further back injuries is improving the overall fitness of the patient and his muscle tone. **Of special note, back support belts, long worn in industry, have equivocal data with most studies being negative.** "Back School" also does not seem to help.

HELPFUL TIP: Physical therapy modalities such as application of heat, cold, and ultrasound, and muscle stimulation may have short-term benefit. Rehabilitation exercises focusing on trunk extensors, abdominal muscles, and aerobic conditioning promote early mobilization, which is critical in treating acute back pain. **The specific exercise does not matter as much as the mobilization.** Sham therapy works as well as specific exercises as long as the patient is mobile.

Objectives: Did you learn to . . .

- Generate a differential diagnosis and understand the etiology of lumbar spine pain?
- Evaluate and treat acute low back pain?
- Recognize warning signs of low back pain?

QUICK QUIZ: BACK PAIN

Spondylolysis commonly occurs in which part of the spine?

A) Cervical spine lateral processes.
B) Thoracic spine pars interarticularis.
C) Thoracic spine lateral processes.
D) Lumbar spine pars interarticularis.

Discussion

The correct answer is "D." Spondylolysis is characterized by bilateral pars interarticularis fractures and most commonly occurs in the lumbar region.

QUICK QUIZ: MORE BACK PAIN

Spondylolysis generally presents with pain:

A) When the slippage is 10–15% and the patient is an early teen (12–14).
B) When the slippage is 25% and the patient is an early teen (12–14).
C) When slippage is 25% and the patient is in the late teens and early 20s.
D) When slippage is 10–15% and the patient is >60 years old.
E) When slippage is 25% and the patient is >60 years old.

Discussion

The correct answer is "C." Spondylolysis is generally a problem in the late teens and 20s. Patients become symptomatic when there is 25% slippage or greater. Predisposing factors include recurrent lumbar hyperextension (gymnasts, football players, etc.), although many patients do not have an identifiable cause. Patients present with back pain that is made worse by hyperextension. Treatment is usually conservative but may require surgical intervention if cord compromise occurs.

QUICK QUIZ: EVEN MORE BACK PAIN

Anterior slippage of one vertebra on another is called:

A) Spondylolysis.
B) Spondylolisthesis.
C) Spondylitis.
D) Spondyloarthropathy.
E) Scheuermann disease.

Discussion

The correct answer is "B." Slippage of one vertebra on another is called spondylolisthesis. "A," spondylolysis, is discussed above. Spondyloarthropathy is a nonspecific term referring to inflammation of the spine and encompasses such diseases as ankylosing spondylitis, Reiter disease, enteropathic arthritis, etc. Spondylitis is a more specific term for the same thing (e.g., ankylosing spondylitis). "E," Scheuermann disease, is a process causing kyphosis by compression of the vertebrae (at least 5 degrees of wedging in 3 consecutive vertebrae). The cause is unknown but it tends to present in adolescence.

QUICK QUIZ: BACK PAIN IN CHILDREN

A 4-year-old boy presents to your office accompanied by his mother who says he has a limp and LBP. This has been getting progressively worse over the past 2 weeks. When the patient sits, he sits in a "tripod" position supporting his weight on his hands. Vitals are normal without a fever and a CBC is normal.

This history is most consistent with:

A) Discitis.
B) Occult fracture.
C) Growing pains.
D) Juvenile rheumatoid arthritis.

Discussion

The correct answer is "A." This history is most consistent with discitis. Discitis is an inflammatory process of the disk usually found in children age infancy to 3 years but may occur at any age. The etiology is usually *Staphylococcus* (low-grade infection) but there may be sterile inflammation. Fever is usually absent in discitis (seen in only 25%), and blood cultures are sterile. The white count is usually normal, although ESR is elevated in 90%. Treatment is not standardized, but most experts would include antistaphylococcal antibiotics. "B," occult fracture, is unlikely in a child this age. "C," growing pains, does not present with back pain (see the discussion of growing pains elsewhere in this chapter). Juvenile rheumatoid arthritis presents with small joint involvement as opposed to back pain.

CASE 12

A 24-year-old male presents to the clinic 2 days after a collision during a softball game in which he fell on his outstretched right hand ("But I made the play!" he exclaims). He reports he could not continue playing and that his pain has not improved. He has some general edema around the right wrist, poor grip strength secondary to pain, point tenderness over the radial aspect of the wrist ("snuff box tenderness"), and decreased ROM. There is no obvious deformity, and he is neurovascularly intact.

Of the following, what would be the most likely diagnosis for this patient?

A) Colles fracture.
B) Scaphoid fracture.
C) Smith fracture.
D) Extensor carpi radialis strain.
E) Scapholunate sprain.

Discussion

The correct answer is "B." Although all of these could be in the differential diagnosis, "B" is the most likely based on mechanism of injury and clinical findings. The scaphoid spans both the proximal and distal carpal row. In this position, it is quite vulnerable to high-impact injuries, such as a fall on an outstretched hand, and is the most commonly fractured carpal bone. The absence of deformity makes a Colles or Smith fracture less likely.

> HELPFUL TIP: Palpating for snuffbox tenderness with the wrist in slight ulnar deviation increases the sensitivity of the physical exam.

> An additional physical exam finding consistent with a scaphoid injury is pain at the scaphoid with axial loading of the thumb.

* *

Plain film radiographs, including AP and lateral of the hand and wrist as well as scaphoid views, are negative for fracture.

What is the most appropriate next step for this patient?

A) Short-arm thumb spica cast with follow-up in 10–14 days.
B) NSAIDs, ice, compression, and elevation followed by physical therapy.
C) Bone scan or CT to rule out an occult fracture.
D) Orthopedic referral.
E) Return to play within the week.

Discussion

The correct answer is "A." Scaphoid fractures are often occult acutely and usually will be evident on plain films after 10–14 days due to bony resorption along the fracture line. If repeat films are negative but suspicion remains high, an MRI or bone scan should be considered.

> HELPFUL TIP: Although not the standard of care, early MRI or CT (neither is definitively superior to the other) to evaluate for occult scaphoid fractures may allow patients to return to full activity sooner than would be possible if they were splinted for 10–14 days. This may be cost-effective for certain patients (i.e., concert violinists or the Iowa Hawkeye's starting quarterback). Both MRI and CT are better at excluding fractures than they are at confirming them (they can be ruled out, but not necessarily ruled in).

* *

Repeat wrist radiographs including scaphoid views 2 weeks postinjury indicate a nondisplaced fracture of the **proximal** pole of the scaphoid.

You recommend which of the following treatment plans?

A) Wrist and thumb spica splint and physical therapy because good blood supply at the proximal pole allows fast healing.
B) Thumb spica cast for 6 weeks then repeat x-rays.
C) Short-arm cast excluding the thumb for 4–6 weeks.
D) Orthopedics referral for open reduction/internal fixation.
E) B or D.

Discussion

The correct answer is "E." It is clear that a spica cast with the thumb included is important; whether a short- or long-arm cast is optimal is still a matter of debate. Open fixation is another option. Generally, treatment of scaphoid fractures should be overseen by an orthopedic surgeon since there is a high rate of complications. A proximal pole fracture has high risk for nonunion and avascular necrosis. **The blood supply to the scaphoid is through the distal pole, putting the proximal pole at high risk for complications.** Evidence of healing may not be well visualized on plain films, and a CT or MRI may be needed to confirm the degree of healing. The closer the fracture line is to the proximal pole, the lower the threshold for orthopedic referral.

HELPFUL TIP: Healing time for a distal pole scaphoid fracture is 6–8 weeks, middle third or waist fractures are 8–12 weeks, and proximal pole fractures can take 12–24 weeks.

Objectives: Did you learn to . . .

- Recognize a patient at risk for scaphoid fracture?
- Manage a patient with a scaphoid fracture?

QUICK QUIZ: HAND INJURIES

A patient presents after "jamming" his index finger while playing basketball. He has mild swelling at the DIP joint. At rest, his DIP is flexed. He has full ROM of all joints except he cannot extend at the DIP.

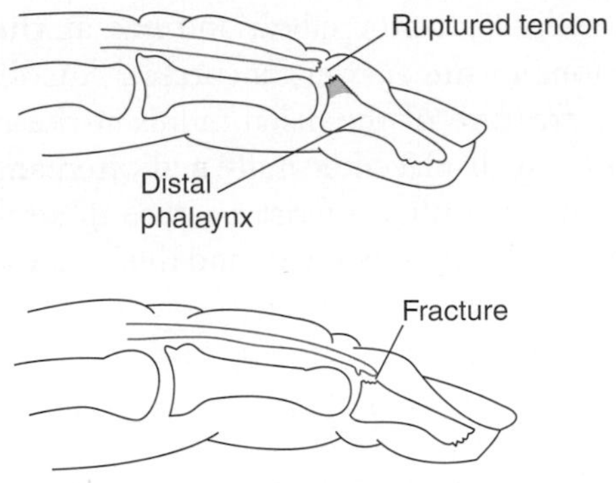

Figure 12–3

What is the appropriate treatment and follow-up?

A) RICE therapy, PRN follow-up.
B) A full extension splint of the DIP joint worn at all times with orthopedic follow-up in 1–2 weeks.
C) A removable aluminum splint to be worn for comfort, follow-up in clinic in 1 month.
D) Ibuprofen and return to full activities, PRN follow-up.

Discussion

The correct answer is "B." The patient has suffered an injury to his extensor tendon mechanism, known as a "mallet finger." X-rays are indicated to evaluate for a bony fracture/avulsion. The initial treatment is an extension splint at the DIP joint, and follow-up with an orthopedic surgeon as surgical correction is sometimes required. The splint must be worn at all times. See Figure 12–3 for the anatomy of a mallet finger.

QUICK QUIZ: FRACTURES

A Colles fracture consists of:

A) A fracture of the midshaft of the radius and ulna.
B) A fracture of the head of radius and ulna that is displaced dorsally and is angulated.
C) A fracture of the head of the radius and ulna that is displaced ventrally and is angulated.
D) None of the above.

Discussion

The correct answer is "D," none of the above. OK, some of you may have chosen "B." However, the **head**

of the radius is at the elbow and **not at the wrist.** Thus, none of the answers is correct. A Colles fracture is a fracture of the distal radius at the metaphysis, which is displaced dorsally and often angulated. It is the most common wrist fracture in adults. The ulnar styloid is often involved, and there may be intra-articular involvement as well.

QUICK QUIZ: DE QUERVAIN TENOSYNOVITIS

Which of the following physical exam findings would be associated with the diagnosis of De Quervain tenosynovitis?

A) Positive Finkelstein test.
B) Positive Phalen test.
C) Positive Tinel sign.
D) Sensory loss over the C7 dermatome.
E) Weakness of the intrinsic muscles of the hand.

Discussion

The correct answer is "A." De Quervain tenosynovitis is a tendonitis of the abductor pollicis longus, the extensor pollicis brevis, and occasionally the extensor pollicis longus. Full flexion of the thumb into the palm and ulnar deviation of the wrist produces exquisite tenderness over the radial aspect of the wrist (positive Finklestein test). Other findings may include soft-tissue swelling and pain over the abductor pollicis longus and extensor pollicis brevis tendons near the radial styloid. Crepitus may also be palpable or audible with ROM.

QUICK QUIZ: DE QUERVAIN TENOSYNOVITIS

The appropriate treatment of De Quervain tendonitis includes which of the following?

A) Thumb spica splint.
B) NSAIDs.
C) Steroid injection.
D) Surgical release of the tendon.
E) All of the above.

Discussion

The correct answer is "E." All of the above treatments have been used successfully for the treatment of De Quervain tendonitis. It is of note that some prefer steroid injection as the first-line therapy rather than NSAIDs. Surgery is obviously a last choice.

QUICK QUIZ: ANGER MANAGEMENT ISSUES

A 19-year-old male was mad at his girlfriend and decided to punch the wall. "He fought the wall and the wall won." Radiographs demonstrate a fifth metacarpal fracture with some angulation.

What is the maximal acceptable angulation and rotation for a boxer fracture, fourth or fifth metacarpal, to maintain full hand function?

A) 10 degrees of dorsal angulation and 10 degrees of rotation.
B) 30 degrees of dorsal angulation and 5 degrees of rotation.
C) 40 degrees of dorsal angulation and 0 degrees of rotation
D) 90 degrees of dorsal angulation and 0 degrees of rotation.

Discussion

The correct answer is "C." **Any degree of rotation**, or **>40 degrees of dorsal angulation**, may result in significant functional deficits. Reduction should be attempted if angulation is >10 degrees. Patients should be advised that with angulations >10–15 degrees, there will likely be a loss of metacarpophalangeal (MCP) prominence, although there should be no loss of function. If this is unacceptable to the patient, referral is recommended.

HELPFUL TIP: Any "scissoring" or crossing of the patient's fingers while they clench their fist should raise your suspicion for a rotational deformity.

HELPFUL TIP: Boxer fractures **are not** caused by a fall on an outstretched hand regardless of what many patients may claim.

CASE 13

The next patient in the ED was trying to break up a bar fight when he was tripped and fell onto his side, landing on the tip of his right shoulder. He states that he can actively move his arm but is limited by pain on the top of his shoulder. He has also noticed a small painful bump on top of the right shoulder and is concerned that he "broke his collarbone."

Based on the mechanism of injury and patient history, the most likely injury would be?

A) Acromioclavicular (AC) sprain.
B) Biceps tendon rupture.
C) Glenohumeral dislocation.
D) Rotator cuff tear.
E) Scapula fracture.

Discussion

The correct answer is "A." Although any of these injuries may be present, an AC sprain is the most likely based on the history and the way the patient fell. A thorough exam should be able to further distinguish between these injuries. "B" is not likely, given the mechanism of injury. The deformity associated with biceps tendon rupture (a defect in tendon with pain and deformity in the muscle belly representing the contracted, detached muscle) would be on the upper arm or at the elbow, not on the "top" of the shoulder. "C" is incorrect. The deformity and loss of ROM of a glenohumeral dislocation (shoulder dislocation) is usually obvious. The mechanism of injury is typically a forced abduction and external rotation. "D" is less likely. A rotator cuff tear will present with pain more laterally over the subacromial space and should not have an associated deformity. The ROM is generally markedly limited by pain. "E" is unlikely. Scapula fractures are uncommon and are usually the result of high velocity blunt trauma such as a blow from a baseball bat or motorcycle accident. Plain film radiographs should be obtained to rule out a clavicle fracture, especially when any deformity is present.

Your patient is worried that he broke his "collarbone." If he did sustain a clavicle fracture, which of the following would be appropriate treatment?

A) External fixation with molded plaster to maintain alignment.
B) A sling for comfort only.
C) A figure 8 splint.
D) B and C.
E) Any of the above choices is appropriate.

Discussion

The correct answer is "B." While the traditional teaching has been that a figure 8 splint is required, it adds nothing to the treatment of a clavicle fracture. Pain control and using a sling work just as well. Additionally, figure 8 splints often increase a patient's pain and can cause a brachial plexus injury. Thus, a sling is preferable.

The proper treatment for a clavicle fracture that is displaced is:

A) Closed reduction and then a sling.
B) Open reduction and immobilization.
C) Open reduction and **early** mobilization.
D) A sling.
E) None of the above.

Discussion

The correct answer is "D." The ends of a displaced clavicle fracture need not be approximated for healing to occur and for function to return. Thus, any reduction is generally not necessary.

> HELPFUL TIP: The paradigm of the treatment of clavicle fractures is shifting with more patients getting an internal fixation. This depends on the degree of displacement and the occupation of the patient (Surgeons? Yes. Car Salesmen? Not so much).

* *

You send the patient for x-rays. AP radiographs show slight widening of the AC joint on the injured side with symmetric distance between the clavicles and coracoid processes. The exam and radiograph confirm your suspicion of an AC injury.

For this patient with an AC sprain, you offer:

A) Sling for comfort, ice, and NSAIDs or analgesics for pain control.
B) Referral for open fixation.
C) Figure 8 strap for 4–6 weeks.
D) Corticosteroid injection followed by physical therapy.
E) Manual reduction, then sling immobilization for 6–8 weeks.

Discussion

The correct answer is "A." Surgical fixation is rarely needed for AC injuries unless an anterior or posterior displacement of the clavicle is present or in injuries in which the coracoclavicular interspace distance is increased >100% more than the distance seen on the uninjured side without weights. Choices "C," "D," and "E" are not appropriate for this type of injury.

Objectives: Did you learn to . . .

- Differentiate between causes of shoulder injuries?
- Treat a clavicular fracture?
- Manage AC injuries?

CASE 14

A 65-year-old male presents with left shoulder pain and weakness that started after he put a new roof on his house. The pain came on gradually and is made worse with abduction and flexion of the shoulder joint. He describes himself active and healthy, and he only takes acetaminophen when needed for shoulder pain. You suspect that he may have a rotator cuff injury.

If this is the case, what do you expect to find on exam?

A) Tenderness to palpation of the greater tuberosity of the humerus.
B) Limited active ROM.
C) Normal passive ROM.
D) Shoulder shrug with attempted abduction.
E) Any of the above.

Discussion
The correct answer is "E." Ok, so this might fit under the category of "trick question," but the shoulder exam can be normal in a patient with rotator cuff tear, or it can include any of the elements listed in "A" through "D."

Which of the following muscles is not a part of the rotator cuff?

A) Supraspinatus.
B) Infraspinatus.
C) Subscapularis.
D) Teres major.
E) Teres minor.

Discussion
The correct answer is "D." The rotator cuff consists of the other four muscles listed and functions to rotate the arm and stabilize the humeral head.

Which of the following muscles is the most commonly torn in the rotator cuff?

A) Supraspinatus.
B) Infraspinatus.
C) Subscapularis.
D) Teres minor.

Discussion
The correct answer is "A." The supraspinatus is generally the point of origin for most tears.

> HELPFUL TIP: Full thickness tears of the rotator cuff are uncommon in individuals below the age of 40, unless associated with trauma.

* *

Based on your history and physical exam, you diagnose a rotator cuff tendonosis.

Appropriate initial management of this 65-year-old male should be:

A) Acetaminophen and physical therapy.
B) Oral corticosteroids and physical therapy.
C) Subacromial injection with corticosteroid and physical therapy.
D) Surgical repair and physical therapy.
E) None of the above.

Discussion
The correct answer is "A." For initial management in an individual >60 years of age, acetaminophen and physical therapy for 6 weeks is the best answer. If they have no improvement or inadequate response, a corticosteroid injection may be used judiciously. Injection will likely cause at least short-term pain relief but is thought to weaken the tendon and may accelerate extension of the tear. Oral steroid administration may provide relief, but it is associated with a higher incidence of systemic side effects. Patients with significant symptoms or failed therapy should be considered for MRI, orthopedic referral, and surgical management. Patients under the age of 60 with acute traumatic tears should be considered for surgery, with best results within 6 weeks of injury.

> HELPFUL TIP: The old adage about corticosteroids causing weakening of the tendon has recently been questioned. It is now thought that the steroid injection provides enough relief of the pain that the patient will start using

the extremity in ways he or she had not done before. This leads to tendon rupture from the additional load. However, the point remains that steroid injections may be associated with, but not causative of, tendon rupture.

* *

Your patient is successful in rehabilitating his left shoulder, but then he returns 2 years later with right shoulder problems. The right shoulder has become progressively stiff and painful, and his ROM is now significantly limited in all directions. Your examination is consistent with "frozen shoulder" or adhesive capsulitis.

Adhesive capsulitis is most commonly associated with which of the following?

A) Diabetes mellitus type 1.
B) Hyperthyroidism.
C) Spondyloarthritis.
D) Nondominant arm.
E) Male gender.

Discussion

The correct answer is "A." Adhesive capsulitis has no clear predilection as to gender, race, arm dominance, or occupation. It is characterized by loss of ROM of the shoulder in all directions, with loss of both passive and active motion. It has a high incidence in patients with type 1 diabetes and tends to be more recalcitrant in those patients, of whom up to 50% will have bilateral involvement—although not necessarily concomitantly. Adhesive capsulitis is not typically related to trauma, but it can be associated with disuse due to pain, osteoarthritis, sling use, etc. Other conditions that are associated with adhesive capsulitis include **hypo**thyroidism, cervical disc disease, and Parkinson disease.

HELPFUL TIP: Adhesive capsulitis is considered to be idiopathic and separate from posttraumatic or postoperative joint stiffness or adhesions.

What initial treatment do you recommend for this patient?

A) Arthroscopic debridement.
B) Oral corticosteroids.
C) NSAIDs and a sling for comfort.
D) Extended progressive physical therapy.
E) Mobilization under anesthesia.

Discussion

The correct answer is "D." A progressive stretching program with heat and NSAIDs or acetaminophen to improve comfort is the most appropriate early treatment. A corticosteroid injection may be beneficial, but should be used cautiously in diabetic patients. Oral steroids have no greater benefit than NSAIDs. "C" is incorrect because a sling will contribute to further immobilization and worsening of the problem. Mobilization under anesthesia may be a last resort in true adhesive capsulitis, but is more commonly used for posttraumatic or postoperative joint stiffness or adhesions that do not respond to conservative treatment.

HELPFUL TIP: The typical clinical course for adhesive capsulitis evolves over 1–2 years with an initial "freezing" phase characterized by progressing pain and stiffness followed by a slow "thawing" phase with decreasing pain and increasing ROM.

Objectives: Did you learn to . . .

- Define the muscles of the rotator cuff?
- Identify, evaluate, and treat a rotator cuff injury?
- Recognize the presentation, associations, and treatment of adhesive capsulitis?

CASE 15

A 58-year-old male presents after sudden onset of right upper arm pain. He was working in the yard, cutting and pulling out some bushes, when he heard a "snap" and felt the pain. He has a history of rotator cuff tendonosis and osteoarthritis.

You should look for all of the following on physical examination EXCEPT:

A) A positive elevated arm stress test ("Roos" test).
B) A palpable biceps muscle defect.
C) Normal grip strength.
D) An asymmetric bulge in the affected arm.

Discussion

The correct answer is "A." The elevated arm stress test is used to evaluate a patient for thoracic outlet syndrome. Have the patient lift both arms with the elbow at shoulder height while pushing the shoulders backward and repeatedly gripping and relaxing the hands. The test is positive if neurological or vascular symptoms are reproduced when the arm is elevated for a prolonged period. This patient's presentation is not consistent with thoracic outlet syndrome. However, the history is consistent with biceps tendon rupture. "B" through "D" would be expected in a patient with biceps tendon rupture. Yes, there is usually normal grip strength. The injury is, of course, in the upper arm.

> **HELPFUL TIP:** Provocative maneuvers for thoracic outlet syndrome (Roos test, etc.) have poor sensitivity and specificity (<60%). They are most helpful if positive and the patient's symptoms are reproduced.

Which portion of the biceps is most commonly involved in ruptures?

A) Distal tendon.
B) Proximal short head tendon.
C) Proximal long head tendon.
D) Mid-muscle belly.
E) Proximal short head belly.

Discussion

The correct answer is "C." The long head is most commonly affected due to its position and risk for weakening secondary to rotator cuff tendonosis and shoulder impingement.

* *

You decide this patient has a rupture of the long head of the biceps tendon.

How is this injury treated initially?

A) Immediate surgical repair.
B) Delayed surgical repair.
C) Immobilization for 4–6 weeks with sling.
D) NSAIDs and physical therapy.

Discussion

The correct answer is "D." For most isolated proximal long or short head tears (with the exception of some young athletes and heavy laborers who would not tolerate the slight decrease in strength), treatment is conservative. Analgesics and physical therapy typically suffice. Surgical repair may be indicated if conservative therapy fails. Of note, you should discuss with patients the cosmetic deformity that will be permanent when these injuries are unrepaired versus scarring associated with surgery. Generally, there is approximately a 10% loss of elbow flexion and supination strength with an isolated proximal tear.

> **HELPFUL TIP:** Although proximal biceps tendon ruptures are treated conservatively, distal ruptures should be referred for early surgical repair, as the continuity of the entire muscle is lost and function at the elbow joint is significantly impaired with a 30–40% loss of strength across the elbow joint.

Objectives: Did you learn to . . .

- Identify the clinical presentation of biceps tendon rupture?
- Manage a patient with biceps tendon rupture?

CASE 16

A 25-year-old male presents to you with a history of a soccer injury. Someone evidently fell on his right foot while trying to steal the ball. The patient rapidly and forcefully twisted around the fixed foot. Since then he has had significant pain and swelling of the foot. His x-ray is shown in Figure 12–4.

This radiographic abnormality is notable for:

A) Its difficulty to detect as a fracture
B) Marked instability.
C) Association with significant pain.
D) All of the above.
E) None of the above.

Discussion

The correct answer is "D," all of the above. This is a Lisfranc fracture, which occurs between the metatarsals and the tarsal bones (the space between the metatarsals and the tarsal bones is known as the Lisfranc joint). Look for a widened space between the first and second and/or second and third metatarsals. There may also be a stepoff between the second metatarsal and middle cuneiform. These fractures may be difficult to identify unless you are looking

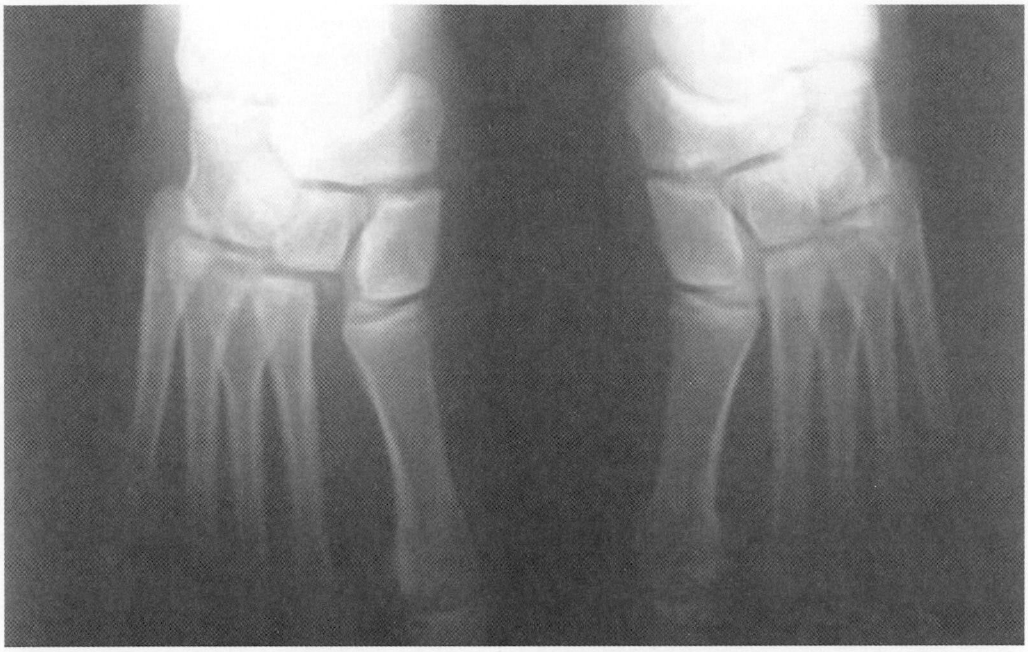

Figure 12–4

for them. Significant foot pain should be a tip off. See Figure 12–5 for further explanation.

HELPFUL TIP: Weight bearing "stress" films may be required in order to identify a Lisfranc fracture.

Appropriate treatment for this type of injury should include:

A) Weight bearing as tolerated in a postop or hard-soled shoe.
B) Rest, ice, compression, elevation, NSAIDs, and activity as tolerated. Will heal well and can be treated like a mid-foot sprain.
C) Orthopedic referral for open reduction/internal fixation (ORIF).
D) Walking boot that can be removed for several weight bearing hours a day.

Discussion

The correct answer is "C." This fracture and dislocation will lead to significant long-term pain if not recognized and treated appropriately. Any significant displacement (>2 mm) should be referred for surgical consideration. These are generally complex injuries prone to poor outcomes and should be managed by an orthopedic consultant.

Objectives: Did you learn to . . .

- Identify a Lisfranc fracture?
- Manage a patient with a Lisfranc fracture?

CASE 17

An 18-year-old female gymnast lands her dismount from the balance beam awkwardly. She reports the knee buckling, hearing a pop, and experiencing immediate right knee pain. She presents to your office 45 minutes after the injury. She is able to bear some weight on the leg but reports it is already swollen and feels loose. On exam, there is a knee effusion present.

Based on the information above, the most likely isolated injury experienced by this athlete is:

A) Medial meniscus tear.
B) MCL sprain.
C) Distal quadriceps/patellar tendon rupture.
D) Anterior cruciate ligament (ACL) rupture.
E) None of the above.

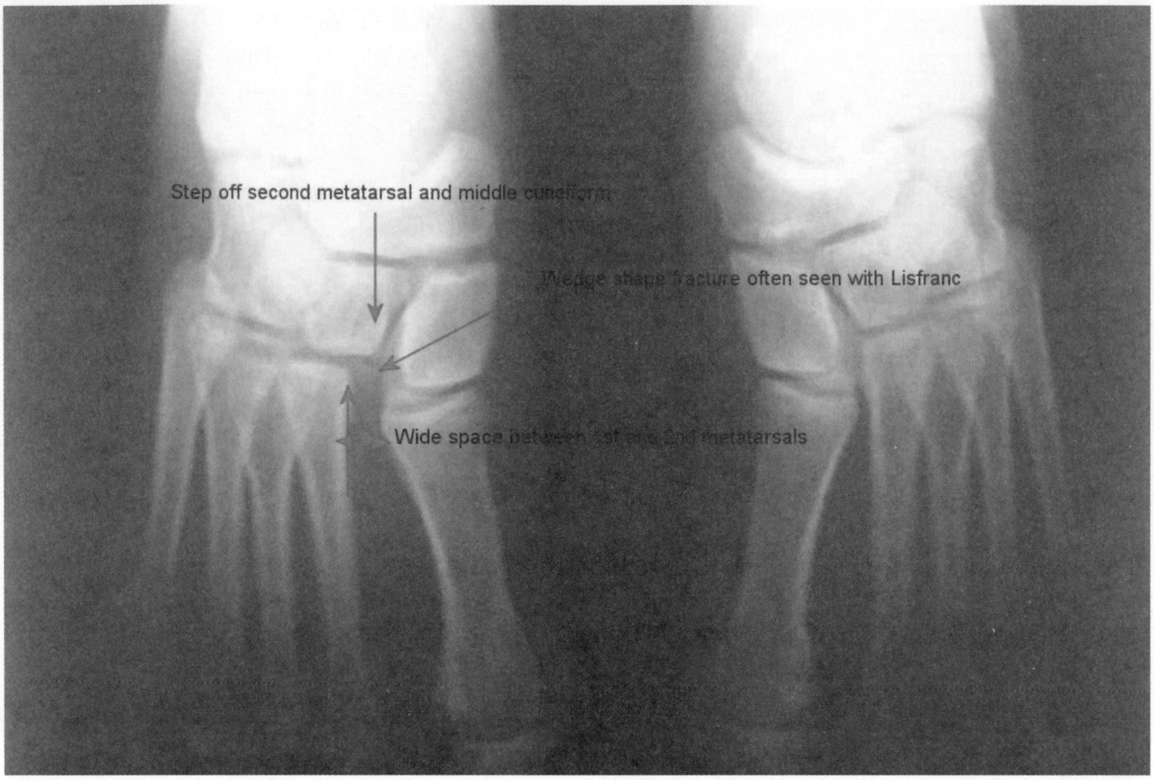

Figure 12–5

Discussion

The correct answer is "D." Did the patient or someone else hear a pop? If yes, suspect ACL tear (80%), meniscal injury (15%), and rarely a fracture. When did you notice swelling? If 0–12 hours after the injury, suspect ACL tear or patellar dislocation/subluxation; if 12–24 hours, suspect meniscal injury. If there is hemarthrosis on aspiration, suspect ACL injury (>75%), patellar subluxation, or intra-articular fracture. A history of, "My knee gives way; buckles; feels loose; or comes apart," may be secondary to patellar subluxation/dislocation, ACL deficiency, or arthritis. Collateral ligament injuries, MCL or LCL, do not typically present with significant effusion and typically feel stable with forward ambulation but are painful with side-to-side movements. Muscle or tendon rupture may cause buckling, but will not typically cause effusion and will generally have an obvious deformity and inability to bear weight.

The best test to confirm the diagnosis of the above injury would be?

A) Plain film radiographs.
B) McMurray test.
C) Lachman test.
D) Anterior drawer test.

Discussion

The correct answer is "C." In **the hands of an experienced clinician**, the Lachman test is the most sensitive test for ACL insufficiency (80–95%). The anterior drawer sign is negative in about 50% of acute ACL tears, and often is negative subacutely. McMurray test is used to evaluate for a meniscal tear. Plain films should be obtained for all patients with acute knee injury with effusion or suspected ACL tear. However, x-rays are rarely positive for more than effusion or Segond fracture (avulsion of the lateral joint capsule from the tibia). Although an MRI may be considered a gold standard test, its sensitivity has been reported as 97% when compared against arthroscopy findings, and is positive in only 82% in cases of complete rupture. An orthopedic consult is generally indicated if ACL injury is suspected, and obtaining one is less expensive than MRI.

HELPFUL TIP: The Lachman test is performed with the knee flexed at 20–30 degrees with the patient in a supine position. The examiner then attempts to anteriorly displace the tibia on the femur while stabilizing the femur.

Always remember to check the contralateral side. Some patients have naturally lax joints.

* *

You feel that this patient is very appropriate for radiographic evaluation, and you obtain x-rays of the knee.

Which of the following is NOT one of the criteria of the Ottawa knee rules predicting the need for knee radiographs?

A) Age <18.
B) Pain isolated to the patella.
C) Tenderness at the head of the fibula.
D) Inability to flex the knee 90 degrees.
E) Inability to bear weight for four steps.

Discussion

The correct answer is "A." The age criterion for the Ottawa knee rules is age >55 years. All of the other options are correct. If **any** of these criteria are present (including a patient >55 years of age), a radiograph should be obtained. These rules have been validated and are 97% sensitive for fracture. The Pittsburgh rules, which are reportedly 99% sensitive, have only two criteria: (1) age <12 years or age >50 and (2) inability to bear weight in the clinic or ED. Of the two, the Ottawa rules are the more commonly accepted.

* *

The x-ray shows no fracture. You prescribe a knee immobilizer, rest, ice, NSAIDs, and refer the patient to an orthopedic surgeon. The patient returns 2 days later with marked effusion and pain. To help relieve the pain, you perform an arthrocentesis and 90 mL of bloody aspirate is obtained. As per your clinic's standard protocol, the joint fluid is sent for analysis. The analysis returns with the only abnormalities being blood and **fat droplets**.

Based on the effusion, you suspect what diagnosis?

A) Complete ACL rupture.
B) Meniscal tear.
C) ACL and PCL tear.
D) Intra-articular fracture.
E) Patellar subluxation.

Discussion

The correct answer is "D." **Fat from bone marrow** may be seen even with a small intra-articular fracture. Consider CT or MRI if fracture is not noted on plain film. If a fracture is still not demonstrated, consider referral for orthopedic consultation.

Objectives: Did you learn to . . .

- Generate a differential diagnosis for knee pain in an athlete?
- Diagnose ACL injury?
- Determine when knee radiographs are appropriate?

QUICK QUIZ: KNEE PAIN

The best clinical test(s) for determining the presence of a meniscal injury is (are):

A) Posterior sag test.
B) Apley test.
C) McMurray test.
D) Pivot shift test.
E) B and C.

Discussion

The correct answer is "C." The McMurray test is the best test for determining meniscal injury. This is done by flexing the knee and then extending the knee while performing internal and external rotation of the tibia/fibula. Keep one hand on the knee. The test is positive when the examiner feels a pop during the maneuver or when there is significant pain during internal or external rotation. The Apley test is done with the patient in a prone position. Move the knee to 90 degrees of flexion. Put downward pressure on the tibia/fibula while internally and externally rotating the lower leg. Pain suggests a meniscal tear. Pain should be relieved by distracting the joint. The posterior sag test is used to detect PCL injury, while the pivot shift test is used to detect ACL injury.

CASE 18

A 24-year-old female presents to the clinic 24 hours after slipping on a patch of ice outside her home. She reports feeling a "pop" and immediate pain on the lateral aspect of the ankle. She reports significant swelling in the first few hours with pain and inability to bear weight initially, but now she is able to walk with a significant limp. She reports no significant past injuries to the foot or ankle. On exam, you note edema/effusion over the lateral ankle, some ecchymosis, tenderness, but no laxity on anterior drawer and inversion stress. There is no bony tenderness on palpation of the foot and ankle, but there is tenderness anterolaterally in the soft tissue.

The most likely injury this patient has suffered is?

A) Fracture of the distal tibia.
B) Fracture of the distal fibula.
C) Sprain of the lateral ligament complex.
D) Sprain of the medial ligament complex.
E) Syndesmosis sprain.

Discussion

The correct answer is "C." A sprain is most likely because there is no bony tenderness. And, since she is tender laterally, the lateral ligament complex is most likely sprained.

In this case, the most likely structure injured would be the:

A) Anterior talofibular ligament.
B) Distal fibula.
C) Distal tibia.
D) Deltoid ligament.
E) Achilles tendon.

Discussion

The correct answer is "A." This is a sprain of the anterior talofibular ligament. This is the first ligament injured with an inversion ankle sprain. It is followed by the calcaneofibular ligament if enough force is involved. "E," Achilles tendon injury (specifically rupture), is of special note. First, this injury presents as pain in the Achilles tendon area. With a complete Achilles tendon tear, the patient will have marked weakness of plantar flexion. A diagnostic test (Thompson test) is to squeeze the posterior calf with the patient lying supine on the bed and the feet dangling off. In response, the foot should plantar flex. If this does not occur, consider Achilles rupture. Operative and nonoperative treatments have been used. Operative treatment carries a lower risk of rerupture.

HELPFUL TIP: The Ottawa criteria reliably predict who needs an ankle radiograph and who does not. The Ottawa foot and ankle criteria are listed in Figure 12–6.

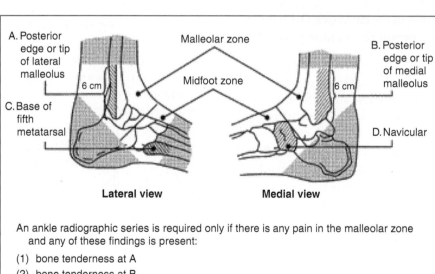

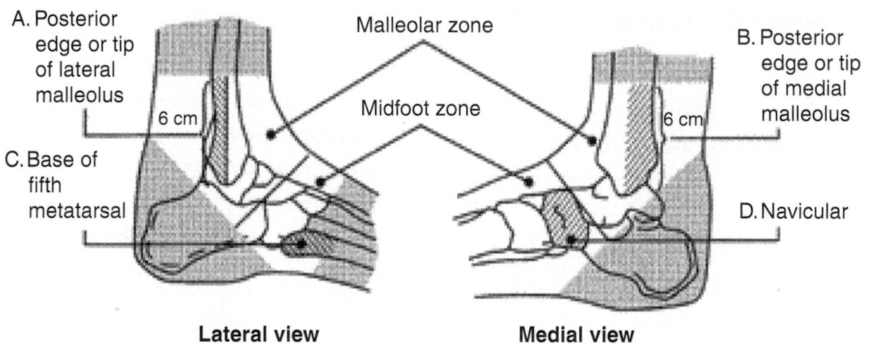

An ankle radiographic series is required only if there is any pain in the malleolar zone and any of these findings is present:

(1) bone tenderness at A
(2) bone tenderness at B
(3) inability to bear weight both immediately and in the ED

A foot radiographic series is required only if there is any pain in the midfoot zone and any of these findings is present:

(1) bone tenderness at C
(2) bone tenderness at D
(3) inability to bear weight both immediately and in the ED

Figure 12–6 **Ottawa foot and ankle x-ray criteria**

Which of the following is the most appropriate management of this patient's sprained ankle?

A) Cast for 4 weeks followed by physical therapy.
B) Crutches, nonweight bearing for 2 weeks, and then progressive physical therapy.
C) Rest, ice, elevation, and early mobilization using external support, crutches or cane if needed. Progress to activity as tolerated.
D) Refer for orthopedic consultation.
E) Immobilization with short-leg walking cast, heat for comfort, analgesics or NSAIDs, and progress to activities as tolerated.

Discussion

The correct answer is "C." Treatment for most grade I and II sprains includes external support, such as an air or gel splint, ice application, and elevation; early mobilization is critical and will hasten recovery. NSAIDs or acetaminophen should be used for pain control. The patient should be allowed partial weight bearing as tolerated with crutches or a cane. Patients with recurrent problems of instability or an acute grade III sprain should be referred to an orthopedist for evaluation.

HELPFUL TIP: Early mobilization and weight bearing reduces the time of disability for ankle sprains. Rest and nonweight bearing should be minimized. Allow the patient to advance activities as tolerated.

Objectives: Did you learn to . . .

- Identify a patient with an ankle sprain?
- Differentiate ankle sprain from fracture based on history and exam?
- Use the Ottawa ankle rules to determine when to obtain an ankle radiograph?
- Manage a patient with an ankle sprain?

CASE 19

A 27-year-old male presents to your clinic following an inversion-type injury to the foot and ankle. He cannot bear weight on the foot on presentation. He complains of pain and swelling laterally on the foot and ankle. There is some soft-tissue swelling but no obvious deformity. There is tenderness over the lateral ankle ligaments as well as over the base of the fifth metatarsal. AP and lateral films of the foot and ankle are obtained and reveal a nondisplaced transverse fracture through the proximal base of the fifth metatarsal. The radiograph is available for your review in Figure 12–7.

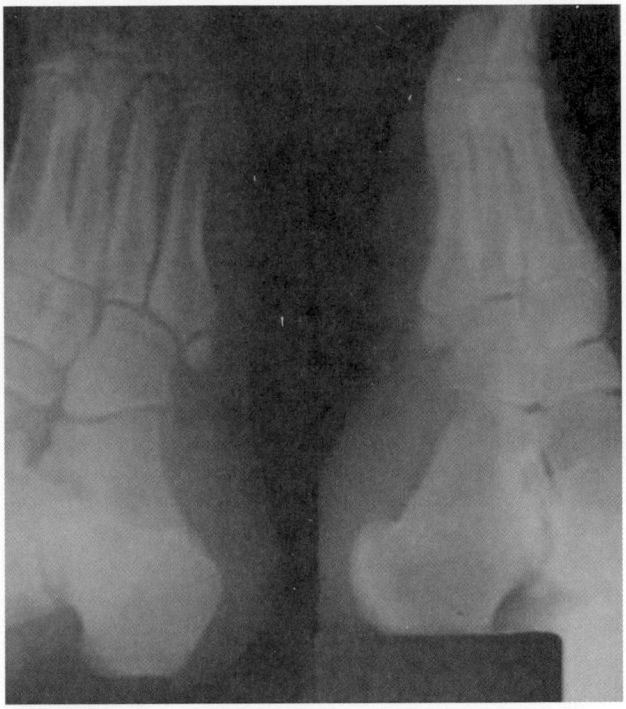

Figure 12–7

What is this injury called?

A) Jones fracture.
B) Maisonneuve fracture.
C) Kirschner fracture.
D) Avulsion fracture of tuberosity, base fifth metatarsal

Discussion

The correct answer is "D." This is an avulsion fracture of the base of the fifth metatarsal that commonly results from an inversion ankle injury. Attempts at dynamic stabilization by the peroneus brevis cause an **avulsion of the proximal portion of the metatarsal base**. This type of fracture generally heals well. If it does not, it is generally asymptomatic. A **Jones fracture** is a transverse fracture through the proximal fifth metatarsal shaft (see Figure 12–8). Jones fractures have a high incidence of nonunion because they occur in a watershed area of blood supply.

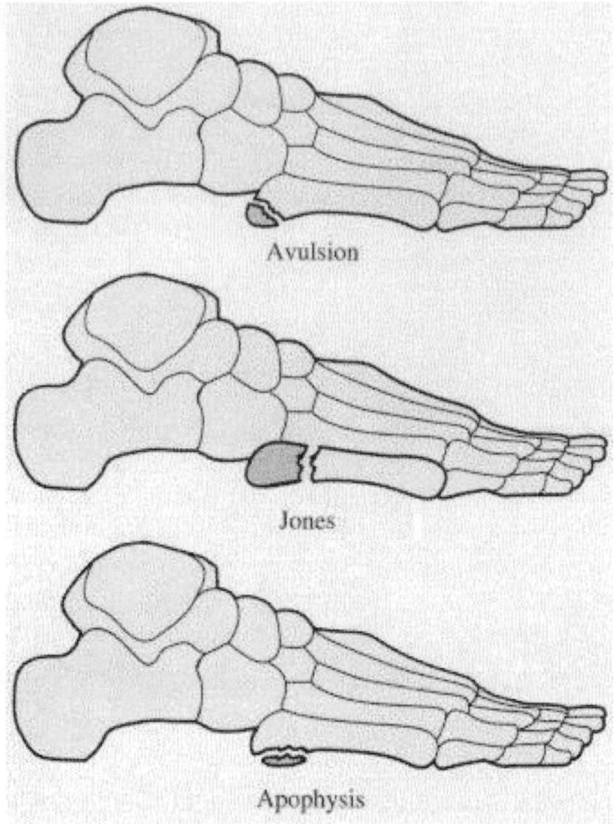

Figure 12–8 **Fractures of the fifth metatarsal bone**

HELPFUL TIP: An unfused apophysis in children and adolescents may be confused with a fifth metatarsal avulsion injury. Tuberosity avulsion fractures are transverse, while the unfused apophysis is oriented vertically along the long axis of the metatarsal.

Appropriate treatment for the fracture described above would be:

A) A wooden postoperative shoe or walking boot, with weight bearing as tolerated for 2–4 weeks.
B) Nonweight-bearing short-leg cast for 6–8 weeks.
C) Operative internal fixation.
D) Rest, ice, compression, elevation, and NSAIDs as needed.
E) None of the above.

Discussion

The correct answer is "A." Nondisplaced tuberosity fractures can be managed with a wooden postoperative shoe or cast fracture boot, with weight bearing as tolerated for 2–4 weeks. For a fracture with a displaced fragment >3 mm, orthopedic referral should be considered. Fractures to the metaphyseal–diaphyseal junction (**Jones fractures**) result from a vertical load placed on the lateral foot, such as an inversion injury or a stress injury. Jones fractures can be managed with 6–8 weeks in a nonweight-bearing short-leg cast if nondisplaced **but are best referred due to high incidence of nonunion.** All displaced Jones fractures and intra-articular tuberosity fractures should be referred for orthopedic management.

HELPFUL TIP: Stress fractures of the forefoot are common in competitive and recreational athletes, especially after a sudden increase in activity, intensity, duration, frequency, or a change in surface type. They may be occult on plain films acutely, but some subtle periosteal change may be evident on close exam in the area of maximal tenderness. If plain films are negative but suspicion remains high, consider an MRI or bone scan (less specific). The same treatment considerations apply to metatarsal stress fractures as to any other nondisplaced forefoot fracture.

Objectives: Did you learn to . . .

- Evaluate foot injuries?
- Describe fifth metatarsal fractures?
- Manage straightforward metatarsal fractures and identify which fractures should be referred?

CASE 20

A 40-year-old female factory worker presents with progressively worsening heel pain. She has pain when she first gets out of bed in the morning. The pain tends to subside after 20–45 minutes but is worsened by standing on the concrete floor of the factory where she works. She has a history of diabetes and hyperlipidemia. On examination, you find an obese female with a normal stance and gait. She has exquisite tenderness to palpation just distal to the heel on the underside of the foot. Pain is exacerbated by dorsiflexion of the toes.

Which of the following is the most likely diagnosis?

A) Tarsal tunnel syndrome.
B) Achilles tendon tear.

C) Charcot foot.
D) Plantar fasciitis.
E) Plantar fascia rupture.

Discussion
The correct answer is "D." Plantar fasciitis, the most common cause of heel pain in adults, is a degenerative condition of the origin of the plantar fascia. "A" is incorrect. Tarsal tunnel syndrome is due to posterior tibial nerve entrapment and presents with diffuse pain at the medial ankle and arch of the foot. Paresthesias and dysesthesias often occur as well. "B," Achilles tendon rupture, is incorrect because the pain should be sudden, stabbing, and located in the calf (not the plantar aspect of the heel). "C" is also incorrect. Charcot foot does occur in diabetics, but it is actually the result of neuropathy and so generally does not present with pain. Instead, Charcot foot presents as an inflammatory condition (e.g., warmth, erythema, and edema) and progresses to joint instability and severe foot deformities. Finally, "E" is incorrect because plantar fascia rupture should have a sudden onset and is related to trauma.

Which of the following is true of plantar fasciitis?

A) It more commonly occurs in individuals with pes cavus.
B) It is more common in women.
C) It is commonly an acute injury.
D) Radiographic identification of a "heel spur" or osteophyte is pathognomonic.
E) None of the above.

Discussion
The correct answer is "B." Plantar fasciitis is not associated with any particular foot type. It is nearly twice as common in women as men. It is also more common in overweight individuals. Although a tear of the plantar fascia may occur acutely, more typically a degenerative or repetitive trauma causes tendonosis. Radiographs are not recommended. Spurring may be seen in up to 50% of patients with plantar fasciitis, but is present in 20% of age matched asymptomatic adults. **Thus, the finding of a spur does not mandate surgical intervention, and radiographs are not diagnostic.**

Appropriate initial treatment for this patient's plantar fasciitis should include:

A) A heel cup or silicon pad.
B) Achilles stretching.
C) Ice or heat.
D) NSAIDs.
E) All of the above.

Discussion
The correct answer is "E," all of the above. Other initial treatments to consider include night splints to maintain ankle dorsiflexion and stretch the Achilles tendon and plantar fascia. Physical therapy modalities such as ultrasound may be helpful as well.

> HELPFUL TIP: Not all heel pain is plantar fasciitis. Remember these others: tarsal tunnel syndrome (described above), painful heel pad syndrome (pain located over the heel secondary to breakdown of fibrous septae from overuse and which may take up to 6 months to heal), and piezogenic papules (pain over medial/inferior aspect of heel, tender papules noted when patient standing).

Objectives: Did you learn to . . .

- Diagnose plantar fasciitis and consider other causes of heel and foot pain?
- Describe the natural history of and treatments for plantar fascitis?

QUICK QUIZ: HAND INJURIES

A "gamekeeper's thumb" would likely be seen as the result of which of the following injuries?

A) Fall on an outstretched hand.
B) Crush injury, for example, between two pieces of machinery.
C) Fall by a skier using a ski pole.
D) Excessive electronic gaming (e.g., Nintendo and Xbox).
E) Fall from a mountain bike.

Discussion
The correct answer is "C." A gamekeeper's thumb is defined as an injury (partial or complete tear) of the ulnar collateral ligament of the first MCP joint. This injury can occur with hyperextension of the thumb, as happens when falling with a ski pole. These injuries do well with casting, or, in the case of a very unstable joint, surgery.

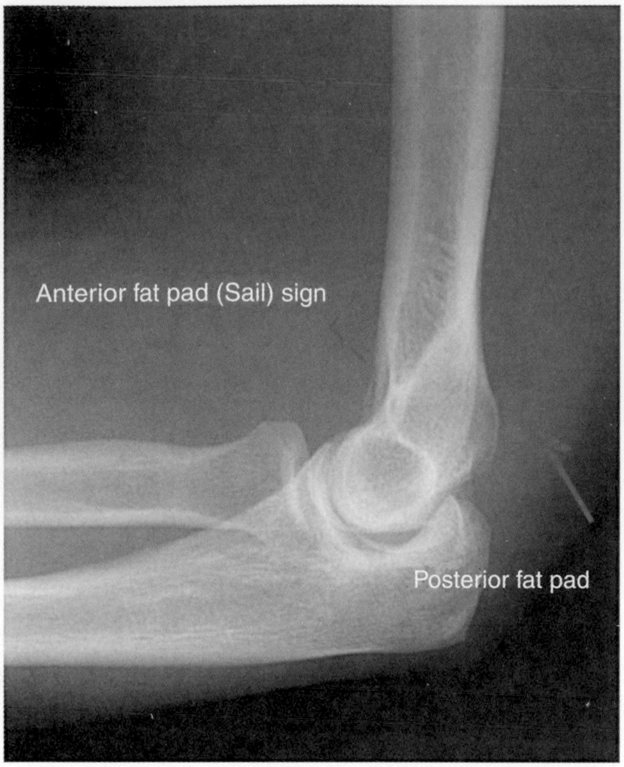

Figure 12–9 **Anterior and posterior fat pads in a radial head fracture**

QUICK QUIZ: FRACTURES

The most specific finding on radiograph for a radial head fracture is:

A) Anterior fat pad sign.
B) Posterior fat pad sign.
C) Trousseau sign.
D) Medial fat pad sign.

Discussion
The correct answer is "B." The posterior fat pad sign, which indicates an effusion in the joint, is the most **specific** of the findings for a radial head fracture. An **anterior** fat pad sign is the most sensitive. Figure 12–9, demonstrates both the anterior and posterior fat pad signs. There is no medial fat pad sign, and Trousseau sign is related to hypocalcemia and is carpal spasm with arterial occlusion (as with a blood pressure cuff).

QUICK QUIZ: RADIAL HEAD FRACTURE

The proper treatment of a nondisplaced, fractured radial head is:

A) Internal fixation.
B) Sling with early mobilization.
C) Short-arm cast.
D) Long-arm cast.

Discussion
The correct answer is "B." For a nondisplaced radial head fracture, the treatment is simply a sling for comfort and early mobilization. Mobilization is especially important to avoid a stiff elbow. Orthopedic referral should be considered if there is any limitation of motion.

QUICK QUIZ: FRACTURES

The most common elbow fracture in the pediatric population with a positive "fat pad sign" but no obvious fracture on x-ray is:

A) Radial head fracture.
B) Supracondylar fracture.
C) Medial condyle fracture.
D) Lateral condyle fracture.
E) Olecranon fracture.

Discussion
The answer is "B" supracondylar fracture. Although in adults the most common occult elbow fracture is of the radial head, in the pediatric population it is a supracondylar fracture. These may be significantly displaced, but if nondisplaced they can be very subtle and the only sign of a fracture may be a displaced posterior (or anterior) fat pad.

QUICK QUIZ: HIP PAIN

A 76-year-old female nursing home resident is brought to clinic after rolling out of bed last night. She is normally able to ambulate independently, but today cannot bear weight due to pain in her hip. She has significant hip tenderness and pain with any movement of her leg. She is unable to perform a straight leg raise secondary to pain. Plain x-rays of her pelvis and hip are read as osteopenia with no obvious fracture.

What is the most appropriate next step?

A) Conservative treatment with acetaminophen and bedrest until able to ambulate.
B) Admission for observation.

C) Hip MRI.
D) Physical therapy.
E) Fentanyl patch.

Discussion
The correct answer is "C." The patient may have an occult hip fracture. Rates of occult hip fractures range for 2–10% of all hip fractures. To miss the diagnosis of a hip fracture may lead to displacement of the fracture and a worse outcome. Both CT and MRI can be used to evaluate for occult fracture, but most studies indicate that MRI has a greater sensitivity.

CASE 21

A 45-year-old female hospital clerk presents with bilateral aching pain in the forearms and thenar eminences. The pain is made worse with driving and typing. She also has intermittent numbness over the same areas. She tried to ignore the symptoms, but today she dropped her coffee mug on her computer keyboard and became alarmed at her loss of strength. She has hypothyroidism and is obese, but she reports that her health is otherwise good.

Based on the history alone, which of the following is the most likely diagnosis?
A) Carpal tunnel syndrome.
B) Osteoarthritis.
C) Ulnar neuropathy.
D) Diabetic neuropathy.
E) Stroke.

Discussion
The correct answer is "A." Carpal tunnel syndrome is due to median nerve entrapment in the carpal tunnel of the wrist. Typical symptoms include numbness, paresthesias, and pain at the palmar/radial aspect of the hand, quintessentially the thenar eminence. In more severe or long-lasting cases, you may see atrophy of the thenar eminence. Patients may also develop weakness of thumb opposition. Osteoarthritis of the wrists does not usually cause nerve symptoms but can cause spondylosis and nerve root impingement on occasion. Ulnar neuropathy involves the ulnar aspect of the hand, especially the 4th and 5th fingers, rather than the radial aspect, which is involved with carpal tunnel syndrome. Diabetic neuropathy typically presents in the feet since they are innervated by the longest nerves in the body. *Note:* **This could represent cervical disk disease as well, especially given that it is bilateral.**

* *

Phalen sign is positive (placing the wrists in a flexed position causes aching and numbness in the median nerve distribution).

What is the best next step in the continuing evaluation and management of this patient?
A) Nerve conduction studies.
B) Radiograph of the wrist.
C) MRI of the cervical spine.
D) Orthopedic referral.
E) Initiation of treatment.

Discussion
The correct answer is "E." In a clear-cut case of carpal tunnel syndrome, there is no need for further studies. If the diagnosis is in doubt, EMG/nerve conduction studies may be of benefit. If the ROM in the wrist is limited, x-rays may be helpful. At this point in time, MRI and orthopedic referral are not likely to add much.

Which of the following IS NOT associated with carpal tunnel syndrome?
A) Hypothyroidism.
B) Diabetes mellitus.
C) Amyloidosis.
D) Polycythemia vera.
E) Rheumatoid arthritis.

Discussion
The correct answer is "D." All of the above are associated with carpal tunnel syndrome except for polycythemia vera. Polycythemia vera can cause erythromelalgia which is a burning pain of the hands and feet associated with erythema, pallor, or cyanosis. It responds to aspirin. Other conditions associated with carpal tunnel syndrome include pregnancy, menopause, obesity, acromegaly, and end-stage renal disease. The point here is that patients with carpal tunnel syndrome should have a systemic cause ruled out, either clinically or with labs.

What is the most appropriate initial treatment?
A) Thumb spica splint.
B) Steroid injection.
C) NSAIDs and neutral position wrist splints.
D) Short-arm casts.

Discussion

The correct answer is "C." Conservative therapy should be initiated first, unless there is some compelling reason for more aggressive therapy (e.g., severe weakness of the hands and loss of function). Most patients respond well to NSAIDs and the use of neutral position splints. The traditional cock-up splints are not as effective as neutral position splints. The splints should be worn at night. The patient may wear the splints during the day, too, but should take them off for several hours per day to avoid disuse muscle atrophy. "A" is incorrect since a thumb spica is not needed. "B," steroid injection, might be tried if initial conservative measures fail. "D" is just wrong—don't cast patients with carpal tunnel syndrome!

> HELPFUL TIP: Oral steroids have been used for carpal tunnel with limited success. Unfortunately most modalities (NSAIDs, splints, steroids, etc.) are no better than placebo in randomized trials.

> HELPFUL TIP: Phalen and Tinel signs are crude tools at best. Tinel sign, which is a painful sensation of the fingers induced by percussion of the median nerve at the level of the carpal tunnel, may be positive, but is only 50% sensitive (flip a coin) and 54% specific. Phalen sign, keeping both wrists in a palmar-flexed position, may reproduce symptoms. Sensitivity varies from 10% to 88% depending on study; its specificity is 80%.

Objectives: Did you learn to . . .

- Diagnose carpal tunnel syndrome and consider other causes of wrist pain?
- Manage a patient with carpal tunnel syndrome?

QUICK QUIZ: CASTING

A few days ago, your partner placed a cast on the arm of a 20-year-old male for a distal radial fracture. He calls your office today, when your partner has gone fishing. The patient is complaining of increasing pain and numbness of his fingers in the casted arm.

Which course of action is most appropriate?

A) Have the patient follow up tomorrow, when your partner is back in the office.
B) Send the patient to the emergency room for compressive Doppler exam of the arm to rule out venous thrombosis.
C) Ask the patient to come to clinic to have the cast replaced.
D) Tell the patient that these are expected symptoms and advise him to take some aspirin.
E) Recommend that he have his cast signed by as many friends as possible to take his mind of these clearly psychosomatic symptoms.

Discussion

The correct answer is "C." This patient has symptoms that are most likely due to an improperly fitted cast. The problem here could be vascular compromise, nerve compression, or a compartment syndrome. He should be seen without delay, and the cast should be adjusted or replaced. The cast can be bivalved or have a window cut into it.

BIBLIOGRAPHY

Anderson BC. *Office Orthopedics for Primary Care: Treatment.* 3rd ed. Philadelphia, PA: Saunders; 2005.

Dixit S, et al. Management of patellofemoral pain syndrome. *Am Fam Physician.* 2007;75(2):194.

Griffin LY, et al., eds. *Essentials of Musculoskeletal Care.* 3rd ed. Rosemont, IL: American Academy of Orthopaedic Surgeons; 2005.

Kindale S. Evaluation and treatment of acute low back pain. *Am Fam Physician.* 2007;75(8):1181-1188.

Margaretten ME, et al. Does this adult patient have septic arthritis?. *JAMA.* 2007;297(13):1478-1488.

McGillicuddy DC, et al. How sensitive is the synovial fluid white blood cell count in diagnosing septic arthritis? *Am J Emerg Med.* 2007;25(7):749-752.

Sawyer JR, Kapoor M. The limping child: A systematic approach to diagnosis. *Am Fam Physician.* 2009;79(3):215.

Simons R, Sherman S, eds. *Emergency Orthopedics.* 6th ed. New York, NY: McGraw-Hill Professional; 2010.

Simpson MR. Tendinopathies of the foot and ankle. *Am Fam Physician.* 2009;80(10):1107.

Steill IG, et al. Prospective validation of a decision rule for the use of radiography in acute knee injuries. *JAMA.* 1996;275:611.

Wilson JJ, Best TM. Common overuse tendon problems: A review and recommendations for treatment. *Am Fam Physician.* 2005;72(5):811-818.

13 Pediatrics

Kelly Wood and Andrew Peterson

CASE 1

A 6-year-old male presents to your office with his mom. He has been soiling his underwear frequently and it is causing stress at home and school. His parents are frustrated and think he is old enough to know better. At school, he is being teased and being called "stinky pants" and he reports feeling embarrassed. Mom asks you if there is something medically wrong with him.

What percentage of chronic encopresis is functional (meaning no underlying medical or organic cause)?

A) 10%.
B) 25%.
C) 50%.
D) 75%.
E) 90%.

Discussion

The correct answer is "E." Ninety percent of chronic encopresis is functional. Functional encopresis is the repeated involuntary passage of stool into underwear in a child who is 4 years of age or older and at a developmental level appropriate for toilet training without an underlying medical cause. The most common reason is retentive constipation with overflow incontinence. Frequently the child has an associated psychological problem. Boys are affected more often than girls. Children with this disorder withhold feces voluntarily thereby avoiding defecating. As stool stays in the colon, more water is absorbed creating harder stool that is more difficult to pass. This leads to a self-perpetuating cycle. The excess stool stretches the rectum with eventual loss of sensation to defecate. Liquid stool may leak around the impacted mass, which parents often mistake as diarrhea. In some, a triggering event such as passage of a painful stool leading to fear of stooling, forced toilet training before the child is ready, or dislike of using public toilets (starting school) may have occurred. A common theme is parental misunderstanding of the problem thinking it is due to an undiagnosed medical problem, attention-seeking behavior, or child laziness.

HELPFUL TIP: Some definitions ... **Nonretentive encopresis** is the voluntary stooling of one's pants. Once a medical cause has been rule out, this is purely a behavioral or psychiatric problem. **Primary encopresis** is when stool continence has never been achieved. **Secondary encopresis** occurs when accidents began after a period of successful toilet training.

Which of the following conditions is associated with encopresis?

A) Urinary tract infections.
B) Enuresis.
C) Social isolation.
D) ADHD.
E) All of the above are associated with encopresis.

Discussion

The correct answer is "E." Encopresis is an independent risk factor for urinary tract infections. Feces in the underwear allows for close contact with the urethra and introduction of bacteria. Chronic contracting of pelvic floor muscles to withhold stool may lead to dysfunctional voiding and urinary stasis. Enuresis occurs in up to 40% of patients with chronic constipation. A mass of stool in the rectum can compress the bladder leading to uncontrolled voiding. The chronic odor of feces makes socialization rough and teasing frequent. ADHD frequently is associated with functional constipation and encopresis due to being too distracted to use the bathroom.

> HELPFUL TIP: Encopresis and daytime enuresis should prompt you to rule out a spinal cord lesion.

Which of the following are medical (organic) causes of constipation?

A) Hypothyroidism.
B) Hypercalcemia.
C) Cystic fibrosis.
D) Lead poisoning.
E) All of the above.

Discussion

The correct answer is "E." All of the above can cause constipation and thus fecal incontinence. Organic causes account for only 5–10% of encopresis cases and can be anatomical (anterior displaced anus), neurological (Hirschsprung disease), metabolic (Celiac disease), or iatrogenic (medications such as narcotics). The first step in evaluating a child with encopresis is to rule out an underlying medical condition starting with a good history and physical exam. Do not forget to ask about timing of meconium passage in the past medical history. Rectal examination is essential. Look at the back for signs of an occult spina bifida such as sacral dimple or hair tuft. Lack of anal wink, cremasteric reflex, or deep tendon reflexes is suggestive of a neurologic cause. Often a painful fissure may initiate a vicious cycle of pain with stooling leading to the withholding of stool leading to even more painful defecation, etc.

> HELPFUL TIP: Fecal impaction is a clinical diagnosis made by feeling a hard stool mass on rectal exam. It is not made by abdominal x-ray.

> HELPFUL TIP: Abuse may be a triggering event for constipation and encopresis. If abuse is suspected, you should contact child protective services.

All of the following are useful in the treatment of functional encopresis EXCEPT:

A) Polyethylene glycol (PEG).
B) Oral sodium phosphate solution (OsmoPrep).
C) Mineral oil.
D) Lactulose.
E) Milk of magnesia.

Discussion

The correct answer is "B." In 2008, the FDA placed a black box warning on oral sodium phosphate solutions due to risk of acute kidney injury from deposition of calcium–phosphate crystals. As a result, nonphosphate-containing medications are used. Treatment begins with disimpaction that can be performed manually, with enemas, or with an oral medication such as PEG or mineral oil. Many treatment guidelines prefer disimpaction using oral PEG solutions over manual disimpaction. It seems like a strange concept but it works and is more humane. Treatment should be individualized. After disimpaction, patients require maintenance therapy (combination of medical, behavioral, dietary, and counseling). Medications such as milk of magnesia (magnesium hydroxide), mineral oil, or PEG should be used daily and incrementally increased until the patient is having regular, soft bowel movements.

Increased fiber and fluid intake should be encouraged to help keep stools soft. Behaviorally, the child should sit on the toilet with active pushing after each meal to make use of the gastrocolic reflex. The child does not have to stool but rather this encourages them to use the toilet. Use of a footstool may improve Valsalva maneuvers. A sticker chart can give visual encouragement. Families need to understand that there is no quick fix and relapse is common (about 50%). It takes months for the rectum to return to normal size and sensation. Patients who fail to improve after 6 months of compliant treatment should be referred to a specialist.

HELPFUL TIP: Remember never to use mineral oil in any child who is at risk of aspiration. It can cause a chemical pneumonitis.

HELPFUL TIP: A Malone antegrade continence enema (MACE) procedure may be performed in extreme cases. This surgical procedure involves creating an appendicostomy by connecting the appendix to skin level at the umbilicus. Antegrade enemas though small catheters then are used to keep the colon washed out.

Objectives: Did you learn to . . .

- Describe encopresis, including its presentation, diagnosis, and causes?
- Differentiate between organic and nonorganic causes of encopresis?
- Medically manage encopresis?

QUICK QUIZ: NEONATAL POLYCYTHEMIA

Causes of neonatal polycythemia (central venous hematocrit of 65% or greater) in the immediate postpartum period include all of the following EXCEPT:

A) Delayed umbilical cord clamping.
B) Twin–twin transfusion.
C) Congenital adrenal hyperplasia.
D) Diabetic mother.
E) Sepsis.

Discussion

The correct answer is "E." Neonatal polycythemia can be caused by all of the above except for sepsis. Other causes include chronic intrauterine hypoxia (e.g., mother is a heavy smoker), intrauterine growth restriction, maternal hypertension, congenital hypothyroidism, and chromosomal abnormalities (e.g., trisomy 21, 18, and 13).

QUICK QUIZ: MORE ON NEONATAL POLYCYTHEMIA

Patients with neonatal polycythemia are at risk for hyperviscosity syndrome including respiratory distress, hypoxia, cyanosis, hyperbilirubinemia, hypoglycemia, etc. Heart failure, stroke, renal vein thrombosis, and necrotizing enterocolitis may also occur.

The best treatment for these patients is:

A) Phlebotomy.
B) Exchange transfusion with normal RBCs.
C) Exchange transfusion using D5W.
D) Exchange transfusion using normal saline.
E) Aspirin.

Discussion

The correct answer is "D." Partial exchange transfusion using normal saline is the treatment of choice. "A" is incorrect since phlebotomy alone will reduce overall circulating volume and may actually exacerbate the problem. "B" is incorrect. If you chose this, back home for you! What is the point of taking out cells and then putting more in, I ask you? "C" is incorrect because large amounts of D5W can cause fluid shifts, electrolyte abnormalities, and hemolysis. Of note, patients with a hematocrit of 65–70% can be observed if they are asymptomatic. There is no one-to-one predictable relationship between hematocrit and blood viscosity. Also of note, there is no evidence that long-term outcomes are improved with partial exchange transfusion versus observation.

CASE 2

Amy, a 4-day-old female, comes to clinic because "she is yellow." She was born at term to a 25-year-old married woman. Maternal lab results are as follows: blood type A+, RPR nonreactive, rubella immune, group B streptococcus (GBS) negative. Amy has been breastfeeding every 3–5 hours. She has had one stool and three urine diapers a day. Her weight is 15% less than her birth weight. On your exam, you notice jaundice from the head to the thighs. Her total bilirubin level is 25.2 mg/dL. The conjugated (direct) fraction is 0.4 mg/dL.

Which of the following statements is correct?

A) She has breastfeeding failure jaundice.
B) She has physiologic jaundice.

C) She has biliary atresia; you must consult pediatric gastroenterology.
D) There is an ABO incompatibility between the mother and child.

Discussion

The correct answer is "A." Amy most likely has breastfeeding failure jaundice. This occurs within the first several days of birth before the mother's milk supply is adequate. This must be distinguished from **breast milk jaundice,** which **usually occurs later** without evidence of dehydration. One sign that Amy is not receiving adequate breast milk feedings—and that this is **breastfeeding failure jaundice** instead of breast milk jaundice—is the fact that she is 15% below birth weight, having fewer than 6 wet diapers per day and fewer than two to five stools a day. You should try to evaluate the mother's milk supply by asking about the mother's feeling of engorgement, if she feels her breasts empty with feeding, if she notices milk on the infant's lips and tongue immediately after feeding, and if she hears the baby swallow with feedings. "B" is incorrect. Even though physiologic jaundice peaks at this age, the level of 25.2 mg/dL is higher than would be expected with physiologic jaundice (which should not be higher than 17 mg/dL in a term infant). "C" is incorrect because biliary atresia presents with **conjugated** hyperbilirubinemia (the liver can appropriately conjugate bilirubin, but there is obstruction to the outflow of the conjugated bilirubin—essentially an obstructive process). "D" is incorrect because ABO incompatibility is unlikely in a mother whose blood type is something other than O. Additionally, Rh incompatibility is impossible due to the mother being Rh+. However, minor antigen incompatibility remains a possibility.

> HELPFUL TIP: **Causes of an elevated direct (conjugated) bilirubin:** infection (including congenital), metabolic abnormalities (cystic fibrosis, Rotor and Dubin Johnson, etc.), anatomic abnormalities (biliary atresia, etc.), and cholestasis (especially from CVN). Note that conjugated bilirubin does not cause kernicterus.
> **Causes of an elevated indirect bilirubin:** increased breakdown of RBCs (ABO/Rh incompatibility, cephalohematoma, thalassemias, etc.), prematurity, hypothyroidism.

All of the following are risk factors for severe neonatal hyperbilirubinemia EXCEPT:

A) Exclusive breastfeeding.
B) Gestational age $\geq$41 weeks.
C) Significant birth trauma.
D) Visible jaundice in first 24 hours of life.

Discussion

The correct answer is "B." Major risk factors for severe hyperbilirubinemia in infants include lesser gestational age rather than greater gestational age. "A" is true, and exclusively formula-fed infants are less likely to have severe hyperbilirubinemia (but this is not a reason to recommend bottle feeding). Cephalohematoma and large bruises result in increased bilirubin production from heme breakdown, so "C" is true. The earlier jaundice occurs, the higher the peak is likely to be, so "D" is also true. Other major risk factors for severe hyperbilirubinemia include a sibling who required phototherapy, East Asian race, and blood group incompatibility.

> HELPFUL TIP: Infants with total serum bilirubin levels >5 mg/dL typically have visible jaundice. The jaundice usually starts at the head and progresses distally to the feet. It resolves in the opposite pattern with the distal extremities resolving first.

> HELPFUL TIP: Jaundice present in the first 24 hours of life is pathologic and usually due to hemolytic disease such as ABO incompatibility.

* *

Amy's CBC is unremarkable and blood type is A+.

Which of the following is the most appropriate initial treatment for this patient?

A) Admission for exchange transfusion.
B) Admission for IV fluids alone to improve hydration.
C) Admission for phototherapy.
D) Discharge to home with recommendations for formula feeding, light exposure, and follow-up bilirubin tomorrow.

Discussion

The correct answer is "C." Amy should be treated with intensive phototherapy given her level of hyperbilirubinemia. "A" is incorrect because phototherapy should be employed first and an exchange transfusion would follow if phototherapy failed to lower the bilirubin level or signs of acute bilirubin encephalopathy developed. "B" is incorrect since phototherapy is the definitive treatment. **Adjunctive** therapy with intravenous fluids is considered if weight loss exceeds 12% of birth weight. "D" is incorrect simply because this patient needs intensive phototherapy. A serum bilirubin level of 25 mg/dL or higher is a medical emergency and requires immediate hospital admission for phototherapy.

> HELPFUL TIP: The American Academy of Pediatrics (AAP) has established threshold values for hyperbilirubinemia treatment with phototherapy and exchange transfusion. Decisions regarding treatment vary depending on the infant's risk, age (in hours after delivery), gestational age, and total bilirubin level. There are graphs, tables, and nomograms to assist with decision making. Decision-making software is available at: http://www.babydoc.co.il/article-364.htm or http://bilitool.org/ (the easier of the two).

* *

You admit Amy for further management. You confirm Amy's current weight, which is indeed down 15% from birth weight. Children often lose about 10% of their weight after birth.

Beyond what point in time is it considered problematic if the patient has not returned to his or her birth weight?

A) 5 days.
B) 7 days.
C) 10 days.
D) 14 days.
E) None of the above. Don't worry, be happy.

Discussion

The correct answer is "D." Children should regain their birth weight by age 2 weeks. Anything beyond this is reason for concern.

* *

Amy does well under your care (and the bili lights . . .) and returns at age 2 months. Mom questions the need for immunizations during the well exam "since we never see these archaic diseases anymore—I mean, come on, I can't even find a chicken pox party." Plus, she's read information on the Internet and has concerns about immunization safety. And wasn't there a study about kids who suffered autism because of thimerosal in a vaccine? And another study that vaccines transformed children into space aliens? Unfortunately, Amy's mother's concerns are not unusual. Parents often bring up several misconceptions about vaccinations.

What is a common side effect that Amy might have after her immunizations at her 2-month visit?

A) Fever to 104° F.
B) Autism.
C) Diabetes.
D) Erythema at the site of immunization.
E) Symptomatic shedding of virus in her stool.

Discussion

The correct answer is "D." Vaccine side effects, such as **low-grade fevers** (not to 104°F as in answer "A"), induration and redness at the site, and fussiness are common. However, they are self-limited. "B" and "C" are incorrect. Autism and diabetes **have not** been linked to vaccines in large, well-designed studies. "E" is incorrect because the DTaP, HIB, and IPV vaccines are inactivated. Thus, the virus or bacteria is killed and purified for a specific component. The hepatitis B vaccine is constructed with genetic engineering in a yeast cell. Thus, one would not shed virus in the stool. The MMR, oral polio, oral rotavirus, and varicella vaccines are live attenuated vaccines. With these immunizations, the virus has been weakened but can still replicate and be shed in stool. In an immunocompetent host, this usually is not of clinical significance. Thus, "E" is incorrect.

> HELPFUL TIP: The article linking MMR vaccine to autism has been withdrawn by the authors (and Lancet) and the lead author has lost his license to practice because of fraudulent data.

HELPFUL (BUT CONFUSING) TIP: Pretreating the child with acetaminophen can increase patient comfort. However, the acetaminophen seems to blunt the immune response leading to lower antibody titers. Whether this is clinically significant is unknown.

* *

Amy's mother accepts that advice but still has concerns.

What other factually correct information can you share with her about vaccines?

A) Giving a child multiple vaccines at the same time weakens her immune system.
B) The fever and rash side effects of the MMR are from the measles component and usually occur 1 week after the vaccine is given.
C) If Amy receives her MMR at a 9-month visit (before she travels to visit Aunt Tilley who has been banished to Outer Mongolia), her MMR immunization would be considered complete after this dose and another one at 5 years old.
D) If Amy had an acute otitis media and fevers of 100.4°F, we should delay her immunizations until she is afebrile.
E) Immunizations are not important, since these diseases are rare in the United States.

Discussion

The correct answer is "B." The measles component can occasionally cause a fever and rash 5–10 days after the immunization. This occurs in 5–15% of infants. Up to 25% of adult women may have arthralgias after the vaccine. The MMR dosing schedule includes two doses of MMR. However, the first must be **after** 1 year of age. It may be given sooner if the child is at risk (such as with travel or with a measles outbreak) but must be repeated after the first birthday. Thus, "C" is incorrect. Minor illnesses should not prevent vaccination. True contraindications include anaphylactic reactions to a vaccine or vaccine constituent, moderate-to-severe febrile illness, and encephalopathy within 7 days of DTaP. Live virus vaccines are contraindicated in immunocompromised patients.

HELPFUL TIP: As a general rule, if a patient misses a vaccine, just start up where you left off. There is no need to increase the number of vaccines given.

* *

Amy continues her scheduled well child exams. At one of those visits, she was babbling and crawling around the office. She poked her fingers at the outlet covers (which thankfully were covered) and could use a pincer grasp to pick up a raisin off the floor (ew, gross!).

These behaviors are appropriate for the development of a child at approximately age:

A) 6 months.
B) 9 months.
C) 15 months.
D) 24 months.

Discussion

The correct answer is "B." Take a moment to review the developmental milestones in Table 13–1.

* *

Amy continues her scheduled well child exams. However, at 14 months old, mom brings Amy for a sick visit because she turned blue. After taking a complete history and doing a complete physical exam, you appropriately diagnose breath-holding spells.

Which of the following statements about breath-holding spells is true?

A) The incidence of breath-holding spells for children between 6 months old and 6 years old is 50%.
B) If a color change occurs, it occurs after loss of consciousness.
C) Seizure-like activity may occur with breath-holding spells.
D) A child typically takes 60–90 minutes to return to her baseline after a breath-holding spell.
E) The evaluation should include an echocardiogram (ECG) and electroencephalogram (EEG).

Discussion

The correct answer is "C." A typical breath-holding spell begins with an inciting event (like Santa did not bring the right toy or mom refused to buy a Happy

Table 13-1 DEVELOPMENTAL MILESTONES

Age	Gross Motor	Visual Motor	Language	Social
1 mo	Raises head slightly from prone, makes crawling movements, lifts chin up	Has tight grasp, follows to midline	Alert to sound (e.g., by blinking, moving, startling)	Regards face
2 mo	Holds head in midline, lifts chest off table	No longer clenches fist tightly, follows object past midline	Smiles after being stroked or talked to	Recognizes parent
3 mo	Supports on forearms in prone, holds head up steadily	Holds hands open at rest, follows in circular fashion	Coos (produces long vowel sounds in musical fashion)	Reaches for familiar people or objects, anticipates feeding
4–5 mo	Rolls front to back and back to front, sits well when propped, supports on wrists, and shifts weight	Moves arms in unison to grasp, touches cube placed on table	Orients to voice; 5 mo: orients to bell (localized laterally), says "ahgoo," razzes	Enjoys looking around environment
6 mo	Sits well unsupported, puts feet in mouth in supine position	Reaches with either hand, transfers, uses raking grasp	Babbles; 7 mo: orients to bell (localizes indirectly); 8 mo: "dada/mama" indiscriminately	Recognizes strangers
9 mo	Creeps, crawls, cruises, pulls to stand, pivots when sitting	Uses pincer grasp, probes with forefinger, holds bottle, finger-feeds	Understands "no," waves bye-bye; 10 mo: "dada/mama" discriminantly; 11 mo: one word other than "dada/mama"	Starts to explore environment, plays pat-a-cake
12 mo	Walks alone	Throws objects, lets go of toys, hand release, uses mature pincer grasp	Follows one-step command with gesture, uses 2 words other than "dada/mama"; 14 mo: uses 3 words	Imitates actions, comes when called, cooperates with dressing
15 mo	Creeps upstairs, walks backward	Builds tower of 2 blocks in imitation of examiner, scribbles in imitation	Follows one-step command without gesture, uses 4–6 words and immature jargon (runs several unintelligible words together)	Indicates some simple needs by pointing, hugs parents
18 mo	Runs, throws toy from standing without falling	Turns 2 or 3 pages at a time, fills spoon and feeds self	Knows 7–20 words, knows 1 body part, uses mature jargon (includes intelligible words in jargon)	Copies parent in tasks (e.g., sweeping, dusting), plays in company of other children
21 mo	Squats in play, goes up steps	Builds tower of 5 blocks, drinks well from cup	Points to 3 body parts, uses 2-word combinations, has 20 word vocabulary	Asks to have food and to go to toilet
24 mo	Walks up and down steps without help	Turns pages one at a time, removes shoes, pants, etc., imitates behavior of others	Uses 50 words, 2-word sentences, uses pronouns (I, you, me) inappropriately, points to 5 body parts, understands 2-step command	Parallel play

(Continued)

Table 13–1 DEVELOPMENTAL MILESTONES (Continued)

Age	Gross Motor	Visual Motor	Language	Social
30 mo	Jumps with both feet off floor, throws ball overhand	Unbuttons, holds pencil in adult fashion, differentiates horizontal and vertical line	Uses pronouns (I, you, me) appropriately, understands concept of "one," repeats 2 digits forward	Tells first and last names when asked, gets drink without help
3 yr	Pedals tricycle, can alternate feet when going up steps	Dresses and undresses partially, dries hands if reminded, draws a circle	Uses 3-word sentences, plurals, and past tense. Knows all pronouns. Minimum of 250 words, understands concept of "two"	Group play, shares toys, takes turns, plays well with others, knows full name, age, sex
4 yr	Hops, skips, alternates feet going downstairs	Buttons clothing fully, catches ball	Knows colors, says song or poem from memory, asks questions	Tells "tall tales," plays cooperatively with a group of children
5 yr	Skips, alternating feet, jumps over low obstacles	Ties shoes, spreads with knife	Prints first name, asks what a word means	Plays competitive games, abides by rules, likes to help in household tasks

Meal). Breath-holding spells occur in up to 4% of children and 80% start before 18 months. The child begins to cry, holds his or her breath, turns blue, and loses consciousness. After loss of consciousness, some rhythmic jerking of the extremities may occur. The loss of consciousness is brief and the child returns quickly to normal activity. The differential diagnosis includes cardiac arrhythmias, seizures, and apnea. If the history is classic for breath-holding spells, no further evaluation is necessary. The treatment is parental reassurance. Parents should be encouraged to ignore the episodes and not to give in to child's requests in attempt to avoid the spells. Iron supplementation may decrease the frequency of spells if anemia or iron deficiency is present.

HELPFUL TIP: This type of spell may be referred to in the literature as an "ALTE" (apparent life-threatening event). The term ALTE is nonspecific and is defined by what the parents observe: apnea, cyanosis, decreased responsiveness, etc. There is no relationship between an ALTE and sudden infant death syndrome (SIDS). The most common causes of an ALTE include lower respiratory track infection, GERD, and seizure. Additional causes include breath-holding spells, electrolyte abnormalities, cardiac dysrhythmias, metabolic diseases, and CNS problems. Always consider child abuse in your differential. Fifty percent of the time no cause is identified. A good history and physical exam are the most important evaluation tools. Diagnostic testing should be guided by history and physical exam findings.

Between 12 and 15 months of age, Amy should receive all of the following vaccines, as per Centers for Disease Control and Prevention (CDC) recommendations, EXCEPT:

A) MMR.
B) Varicella.
C) Hepatitis A.
D) Rotavirus.
E) Influenza.

Discussion

The correct answer is "D." Vaccination schedules and recommendations seem to represent quickly moving targets, so a regular review is required to keep up to date. At 12–15 months, the CDC recommends initial MMR, varicella, and hepatitis A vaccinations for all US children. Influenza recommendations are

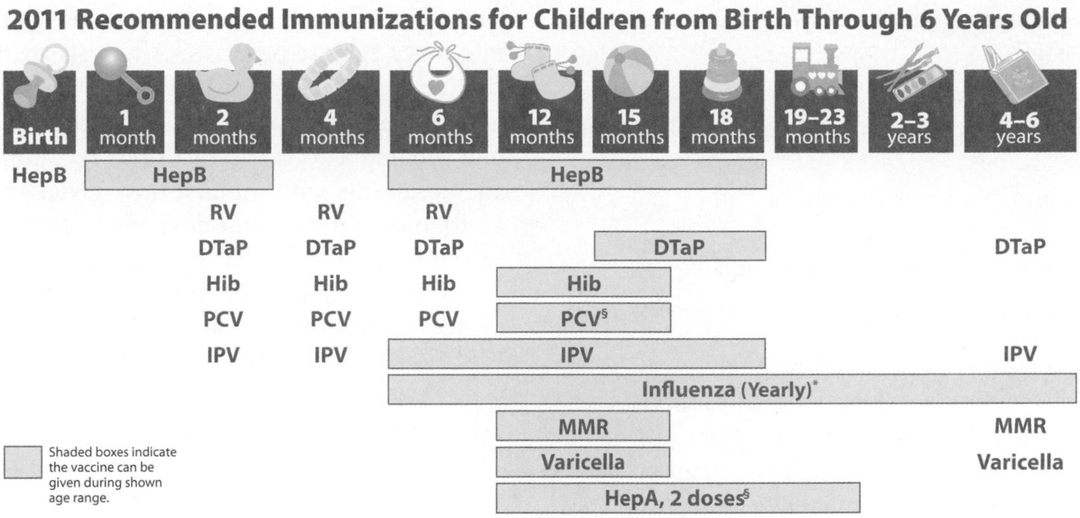

Figure 13–1 ***Take a moment to review the current (2011) immunization recommendations. RV, rotavirus; PCV, pneumococcal conjugated vaccine; IPV, intramuscular polio vaccine.*** **(Centers for Disease Control and Prevention, U.S. Department of Health and Human Services: http://www.cdc.gov/vaccines/parents/images/parent_ver_sch_0_6yrs_view.jpg)**

updated annually and have become progressively more inclusive over time. The CDC recommends that all children ages 6 months through 18 years receive the influenza vaccine annually during the appropriate season. Of note, rotavirus vaccine should not be administered to children older than 32 weeks, and the first dose should not be given after 15 weeks. See Figure 13–1 for the most recent guidelines available at the time of publication.

* *

Amy's breath-holding spells resolve by the time she is 3 years old, and she continues to grow and develop normally. Amy's next issue comes when she is 5 years old and in your office for her prekindergarten physical.

You notice a new murmur. Of the following, which suggests that this is a benign murmur?

A) Murmur is grade II/VI.
B) Murmur has a thrill.
C) Murmur radiates to the apex.
D) Murmur is diastolic.
E) Murmur is holosystolic.

Discussion

The correct answer is "A." Not all murmurs need to be referred to a cardiologist. There are features that can help differentiate pathologic from benign murmurs. A murmur that is diastolic, grades III–VI, pansystolic, or associated with cardiac symptoms is likely pathologic and requires further investigation. A benign murmur typically is systolic, soft (grades I–II, occasionally III), nonradiating, and short. A "benign" murmur is not a diagnosis of exclusion. You should try to make a decision about which innocent murmur it is. See Table 13–2.

* *

On Amy's exam, you hear a grade III/VI **systolic** murmur in the pulmonic area with **fixed** splitting of the second heart sound. She is otherwise healthy without any cardiac symptoms.

Table 13–2 "BENIGN" CARDIAC MURMURS OF CHILDHOOD[a]

Still's murmur: A grade I–III murmur heard best in left middle sternal border or between left lower sternal border and apex. It is a "musical," vibratory or buzzing systolic ejection murmur, which is louder when the patient is supine, compared with when upright. A Still's murmur may get louder as blood flow increases with fever, exercise, or excitement.
Venous hum: A grade continuous I–III murmur heard best in the supraclavicular area. It should resolve when the patient is recumbent or with pressure over the jugular vein.
Pulmonic murmur: Heard as a grade I–III systolic ejection murmur in the first half of systole. It is generally best heard in the left upper sternal border.

[a]Murmurs that change with respiration are generally, but not always, benign.

What is the appropriate next step in management of this issue?

A) Family reassurance.
B) Endocarditis prophylaxis at the dental visit next week.
C) ECG and chest radiograph.
D) Limit physical activity.
E) Refer for immediate operative repair.

Discussion

The correct answer is "C." Most likely, Amy has an ASD or atrial septal defect. The murmur is a systolic ejection murmur heard best at the upper left sternal border. The sound you hear is caused by increased flow across the pulmonic valve creating a relative stenosis (more volume needs to get through a relatively fixed outlet) and NOT from flow across the ASD. The increased flow across the pulmonic valve causes a wide, fixed split S2. There may be a mid-diastolic rumbling murmur at the lower left sternal border from increased flow across the tricuspid valve if the ASD is very large. The chest x-ray may demonstrate cardiomegaly with increased pulmonary vascular markings. The ECG can be normal or may show mild right ventricular hypertrophy, right axis deviation, and/or right bundle branch block with the characteristic rsR′ pattern in the right precordial leads. Children with an ASD do NOT need endocarditis prophylaxis (except for the first 6 months after their surgical repair) and rarely need to limit their physical activity. Most small ASDs will close spontaneously by age 4 years. Closure by one of a variety of methods is recommended for symptomatic and significant left-to-right shunts with right ventricular enlargement.

Thinking ahead to when Amy becomes an adolescent, what immunizations are currently recommended by the CDC for ages 11–12 years assuming all other immunizations are caught up?

A) Influenza.
B) Tdap.
C) HPV (human papillomavirus vaccine).
D) MCV4 (quadrivalent meningococcal conjugate vaccine).
E) All of the above.

Discussion

The correct answer is "E." Tdap is used in patients older than 7 years. A single booster dose is needed because the DTaP series does not provide life-long immunity against pertussis. Afterward patients may receive booster doses of Td every 10 years. Influenza is recommended yearly for all children >6 months old. Meningococcal vaccination is recommended for all adolescents with the first dose given at age 11 or 12 followed by a booster dose at age 16 per the 2010 recommendations. HPV vaccination is a three-shot series recommended for all girls beginning at age 11 or 12 to prevent cervical cancer and genital warts. HPV vaccine series has been approved for boys aged 9–18 to prevent genital warts. The upper age limit for HPV vaccine in women is age 26.

Objectives: Did you learn to . . .

- Describe the causes of neonatal hyperbilirubinemia?
- Manage an infant with breastfeeding failure jaundice?
- Identify risk factors for severe hyperbilirubinemia?
- Identify vaccine misconceptions, list MMR side effects, and identify contraindications to immunization?
- Recognize stages of infant development?
- Describe and manage ALTEs?
- Differentiate benign from pathologic cardiac murmurs in childhood?
- Recommend vaccines for children in accordance with CDC guidelines?

QUICK QUIZ: JAUNDICE

The current recommendation for the treatment of breast milk jaundice (NOT breastfeeding failure jaundice) is:

A) Continue to breastfeed.
B) Stop breastfeeding and change to a cow's milk formula.
C) Stop breastfeeding and change to soy milk formula.
D) Stop breastfeeding and treat with rehydration solution (e.g., Pedialyte).

Discussion

The correct answer is "A." Patients with hyperbilirubinemia due to breast milk jaundice should continue to breastfeed. Breast milk jaundice begins on days 5–7 of life, peaks by 2 weeks of age, and usually resolves by 10 weeks of age. Bilirubin levels will gradually decline while breastfeeding is continued. If breastfeeding is discontinued, serum bilirubin levels decline rapidly. Kernicterus is a rare. The etiology is unclear but glucuronidase in breast milk resulting in deconjugation and increased enterohepatic recirculation of bilirubin has been proposed.

CASE 3

A family has moved into the area and brings their 1-year-old girl in for a well child check. They bring her medical records with them. Her parents have no concerns, and she has been healthy. Her growth chart concerns you, however. Her length tracks along the 25th percentile. But her weight has gone gradually from around the 25–50th percentile at 0–6 months old to the 10th percentile at 9 months old, and now is at the 5th percentile at 1 year.

Which of the following most likely explains her pattern of growth?

A) Normal.
B) Familial short stature.
C) Prenatal insult such as exposure to drugs or infection.
D) Hypothyroidism.
E) Inadequate nutrition.

Discussion

The correct answer is "E." This patient's pattern of growth is consistent with failure to thrive. The criteria for diagnosis include weight less than the 3rd–5th percentile (depending on the source) **or** a fall of weight of >2 major percentile lines in 6 months **or** weight less than 80% of ideal weight for age **and/or** weight for height less than 5th percentile. The patient meets more than one of these criteria, so "A" is incorrect. In "B," height would be affected. In this child, only the weight (and not the height) is affected. "C" is incorrect because a child with a prenatal insult tends to be smaller globally in both height and weight, and the weight percentile would not be expected to drop so dramatically from birth. "D" is unlikely because in general, the endocrinologic causes result in "stunting" where a child stops gaining height but continues to gain weight. Thus, "E" is the most likely cause of this patient's failure to thrive. Failure to thrive is a clinical description not a diagnosis; therefore, the underlying cause must be identified.

* *

Taking more history, you discover that the patient eats mostly rice and fruit. She does not like meat (happily supported by one of your editors who is vegetarian!). She is picky. She drinks about 12 ounces of whole milk and 12 ounces of apple juice each day. She is active and developmentally appropriate. Her review of systems is negative as is her past medical history.

What is the *LEAST* appropriate way to proceed with evaluation and management of this patient?

A) Allow the child to feed herself whenever she is hungry or thirsty. Parents should offer food and drink frequently throughout the day.
B) Obtain CBC, iron studies, and urinalysis.
C) Limit juice intake.
D) Consult a nutritionist.
E) Prescribe a multivitamin.

Discussion

The correct answer (and least appropriate approach) is "A." The goal of management of failure to thrive is to increase caloric intake, identify treatable causes of failure to thrive, and look for effects of her malnutrition. Thus, a CBC, iron studies, electrolytes, bicarbonate, glucose, and urinalysis may be helpful to investigate possible iron deficiency, anemia, or renal tubular acidosis. Juice should be limited (due to its low nutritional value), meals scheduled, and caloric intake boosted. Although children should feed themselves, they take in more calories when given a set schedule for meals and snacks instead of being allowed to graze on food or drink throughout the day. A nutritionist can help educate the family on appropriate food choices for an infant and ways to boost calories. A child with a restrictive eating pattern, especially poor in iron-containing foods, may benefit from a multivitamin with iron.

HELPFUL TIP: For infants with failure to thrive, encourage the parents to increase caloric density of foods and drinks. Ask them to use whole milk rather than reduced fat milk, to increase the concentration of formula (adding less water), to add butter to food, etc.

* *

Your patient presents to the emergency department (ED) at 14 months old. Mom states that she has had several episodes of emesis over the last 48 hours and today began to have watery, foul-smelling diarrhea. Mom has lost track of number of episodes of emesis and diarrhea. She cannot tell if the child has had urine output because of the watery diarrhea. On your exam, the temperature is 102.5°F, heart rate 180, respiratory rate 50, blood pressure 80/50. Her weight is 8 kg. She has dry, cracked lips and dry skin. She lies in her mom's arms and is not very interested in your exam. Her capillary refill is about 4 seconds with some mottling of the extremities.

What is the *MOST* appropriate next step in the management of this patient's condition?

A) Evaluate for underlying bacterial infection with blood, urine, and stool cultures.
B) Admit to an inpatient unit and begin maintenance IV fluids.
C) Infuse 20 mL/kg normal saline IV over 20 minutes.
D) Begin oral rehydration.
E) Infuse 10 mL/kg D5½ normal saline over 2 hours.

Discussion

The correct answer is "C." This patient is severely dehydrated (estimated 15%) with signs of compromised tissue perfusion; therefore, she should have parenteral fluid resuscitation quickly with a 20 mL/kg isotonic fluid bolus. Although she might need admission, she should be stabilized in the ED before transfer to the inpatient unit; additionally, starting with maintenance fluids is inappropriate. Oral rehydration is cost-effective in less severe dehydration without compromised tissue perfusion. There are several tables published listing the clinical exam associated with various degrees of dehydration. See Table 13–3 for clues in determining the degree of dehydration.

HELPFUL TIP: Dehydration is a clinical diagnosis but laboratory findings can be helpful. The serum sodium classifies the dehydration as hypotonic, isotonic, or hypertonic. Metabolic acidosis is often present and calculation of the anion gap helps determine the cause. Blood urea nitrogen and serum creatine concentrations can be helpful but may be affected by other conditions.

* *

After completing the initial management, the patient is more interested in her surroundings. Her vital signs are pulse 160, respiratory rate 36, and blood pressure 80/50. Her lips are still dry and she is irritable. The capillary refill is 2–3 seconds. She is more interactive with her mother.

What further treatment is indicated for her dehydration?

A) 80 mL/hr × 2 hours of D5¼ NS.
B) 33 mL/hr × 24 hours of D5½ NS with 20-mEq KCl.
C) 50 mL/hr × 24 hours of D5¼ NS.
D) 20 mL/kg NS over 20 minutes.
E) 10 mL/kg D5½ NS over 2 hours.

Discussion

The correct answer is "D." After an initial bolus, the patient should be reassessed. This patient is still moderately dehydrated. Although she has responded to her initial bolus of normal saline, she still has abnormal vital signs as well as signs of dehydration on exam. Therefore, the normal saline bolus should be repeated. Hypotonic solutions (e.g., ½ NS) or those containing glucose and/or potassium should never be used as a bolus. Also, potassium should be withheld until the patient urinates and has better hydration status.

Table 13–3 SIGNS AND SYMPTOMS OF DEHYDRATION

Mild (5% in an infant, 3% in a child): Normal skin turgor, moist lips, tears present, normal vital signs, consolable
Moderate (10% in an infant, 6% in a child): Dry skin and lips, skin tenting, slightly increased pulse, decreased urine output, normal capillary refill
Severe (15% in an infant, 9% in a child): Parched lips, sunken eyes, decreased or no urine output, cool skin, elevated pulse, prolonged capillary refill, lethargic or obtunded

HELPFUL TIP: Maintenance fluids can be calculated using the Holiday-Segar method: daily water needs for the first 10 kg of body weight is 100 mL/kg/day; water needs for 11–20 kg is 50 mL/kg/day; each additional kg over 20 kg is 20 mL/kg/day. Do not forget to account for dehydration, which will require additional fluids to replace the fluid deficit. Also, replace ongoing losses from diarrhea, emesis, etc. You can also calculate the hourly fluid requirement by the 4, 2, 1 method. Children should get 4 ml/kg/hr for the first 10 kg body weight, 2 ml/kg/hr for the next 10 kg and 1 ml/kg/hr for every kg over 20 kg.

$$\text{Fluid deficit (L)} = \text{usual weight (kg)} - \text{current weight (kg)}$$

* *

The patient recovers well from her GI illness, but she returns a few months later to your clinic with a new illness. She has had temperatures of 103°F at home for 2–3 days. She has had no upper respiratory symptoms. Her oral intake has decreased, but she is maintaining good urine output. She has had no vomiting or diarrhea. Your exam reveals a febrile child that is slightly irritable. She is nontoxic and not dehydrated. Her oral cavity shows increased tonsil size with **ulcers on her tongue and lips** but not on the tonsillar pillars. Her anterior cervical lymph nodes are enlarged. The rest of her exam is noncontributory.

What is the most likely diagnosis?

A) Streptococcal pharyngitis.
B) Hand, foot, and mouth disease (coxsackie virus).
C) Herpetic gingivostomatitis.
D) Varicella.
E) Infectious mononucleosis.

Discussion

The correct answer is "C." Primary oral herpes (herpetic gingivostomatitis) is associated with a relatively high fever and anteriorly placed ulcerations and vesicles (gums, tongue, and lips). Symptoms tend to start relatively abruptly with pain, salivation, refusal to eat, and fever. Herpes gingivostomatitis may recur during life in the form of "cold sores." "B" is incorrect because the patient does not have hand and foot lesions. "D," varicella, can occur in the oral pharynx but would have lesions elsewhere in various stages and respiratory symptoms as well. Infectious mononucleosis is not associated with vesicular lesions or mucosal ulcerations.

HELPFUL TIP: The poorly named "**herpangina**" caused by enteroviruses (usually coxsackie A) is another consideration here. Herpangina is associated with fewer vesicles and **ulcers located in the posterior oropharynx along the posterior soft palate and tonsillar pillars and fossa.** Headache, vomiting, and abdominal pain may be present with fever and mouth lesions. Note that this is a different clinical entity from hand, foot, and mouth disease.

* *

Next, you see the patient's sister who is age 10 and presenting for a school physical. Her mother is concerned because this patient has pubic hair, which her mother thinks is premature (and scary . . . her baby is not growing up yet!). On your exam, she has enlarged areola and a small amount of breast tissue. She also has sparse, dark, but mostly straight pubic hair.

This patient is sexual maturity rating or Tanner stage:

A) 1.
B) 2.
C) 3.
D) 4.
E) 5.

Discussion

The correct answer is "B." Breast buds and sparse, downy pubic hair put the patient in Tanner stage 2. Tanner stage 1 is prepubertal. Any sign of puberty moves a child from Tanner 1 to Tanner 2. Tanner stage 5 is adult or fully matured secondary sexual characteristics. See Table 13–4 for details.

* *

The mom has a lot of questions about puberty. She is nervous about beginning to discuss sexual development with her daughter.

Table 13–4 TANNER STAGES

Stage 1: Prepubertal

Stage 2: Sparse growth of downy hair at base of penis or along labia

- Girls: Breast bud development.
- Boys: Enlargement of scrotum and testes with reddening and thickening of scrotal skin

Stage 3: Darkening, coarse hair sparsely in pubic area

- Girls: Enlargement of breasts (primary mound)
- Boys: Elongation of penis and increased size of testes.

Stage 4: Adult pubic hair distribution (triangle) but smaller area covered with no extension to medial thighs

- Girls: Areola and papilla begin to mound above the level of the breast (secondary mound)
- Boys: Increase in breadth and development of penis, darkening of scrotal skin, enlargement of tests

Stage 5: Adult breasts, genitals, and hair distribution.

What is a developmental fact that you can provide the mom for discussion with her daughter?

A) Typically, in females, the first sign of puberty is pubic hair.
B) At 10 years old, the patient is experiencing premature puberty.
C) The height spurt occurs early during puberty and is almost complete at menarche.
D) Menarche occurs approximately 1 year after breast budding.
E) Schools discuss puberty and relieve mom of that duty (whew!).

Discussion

The correct answer is "C." In girls, the growth spurt occurs early and is almost complete at menarche. Females begin puberty about 1–2 years before males. "A" is incorrect as thelarche, or breast budding marks female onset of puberty. "B" is incorrect. The average age of breast budding is 10.9 years. Thus, Sara is appropriate in her pubertal timing. "D" is incorrect. Menarche typically begins 2 years after breast budding. "E" is incorrect. Although schools may discuss puberty, they are often limited in the time and content. It is important for the child to hear her mother's opinions on puberty and sex.

HELPFUL TIP: Precocious or early puberty is defined as the onset of secondary sexual characteristics before age 8 for girls and age 9 for boys. Delayed puberty is the lack of such changes by age 14.

Objectives: Did you learn to . . .

- Define failure to thrive in a child?
- Evaluate a child with failure to thrive?
- Evaluate a dehydrated child and determine severity of dehydration?
- Manage dehydration in the ED?
- Calculate rehydration fluids for a dehydrated child?
- Generate a differential diagnosis for pharyngitis with blisters?
- Describe changes of puberty and Tanner staging in a female?

QUICK QUIZ: FEEDING INFANTS

Which is not an indication for use of soy formula in an infant?

A) Galactosemia.
B) Congenital lactase deficiency.
C) Cow milk protein intolerance.
D) Parental desire for a vegan diet.

Discussion

The correct answer is "C." Few indications exist for use of soy-based formula over cow milk–based formula. Soy formula is lactose free and therefore should be used in conditions "A," "B," and "D." Galactosemia is a metabolic disorder characterized by the inability to breakdown galactose. Dietary galactose comes from lactose found in human and cow milk. An extensively hydrolyzed or amino acid formula should be used for cow milk protein intolerance as infants are often sensitive to both cow milk and soy proteins. Reflux deserves special note. There is no data supporting the use of soy formula for reflux.

CASE 4

A 2-year-old male presents to your office with his father complaining that the patient has had intermittent crying followed by episodes of profound lethargy during which he is difficult to arouse. The father relates that the patient will sometimes clutch at his abdomen and roll into the fetal position during episodes. These episodes have been going on for about 4 hours. He has had no fever, no vomiting, and no diarrhea. Nobody else at home has been sick. He is developmentally normal and has no significant past medical history. His exam reveals that he is afebrile and lethargic but can be aroused. His abdominal exam is benign. The rest of the exam is unremarkable.

Given his presentation, your clinical suspicion is for:

A) Meningitis.
B) Renal colic.
C) Intussusception.
D) Gastric outlet obstruction.
E) Appendicitis.

Discussion
The correct answer is "C." The patient may have intussusception. The combination of abdominal colic **plus** mental status changes should suggest intussusception. The etiology of the mental status changes is not clear, but mental status changes are one of the classical findings of intussusception. "A," meningitis, should still be a consideration in a patient with mental status changes, but abdominal pain is not usually part of the presentation. Additionally, the patient is afebrile and his symptoms are intermittent, making meningitis less likely. "B" is not associated with mental status changes. "D" and "E" usually present with some abnormal findings on abdominal exam.

HELPFUL TIP: Fewer than 15% of patients with intussusception present with the classic triad of colicky abdominal pain, palpable sausage-shaped abdominal mass, and currant jelly stool.

Which laboratory finding will help you to confirm the diagnosis of intussusception?

A) CBC.
B) Urinalysis.
C) Glucose.
D) Serum lactate.
E) None of the above.

Discussion
The correct answer is "E." None of the above will help to make the diagnosis of intussusception. Early in the course, the CBC may be normal and only 75% will have heme positive stools.

HELPFUL TIP: "Currant jelly stools" are a late finding in intussusception and are a reflection of mucosal ischemia. You really want to make the diagnosis before you see "currant jelly" per rectum. (Hey, have you ever actually seen currant jelly? It is bright red and gloopy, kind of like grandma's cranberry sauce.)

* *

You decide that this patient probably has intussusception based on your history and physical exam.

The next step in diagnosing this patient is:

A) Upper GI with barium.
B) A plain film of the abdomen.
C) An air enema.
D) An abdominal ultrasound.
E) C or D.

Discussion
The correct answer is "D." In general, an ultrasound is the diagnostic modality of choice. An ultrasound may show a typical "bull's eye" lesion helping to make the diagnosis. "C," an air enema, is a diagnostic and therapeutic intervention. An air enema can be used to reduce the intussusception obviating the need for surgery. In general, however, a diagnosis is first made by ultrasound. An upper GI will be of no use since intussusception is a distal process. A plain film of the abdomen will most likely be nondiagnostic as is the case in most abdominal processes (except perhaps bowel obstruction).

HELPFUL TIP: For intussusception, an air or water-soluble contrast enema is preferred over traditional barium enema. Bowel perforation is the main risk of nonoperative reduction. Air and water-soluble contrast are much less harmful than barium if leaked into the peritoneum.

* *

Well, the ultrasound tech is in the Cayman Islands, so you opt for an air enema, which simultaneously diagnoses and reduces the intussusception. The patient appears well with no signs of perforation. He is eating goldfish crackers by the fistful in the ED.

Which of the following is the next step in the treatment of this patient?

A) Discharge to home with good discharge instructions including signs and symptoms to monitor for recurrence or complications requiring return.
B) Admission for IV antibiotics to treat any microperforation that may have occurred with the enema.
C) Discharge to home, planning for elective surgery to fix the area of intussusception to the posterior peritoneal cavity to prevent recurrence.
D) Admission to the hospital for observation.
E) Admission to the hospital with surgery within the next 24 hours to fix the area of intussusception to the posterior peritoneal cavity to prevent recurrence.

Discussion

The correct answer is "A." No further treatment needs to be undertaken at this point or, necessarily, ever, if the patient does well. In hospital observation for 24–48 hours after successful reduction had been the standard of practice but it had never been validated. The purpose of observation admission was to monitor for recurrent intussusception that happens in approximately 10% of cases within the first 24 hours. Children who have undergone successful reduction with no signs of perforation and are tolerating oral intake may be discharged home after a short observation period in the ED. Caregivers should be given good instructions on what to monitor for and where to go if symptoms return.

HELPFUL TIP: Most cases of intussusception are idiopathic. Less than 10% of patients have a pathologic lead point such as a Meckel diverticulum, intestinal polyp, or lymphoma. Increased age of child increases the risk of a lead point.

HELPFUL TIP: Different types of intestinal obstructions occur at different ages. Obstruction at birth is typically an anatomic atresia, meconium ileus, or Hirschsprung disease. Volvulus due to malrotation can occur at any age, but most commonly appears in infancy. Between birth and 5 weeks of age, hypertrophic pyloric stenosis appears. Intussusception is the most common cause of GI obstruction between 3 months and 6 years of age.

Objectives: Did you learn to . . .

- Recognize the clinical presentation of intussusception?
- Evaluate and treat a child with intussusception?

CASE 5

Benjamin, a 4-month-old male, comes to your office for a well baby check. His parents have no concerns. Development and feeding are progressing as expected. On your exam, his head is >95th percentile, but his weight and height are still at the 50th percentile. His previous head circumferences have all been at the 50th percentile. He is a social infant but is having difficulty supporting his large head.

What is the imaging study *LEAST* likely to assist in the diagnosis of the macrocephaly?

A) X-ray.
B) CT scan.
C) MRI scan.
D) Ultrasound.

Discussion

The correct answer is "A." Because the change of head size is so dramatic, an imaging study is needed, but skull radiographs are not likely to assist you in arriving at a diagnosis. The other modalities are used in this setting, and each has its benefits and detractions. Ultrasound or CT scan is frequently obtained first. Ultrasound offers the advantage of no radiation exposure, but it is limited in its application. Ultrasound is primarily used to assess fluid-filled spaces (ventricles in hydrocephalus, subdural hematoma, etc.). CT scan is a rapid and readily available test that can detect hemorrhages, intracranial calcifications, skull fractures, Chiari malformations, and more. CT is limited in its ability to delineate soft-tissue problems, which is where MRI becomes important.

HELPFUL TIP: The differential diagnosis of macrocephaly is long and includes hydrocephalus, brain tumor, benign familial macrocephaly, neurocutaneous disorder (e.g., neurofibromatosis, tuberous sclerosis), hemorrhage, and metabolic disorders (e.g., Tay–Sachs disease, mucopolysaccharidoses).

* *

You order a CT scan, which shows subdural hematomas.

What is your next step in managing Benjamin?

A) Admit to the hospital.
B) Exam of eyes in an ophthalmologist's office.
C) "Babygram" to view entire skeleton of infant for fractures.
D) Alert the department of human services within the next week.
E) Send the patient to a neurosurgeon's office for the next available appointment.

Discussion

The correct answer is "A." Subdural hematomas in an infant are highly suspicious of abusive head trauma. **Your first priority is to protect the child by admission to the hospital.** A retinal exam and skeletal survey are important in the evaluation but are secondary to protection of the child. A "babygram" should never be done to evaluate for skeletal trauma. There is a specific procedure for performing a skeletal survey for abuse. Your state agency responsible for investigating child abuse must be notified within **24 hours** (although clinicians are encouraged to know their legal responsibilities in the state in which they practice). Protection of the child is most important; if the family flees, calling the police or the appropriate state agency would be the first step. Suspicion of abuse, especially abusive head trauma, is an emergency, and it should not wait for a neurosurgeon's next available appointment.

HELPFUL TIP: Retinal hemorrhages, especially when extensive and involving multiple layers, are highly suspicious for abuse. Nonabusive causes of retinal hemorrhages are very rare. Vaccinations, mild head trauma, CPR, seizures, and routine play do **not** cause retinal hemorrhages.

* *

As you have done in this case, radiological studies should always be obtained in the evaluation of suspected child abuse. However, the cause of fractures has a broader differential than abuse.

Which patient's injuries and/or radiological studies would be pathognomonic of abuse?

A) A 9-month-old male with widened distal radius and ulna with fraying and cupping evident on radiograph.
B) A 21-month-old female with multiple fractures at different ages on radiograph. She has delayed tooth eruption and sparse hair.
C) A colicky 1-month-old male infant with callus on the left clavicle.
D) A 2-year-old female with a spiral fracture of the distal right tibia.
E) None of the above.

Discussion

The correct answer is "E." None of these injuries is diagnostic of abuse. Although each of these children would make you think of possible abuse, none of them have been abused. Answer "A" is a child with rickets. Answer "B" is a child with osteogenesis imperfecta. Answer "C" is a child who sustained a clavicle fracture at birth. Answer "D" is a child with a "toddler's fracture." A toddler's fracture is a spiral tibial fracture found in children age 9–36 months (see Chapter 12). These fractures are found in the distal one-third of the tibia.

* *

Benjamin's evaluation shows bilateral subdural hemorrhages and retinal hemorrhages. His skeletal survey is negative. The state agency removes him from the home and places him in foster care. Benjamin then returns for his 6-month well child exam. He has been in foster care since you last saw him. His vision is being followed by an ophthalmologist. He smiles and squeals. His foster mother says, "Looks like he's right-handed. Does that mean that he's advanced for his age?" He rolls both ways. He has started on rice cereal and bananas. He sleeps well. On your exam, he continues to have macrocephaly but a soft fontanelle. His left hand is fisted. The rest of the exam is unremarkable.

What is your assessment and plan for Benjamin?

A) Normal 6 months old: Routine anticipatory guidance and immunizations.
B) Infant with history of head trauma: Delay pertussis vaccination.
C) Infant with history of head trauma: Perform Denver Developmental Screening Test and document findings; repeat in 3 months.
D) Hypertonic left upper extremity: Monitor progress at next well child check.
E) Hypertonic left upper extremity: Refer for further evaluation and treatment of his delay.

Discussion

The correct answer is "E." Benjamin has a risk of developmental delays due to his abusive head injury. He should be monitored closely for delays. One way to monitor for delays is by performing a screening test, such as the Denver Developmental Screening Test. However, Benjamin has concerns that go beyond screening. The concerns are the tightly fisted left hand with corresponding favoring of his right hand suggestive of spastic hemiplegia. Early hand preference is a worrisome sign. Typically hand preference is not definite before 18–24 months. Hand preference should prompt the physician to examine the other extremity. In this case, there is hypertonicity resulting from his trauma. Any child with concern of developmental delay should be referred for further evaluation. Some local and state agencies offer a free service to families to evaluate development and offer therapy. Do NOT watch and wait with a suspected delay. The earlier intervention begins, the better the outcome.

Objectives: Did you learn to . . .

- Recognize and evaluate macrocephaly in an infant?
- Generate a differential diagnosis of macrocephaly in an infant?
- Determine when child abuse should be included in the differential diagnosis?
- Describe some aspects of developmental delay and its management?

QUICK QUIZ: DEVELOPMENTAL DELAY

A mother brings her 18-month-old son in for a routine visit but is concerned that he is not as verbal as he was 3 months ago. She reports that he eats well. He just started walking. You wish to screen him for a pervasive developmental disorder.

What is the most appropriate office tool to use with this patient given his age and presenting symptoms?

A) Ages and Stages Questionnaire.
B) Conner's Rating Scale—Revised Short Form.
C) Denver Developmental Screening Test.
D) Modified Checklist for Autism in Toddlers.
E) All of the above questionnaires are equally valid choices.

Discussion

The correct answer is "D." The Modified Checklist for Autism in Toddlers (M-CHAT for short) is a validated office-screening tool for autism spectrum disorders. It would be the most appropriate tool of the options given. However, there are other tools that you could employ for the same indication (e.g., Screening Tool for Autism at Two Years, Infant Toddler Checklist). "A" is incorrect as the Ages and Stages Questionnaire is a broad-based developmental screening tool, as is the Denver Developmental Screening Test (which also takes much more time). "B" is incorrect because this test is used to detect ADHD. Of note, the AAP recommends screening for autism spectrum disorders using a standard screening tool such as the M-CHAT at ages 18 and 24 months.

CASE 6

A 5-year-old male presents to your clinic with his mother with a complaint of enuresis. Evidently, this child has **never** been completely continent at night, wetting his bed several times per week. This has become somewhat of a problem for him now that his friends are having sleepover birthday parties. Plus, his mother confides that she's tired of paying for pull-ups and cleaning sheets. His incontinence is monosymptomatic (meaning no overactive bladder symptoms or daytime wetting).

What percent of 5-year-olds continue to have enuresis?

A) 1%.
B) 10%.

C) 20%.
D) 40%.
E) 75%.

Discussion

The correct answer is "B." About 10% continue to have enuresis at age 5 years. Even though this would suggest that it is a variant of normal, there is extreme social pressure on children this age to remain dry at night. Parental expectations may depend on their experience with other children. For example, if an older sibling was dry at night at age 3 or if a younger sibling is dry while an older child has enuresis, parents may not accept the bed wetting as normal. Age 5 is considered the cutoff for "normal" enuresis; therefore, at age 6, it is considered a problem.

HELPFUL TIP: Note that the child in this case is male. Enuresis affects twice as many males as females.

* *

Because he has had no period of nocturnal dryness, this patient has primary enuresis.

Which of the following is likely to be part of this child's history?

A) A family history of enuresis.
B) A stressful event in the family such as the birth of a new child or parental divorce.
C) Increased fluid intake over the past 2 months.
D) History of urinary tract infections.

Discussion

The correct answer is "A." Enuresis is divided into primary and secondary enuresis. Primary enuresis occurs in cases where there is **never** a consistent period of dryness at night. Secondary enuresis occurs when there is a period of dryness (by convention, 6 months) before the patient develops enuresis. "B," "C," and "D" would more likely be seen in children with **secondary** enuresis. Primary enuresis tends to be a familial trait.

HELPFUL TIP: About 15% of patients with enuresis become dry each year. The longer enuresis persists, the less likely it is to resolve.

One percent of patients older than 15 years continue to have primary enuresis.

* *

This patient's exam is essentially normal including neurologic evaluation.

Further evaluation of this patient should include all of the following EXCEPT:

A) Asking about a history of bowel problems.
B) Assessment of growth and development.
C) Investigation into family history of nocturnal enuresis.
D) Spine MRI to rule out pathologic lesion.
E) Urinalysis.

Discussion

The correct answer is "D." Patients with enuresis who have an otherwise normal neurologic exam need not have an MRI done. If on exam this child had neurologic findings, an MRI would be indicated. All of the remaining options are part of a thorough evaluation of nocturnal enuresis. Of particular note is the assessment of growth and development (is this child neurologically delayed leading to enuresis?). Attention to bowel problems is also important. Fecal impaction can lead to incontinence. Asking about snoring can help to identify obstructive sleep apnea, which can be associated with enuresis.

* *

You find no indication of an underlying cause, and you decide that this is primary enuresis. The parents are desperate for some sort of intervention to fix the problem, since it is becoming a major source of anxiety in the home and of teasing at school.

Which of the following should constitute *INITIAL* treatment of this patient's primary enuresis?

A) Patient education and motivational training (e.g., rewards for staying dry).
B) Over-learning.
C) Enuresis alarm.
D) Nasal desmopressin (DDAVP).
E) Oral desipramine.

Discussion

The correct answer is "A." All of the above have been found to be useful in the treatment of enuresis; however, the best initial approach includes education. Patients and parents should be informed of how common this condition is, how to reduce fluid intake in the evening without getting dehydrated, and how to schedule voiding. Motivational training plays a role as well. The other interventions are secondary. "B," over-learning, is thought to help prevent relapses in patients who have been successful with an enuresis alarm. Once continence is achieved with the alarm, the child drinks a set amount of fluid before bedtime. The amount is successively increased once dryness is achieved until a maximum is reached. The idea is that the patient is conditioned to respond to his increasing bladder capacity.

"C," an enuresis alarm, is an effective treatment but relatively expensive and requires significant motivation on the part of the family. The enuresis alarm increases success of the other options when used in combination and has shown the best long-term results. "D" and "E" are incorrect in this scenario although they are used to treat enuresis. Relapse is more common when pharmacologic therapy is discontinued than with the other modalities. However, medications are effective as a short-term treatment option but are felt to be second tier to be used when the urine alarm fails or is impractical (think sleepover or summer camp). Of note, "D" is wrong for another reason: **nasal** DDAVP is no longer approved for nocturnal enuresis due to problems with hyponatremia. Oral DDAVP still carries the enuresis indication, but it can cause hyponatremia as well—it just occurs less often.

> HELPFUL TIP: Retention control training is no longer recommended as it was not found to significantly decrease wetting. Retention-control training was based on the (faulty) premise that enuretic children had smaller bladder capacities. The child would hold in urine in an attempt to stretch the bladder and increase capacity. Retention control training can increase bladder capacity but does not improve enuresis. But maybe if you are a truck driver...

Objectives: Did you learn to . . .

- Define primary and secondary enuresis?
- Describe some of the epidemiologic characteristics of enuresis?
- Evaluate a patient with enuresis?
- Develop a management strategy for enuresis?

QUICK QUIZ: MECONIUM

Delayed meconium passage occurs in which of the following conditions?

A) Encopresis.
B) Hirschsprung disease.
C) Cystic fibrosis.
D) Hyperthyroidism.
E) B and C.

Discussion

The correct answer is "E." Seventy percent of newborns will pass meconium within the first 12 hours of life. More than 90% of newborns pass meconium within the first 24 hours. In those with delayed passage of meconium (generally defined as >24 hours of life), consider Hirschsprung disease, cystic fibrosis, **hypo**thyroidism, sepsis, intrauterine narcotic exposure, or imperforate anus.

QUICK QUIZ: RASH

Your next patient in the ED is a 3-year-old female with a rash. After playing outside (could playing outside be a red herring? The editors think so . . .), her father found spots on her legs, and she did not want to walk because her knees hurt. On exam, she is afebrile with normal vitals and slightly irritable but otherwise interactive. She has slight nasal drainage, which her father says is a residual from a cold last week. Her legs and buttocks have palpable purpura. Her knees are mildly swollen and are painful with range of motion. Her CBC (including platelets) and coagulation studies are normal, and her urinalysis is significant for 2+ hematuria.

The most likely diagnosis in this patient is:

A) Acute exposure to lawn chemicals.
B) Henoch–Schönlein purpura (HSP).

C) Juvenile idiopathic arthritis (JIA).
D) Meningococcemia.
E) Rocky Mountain spotted fever.

Discussion

The correct answer is "B." This is classic HSP, an IgA-mediated, self-limited, leukocytoclastic vasculitis. The symptoms and signs of HSP are a rash (typically nonthrombocytopenic purpura), abdominal pain (from submucosal hemorrhage and edema), arthritis/arthralgia, and renal disease. Typically, the vasculitis follows an upper respiratory infection or streptococcal pharyngitis, such as in this case. Treatment for HSP is supportive.

"A," lawn chemical exposure, usually results in nothing but may cause acute cholinergic symptoms if organophosphates are used. "C," JIA, is not likely because the rash of systemic onset JIA is evanescent salmon-pink rash on the trunk and axilla that classically occurs when the patient spikes a fever. "D," meningococcemia, is incorrect because the patient is afebrile, alert, and nontoxic appearing without laboratory evidence of disseminated intravascular coagulopathy. "E" is unlikely because Rocky Mountain spotted fever presents with headache, high fever, petechial rash involving the palms and soles, and the patients will appear toxic. Additionally, patients with Rocky Mountain spotted fever have thrombocytopenia when their petechiae appear.

HELPFUL TIP: The rash of HSP is frequently initially urticaria with surrounding edema. The rash tends to be symmetric and occur in dependent areas developing first on the legs or on pressure points (buttocks).

CASE 7

A 7-month-old fully immunized female presents to the office with fever. Mom reports she has "not been herself" and felt "a bit warm on the forehead." Vitals reveal a temperature of 39.2°C. Physical exam reveals a mildly toxic infant. You perform a complete history and physical but are unable to identify a source of the fever.

What is the first step in your approach to this child?

A) Obtain a urinalysis and urine culture.
B) Admit for observation and perform blood, urine, and CSF for culture.
C) Give an intramuscular dose of ceftriaxone.
D) Order acetaminophen 30 mg/kg and discharge the patient if the temperature comes down.
E) Admit for IV fluids overnight.

Discussion

The correct answer is "A." At this age, occult serious bacterial infection is less likely than during the neonatal period especially when vaccinated against *Haemophilus influenzae* type b and *Streptococcus pneumoniae*. In a well-appearing child older than 90 days with a fever without a focal source, most experts recommend a screening urinalysis and urine culture as the initial diagnostic test. "B" is overly aggressive, and "C" is not indicated and can make diagnostic tests more difficult to interpret should this child become sicker. "D" might be appropriate although the dose of acetaminophen is wrong (it should be 15 mg/kg/dose by mouth every 4–6 hours). Since you are not seeing signs of dehydration, "E" is inappropriate.

HELPFUL TIP: Studies have shown that the incidence of occult bacteremia is less than 1% in well-appearing **fully immunized** infants 3–36 months of age presenting with fever without localizing signs. Often, a positive blood culture is due to contamination, which results in unnecessary additional testing, treatment, and cost. Some of you may be thinking, "What about a CBC?" In this type of patient, the WBC count can be equally misleading. The most important factors in decision making are the patient's age, immunization status, and clinical appearance.

HELPFUL TIP: Some suggest a single **rectal *loading*** dose of acetaminophen dosed at 30 mg/kg. Subsequent rectal doses should be 10–15 mg/kg/dose every 4–6 hours. The maximum daily dose of 75 mg/kg should not be exceeded.

What is the most appropriate manner in which to obtain a urine specimen in this child?

A) Midstream "clean-catch."
B) Bag specimen from sterile plastic bag taped to the perineal region.
C) Bladder catheterization.
D) Suprapubic aspiration.
E) C or D.

Discussion

The correct answer is "C." The gold standard test for the diagnosis of urinary tract infection is a quantitative urine culture. While the urinalysis and microscopy may suggest UTI, no component, or combination of components, is as sensitive or specific as culture. Therefore, if a child is likely to require antimicrobial therapy, one should attempt to obtain urine for culture in a manner not likely to cause contamination. The mid-stream "clean-catch" may be obtained in older children who are toilet trained, making certain that the perineum is cleansed first. Bag specimens are prone to contamination and should be avoided in toxic patients who are likely going to need antibiotics. Suprapubic aspiration is generally not necessary though it is the gold standard.

HELPFUL TIP: Guidelines suggest that one option in a **nontoxic** infant is to get a bag urine. If this is positive, it must be followed up with a urine obtained by catheterization or suprapubic aspirate. This should then be sent for culture. Any child who will need antibiotics on a relatively emergent basis should have a urine obtained by catheterization or suprapubic aspiration sent.

The patient has 20 WBC/hpf on UA. Without knowing the culture and susceptibility results, which antibiotic would be the LEAST appropriate choice for the treatment of a UTI in this child?

A) Trimethoprim/sulfamethoxazole.
B) Amoxicillin.
C) Cefdinir.
D) Cefixime.

Discussion

The correct answer is "B." The resistance rate to amoxicillin is high. Thus, amoxicillin is not a good choice for treating a UTI in children (or anybody with a UTI). The usual choice for empiric oral antibiotic treatment of UTI in children includes, sulfonamides, or third-generation cephalosporins. Fluoroquinolones may be considered in adolescents or children older than 1 year with a complicated UTI. The duration of treatment should be 7–10 days for uncomplicated UTI. If the child appears clinically ill suggesting pyelonephritis, initial parenteral treatment with ceftriaxone would be an appropriate first-line agent. Many experts prefer a 14-day course for those with pyelonephritis.

* *

Her urine culture reveals *Escherichia coli* susceptible to trimethoprim/sulfamethoxazole, and you treat her appropriately.

Following her initial treatment, what diagnostic study should be performed next?

A) Abdominal supine and upright radiographs.
B) Renal ultrasound and voiding cystourethrogram (VCUG).
C) Spiral CT of abdomen and pelvis.
D) Urology consultation for urodynamic studies.
E) None of the above.

Discussion

The correct answer is "E." In **febrile infants** with UTI, it is important to look for anatomic abnormalities of the urinary tract. Ultrasound imaging is recommended following a first febrile UTI to identify those at risk for recurrence and subsequent damage to renal parenchyma (male or female). So, "B" would be correct if not for the inclusion of VCUG. Urinary tract ultrasonography should be performed at the earliest convenient time. Ultrasound is useful in the evaluation for kidney size and hydronephrosis, but it is limited in the evaluation of vesicoureteral reflux (VUR), a common abnormality associated with recurrent UTI. VUR is evaluated with a VCUG or radionuclide cystogram (RNC). VCUG should be done after a first febrile UTI **only when there is evidence of renal abnormality on the ultrasound including scaring, hydronephrosis, abnormal anatomy, etc.** Routine VCUG **is not** recommended. Thus, choice "B" is incorrect. **To repeat: Routine VCUG is not indicated after a first febrile UTI** unless there is an abnormality on the ultrasound.

Table 13–5 INTERNATIONAL REFLUX STUDY COMMITTEE GRADING OF VESICOURETERAL REFLUX

Grade I: Involves the ureter only.
Grade II: Involves the ureter, pelvis, and calyces without dilatation.
Grade III: Involves the ureter, pelvis, and calyces with mild ureter and pelvis dilatation.
Grade IV: Involves the ureter, pelvis, and calyces with significant dilatation and blunting of the calyceal fornices.
Grade V: Demonstrates dilatation and tortuosity of the ureter as well as loss of the calyceal fornices.

* *

For some unknown reason, a VCUG is done (you said "Is it time for tea?" and it got transcribed as "do a VCUG") and Olivia is found to have grade II reflux (see Table 11–5).

Which of the following would be the most appropriate initial management of her reflux?

A) Prescribe prophylactic antibiotics.
B) Refer for surgical intervention.
C) Perform GFR to assess renal scarring.
D) Observe for now with repeat VCUG in 6 months.
E) None of the above.

Discussion

The correct answer is "E." **There is no evidence that antibiotics are effective at preventing recurrent UTI in patients with grades I–IV reflux. Don't do it.** Studies are ongoing about grade V reflux. Mild reflux tends to resolve with maturity. Renal scarring is best detected by radioisotope scanning with 99m-technetium dimercaptosuccinate. Doing a GFR looks at kidney function and does not assess for renal scarring. Therefore, "C" is incorrect. "D" is incorrect because a VCUG was not indicated in the first place!

HELPFUL (OR CONFUSING) TIP: We don't know what the board exam will want as an answer. Traditionally, ultrasound and VCUG have been done after a first UTI in a male infant and a second UTI in a female infant. Surgical intervention is generally reserved for those with severe reflux (grades IV–V) or recurrent UTI despite prophylactic antibiotics (although as noted above, prophylactic antibiotics are not really helpful in grade IV reflux). See Pediatrics, Aug 28, 2011; DOI:1542/peds.2011-1330 for more information.

Objectives: Did you learn to . . .

- Evaluate an older (>3 months old) infant with fever?
- Diagnose and treat a child with an initial urinary tract infection?
- Recognize that urinary tract infection is often a marker for urinary tract abnormalities in children?
- Manage a patient with VUR?

CASE 8

Anthony is a 2300-g male infant born at 35 weeks' gestation to a 23-year-old G2P2 single female. The mother did not seek prenatal care and routine screening labs were not available. She presented to the ED in active labor shortly following spontaneous rupture of membranes at home. Upon transfer to the obstetric ward, she was noted to be febrile (38.8°C) and received intravenous antibiotics. Five hours later, the infant was delivered via spontaneous vaginal delivery.

Management of this newborn infant whose mother probably has chorioamnionitis (not simply GBS screen positive) should include which of the following?

A) Empiric therapy with gentamicin.
B) Empiric therapy with ampicillin.
C) Empiric therapy with vancomycin.
D) A and B.
E) All of the above.

Discussion

The correct answer is "D." Maternal chorioamnionitis is an important risk factor for early onset sepsis in the newborn. The 2010 CDC guideline on the prevention of perinatal group B streptococcal disease recommends that all infants born to mothers with chorioamnionitis have screening labs and blood cultures at birth followed by minimum of 48 hours of antibiotic therapy. Antibiotic therapy may be extended and/or modified depending on the clinical course and culture results. A lumbar puncture for CSF culture and analysis should be performed if the child is septic appearing. Ampicillin and gentamicin as empiric therapy cover the most likely organisms including GBS and gram-negative pathogens, respectively.

* *

Anthony is started on appropriate antibiotics. Examination of this neonate reveals hepatosplenomegaly, lymphadenopathy, petechiae, and white mucocutaneous patches in the infant's mouth. His CBC reveals a hemoglobin of 12 g/dL and a platelet count of 85,000/mm^3 with evidence of hemolysis on the peripheral smear.

The most likely pathogen infecting this infant is:

A) Rubella.
B) Cytomegalovirus.
C) *Toxoplasma gondii.*
D) *Treponema pallidum.*
E) *Candida albicans.*

Discussion

The correct answer is "D." Neonatal manifestations of congenital syphilis include hepatosplenomegaly, lymphadenopathy, jaundice, rash, hemolytic anemia, and thrombocytopenia. Unfortunately, these findings overlap considerably with many of the other congenital TORCH (toxoplasmosis, rubella, CMV, herpes) infections. Abnormalities more specific to congenital syphilis include white, patchy mucocutaneous lesions, edema, rhinitis (snuffles), osteochondritis, and pseudoparalysis. Congenital syphilis is caused by transplacental transmission of the spirochete *T. pallidum* ("D"). Intrauterine infection can result in stillbirth, hydrops fetalis, or prematurity.

> HELPFUL TIP: Late sequelae of congenital syphilis involve the bones and joints, teeth, eyes, and CNS and include bowed shins (Saber shins), frontal bossing, saddle nose, pegged central incisors, interstitial keratitis, and sensorineural deafness. The Hutchinson triad includes interstitial keratitis, deafness, and notched, peg-shaped teeth.

* *

In addition to the laboratory data obtained above, you order an ultrasound of the patient's head, which appears normal.

Intracerebral calcifications are CLASSICALLY associated with which congenital infection(s)?

A) Cytomegalovirus.
B) Toxoplasmosis.
C) *T. pallidum.*
D) Rubella.
E) A and B.

Discussion

The correct answer is "E." The clinical manifestations of congenital cytomegalovirus and toxoplasmosis are often similar. Infants are typically asymptomatic at birth, but a significant number ultimately develop visual impairment, learning disabilities, and mental retardation months to years later. Those infants who are symptomatic at birth may demonstrate intrauterine growth retardation, hepatosplenomegaly, jaundice, hemolytic anemia, and thrombocytopenia. Intracerebral calcifications also occur in both CMV and toxoplasmosis. The calcifications tend to be periventricular in CMV (remember this by the fact that the calcifications look like a "C" in CMV) and more dispersed throughout the cortex in toxoplasmosis (remember by noting the X in both cortex and toxoplasmosis). Additional central nervous system abnormalities include microcephaly, chorioretinitis, and sensorineural hearing loss.

Objectives: Did you learn to . . .

- Appropriately manage the neonate born to a mother who has evidence of chorioamnionitis?
- Recognize that many congenital TORCH infections may have overlapping signs and symptoms?
- Recognize that many infants with congenital TORCH infections are asymptomatic at birth?

QUICK QUIZ: CONGENITAL INFECTIONS

A small for gestational age newborn infant is found to have hepatosplenomegaly, jaundice, and thrombocytopenia. Cardiac examination reveals a grade II/VI continuous murmur heard best at the left upper sternal border. An ophthalmologic examination demonstrates micro-ophthalmia and cataracts.

The result of which maternal prenatal screening lab is likely to have been concerning in the above case?

A) VDRL.
B) Rubella immunity status.

C) HIV status.
D) Varicella zoster immunity status.
E) GBS cultures.

Discussion

The correct answer is "B." Cardiac, ophthalmologic, auditory, and neurologic findings predominate in the symptomatic infant with congenital rubella. Up to 85% of infants infected during the first 12 weeks of gestation will have some form of congenital defect. This decreases to 5% when the primary infection occurs after the third to fourth month of gestation. Ophthalmologic findings include microphthalmia, cataracts, glaucoma, and salt and pepper retinopathy. Infants are often microcephalic and develop sensorineural hearing deficits, meningoencephalitis, and mental retardation. Additional findings of hepatosplenomegaly, thrombocytopenia, and osteitis may be present. A characteristic "blueberry muffin" appearance may be present due to the combination of jaundice and extramedullary (skin) hematopoiesis. Syphilis and GBS infections are described above and they do not typically cause the ophthalmologic findings described in this case. "C" is incorrect because congenital HIV infection is commonly asymptomatic. Evidence of immune deficiency may present later in the child's life with failure to thrive, generalized lymphadenopathy, hepatosplenomegaly, and recurrent infections. "D" is incorrect because congenital herpes infections do not cause cardiac abnormalities.

HELPFUL TIP: USPSTF recommends universal hearing screening for newborns.

QUICK QUIZ: CONGENITAL INFECTIONS

Which of the following cardiac lesions is likely to be found in an infant with congenital rubella?

A) Patent ductus arteriosus (PDA).
B) Tetralogy of Fallot.
C) Transposition of great vessels.
D) Coarctation of aorta.
E) Bicuspid aortic valve.

Discussion

The correct answer is "A." The most common cardiac lesions associated with congenital rubella are PDA and peripheral pulmonary artery stenosis. PDA is characterized by a continuous "washing machine" murmur heard best over the left upper sternal border. Tetralogy of Fallot and transposition of great vessels are classically cyanotic heart defects that have no known association with congenital infections. (See the Web-based cases for a more complete discussion of congenital heart disease.) Coarctation of the aorta and bicuspid aortic valve both cause harsh systolic murmurs. The murmur of coarctation radiates to the back. Both coarctation and bicuspid aortic valve are commonly found in females with Turner syndrome.

CASE 9

A term newborn infant is noted to have a solitary, tense bulla located on the dorsum of his wrist. The underlying skin is nonerythematous. Pregnancy was uncomplicated; however, the infant was delivered via cesarean section for failure to progress. The infant appears to be a vigorous feeder and is noted to frequently suck on his hands and wrists while in the nursery. He is otherwise asymptomatic.

Which of the following is MOST appropriate at this time?

A) Start acyclovir.
B) Perform lumbar puncture and send a sample of the CSF for HSV PCR.
C) Perform a Tzanck smear of the bulla fluid.
D) All of the above.
E) Observation with no intervention at this time.

Discussion

The correct answer is "E." Nothing needs to be done at this time. The appearance and location of the bulla is consistent with a sucking blister. A solitary bulla or blister on normal-appearing skin located on the upper limbs may be present at birth from in utero sucking. Often when presented with the affected extremity, the infant will demonstrate the sucking behavior in that location. Such blisters are often mistaken for herpes simplex, but the solitary nature and location help to establish the correct diagnosis—although there may be multiple blisters at times. Additional history of cesarean section makes HSV less likely in this scenario. Nonetheless, a sucking blister is a diagnosis of exclusion, and other more serious diagnoses should be ruled out by history and exam and further testing as indicated.

The FALSE statement regarding neonatal herpes simplex virus infection is:

A) The majority of infants with neonatal HSV are born to mothers with symptomatic herpetic lesions.
B) The incidence of neonatal transmission is higher when the pregnant woman experiences primary infection versus secondary reactivation.
C) Most neonatal HSV infections are caused by HSV 2.
D) Intrauterine exposure accounts for the minority of perinatal HSV infection.
E) Herpetic skin lesions are often present in infants with CNS or disseminated HSV.

Discussion

The correct answer is "A." Less than one-third of infants with neonatal HSV are born to mothers with active genital lesions. In fact, most cases of neonatal HSV are found in infants of asymptomatic mothers who are shedding the virus. Neonatal herpes simplex virus often results in serious morbidity and mortality. Infants with HSV present with one of the following three disease patterns with overlapping features: localized disease involving the skin, eyes, and mouth; CNS disease; or disseminated infection. Encephalitis may occur with or without skin involvement; therefore, HSV infection should be suspected in any infant from birth to approximately 4 weeks of age that presents with fever, seizure, or mental status abnormalities such as lethargy, irritability, or poor feeding.

The other options are correct. A woman who contracts a primary infection during the pregnancy has a greater than 30% chance of transmitting the virus to her infant. There is less than 2% transmission if she experiences a secondary reactivation intrapartum. The majority of neonatal HSV is due to infection with HSV 2. Only 5% of congenital infections occur in utero, as the majority occurs via exposure to infected cervical secretions during birth. Skin lesions are present in 60% of CNS cases and about 75% of disseminated cases.

HELPFUL TIP: Most neonates with HSV infection do not present with skin findings at birth. It is more typical for neonates to develop HSV skin lesions 5–14 days after delivery.

HELPFUL TIP: Infants born vaginally or via cesarean delivery to moms with active genital HSV lesions need HSV cultures of the mouth, nasopharynx, conjunctiva, and rectum obtained at 12–24 hours of age. In infants born to moms with a primary outbreak at time of delivery, some experts recommend empiric acyclovir therapy after obtaining the appropriate cultures. Infants of mothers with a recurrent outbreak do not require empiric acyclovir treatment but still should be monitored closely for signs of infection.

Objectives: Did you learn to . . .

- Differentiate between a herpes lesion and a sucking blister?
- Recognize rates and modes of transmission of herpes in neonates?
- Identify some of the clinical manifestations of neonatal herpes?

CASE 10

A bunch of parents in your neighborhood decide to have a "chickenpox" party (prompting you to consider moving to a place where people believe in modern medicine). They want to synchronize their kids' chickenpox outbreaks with their busy schedules (heaven forbid we should get immunized—after all, it isn't natural!). One of the mothers, who has never herself had chickenpox, finds out that she is pregnant the day after being exposed to chickenpox. She is not yet symptomatic (from the pregnancy or the chickenpox).

The best advice for this potential mother about her pregnancy is:

A) Consider termination since it is likely that the child will have congenital varicella.
B) Get treated within 48 hours of exposure with varicella immune globulin.
C) Get treated within 48 hours of exposure with varicella immune globulin plus varicella vaccine.
D) Get treated within 48 hours of exposure with IVIG plus varicella vaccine.

Discussion

The correct answer is "B." Women who are varicella susceptible (not immune), are pregnant, and are exposed to chickenpox should be treated with varicella immune globulin (VariZIG) within 96 hours of exposure. If VariZIG is unavailable, IVIG may be given instead. **The vaccine should be avoided during pregnancy. It is a live, attenuated, virus and still carries some risk to the fetus (although the degree of risk is unknown).**

You can let the mother know that:

A) Varicella immune globulin has been shown to reduce the risk of congenital varicella.
B) Varicella immune globulin is aimed mostly at attenuating the case in the mother should she be infected.
C) Varicella immune globulin has not been shown to prevent congenital varicella.
D) A and B.
E) B and C.

Discussion
The correct answer is "B." Varicella immune globulin is aimed at reducing the symptoms in the mother and attenuating her case of varicella. Both "A" and "C" are false. There are no good data either way about how varicella immune globulin will affect the child's outcome vis-à-vis congenital varicella.

Manifestations of intrauterine infection with varicella zoster include all of the following defects EXCEPT:

A) Optic atrophy.
B) Congenital cataracts.
C) Cardiac abnormalities.
D) CNS abnormalities.
E) Limb hypoplasia.

Discussion
The correct answer is "C." Cardiac abnormalities are not seen with varicella zoster exposure in utero. In addition to the findings above, patients with congenital varicella zoster will have cutaneous scarring called cicatrix.

* *

Now that all of these children have been infected with varicella zoster, the question arises about how long they should be kept out of school.

These children are considered infectious until:

A) 5 days after the first lesion appears.
B) 10–14 days after the first lesion appears.
C) New lesions are no longer forming.
D) All lesions are crusted over.
E) They are no longer febrile.

Discussion
The correct answer is "D." Patients are considered infectious until all lesions are crusted over. Lesions need not have healed entirely, only crusted over.

Objectives: Did you learn to . . .

- Offer treatment for varicella exposure to a pregnant nonimmune female?
- Recognize the uses of varicella immune globulin?
- Identify symptoms of congenital varicella infection?

CASE 11

A 3-year-old child presents to your office with a history of bright red cheeks. Over the past several days, she has had mild fever with mild muscle aches. Except for the rash, the child is now asymptomatic.

The most likely cause of this patient's illness is:

A) Parvovirus B-19.
B) Herpes virus 6.
C) Rubeola.
D) Rubella.
E) Influenza virus.

Discussion
The correct answer is "A." A mild systemic illness followed by red, "slapped cheeks" is typical of erythema infectiosum or "fifth disease," caused by parvovirus B-19. The red, slapped cheeks are generally followed by a lacy, reticular rash on the extremities and trunk. This is generally a self-limited illness in children.

Complications of parvovirus B-19 infection—either congenital or acquired—include all of the following EXCEPT:

A) Aplastic anemia.
B) Birth defects, including CNS and limb disease.
C) Hydrops fetalis.
D) Inflammatory arthritis.
E) Intrauterine fetal death.

Discussion

The correct answer is "B." Parvovirus B-19 causes all of the above except for birth defects. Fetal death, anemia, or nonimmune-mediated hydrops fetalis are potential outcomes of intrauterine exposure (one-third of infected women will pass the virus to their fetus). Most infants infected in utero are born normally at term, including those with evidence of hydrops earlier in the pregnancy. A small subset will acquire chronic or prolonged postnatal infection of unknown significance. "A," transient aplastic crisis, can occur in those with chronic hemolytic conditions such as sickle cell anemia. "D," inflammatory arthritis, is common in adults and adolescents with females more commonly affected.

* *

The question of whether or not to exclude this child from preschool is raised. The patient still has the rash. There are a couple of pregnant teachers at the preschool.

You can tell the child's mother that:

A) This child is infectious and should be excluded from preschool until the rash resolves.
B) Since almost all adult women are already immune, there is no need to worry about transmission to the teachers.
C) Since this virus is an enterovirus, careful hygiene in the school will prevent spread.
D) This child can be allowed back into preschool and is no longer infectious.

Discussion

The correct answer is "D." Once the rash is present, this child is no longer infectious and can be allowed back into school. "B" is incorrect because only about 50% of adult women are immune. "C" is incorrect. First, this is not an enterovirus. Second, the exact mechanism of transmission is not known.

> HELPFUL TIP: Just try getting this child with a rash back in school and past the school nurse. It is impossible... On the other hand, schools are well aware that there is a magical effect of topical antibiotics in preventing the spread of viral conjunctivitis.

Objectives: Did you learn to...

- Recognize the clinical manifestations of parvovirus B-19 infection ("fifth disease")
- Identify complications of parvovirus B-19 infection?

QUICK QUIZ: CHILDHOOD INFECTIONS

Which of the following is characterized by a high fever, possibly over 40°C, a bulging fontanelle, a maculopapular rash that begins *after* the fever abates, conjunctivitis, and upper respiratory symptoms?

A) Roseola infantum (erythema subitum).
B) Rubeola (measles).
C) Rubella (German measles).
D) Varicella (chicken pox).
E) Meningococcal meningitis.

Discussion

The correct answer is "A." Such a clinical presentation is typical of roseola infantum. Roseola infantum, which is caused by the human herpes 6 (and rarely herpes 7) virus, is characterized by a high fever for 3–5 days (often over 40°C), generalized malaise, a bulging fontanelle in up to 26% of infants, conjunctivitis, perhaps oral mucosal ulcers, and a rash that appears as the fever begins to defervesce. Children usually look amazingly well for the height of the fever.

QUICK QUIZ: GASTROINTESTINAL SYMPTOMS

A young couple brings in their 18-month-old female for a 12-hour history of vomiting and diarrhea. The patient has felt warm, and her oral intake has been depressed. However, she continues to make tears with crying and has wet diapers. Her medical history is unremarkable. On exam, you find a tired-looking female who perks up slightly when you open a bag of toys (who *are* you anyway... Santa?). Her temperature is 38.5°C, and her capillary refill is less than 3 seconds. The remainder of the exam is nonfocal. You think that she has a viral gastroenteritis, and give the parents some advice regarding rehydration.

Which of the following is the most appropriate advice for this patient?

A) Avoid all solid food for the next 24–48 hours.
B) Use milk as the primary rehydration solution.
C) Use only watered-down tea for rehydration.
D) Use a commercially prepared oral rehydration solution and reintroduce foods as tolerated.
E) Use cola beverages (e.g., Coca-Cola or Pepsi) because they contain more sodium than commercially available oral rehydration solutions.

Discussion

The correct answer is "D." Effective oral rehydration can be accomplished with any one of the rehydration solutions on the market (e.g., Pedialyte). "A" is incorrect. There is no need to limit the food intake of patients with vomiting or infectious diarrhea. They can have whatever they can tolerate. The concept of "gut rest" is obsolete and leads to increased bowel permeability and prolonged diarrhea. So, early feeding is optimal and recommended. There is no need to avoid lactose-containing products. Transient lactase deficiency after gastroenteritis is usually self-limited and does not require treatment unless symptoms are prolonged or severe after dietary reintroduction. "C" and "E" are incorrect. There is no role for weak tea, flat soda, "Jello water," sports drinks, juice, etc., in the management of gastroenteritis. The most common cause of hyponatremic seizures in the child is improper rehydration during gastroenteritis. Many commercial drinks, such as cola beverages and sports drinks, are not specifically designed for oral rehydration, and the sodium concentration is typically much lower, risking hyponatremia (in other words, the reverse of "E" is true). Additionally, these drinks usually have a high sugar content, which can worsen diarrhea due to osmotic effects.

> HELPFUL TIP: In the exclusively breastfed infant with vomiting and/or diarrhea, breastfeeding should be encouraged and not replaced with oral rehydration solutions.

> HELPFUL TIP: During a GI illness, advise parents to avoid nonabsorbable sugars, like those found in apple or grape juice. These can promote an osmotic diarrhea.

CASE 12

A new mother and father bring their 2-month-old infant to your office with a complaint of inconsolable crying. This started at about 3 weeks of age and occurs about the same time every day. The crying will last for hours and is becoming quite disruptive. The child will draw up his knees and seem to be in quite a bit of pain. They have tried pretty much everything that they can think up including car rides, swings, swaddling, various types of music, etc., but to no avail. Shivers run up and down your spine as you recall your own early parenting experiences . . . or as you remember why you don't have kids (please apply the appropriate phrase for your personal experience).

The most likely diagnosis is:

A) Colic.
B) Intussusception.
C) Hair around the penis or toes or corneal abrasion.
D) Constipation.
E) Cluster headache.

Discussion

The correct answer is "A." Colic generally begins at 3 weeks of age, peaks at about 6 weeks of age, and abates by 3 months of age. It is defined by a rule of 3s: intense crying for 3 hours per day for 3 days per week for 3 weeks. However, most parents, grandparents, nosy aunts, and pediatricians will describe any particularly fussy baby as "colicky." The cause is unknown. "B" is incorrect. While intussusception can certainly present with colicky abdominal pain, it is not likely to be recurrent for several days or weeks without a more significant problem (e.g., bloody stools) developing. "C," a hair or thread around a child's toes or penis or corneal abrasion, should be considered in any child with inconsolable crying. Again, this is not likely to result in crying that is daily and episodic. "D" is incorrect as this history is not consistent with constipation. And "E," a cluster headache, does not occur in this age group.

> HELPFUL TIP: While inconsolable crying has often been attributed to a corneal abrasion, recent data calls this into question. Just as many children who were NOT crying had corneal abrasions.

You can advise the parents that:

A) Phenobarbital is safe and effective for controlling infant colic (when given to the parents to help them "chill out").
B) Elimination of cruciferous vegetables from the diet of breastfeeding mothers has been shown to reduce infant colic.
C) Simethicone has been shown to be effective in infant colic.
D) Anticholinergic drugs are effective in treating infant colic, but the risks are unacceptable.
E) Children who breastfeed are less likely to develop colic.

Discussion

The correct answer is "D." Anticholinergic drugs have been shown to be effective in the treatment of colic. However, the risks associated with the use of these drugs are generally considered unacceptable. The rest of the answers are incorrect. It does not seem as though breastfed infants are any less likely to develop colic than are bottle-fed infants. The evidence for elimination of cruciferous vegetables is inconclusive. Simethicone **is not** effective in treating infantile colic, but it gives the parents something to do.

HELPFUL TIP: The cause of colic is unknown and likely multifactorial. Rarely a medical explanation is found. **It is important to identify alternative caregivers, since infant colic can be a major stress on parents and can possibly lead to abuse.**

HELPFUL TIP: There is evidence to support a trial of a hypoallergenic diet in infants with colic. Formula-fed infants may try an extensively hydrolyzed or amino acid formula. Use of partially hydrolyzed or lactose-free formulas is of no benefit. Maternal elimination diet avoiding cow and soy milk proteins may be tried for breastfed infants.

HELPFUL TIP: Alternative therapies such as probiotics may be considered in severe cases. Evidence for spinal manipulation in treating colic is inconclusive. In a crossover study, 24% sucrose has been shown to be beneficial (Tootsweet and other brands... or make it yourself).

* *

You next see the same child when he is 2 years old. His parents bring him to your ED with a history of a "barky" cough. He has had an antecedent upper respiratory infection for a couple of days with a runny nose and a temperature of 38.2°C. On arrival in the ED, he has retractions and stridor but does not look toxic. He's barking like a seal... a sick seal. He also has vomiting after episodes of coughing.

The MOST LIKELY diagnosis in this child is:

A) Epiglottitis.
B) Laryngotracheobronchitis.
C) Bacterial tracheitis.
D) Retropharyngeal abscess.
E) Gastroenteritis.

Discussion

The correct answer is "B." This represents laryngotracheobronchitis, also known as "croup." Typically, patients have an antecedent URI with a low-grade fever, a barky cough, and stridor, which are usually worse at night. "A" is incorrect because patients with epiglottitis generally do **not** have an antecedent URI, but they do have a much higher temperature with sudden onset of symptoms and a toxic appearance. "C" is incorrect. Patients with bacterial tracheitis do have an antecedent URI but then develop a second stage of the illness (e.g., a biphasic illness) with sudden onset of high fever, purulent sputum production, and stridor. These patients look toxic. "D," a retropharyngeal abscess, occurs in conjunction with high fever, drooling, refusal to swallow, and toxic appearance. "E" is incorrect. This child has posttussive emesis. Gastroenteritis does not include the other features found in this child with croup.

* *

You decide to treat this patient in the ED.

All of the following are appropriate treatments EXCEPT:

A) Nebulized racemic epinephrine.
B) Antibiotics.

C) Nebulized L-epinephrine 5 mL of 1:1000.
D) Dexamethasone 0.6 mg/kg IM or PO.
E) Oxygen.

Discussion
The correct answer is "B." One would not want to use antibiotics in this patient. This is a viral illness, usually parainfluenza. All of the other answers are correct. Hypoxic patients should receive oxygen. Of particular note is "C." While classically we have used racemic epinephrine, the "D" isomer is inactive. Additionally, racemic epinephrine is more expensive and must be kept refrigerated if a multidose vial is used. L-epinephrine, 5 mL of 1:1000, delivered by nebulizer is as effective as racemic epinephrine, is cheaper, and is the same dose for everyone (and our favorite since we can't do simple math!).

> HELPFUL TIP: The AAP has no guidelines regarding the management of croup. Humidified air was a mainstay of treatment (have you ever spent a winter night holding a coughing child in a bathroom with the shower on full blast?). Recent literature shows little clinical effectiveness, but the studies were small and may have had a type II error (i.e., not enough patients to find a difference if one is present).

* *

You give the patient nebulized epinephrine and his stridor resolves. You now need to decide what to do with this patient.

You tell the parents that since the child had nebulized epinephrine:

A) He needs to be admitted because of the "rebound" effect seen with epinephrine in croup.
B) He needs to be observed in the ED for 6 hours to make sure his symptoms do not recur.
C) He must be observed for 2 hours in the ED to make sure his symptoms do not recur.
D) He can be discharged immediately with follow-up tomorrow.

Discussion
The correct answer is "C." The patient should be observed for 2 hours. The thinking about this has changed. Admission after nebulized epinephrine was the rule. Now, 2-hour observation is considered sufficient. There is no "rebound effect." The patient may return to his pretreatment state but will not get worse as the result of the epinephrine treatment. If stridor at rest returns during the observation period requiring additional treatments, admission is warranted.

* *

The patient is breathing a little easier after the nebulized epinephrine and has received acetaminophen for his fever. He is drinking a little and does not appear significantly dehydrated.

Which of the following *is the most appropriate* treatment for this patient?

A) Prednisone 1 mg/kg PO once.
B) Prednisone 2 mg/kg PO followed by a taper.
C) Dexamethasone 0.2 mg/kg IV once.
D) Dexamethasone 0.6 mg/kg PO once.
E) Dexamethasone 5 mg/kg IM once.

Discussion
The correct answer is "D." Steroids have been proven to be beneficial in the treatment of croup. The best of the choices is dexamethasone 0.6 mg/kg with a maximum dose of 10 mg. Dexamethasone is chosen because of its relatively long half-life that allows it to remain active during the duration of the illness (about 3 days). The least invasive route is recommended, and oral dexamethasone is appropriate in patients tolerating PO intake. The other answers are not correct for treating croup.

> HELPFUL TIP: Dexamethasone given as single 0.6 mg/kg dose is the most studied regimen, but 0.3 and 0.15 mg/kg single dosages are as effective. For some reason, the authors just cannot make the leap to 0.15 mg/kg, so we use 0.3 mg/kg. Multiple dose regimens have not been proven more effective and may increase the risk of infectious complications.

Objectives: Did you learn to . . .

- Evaluate a patient with colic and offer management strategies to the parents?
- Diagnose laryngotracheobronchitis ("croup")?
- Manage a patient with laryngotracheobronchitis?

QUICK QUIZ: EPIGLOTTITIS

You have a child in the ED who is toxic appearing with the sudden onset of high fever, drooling, and stridor. You suspect epiglottitis.

What is the FIRST step in the treatment of this patient?

A) Draw blood work including a CBC.
B) Place an IV for access and fluids.
C) Give a dose of IM steroids (e.g., dexamethasone 0.6 mg/kg) to help shrink the epiglottis.
D) Put a face mask on the child and administer albuterol via face mask.
E) Leave the child on the mothers lap and don't upset the child (you don't want a temper tantrum in the ED . . .).

Discussion

The correct answer is "E." Anything that upsets the child can lead to increased airway obstruction. Leave the child in the parent's lap and do not upset him. "A" and "B" are incorrect because they may upset the child, leading to increased work of breathing and increased obstruction. "C," dexamethasone, is indicated for croup and not for epiglottitis. "D" is also incorrect. However, it would **not** be wrong to give blowby oxygen or blowby nebulized epinephrine **if it did not agitate the child.**

QUICK QUIZ: EPIGLOTTITIS

Which of the following IS NOT needed in the optimal diagnosis and treatment of epiglottitis?

A) "Thumb sign" on radiograph.
B) Antibiotics to cover *H. influenzae.*
C) Antibiotics to cover *S. pneumoniae.*
D) An operating room.
E) Personnel able to emergently manage the airway.

Discussion

The correct answer is "A." The use of radiographs in suspected epiglottitis is fraught with problems and delays potentially life-saving therapy. **DON'T DO IT.** Epiglottitis is a clinical diagnosis that requires visualization of the epiglottis. This is preferably done in the operating room with a setup for both intubation and tracheostomy should that become necessary. If the child is mildly ill, looking at the epiglottis in the ED is permissible. However, be prepared to manage the airway. "B" and "C" are both correct. Since the advent of *H. influenzae* vaccine, there is no longer a single organism causing most cases of epiglottitis. Bacteria that can cause epiglottitis include *H. influenzae, S. pneumoniae, S. aureus,* and groups A, B, and C beta-hemolytic streptococci. Epiglottitis may also be of viral origin.

QUICK QUIZ: NEONATAL INFECTIONS

What is the most likely etiologic agent in this child: 2-week-old male with conjunctivitis, cough, rales, nasal congestion, infiltrate on radiograph, but no fever or wheezes?

A) Influenza.
B) Chlamydia.
C) RSV.
D) Parainfluenza.
E) Gonorrhea.

Discussion

The correct answer is "B." This is a classic description of Chlamydia infection in the newborn. Patients usually present between 5 and 14 days with exudative conjunctivitis and pneumonia. Nucleic acid amplification of a conjunctival scraping is the new gold standard for diagnosis. Conjunctival cells must be present for an adequate specimen because Chlamydia is an intracellular pathogen. Treatment is with systemic antibiotics **even if conjunctivitis is the only symptom present.** Erythromycin is the drug of choice. Azithromycin is an alternative. Topical treatment is not indicated for the conjunctivitis and alone is not sufficient for treatment of this patient.

CASE 13

A 12-month-old presents to your office in January (in the northern hemisphere . . . we hear this book is huge in New Zealand . . . cheers, mates!) with a 2-day history of runny nose and cough. The child now has wheezing with nasal flaring and retractions, and his oxygen saturation is 89%. There has been no fever, and several of the other children and adults in the family have had "a cold" over the past several weeks.

On exam, you hear scattered wheezes and rales. You diagnose bronchiolitis.

The MOST LIKELY organism involved in this child's illness is:

A) Rhinovirus.
B) Adenovirus.
C) Respiratory syncytial virus (RSV).
D) Parainfluenza.
E) Human metapneumovirus.

Discussion

The correct answer is "C." The **most common** cause of bronchiolitis in children is RSV. All of the others can also cause bronchiolitis, as can influenza virus, but less commonly than RSV.

Which of the following treatments has been unequivocally shown to be effective in bronchiolitis?

A) Nebulized albuterol.
B) Nebulized epinephrine.
C) Corticosteroids such as prednisone or dexamethasone.
D) All of the above.
E) None of the above.

Discussion

The correct answer is "E." None of the above has been shown to be effective in bronchiolitis. The mainstay of treatment is supportive care. Albuterol may cause worsening hypoxia due to induction of V/Q mismatch.

> **HELPFUL TIP:** Nebulized hypertonic saline (3%) has been shown to be mildly beneficial in hospitalized patients by decreasing clinical bronchiolitis score and shortening length of stay. This makes sense. The hypertonic saline will draw fluid from the bronchi and shrink tissues thereby reducing obstruction.

RSV is usually diagnosed by:

A) Nasal wash using immunofluorescence or antigen detection.
B) Baseline and convalescent antibody titers.
C) Blood culture for RSV.
D) Sputum Gram stain.
E) Induced sputum culture.

Discussion

The correct answer is "A." A nasal wash for RSV immunofluorescence or antigen detection is used to diagnose RSV. Reverse transcription-polymerase chain reaction (RT-PCR) assays may also be used. The other options are incorrect.

> **HELPFUL TIP:** Bronchiolitis is a clinical diagnosis that does not require any diagnostic testing.

> **HELPFUL TIP:** Never give ribavirin for RSV. It doesn't work.

Which of the following is indicated for the prevention of RSV in high-risk infants?

A) Vaccination against RSV.
B) Oral ribavirin.
C) Rimantadine or oseltamivir.
D) Palivizumab (Synagis®)
E) RSV–IVIG (RespiGam)

Discussion

The correct answer is "D." Palivizumab is a licensed prophylactic monoclonal antibody against RSV that is given via monthly intramuscular injection to high-risk patient populations during the RSV season. Potential qualifying infants include those with associated prematurity, significant congenital heart disease, and or chronic lung disease. RSV–IGIV, or RespiGam, is no longer used. There is no current RSV vaccine. None of the other answers are correct.

Objectives: Did you learn to . . .

- Recognize the clinical presentation of a patient with RSV bronchiolitis?
- Diagnose and treat RSV bronchiolitis?
- Describe what patients may possibly benefit from ribavirin and RSV prophylaxis?

CASE 14

A 4-week-old infant presents to your office with his parents. The parents note that he has had vomiting every time he eats. His vomitus is mostly formula and nonbilious. He seems to be hungry and is demanding to be fed often. Except for the vomiting, he seems to be well without diarrhea. Exam reveals an afebrile infant in no distress with normal cardiac and pulmonary exams and a relatively benign abdomen. There is no "olive" palpable.

Your working diagnosis is:

A) Midgut volvulus.
B) Gastroenteritis.
C) Pyloric stenosis.
D) CNS injury with increased intracranial pressure.

Discussion

The correct answer is "C." This most likely represents idiopathic hypertrophic pyloric stenosis. The classic presentation of pyloric stenosis is nonbilious vomiting immediately after feeding, followed by a demand to feed again soon after (much the same as a teenager... the demand of feeding, not the vomiting). The symptoms are progressive. Initially, the vomiting may or may not be projectile and may occur after every feed or intermittently. Classically, pyloric stenosis occurs in infants 2 weeks to 2 months of age. "A," midgut volvulus, is unlikely because these patients have bilious vomiting. Our patient has nonbilious vomiting. "B," gastroenteritis, is not likely because there is no diarrhea, fever, or appetite loss. "D" is unlikely. While CNS injury with increased intracranial pressure and vomiting is a possibility, you would expect to see other evidence of CNS injury such as lethargy, possibly signs of head injury, etc.

Which of the following patients is most likely to present with pyloric stenosis?

A) A first born male.
B) A first born female.
C) A second born male.
D) A second born female.
E) The rate of pyloric stenosis is equal in all of these groups.

Discussion

The correct answer is "A." There is a 4:1 male:female preponderance, and about 30% of all cases occur in a first born child. Thus, first born males are at a particular risk for pyloric stenosis. Also, family history is important as infants born to a mother or father who had pyloric stenosis are at increased risk. Do you think Pharaoh didn't like pyloric stenosis?

* *

You give the patient a bolus of IV normal saline and decide to confirm the diagnosis with a Gastrografin test.

What are you most likely to see on radiograph if this patient has pyloric stenosis?

A) "Bullseye" or "target" lesion.
B) Corkscrew pattern of small bowel.
C) Ulcerations of the gastric mucosa.
D) String sign.
E) Rapid filling of the bowel distal to the pylorus.

Discussion

The correct answer is "D." The string sign is formed when contrast material trickles through the elongated pyloric channel (and thus looks like a thin string on x-ray). "A," "Bullseye" or "target" lesion, is seen on ultrasound with intussusception. "B," a corkscrew pattern, is seen with midgut volvulus. Ulcerations of the gastric mucosa are seen, of course, with gastric ulcers. "E" is obviously not true. The whole problem with pyloric stenosis is that little or anything can get from the stomach to the small bowel. Ultrasound can also be used to make the diagnosis of pyloric stenosis. Ultrasound is often the first test followed by a contrast study if needed.

> **HELPFUL TIP:** Previously the diagnosis of pyloric stenosis was made based on physical exam findings of a palpable pyloric mass, "palpable olive," with occasional visible gastric peristaltic waves. Due to increased awareness, the diagnosis is frequently made before physical exam findings are apparent.

> **HELPFUL TIP:** The definitive treatment for pyloric stenosis is surgical. However, it is an urgent, but not emergent, surgical indication. Make sure to take the time to correct fluid and electrolyte abnormalities prior to surgery.

* *

You have a surgical consultant see the patient, pyloromyotomy is done, and everybody is happy.

Objectives: Did you learn to . . .

- Identify clinical manifestations of pyloric stenosis?
- Diagnose and manage pyloric stenosis?

QUICK QUIZ: PEDIATRIC BELLY PAIN

The treatment for midgut volvulus is:

A) Watchful waiting.
B) Maneuver of Leopold.
C) Emergent surgery.
D) Air enema.
E) Nasogastric suction and bowel rest.

Discussion

The correct answer is "C." Midgut volvulus is a surgical emergency. None of the others are correct. Watchful waiting is dangerous and risks ischemic bowel with perforation, so "A" and "E" are wrong. Leopold maneuvers are used to move a breech pregnancy to vertex and have nothing to do with the bowel. "D," air enema, can be used to reduce an intussusception but has no role in the treatment of midgut volvulus.

CASE 15

A 5-year-old male who was recently diagnosed with influenza presents to your ED with complaints (via the parents) of intractable vomiting and mental status changes. On exam, the child is febrile and is vomiting but has neither meningeal signs nor focal neurologic findings. His liver is palpable.

Influenza is associated with which of the following complications?

A) Pneumonia.
B) Rhabdomyolysis.
C) Myocarditis.
D) Encephalitis
E) All of the above.

Discussion

The correct answer is "E." All of the above can be a result of influenza. Pneumonia may be viral or due to bacterial superinfection.

* *

You get labs on this patient. He is noted to be hypoglycemic and to have markedly elevated liver enzymes. His bilirubin is normal. The patient's white blood cell count and differential suggest a viral illness.

The MOST LIKELY diagnosis based on this patient's history, physical, and laboratory findings is:

A) Reye syndrome.
B) Bacterial meningitis.
C) Transverse myelitis.
D) Hepatic encephalopathy secondary to hepatitis.
E) Diabetes mellitus in the "honeymoon" period with Somogyi phenomenon.

Discussion

The correct answer is "A." This patient most likely has Reye syndrome (encephalopathy with fatty liver degeneration). Reye syndrome presents with intractable vomiting, elevated transaminases with a normal bilirubin level, hypoglycemia, and mental status changes (excitability, delirium, coma). Reye syndrome generally occurs in a genetically susceptible person associated with a viral illness such as influenza or chickenpox. This patient is not likely to have meningitis given the absence of an elevated white count and lack of meningeal signs. Also, he clearly does not have transverse myelitis, an autoimmune condition producing rapidly progressive weakness and sensory disturbance. "E" is incorrect since the Somogyi phenomenon refers to stress hormone-induced morning hyperglycemia in a patient on insulin who is having unrecognized hypoglycemia at night (and which does not exist . . . see Chapter 10).

The medication MOST associated with Reye syndrome is:

A) Ibuprofen.
B) Celecoxib (Celebrex).
C) Aspirin.
D) Acetaminophen.
E) Naproxen.

Discussion

The correct answer is "C." The use of aspirin in a child with a viral illness, classically influenza or chickenpox, has been associated with the development of Reye syndrome. Of note, the incidence of Reye syndrome has been steadily declining now that parents are aware that they should avoid aspirin use in children. Reye syndrome is now a very rare disease.

HELPFUL TIP: The treatment of Reye syndrome is supportive and includes controlling hypoglycemia and treating cerebral edema. There is no specific treatment of this illness. The mortality rate remains high. Surviving patients should be screened for an underlying fatty acid oxidation defect.

* *

For some reason, you found heme positive stool in this patient. You must have been thinking that every patient deserves at least one rectal exam.

All of the following are relatively common causes of heme positive stools in children 1–5 years of age EXCEPT:

A) Colon polyps.
B) Ulcers.
C) Swallowed epistaxis.
D) Gangrenous bowel.
E) Intussusception.

Discussion

The correct answer is "D." Gangrenous bowel tends to be found in neonates and younger infants as a result of necrotizing enterocolitis, midgut volvulus, etc. All of the others are correct. See Table 13–6 for more causes of occult GI blood loss in children.

Objectives: Did you learn to . . .

- Recognize sequelae of influenza infection?
- Describe Reye syndrome?
- Manage a patient with Reye syndrome?
- Identify some causes of heme positive stools in children?

Table 13–6 CAUSES OF HEME POSITIVE STOOLS IN CHILDREN

Less than 1 year: Swallowed maternal blood (especially if the child is a vampire), anal fissure, intussusception, duodenal or gastric ulcers, gangrenous bowel, Meckel diverticulum, cow milk protein intolerance
More than 1 year: Colon polyps, ulcers, anal fissure, esophageal varices, intussusception, hemorrhoids, swallowed epistaxis, Mallory-Weiss tears, bacterial enteritis.

CASE 16

A mother comes to you with concerns about SIDS in her infant. Evidently, her sister had a child who died of SIDS, and she is concerned that her child is now at elevated risk.

You can tell her which of the following?

A) Twin concordance studies suggest SIDS is a genetic disorder.
B) Since her child is now 5 months old, there is no risk of SIDS since SIDS generally occurs before 3 months of age.
C) Siblings of an infant with SIDS have a fivefold increase in the risk of SIDS.
D) SIDS is more likely to occur in female infants.
E) Young maternal age (<20 years old) is associated with reduced risk of SIDS.

Discussion

The correct answer is "C." A sibling of child who died with SIDS has a fivefold increased risk of dying of SIDS (although the absolute risk is still less than 1%). "A" is incorrect. The cause of SIDS is unknown with interaction between genetic and environmental risk factors. Abnormal arousal may play a role. SIDS does not seem to be an isolated genetic disorder. "B" is incorrect. SIDS generally occurs between 2 and 4 months (median age 11 weeks). However, 90% of cases occur before 6 months of age, so a 5-month-old child is still at risk. "D" is incorrect as it is more common in males with a ratio of 3:2. Finally, the opposite of "E" is true: maternal age <20 years old is a risk factor as is maternal smoking and the infant's sleeping position.

All of the following have been associated with an increased incidence of SIDS EXCEPT:

A) Side-sleep positioning.
B) Prone-sleep positioning.
C) Early introduction of solid foods.
D) Premature birth.
E) Intrauterine exposure to drugs.

Discussion

The correct answer is "C." The introduction of solid foods has nothing to do with the development of SIDS. All of the other factors increase the rate of SIDS. Of note, any nonsupine sleeping position is associated with an increased incidence of SIDS.

The most important advice you can give to prevent SIDS is:

A) Avoid feeding close to bedtime to reduce aspiration risk.
B) Place the child in the prone position (stomach and face down) when sleeping.
C) Use a child alarm in the room to alert the parent(s) if something is wrong.
D) Place the child in the supine position (stomach and face up) when sleeping.
E) Use sheepskin or polystyrene bedding to prevent suffocation.

Discussion

The correct answer is "D." Having the infant sleep in a supine position ("**back** to sleep") reduces the risk of SIDS by up to 50%. "B" (prone sleeping position) and "E" (polystyrene or sheepskin bedding) **increase the risk** of SIDS. Smoking cessation is important as smoking during pregnancy or after increases the risk of SIDS. Co-sleeping should be discouraged as it increases the risk of SIDS.

HELPFUL TIP: The use of pacifiers in bed actually decreases the risk of SIDS as well. Give it to the child when he or she is put down for sleep. Do not reinsert it once the child is asleep if he/she spits it out.

HELPFUL (AND SCARY) TIP: Nothing is free (especially the board exam... how much are you paying for that sucker?). Supine sleeping has increased the rate of positional plagiocephaly (flattening of the head, in this case in the occipital region). This risk can be minimized by placing the child in a **prone** position **while awake and supervised** (commonly referred to as "tummy time").

Objectives: Did you learn to...

- Identify risks of SIDS?
- Give advice on how to reduce the risk of SIDS?

CASE 17

The parents of a 1-month-old female are in your office for a routine checkup. They are first time parents and are concerned about feeding. Evidently, one of the grandmothers is "from the old country." Back in her day in the "old country," they would start children on solid foods at 2 months of age—usually starting with strained liver (lots of vitamins and stuff plus it is disgusting and the adults wouldn't eat it...). This grandmother also cannot figure out why the couple is wasting their money on formula when cow's milk (better yet, goat's milk when available) "worked just fine for me." They would like your advice about feeding.

You let them know that:

A) Solid foods should be introduced at 3 months for all children. Two months of age is too soon. And grandma's right. Start with liver.
B) Cow's milk is considered adequate only after 6 months of age.
C) Early introduction of cow's milk has been irrefutably linked to type 1 diabetes mellitus.
D) The first foods introduced should be strained meats.
E) Children should have good head control before solid foods are introduced.

Discussion

The correct answer is "E." Doesn't "E" just sound best? We mean, even if you hadn't a clue, you would still pick "E," right? Children should have good head control before starting solid foods. "A" is incorrect for several reasons. First, solid foods are generally not recommended until 4 months of age. Second, note that the answer says "all children." Third, the answer involves liver. Liver is disgusting no matter what age... don't foist it on a trusting, unsuspecting, infant. Some children do not want solid foods until 6 months of age. "B" is incorrect. Cow's milk should be avoided for the first year of life. Breastfeeding is optimal. This failing, infant formula contains additional nutrients not found in cow's milk. Additionally, the use of cow's milk has been linked to an increase in gastrointestinal blood loss and iron deficiency anemia. "C" is incorrect. There has been some observational evidence to suggest a connection between diabetes type 1 and cow's milk, but the data are quite suspect. "D" is incorrect. Foods should be introduced one at a time, but there is no requirement as to what the first food should be. Usually, iron fortified cereals are introduced first.

HELPFUL TIP: AAP guidelines recommend 400 IU/day of vitamin D from birth through the teenage years, no exceptions. This can come either from supplements or foods. Breast milk does not contain enough vitamin D and these infants should be supplemented in the first few days of life.

* *

The parents manage to fend off this grandmother (quite an accomplishment, eh?). The child continues on formula feedings. However, the child gets somewhat fussy on occasion and has occasional bouts of diarrhea. The family wants to know what to do.

Your advice is to:

A) Change formulas because this represents an allergy to the cow's milk formula.
B) Do not change formulas.
C) Change formulas because this likely represents lactase deficiency.
D) Switch to a formula based on short chain fatty acids since this likely represents an inability to absorb and metabolize fats.

Discussion

The correct answer is "B." Children will occasionally be fussy and have occasional diarrhea. This does not indicate a formula allergy or intolerance. Reflux and spitting up are also common in infants. Again, this does not indicate a formula allergy. The parents should be reassured that as long as the child is growing and is not having significant difficulties, continuing the current formula is acceptable.

HELPFUL TIP: Remember, as noted above, reflux or spitting up does not mean formula intolerance. **Do not make multiple formula changes!** This medicalizes a normal pattern in children. The majority of spitting up and reflux will resolve by 1 year of age. If the child looks well and is growing, there is no need to change the formula.

* *

The parents decide that you are correct and continue to feed the child the cow's milk formula. Much as you predicted, the child does well on this formula. However, the child is now becoming "constipated" and the grandmother would like to give this child a laxative (preferably some concoction from the "old country" that no one else can pronounce or formulate). She (the infant, not the grandmother) is having only one bowel movement per day rather than the 3–4 per day that occurred during the first several months of life.

You let the parents know that:

A) One stool a day is likely normal for this infant.
B) An infant having less than 2–3 bowel movements per day is likely constipated since bowel transit time is only 8.5 hours or so.
C) Infants fed soy-based formula tend to have softer stools than those fed cow's milk formula.
D) Breastfed infants may normally have up to 10 stools per day.
E) A and D.

Discussion

The correct answer is "E." The number of bowel movements in a normal infant can vary widely from 10 per day in a breastfed infant to 1 per day or every other day in a formula-fed infant. What is more important is whether the child has to strain to pass stool, how hard the stool is, etc. The number of stools per day is less important.

* *

On further questioning, it becomes clear that the grandmother may be correct. This child is having a hard time passing stool and passes only small amounts of hard stool with great effort (red-purple face, lots of crying, etc.). The parents would like some advice.

All of the following are reasonable suggestions EXCEPT:

A) Change to a formula with a preponderance of whey protein such as Carnation Good Start.
B) Treat with corn syrup.
C) Add fruit juices if the child is older than 2 months.
D) Treat with lactulose.
E) Use a glycerin suppository for occasional constipation.

Discussion

The correct answer is "C." Fruit juices should not be used under the age of 4 months. Beyond that age, sorbitol-containing juices such as pear, prune, or apple may be used to treat constipation. Of particular note is "B." There was concern a number of years ago that corn syrup caused infant botulism. This has since been shown to be unfounded. All of the remaining answers are viable options.

* *

The child does well after the parents implement your plan, but she continues to have some reflux symptoms. This is getting worrisome to the parents although the child is growing well.

Which of the following IS recommended as standard therapy in treating this child's reflux?

A) Prone positioning of the child when sleeping.
B) Trial of hypoallergenic diet.
C) Use of a proton pump inhibitor.
D) Elevating the head.
E) Thickening the formula with rice cereal.

Discussion

The correct answer is "E." Thickening the formula may be helpful. Placing the child in prone position while sleeping increases the risk of SIDS. Neither a hypoallergenic diet, an H2 blocker, a proton pump inhibitor, nor elevating the head has been shown to reduce reflux. In fact, elevating the head may increase reflux.

HELPFUL TIP: In infants with gastroesophageal reflux **disease** (not just physiologic reflux), a trial of milk and soy protein free diet for 1–2 weeks is reasonable. H2 blockers and PPIs have also been used but with very limited success. Prokinetic agents such as metoclopramide and erythromycin help improve gastric emptying, but studies have failed to show much efficacy for GERD. In 2009, the FDA issued a black box warning linking chronic metoclopramide use with tardive dyskinesia.

Objectives: Did you learn to...

- Give appropriate advice for nutrition and feeding during infancy?
- Diagnose and manage constipation in infancy?
- Treat an infant with significant gastroesophageal reflux?

CASE 18

A 23-year-old G2P1 female at 31 weeks of gestation presents to the ED and delivers precipitously. Her pregnancy was uncomplicated. The neonate is a 1.25-kg male. The helicopter is on its way to transport this premature infant to your regional pediatric hospital.

In the meantime, the BEST treatment for this newborn is:

A) Antibiotics.
B) Corticosteroids.
C) High-pressure 100% oxygen.
D) Routine care (warmth, stimulation, etc.) and nothing else.
E) Surfactant.

Discussion

The correct answer is "E." Without any further information, you must assume that this patient is at significant risk for neonatal respiratory distress syndrome (RDS). The appropriate treatment is surfactant. The dose of surfactant depends on the preparation, and the timing of administration varies by source (some authors favor immediate administration "prophylaxis," while others recommend "early rescue" treatment—usually within 2 hours of delivery). Surfactant therapy has good evidence for decreasing morbidity and mortality and should be used in all premature infants who are at risk for RDS (see next question) or acutely symptomatic. On the basis of synergistic interactions, experts recommend combination therapy with **antenatal** corticosteroids for the mother (if possible... see Chapter 15) and surfactant for the premature infant. "A" is incorrect as it is not the most important initial therapy although empiric antibiotic therapy is often indicated in premature infants due to difficulty in distinguishing between RDS and sepsis. "B" is incorrect because **postpartum steroids for the infant are associated adverse neurodevelopmental outcomes.** As for "C," excessive oxygen can be toxic to premature infants and currently initial resuscitation should begin with blended oxygen or room air. "D" might be the second best option if surfactant were unavailable.

HELPFUL TIP: Surfactant has been shown to decrease air leaks and mortality from RDS but does not decrease the incidence of chronic lung disease or bronchopulmonary dysplasia.

All of the following are risk factors for neonatal RDS EXCEPT:

A) Cesarean section.
B) Gestational diabetes.
C) Male sex of infant.
D) Prolonged rupture of membranes.

Discussion

The correct answer is "D." Prolonged rupture of membranes is associated with a **decreased** risk of neonatal RDS. All of the others are associated with an increased risk. Of course, increasing prematurity is associated with increasing risk of RDS as is multifetal pregnancy, especially in the second fetus delivered in a twin pregnancy.

> HELPFUL TIP: The lecithin/sphingomyelin (L/S) ratio is the traditional method for assessing fetal lung maturity. If the L/S ratio is >2, the risk of RDS is low. Other options include phosphatidylglycerol level and direct surfactant measures. It is important to realize that these tests have fairly low-positive predictive values.

> HELPFUL TIP: As premature infants grow into adults, keep an eye on their blood pressures and glucose levels. Infants who were born prematurely and at very low birth weight (<1.5 kg) have more problems with hypertension and glucose intolerance as adults.

* *

Because of your congenial bedside manner and amazing command of medical knowledge, this family returns to see you many times over the ensuing years. After reflecting on how awesome you are, you turn your attention to the newest addition to the family, a 4-day-old male infant you delivered—this time in the labor and delivery unit. He is the product of a full-term, uncomplicated pregnancy. He is breastfed and was doing well until this morning. Unfortunately, his mother noticed today that he is breathing harder, eating poorly, and looking more yellow. You note a respiratory rate of 72 and crackles on lung exam, so you order a chest x-ray.

Which of the following diagnoses is most likely?

A) Neonatal RDS.
B) Persistent pulmonary hypertension.
C) Pneumonia.
D) Pneumothorax.
E) Transient tachypnea of the newborn.

Discussion

The correct answer is "C." Pneumonia is more likely than the other options because of the timing of the symptoms. Neonatal pneumonia may be early (within the first week of life) or late onset. The pathogenic organisms involved are different for early and late disease. Patients presenting with early onset pneumonia are more likely to have acquired the infection in utero or during delivery; GBS is the most common pathogen in these cases. Patients presenting with late pneumonia may have acquired the disease during delivery, during hospitalization, or while in the community; GBS, *E. coli*, *S. aureus*, *Listeria*, HSV, and Chlamydia may all cause pneumonia in these patients. "A" is incorrect since RDS should not occur in a full-term infant nor present this late. "B" is incorrect because persistent pulmonary hypertension should present shortly after birth with hypoxemia and cyanosis. "D," pneumothorax, is a common result of the trauma of birth, and up to 2% of infants may sustain a pneumothorax during delivery. However, very few infants with a pneumothorax are symptomatic, and you would expect the symptoms to occur shortly after delivery. "E" is incorrect because transient tachypnea of the newborn occurs with 1–2 hours of birth and resolves on its own.

* *

You found your thermometer, and it turns out that your patient is febrile. The chest x-ray shows a left lower lobe infiltrate.

Which of the following antibiotics is LEAST appropriate in this setting?

A) Ampicillin.
B) Ceftriaxone.
C) Gentamicin.
D) Vancomycin.

Discussion

The correct answer is "B." Ceftriaxone is contraindicated in neonates. Ceftriaxone displaces bilirubin from albumin-binding sites resulting in more severe hyperbilirubinemia and risk of bilirubin encephalopathy (this infant is jaundiced) and may cause fatal precipitates in the lung and kidney when coadministered with calcium (perhaps not an immediate concern for this patient). Cefotaxime may be used, but this is not a choice. It would be prudent to provide empiric antibiotic coverage for all likely bacterial pathogens. The combination of ampicillin and gentamicin is preferred for coverage of GBS, gram-negative enteric bacteria, and *Listeria*. Due to the potential for MRSA to cause pneumonia in the neonatal period, vancomycin is reasonable but should not be used alone.

> HELPFUL TIP: Remember the possibility of sustained paroxysmal supraventricular tachycardia with CHF in the patient who is tachypneic, has rales, and is feeding poorly. Not all rales in infants are from an infectious cause.

Objectives: Did you learn to . . .

- Provide appropriate treatment to an infant at risk for neonatal RDS?
- Identify risk factors for neonatal RDS?
- Describe causes of respiratory distress in the neonatal period?

CASE 19

A 20-day-old former term male infant is brought to the clinic for evaluation of fever. He was born via uncomplicated vaginal delivery. Mom was GBS negative. In clinic, the infant has a temperature of 38°C but is otherwise vigorous with normal vital signs.

What should be done next?

A) Discharge home with follow-up the next day.
B) Treat with empiric antibiotics. Cultures are not necessary for this age group.
C) Obtain a chest x ray.
D) Admit to the hospital.
E) Treat with ibuprofen.

Discussion

The correct answer is "D." Fever in a neonate (younger than 28 days) or young infant (age 29–90 days) is defined as a temperature ≥38°C or 100.4°F (rectal). Up to 15% of febrile neonates and young infants will have a serious bacterial infection such as bacteremia, urinary tract infection, meningitis, pneumonia, osteomyelitis, septic arthritis, omphalitis, mastitis, or scalp abscess. UTI is the most common. The infant may appear well with fever being the only manifestation of a serious infection. Risk stratification is based on age, comorbidities, laboratory studies, and the presence of viral infection such as bronchiolitis. Protocols including Boston, Philadelphia, Pittsburgh, and Rochester help to classify the infant as low risk for serious bacterial infection based on clinical appearance and laboratory investigation. If an infant qualifies as low risk, hospitalization, empiric antibiotics, and lumbar puncture may not be indicated. Two of the three protocols only apply to infants older than 29 days. There is no clear consensus on the best approach to evaluating and managing febrile infants younger than 90 days. Currently, all febrile neonates, ill appearing infants, or those not meeting low-risk criteria should be admitted for a full evaluation and empiric antibiotic therapy. "B" is incorrect as cultures should be obtained prior to antibiotic therapy. You may obtain a chest x-ray as part of your evaluation, but the best answer is admission. Ibuprofen is not approved for use in infants younger than 6 months.

* *

The patient is admitted. Blood work including a complete blood count and blood culture is obtained. Urinalysis and urine culture are obtained via sterile catheterization. A lumbar puncture is performed after obtaining consent (of course) and cerebrospinal fluid is sent for culture and analysis.

While waiting for your laboratory testing results what empiric antibiotics will you start?

A) Ampicillin.
B) Cefotaxime.
C) Metronidazole.
D) B and C.
E) A and B.

Discussion

The correct answer is "E." The choice of empiric antibiotics is based on most likely infecting bacterial organisms in a patient of this age. Bacterial infections in neonates likely were acquired during delivery. The most common organisms are GBS, *E. coli*, and *Listeria monocytogenes*. Empiric treatment should be with ampicillin and cefotaxime or ampicillin and gentamicin. Ampicillin provides coverage for *Listeria* and enterococci. If gram-positive cocci are seen on CSF Gram stain, vancomycin should be used instead of ampicillin. Empiric acyclovir treatment should be considered if signs and symptoms of HSV infection are present.

* *

While examining the patient, you notice he is not moving his right arm. When you ask the mom she believes that is new but is unsure when he stopped using it. Examination reveals tenderness over the right proximal humerus with overlying redness, swelling, and pain with moving the shoulder joint, a symmetric Moro reflex, and intact grasp reflex.

What is the likely cause?

A) Erb palsy.
B) Klumpke palsy.
C) Humerus fracture.
D) Osteomyelitis.
E) Cerebral vascular incident.

Discussion

The correct answer is "D." Fever, pseudoparalysis (reluctance to move affected limb) and swelling with erythema of the affected area is concerning for osteomyelitis with associated septic arthritis. Osteomyelitis, an infection of the bone, usually results from hematogenous seeding. Infants have blood vessels that cross the growth plate allowing for bone infections to spread to the adjacent joint resulting in septic arthritis. *S. aureus* is the most common cause of osteomyelitis in all pediatric age groups. *H. influenzae* is less common since immunizations were begun; however, until culture results are available, it should be covered empirically in children aged 6 months to 4 years who have not yet completed their immunization series. GBS and gram-negative rods such as *E. coli* are seen in neonates and should be covered empirically. "A" and "B" are types of brachial plexus injuries from birth trauma that result in paralysis and an asymmetric Moro reflex due to peripheral nerve injury. "C," a humerus fracture, though rare can occur as a result of birth trauma but is unlikely based on delayed presentation. "E" is incorrect as most neonatal strokes present with seizures and or altered mental status.

HELPFUL TIP: Neonates with osteomyelitis commonly are afebrile and present with nonspecific symptoms such as irritability, decreased movement of a limb (pseudoparalysis), or pain with moving the affected extremity (think diaper changes). Often the diagnosis is delayed and misdiagnosed at first as a traumatic injury.

HELPFUL TIP: Neonatal osteomyelitis often involves multiple bones.

* *

You discuss your concerns with the mother.

She asks you how do you diagnose a bone infection? Your response is:

A) Clinically.
B) With cultures.
C) With x-ray.
D) With MRI.
E) All of the above.

Discussion

The correct answer is "E." Osteomyelitis is a clinical diagnosis requiring you to think about it in your differential. Cultures and imaging confirm the diagnosis. There is no specific laboratory test. Frequently, a leukocytosis with left shift and reactive thrombocytosis is present. Inflammatory markers including C-reactive protein and erythrocyte sedimentation rate are usually elevated and can be followed to document response to therapy. Cultures of the blood, joint fluid, and/or bone are positive in 50–80%. Plain x-rays can rule out other causes such as a fracture but are often not useful in early osteomyelitis as it can take up to 10 days to see changes such as a lytic lesion. MRI is the best imaging study allowing for abscess detection and differentiation between bone and soft-tissue infection. MRI often requires sedation and is expensive. A radionuclide bone scan is helpful for poorly localized pain and or concerns about multiple bone involvement. Ultrasound can be helpful in septic arthritis.

* *

You consult your pediatric orthopedic colleagues who take the infant to the operating room to wash out the joint and obtain cultures. An x-ray shows a lytic lesion in the proximal humerus.

Cultures of the joint and bone grow GBS. What is the length of antibiotic treatment?

A) 7 days.
B) 10 days.
C) 4 weeks.
D) 3 months.
E) 1 year.

Discussion

The correct answer is "C." Acute osteomyelitis is treated with antibiotics for a minimum of 3 weeks with most courses lasting 4–6 weeks. The majority of patients may be treated initially with intravenous antibiotics followed by transition to oral antibiotics after clinical improvement and lack of contraindication to oral therapy. In neonates, the entire course is frequently completed intravenously due to lack of clinical trials. Even with appropriate treatment, neonatal osteomyelitis may result in permanent deformities to the bone or joint with resulting decreased range of motion, asymmetric limb length, and abnormal gait; therefore, long-term follow-up is mandatory.

* *

The mom asks you about future pregnancies and if there is anything she should do differently especially regarding her GBS status. She tested negative with above pregnancy. You discuss indications for GBS prophylaxis during labor.

All are indications for maternal intrapartum antibiotic prophylaxis EXCEPT:

A) GBS positive at 35–37 weeks' gestation.
B) Unknown GBS status with no risk factors.
C) GBS bacteriuria during current pregnancy.
D) History of a previous infant with invasive GBS infection.
E) Unknown GBS status with rupture of membranes $\geq$18 hours.

Discussion

The correct answer is "B." Per the 2010 CDC guidelines, intrapartum antibiotic prophylaxis is indicated for females in labor if they have (1) GBS positive culture at 35–37 weeks' gestation, (2) GBS bacteriuria anytime during current pregnancy, (3) a history of previous infant with GBS disease, and (4) an unknown GBS status with one or more risk factors. The risk factors include (1) less than 37 weeks' gestation, (2) rupture of membranes for $\geq$18 hours, (3) temperature during labor $\geq$100.4°F or 38°C. As this mom now has had an infant with invasive GBS disease, she requires prophylactic antibiotics during labor with all future pregnancies regardless of her culture results.

> HELPFUL TIP: Antibiotic prophylaxis during labor decreases the incidence of early onset GBS disease (within the first 7 days of life) but does not affect late onset GBS disease (7 days to 3 months of age).

Objectives: Did you learn to . . .

- Initiate a diagnostic investigation and management strategy for a febrile infant younger than 90 days?
- Diagnose and manage osteomyelitis?
- Describe indications for maternal intrapartum antibiotic prophylaxis for GBS?

QUICK QUIZ: FEBRILE SEIZURE

You are evaluating a 10-month-old fully immunized child after a simple febrile seizure. The child is previously healthy and has not taken antibiotics recently. Physical exam is unremarkable with no meningeal signs and a normal neurologic exam.

What diagnostic testing should be performed?

A) Lumbar puncture.
B) EEG.
C) Neuroimaging such as head CT or MRI.
D) Serum electrolytes.
E) None of the above.

Discussion

The correct answer is "E." Per the 2011 AAP guidelines, evaluation of a simple febrile seizure should focus on identifying the cause of the fever. Meningitis should always be considered and a lumbar puncture should be performed if meningeal signs or symptoms are present. Lumbar puncture is an **option** in infants 6–12 months of age who are not fully immunized or immunization status is unknown and in patients pretreated with antibiotics as meningitis signs may be masked. Routine evaluation with EEG, neuroimaging, serum electrolytes, or complete blood cell count should not be done if the only reason is to identify the cause of the febrile seizure. Previous recommendation was to perform a lumbar puncture on all infants younger than 12 months who presented with a simple febrile seizure. This recommendation was made before the widespread immunization against *H. influenzae* type b (Hib) and *S. pneumoniae*.

BIBLIOGRAPHY

Berg MD, et al. Part 13: Pediatric basic life support. *Circulation*. 2010;122(18, Suppl 3):S862-S875.

Brown ML, et al. Treatment of primary nocturnal enuresis in children: A review. *Child Care Health Dev*. 2011; 37(2):153-160.

Cohen-Silver J, Ratnapalan S. Management of infantile colic: A review. *Clin Pediatr (Phila)*. 2009;48(1): 14-17.

Committee on Infectious Diseases, American Academy of Pediatrics. *Red Book: 2009 Report of the Committee of Infectious Diseases*. 28th ed. Elk Grove, IL: American Academy of Pediatrics; 2009.

Fu LY, Moon RY. Apparent Life-threatening Events (ALTEs) and the Role of home monitors. *Pediatr Rev*. 2007;28(6):203-208.

Gerber JS, Offit PA. Vaccines and Autism: A tale of shifting hypotheses. *Clin Infect Dis*. 2009;48(4):456-461.

Kattwinkel J, et al. Part 15: Neonatal resuscitation. *Circulation*. 2010;122(18, Suppl 3):S909-S919.

Kliegman RM, et al. *Nelson Textbook of Pediatrics*. 19th ed. Philadelphia, PA: Elsevier Saunders; 2011.

Lauer BJ, Spector ND. Hyperbilirubinemia in the Newborn. *Pediatr Rev*. 2011;32(8):341-349.

Moon RY, Fu LY. Sudden infant death syndrome. *Pediatr Rev*. 2007;28(6):209-214.

NCIRD. Recs/Schedules/Child Schedule main page. Available at: http://www.cdc.gov/vaccines/recs/schedules/child-schedule.htm#hcp. Accessed August 12, 2011.

NCIRD. Recs/Vac-Admin/Contraindications to Vaccines Chart. Available at: http://www.cdc.gov/vaccines/recs/vac-admin/contraindications-vacc.htm. Accessed August 12, 2011.

Rappaport D, et al. Should blood cultures be obtained in all infants 3 to 36 months presenting with significant fever? *Hosp Pediatr*. 1(1):46-50.

Russell KF, et al. Glucocorticoids for croup. *Cochrane Database Syst Rev*. 2011;(1):CD001955.

Zaoutis L, Chiang V. *Comprehensive Pediatric Hospital Medicine*. Philadelphia, PA: Mosby, Inc. 2007.

14

Adolescent Medicine

Jason Powers and Jason K. Wilbur

CASE 1

A 14-year-old male presents to your clinic with his mother for a routine well-child examination. The patient's mother has some questions about puberty. Her son enjoys playing sports, and she is concerned that he may be too small to play football. The past medical history is unremarkable.

Which of the following can you tell the mother will likely be the first sign of puberty in this boy?

A) Increase in penile length.
B) Enlargement of the testes.
C) Deepening of the voice.
D) Rapid increase in linear growth.
E) Coarsening of pubic hair.

Discussion
The correct answer is "B." Increase in the volume of the testes is the first sign of pubertal development in boys, with average age of onset of 12 years (range 10–14). "E" is of special note. While pubic hair appears shortly after the onset of puberty, it is initially long and straight and not in a mature distribution. Coarsening of the pubic hair is a more advanced pubertal stage, occurring approximately 1.5 years after the onset of puberty; an increase in penile length occurs simultaneously. The maximal growth spurt occurs on average at age 14, or approximately 2 years after onset of puberty. Changing of the voice is a secondary hormonal effect that is quite variable in nature.

* *

From the mother, you learn that the patient's father began going through puberty during high school, and he did not reach his adult height until he was in college at about age 20. The patient's father is 5′10″ tall (~178 cm). The mother is 5′3″ tall (~160 cm). Physical examination reveals that your patient is Tanner stage I for genitalia and pubic hair. His height and weight continue to track along their previously established curves on the growth chart, both at approximately the fifth percentile. The remainder of the examination is unremarkable.

What is your next step in evaluation of this patient's short stature?

A) Obtain hand radiographs to assess bone age.
B) Draw blood to test for growth hormone and testosterone levels.
C) Obtain an endocrinology consult.
D) Order computed tomography (CT) imaging of the brain to rule out hypothalamic tumors.
E) Order magnetic resonance imaging (MRI) of the brain to rule out hypothalamic tumors.

Discussion
The correct answer is "A." In the face of a normal physical examination and appropriate linear growth velocity, the likelihood of an intracranial process is very low. An assessment of bone age can be obtained easily, and relatively inexpensively, and would be useful prior to performing other tests.

* *

You decide to obtain a bone age, and the radiologist reports bone age as 12 years, 3 months (remember that out-patient is 14 years old).

What is the most likely diagnosis for your patient?

A) Growth hormone deficiency.
B) Sella turcica tumor.
C) Constitutional delay.
D) Idiopathic testicular atrophy.
E) Testosterone receptor abnormality.

Discussion

The correct answer is "C." The bone age of 12 years, 3 months is reassuring. His bones are immature and still have the ability to grow; there is no fusion of the growth plates. Had the bone age been 14, it is likely that his adult height would be short: the bones would no longer have the inherent ability to grow. Bone age assessment is an accurate tool for determination of expected growth. Constitutional delay is the most common diagnosis for short stature, and it is often associated with a delayed onset of puberty. Constitutional delay is a diagnosis of exclusion; a complete history and physical often rules out other diagnoses. Family history often reveals a parent who was a "late bloomer" but eventually had normal pubertal development. This adolescent's history of normal linear growth velocity (albeit along the fifth percentile) is reassuring for the absence of growth hormone deficiency or intracranial abnormalities. The combination of appropriate linear growth velocity, appropriate adjustment for bone age, and paternal history of late pubertal development is classic for constitutional delay.

* *

When your patient's height is plotted on a growth curve and adjusted for bone age rather than chronological age, the height now plots just below the 50th percentile. Your patient now has a question of his own. His biggest concern is that some of his classmates are starting to get taller, and he is afraid he will be too short to continue competing in sports. The mother is 5′3″ tall and the father is 5′10″ tall.

Based on what you know today, what is your best estimate of this patient's adult height?

A) 5′3″ ± 2″ (160 ± 5 cm).
B) 5′5″ ± 2″ (165 ± 5 cm).
C) 5′7″ ± 2″ (170 ± 5 cm).
D) 5′9″ ± 2″ (175 ± 5 cm).
E) 5′11″ ± 2″ (180 ± 5 cm).

Discussion

The correct answer is "D." You can provide a rough estimate of the patient's adult height using the calculation for mid-parental height (MPH). Remember that the parent of the opposite gender—the mother in this case—must have the height adjusted for this calculation. For boys, add 5 inches to the mother's height (12.5 cm); then average this corrected maternal height and the paternal height to determine the MPH. For girls, subtract 5 inches from the paternal height; then average this corrected paternal height and the maternal height to calculate the MPH. In our patient's case, his mother's corrected height is 68 inches, averaged with his father's height of 70 inches to get an MPH of 69 inches. A margin of error of ± 2 inches (5 cm) is often given with MPH estimates.

Objectives: Did you learn to . . .

- Evaluate a patient with growth concerns?
- Identify the clinical presentation of constitutional delay?
- Calculate MPH?

CASE 2

Your next patient is a 16-year-old female cross-country runner who you are seeing in follow-up for right shin pain. She was diagnosed in the local emergency department 1 week ago with "shin splints" and told to limit her activities. In your office, she tells you that the pain has been worsening over the last 3 months, and she has progressively decreased the distance and time of her runs (but, of course, she's a runner, so she hasn't quit). She denies fever, swollen joints, or other systemic symptoms. She normally has regular menses but notes that she has irregular menses during cross-country season. The patient's past medical history is significant for a stress fracture in her left foot 18 months ago. Your exam reveals tenderness at the middle one-third of the right tibia. Also, she has pain on a single-leg hop. You are able to review her x-rays from the emergency department, which do not reveal any fractures or other abnormalities.

What is the most appropriate next step to diagnose your patient's leg pain?

A) Ultrasound of the lower extremity.
B) MRI of the lower extremity.
C) Dual-energy x-ray absorptiometry (DEXA) scan.
D) Thyroid-stimulating hormone (TSH) level
E) Urine pregnancy test.

Discussion

The correct answer is "B." MRI is sensitive and specific for stress fractures and has become the preferred study. The patient's history and examination are concerning for the presence of a tibial stress fracture. Stress fractures often present insidiously and cause gradual progression in symptoms over time until a critical point is reached in terms of sports participation. Half of stress fractures are not visible on plain radiographs. Ultrasound can help in evaluating soft tissue masses, but it does not play a role in evaluating stress fractures. DEXA scan can provide whole-body and site-specific measurement of bone mineral density, which may be related to the pathophysiology of stress fractures, but does not help diagnose a site of injury. Radionuclide bone scans are often less expensive than CT or MRI, and they demonstrate sites of injury based on increased uptake of the radionuclide material. However, bone scans are not specific for stress fractures and are often falsely positive. Given the patient's other complaints, TSH and urine pregnancy test may be warranted but will not assist in the diagnosis of her leg pain.

* *

An MRI is obtained and confirms the presence of a stress fracture in the middle one-third of the right tibia. Because of your patient's history, especially that of multiple stress fractures, you are concerned she may be suffering from the female athlete triad.

What are the components of the female athlete triad?

A) Disordered eating, menstrual dysfunction, altered bone mineral density.
B) Depression, weight loss, sports-related injury.
C) Poor sports performance, low self-esteem, injury.
D) Weight gain, bony injury, mood changes.
E) Fanatical attachment to sports, testosterone abuse, anger management issues.

Discussion

The correct answer is "A." The female athlete triad was first identified in the early 1990s and originally characterized as anorexia, amenorrhea, and osteoporosis. As more has been learned about the triad, the realization has been made that the triad likely represents a broader spectrum disorder within each category. Many young women with the triad will exhibit disordered eating behaviors, such as caloric restriction or use of diuretics and diet pills, but would not meet the criteria for anorexia or bulimia nervosa. Menstrual dysfunction may include oligomenorrhea or irregular, intermittent menses, as well as amenorrhea. These young women may also have abnormal bone mineral density, with predisposition to bony injury, without having reached the strict criteria of osteoporosis.

* *

The patient comes back to the office to receive her test results, and you take the opportunity to obtain more history. The patient admits that she is very concerned about her diet during her cross-country season, and she is very careful to choose foods that have very little fat but are often high in protein. She will occasionally "go overboard" and eat a lot, for which she compensates by taking part in extra workouts. She has also used laxatives in the past "to not gain weight when I eat too much."

Which of the following findings is NOT classically found in bulimia nervosa?

A) Loss of dental enamel.
B) Enlarged parotid glands.
C) Metabolic acidosis.
D) Skin changes over the dorsum of the hands.
E) Weight less than 85% of expected.

Discussion

The correct answer is "E." Loss of dental enamel, skin changes over the dorsum of the hands, and enlarged parotid glands may be seen as a result of repetitive self-induced vomiting. While self-induced vomiting would cause a metabolic alkalosis through loss of stomach acid, repetitive use of laxatives can cause gastrointestinal losses of bicarbonate, resulting in a metabolic acidosis. **Individuals with bulimia nervosa often maintain a normal weight,** while anorexia nervosa has strict diagnostic criteria requiring maintenance of body weight at less than 85% of ideal body weight.

* *

Your patient also relates that she began having her periods around age 12. While they were initially irregular, they seemed to become more regular prior to starting high school. However, as she became more involved in high school sports, her periods became more irregular. During her off-season, her menses are "more regular," though she cannot predict when they will occur. She recalls that her last period was about 7 weeks ago.

In evaluating your patient's menstrual dysfunction, what would be your next course of action?

A) Obtain serum LH, follicle-stimulating hormone (FSH), and estradiol levels.
B) Order an abdominal and pelvic ultrasound.
C) Perform a speculum-assisted pelvic exam with Papanicolaou smear.
D) Confirm urine beta-hCG levels.
E) Prescribe a oral progestin-only pill (progestin challenge).

Discussion
The correct answer is "D." The most common cause of secondary amenorrhea in women of childbearing age remains pregnancy. If pregnancy has been excluded, and the history and physical are reassuring, a progestin challenge can be helpful to determine if adequate estrogen is present; the progestin challenge should induce menses if adequate estrogen exists. Imaging studies and hormonal levels may help in excluding other diagnoses or if warranted by exam. "Pap and pelvic" exams are recommended for sexually active women over age 21, but may not be necessary in the initial evaluation of menstrual dysfunction in this setting.

* *

Your patient's pregnancy test is negative, and a progestin challenge induced menses. A comprehensive plan is developed that includes psychological counseling, dietary modification, physical therapy, consultation with a nutritionist, and frequent follow-up. Over the next several months, the patient recovers from her injury, and returns to running on a modified schedule. However, she now complains of heavy, painful menses and wants to go on the "shot" to stop them.

In your counseling about birth control options, which of the statements below is FALSE?

A) The birth control pill can be used to treat irregular menses of the female athlete triad and will also increase bone deposition.
B) The effect of Depo-Provera (medroxyprogesterone) is to suppress the hypothalamic–pituitary–ovarian axis, creating a low estrogen state akin to peri-menopause.
C) The FDA issued a "Black Box" warning on Depo-Provera that states "prolonged use ... may result in loss of bone density that may not be completely reversible after discontinuation of the drug."
D) The risk of future fracture using Depo-Provera is unknown, as bone density is an incomplete measure of bone strength, and remodeling and recovery are significant.

Discussion
The correct answer is "A." The other statements are all true. Starting a combined estrogen/progesterone contraceptive pill will restart a menstrual cycle but may not increase bone density. Insulin-like growth factor-1 (IGF-1) **can** increase bone density, and **endogenous** IGF-1 levels increase when caloric intake increases (see Grinspoon, et al. J Clin Endocrinol Metab 2002;87(6):2883-2891).

* *

In your routine anticipatory guidance, you discover that she avoids most dairy products due to a combination of prior concerns about fat content and lactose intolerance.

What do you recommend for her daily intake of calcium?

A) 900 mg.
B) 1100 mg.
C) 1300 mg.
D) 1700 mg.
E) 2100 mg.

Discussion
The correct answer is "C." While the absolute best intake of calcium for individuals is unknown, studies have shown positive calcium balance for adolescents with an intake of 1200–1500 mg daily. In its 2010 report, the Institute of Medicine (IOM) set 1300 mg/day as the "adequate" dietary intake for boys and girls 9–18 years of age. This guideline was set to meet the needs of 95% of healthy children, with the upper limit of calcium intake set at 2500 mg/day.

For most persons, 1300 mg/day of calcium intake can be accomplished with four servings of dairy products (8 oz of milk = 8 oz of yogurt or cottage cheese = 1 inch cube of cheese) plus a varied diet that includes other calcium-rich foods (e.g., broccoli, collard greens, and turnip greens). Despite widespread non- and low-fat dairy options and numerous supplements, concern over fat intake has resulted in an average adolescent intake of only 700–800 mg/day for girls and about 1000 mg/day for boys—and yet, we have an obesity epidemic. Ironic but not funny.

On average, what percentage of total body mineral content has a young woman deposited by the time she reaches 12 years of age?

A) 20–30%.
B) 40–50%.
C) 70–75%.
D) 80–85%.
E) 95–100%.

Discussion
The correct answer is "D." Research suggests that by age 12, a young woman has reached approximately 83% of her peak bone mineral content, with 50% deposition happening from the time of "peak height velocity," which is premenarchal, through 1 year postmenarche. The ability to absorb calcium from the diet is also enhanced during this period. Rates of deposition begin to decline approximately 2 years postmenarche, and no significant gains are seen after the age of 17. These statistics emphasize that osteoporosis, while manifesting in older adults, is truly an issue of adolescent preventive medicine.

* *

Your patient returns from a high-powered sports medicine clinic in Palm Springs (... or Laguna Beach... or anywhere more likely to make MTV than Iowa). She brings you her DEXA results consistent with osteopenia. She looks at you over her designer shades and asks, "So, what are we gonna do about that, Doc?"

You scour the literature and recommend:

A) Alendronate.
B) Calcium and vitamin D.
C) Vigorous weight-bearing exercise.
D) Dehydroepiandrosterone (DHEA).
E) All of the above.

Discussion
The correct answer is "B." Alendronate has no proven benefit in adolescent osteopenic females. Recommending exercise is the usual course for older patients with osteopenia, but you need to be careful in the adolescent with weight concerns who may exercise excessively at baseline. DHEA is investigational and has not been shown to increase bone mineral density. Stick with the standard of care: calcium in the daily doses recommended above and **vitamin D 600 IU daily** (note that this recommendation is a change in the 2010 IOM guideline).

Objectives: Did you learn to...

- Evaluate leg pain in a runner?
- Identify the "female athlete triad?"
- Recognize the importance of calcium and vitamin D intake and osteoporosis prevention in adolescence?

QUICK QUIZ: ADOLESCENT ATHLETES

For adolescent athletes, what is the number one cause of sudden cardiac death (SCD)?

A) Marfan syndrome.
B) Coronary artery disease.
C) Congenital malformation of coronary arteries.
D) Hypertrophic cardiomyopathy.
E) Long QT syndrome.

Discussion
The correct answer is "D." Hypertrophic cardiomyopathy is an autosomal-dominant trait with highly variable penetrance that results in asymmetric septal wall hypertrophy. This may cause functional aortic outflow tract obstruction as well as predispose the athlete to arrhythmias. Unfortunately, this condition is often asymptomatic prior to the terminal event and screening tests such as electrocardiographs and echocardiograms have not been proven effective at early detection of this condition. Aberrant coronary arteries are the second leading cause of SCD in young athletes. Marfan syndrome and long QT syndrome are less common.

CASE 3

As part of your group's community outreach, you are participating in a sports participation physical screening. (Somehow your partner got to throw out the first pitch at a baseball game, and you got this... we're guessing you must be new.) One of the students is noted to be hypertensive with a blood pressure of 143/95. There is no family history of sudden death or early heart attack. He has never experienced any symptoms with exercise. His parents indicated on the form that they did not recall any history of previous heart murmur or high blood pressure. The athlete passes through the remaining stations, and a I/VI systolic murmur is heard. The examiner asks the athlete to perform a Valsalva maneuver by holding his breath and bearing down while auscultation is repeated.

Which of the following correctly describes the relationship between murmur intensity and the likely type of murmur?

A) Valsalva maneuver increases flow murmur, decreases outflow tract obstruction murmur.
B) Valsalva maneuver increases both flow murmur and outflow tract obstruction murmur.
C) Valsalva maneuver decreases both flow murmur and outflow tract obstruction murmur.
D) Valsalva maneuver decreases flow murmur, increases outflow tract obstruction murmur.

Discussion

The correct answer is "D." The Valsalva maneuver decreases venous return to the heart, resulting in decreased diastolic filling. You would expect this to cause decreased flow through the outflow tract and thus a softer flow murmur. However, the decreased flow exacerbates the **functional** outflow tract obstruction of hypertrophic cardiomyopathy (there is less volume to push the septum out of the way resulting in a tighter functional stenosis), resulting in a louder murmur. In summary, **benign flow murmurs will decrease in intensity with Valsalva maneuver, while the murmur of hypertrophic cardiomyopathy will increase with a Valsalva maneuver.**

HELPFUL TIP: The systolic crescendo–decrescendo murmur of hypertrophic cardiomyopathy increases in intensity when the patient moves from a supine to an upright position. S4 may be heard as well.

* *

Reassured by a murmur that disappears with Valsalva maneuver and an otherwise unremarkable exam, you are now faced with an adolescent athlete with an elevated blood pressure confirmed by manual retesting.

What is the best recommendation for this athlete regarding sports participation and follow-up of his elevated blood pressure?

A) Qualified participation pending serial blood pressure checks over the next 3 weeks.
B) Complete disqualification for 2 months, followed by return if ECG and echocardiogram are normal.
C) Disqualification from competition only for 1 month, but allowed to practice once seen by a nephrologist.
D) Full participation with no required follow-up based on reassuring history and examination.
E) Full participation with blood pressure recheck prior to the next competitive sport season.

Discussion

The correct answer is "A." It is important to remember that the diagnosis of hypertension cannot be made at a single screening visit. The screening test may be affected by patient anxiety ("white coat hypertension" or standing half naked in front of all of his peers), recent caffeine ingestion, drugs, or a number of other factors (including a common occurrence of scheduling PPEs for right after practice). Most recommendations include three separate recordings of blood pressure on different occasions after several minutes at rest, sitting comfortably.

Because exercise is beneficial for blood pressure control, continued aerobic activity is encouraged while the serial blood pressure readings are obtained. Debate exists as to recommendations regarding static exercises, such as weightlifting. While lifting of heavy weights can exacerbate high blood pressure, there is some evidence to suggest that use of light-to-moderate weights with repetition is beneficial. Certainly, the presence of any additional symptoms with exercise, such as headache or lightheadedness, would require more significant limitations in activity.

Objectives: Did you learn to . . .

- Identify important issues to address at the preparticipation physical exam?
- Evaluate an adolescent athlete with elevated blood pressure?
- Evaluate a cardiac murmur revealed on preparticipation physical exam?

CASE 4

A 15-year-old female presents to your office for a well-adolescent examination. She is a healthy teenager with no complaints. You have incorporated into your routine a screening tool, the Guideline for Adolescent Preventive Services (GAPS), one of many such tools available. The questions cover all areas of adolescent development and are designed so that areas of concern are easily identified.

What are the three leading causes of mortality for adolescents?

A) Leukemia, suicide, accidental drowning.
B) Childhood cancers, perinatally acquired HIV, suicide.
C) Congenital malformations, childhood cancers, suicide.
D) Accidental injury, homicide, suicide.
E) Childhood cancers, SCD, suicide.

Discussion
The correct answer is "D." Accidental injury, homicide, and suicide are the three leading causes of death for adolescents and should be addressed during preventive health visits. Accidental injuries often involve the use of alcohol or other substances in combination with motor vehicle operation or other risk-taking behaviors. Ask not only about personal use of alcohol, but also if they are ever passengers of another teenager (or adult) who drives while impaired or intoxicated.

* *

You also noticed that your patient checked "yes" for a history of use of alcohol and marijuana.

What is the approximate frequency of lifetime use of these substances among 9th–12th grade students according to the Centers for Disease Control and Prevention (CDC's) 2005 Youth Risk Behavioral Survey?

A) Alcohol 30–40%; marijuana <5%.
B) Alcohol 40–50%; marijuana 5–10%.
C) Alcohol 50–60%; marijuana 10–20%.
D) Alcohol 60–70%; marijuana 20–30%.
E) Alcohol 70–80%; marijuana 30–40%.

Discussion
The correct answer is "E." The survey found 74.3% of adolescents reporting use of alcohol at some point in their lives, and 38.4 % reporting use of marijuana; and incidentally, 54.3% have tried cigarettes.

HELPFUL TIP: Screening tools for adolescent substance use include the "CRAFFT" questions, developed by the "Center for Adolescent Substance Abuse Research" (CeASAR), Children's Hospital Boston. Similar to the "CAGE" tool for adult alcohol assessment, the letters stand for:

Cars (Have you ever gotten into a CAR under the influence, or with a driver who is?)

Relax (Do you use a substance to help you RELAX?)

Alone (Do you use a substance ALONE?)

Forget (Have you ever had spells of FORGETfulness/blackouts when using?)

Friends (Are your FRIENDS concerned about your use?)

Trouble (Have you gotten into TROUBLE from your use?)

* *

After eliciting a positive response to questions about drug use, you ask the patient about depression, and she states that she has been feeling "down" for several months now.

What would your next step be?

A) Call the police and report the illegal use of substances by a minor.
B) Reassure the patient about her confidentiality rights, counsel her to quit using drugs, and see her back annually.
C) Begin the patient on an SSRI and see her back in a month.

D) Negotiate next steps to guarantee the patient's safety and consider counseling referral.
E) Obtain a nonconsented urine drug screen to document recent use.

Discussion

The correct answer is "D." Most states and HIPAA guarantee teenagers confidentiality, to be broken only when there is an issue of personal danger to self or others or physical/sexual abuse. It is recommended that the patient be involved and consent to who and how the information is shared. Rarely is there a need to involve police, unless there is an issue of abuse requiring a report or concern over safety if the patient is returned to the home environment.

Answer "C" is incorrect. If an SSRI is started, close supervision is required for adolescents. Studies suggest increased suicidality in teenagers treated with SSRIs. There are also increased attempts at suicide but not an increase in successful suicide. The American Academy of Child and Adolescent Psychiatry website has resources outlining patient and parent information about the risks and benefits of pharmacologic treatments. Cognitive behavioral therapy (CBT), along with talk therapy, has been shown to be the best first-line treatment for adolescents with mood disorders. In any case, close follow-up of a depressed adolescent (weekly visits or phone calls) is recommended.

> HELPFUL TIP: SSRIs are not that effective for pediatric/adolescent depression. The NNT to benefit one patient is 10. Fluoxetine has the most favorable benefit/risk profile **in adolescents** and is recommended as first-line therapy by most published guidelines.

> HELPFUL TIP: The American Academy of Pediatrics has a position statement against the use of nonconsented urine drug screens as a "screening" tool due to the lack of accuracy and the violation of patient trust.

Objectives: Did you learn to . . .

- Identify and employ useful screening tools for routine adolescent exams?
- Recognize the importance of depression in adolescents?
- Describe causes of death in adolescents?
- Understand the common lifetime experience use of alcohol, tobacco, and marijuana?
- Describe screening and treatment options for mood disorders and substance abuse?

CASE 5

Your afternoon has a number of patients with sports-related complaints. A 14-year-old wrestler has arrived in the office complaining of a rash on his left shoulder. The rash appears to consist of several small lesions with a vesicular appearance but no purulence and minimal erythema. There is neither tenderness to palpation nor tactile warmth in the affected area.

What would be your best test to confirm your diagnosis of these lesions?

A) Microscopic evaluation with potassium hydroxide (KOH) preparation of the contents of one of the lesions.
B) Gram stain of the contents of one of the lesions.
C) Culture of the contents of one of the lesions.
D) Tzanck smear of the contents of one of the lesions.

Discussion

The correct answer is "D." A Tzanck prep will give you immediate information about whether this represents herpes simplex. This is important information when deciding whether or not this patient can return to wrestling.

* *

The lesions have appeared within the past day, and your laboratory testing confirms that the diagnosis is herpes simplex. Your patient does not recall any previous lesions like these. He denies any systemic symptoms.

What would be the best course of treatment for this patient?

A) Cover the involved area to allow return to wrestling.
B) Treat with topical acyclovir and return to wrestling when lesions have crusted over.
C) Treat with oral acyclovir and return to wrestling when lesions have crusted over.
D) Treat with oral steroids to suppress the response and promote quicker return to wrestling.
E) Treat with topical antifungal medication and allow return to wrestling.

Discussion

The correct answer is "C." Cutaneous herpes, also referred to in wrestling as *herpes gladiatorum*, is a highly contagious illness. Answer "B" is incorrect because topical acyclovir is **not** effective in treating herpes simplex. Most state high school athletic associations have specific rules regarding the treatment of cutaneous disorders in wrestling, including herpes, tinea corporis, and impetigo. With regard to herpes simplex, all lesions must be fully crusted over **and** the athlete must have had at least 3 days of oral antiviral therapy prior to returning to competition. "D" is incorrect because oral steroids would suppress the athlete's immune response, which would allow for further spread of the lesions.

* *

Your next patient is a 15-year-old male who is here for a sports physical. You review your patient's chart and scan his immunizations. The patient's mother remembers her son receiving his "kindergarten shots"; he has had no immunizations since. His records reveal the following vaccines: 5 doses of diphtheria–tetanus–acellular pertussis (DtaP), 2 doses of oral polio vaccine (OPV), 2 doses of injectable polio vaccine (IPV), 4 doses of *Haemophilus Influenzae* Type B (HiB), 2 doses of measles–mumps–rubella (MMR), and a clinical history of chicken pox.

Which, if any, immunizations would you offer today?

A) None; the patient is up-to-date for all immunizations.
B) Conjugate pneumococcal vaccine.
C) Hepatitis A/B vaccine; conjugate meningococcal vaccine; OPV.
D) Hepatitis A/B vaccine; tetanus, diphtheria and pertussis (Tdap) vaccine; conjugate meningococcal vaccine.
E) Human papillomavirus (HPV) vaccine; Tdap; varicella vaccine.

Discussion

The correct answer is "D." Universal vaccination for hepatitis B is now the standard recommendation, and the vaccine is included in the primary immunization series for infants. Since adolescence is a time when experimentation with drugs and sexual activity becomes more prevalent, vaccination for hepatitis B becomes even more relevant. Hepatitis A vaccine is now being required in many states before entry to school and is universally recommended for all children ages 12 months–2 years. A catch-up vaccination schedule is now recommended for ages 2–18 years. For those not vaccinated against hepatitis B, a combined hepatitis A/B vaccine exists.

Most children receive their last DTaP prior to entering preschool or kindergarten (age 4–5 years). Beginning in 2005, the CDC recommended giving the tetanus booster **with pertussis** at entry to middle school/junior high (ages 11–12). A Tdap "catch-up" vaccination is recommended for those who missed the pre-junior high school booster, and the Tdap can be given within 2 years of the last Td vaccine for those who want pertussis protection (and has been safely administered within 18 months of Td). For protection against some serotypes of *Neisseria meningitidis*, the CDC recommends universal vaccination with the conjugate vaccine (e.g., Menactra) for teens. "E" is incorrect because he has already had chicken pox.

HELPFUL TIP: In December 2011, the Advisory Committee for Immunization Practices (ACIP) recommended that the HPV vaccine be given to adolescent males as well as females. The ACIP based this recommendation on the vaccine's known efficacy in preventing HPV-associated cancers (anal, cervical, penile, and oropharyngeal) and anal and genital warts. But as of this writing, the recommendation has not been approved by the CDC (although ACIP recommendations almost always are approved by the CDC).

Which statement does NOT accurately describe how the conjugate meningitis vaccine (Menactra) differs from the older polysaccharide meningitis vaccine (Menomune)?

A) Menactra elicits a T-cell immune response that gives long-term immunity and allows for herd immunity.
B) Menactra protects against all the types of *N. meningitidis*: A, B, C, Y, W-135.
C) Menomune does not elicit a booster effect, may only be given once, and is recommended only at the onset of high-risk activity, such as living in dorms or being a military recruit.

D) Menactra should be offered at entry to middle school/junior high (11–12), as the highest incidence of mortality for *N. meningitidis* is for individuals 15–25, and may be given again at entry to college.

Discussion

The correct answer is "B." Unfortunately neither the Menomune nor Menactra protects against serogroup Type B. *N. meningitidis* Type B is endemic in North America; so statistically, the CDC expects to prevent about 75% of *N. meningitidis* cases with the Menactra vaccine.

Objectives: Did you learn to . . .

- Identify herpes gladiatorum and describe its treatment?
- Prescribe vaccines appropriately for adolescents?

CASE 6

A 15-year-old female returns for her annual well-child check and sports physical. She is well known to your clinic, and over the years she has steadily gained weight. Her parents and a younger sibling are overweight, and now she has become obese by measure of the pediatric BMI percentages. In recent years, you have become more diligent with watching the BMI on her growth curve. She is aware of her weight problem, yet has not voiced any plan for attempting weight loss.

What defines "obesity" in adolescents?

A) A BMI in the 85th–94th percentile for age-specific measures.
B) A BMI ≥95th percentile for age-specific measures.
C) The child has the appearance of being heavy.
D) The child complains of being fat or overweight.
E) The parents have concerns that the child is too heavy.

Discussion

The correct answer is "B." A BMI in the range of 85–94% is considered "overweight," and a BMI at or above 99% is considered "severe obesity." The use of BMI allows for an objective measure, and although not perfect, can give a picture on the growth curve to patients and parents where they stand relative to age-related norms. A subjective concern about weight is important, and does warrant more evaluation.

Her BMI is now at the 97th percentile, having jumped from the 86th percentile last year. What additional workup is needed?

A) Fasting glucose level.
B) Fasting lipids.
C) Renal function testing with BUN and creatinine.
D) Liver function testing with AST and ALT.
E) All of the above.

Discussion

The correct answer is "E." Once a child reaches a BMI of 85–94%, a lipid panel is recommended to evaluate for hyperlipidemia. Screening should be done for early onset type 2 diabetes. When the BMI reaches the 95th percentile, renal function and blood pressure should be monitored, and liver function should be checked (looking for signs of fatty liver). Fatty liver disease is possible at an early age and is reversible if weight loss can be achieved. Close attention to family history is essential, too. If family members are obese or have obesity-related comorbidities, then early intervention and workup is more crucial. For females who have started menses, it is important to assess for any changes in menstrual patterns.

Which of the following is NOT a recommended early childhood intervention to prevent and/or treat obesity?

A) Encouraging breast-feeding.
B) Decreasing screen time on TV or computer.
C) Planning fewer family meals.
D) Restricting calories from sweets and fast foods.
E) Improving efforts for exercise and outdoor activity.

Discussion

The correct answer is "C." Helping with food preparation, and sitting down as a family for meals, can lead to consumption of more nutritious and lower calorie dense foods. Breast-feeding can lead to protection against obesity even into the teenage years. Formal recommendations suggest limiting TV, computer use, and video games to less than 2 hours per day. Fast food, sweets, and desserts need to be limited to small servings or few servings per week. Finally, 60 minutes of exercise should be encouraged every day—doing a variety of activities will keep children more engaged and interested.

HELPFUL TIP: If children do become overweight or obese, directed weight loss should be implemented. For kids with a BMI at 85–94%, the goal is weight maintenance until they reach a BMI 84% or less. Weight loss at a rate of one pound per week is recommended for kids who have BMI at 95–99%. And for those who are at or above a BMI of 99%, the recommended weight loss is two pounds per week.

* *

During the exam of the patient, you notice more acne than the past, some coarse facial hair, and dark skin pigmentation around the base of her neck.

What is another finding you may expect to see with further questions and tests?

A) Normal menses.
B) Low free testosterone level.
C) Low dehydroepiandrosterone sulfate (DHEA-S).
D) Hypoglycemia.
E) Abnormal hypothalamic–pituitary axis hormones.

Discussion

The correct answer is "E." She is showing signs of possible polycystic ovarian syndrome (PCOS). This can be associated with elevated prolactin, low TSH, and a marked elevation of FSH relative to lutenizing hormone. PCOS can be associated with early menarche, dysmenorrhea, and amenorrhea. A pregnancy test should be done in any case of unexplained amenorrhea. PCOS is also associated with **elevations** of testosterone, DHEA-S, and androstenedione. If there are other significant physical exam findings such as elevated blood pressure, purple striae, and a "buffalo hump," consider screening for Cushing syndrome.

* *

Her obesity is discussed openly during the office visit. As expected, she is ashamed and embarrassed about her weight gain. She admits to not knowing what to do and she asks if anything can be done to quickly lose weight.

Which of these medications have shown promise as a first-line therapy?

A) Topiramate (Topamax).
B) Bupropion (Wellbutrin).
C) Orlistat (Xenical).
D) Sibutramine (Meridia).
E) None of the above.

Discussion

The correct answer is "E." No medication is approved for children or adolescents as a first-line therapy. Antidepressants are not helpful if used primarily for weight loss. If there is comorbid depression, which is more common in obese children, a "weight loss" or "weight neutral" antidepressant may be appropriate. Antiepileptic medications have not proven helpful. Sibutramine was pulled off the market in 2010 due to troubling cardiac side effects, but was not approved for use in children anyway. Orlistat is approved for children age 12 and older. Yet, the benefits are limited to an additional 2–3 kg of weight loss. Side effects are often intolerable and include loose, oily stools and stool urgency (just mention the phrase "fecal incontinence" to a teenager and see how far you get). Experts agree that orlistat is only appropriate for adolescents with comorbidities caused by obesity.

HELPFUL TIP: The risk of becoming overweight can decrease by 4% for each month of breast-feeding up to age 9 months.

HELPFUL TIP: Recent data suggests that weight loss in adolescence will lead to decreased cardiovascular disease as an adult (N Engl J Med 2011;365:1876-1885).

(ONE MORE) HELPFUL TIP: Adolescent self-harm (cutting, burning, etc.) occurs in about 10% of adolescents. However, you can reassure parents that this declines to 3% as a young adult (The Lancet, Early Online Publication, 17 November 2011 doi:10.1016/S0140-6736(11)61141-0).

HELPFUL TIP: Recent data links childhood metabolic syndrome to lower IQ scores and impaired cognition. Whether metabolic syndrome is causal and whether this is reversible is not yet known (Pediatrics 2012;130:1-9).

Objectives: Did you learn to . . .

- Define "overweight" and "obesity" in an adolescent?
- Identify risk factors associated with obesity in an adolescent?
- Manage an adolescent with a weight problem?

CASE 7

You have watched your patient transform over the years from a rather normal-appearing boy into a very large, muscular, and intense young man. He is now 17 years old, and he has gained almost 45 pounds in the last year alone as he prepares for his senior year of football and attempts to attract the attention of college recruiters. Without a doubt he has worked very hard on the field and in the weight room, but you also must raise the question of whether or not he has used some kind of supplement to help him change so drastically.

Which of these substances is NOT prohibited by high school athletic associations or the NCAA?

A) Erythropoietin.
B) Creatine.
C) Androstenedione.
D) Ephedrine.
E) DHEA.

Discussion

The correct answer is "B." Creatine is allowed for use as a dietary supplement for athletes. However, the American College of Sports Medicine does not recommend the use of creatine in any athlete less than 18 years old. An estimated 8% of children 14–18 years old take creatine routinely. All the other listed supplements are prohibited for use as performance-enhancing supplements. Other prohibited substances include anabolic steroids, pseudoephedrine, and blood transfusions.

* *

Your patient does admit to using regular protein shakes and taking creatine. He denies the use of any illegal or prohibited substances and says he would never do anything dangerous. During his exam, his blood pressure is 146/92 and his lab results show normal electrolytes, normal TSH, normal urinalysis, BUN 22, and creatinine 1.6 (marked elevation for age 17).

What is a possible side effect from the use of creatine?

A) Gastrointestinal discomfort.
B) Edema.
C) Muscle cramps.
D) Acute renal insufficiency.
E) All of the above.

Discussion

The correct answer is "E." All are potential adverse effects from creatine use. Most importantly, if used carelessly, creatine can lead to acute renal insufficiency. Creatine is excreted via the kidneys, and if overconsumed in the setting of dehydrating exercise, it can cause renal injury. Seventy-five percent of adolescent athletes who take creatine are either unaware of the proper dose or knowingly take too much. If used, plenty of water is required to help avoid troubling side effects.

All of the following substances can provide potential athletic performance benefits, except:

A) Human growth hormone (HGH).
B) Caffeine.
C) Creatine.
D) Electrolyte replacements.
E) Sodium bicarbonate.

Discussion

The correct answer is "A." HGH has no proven benefits for enhancing sports performance. Other substances with no proven benefits include amino acids, beta-hydroxy-beta-methylbutyrate, androstenedione, DHEA, chromium, and iron (when not iron deficient). The other substances can provide short-term or long-term benefits. Caffeine has only a transient effect to help sharpen focus and intensity for brief periods of activity. Creatine can improve strength for those sports that require very short bursts of intense effort. Electrolyte replacement drinks (or tablets) and sodium bicarbonate can help for more prolonged endurance activities where dehydration and resulting electrolyte imbalances are common.

* *

Your patient denies using "steroids," but does know of older guys in the gym where he trains who have routinely used anabolic steroids.

Besides the obvious added muscle girth, what are some other potential benefits of anabolic steroids for athletes?

A) Improved lipid profile.
B) Taller stature.
C) Anxiety relief.
D) Lower blood pressure.
E) None of the above.

Discussion

The correct answer is "E." There are no other clear benefits if used for athletics only. Potential negative effects include lower HDL, elevated blood pressure, left ventricular hypertrophy, gynecomastia, aggressive or even suicidal behavior, azoospermia, virilization of females, premature physeal closure in adolescents that could lead to shorter stature, and acute myocardial infarction. Approximately 33% of anabolic steroid users are not even athletes and use the substance to help improve physical appearance. Recent estimates in high school athletes show steroid use to be 4–11% in males and 3% in females. The temptation to use the illegal substance is driven by pressures to be better than peers, to fulfill one's "full potential," to live up to sports idols, and to help acquire college scholarships and/or sports contracts at a young age.

Objectives: Did you learn to . . .

- Describe the effects of some common performance-enhancing drugs?

CASE 8

A 14-year-old female comes into the office with a chief complaint of headache. She says the headache began after her soccer game yesterday. She recalls striking her head against an opponent when trying to head the soccer ball. During the remainder of the game, she began to feel a headache, and the harder she ran, the more "woozy" she felt. She denied any loss of consciousness, vomiting, visual symptoms, or neck pain. Today, she also has poor concentration and feels excessive fatigue.

Which of the following is NOT a feature of an acute concussion?

A) Caused by an impulsive force transmitted to the brain.
B) Symptoms usually resolve spontaneously.
C) There is a functional disturbance to the body.
D) Neuroimaging shows abnormalities.
E) Clinical symptoms are highly variable and inconsistent.

Discussion

The correct answer is "D." There is no evident structural brain injury with an acute concussion. Evidence is now showing that multiple concussions, or even less severe, minor traumas to the brain can eventually lead to structural tissue damage. Concussions have a rapid onset of symptoms, and can vary from short-lived impairment to prolonged postconcussive symptoms. Symptoms show a graded functional disturbance and can affect persons in very different ways. Studies are showing that younger athletes tend to have more severe symptoms and recover more slowly than older, college-aged athletes. This is likely due to the more dynamic brain growth in younger children and adolescents.

HELPFUL TIP: Concussion is defined as a disturbance in brain function caused by trauma to the head. It does not require loss of consciousness or amnesia. Lightheadedness and nausea, etc., after a head injury are signs of concussion.

Which of the following treatments is key for your concussion patient?

A) Early return to aerobic exercise—today if possible.
B) Ibuprofen 800 mg every 8 hours as needed.
C) Avoiding excessive sleep.
D) Aspirin 325 mg daily as needed.
E) Full cognitive rest, even missing school if needed.

Discussion

The correct answer is "E." The initial and key step in caring for the concussion patient is full physical **and** cognitive rest. Very often, a return to the classroom can aggravate or prolong concussive symptoms. Once symptoms are clearly improving at rest, the student-athlete can get back to class. Sleep can provide a means of allowing the brain to rest and heal. No medications have proven helpful in alleviating the effects of a concussion. NSAIDs, aspirin, or acetaminophen may help with headache or pain.

In which case of head injury would neuroimaging be appropriate?

A) Ongoing mild headache for several days.
B) Poor memory of the recent game and the events of the injury.
C) Any new seizure activity.
D) Loss of consciousness for less than 30 seconds.
E) Mild irritability, depressed mood, and insomnia.

Discussion

The correct answer is "C." Seizure activity after head trauma or concussion requires imaging. Other symptoms that should prompt a head CT include severe headache, focal neurological symptoms, repeated emesis, difficulty arousing, slurred speech, prolonged poor orientation, concurrent neck pain, significant irritability, loss of consciousness for over 30 seconds, and any new neurologic or escalating symptoms. The initial study is normally a head CT, but if presenting after 48 hours from injury, a brain MRI is more suitable. Remember that the vast majority of concussion cases will **not** require imaging.

Which of the following elements of past medical history may be relevant for this adolescent patient following her concussion?

A) Depression.
B) Generalized anxiety disorder.
C) Attention-deficit hyperactivity disorder (ADHD).
D) Migraine headaches.
E) All of the above.

Discussion

The correct answer is "E." All of these conditions could be negatively affected by a concussion. Concussions can cause a temporary mood disorder and certainly aggravate depression and anxiety. Commonly, concussions will cause decreased concentration and inattentiveness. Teens who already have ADHD will likely have worsened symptoms and may need modification of their treatment. The headache of post concussive syndrome may overlap or intensify an underlying headache diagnosis. Concussion may act as a trigger causing an increase in pre-existing migraines.

* *

Your patient is an accomplished soccer player and feels a lot of pressure to return to action. She wants to play in the next game, and her coach and teammates are asking if she'll be back to practice this afternoon—which explains why your waiting room is so full of teenage girls wearing shin guards.

What is your best advice about her return to practice and play?

A) Go back to practice today, but take it slow and avoid full speed play.
B) Try to participate in simple drills and just cheer on your teammates.
C) Go home and rest. No school or practice today.
D) Be ready to play soon because your team needs you.
E) Whatever it takes to get the soccer team out of the office.

Discussion

The correct answer is "C." Her return to participation needs to be a graded return to activity. Each step of the recovery may be 24 hours. With each stage, if the athlete has continued symptoms, she is not ready to advance to full recovery. If she advances her activity to the next level and has recurrence of symptoms, then she needs to go back to the prior recovery step.

The first stage of recovery is no activity—complete physical and cognitive rest. The next step is return to full academic activities. Step three is light aerobic activity, followed by step four, sport-specific drills. Next, the player can return to noncontact practice. If still symptom free, then she can return to full speed, contact practice. Finally, she can return to game action. If exertion causes any return of symptoms, then she is not ready. Even with normal neuropsychiatric tests, symptomatic athletes should not play. The steps should be followed with the assistance of a healthcare provider or a qualified athletic trainer. The athlete cannot be put in the position of making the decision about how fast to return to regular play. After a first concussion, the player needs to be watched for other episodes. Two or more concussions have been shown to lower grade point averages; and three or more concussions may cause prolonged symptoms over 3 months in duration.

HELPFUL TIP: If a concussion occurs, please do not allow return to play the same day. The risk for second-impact syndrome is much greater if a player returns to play too early after a concussion. This is most likely to occur when a player does not report symptoms (more common in male athletes) after sustaining a concussion, and then has another head trauma. The rare second-impact syndrome can lead to cerebral vascular congestion, cerebral edema, and even death. The greatest risk athletes are those under age 20.

HELPFUL TIP: "Cognitive rest" after a concussion may need to include no reading, no computer games, no Internet, no smart phone use, no homework or school attendance, and avoidance of driving. Here's the simple idea: the brain is hurt, so don't overuse it too early. Prevention of concussions is best accomplished by education of athletes and coaches, and by early recognition of more minor symptoms. Mouth guards do not have any proven benefit in preventing concussion, and helmets do not lessen the incidence of concussions; they just prevent more severe traumatic brain injuries.

Objectives: Did you learn to . . .

- Define concussion and recognize its importance in adolescent athletes?
- Treat a patient with concussion?

BIBLIOGRAPHY

Barlow et al., for the Expert Committee. The Expert Committee on the Assessment, Prevention, and Treatment of Child and Adolescent Overweight and Obesity. *Pediatrics*. 2007;120(S4):5164-5192.

Halsted ME, et al. Clinical Report: Sport-related concussion in children and adolescents. *Pediatrics*. 2010; 126(3):597-615.

Jenkinson DM, Harbert AJ. Supplements and sports. *Am Fam Physician*. 2008;78(9):1039-1046.

Kliegman RM, et al., eds. *Nelson Textbook of Pediatrics*. 17th ed. Philadelphia, PA: W.B. Saunders Co.; 2007.

McDowall JA. Supplement use by young athletes. *J Sports Sci Med*. 2007;6:337.

Rao G. Childhood obesity: Highlights from the AMA expert committee recommendations. *Am Fam Physician*. 2008;78(1):56-63.

Samuels RC, Cohen LE. Understanding growth patterns in short stature. *Contemp Pediatr*. 2001;18:94-122.

Scorza KA, et al. Current concepts in concussion: Evaluation and management. *Am Fam Physician*. 2012; 85(2):123.

Stephens MB. Preventive health counseling for adolescents. *Am Fam Physician*. 2006;74(7):1151-1156.

Tanner JM, et al. Standards for children's heights at ages 2 to 9 years allowing for height of parents. *Arch Dis Child*. 1970;45:755.

Thein-Nissenbaum JM, Carr KE. Female athlete triad syndrome in the high school athlete. *Phys Ther Sport*. 2011;12(3):108-116.

15

Obstetrics and Women's Health

Sandra Rosenfeld-O'Tool and Mark A. Graber

CASE 1

A 24-year-old nulligravida female presents for her annual exam. Her gynecologic history is remarkable for irregular menses, menstruating every 4–8 weeks. She would like a more reliable form of contraception (currently using condoms) and would like to have predictable menses, but is very concerned regarding weight gain with various contraception methods.

How would you counsel her regarding weight changes and contraception?

A) Studies show there is no significant difference in weight gain of women initiating oral contraceptive pills (OCPs) versus placebo.
B) Weight gain of 10 pounds is expected during the first year of use with any type of OCPs.
C) Weight gain of 10 pounds is expected during the first year of use with monophasic pills, but not with triphasic formulations.
D) Weight loss of 10 pounds is expected during the first year of use with Depo-Provera (medroxyprogesterone acetate).

Discussion

The correct answer is "A." Studies have shown no significant weight gain with OCP use when compared with placebo. Trials have been conducted evaluating estrogen components of 20–50 μg, both monophasic and triphasic. **There is no evidence to support the premise that triphasic formulations offer improvement in weight changes.** Depo-Provera has variable effects on weight gain. Several studies have shown a weight gain of 3–6 kg in the first year of use; however, other studies have shown no difference in weight gain between Depo-Provera and placebo.

After reassuring her regarding the concerns of weight gain, you tell her about the additional potential benefit(s) of OCPs, which include:

A) Improvement in acne.
B) Decreased dysmenorrhea.
C) Decreased menstrual flow.
D) Decreased risk of ovarian cancer.
E) All of the above.

Discussion

The correct answer is "E." Besides these, additional benefits of OCP use include regulation and predictability of menses, decreased anemia, decreased hirsutism, and decreased risk of endometrial and colon cancers. (*Note*: the cancer risk reduction is based on epidemiologic studies, not randomized controlled trials.)

HELPFUL TIP: In general, patients should be followed up within a few months for blood pressure checks, etc., after starting OCPs.

* *

After further discussion, she reports that she has headaches every 1–2 months. She has never been evaluated for migraines, but reports that her headaches are bilateral, posterior, throbbing, and relieved with sleep and over-the-counter medication. She denies associated aura, nausea, or focal neurologic changes.

How would you counsel her regarding OCPs and headaches?

A) Headaches are an uncommon reason for discontinuation of OCPs.
B) She should not use OCPs, because they are contraindicated in anyone with headaches.
C) She should use progestin-only pills.
D) She should use OCPs, as it is hard to predict whether her headaches will be affected.

Discussion
The correct answer is "D." Although headache is a frequently cited reason for women to discontinue OCPs, there is not a strong correlation between headache frequency and intensity for most women. There is no evidence that the type of progestin or amount of estrogen will alter the headaches, except in women with menstrual migraines. Among women with migraines, headaches improve, worsen, or are unchanged after initiation of OCPs (helpful, no?). **There is an increased risk of stroke in women with a history of pseudotumor cerebri or migraines with aura or focal neurologic changes; therefore, OCPs are CONTRAINDICATED in this group of women. There is also an increased risk of thromboembolic events with drospirenone containing OCPs (Yaz, etc.).**

> HELPFUL TIP: Additional contraindications to OCP use include any previous thromboembolic event or stroke, a history of estrogen-dependent tumor (e.g., some breast cancers), active liver disease, pregnancy (although accidental use of OCPs early in pregnancy has not been definitively linked to adverse outcomes), undiagnosed abnormal uterine bleeding, women older than 35 years who smoke (due to increased risk of cardiovascular disease), and **first 3 weeks postpartum** (2011 CDC recommendation based on increased venothromboembolism risk in the immediate postpartum period).

* *

The patient wants to know how long she should use a backup method of contraception after starting the pill.

You tell her to use a backup method for:

A) 1 week.
B) 1 month.
C) 2 months.
D) The OCP provides effective contraception immediately.

Discussion
The correct answer is "B." OCPs must be taken for 1 month before they become effective. As to "D," tell her this and you will likely be making child support payments for 18 years.

> HELPFUL TIP: Rifampin is the only antibiotic that reduces the effectiveness of OCPs. There is no need for a backup method when giving a course of amoxicillin, for example.

> HELPFUL TIP: Women on OCPs are recommended to have Pap smears every 2 years. (American College of Obstetricians and Gynecologists [ACOG], 2009).

* *

Eight months later, the patient calls to speak with your nurse regarding nausea and vomiting. Apparently, she decided to stop taking her OCP. Her last menstrual period was 10 weeks earlier, and she had a positive home pregnancy test 5 weeks ago. Over the last week, she has been vomiting once every day, at various times, but is nauseated throughout most of the day. She wants to know if there is anything else that is "safe" that she can do to decrease the nausea.

What is your most appropriate response?

A) "This level of nausea and vomiting is abnormal and needs an immediate workup to rule out other pathology."
B) "This level of nausea and vomiting is very common, and there are several modifications and over-the-counter medications that are safe."
C) "This level of nausea and vomiting is very common; however, there are no medications that can be initiated in the first trimester."

D) "This level of nausea and vomiting is very common. Metoclopramide, promethazine, and ondansetron are our first-line therapies."
E) "Deal with it. Office hour are only 8–5."

Discussion

The correct answer is "B." Mild-to-moderate nausea and vomiting are very common in the first trimester of pregnancy, often improving by 16 weeks of gestation. Several modifications can improve symptoms, including small, frequent meals, avoiding fatty foods, and avoiding environmental triggers (perfumes, smoking, position changes, or certain movements). Over-the-counter remedies include ginger ale, vitamin B6 (10–25 mg three to four times daily), and doxylamine (10–12.5 mg three to four times daily). Vitamin B6 and doxylamine may be used together. For those who do not respond, antiemetics including metoclopramide or promethazine should be considered (thus, "D" represents a next step, not a first step). Up to 2% of the time, nausea and vomiting represent hyperemesis gravidarum, which involves weight loss of more than 5% of prepregnancy weight or dehydration and ketonuria.

If the patient had instead presented with 6–8 episodes of emesis daily, an 8-pound weight loss since her last menses, and a urine specific gravity of >1.030 and ketonuria, your workup should have included:

A) Quantitative beta-human chorionic gonadotropin (beta-hCG).
B) Serum electrolytes, BUN, and creatinine.
C) Thyroid-stimulating hormone (TSH).
D) Pelvic ultrasound.
E) All of the above.

Discussion

The correct answer is "E." As with any other severely nauseated and vomiting patient, it is reasonable to check for electrolyte imbalances. Severity of nausea and vomiting correlates with higher levels of hCG, as would be seen with a molar or twin pregnancy. Gestational trophoblastic disease, although rare, should be evaluated for with an hCG level. The ultrasound would confirm a twin pregnancy and could provide evidence of a molar pregnancy. TSH can exclude hyperthyroidism.

* *

Fortunately, your patient's symptoms improved with dietary changes, vitamin B6, and doxylamine. She presents for her initial prenatal visit at 12 weeks gestation.

You offer her the routine prenatal tests at this visit, which include all of the following EXCEPT:

A) Syphilis testing.
B) HIV testing.
C) 1-hour postcarbohydrate load serum glucose level.
D) Blood type and antibody screen.
E) Fetal nuchal translucency with maternal hCG and plasma-associated pregnancy protein A (PAPP-A).

Discussion

The correct answer is "C." Diabetes screening (50-g carbohydrate load with blood glucose obtained at 1 hour) is typically not completed until 24–28 weeks gestation. Patients with a history of gestational diabetes or those who are suspected to have diabetes may be candidates for earlier screening. Syphilis and HIV testing is completed to decrease the risk of perinatal transmission. The blood type and antibody screen is used to identify mothers with blood antibodies that could cause hemolytic disease of the fetus. Mothers who are Rh negative will subsequently receive RhoGAM as well.

HELPFUL TIP: For those of you who don't do OB (like your editors), nuchal translucency looks at fluid collections in the cervical spine area. Increased translucency suggests increased fluid collection and is associated with abnormalities such as Down syndrome, Turner syndrome, and hemodynamic problems (cardiac abnormalities).

Two maternal serum markers, hCG and PAPP-A, and one fetal marker (nuchal thickness) should be used between 11 and 14 weeks to evaluate for Down syndrome. This method offers a Down syndrome detection rate of approximately 85% with a 5% false-positive rate (see ACOG Practice Bulletin No. 77: Screening for Fetal Chromosomal Abnormalities. *Obstet Gynecol* 2007;109:217.).

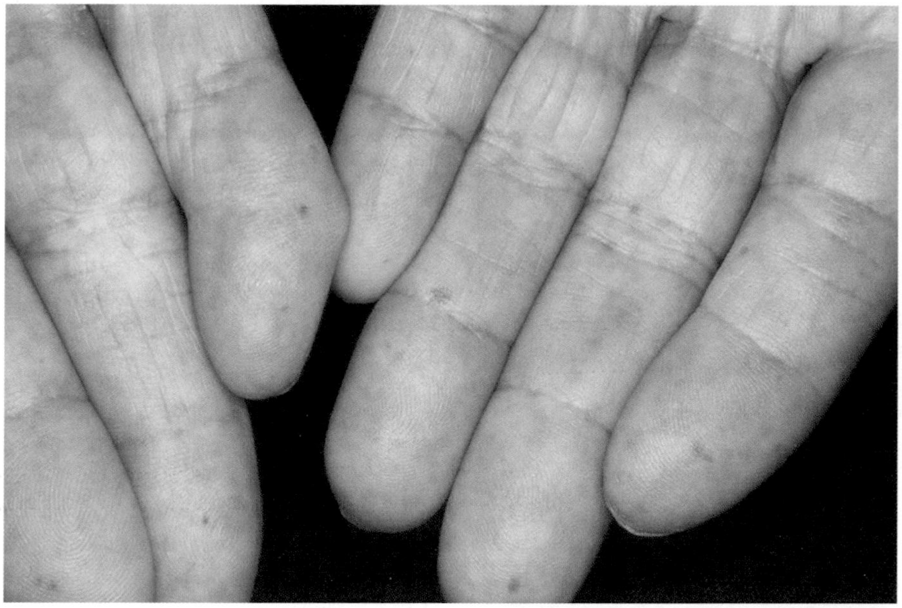
Figure 7–1

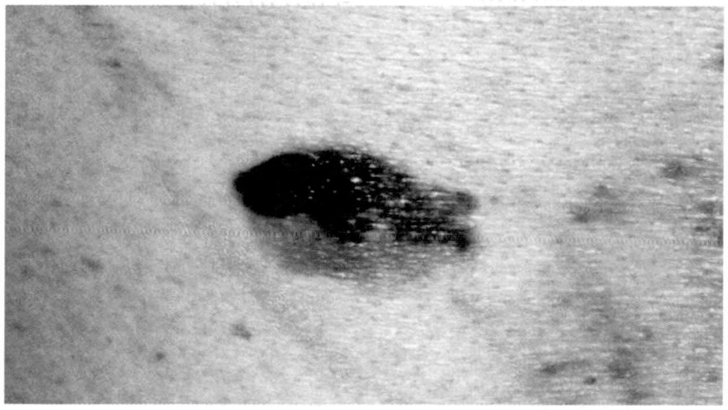
Figure 17–1

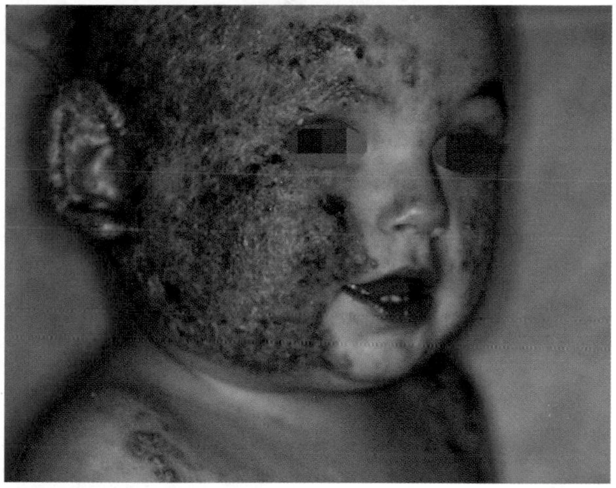
Figure 17–2

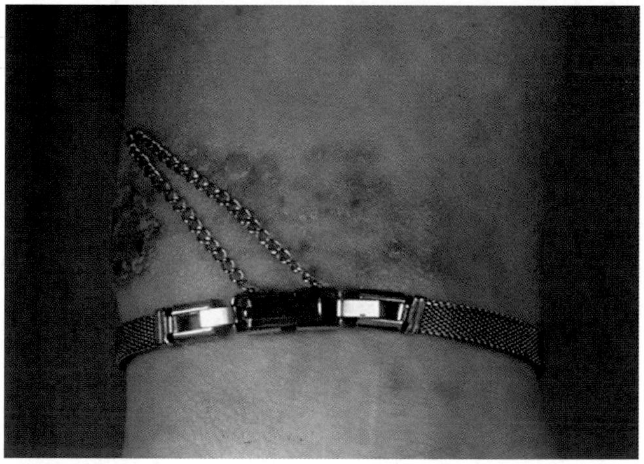
Figure 17–3

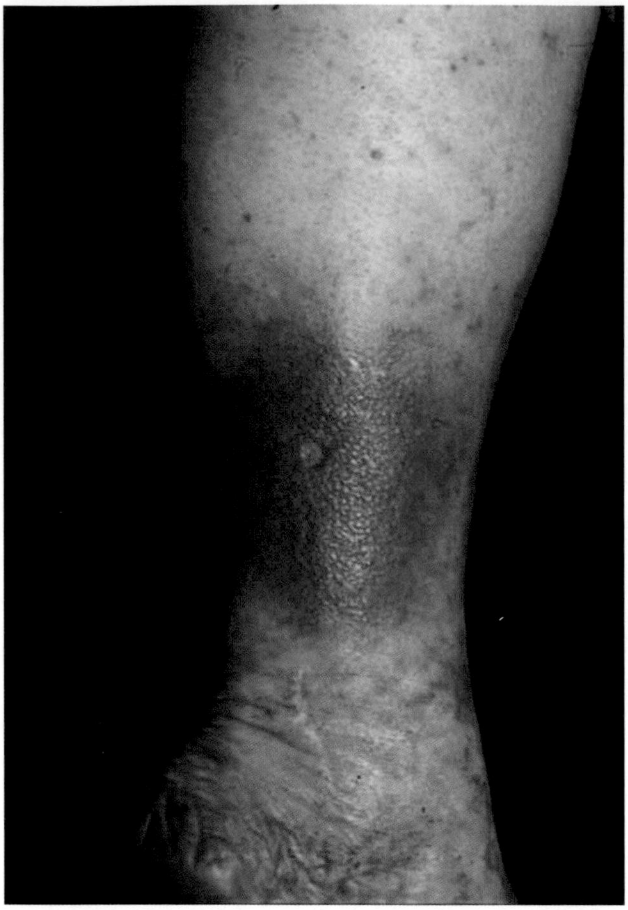

Figure 17–4

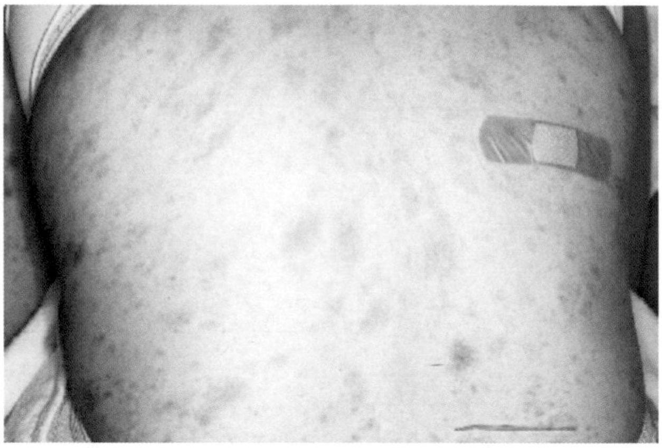

Figure 17–6 Knoop KJ, Stack LB, Stack LB, Storrow AB: *Atlas of Emergency Medicine,* 2nd Edition: http://www.accessemergencymedicine.com.

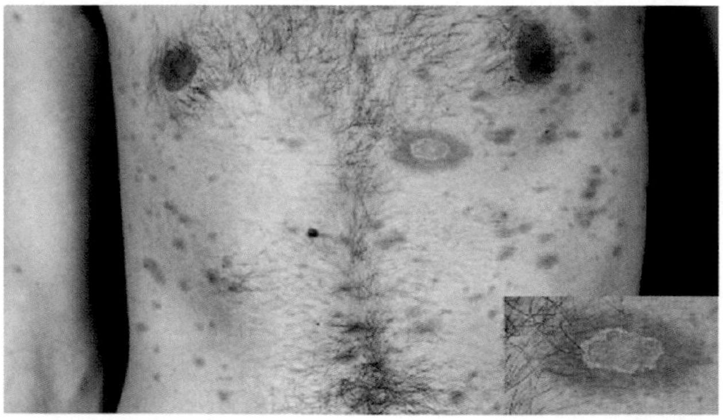

Figure 17–5 Wolff K, Johnson RA, Suurmond, D: *Fitzpatrick's Color Atlas & Synopsis of Clinical Dermatology,* 5th Edition: http://www.accessmedicine.com.

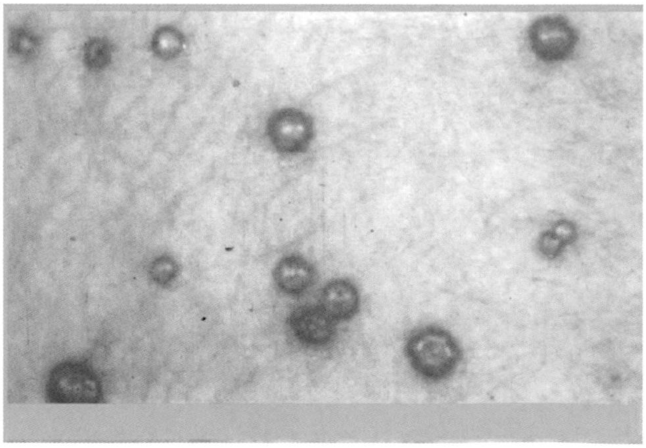

Figure 17–7

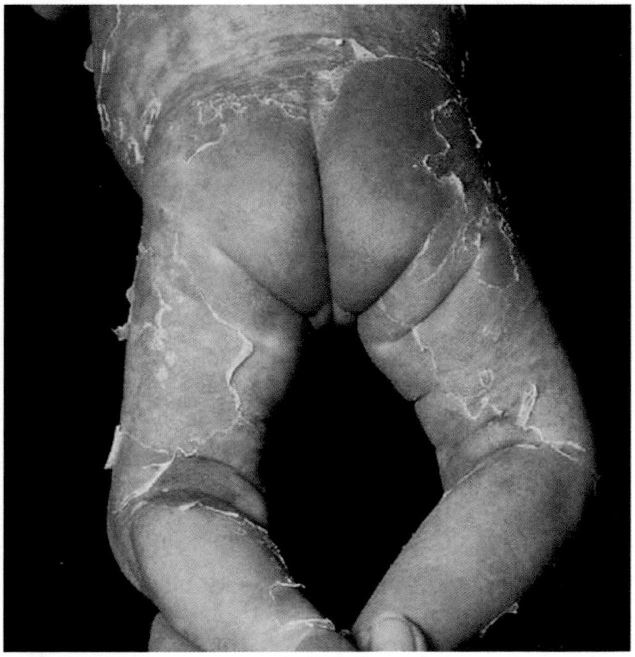

Figure 17–10 **Wolff K, Johnson RA, Suurmond, D: *Fitzpatrick's Color Atlas & Synopsis of Clinical Dermatology*, 5th Edition: http://www.accessmedicine.com.**

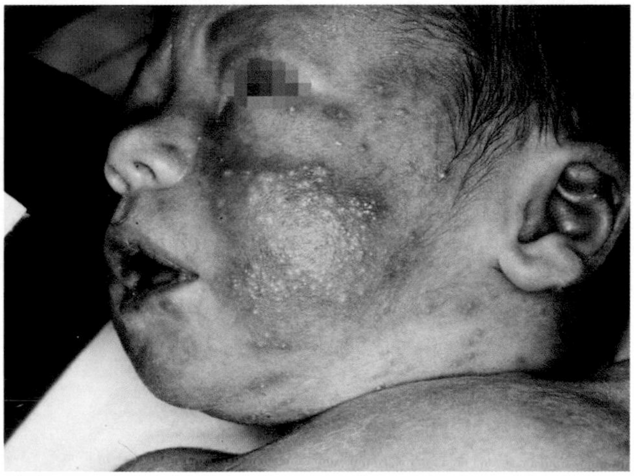

Figure 17–8

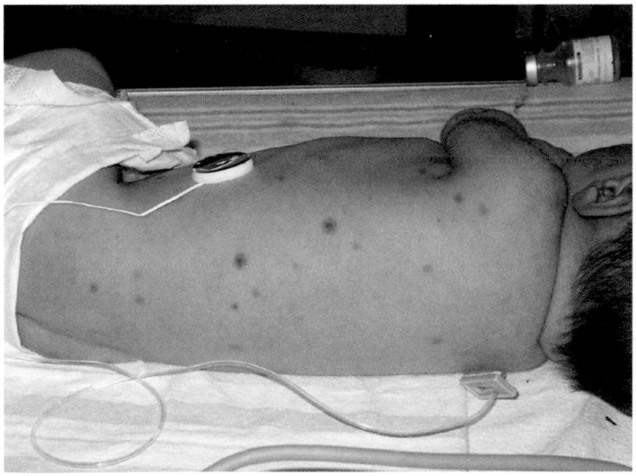

Figure 17–9

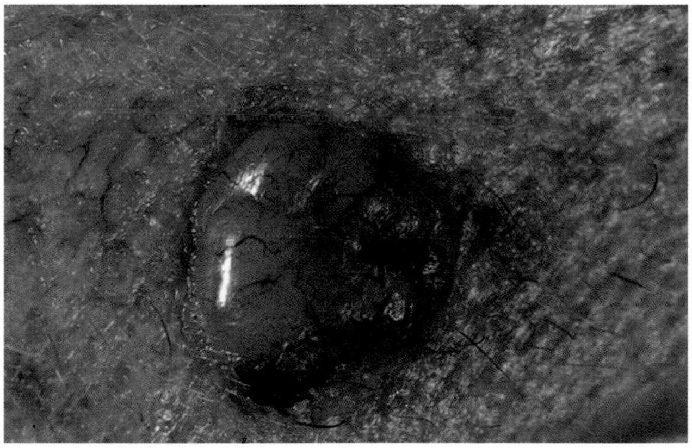

Figure 17–11

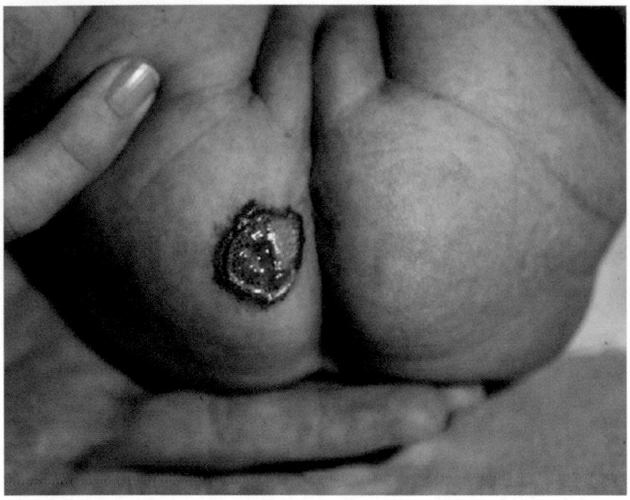

Figure 17–12

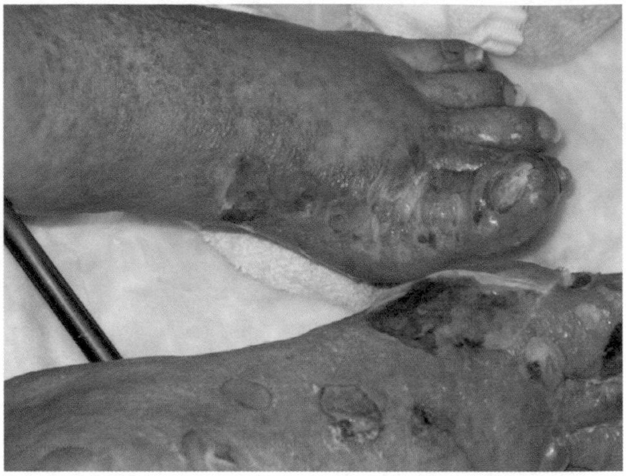

Figure 17–14

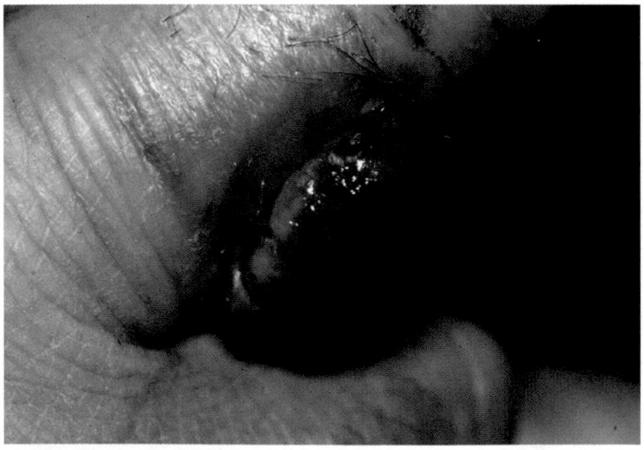

Figure 17–13

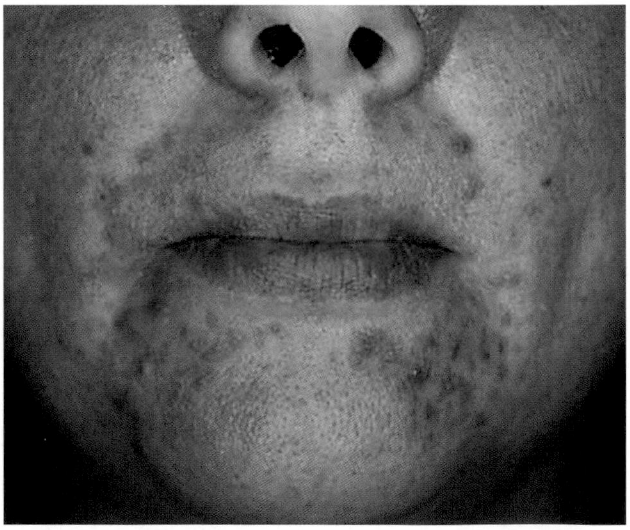

Figure 17–15

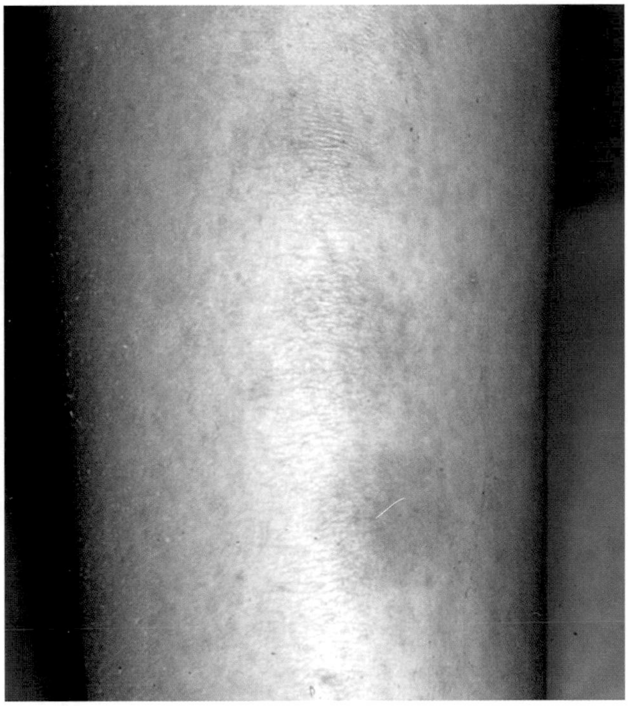

Figure 17–16

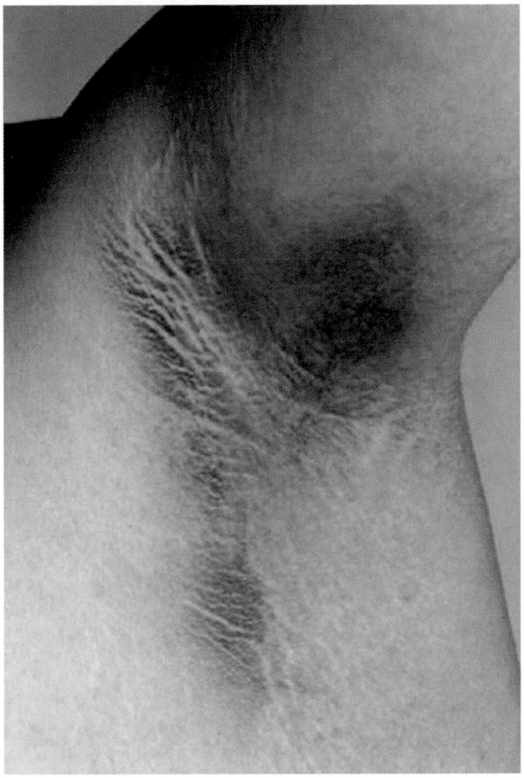

Figure 17–18 **Wolff K, Johnson RA, Suurmond, D: *Fitzpatrick's Color Atlas & Synopsis of Clinical Dermatology*, 5th Edition: http://www.accessmedicine.com.**

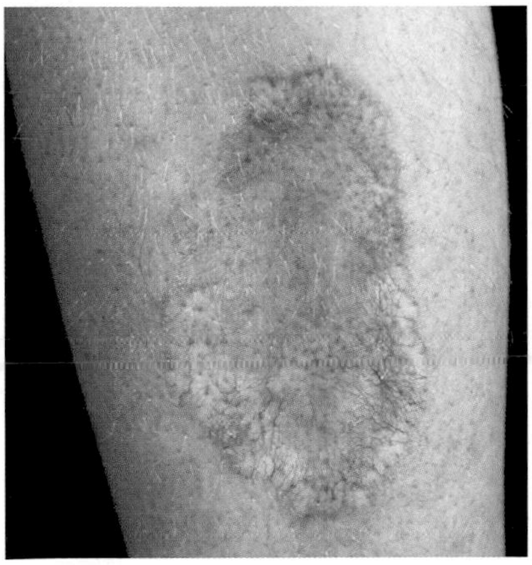

Figure 17–17 **Wolff K, Johnson RA: *Fitzpatrick s Color Atlas & Synopsis of Clinical Dermatology*, 6th Edition: http://www.accessmedicine.com.**

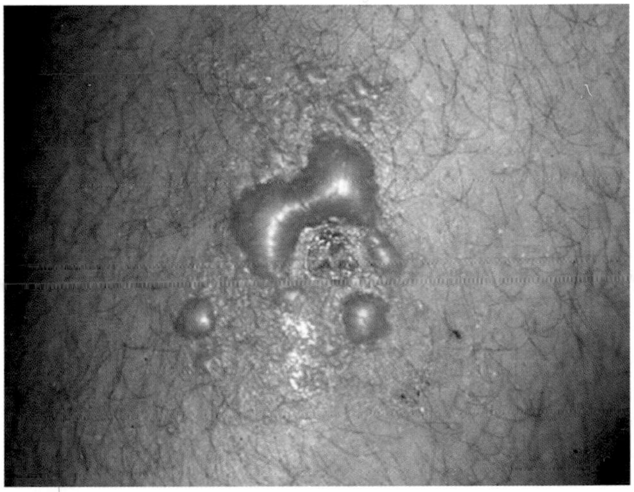

Figure 17–19

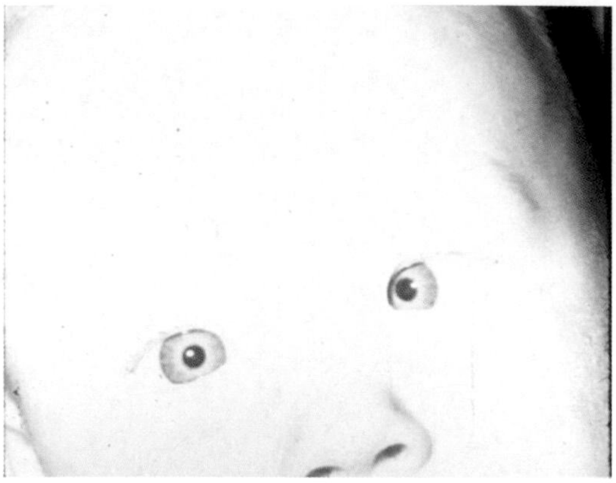

Figure 19–1 **Congenital esotropia. Note the large deviation with abnormal corneal light reflexes. The corneal light reflex of the left eye appears more temporal than that of the right eye. Therefore, the eye is deviated inwards.**

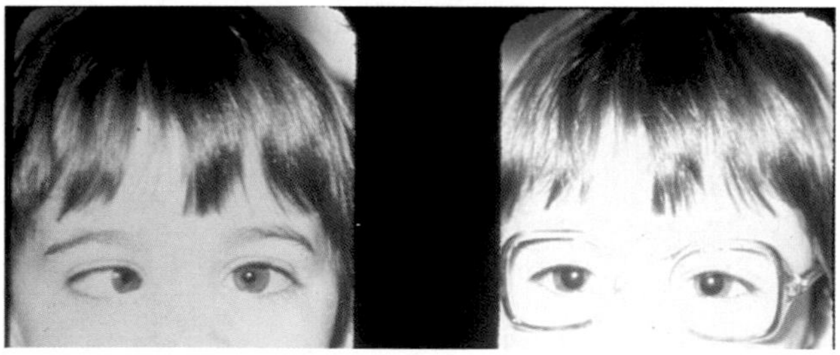

Figure 19–2 **Accommodative esotropia improves when vision is corrected.**

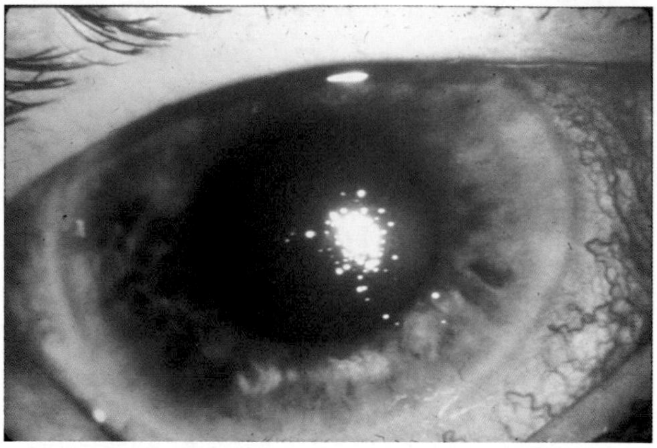

Figure 19–3 **Acute Angle Closure Glaucoma. Note the injection, hazy corneal reflex, and mid-dilated pupil.**

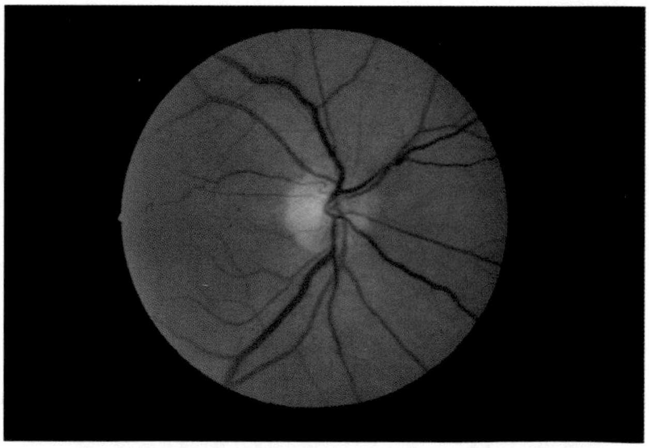

Figure 19–4 **Normal optic nerve.**

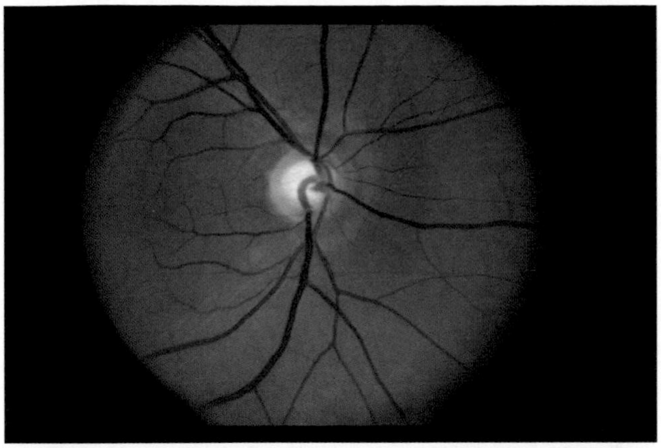

Figure 19–5 ***Glaucomatous optic nerve. Observe the cupping of the optic nerve head.***

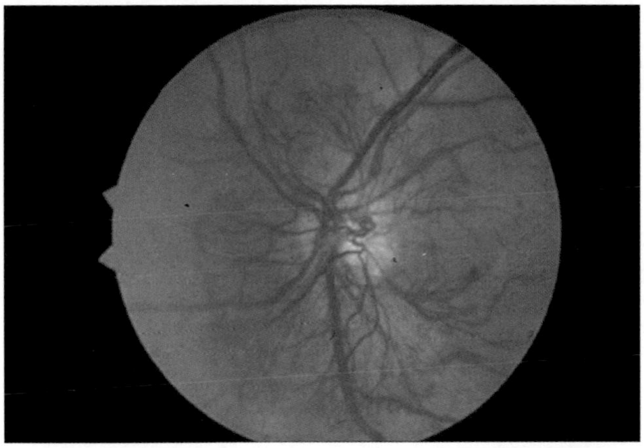

Figure 19–6 ***Proliferative diabetic retinopathy. Neovascularization of the optic nerve.***

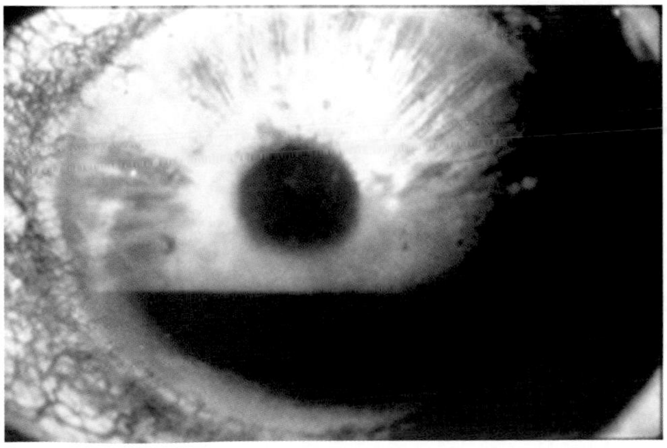

Figure 19–7

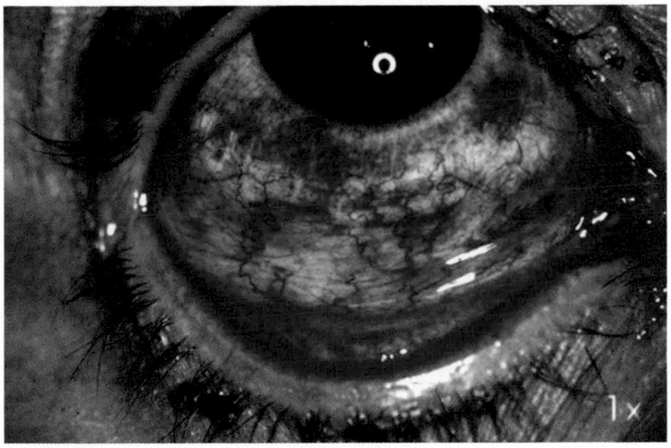

Figure 19–8 ***Viral conjunctivitis.***

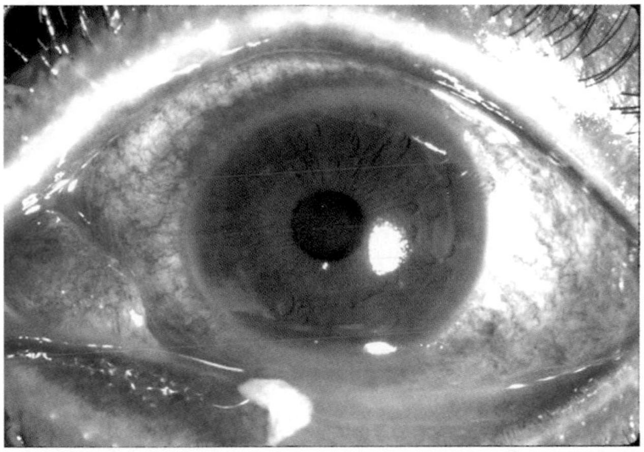

Figure 19–9 ***Bacterial conjunctivitis. Note the mucopurulent discharge.***

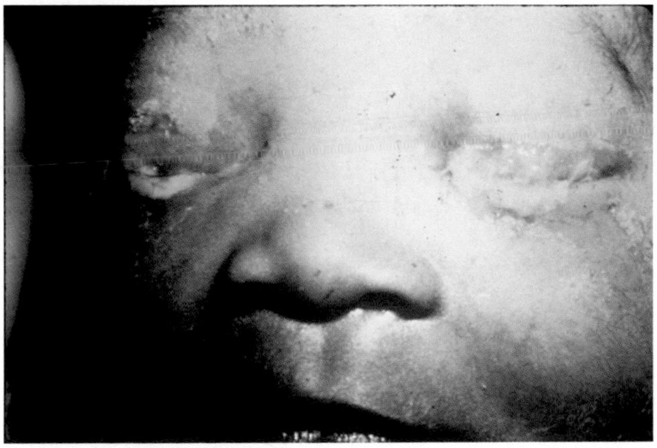

Figure 19–10 ***Ophthalmia neonatorum. Note the severe mucopurulent discharge.***

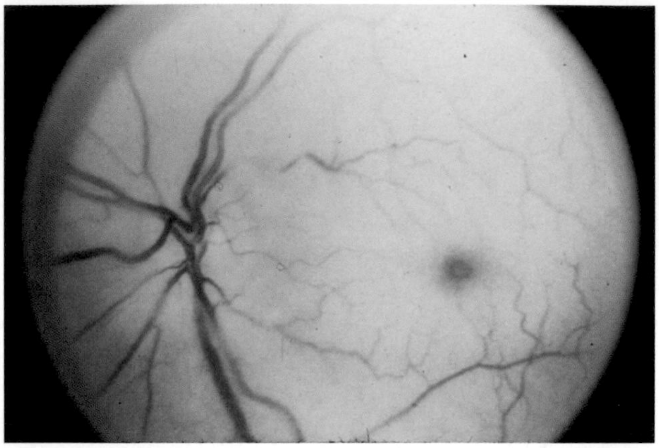

Figure 19–11

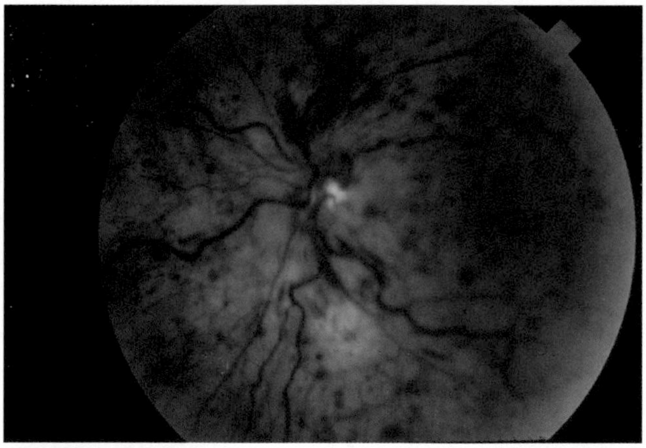

Figure 19–12 ***Central retinal vein occlusion. Note the dilated tortuous veins, optic disc edema, and retinal hemorrhage/edema.***

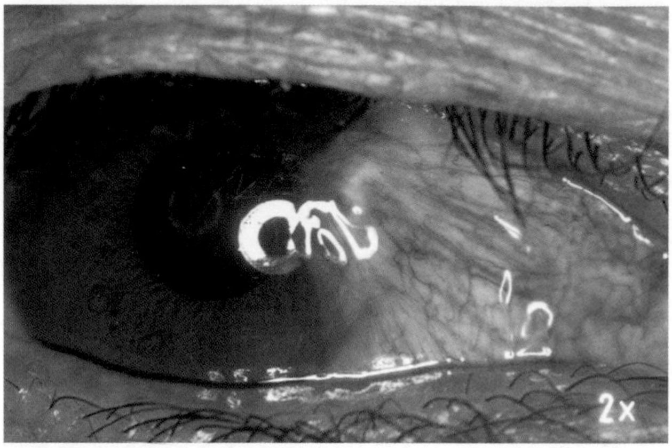

Figure 19–13

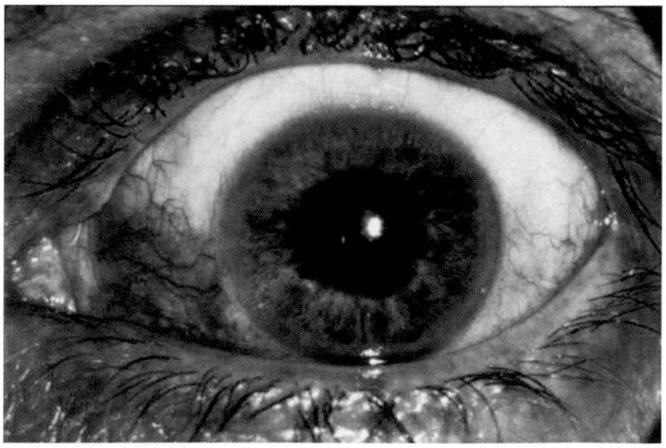

Figure 19–14

HELPFUL (AND IMPORTANT) TIP: Since it does not screen for neural tube defects, first trimester screening does not negate the need for a second trimester maternal serum triple or quad screen, including AFP (alpha fetal protein), hCG, uE3 (unconjugated estriol), and inhibin A, which is done between 15 weeks 0 days and 19 weeks 6 days of gestation.

* *

The patient has passed all of her screening tests with flying colors so far. She returns at 36 weeks of gestation.

What additional screening test(s) is/are obtained near 36 weeks gestation?

A) Amniocentesis.
B) 3-hour glucose tolerance test.
C) Fetal fibronectin (FFN).
D) Group B streptococcus (GBS) culture.
E) All of the above.

Discussion

The correct answer is "D." The CDC recommends maternal screening for GBS between 35 and 37 weeks gestation. The only persons who should be excluded are women who had bacteruria with GBS during the current pregnancy or those who had an infant previously infected with GBS. These mothers are treated empirically with antibiotics in labor and do not need screening. Mothers whose culture status is unknown should receive antibiotic prophylaxis **in labor** only if one of the following exists: (1) intrapartum fever (>38°C), (2) preterm labor (<37 weeks gestation), or (3) prolonged rupture of membranes (>18 hours). FFN is not recommended as a routine screening test, but you will see more on this later.

Objectives: Did you learn to . . .

- Describe contraception options?
- Provide appropriate routine prenatal care?
- Recognize nausea and vomiting of pregnancy and describe its appropriate management?

CASE 2

You are taking obstetric calls for your group this weekend. Labor and delivery calls you about a 27-year-old G1P0 at 38 weeks gestation who awoke this morning complaining of wetness. However, when she went to the bathroom she discovered significant vaginal bleeding that had soaked her bed. She denies any cramping or abdominal pain. She is on her way to the hospital.

You tell the nurses to initiate all of the following interventions immediately upon the patient's arrival EXCEPT:

A) Obtain IV access.
B) Draw blood for type and screen.
C) Perform a digital vaginal exam.
D) Initiate fetal monitoring.
E) Draw blood for complete blood count.

Discussion

The correct answer is "C." A small-to-moderate amount of bleeding is not unexpected during labor; however, the profuse bleeding described by the patient is an obstetric emergency. The first priorities are to obtain IV access and ensure that the mother is hemodynamically stable. Baseline laboratory evaluation will give some indication of the amount of blood loss and establish that blood is available for transfusion if necessary. Monitoring of the fetal heart rate (FHR) will establish viability. Also, an ultrasound should be done to evaluate for placenta previa. A digital vaginal examination should NOT be performed until the diagnosis of placenta previa has been excluded. A consultation with someone skilled in cesarean section should be obtained if the initial evaluation suggests that immediate fetal delivery is necessary.

HELPFUL TIP: Classically, placenta previa presents as painless third trimester bleeding, whereas, placental abruption classically presents as painful third trimester bleeding. Note that these are the "classic" presentations, not pathognomonic.

* *

When the patient arrives at the hospital, she alters her recollection of events to say that the fluid soaking the bed sheets was blood-tinged and pink in color and first occurred 2 hours ago. She continues to have vaginal leakage but denies any bright red bleeding or contractions. Ultrasound reveals a fundal (not previa, over the cervix) placenta without any evidence of abruption. Fetal heart tones are in the 140s and reactive. Sterile speculum examination reveals fluid, which is Nitrazine and ferning positive. Her GBS culture performed 3 weeks ago is negative.

What is the most appropriate next step in the management of this patient?

A) Begin an induction of labor.
B) Send her home after 4 hours of reassuring fetal monitoring.
C) Treat her with IV penicillin for GBS prophylaxis.
D) Repeat her GBS culture.

Discussion

The correct answer is "A." And "B" is not a good choice. A patient should not be sent home after rupture of membranes. She is at risk for intrauterine infection, and induction is indicated to reduce the risk of infection. Induction of labor, even with an unfavorable cervix, is not associated with an increase in cesarean or operative vaginal delivery, but it is associated with fewer maternal infections and fewer neonatal intensive care unit admissions. (However, any unfavorable cervix is more likely to require operative delivery—regardless of induced or spontaneous onset of labor.) "C" and "D" are incorrect. Her GBS culture was negative 3 weeks ago. Although GBS colonization can be transient, since the culture was completed within 5 weeks, it should be reliable. Even if her membranes were ruptured for more than 18 hours, she would not require treatment with antibiotics unless she developed a fever. **If a fever develops, think chorioamnionitis to choose antibiotic therapy.**

* *

Sterile vaginal exam reveals a cervix that is 1 cm dilated, 3-cm long (effacement), and vertex at −1 station. The patient agrees to an induction of labor.

The best method for this patient is to:

A) Insert intracervical laminaria.
B) Begin IV oxytocin at 2 milliunits per minute.
C) Insert intravaginal dinoprostone.
D) Have her partner sit on her abdomen.

Discussion

The correct answer is "B." The use of intravaginal and intracervical methods for cervical ripening may increase the risk of infection after membranes have ruptured. Thus, "A" and "D" are not the best choices (although they are used with intact membranes). Oxytocin should be closely titrated via IV route for labor induction or augmentation. The general starting doses are 0.5–6 milliunits per minute, increased by 1–6 milliunits every 20–40 minutes, to a maximum dose rarely exceeding 40 milliunits per minute.

* *

The patient is currently in labor (success!), and now her cervical exam is 6-cm dilation, 1-cm effaced, and −1 station. The amniotic fluid is still clear, having ruptured approximately 22 hours ago. She has an epidural for analgesia. The FHR baseline has increased to 165 beats per minute with minimal variability. Contractions occur every 3 minutes. Maternal temperature is now 38.6°C, and her pulse is 110. The patient denies any complaints.

Given the history of prolonged rupture of membranes and fever, which of the following is the diagnosis of most concern at this point?

A) Normal labor.
B) Epidural fever.
C) Nosocomial infection.
D) Chorioamnionitis.

Discussion

The correct answer is "D." Chorioamnionitis is the most likely diagnosis and the diagnosis of most concern given the prolonged rupture of membranes. Treatment should be initiated immediately. "A" is incorrect as fever is not a normal part of labor. "B" is possible, but not as likely and a dangerous assumption. There is an association between the use of epidural analgesia and a rise in maternal temperature. Etiologies proposed for this temperature increase include lack of pain-induced hyperventilation and decreased perspiration due to sympathetic blockade. "C" is extremely unlikely given her brief time in the hospital.

What is the next step in the care of this patient?

A) Stop the oxytocin.
B) Remove the epidural.
C) Initiate broad-spectrum antibiotics.
D) Call the your backup for cesarean section (or do it yourself).

Discussion

The correct answer is "C." Initiation of antibiotics is associated with a decrease in both maternal and neonatal morbidity. Multiple organisms are isolated in more than 66% of cases; therefore, antibiotics should be broad. Approved regimens include ampicillin and gentamicin, ticarcillin/clavulanate, or piperacillin. There is no need to stop the oxytocin and proceed with a cesarean delivery unless there is another indication. Although epidural anesthesia is associated with increased maternal temperature, it should only be removed if it is felt to be contributing to maternal pathology (e.g., meningitis, epidural abscess, or epidural bleed).

* *

The patient's labor is progressing. Her cervix is 9 cm dilated, completely effaced, and station is +3. Her temperature is 39.0°C. The FHR pattern is shown in Figure 15–1.

What is the FHR interpretation?

A) Baseline 165 beats per minute, reactive.
B) Baseline 165 beats per minute, with periods of bradycardia.
C) Baseline 165 beats per minute, with late decelerations.
D) Baseline 165 beats per minute, with variable decelerations.

Discussion

The correct answer is "C." The FHR pictured is about 165 beats per minute. There is moderate variability present. Following each contraction, there are late decelerations to the 110s. "A" is incorrect since "reactive" refers to a nonstress test, not fetal monitoring during labor. (See the following "Helpful Tip.") "B" is incorrect as fetal bradycardia is defined as a FHR of less than 110 beats per minute for at least 10 minutes. "D" is incorrect. Variable decelerations vary with respect to timing, duration, and depth.

HELPFUL TIP: A reactive nonstress test is defined as 2 accelerations of at least 15 beats above baseline and lasting at least 15 seconds within a 20-minute interval in gestations **greater than 32 completed weeks.** In gestations less than 32 weeks, reactive is defined as 2 accelerations at least 10 beats above baseline and lasting at least 10 seconds.

What is the likely etiology of the FHR tracing in Figure 15–1?

A) Head compression.
B) Placental insufficiency.
C) Cord compression.
D) Any of the above is equally likely to cause the tracing.

Discussion

The correct answer is "B." Late decelerations are believed to be secondary to transient fetal hypoxia in response to decreased placental perfusion. Prompt evaluation and intervention is warranted. Early decelerations are generally reassuring and attributed to fetal head compression. Variable decelerations are the most common decelerations seen in labor and indicate cord compression. Variable decelerations can sometimes be relieved by maternal repositioning or amnioinfusion.

What is the LEAST appropriate course of action now?

A) Administer maternal oxygen.
B) Stop oxytocin.
C) Forceps or vacuum-assisted vaginal delivery.
D) Consider cesarean delivery.
E) Reposition mother (roll to one side or knee–chest).

Discussion

The correct answer is "C." Increasing maternal O_2 may improve fetal oxygenation. Oxytocin can decrease placental blood flow via uterine stimulation, and hence should be decreased or stopped if nonreassuring FHR changes are present. If there is evidence of maternal hypotension, maternal hydration may be indicated. Another option is position changes (left lateral) to improve placental perfusion. Maternal position can affect uterine blood flow and placental perfusion. The gravid uterus may compress the vena cava while supine. Because the patient is 9 cm dilated, forceps or vacuum-assisted vaginal delivery (also known as "operative vaginal delivery") is NOT indicated.

* *

The FHR changes resolve with your appropriate interventions. The patient progresses to complete dilation and delivers vaginally 1 hour later. No antibiotics are continued following delivery, and the maternal temperature 2 hours after delivery is 37.0°C. On postpartum day 1, your patient complains of sore

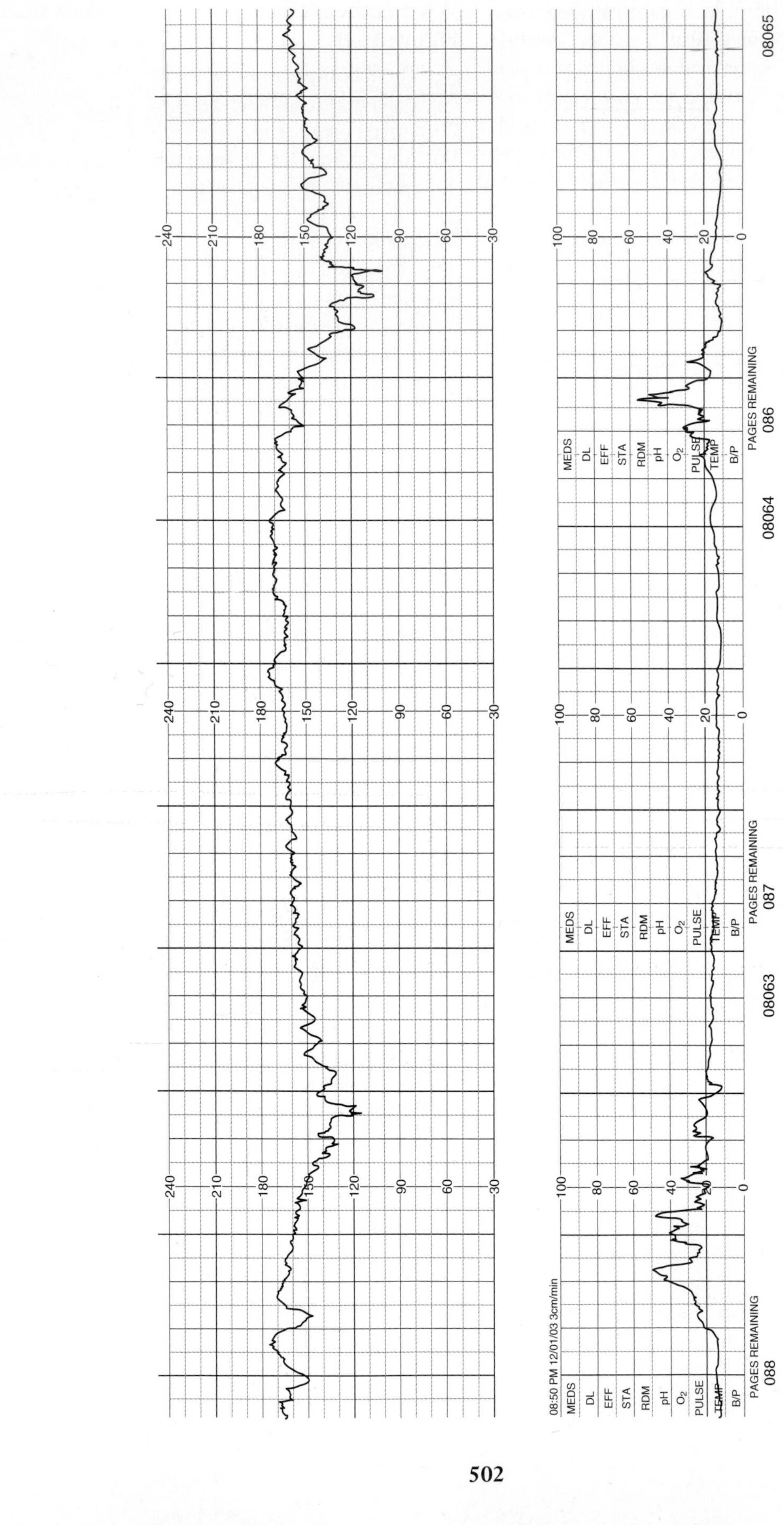
08:50 PM 12/01/03 3cm/min
MEDS
DL
EFF
STA
RDM
pH
O_2
PULSE
TEMP
B/P
PAGES REMAINING
088
PAGES REMAINING
087
PAGES REMAINING
086
08063
08064
08065
240
210
180
150
120
90
60
30
100
80
60
40
20
0

Figure 15–1

breasts from breast-feeding but no particular swelling of the breast (beyond what is expected postpartum), and her abdomen is sore "all over." She is having a moderate amount of lochia, and her temperature is 38.4°C.

The most likely cause of the fever at this time is:

A) Endometritis.
B) Mastitis.
C) Deep vein thrombosis.
D) Septic pelvic thrombophlebitis.

Discussion

The correct answer is "A." Whenever fever occurs in the immediate postpartum period, endometritis should be suspected. The presence of intra-amniotic infection increases the risk of postpartum endometritis to 13%. Antibiotics are not routinely continued for chorioamnionitis after a vaginal delivery because the "source" of the infection (the placenta) has been removed.

Mastitis is characterized by a swollen, firm, tender breast with systemic symptoms including fevers, chills, and flu-like symptoms. However, it was stipulated that the breasts were normal for a postpartum patient. *Staphylococcus aureus* is the typical pathogen. Pregnancy and the postpartum period increase a woman's risk of thrombogenesis. However, DVT is not a likely source of the fever. Septic pelvic thrombophlebitis is a diagnosis of exclusion and is usually entertained when fever spikes continue following treatment for endometritis.

* *

You start appropriate antibiotics and the patient does well. The family, in gratitude, names the child after you and makes you the godparent necessitating gifts for the next 18 years on the infant's birthday.

> HELPFUL TIP: Infants born to women with chorioamnionitis have a fourfold increase in neonatal mortality and a threefold increase in the incidence of respiratory distress, neonatal sepsis, and intraventricular hemorrhage.

Objectives: Did you learn to . . .

- Triage and manage third trimester bleeding?
- Recognize and treat a patient with premature rupture of membranes?
- Evaluate and manage intrapartum fever?
- Interpret FHR patterns and manage abnormal patterns?
- Appreciate the risk factors, evaluation, and management of postpartum infection?

CASE 3

You are seeing a 31-year-old G2 P1 at 41 weeks gestation by definite last menstrual period and 16-week ultrasound. She continues to note fetal movement and her examination is normal: BP 120/68, urine dipstick negative for protein and glucose, fundal height 42 cm, vertex, FHR 156. Her cervix is soft, anterior, 2–3 cm dilated, 50% effaced, and +1 station. She was induced with her first pregnancy, and this time she wants to have a "natural labor." You decide to check a Bishop score.

The Bishop score helps to determine:

A) The health of the fetus.
B) The likely success with induction.
C) The maturity of the fetal lungs.
D) The results of a Catholic Intramural Baseball game.

Discussion

The correct answer is "B." The Bishop score, which takes into account cervical dilation, cervical effacement, station of the infant, and cervical consistency, can be used to predict the likelihood of a successful induction.

* *

The Bishop score is favorable.

Which of the following are the most appropriate recommendations at this point?

A) She should be induced at once; there is a high chance of fetal mortality after 41 weeks gestation.
B) Since her antepartum course has been uncomplicated to date, it is safe for her to await spontaneous labor until 43 weeks gestation.
C) She should undergo a nonstress test and ultrasound for amniotic fluid index.
D) She should plan for a cesarean section.

Discussion

The correct answer is "C." By definition, a term gestation is one completed in 38–42 weeks. There is no significant increase in fetal mortality in an uncomplicated pregnancy at term. Virtually all reports suggest an increase in perinatal morbidity and mortality when pregnancy goes beyond 42 weeks gestation. Antenatal surveillance of postterm pregnancies should be initiated at 41 weeks gestation.

> HELPFUL TIP: Accurate determination of conception is important in reducing the false diagnosis of postterm pregnancy. The estimated date of delivery is most reliably and accurately determined early in pregnancy.

Which of the following nonpharmacologic methods of augmenting or inducing labor is LEAST likely to be effective?

A) Stripping the amniotic membranes.
B) Prolonged walking.
C) Amniotomy.
D) Nipple stimulation.

Discussion

The correct answer is "B." Stripping membranes appears to be effective in initiating spontaneous labor within 72 hours. Amniotomy may be used for labor induction, especially if the Bishop score is favorable, but oxytocin is more effective. Nipple stimulation causes release of oxytocin and may be utilized for labor induction, but its marginal benefit is only seen in patients with a favorable Bishop score. Walking does not result in labor induction or augmentation, but it's not harmful either.

> HELPFUL TIP: Sexual intercourse is sometimes recommended to induce labor. Studies are of low quality and use various endpoints . . . also, it is difficult to standardize the intervention (we could make a joke here but won't). One of the better quality studies (Tan et al., 2006) did find that coitus was associated with reduced need for labor induction at 41 weeks.

If induction becomes necessary, which of the following pharmacologic interventions would be the best approach to your patient who has a cervix that is soft, anterior, 2–3 cm dilated, 50% effaced, and +1 station?

A) IV oxytocin.
B) Intracervical PGE2 (dinoprostone).
C) Intravaginal PGE2 (dinoprostone).
D) Intravaginal PGE1 (misoprostol).
E) None of the above. All pharmacologic interventions are contraindicated.

Discussion

The correct answer is "A." This patient does not need further cervical ripening but is a candidate for induction of labor. PGE2 gel (dinoprostone, brand name Cervidil or Prepidil) is administered vaginally—not intracervically—and is used for cervical ripening when induction is indicated but the status of the cervix is unfavorable. PGE2 gel is not indicated for induction of labor. PGE1 (misoprostol, option "D") can be administered intravaginally or orally and has been found to be effective for both cervical ripening and labor induction. However, the Food and Drug Administration (FDA) has not approved it for use in pregnancy. Because the cervix is favorable in this case, proceeding with oxytocin is the best option.

* *

Your patient's husband is called up for active duty in Iraq (or Afghanistan . . . or Libya or . . . insert appropriate country at the time you are reading this) and is due to report in the next few days. She is now 41 2/7 weeks gestation and desires induction so he can be with her for the delivery. You admit her to labor and delivery the following morning. The initial FHR monitoring **before any induction (also known as a nonstress test)** is shown in Figure 15–2.

What is the correct interpretation?

A) Baseline = 150 beats per minute; not reactive.
B) Baseline = 150 beats per minute; reactive.
C) Baseline = 180 beats per minute; decelerations to 150s.
D) Baseline = 180 beats per minute; moderate variability.

Discussion

The correct answer is "B." The baseline is about 150 beats per minute. There are two accelerations greater than 15 beats and lasting longer than 15 seconds, which meets the criteria for a reactive nonstress test. There is one contraction and evidence of uterine irritability noted as well.

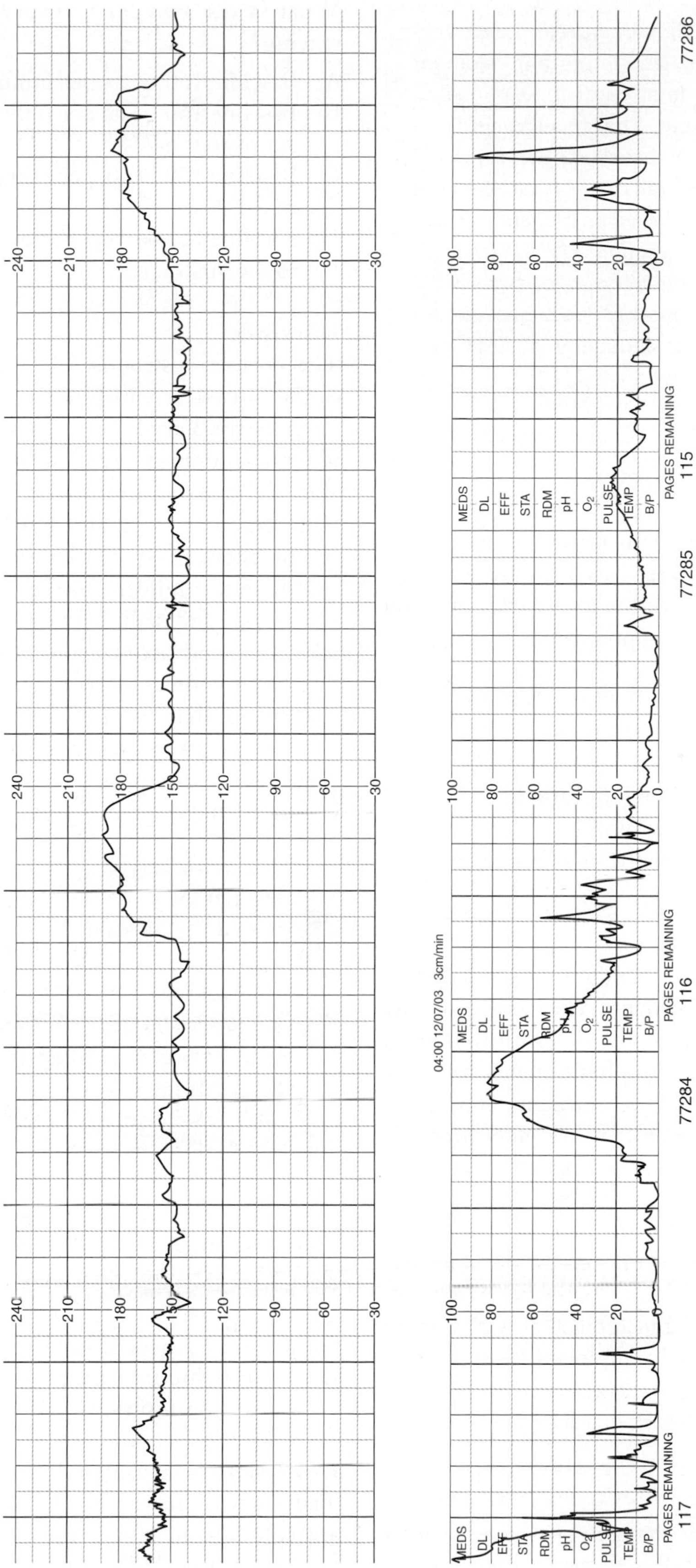

04:00 12/07/03 3cm/min
PAGES REMAINING
117
116
115
77284
77285
77286
MEDS
DL
EFF
STA
RDM
pH
O_2
PULSE
TEMP
B/P

Figure 15–2

HELPFUL TIP: When interpreting FHR tracings, variability is an important element that demonstrates fetal cardiac response to parasympathetic input. The small wave form fluctuations within the baseline heart rate tracing represent the FHR variability. After 28 weeks gestation, variability should be present. It is categorized as absent (no amplitude, flat tracing), minimal (0–5 beat amplitude), moderate (6–25 beat amplitude), or marked (>25 beat amplitude). The absence of variability is associated with fetal decompensation.

* *

You perform amniotomy with return of particulate meconium-stained fluid. Her cervix is now 5 cm dilated, 80% effaced, with vertex at +1 station. You elect to continue monitoring progress.

Which of the following choices of labor analgesia is MOST appropriate at this point?

A) Epidural analgesia.
B) Local perineal anesthetic infiltration.
C) Bilateral pudendal nerve block.
D) All of the above are equally appropriate.

Discussion

The correct answer is "A." Epidural analgesia offers the most effective form of pain relief and generally may be utilized once the patient is determined to be in active labor. Various local anesthetic agents are available for local infiltration of the perineum and vagina to provide analgesia for **episiotomy or laceration repair following delivery but not for labor.** Bilateral pudendal nerve blocks are useful during the **second** stage of labor, as a supplement to epidural analgesia for anesthesia of the sacral nerves, or as an option for operative vaginal delivery anesthesia (forceps, vacuum). Opioid agonists and agonist–antagonists are also available and commonly employed. However, recent reports suggest that the analgesic effect of opioids in labor is limited when using doses that won't effect the fetus.

* *

The nurse notices some changes on the fetal heart monitor. The current FHR is shown in Figure 15–3.

What is the correct interpretation of this FHR tracing?

A) Baseline 160 beats per minute; reactive.
B) Baseline 160 beats per minutes; variable decelerations to the 90s.
C) Baseline 160 beats per minute; late decelerations to the 90s.
D) Baseline 160 beats per minute; early decelerations to the 90s.

Discussion

The correct answer is "B." Variable decelerations to the 90s occur with the first and last contractions on this strip. Variable decelerations vary with respect to timing, duration, and depth—thus, the name "variable." They are not uniform. Variable decelerations represent changes in the FHR in response to cord compression. Early decelerations are typically more repetitive and uniform and begin with the onset of the contraction and nadir with the contraction peak (mirroring the contraction). Early decelerations represent fetal head compression. Late decelerations are also repetitive and uniform. They begin after the contraction peak and represent placental insufficiency. Late decelerations are more concerning and should be investigated and treated aggressively.

HELPFUL TIP: In 2008, the National Institute of Child Health and Human Development along with the ACOG and the Society for Maternal Fetal Medicine developed new recommendations for intrapartum electronic FHR monitoring. These can be found in *Rev Obstet Gynecol* 2008;1(4):186-192 or at http://www.ncbi.nlm.nih.gov/pmc/articles/PMC2621055/

Given the findings in Figure 15–3, which of the following should be performed next?

A) Check the patient's cervix.
B) Place a fetal scalp electrode.
C) Begin IV oxytocin infusion.
D) Place an intrauterine pressure catheter and begin an amnioinfusion.

Discussion

The correct answer is "A." Variable decelerations are common in labor, and brief variable decelerations are benign. When variable decelerations become

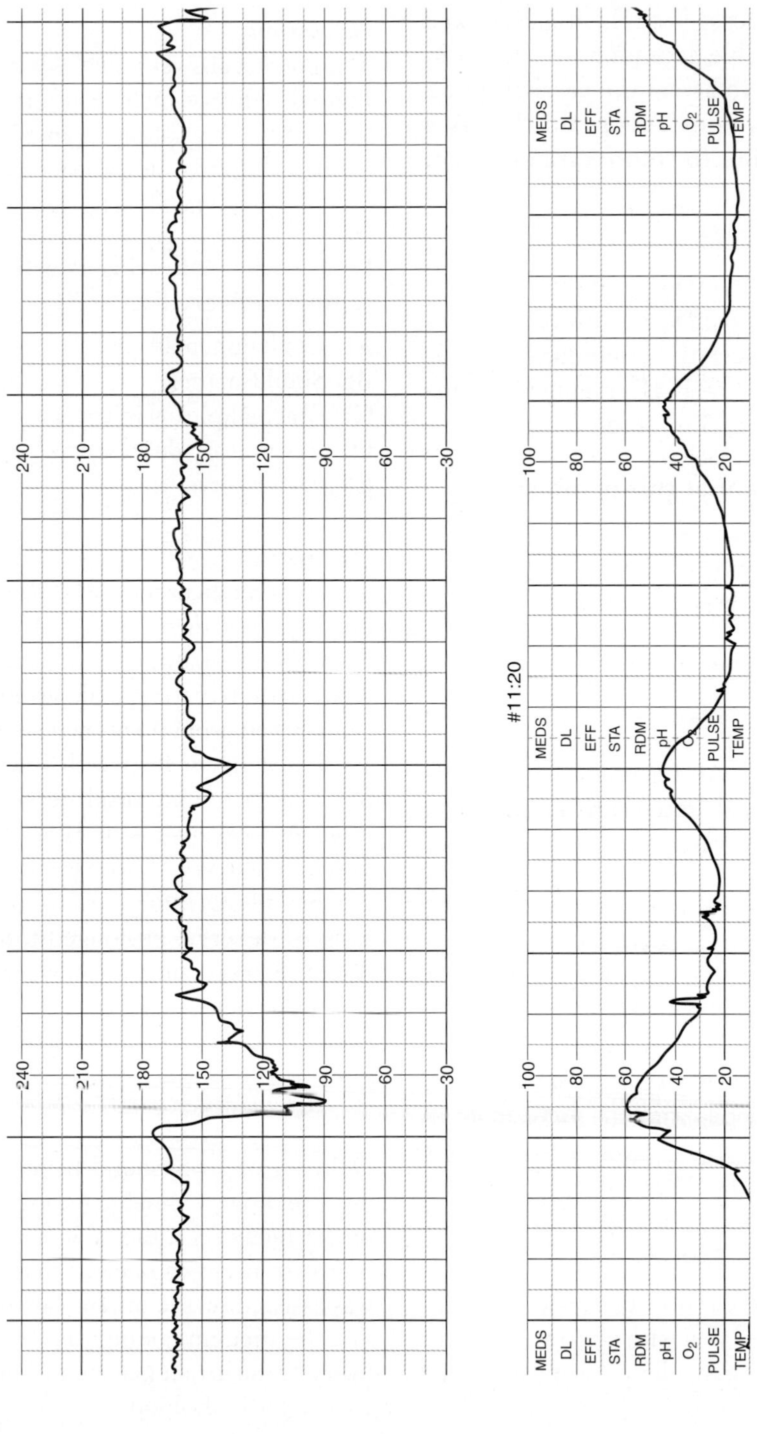
240
210
180
150
120
90
60
30
100
80
60
40
20
#11:20
MEDS
DL
EFF
STA
RDM
pH
O_2
PULSE
TEMP

Figure 15–3

recurrent, progressively deeper, longer lasting, and with delayed return to baseline, they are nonreassuring and may reflect hypoxia. A pelvic examination should be performed to determine if the umbilical cord is prolapsed or if there has been rapid descent of the fetal head or rapid progression of labor. Oxytocin should not be considered since she is having adequate contractions. Replacement of the amniotic fluid with normal saline infused through a transcervical catheter has been reported to decrease both the frequency and severity of repetitive variable decelerations. However, it would first be helpful to assess the cervical status. **Amnioinfusion is no longer recommended as a prophylactic intervention for moderate or severe meconium.**

* *

Labor progresses without incident. Your patient is now completely dilated and effaced, with vertex at +3 station. She is comfortable with her epidural and able to push with good effort. The FHR tracing is reassuring. Contractions are every 3 minutes.

Appropriate management at this point is:

A) Continue pushing.
B) Vacuum-assisted delivery.
C) Forceps-assisted delivery.
D) Midline episiotomy.
E) Augment with oxytocin.

Discussion
The correct answer is "A." At this point, labor is progressing and maternal–fetal status is reassuring. You should continue expectant management. No intervention is indicated.

HELPFUL TIP: Episiotomies should not be performed routinely. Indications for episiotomy are typically related to nonreassuring fetal status and dystocia. **There is no evidence that episiotomies reduce perineal trauma, postpartum dyspareunia, etc.**

* *

She pushes for 3 hours. She is now exhausted. The fetal head now separates the labia with contractions, and then recedes slightly. You consider offering assistance with delivery.

In counseling your patient and her husband about the maternal risks of operative vaginal delivery, which of the following should you discuss?

A) Vaginal trauma.
B) Shoulder dystocia.
C) Fetal injury.
D) Perineal and rectal trauma.
E) All of the above.

Discussion
The correct answer is "E." Maternal risks of operative vaginal delivery include injury to the lower genital tract and rectal sphincter involvement in the case of a third- or fourth-degree laceration. In addition, fetal complications need to be discussed as well.

Each of the following is a fetal risk of operative vaginal delivery EXCEPT:

A) Cephalohematoma.
B) Skull fracture.
C) Brachial plexus injury.
D) Respiratory distress syndrome.
E) Facial nerve palsy.

Discussion
The correct answer is "D." Respiratory distress syndrome is not increased by assisted delivery. Neonatal cephalohematoma, retinal hemorrhage, and jaundice (secondary to breakdown and reabsorption of the cephalohematoma) are more common with vacuum-assisted delivery than with forceps-assisted delivery. Skull fracture and facial nerve injury is more common with forceps-assisted delivery than with vacuum-assisted delivery. Shoulder dystocia with resultant brachial plexus injury is more common with vacuum-assisted delivery, prolonged time required for delivery, and increasing birth weight. Note that injury can occur before operative delivery as a result of abnormal labor forces (has anyone told the malpractice attorneys?).

* *

Delivery of an 8-pound baby is accomplished without operative vaginal assistance. The mere presence of the vacuum on the table was enough to entice the uterus to perform one last massive contraction. This was assisted by the infant clawing its way out when it saw the vacuum coming. Following spontaneous delivery of the **intact** placenta 15 minutes later, you note a large gush of blood.

Which of the following is the most likely source of the bleeding?

A) Uterine atony.
B) Vaginal laceration.
C) Cervical laceration.
D) Retained placenta.

Discussion

The correct answer is "A." Postpartum hemorrhage is most commonly associated with uterine atony. Risk factors include prolonged labor, over-distended uterus (such as from 2 . . . or 8 . . . gestations), very rapid labor, high parity, chorioamnionitis, retained placental tissue, poorly perfused myometrium, halogenated hydrocarbon anesthesia, and previous atony. Maternal trauma to the genital tract may result in postpartum hemorrhage and should be routinely investigated following assisted delivery. A retained placenta cotyledon is another common source for postpartum hemorrhage. The placenta should be inspected, and if there is any question of retained products of conception, the uterus should be manually explored.

Which of the following should be undertaken next?

A) Obtain IV access and initiate hydration.
B) Begin bimanual uterine compression.
C) Inspect vagina and cervix for lacerations.
D) Obtain blood for type and screen for possible blood transfusion.
E) All of the above.

Discussion

The correct answer is "E." Postpartum hemorrhage is an obstetrical emergency and must be addressed immediately. The gravid uterus receives 500 mL of blood per minute, which can lead to massive hemorrhage if not addressed quickly. Additional personnel should be notified to help with obtaining IV access and blood draws, while you quickly try to identify the source of bleeding.

* *

After thorough exploration of the vagina and uterus, you suspect uterine atony is the cause of bleeding. While continuing uterine massage, you think about your options.

Which of the following is/are options in treating this patient's bleeding?

A) Dilute oxytocin IV.
B) Methylergonovine (Methergine) IM.
C) Carboprost tromethamine (Hemabate) IM.
D) Misoprostol PR.
E) All of the above.

Discussion

The correct answer is "E." Oxytocin can be given as a dilute IV solution or IM. It should never be administered as an undiluted IV bolus, due to the risk of hypotension and cardiac arrhythmia. Methergine (methylergonovine) may be administered orally or intramuscularly (**not intravenously**). Caution should be used in women with hypertension, as Methergine can cause hypertension. Hemabate (carboprost tromethamine) is an F-2α prostaglandin analog that is administered IM or directly into the uterine myometrium. Caution should be used in women with asthma, as Hemabate can cause bronchoconstriction. Misoprostol is a prostaglandin E1 analog that can be administered to women with asthma or hypertension. Rectal or oral administration can be used, but rectal administration is preferred in a patient with potential hemodynamic instability. This can be a life saver especially in the third world countries where other options may not exist.

HELPFUL TIP: Methergine (an ergot alkaloid), oxytocin, Hemabate, and misoprostol all cause smooth muscle contraction in the uterus.

* *

She requires IV crystalloid and 4 units of packed red cells for symptomatic anemia following delivery. Both mother and infant do well, however, and the patient and baby are discharged on postpartum day 2. You schedule a follow-up appointment in 2 days. You are concerned about Sheehan syndrome given the severe postpartum hemorrhage.

All of the following are characteristic of Sheehan syndrome EXCEPT:

A) Failure in lactation.
B) Amenorrhea.
C) Desire to be a punk rocker.
D) Decreased LH/follicle-stimulating hormone (FSH).
E) Adrenal cortical insufficiency.

Discussion

The correct answer is "C." Severe intrapartum or postpartum hemorrhage may result in pituitary necrosis due to hypovolemia and hypoperfusion. This leads to a global hypopituitarism known as Sheehan syndrome. Initial symptoms may be vague (lethargy, anorexia, weight loss, difficulty with lactation), and the syndrome can go unrecognized. It is characterized clinically by endocrine deficiency syndromes as a result of loss of anterior pituitary function. Characteristic manifestations include failure of lactation, amenorrhea, breast atrophy, loss of pubic and axillary hair, adrenal cortical insufficiency, and hypothyroidism. Desire to be a punk rocker is "Sheena syndrome." If you don't get it, you missed the Ramones.

Objectives: Did you learn to . . .

- Recognize the risks of prolonged pregnancy and identify appropriate timing of intervention?
- Describe the indications and risks associated with induction of labor?
- Interpret intrapartum fetal hearth rate patterns and choose appropriate management options?
- Evaluate analgesia options, contraindications, and risks during labor and delivery?
- Recognize the indications for and management of operative vaginal and abdominal delivery?
- Evaluate and manage postpartum hemorrhage?

CASE 4

While on call for your small community hospital, a nurse on the labor and delivery ward calls you about a patient with preterm contractions. You come in to see the patient and find a 33-year-old G1 at 26 weeks gestation by in vitro fertilization. She is usually followed at an academic hospital 400 miles away. She looks worried and says, "I'm going to have twins. But not now!" She has a copy of her prenatal record (you nearly fall over backward at her foresight and planning), and her prenatal lab results are unremarkable. Her most recent ultrasound was 1 week ago, confirming a dichorionic, diamniotic gestation with concordant growth.

All of the following risks are increased with a multifetal gestation EXCEPT:

A) Preterm labor.
B) D-isoimmunization (Rh isoimmunization).
C) Preterm rupture of membranes.
D) Intrauterine growth restriction.
E) Twin–twin transfusion syndrome.

Discussion

The correct answer is "B." The most significant complication of multiple gestations is preterm labor resulting in preterm delivery. Preterm rupture of membranes and intrauterine growth restriction also occur more frequently in multiple gestations than singleton pregnancies. The risk of all these complications is directly proportional to the number of fetuses. Twin–twin transfusion syndrome rarely occurs and is associated with monochorionic gestations. A greater risk of D-isoimmunization is not associated with a multifetal gestation.

* *

The nurse asks if you want to check fetal fibronectin (FFN).

A negative fetal fibronectin is associated with:

A) Fetal lung immaturity.
B) Ruptured fetal membranes.
C) A decreased risk of preterm birth.
D) An increased risk of preterm birth.

Discussion

The correct answer is "C." FFN is a basement membrane protein produced by the fetal membranes. A negative test is useful in assessing the risk of preterm delivery during the following 2-week period. A negative test is reassuring. A positive test is not useful as the test has low positive predictive value. The test is performed on a sample from the posterior vaginal fornix or the external cervical os. In performing FFN testing, the following criteria must be met: intact amniotic membranes, minimal cervical dilation (<3 cm), and sampling between 24 0/7 and 34 6/7 weeks. FFN does not assess fetal lung maturity. Ruptured membranes would cause a positive FFN (but, of course, then you don't need it... labor is going to happen one way or another).

> HELPFUL TIP: The main use for fetal fibronectin lies in its high negative predictive value. With a properly performed test in a symptomatic patient, up to 99.5% of patients with a negative FFN will not deliver in the subsequent 7 days.

* *

You are wondering if this patient is a good candidate for corticosteroid therapy.

Regarding the risks and benefits of corticosteroid therapy for fetal lung maturation, which of the following is FALSE?

A) Corticosteroid therapy is recommended for all pregnant women between 24 and 34 weeks gestation who are at risk of preterm delivery within 7 days.
B) Corticosteroid therapy has been associated with an increased risk of neonatal infection.
C) Multiple courses of corticosteroids have been associated with fetal adrenal suppression.
D) Corticosteroids accelerate the appearance of pulmonary surfactant in the fetal lungs.

Discussion

The correct answer is "B." There is no evidence that antenatal corticosteroid therapy increases the risk of neonatal infection. However, maternal infection is a **relative** contraindication to corticosteroid therapy. Corticosteroids are recommended for all pregnant women between 24 and 34 weeks gestation who are at risk of preterm delivery within 7 days. Corticosteroids may be given after 34 weeks if there is documented fetal lung immaturity and delivery will likely occur before lung maturation. Multiple courses have been associated with fetal adrenal suppression and are no longer recommended because they offer no additional clinical benefit.

> HELPFUL TIP: Antenatal corticosteroids not only reduce the incidence of neonatal respiratory distress in preterm infants but also reduce the rates of intraventricular hemorrhage, necrotizing enterocolitis, and overall mortality. **Thus, it is imperative that mothers who fall into the 24–34 weeks gestation window and who are at risk of imminent delivery receive steroids.**

Which of the following agents has been approved by the FDA for tocolysis?

A) Nifedipine.
B) Magnesium sulfate.
C) Prostaglandin inhibitors.
D) Ritodrine.
E) Terbutaline.

Discussion

The correct answer is "D." The only FDA-approved agent for use as a tocolytic is ritodrine, a beta-adrenergic receptor agonist, which is no longer marketed in the United States (so, yes, this is historical trivia, but you still need to stay awake for the bigger issue of tocolytics!). Thus, other agents have been investigated not only to identify a more reliable tocolytic but also to minimize the side effects. Terbutaline, magnesium sulfate, prostaglandin inhibitors, and calcium channel blockers have all been studied and may be utilized in select cases for tocolysis—but realize that these drugs are not approved by the FDA for this indication.

> HELPFUL TIP: Tocolysis only prolongs labor by 48 hours at best, so the real goal should be to prolong the pregnancy until steroids have time to be effective. Contraindications to tocolysis include evidence of fetal distress, fetal anomalies, abruptio placentae, placenta previa with heavy bleeding, and severe maternal disease.

* *

You examine the patient after collecting a fetal fibronectin. Her cervix is 1 cm dilated at the external os and closed at the internal os, long, and posterior. Ultrasound shows that the first infant is vertex. The monitor shows FHR baselines of 140 and 145. Contractions are irregular, occurring every 4–9 minutes. Urine dipstick shows a specific gravity of 1.030.

The LEAST appropriate intervention is:

A) Continuation of monitoring.
B) Oral hydration.
C) Obstetrical consult for cerclage placement.
D) Cultures for group B streptococci, gonorrhea, and chlamydia.
E) Administration of corticosteroids.

Discussion

The correct answer is "C." Cerclage (stitch to hold the cervix closed) is indicated for incompetent cervix, not preterm labor. A cerclage is typically placed in the first part of the second trimester after fetal viability has been established. It would not be used at 26 weeks. The patient should be evaluated carefully and the frequency of uterine contractions should be assessed during the initial management. Because dehydration may result in uterine irritability, rehydration may stabilize the uterus. There is no proven benefit of hydration in the patient who is euvolemic. Get cultures to prevent perinatal transmission even though treatment of positive cultures has not been established to aid in the prevention of preterm birth. Corticosteroids are discussed earlier.

HELPFUL (AND USELESS IF NOT AT LEAST INTERESTING) TIP: Delivery rates in Israel go up around Jewish holiday fast days likely because of the relative dehydration.

Objectives: Did you learn to . . .

- Identify risks and evaluate a multifetal pregnancy?
- Recognize preterm labor and manage it appropriately?
- Understand the indications, contraindications, risks, and benefits of tocolytics and corticosteroids?

CASE 5

A 33-year-old G1 at 35 2/7 weeks presents to labor and delivery. Her pregnancy has been complicated by preterm labor. Her GBS status is unknown. On admission, she is uncomfortable with regular contractions every 3–4 minutes. The FHR baseline is 135 with moderate variability. Her cervix is 6 cm dilated, completely effaced, with a bulging bag of water and fetus in vertex presentation.

Which of the following is your best course of management?

A) Administer corticosteroids.
B) Administer tocolytics.
C) Initiate GBS prophylaxis.
D) Discharge her to home until she is in active labor.
E) A, B, and C.

Discussion

The correct answer is "C." GBS prophylaxis is indicated for preterm delivery if GBS status is unknown. Appropriate antibiotics include penicillin or ampicillin, or alternative intravenous agent if the patient has a penicillin allergy. For corticosteroid administration (24–34 weeks), 35 2/7 weeks gestation is outside of the window. Given the gestational age (>34 weeks), advanced cervical dilation, and high likelihood of imminent delivery, tocolysis should be avoided.

HELPFUL TIP: Indications for GBS prophylaxis: (1) GBS screen positive during current pregnancy; (2) GBS bacteriuria anytime during current pregnancy; (3) prior history of giving birth to a neonate with GBS disease; (4) unknown GBS status **plus** fever, preterm labor, or prolonged rupture of membranes. No GBS prophylaxis is indicated in women who are **culture negative** with fever, preterm labor, or prolonged rupture of membranes.

HELPFUL TIP: The risk for recurrent premature delivery in subsequent pregnancies is about 15%. 17α-Hydroxyprogesterone caproate significantly reduces the incidence of preterm birth when started at 16–20 weeks.

Objective: Did you learn to . . .

- Describe indications for GBS prophylaxis?

QUICK QUIZ: PRETERM BIRTH

Risk factors for preterm birth include each of the following EXCEPT:

A) Multiple gestation pregnancy.
B) Maternal bacteriuria.
C) Maternal history of preterm contractions, with term birth.
D) Maternal smoking.
E) Maternal hypertension.

Discussion

The correct answer is "C." While preterm contractions are concerning, a maternal history of preterm contractions with term birth does not increase the risk of preterm delivery in a subsequent pregnancy. Multiple gestations, history of preterm birth, smoking, cocaine use, asymptomatic bacteriuria, and hypertension are all risk factors for preterm birth.

CASE 6

A 37-year-old G3 P0111 (full term, preterm, abortions, living children) presents for routine obstetric care at 10 weeks gestation. Her second pregnancy was complicated by severe preeclampsia at 35 weeks requiring induction of labor and magnesium sulfate therapy. Her past medical history is uncomplicated. Her blood pressure is 132/86, urine protein is negative, and physical exam is unremarkable. Uterine size is consistent with dates and fetal heart tones are auscultated. The patient wonders if she will deliver early and need that "magnesium medicine" again.

You counsel her that her risk of recurrent severe preeclampsia is in the range of:

A) <5%.
B) 20–30%.
C) 50–60%.
D) >90%.

Discussion

The correct answer is "B." The risk of recurrence of preeclampsia is affected by both gestational age at diagnosis and the severity of preeclampsia. Preeclampsia at an early gestational age or preeclampsia that is severe increases the risk of recurrence. The overall recurrence risks are estimated at less than 10% for mild preeclampsia and greater than 20% for severe preeclampsia. Risk factors for preeclampsia include young maternal age, advanced maternal age, diabetes, and chronic hypertension, among many others.

* *

The patient would like to do anything reasonable to prevent preeclampsia again.

In addition to obtaining baseline laboratory evaluation (CBC, AST, ALT, creatinine, 24-hour urine for protein) to aid in early diagnosis, you recommend the following therapy:

A) Low-sodium diet.
B) Diuretic for hypertension and edema.
C) Aspirin 81 mg daily.
D) Subcutaneous heparin therapy at prophylactic doses.
E) None of the above.

Discussion

The correct answer is "E." There is currently no approved therapy to reduce the risk of preeclampsia in a subsequent pregnancy. Management includes early identification of patients with preeclampsia. The diagnosis of preeclampsia can often be challenging, so the additional knowledge of liver, renal, and platelet function at the beginning of pregnancy can help clarify the diagnosis, especially in someone with chronic hypertension.

* *

Because of her age (37), the patient also inquires about her risk for delivering a baby with Down syndrome.

What is her estimated risk of a Down syndrome baby with this pregnancy?

A) 1/9000.
B) 1/1200.
C) 1/150.
D) 1/12.

Discussion

The correct answer is "C." The risk of Down syndrome begins to rise rapidly at age 35, with an estimated risk of 1/250 at age 35, 1/150 at age 37, and 1/70 at age 40.

* *

After hearing her age-related risk for Down syndrome, the patient asks about what tests she should have to screen for Down syndrome.

You counsel her regarding various tests and offer:

A) First trimester triple screening (PAPP-A, hCG, and nuchal lucency).
B) Chorionic villus sampling (CVS).
C) Amniocentesis.
D) Second trimester quadruple screening (hCG, maternal serum alpha fetal protein [MSAFP], estriol, inhibin-A).
E) All of the above.

Discussion

The correct answer is "E." All patients should be offered first trimester screening, and if declined, they should be offered second trimester quadruple screening. Because of her advanced age (>35 years at the time of delivery), the patient should be offered CVS and amniocentesis as well. Patients should understand that the first and second trimester screening tests are just that—**screening methods**. However, both CVS and amniocentesis can diagnose Down syndrome, in addition to other chromosomal abnormalities. CVS is typically completed between 10 and 13 weeks gestation, whereas amniocentesis is performed after 15 weeks. Both are invasive procedures, which carry risks, including pregnancy loss, rupture of membranes, and fetal injury.

* *

The patient undergoes first trimester screening, which decreases her Down syndrome risk to 1/800. She declines an amniocentesis. You draw her MSAFP only at 17 weeks, because you know that the first trimester screening does not evaluate for neural tube defects. The AFP is normal. She subsequently undergoes diabetes screening with a 1-hour post-50-g glucose test, which shows a glucose level of 170 mg/dL.

The next step is:

A) Order a 3-hour glucose tolerance test.
B) Set up diabetes teaching and a consult with a nutritionist/dietician.
C) Start glyburide.
D) Start insulin.
E) All of the above.

Discussion

The correct answer is "A." The 1-hour 50-g glucose load (Glucola) test is a screening test for gestational diabetes. Since hers is $\geq$140 mg/dL, it is considered a positive screen (see accompanying "Helpful Tip"). The next step is to perform a more specific test, which is the 3-hour glucose tolerance test, utilizing a 100-g glucose load.

> HELPFUL TIP: The cutoff for the 1-hour 50-g glucose load (Glucola) test is either $\geq$130 mg/dL or $\geq$140 mg/dL, and either is currently acceptable. This test is the most commonly used screening method in the United States. The International Association of Diabetes in Pregnancy Study Group has proposed new screening guidelines for gestational diabetes. These would be more aggressive, including universal screening (with fasting glucose or A_{1c}) at the initial visit and a glucose level 2 hours after a 75-g glucose load in the second trimester that would be used for screening and diagnosis. As of 2011, the ADA endorsed this method of screening but ACOG had not.

* *

The patient completes her glucose tolerance test with values of:

Fasting: 92 mg/dL
1 hour: 194 mg/dL
2 hour: 169 mg/dL
3 hour: 148 mg/dL

The next step in management is:

A) Continue routine prenatal care.
B) Set up diabetes teaching and a consult with a nutritionist/dietician.
C) Start glyburide.
D) Start insulin.

Discussion

The correct answer is "B." The recommended upper limit of normal serum glucose levels for the 3-hour glucose tolerance test are:

- Fasting: 95 mg/dL.
- 1 hour: 180 mg/dL.
- 2 hour: 155 mg/dL.
- 3 hour: 140 mg/dL.

If a patient has two or more glucose levels that are above these, she is diagnosed with gestational diabetes (GODM). Your patient fails on three of four of her results. The recommendation is to initiate dietary modifications including carbohydrate restriction with frequent blood sugar monitoring. Insulin should be started only if the patient fails to control her diabetes with dietary changes. Some practitioners are using glyburide in GODM, but this is not FDA approved.

* *

The patient is seen for her 32-week visit and her fundal height is only 28 cm (which surprises you, given her diagnosis of gestational diabetes!). She has been compliant with the dietary changes and her blood sugars are usually 80s fasting and 120s 2-hour postprandial. She has gained 20 pounds so far in the pregnancy. You send her for an ultrasound, which reveals an infant measuring only 28 3/7 weeks gestation, weighing

1168 g (<10th percentile). Amniotic fluid volume and umbilical artery Dopplers are normal.

Appropriate follow-up includes:

A) Changing the estimated due date.
B) Scheduling an induction.
C) Repeating the ultrasound for growth in 1 week.
D) Repeating the ultrasound for growth in 3–4 weeks.

Discussion
The correct answer is "D." Current ultrasound techniques are not sensitive enough to assess growth at weekly intervals ("C"), and therefore waiting at least 3 weeks would give a better assessment of growth rate. This infant demonstrates intrauterine growth restriction. The patient had a first trimester ultrasound with her first trimester screening, which establishes her due date. **It is inappropriate to change her due date based on a 32-week ultrasound.** Initiating an induction would be inappropriate without further investigation, given the early gestational age. You could do an ultrasound at 1–2 weeks to assess amniotic fluid and umbilical Doppler but not fetal size. A nonstress test would also be indicated at this point.

* *

The patient continues with weekly nonstress tests and her ultrasound at 35 weeks reveals appropriate interval growth, but remains growth restricted at a weight of 1846 g (<10th percentile). Today her blood pressure is 146/88 and urine protein on dipstick is +1.

At this time, appropriate intervention includes:

A) Administering corticosteroids.
B) Obtaining a 24-hour urine for protein.
C) Following up with a routine appointment in 1 week.
D) Starting labetalol.
E) All of the above.

Discussion
The correct answer is "B." Given the patient's elevated blood pressure and proteinuria, you need to be concerned about recurrent preeclampsia. Urinary excretion of protein is transient, and a 24-hour urine protein level is a more accurate reflection of proteinuria and the preferred method to diagnose preeclampsia. The patient is at 35 weeks gestation (although measuring smaller), which is beyond the recommended gestation at which corticosteroids are administered. This patient must be followed up in a couple of days so that you don't miss the diagnosis of preeclampsia. Although antihypertensives such as labetalol can be utilized in pregnancy, they are not routinely initiated for mild elevations in blood pressure at later gestations.

* *

Serial blood pressure measurements in the clinic reveal no blood pressures greater than 146/88. Her nonstress test is reactive. The patient is sent home to collect her 24-hour urine and returns in 2 days. Her blood pressure is now 148/90 and she has trace protein on urine dipstick. The 24-hour urine returns at 180 mg (her baseline 24-hour urine protein at the beginning of the pregnancy was 116 mg). She denies any headache, visual changes, nausea, or abdominal pain.

Your diagnosis is:

A) Gestational hypertension.
B) Mild preeclampsia.
C) Severe preeclampsia.
D) Acute renal failure.

Discussion
The correct answer is "A." She now has two blood pressure readings greater than 140/90 and more than 6-hour apart, which satisfies the criteria for hypertension. Given that this elevation in blood pressure started after 20 weeks gestation, it is likely pregnancy related. She does not have protein >300 mg in a 24-hour urine collection, so she does not meet that diagnostic criterion for mild preeclampsia. Nor does she qualify for severe preeclampsia. Criteria for mild and severe preeclampsia are outlined in Table 15–1.

* *

She returns to the office for her appointment 5 days later, after having felt well over the weekend. However, today she developed a headache. Her blood pressure is 166/112 and her urine dipstick reveals 3+ protein.

Your next step is to:

A) Start oral labetalol and see the patient back in 2 days for a blood pressure check.
B) Repeat the 24-hour urine for protein.
C) Admit to labor and delivery for blood work and monitoring, with plans to move toward delivery.
D) Administer corticosteroids.

Table 15–1 PREECLAMPSIA CRITERIA

Criteria for preeclampsia

- Proteinuria ≥300 mg in a 24-hour specimen AND
- Systolic blood pressure of 140 mm Hg or higher OR
- Diastolic blood pressure of 90 mm Hg or higher that occurs after 20 weeks of gestation in a woman with previously normal blood pressure

Criteria for severe preeclampsia

The above listed criteria for preeclampsia are met plus one or more of the following:

- Severe hypertension (systolic blood pressure >160 mm Hg or diastolic blood pressure >110 mm Hg). BP must be obtained on two occasions at least 6 hours apart while the patient is on bed rest.
- Proteinuria of 5 g or higher in a 24-hour urine specimen
- Oliguria
- Cerebral or visual disturbances, including headache
- Pulmonary edema
- Epigastric pain or right upper quadrant pain
- Impaired liver function
- Thrombocytopenia
- Fetal growth restriction

Discussion

The correct answer is "C." The clinical picture is now developing into severe preeclampsia (headache, systolic BP >160, diastolic BP >110, and 3+ proteinuria). The patient needs to be admitted for further monitoring of blood pressure and symptoms. In addition, blood work should be obtained for CBC and liver and renal function. Starting oral labetalol would treat the patient's hypertension, but this step alone is not prudent for a patient who probably has severe preeclampsia. The 24-hour urine protein collection may be helpful in meeting the technical criteria to diagnose preeclampsia and can be done during admission; however, the results would not change the immediate management of the patient. The patient is at 36 weeks gestation, and corticosteroids are not indicated.

HELPFUL TIP: The blood pressure can be controlled with labetalol or hydralazine: avoid nitroprusside. The down side of BP control is that it reduces placental flow. And, treated BP has no effect on the course of pre-eclampsia. Therefore, treat BP only if >160/100 **or** the patient is having end-organ symptoms.

* *

You admit her to the hospital. Repeat blood pressure is 164/98 and urine dipstick shows 3+ protein. Her cervix is soft, 2 cm dilated, 50% effaced, with fetus vertex at −2 station.

What is the most appropriate intervention at this point?

A) Begin induction for vaginal delivery.
B) Start magnesium sulfate.
C) Prepare for a cesarean delivery in case it is needed.
D) All of the above.

Discussion

The correct answer is "D." All of these options are important to consider at this time. Induction with oxytocin and treatment of preeclampsia with magnesium are appropriate at this point. Obstetrical backup should be involved earlier rather than later unless you possess the skill to do the cesarean section yourself.

HELPFUL TIP: Delivery of the baby (baby and placenta, really) is the ultimate treatment for preeclampsia and should be affected as soon as feasible when the mother's condition demands it.

* *

You begin magnesium sulfate for the preeclampsia and oxytocin for induction. The induction proceeds without incident, and she delivers a viable male infant.

How long will you continue the magnesium sulfate?

A) Until delivery.
B) For 12 hours after delivery.
C) For 24 hours after delivery.
D) Until the urine protein dipstick is negative.
E) Until discharge.

Discussion

The correct answer is "C." Treatment should be continued for 24 hours following delivery.

HELPFUL TIP: Monitor deep tendon reflexes, level of consciousness, and urine output for all patients on magnesium. Turn off the magnesium infusion if signs of toxicity emerge (e.g., decreased mental status, hyporeflexia) or if the patient is at risk for impending toxicity (e.g., from renal failure).

Objectives: Did you learn to . . .

- Screen for, diagnose and manage gestational diabetes?
- Evaluate, diagnose, and manage hypertension in pregnancy?
- Define and manage preeclampsia?
- Identify intrauterine growth restriction?

CASE 7

Now, you have to rush from L&D back to clinic (this never happens, right?) where you meet a 31-year-old woman for pre-pregnancy counseling. She has a history of stage I hypertension and a heart murmur. She has dyspnea when climbing stairs but performs normal activities of daily living with minimal difficulty. She takes lisinopril 10 mg daily for her blood pressure. On physical examination, heart rate is 82 bpm and blood pressure is 138/90 mm Hg. Height is 5′6″ and weight is 160 lb. She appears well.

Regarding the management of her chronic hypertension during pregnancy, which is the most appropriate next step?

A) Discontinue lisinopril and begin methyldopa and recheck blood pressure in 2 weeks.
B) Increase lisinopril to 20 mg daily and recheck blood pressure in 2 weeks.
C) Make no changes at this time.
D) Discontinue lisinopril; recheck blood pressure in 2 weeks.
E) Either A or D is correct.

Discussion

The correct answer is "E." ACE inhibitors are contraindicated in pregnancy; therefore, a woman contemplating pregnancy should discontinue the medication or replace it with a safer alternative. In fact, for a woman capable of conceiving, ACE inhibitor use is discouraged unless no better alternative exists. Women with chronic hypertension, which is mild (systolic blood pressure 140–160 mm Hg), have a low risk for cardiovascular complications during pregnancy and can be managed with nondrug therapy. In 2 weeks, when she visits, if she is hypertensive, select a medication regarded as safe during pregnancy; methyldopa, nifedipine, or labetalol would be preferred. You could start this at the current visit while discontinuing the ACE.

Which of the following statements about cardiovascular physiology in pregnancy is *INCORRECT*?

A) Blood volume and cardiac output increase by approximately 50% during pregnancy.
B) Heart rate increases by 10–20 beats per minute, peaking in the third trimester.
C) Systemic arterial pressure increases during the first trimester, reaches a peak in midpregnancy, and remains at that level until labor and delivery.
D) Left ventricular ejection fraction remains constant or increases slightly throughout pregnancy.
E) A temporary rise in venous return immediately following delivery may lead to a substantial rise in left ventricular filling pressure and cardiac decompensation in women with certain types of heart disease.

Discussion

The correct answer is "C." Systemic arterial pressure decreases during the first trimester, reaches a nadir during the second trimester, and returns to prepregnancy levels in the third trimester. The other statements are true. Answer "E" should receive special mention. Immediately following delivery, relief of caval compression may cause a rise in venous return, despite blood loss, leading to clinical deterioration in some women with heart disease.

Objectives: Did you learn to . . .

- Manage stage I hypertension during pregnancy?
- Recognize normal cardiac physiological changes associated with pregnancy?

CASE 8

Enough OB for a while. You are seeing a 28-year-old female whose LMP was approximately 7 days ago. She is complaining of vaginal bleeding and states that she is going through one pad every 20 minutes. Needless to say she is concerned. She is not using anything for contraception. Her vital signs and exam are unremarkable except for blood at the os.

After ruling out pregnancy and assuring that her H&H are stable, what is your next step?

A) Fresh frozen plasma.
B) Medroxyprogesterone 10 mg a day for 10 days.
C) DDAVP to maximize platelet function.
D) Observation: nonintervention is the best policy if the H&H are normal.

Discussion

The correct answer is "B." This patient likely has dysfunctional uterine bleeding. One popular regimen is medroxyprogesterone 10 mg/day for 10 days. This should be followed by a withdrawal bleed. This regimen can be repeated for the first 10 days of the next 3 months. Other options include starting a monophasic OCP (three pills twice a day for 1 day, two pills twice a day for 1 day, one pill twice a day for 1 day and then finish out the pack). Conjugated estrogens are a third option.

The most common side effect of medroxyprogesterone in this dose includes:

A) Bone marrow suppression.
B) Thromboembolic disease.
C) Depression.
D) Sore breasts.

Discussion

The correct answer is "C." Many women will become depressed when taking this dose of medroxyprogesterone. They should be made aware of this ahead of time. The major side effect of the OCP regimen is nausea and vomiting. The OCP regimen should be given with an antiemetic.

> HELPFUL TIP: You will see multiple regimens of medroxyprogesterone for this indication depending on the source; 10 mg/day is one of the most common.

Other causes of this patient's bleeding could include all of the following EXCEPT:

A) Hypothyroidism.
B) Von Willebrand disease.
C) Prolactinoma.
D) Parathyroid disease.
E) Uterine cancer.

Discussion

The correct answer is "D." All of the remaining can cause abnormal bleeding. Obviously, uterine cancer would be unlikely in a 28-year-old. Evaluation of the other causes of bleeding is premature: see if you can fix it first with one of the regimens noted above. If abnormal bleeding persists or recurs, further evaluation is indicated. Other sources of bleeding include a submucosal fibroid, a polyp, or other bleeding disorder.

Objective: Did you learn to . . .

- Evaluate a patient with dysfunctional uterine bleeding?

CASE 9

A 37-year-old G3 P1112 (full term, preterm, abortions, living children) presents for an annual gynecologic exam and has questions regarding contraception. She is wondering if she is a candidate for an intrauterine device (IUD).

All of the following are contraindications to IUD placement EXCEPT:

A) Pregnancy.
B) Acute pelvic infection.
C) Undiagnosed vaginal bleeding.
D) History of chlamydia infection.

Discussion

The correct answer is "D." Although active cervicitis and acute pelvic inflammatory disease (PID) are contraindications to placement of an IUD, a prior Chlamydia infection does not exclude a patient from obtaining an IUD. Undiagnosed vaginal bleeding can be a sign of either endometritis or structural abnormalities of the uterine cavity, which must be addressed prior to considering an IUD. If you chose "A," some goons from the Board are coming to relieve you of your certification.

* *

Your patient has none of these contraindications, and she would like to proceed with the IUD. Her friends have told her that all IUDs cause abortions, and she is unsettled by this idea.

The mechanism of action of IUDs (copper or progesterone) is:

A) Abortifacient.
B) Causes a sterile inflammatory reaction to a foreign body.

C) Impairs sperm transport from the cervix to the fallopian tube.
D) B and C.
E) All of the above.

Discussion

The correct answer is "D." Studies detecting levels of hCG reveal that this hormone is not present in IUD users during the luteal phase. Thus, the IUD is NOT an abortifacient. Studies suggest that the mechanism of action of IUDs includes interference with sperm transport from the cervix to the fallopian tube, inhibition of sperm capacitation or survival, and endometrial inflammatory changes that inhibit implantation.

HELPFUL TIP: Compared with a traditional copper IUD, the progesterone-releasing Mirena® offers the benefit of immediate resumption of menses and fertility following discontinuation. However, the progesterone-releasing IUD is approved for only 5 years of contraception versus 10 years for the copper IUD.

* *

After all of that counseling (that you can't bill for), her husband undergoes a vasectomy. During a routine appointment 2 years later, she complains of worsening menorrhagia. She denies intermenstrual spotting. She has not noticed any lightheadedness or dizziness, but does complain of generalized fatigue. On physical exam, you find a normal sized thyroid and an enlarged, irregular uterus measuring 10–12 weeks in size. There are no distinct adnexal masses, but this is somewhat difficult to discern due to the irregular uterus.

Your initial workup in this 39-year-old female should include all of the following EXCEPT:

A) CBC.
B) TSH.
C) CA-125.
D) Pelvic ultrasound.

Discussion

The correct answer is "C." A CBC will provide information regarding the hematocrit (and therefore the level of anemia) and platelet count—important information for someone with heavy menstrual bleeding. TSH will screen for hypothyroidism, which is a common cause of menorrhagia in a 39-year-old female. A pelvic ultrasound will aid in the evaluation of the mass palpated on examination and characterize the location and size of any uterine fibroids that may contribute to the bleeding; it will also evaluate for any adnexal masses. CA-125 is a nonspecific tumor marker that has a high false-positive rate in premenopausal women. Thus, CA-125 is not recommended as a screening test for ovarian cancer. It can be used as an adjunct to pelvic ultrasound when a complex adnexal mass is identified.

* *

The patient returns in 2 weeks following her ultrasound. Her hematocrit was 31% (indices are consistent with iron-deficiency anemia), platelets 195,000, and TSH 2.8 mU/L (nL). The ultrasound reveals a uterus measuring 12 × 8 × 6 cm, with multiple small intramural fibroids measuring less than 2 cm in diameter. There is one subserosal, pedunculated fibroid measuring 3.5 cm at the fundus.

What is the most appropriate initial management?

A) Expectant management and reassurance.
B) Nonsteroidal anti-inflammatory drugs (NSAIDs).
C) Gonadotropin-releasing hormone (GnRH) agonists.
D) Blood transfusion.
E) Hysterectomy.

Discussion

The correct answer is "B." Most fibroids are asymptomatic, although the most common symptom associated with leiomyomata (fibroids) is abnormal bleeding. This patient's fibroids are not impinging on the uterine cavity but may be contributing minimally to the patient's menorrhagia. Given the presence of anemia, the menorrhagia should be treated in this case. Initial treatment of menorrhagia may include NSAIDs that inhibit prostaglandin synthesis in appropriate doses. NSAIDs have been shown to reduce menstrual blood loss by 30–50% in women with menorrhagia. GnRH agonists may be utilized to produce a medical menopause. However, they are expensive, and long-term usage is associated with significant side effects. Hysterectomy is the definitive treatment for leiomyomata in symptomatic women who have completed childbearing. The mortality associated with hysterectomy is approximately 1/1,000, however. It is generally reserved for women who have failed medical management or have symptoms or signs related to fibroid size.

* *

You start an NSAID. She responds moderately well. You add an OCP, which adequately controls her symptoms. If the patient had not responded to medical therapy, might consider referral to a gynecologist for potential surgical therapy.

What other characteristic(s) would have prompted evaluation for surgery?

A) Prolapsing fibroid through the cervix.
B) 5-cm submucosal myoma protruding 50% into the uterine cavity.
C) Rapidly enlarging uterus.
D) 20-week sized uterus and pelvic pressure.
E) All of the above.

Discussion

The correct answer is "E." A fibroid prolapsing through the cervix has a potential for necrosis and infection and may require surgical removal. A submucosal myoma, especially one that distorts the uterine cavity, can contribute to menorrhagia. A rapidly enlarging uterus would be concerning for a uterine malignancy and would require further investigation. Larger uterine fibroids are more likely to contribute to symptoms of pelvic pressure and pain, which may only respond to surgical correction.

* *

The patient returns in 1 year for her annual exam, and her pelvic exam is unchanged. However, she expresses concern that these fibroids could become cancerous.

What is the risk of uterine malignancy (leiomyosarcoma) in a patient with fibroids?

A) <1%.
B) 5–10%.
C) 40–50%.
D) 90–95%.

Discussion

The correct answer is "A." The estimated incidence of leiomyosarcoma discovered at the time of surgery for fibroids is less than 1%. A leiomyosarcoma is a malignant tumor that does **not** arise from preexisting benign leiomyomata. Leiomyosarcomas typically arise in the fifth or sixth decade of life and arc usually associated with abnormal bleeding or a rapidly enlarging uterus.

Objectives: Did you learn to . . .

- Treat menorrhagia?
- Describe management principles for uterine leiomyomas?
- Recognized contraindications to IUD use?

CASE 10

A 20-year-old nulligravid female presents for evaluation of irregular menstrual cycles. Her past medical history is uncomplicated. Her gynecologic history is remarkable for menarche at age 12 years, irregular menses occurring every 21–40 days, and lasting 5 days, **with last menstrual period 6 months ago.** Her exam reveals no abnormal hair growth, no acne, normal Tanner stage V breast development, normal external genitalia and cervix, with a slightly enlarged uterus at 10 weeks size, and no adnexal masses.

What is the first test you should order?

A) Pelvic ultrasound.
B) Serum prolactin level.
C) Urine hCG.
D) Serum FSH.
E) Serum TSH.

Discussion

The correct answer is "C." Amenorrhea may be either primary or secondary and is defined as the absence of menarche by 16 years (primary amenorrhea) or the absence of periods for 3 cycles or 6 months in a woman who previously had menses (secondary amenorrhea). Pregnancy is the most common cause of secondary amenorrhea and thus must always be ruled out. After pregnancy has been excluded, the diagnostic focus is on differentiating between anatomic cause, ovarian failure, and endocrine abnormalities. The other tests may be done at some point, but a pregnancy test is first.

* *

The urine pregnancy test is positive. Because of her irregular menses, you schedule her in 1–2 weeks for a vaginal ultrasound to confirm her gestational age.

However, she calls your nurse in 3 days with vaginal spotting and lower pelvic cramping.

The most important diagnosis to confirm or exclude is:

A) Spontaneous abortion.
B) Incomplete abortion.
C) Inevitable abortion.
D) Ectopic pregnancy.
E) Twin gestation.

Discussion

The correct answer is "D." Ectopic pregnancy is the leading cause of pregnancy-related death during the first trimester in the United States. Risk factors for ectopic pregnancy include prior PID, prior ectopic pregnancy, and prior tubal or other pelvic surgery. Spontaneous, incomplete, inevitable, threatened, and missed abortions (or miscarriages) are terms to describe pregnancy loss occurring before 20 weeks. Each can result in significant maternal morbidity (including hemorrhage and infection) or death.

Which of the following tests is/are next in the management of this patient?

A) Progesterone level.
B) Serum quantitative beta-hCG.
C) Hematocrit, blood type, and screen.
D) Pelvic ultrasound.
E) All of the above.

Discussion

The correct answer is "E." "A," progesterone level, helps to assess the viability of the pregnancy. A progesterone level <5 ng/mL is nonreassuring (85% spontaneous abortion, 14% ectopic pregnancy), and a level >25 ng/mL is reassuring (<2% ectopic pregnancies). Two serum quantitative beta-hCGs obtained 48 hours apart help assess viability. A rise in level >66% will occur in 85% of normal pregnancies, but only 17% of ectopic pregnancies. Transvaginal ultrasounds should be able to detect an intrauterine pregnancy at hCG levels of 1500–2000 IU. With hCG levels below 1500 IU, an ultrasound is often still helpful for identifying an adnexal mass and potential ectopic pregnancy. A blood type and screen and hematocrit are important to evaluate for Rh status and anemia and prepare for transfusion should the hemorrhage be significant.

* *

Upon presentation, the patient has normal vitals and appears clinically stable. The blood work returns with a hematocrit of 38% and blood type A negative, **antibody screen positive for anti-D**. The hCG level is 5500 IU and progesterone is 18 ng/mL. She has not received any treatment for this bleeding prior to coming to your office.

While waiting for her ultrasound, you counsel her regarding her blood work, which indicates:

A) She should receive RhoGAM immediately, given that she is Rh negative.
B) She has previously been exposed to the D antigen and has developed antibodies.
C) This infant is D antigen positive.
D) She should receive RhoGAM only after confirming that she has an intrauterine pregnancy.

Discussion

The correct answer is "B." Rh "negative" or "positive" refers to the D antigen, as this is the antigen that is responsible for most cases of Rh sensitization. RhoGAM, or anti-D immune globulin, is used to prevent the development of Rh-D antibodies. If Rh-D antibodies are already present (i.e., the patient has already been sensitized), RhoGAM is not effective. This is why options "A" and "D" are incorrect. This patient has evidence of antibodies and has previously been exposed to the Rh-D antigen. "C" is incorrect because not enough time has elapsed with her current bleeding to have induced antibody production to the D antigen. Without RhoGAM, 17% of mothers become sensitized. RhoGAM is recommended with ectopic pregnancies, spontaneous abortions, induced abortions, threatened abortions, amniocentesis, antepartum hemorrhage, and routinely at 28 weeks gestation for Rh-D-negative women who are not sensitized.

HELPFUL TIP: If the Rh-D-negative woman is positive for D antibody, either she has previously been exposed to the D antigen and mounted a response or she was given anti-D immune globulin during the previous 12 weeks (and it is still present).

* *

The patient returns after her ultrasound, which reveals an intrauterine pregnancy measuring 6 weeks, 5 days gestation with cardiac activity at 110 beats per minute. The laboratory staff called you to let you know that the antibody screen was in error, and in fact the patient is A negative, antibody screen *negative*. Therefore, you administer RhoGAM.

You counsel the patient that her diagnosis at this time is:

A) Threatened abortion.
B) Missed abortion.
C) Complete abortion.
D) Ectopic pregnancy.
E) All remain in the differential.

Discussion

The correct answer is "A." Threatened abortion is defined as any vaginal bleeding in the first trimester or up to 20 weeks gestation, which accompanies a **currently** viable intrauterine pregnancy with a closed cervix. A missed abortion is retention of nonviable products of conception in utero for several weeks. A complete abortion indicates the pregnancy and all products of conception have passed from the uterus.

* *

Over the next 2 days, her cramping and bleeding increase and she passes tissue (complete abortion). The patient is somewhat anxious regarding her fertility and is concerned that she may have something "wrong" with her that led to the miscarriage.

What is the most likely etiology of this miscarriage?

A) Uterine anomalies.
B) Maternal infection.
C) Undiagnosed maternal diabetes.
D) Embryonic chromosomal abnormality.
E) Bad karma or mistakes in a past life.

Discussion

The correct answer is "D." Approximately 50% of first trimester spontaneous miscarriages are due to chromosomal abnormalities. Some of these occur prior to clinical recognition of the pregnancy and will go unrecognized by the patient. All of the others can be responsible for a first trimester miscarriage as well but are less common.

HELPFUL TIP: The rate of spontaneous abortion increases with advancing maternal age. For women younger than 20 years with recognized pregnancies, the rate of spontaneous abortion is about 12%; the rate increases to 26% in women older than 40 years.

The next step in the care of this patient is:

A) Hysterosalpingogram.
B) Gonorrhea and chlamydia cultures.
C) Glucose screening.
D) Paternal chromosome testing.
E) Counseling and reassurance.

Discussion

The correct answer is "E." Evaluation to determine the cause of this patient's pregnancy loss is not recommended. In general, evaluation is not recommended for a single first-trimester spontaneous loss if the woman is otherwise healthy. Patients with two or more *consecutive* spontaneous pregnancy losses are candidates for an evaluation to determine the etiology.

Objectives: Did you learn to . . .

- Maintain a high degree of suspicion for pregnancy in a patient presenting with secondary amenorrhea?
- Identify causes of first trimester bleeding?
- Define terminology used in spontaneous abortion (e.g., missed, completed, and threatened)?
- Manage early pregnancy loss?
- Describe Rh-D isoimmunization and its management?

CASE 11

You are now assuming care of a 28-year-old G3 P2002 at 38 3/7 weeks. Her pregnancy has been uncomplicated. On examination, you note her blood pressure is 102/66, urine dipstick is negative for protein and glucose, fetal heart tones are 154 beats per minute, and the fundal height is 44 cm. In reviewing her antepartum record, you note that her previous babies weighed 8.8 and 9.6 pounds at delivery. She has no history of shoulder dystocia. During this pregnancy, her lab results have been normal, and her 1-hour post-Glucola blood glucose was 127 mg/dL at 28 weeks.

Noting that she has a size-date discrepancy, what is your next step in the evaluation and management of this patient?

A) 3-hour glucose tolerance test.
B) Nonstress test.
C) Fetal ultrasound with amniotic fluid index.
D) Immediate induction of labor.
E) Contraction stress test (CST).

Discussion

The correct answer is "C." Size-date discrepancy can be caused by numerous maternal–fetal factors. Given the patient's history, the likely etiologies are either fetal macrosomia or polyhydraminos. Additionally, her body habitus could render the fundal height measurement inaccurate (her weight is not noted). To best determine the etiology, an ultrasound with amniotic fluid index is warranted. A 3-hour glucose tolerance test is not indicated since her screening test (1-hour post-Glucola test) was normal. A nonstress test may be warranted depending on the outcome of the fetal ultrasound and amniotic fluid index. However, if growth and fluid were normal, a nonstress test would not be indicated. The CST is utilized to assess fetal well-being in utero. A CST is done by administering oxytocin to induce contractions and observing the resulting fetal heart rate tracing. If the fetal growth and fluid are normal, a CST is not warranted at this time.

> HELPFUL TIP: Controversy surrounds the issue of induction for fetal macrosomia. Induction has not been shown to improve maternal or fetal outcomes.

Risk factors for fetal macrosomia include all of the following EXCEPT:

A) Gestational age.
B) Maternal smoking.
C) Excessive maternal weight gain.
D) Multiple prior gestations.
E) Macrosomia in a prior infant.

Discussion

The correct answer is "B." Maternal smoking is associated with restricted fetal growth. All of the others are associated with macrosomia. Additionally, male fetus and high maternal birth weight are associated with macrosomia.

* *

Ultrasound findings demonstrate a fetus in the vertex presentation with an estimated fetal weight of 4200 g (9.2 pounds) and an amniotic fluid index of 12.6 cm (normal). You check her cervix and note that she is 1 cm dilated, 50% effaced, with vertex at 0 station.

The optimal management at this time is:

A) Induction of labor.
B) Cesarean section.
C) Expectant management.
D) Repeat the ultrasound weekly.
E) Initiate a weight loss program.

Discussion

The correct answer is "C." Fetal macrosomia is generally defined as a birth weight greater than 4500 g. Large for gestational age implies a birth weight greater than the 90th percentile for a given gestational age (or 4000 g at delivery). Expectant management with spontaneous labor onset generally has been shown to have the best outcomes; all interventions entail an increase in fetal and maternal morbidity.

> HELPFUL TIP: According to ACOG (2009), prophylactic cesarean section should be considered for estimated fetal weight >5000 g in nondiabetic pregnancies and >4500 g in diabetic pregnancies.

> HELPFUL TIP: Maternal risk from macrosomia is primarily related to labor abnormalities and includes postpartum hemorrhage, significant vaginal lacerations, cesarean delivery, and infection.

* *

Shortly after arrival to labor and delivery, your patient has spontaneous rupture of membranes with clear fluid and requests an epidural for management of labor pain. Her cervical exam shows 5 cm dilated, 90% effaced, and 0 station. FHR baseline is 145 with moderate variability and no decelerations (a Category I tracing). **Four hours later, she is comfortable. Her cervix is unchanged.**

Appropriate intervention at this time is:

A) Induction of labor.
B) Augmentation of labor.

C) Cesarean section.
D) Expectant management.
E) Ultrasound to confirm vertex presentation.

Discussion

The correct answer is "B." Her labor has suffered from arrest of dilation and descent. At this time, the appropriate management is augmentation of labor. Induction of labor is the technical term for initiating labor before active labor onset, so "A" is incorrect. While expectant management may be acceptable at this point after counseling the patient, there is a risk of prolonged rupture of membranes and chorioamnionitis. Cesarean section at this point would be premature and unnecessary.

* *

With IV oxytocin, she proceeds to complete and after 2 hours pushing is ready to deliver. You anticipate a shoulder dystocia.

Appropriate maneuvers to reduce a shoulder dystocia include all of the following EXCEPT:

A) McRoberts maneuver (flexing the knees up against the abdomen).
B) Suprapubic pressure.
C) Fundal pressure.
D) Delivery of the posterior arm.
E) Woods corkscrew.

Discussion

The correct answer is "C." Fundal pressure may further worsen impaction of the shoulder and may result in uterine rupture—generally considered bad outcomes. All the others may be used to help relieve shoulder dystocia. Risk factors include previous shoulder dystocia, gestational diabetes, post-dates pregnancy, maternal short stature, abnormal pelvic anatomy, suspected macrosomia, protracted active phase of first stage of labor, protracted second stage of labor, and assisted vaginal delivery. The ALSO course (Advanced Life Support for Obstetrics) uses the HELPERR mnemonic: H—call for help, E—evaluate for episiotomy, L—legs flexed at the hip and knee (McRoberts maneuver), P—suprapubic pressure, E—enter to rotate fetus (Rubin II, Woods corkscrew maneuver, reverse corkscrew maneuver), R—remove posterior arm, and R—roll the patient. There is no evidence that any one maneuver is superior to another in releasing an impacted shoulder or decreasing the chance of injury. Typically, McRoberts maneuver is used first. Last resort techniques include intentional fracture of the fetal clavicle, cephalic replacement (aka, the Zavanelli maneuver—pushing the head back up into the pelvis and performing a cesarean section), and transcutaneous symphysiotomy.

* *

In the same way that carrying an umbrella prevents a thunderstorm, merely being prepared for dystocia obviates the need for special maneuvers. During her prenatal care, you discussed breastfeeding.

You told her the benefits of breastfeeding that include all the following EXCEPT:

A) Species-specific and age-specific nutrients for infants.
B) Adequate iron for premature newborns.
C) High level of immune protection from colostrum.
D) Decreased risk of breast and ovarian cancer in mothers who breastfeed.
E) Fewer illnesses while the infant is breastfed.

Discussion

The correct answer is "B." The benefits of breastfeeding for infants, women, families, and society are well documented. However, human milk may not provide adequate iron for **premature** newborns, infants whose mothers have low iron stores, and infants older than 6 months. All the other choices are correct.

> HELPFUL TIP: Breast milk should only be kept at room temperature for 6 hours. However, it is safest to refrigerate it for 2 days maximum or freeze immediately. Do not heat refrigerated breast milk in the microwave, as it will destroy valuable micronutrients. Warming in hot water is a better way of reheating.

* *

Your patient and her infant do well and are discharged home on postpartum day 2. She returns for her postpartum examination in 6 weeks. She notes incontinence of urine several times a day, especially with coughing, laughing, and sneezing. She has not experienced nocturia, dysuria, or hematuria.

These symptoms are indicative of which type of incontinence:

A) Stress incontinence.
B) Urge incontinence.
C) Overflow incontinence.
D) Functional incontinence.
E) Psychogenic incontinence.

Discussion

The correct answer is "A." Stress incontinence is the involuntary loss of urine during physical activity such as coughing, laughing, jumping, running, and sneezing. Urge incontinence is the involuntary loss of urine associated with an abrupt and strong desire to void (detrusor overactivity). Overflow incontinence is the involuntary loss of urine due to underactivity of the detrusor muscle (e.g., neurogenic bladder) or obstruction (e.g., BPH in men but this is becoming more common in women [not BPH, obstruction]). Functional incontinence is loss of urine associated with physical limitations (e.g., mobility restriction, arthritis, and dementia) in persons who have otherwise adequate bladder control. Psychogenic incontinence is a rare disorder and should be considered a diagnosis of exclusion.

Which of the following is most important to perform prior to initiating incontinence therapy?

A) Evaluate for a vaginal fistula using a dye instillation test.
B) Obtain urinalysis followed by urine culture if abnormal.
C) Refer for cystoscopy.
D) Order urodynamic studies.

Discussion

The correct answer is "B." The first step in the diagnosis of incontinence is a detailed history and physical examination. A urinalysis and urine culture should be obtained to exclude urinary tract infection. Bacteriuria should be treated because the endotoxin produced by *Escherichia coli* may trigger abnormal detrusor activity or act as an alpha-adrenergic blocker. Additional diagnostic tools may include voiding diary, stress test, pad test, cystometry, and cystourethroscopy. If there is concern for a vaginal fistula elicited by the history and physical examination, dye instillation testing may be warranted (IV dye to evaluate for a ureteral fistula, bladder instillation to evaluate for a bladder fistula).

HELPFUL TIP: Bariatric surgery (gastric banding, etc.) reduces the rate of urinary incontinence in women who qualify: Body mass index (BMI) >40 or BMI >35 + comorbidities (DM, sleep apnea, severe joint disease, weight-related cardiomyopathy).

* *

When you have completed your evaluation, you determine that she has stress urinary incontinence.

The best initial treatment option is:

A) Pelvic muscle exercises.
B) Trial of oxybutynin hydrochloride.
C) Fitting of a pessary.
D) Surgical consult.

Discussion

The correct answer is "A." Pelvic muscle exercises (e.g., Kegel exercises) facilitate improved urinary control in 40–75% of patients. The correct method can be taught during a routine pelvic examination. Pelvic physical therapy can by used to provide feedback on the patient's success with these exercises. "B" is incorrect. Oxybutynin hydrochloride is approved for detrusor instability and does not appear to be effective for stress incontinence. It has significant anticholinergic side effects. "C" is incorrect. Several vaginal pessaries have been designed with the intent of providing differential support to the urethrovesical junction for treatment of stress urinary incontinence. This is an option for many women, especially those who want to avoid surgery, but a pessary would not be the initial treatment. "D" is incorrect. Surgical correction is typically reserved until 6–12 months postpartum, as the symptoms may continue to improve during that time.

Objectives: Did you learn to . . .

- Evaluate and manage fetal macrosomia?
- Manage a delivery complicated by dystocia?
- Recognize the ramifications of labor augmentation?
- Discuss the benefits and contraindications for breast-feeding?
- Classify urinary incontinence and treat stress-type incontinence?

CASE 12

A 31-year-old nulligravid single female presents for an annual exam. She has no gynecologic concerns, and her last menstrual period was 3 weeks ago. She uses oral contraception and has regular cycles. Her examination is unremarkable. The Pap smear returns with high-grade squamous intraepithelial neoplasia (HSIL).

You notify her of the Pap smear findings and explain this indicates:

A) She has cervical cancer.
B) She needs further diagnostic testing including colposcopy and possible biopsy.
C) She needs treatment with cryotherapy or laser ablation.
D) She should have the Pap smear repeated in 3–4 months.
E) She should be enrolled in a hospice program.

Discussion

The correct answer is "B." Cervical cytology is the most effective cancer-screening program ever implemented. However, it is not a diagnostic test. The sensitivity is estimated to be about 50% (range of 30–87%), and the specificity is about 95% (range of 86–100%). Liquid based and traditional Pap smears have the same accuracy, and both types are endorsed for screening. Positive Pap smear findings require further investigation with colposcopy and directed biopsy if indicated. Given the finding of high-grade intraepithelial neoplasia on the Pap smear, repeating the Pap smear in 3 months is inappropriate. An endocervical specimen (Pap smear or endocervical curettage) will need to be performed regardless of the appearance of the ectocervix to exclude endocervical pathology. Treatment with a nonexcisional procedure (option "C") is not acceptable and premature without a biopsy to confirm the diagnosis first.

* *

You perform a colposcopy, and the cervix appears grossly normal. An endocervical Pap smear is obtained. There are acetowhite changes with areas of mosaicism at the squamocolumnar junction from the 4 o'clock to 11 o'clock position. The colposcopy is adequate.

When you discuss the cervical findings you explain that:

A) She needs a biopsy of the abnormal area.
B) Given the previous Pap smear, you recommend a "see and treat" loop electrosurgical excision procedure (LEEP).
C) The findings are consistent with dysplasia; no further therapy is warranted.
D) She needs a repeat Pap smear in 3–4 months.
E) Either A or B would be acceptable choices.

Discussion

The correct answer is "E." When acetic acid is applied to the cervix, abnormal cells tend to turn white ("acetowhite"), and as the acetowhite fades, the degree of vascularity can be appreciated. Mosaicism or mosaic changes refer to areas with increased vascularity and are indicative of abnormal changes, often dysplasia. However, "visual" findings at colposcopy are no more than suggestive, so "C" is incorrect. Biopsy of the area is warranted to obtain a tissue diagnosis. The see-and-treat approach ("B") was first advocated for use in women who were felt to be unlikely to comply with follow-up recommendations.

* *

The endocervical Pap smear is negative for dysplasia. You also performed a biopsy of the acetowhite change area, which revealed high-grade cervical intraepithelial neoplasia, in this case CIN III.

Which of the following do you recommend?

A) Hysterectomy.
B) Trachelectomy.
C) Cytological follow-up.
D) LEEP or LASER ablation.
E) 5-fluorouracil intravaginally.

Discussion

The correct answer is "D." While some patients with severe dysplasia (CIN III) may be candidates for a hysterectomy, it would be an overly aggressive approach in this 31-year-old female who has never been pregnant and may wish to conceive in the future. Additionally, women who had high-grade CIN before hysterectomy can develop recurrent vaginal dysplasia (VaIN) or cancer at the vaginal cuff. Likewise, trachelectomy (removal of the entire cervix) would be overly aggressive with no added benefit over a simple cone excision or destructive procedure. Cytological follow-up or "expectant management" is **not** recommended for high-grade dysplasia. The likelihood of regression is low, while the likelihood of persistence or progression to cancer is unacceptably high. A conization or destructive procedure would be the best recommendation in this patient. The advantage of a cone procedure is that it provides further tissue for evaluation. The use of 5-fluorouracil intravaginally is typically not recommended for initial treatment of **cervical dysplasia.** It is used instead for **vaginal dysplasia**, when the extent of disease precludes complete excision or destruction.

* *

Your patient wants to know the likelihood of regression to "normal" without treatment.

What will you counsel?

A) About 90% of CIN III lesions will become invasive cancer without aggressive treatment.
B) About one-third of CIN III lesions spontaneously regress.
C) About two-thirds of CIN III lesions spontaneously regress.
D) About 90% of CIN III lesions will remain CIN III on follow-up after 10 years.

Discussion

The correct answer is "B." About 32% of untreated CIN III lesions will spontaneously regress, while about 56% will persist and 14% will progress to invasive carcinoma.

* *

She is concerned about future childbearing if she undergoes a LEEP.

All of the following are possible complications of LEEP EXCEPT:

A) Cervical incompetence.
B) Cervical stenosis.
C) Cervical ectopy.
D) Decreased fertility.
E) Premature rupture of membranes.

Discussion

The correct answer is "C." Cervical incompetence, stenosis, decreased fertility, and premature rupture of the membranes have been identified following all types of cone procedures, including LEEP, and are estimated to occur following less than 1% of procedures. Each of these complications seems to be related to the volume of tissue removed with the procedure rather than the procedure itself. Cervical ectopy or ectopic cervical pregnancy is quite rare and has NOT been associated with cone or LEEP procedures.

* *

She undergoes treatment as recommended. The pathology reveals CIN III with margins uninvolved.

What do you counsel her about follow-up?

A) She should return for a Pap smear and pelvic exam in 1 year.
B) She should return for a Pap smear in 6 months.
C) She should return for a Pap smear in 2–3 months.
D) She should return for a colposcopy and Pap smear in 2–3 months.
E) She should just "chill"; no follow-up is indicated.

Discussion

The correct answer is "B." The current recommendations for follow-up include Pap smears every 6 months until three sequential Pap smears return as normal following treatment. Then, the patient may resume yearly cytological follow-up. If any of the Pap smears reveal atypical squamous cells (ASC) or higher grade dysplasia, the patient should undergo repeat colposcopy.

* *

At the follow-up evaluation, her cervix appears normal, without lesions or discharge. The Pap smear returns as normal, limited by absence of endocervical cells.

What is the best recommendation for management of this patient now?

A) Repeat the endocervical portion of the Pap smear at her convenience in the next month.
B) Cervical dilation and endocervical curettage.
C) Cervical dilation and endocervical Pap smear.
D) Repeat LEEP.
E) Repeat the Pap smear in 6 months.

Discussion

The answer is "A." Since the Pap smear was limited by the absence of endocervical cells, the patient should have a repeat Pap smear within the next month to exclude abnormality. The additional Pap smear would not "count" as one of the required follow-up evaluations (the Pap and repeat Pap count as one).

HELPFUL (MAYBE) TIP: The new guidelines for Pap smears are ridiculously complex and include differences based on patient age, pregnancy status, etc. Here is a quick guide, which is simplified. If you want to review the actual documents, they are available at http://www.asccp.org/consensus.shtml.

Atypical squamous cells (ASC): Does not in itself indicate dysplasia or a precancerous lesion. It may be secondary to infection or reparative changes (e.g., after pregnancy). ASC is categorized further as the following:

- **ASC-US (unknown significance):** Do human papilloma virus (HPV) testing only if >20 years old (see note below). If this is negative, repeat Pap in 12 months. If this is positive, proceed to colposcopy. If cannot do HPV testing, repeat the Pap in 6 and 12 months. If these are both negative, resume normal screening intervals.
- **ASC-H (favor high grade):** Proceed directly to colposcopy. If no CIN2 or CIN3, do repeat Pap at 6 and 12 months **or** HPV testing at 12 months. If either abnormal, repeat colposcopy. If negative, resume routine screening.
- **LGSIL/LSIL (low-grade squamous intraepithelial lesion that encompasses HPV and CIN I):** Proceed to colposcopy and endocervical Pap smear (although recommendations vary depending on patient age, pregnancy, etc.). If no CIN2 or CIN3, do repeat Pap at 6 and 12 months **or** HPV testing at 12 months. If either abnormal, repeat colposcopy. If negative, resume routine screening.
- **Pap reads HGSIL/HSIL (high-grade squamous intraepithelial lesion that encompasses CIN II, CIN III, CIS (carcinoma in situ):** Options include immediate LEEP **or** colposcopy and endocervical assessment (preferred). If no CIN2 or CIN3 is found in your biopsy specimens (from colposcopy or excision), you have the option of Pap + colposcopy every 6 months for a year or diagnostic excision of lesions. If you choose Pap + colposcopy and both the 6 and 12 month exams are normal, resume routine screening intervals.
- **AGUS (atypical glandular cells of undetermined significance):** Do endometrial sampling (Pipelle for example) + colposcopy + HPV testing. Another option is to just do endometrial **and** endocervical sampling and if this is negative to proceed to colposcopy.

Objectives: Did you learn to . . .

- Manage an abnormal Pap test?
- Recognize the indications and for colposcopy?
- Interpret colposcopic findings?
- Evaluate and manage cervical dysplasia?
- Recognize the risks and potential complications of LEEP?
- Manage the absence of endocervical cells on a Pap test?

CASE 13

You are called to the emergency department to evaluate a patient with a 2-day history of abdominal pain. She is a 24-year-old G1 P1 female whose LMP was 1 week ago. On the "1–10" scale, her pain is a "12." She is on oral contraceptives for birth control. She has "never missed a pill" and "could not possibly be pregnant." Her pain is across her lower abdomen and a little more on the right side than the left. She has felt feverish. She has had some nausea but no vomiting. She denies bowel or bladder problems. Her pain improves with acetaminophen and worsens with activity.

On examination, she appears uncomfortable but not toxic. Her temperature is 38°C, but the rest of her vitals are normal. Her abdominal examination reveals decreased bowel sounds, with tenderness to palpation primarily across the lower quadrants. She has minimal guarding and no rebound tenderness. Her pelvic examination is remarkable for cervical motion tenderness. The uterus is of normal size and consistency with no masses.

Which of the following diagnoses can be absolutely excluded from your differential at this point?

A) Ectopic pregnancy.
B) Appendicitis.
C) PID.
D) Pyelonephritis.
E) None of the above diagnoses should be excluded based on the information available.

Discussion

The correct answer is "E." The differential for lower abdominal pain in a young female includes all of the above and more. Even though your patient seems unlikely to be pregnant due to her consistent use of contraceptives and recent menses, you should not exclude pregnancy without a negative urine hCG.

* *

You obtain cultures/PCR for chlamydia and gonorrhea. The urine pregnancy test is negative ("I told you not to waste healthcare dollars—especially in this economy," your patient complains). The urinalysis is negative for nitrites and leukocytes, and the WBC is 15,600/mm^3 with an increase in bands.

What is the most appropriate next step?

A) Consult surgery and gynecology to confirm your findings.
B) Admit for IV antibiotics and IV hydration.
C) Treat as an outpatient with antibiotics and schedule follow-up for 36–48 hours.
D) Treat with IV antibiotics on an outpatient basis utilizing visiting nurse care.
E) Obtain cultures, discharge the patient, and treat based on culture results.

Discussion

The correct answer is "C." The patient's history, examination, and diagnostic tests are most consistent with PID. PID is a clinical syndrome caused by the ascent of microorganisms from the lower genital tract (e.g., vagina) to the upper genital tract (e.g., endometrium). Most cases of PID can be managed in the outpatient setting. Indications for hospitalization are listed in Table 15–2.

Table 15–2 CRITERIA FOR ADMISSION FOR THE TREATMENT OF PID

- Uncertain diagnosis
- Surgical emergencies (e.g., appendicitis) cannot be excluded
- Suspected pelvic abscesses
- Concurrent pregnancy (due to high risk of maternal mortality, fetal wastage, and preterm delivery)
- Adolescent patient with uncertain compliance with therapy
- Severe illness
- Patient cannot tolerate outpatient regimen (e.g., severe vomiting)
- Lack of response to 72 hours of treatment
- Concurrent HIV infection
- Clinical follow-up cannot be arranged within 72 hours

HELPFUL TIP: The diagnosis of PID is a **clinical** one and not laboratory based! As untreated PID has significant morbidity and mortality, empiric treatment is recommended if the patient meets the following minimal diagnostic criteria:

- Uterine/adnexal tenderness **or**
- Cervical motion tenderness **and**
- No other cause for illness identified

Other helpful (but not necessary) criteria include:

- Temperature $\geq$38°C
- WBC $\geq$10,500/mm^3
- Adnexal mass
- Laboratory evidence of gonorrhea or chlamydia infection
- Elevated C-reactive protein and/or ESR

For empiric antibiotic therapy for PID in this patient, you prescribe:

A) Amoxicillin 500 mg PO TID for 14 days.
B) Ceftriaxone 250 mg IM × 1 *plus* azithromycin 1 g.
C) Ceftriaxone 250 mg IM plus doxycycline 100 mg PO BID for 14 days.
D) A and B.
E) B and C.

Discussion

The correct answer is "C." Recommendations for treatment of PID include ceftriaxone (Rocephin) 250 mg IM ***plus*** doxycycline 100 mg PO BID for 14 (yes, 14) days. Metronidazole may be added to this regimen to cover anaerobic bacteria. **Note that single-dose azithromycin is not indicated for the treatment of PID, only for cervicitis. Thus, 14 days of doxycycline are indicated.**

The current (2011) CDC treatment guidelines for rectal, oral, cervical, or penile gonorrhea include ceftriaxone 250 mg PLUS azithromycin 1 g or 7 days of doxycycline. This is true even if the patient has ONLY gonorrhea. This is to prevent the development of resistant gonorrhea. Note also that the ceftriaxone dose has been changed from 125 to 250 mg (again, this is for an uncomplicated gonorrheal infection). Oral cefixime can be substituted for ceftriaxone but is less effective.

Note: As of July 2012 cefixime is no longer recommended leaving us with no oral regimens. We don't know if this change will make it to thc test or not.

* *

On recheck, she is vomiting her medications and requires admission. She does well and is discharged when she is tolerating oral intake and has been afebrile for 48 hours. You instruct her to finish a 14-day course of doxycycline. She presents for follow-up a week later, at which time her symptoms have completely resolved.

Which of the following is a potential consequence of PID?

A) Infertility.
B) Chronic pelvic pain.
C) Increased risk for ectopic pregnancy.
D) Recurrent PID.
E) All of the above.

Discussion

The correct answer is "E." All the choices above are potential sequelae of PID. Additionally, a tubo-ovarian abscess may develop.

HELPFUL TIP: The etiology of PID is polymicrobial, although sexually transmitted infections, predominantly gonorrhea and/or Chlamydia, are implicated in up to two-thirds of cases. Antibiotic regimens are chosen for broad coverage. The CDC no longer recommends the use of fluoroquinolones for treatment of PID/gonorrhea due to increasing resistance. And, there is ceftriaxone-resistant gonorrhea in Japan with intermediate-resistant gonorrhea in the United States.

* *

You see her next for her annual examination. She quit taking her oral contraceptive 5 months ago after separating from her husband (the jerk gave her Chlamydia, after all!). Subsequently, her periods have been irregular. She is not obese, has minimal acne, and no hirsutism or galactorrhea. Her physical examination is essentially normal.

Urine hCG is negative (you ***did*** immediately think of an hCG, didn't you?) and a serum TSH is normal.

What is the most likely etiology of the irregular cycles?

A) Anovulation.
B) Pituitary tumor.
C) Polycystic ovarian syndrome.
D) Premature ovarian failure.
E) Androgen-secreting tumor.

Discussion

The correct answer is "A." OCPs work by suppressing ovulation. Resumption of ovulation after pill cessation can take several months. In the absence of abnormal history, physical exam, or laboratory findings, the other choices are unlikely to be the etiology of the irregular cycles in this patient.

Each of the following is appropriate initial management of this patient's irregular menses, EXCEPT:

A) Expectant management.
B) Reestablishment of cycle regulation with OCPs.
C) Progestin induced withdrawal cycles.
D) Colposcopy with cervical and endometrial biopsies.

Discussion

The correct answer is "D." Anovulation is expected following OCP cessation; thus, expectant management is a reasonable option, as most people will resume regular cycling within 6 months. She could also opt to resume OCPs for cycle regulation if that is her goal. Withdrawal bleeds could be induced by cyclical progestin challenges. Colposcopy is not indicated in this patient as she has no cytologic abnormalities noted that would require follow-up with colposcopy and biopsy.

* *

The patient is reluctant to resume "the pill." You next evaluate her 8 months later. Her last period was 7 weeks before. A urine pregnancy test is positive. Given her history of PID, you request a quantitative serum beta-hCG and are considering a pelvic ultrasound to confirm intrauterine pregnancy.

What is the minimum expected increase in quantitative hCG in early gestation in a normal pregnancy?

A) 20% increase in 24 hours.
B) 66% increase in 48 hours.

C) 200% increase in 24 hours.
D) 10% increase in 48 hours.
E) 75% increase in 72 hours.

Discussion
The correct answer is "B." hCG typically doubles (increases by 100%) every 48 hours in normal gestation. The minimum increase considered to be compatible with a viable pregnancy is 66% in 48 hours.

If the quantitative serum beta-hCG is 8000 ng/mL and the pelvic ultrasound reveals no intrauterine pregnancy but a probable right tubal pregnancy (no FHR), what would be the most appropriate management option?

A) Medical management with methotrexate.
B) Laparoscopic surgery with evacuation of the products of conception.
C) Consultation with someone able to do a salpingectomy if necessary.
D) Dilation and curettage.
E) Hysterectomy.

Discussion
The correct answer is "C." An ectopic pregnancy may rupture and become a life-threatening event at any point before complete resolution. If the patient becomes hemodynamically unstable, she will need emergent surgery. Thus, an early referral for management is warranted. Medical treatment with methotrexate may be indicated but should be done under close supervision with surgical consultation available.

If the quantitative serum beta-hCG had come back at 1000 ng/mL and no ultrasound were available, how would you have counseled the patient?

A) Given the history of PID, this is most likely an ectopic pregnancy. She should abort the pregnancy at once.
B) Given the history of PID, she should remain on bed rest until a definitive diagnosis is made.
C) She should be given ectopic pregnancy and miscarriage precautions.
D) She should have an urgent surgical consultation today for exploratory laparotomy.
E) She should read the patient education material entitled "So, You Might Be Having an Ectopic Pregnancy."

Discussion
The correct answer is "C." This beta-hCG level is consistent with an early gestation given her history of irregular cycles. However, with her history of PID, she is at risk for ectopic pregnancy. Thus, she should be given ectopic pregnancy and miscarriage precautions. While a history of PID increases the risk of ectopic pregnancy by 7–10-fold, only 8% of such patients will ever have an ectopic. So, it is still highly probable that the patient has a normal intrauterine pregnancy. If you chose "E," you may also want to hand her the pamphlet entitled "So, Your Doctor Has a Horrible Bedside Manner."

* *

In reality, her quantitative serum beta-hCG is 6000 ng/mL. A pelvic ultrasound confirms a viable intrauterine pregnancy at 8 4/7 weeks gestation. She wins the ectopic lottery.

> HELPFUL TIP: Assisted reproductive technology substantially increases the risk of a heterotopic pregnancy (two pregnancies with only one inside the uterus) to about 1%, and in these patients, the rate of ectopic pregnancy is 4–8%, which is about fourfold higher than the general population. Having one ectopic pregnancy predisposes to having a subsequent one.

Objectives: Did you learn to . . .

- Evaluate a patient with pelvic pain?
- Diagnose and treat PID?
- Evaluate and treat irregular menses?
- Diagnose and manage ectopic pregnancies?

CASE 14

A 52-year-old female patient of yours presents for an annual exam and Pap smear. Her last menstrual period was 3 months ago. She has intermittent hot flashes and night sweats. Her examination is remarkable for mild vaginal atrophy. She wonders about "estrogen testing" to see if she needs hormone replacement therapy.

How will you counsel her about the role of estrogen testing?

A) Recommend against estrogen testing.
B) Recommend buccal swab testing as it is the most accurate.

C) Recommend fasting morning serum estradiol testing.
D) Recommend estrogen testing with FSH to ensure menopause status.
E) Recommend initiating annual estrogen testing after the age of 55 years.

Discussion
The correct answer is "A." In a person of the right age with symptoms consistent with menopause, no testing is recommended. Testing is only recommended if the diagnosis is unclear (e.g., a patient younger than 35). It can also be useful when a patient on OCPs presents with a symptoms suggestive of menopause. In this case, an FSH could be done after the patient has discontinued hormonal contraception for 1 week (or on the last day of her placebo pills).

* *

She jokes that you're probably getting kickbacks from the insurance company for ordering fewer tests, and then she asks, "How will you know if I'm going through menopause without an estrogen level?"

How will you counsel her about menopause and its diagnosis?

A) FSH is the definitive test.
B) There is no definitive test of menopause.
C) 6 months amenorrhea, elevated FSH, and decreased estradiol confirm the diagnosis.
D) 12 months amenorrhea, elevated FSH, and decreased estradiol are the definitive test.
E) 2 years of mood swings and hot flashes will clinch the diagnosis.

Discussion
The correct answer is "B." Menopause is a clinical syndrome characterized by the cessation of spontaneous menstrual periods along with associated symptoms of estrogen deficiency such as hot flashes, vaginal atrophy, and psychological symptoms. As such, there is no definitive test.

* *

She is concerned about menopause and wonders if she needs hormone replacement therapy.

All the following are benefits of estrogen-containing hormone therapy (HT) EXCEPT:

A) Osteoporosis prevention.
B) Decrease in colon cancer risk.
C) Decrease in hot flashes and vasomotor symptoms.
D) Decrease in stroke risk.

Discussion
The correct answer is "D." We have learned a lot about HT in postmenopausal women with data from the Women's Health Initiative. Here's a quick summary.

Proven benefits of HT are limited to the following:

- Reduced risk of osteoporosis and related fractures
- Decreased colon cancer risk (**not** seen in estrogen-only arm)
- Improvement of vasomotor symptoms such as hot flashes

HT may increase the risk of the following (variable findings):

- Breast cancer (estrogen-only arm showed a paradoxical **reduction** in risk of breast cancer)
- Myocardial infarction (estrogen-only arm showed no increase risk)
- Venous thromboembolic events
- Stroke

Only women with vasomotor symptoms appear to have improved overall quality-of-life scores with HT. Given the significant excess risks with HT usage, many practitioners now recommend short-term HT use only for vasomotor symptoms and not for osteoporosis or other purported benefits.

An absolute contraindication to use of HT is:

A) Heart disease.
B) Breast cancer.
C) Endometrial cancer.
D) Previous thromboembolic event.
E) All of the above.

Discussion
The correct answer is "D." Previous thromboembolic disease is the only **absolute** contraindication to HT. The others are **relative** contraindications. While HT is not routinely recommended for women who have heart disease or a history of breast or endometrial cancer, it may be useful in women who have significant impairment in their quality of life from vasomotor symptoms refractory to other management methods.

* *

You discuss menopause and the potential risks and benefits of HT with your patient. She decides against

HT for now, but returns in 6 months with continued amenorrhea, hot flashes, and vaginal dryness—which seems to bother her the most.

Options to treat the vaginal dryness include which of the following?

A) Systemic HT.
B) Vaginal estrogen.
C) Lubrication.
D) All of the above.

Discussion

The correct answer is "D." Systemic and local estrogen administration are both effective for treating vaginal dryness. Lubrication with vegetable oil and specifically manufactured lubricants can be effective.

How is vaginal atrophy most rapidly and *accurately* diagnosed?

A) Biopsy of vaginal mucosa.
B) Culture of vaginal swab.
C) Vaginal swab for wet mount microscopic evaluation.
D) Direct visualization of the mucosa during exam.
E) KOH prep of vaginal swab.

Discussion

The correct answer is "C." Vaginal atrophy is most easily diagnosed with microscopy. With atrophic tissue, the wet mount will reveal an abundance of basal and parabasal cells and a paucity of mature squamous epithelium. A biopsy is a bit extreme. "B" and "E" are incorrect since atrophy is not an infectious issue. "D," direct visualization, may aid in the diagnoses but is not as reliable as microscopy.

* *

She decides to try HT to reduce hot flashes.

Assuming the initial hormone replacement fails to resolve her symptoms, further options to treat symptomatic hot flashes include which of the following?

A) Increase the estrogen component.
B) Increase the progestin component.
C) Trial of an SSRI.
D) All of the above.

Discussion

The correct answer is "D." HT is the most efficacious treatment for vasomotor symptoms with almost 90% of women responding. Other options include progestins such as medroxyprogesterone (Provera) or megestrol (Megace), SSRIs, clonazepam, gabapentin (Neurontin), venlafaxine (Effexor), clonidine, exercise, and environmental modifications (e.g., thermostat settings, fans). While there is conflicting evidence for the efficacy of vitamin E and black cohosh, there is no good data to suggest that propranolol or phytoestrogens, such as soy, are effective in treating vasomotor symptoms.

Objectives: Did you learn to . . .

- Evaluate menopausal symptoms?
- Describe hormone replacement therapy, including risks, benefits, and contraindications for its use?
- Diagnose and manage atrophic vaginitis?
- Treat menopausal symptoms?

CASE 15

A 57-year-old postmenopausal patient presents for her annual examination. She is experiencing hot flashes and night sweats, as well as continued vaginal bleeding. Her medical history is otherwise unremarkable. She wants your opinion about resuming hormone replacement.

Her pelvic examination is remarkable for atrophic vaginal mucosal changes, a stenotic cervix without lesions, normal size uterus, no adnexal masses, and no masses palpable on rectovaginal examination.

All of the following are possible causes of her vaginal bleeding EXCEPT:

A) Cervical cancer.
B) Uterine polyp.
C) Polycystic ovary disease.
D) Atrophic vaginitis.
E) Endometrial cancer.

Discussion

The correct answer is "C." Polycystic ovarian disease does not cause vaginal bleeding in postmenopausal women. All the other choices are diagnostic considerations in a postmenopausal female with vaginal bleeding or spotting.

Which of the following studies should you consider obtaining?

A) Urinalysis.
B) Pap smear.
C) Endometrial biopsy.

D) Stool guaiac.
E) All of the above.

Discussion
The correct answer is "E." The patient could easily mistake the source of the bleeding; thus, it is prudent to rule out a rectal or urinary source. Cervical and endometrial evaluations are necessary to rule out gynecological pathology, such as endometrial polyp, hyperplasia, or cancer.

All of the following increase the risk of endometrial cancer EXCEPT:

A) Smoking.
B) Obesity.
C) Unopposed estrogen.
D) Diabetes.
E) Hypertension.

Discussion
The correct answer is "A." Endometrial cancer is believed to be caused by overexposure to unopposed estrogen stimulation of the endometrium. Smoking decreases luteal phase estrogen and is epidemiologically linked to a **decrease** in the risk for endometrial carcinoma (of course, this risk is offset by the other adverse health effects of smoking—go figure!). Risk factors and protective factors are listed in the Tables 15–3 and 15–4.

* *

You review your patient's test results: normal Pap smear and urinalysis, stool guaiac negative for blood, and endometrial biopsy with fragments of benign polyp.

Table 15–3 RISK FACTORS FOR ENDOMETRIAL CANCER

Advancing age
Obesity[a]
Nulliparity
Early menarche
Late menopause
Chronic anovulation (e.g., PCOS)
Unopposed exogenous estrogen use
Tamoxifen
Hypertension
Diabetes

[a]Obesity leads to increased estrogen levels from peripheral conversion of androstenedione. The presence of DM and HTN as risk factors may simply reflect the high incidence of obesity in patients with these disorders.

Table 15–4 PROTECTIVE FACTORS FOR ENDOMETRIAL CANCER[a]

Progesterone
Oral contraceptives
Cigarette smoking
Multiparity

[a]All reduce exposure to unopposed estrogens.

Over the next 3 years, she continues to have rare occurrences of vaginal spotting. She has declined further evaluation given the infrequency of the episodes. However, over the last several months, she has experienced an increase in the amount and frequency of the bleeding. Other than an interval weight gain of 27 pounds, there has been no change in her examination. Repeat endometrial biopsy reveals **complex hyperplasia with atypia,** and the pathologist cannot rule out endometrial cancer.

Of the following, the most appropriate intervention is:

A) Repeating the endometrial biopsy.
B) Performing a transvaginal ultrasound to assess endometrial thickness.
C) Starting high-dose progestin therapy.
D) Starting high-dose selective estrogen-receptor modulator therapy (e.g., tamoxifen).
E) Arrange for definitive management (hysterectomy if carcinoma found on further evaluation).

Discussion
The correct answer is "E." Her biopsy findings are highly abnormal and may indicate already existing carcinoma that was not contained in the sample examined. Referral to a gynecologist for definitive management is warranted at this time.

HELPFUL TIP: In postmenopausal women, an endometrial stripe of greater than 5 mm on ultrasound is suggestive of endometrial cancer. In the editor's opinion, this is too insensitive a test and an in-office endometrial biopsy should be done in cases of postmenopausal bleeding. Others would disagree. Ultrasound for endometrial stripe is as little as 63% sensitive when the false-positive rate is $<10\%$. If you want to be 96% sensitive, the false-positive rate is 50%.

Objectives: Did you learn to . . .

- Evaluate postmenopausal bleeding?
- Manage a patient with postmenopausal bleeding?
- Assess a patient for risk of endometrial cancer?
- Evaluate, diagnose, and manage endometrial hyperplasia?

CASE 16

A 15-year-old nulligravid female presents with her mother for evaluation of painful periods. Menarche was at age 14. Her periods are typically every 4–8 weeks and are associated with severe cramping. She has missed 1–2 days of school with each menses because of pain. She denies intercourse. She has never had a pelvic examination. Her review of systems is otherwise negative.

What is the MOST LIKELY etiology of her irregular cycles?

A) Pregnancy.
B) Endometriosis.
C) Anovulation.
D) Hyperthyroidism.
E) Imperforate hymen.

Discussion

The correct answer is "C." Dysfunctional uterine bleeding is common among adolescent girls who have reached menarche. The first few years of menstruation are often characterized by irregular cycles as a result of anovulation. Pregnancy and imperforate hymen lead to absence of menses, not irregular menses. While hyperthyroidism may lead to irregular cycles, it does not typically cause dysmenorrhea, is usually associated with other systemic complaints, and would be unusual in a patient of this age. Endometriosis may cause dysmenorrhea, but is unlikely to occur in a patient this young; most cases of endometriosis present in patients aged 20s–30s.

What is the etiology of her dysmenorrhea?

A) Prostaglandin release.
B) Streptococcal endotoxin release.
C) Estrogen release.
D) Excessive testosterone production.

Discussion

The correct answer is "A." Dysmenorrhea is the term that describes excessive pain in association with menstruation. It is the most common gynecologic compliant, affects about half of all adolescent females, and is the leading cause of periodic school absenteeism. The pathogenesis of dysmenorrhea involves excess prostaglandin release, which causes prolonged, painful uterine contractions. It can be divided in two main subtypes: primary and secondary. Primary dysmenorrhea usually starts before the age of 20 and has a tendency to occur with menarche. It is caused by prostaglandin stimulation of the myometrium. Secondary dysmenorrhea typically arises after the age of 20 and is associated with pelvic pathology or other organic disease.

* *

You perform a physical examination, revealing normal vital signs, normal weight, a benign abdomen, Tanner stage V, and no signs of androgen excess.

Which of the following is the best next step in caring for this patient?

A) Offer reassurance and observation.
B) Initiate combined hormonal contraception.
C) Initiate a GnRH agonist.
D) Prescribe a narcotic analgesic.
E) Refer for diagnostic laparoscopy.

Discussion

The correct answer is "B." OCPs offer cycle regulation and reduction in dysmenorrhea. Option "A," expectant management, is inappropriate given the severity of symptoms and availability of safe and effective treatment. A further workup is not needed at this stage, as her history is straightforward and her physical exam is reassuring, and she certainly does not need surgery now (option "E"). "C" is incorrect. GnRH agonists will induce amenorrhea, hot flashes, accelerated bone loss, are expensive, and require add-back estrogen when utilized longer than 6 months. Narcotic analgesics do not help reduce prostaglandin levels and are not appropriate for pain control in this case, so "D" is incorrect. ***Note*: Although not listed in the answers, NSAIDs are also quite effective at treating dysmenorrhea and should be considered as a first-line drug. Anecdotal evidence suggests that mefenamic acid (Ponstel) may be more effective for dysmenorrhea than other NSAIDs.** Acetaminophen is not as effective as NSAIDs.

HELPFUL TIP: The average age of menarche is 12.8 years in the United States, with the range from 10 to 15 years. Primary amenorrhea is defined as (1) the absence of menses with no secondary sexual characteristics by age 14 or (2) the absence of menses by age 16 regardless of the development of secondary sexual characteristics (or lack thereof).

* *

Your patient and her mother opt to try hormonal regulation with birth control pills. She returns for follow-up in 4 months and is doing well. She admits to being sexually active.

In addition to reviewing the use of birth control pills, she should be questioned or counseled about which of the following?

A) Knowledge of sexually transmitted diseases and use of condoms.
B) Age of her boyfriend.
C) Consensual nature of her relationship.
D) HPV vaccination.
E) All of the above.

Discussion

The correct answer is "E." Visits for contraception are great opportunities for you to discuss safe sexual practices with the patient. Such an interview should include evaluation for sexual assault, coercion, or abuse. The quadrivalent HPV vaccination (brand name Gardasil) was approved by the FDA for use in women aged 9–26 years (and now for males as well). This vaccination prevents infection by HPV types 6, 11 (which are responsible for 90% of genital warts), and types 16 and 18 (which are responsible for 70% of cervical cancer) and is administered in a series of three injections at 0, 2, and 6 months. There is also a bivalent vaccine (brand name Cervarix) that protects against HPV types 16 and 18 only and is approved for use in females aged 11–25 years. It is given as a three-injection series as well at 0, 1, and 6 months.

HELPFUL TIP: HPV is the most common viral sexually transmitted infection in the United States with point prevalence in females ranging from 26% to 64%. Many patients have serial infections with different HPV types. A two shot series may be as effective as a three shot series but has not yet been endorsed as official policy.

HELPFUL TIP: The best time to check a pregnancy test is after the first missed menses. Otherwise, you risk having a false-negative test. Even on day 1 of a missed menses, the sensitivity is only 90% (thus, patients can present with an ectopic pregnancy with a negative urine pregnancy test).

* *

You lose touch with the patient, and she discontinues her OCP. Years later when she returns for a physical examination—and you're still paying off your student loans—she complains of increasing irritability along with intermittent bloating and swelling during the week before her period each month. Although she is annoyed by these symptoms, they are not so severe as to interfere with her usual activities. Her menses now occur monthly without intermenstrual spotting or missed periods.

What is her most likely diagnosis?

A) Major depression.
B) Premenstrual dysphoric disorder (PMDD).
C) Premenstrual syndrome (PMS).
D) Polycystic ovary syndrome (PCOS).
E) Hypothyroidism.

Discussion

The correct answer is "C." PMS is a constellation of physical, emotional, and behavioral symptoms. It is cyclical in nature, occurs during the second half of the menstrual cycle (luteal phase, 7–10 days before menses), and resolves soon after menses. A symptom-free interval occurs during the first half of the cycle (follicular phase). PMDD is more severe but occurs during the same time frame as PMS. Symptoms of PMDD include labile mood, depressed mood, irritability, feelings of hopelessness, hypersomnia or insomnia, and decreased interest in usual activities. PMDD is diagnosed by DSM-IV criteria and some functional impairment must be present.

> HELPFUL TIP: Premenstrual symptoms exist on a continuum with up to 90% of women affected by minimal PMS symptoms while 10% are affected severely. This group with more severe symptoms can be categorized as having PMDD.

Each of the following is a key element of the diagnosis of PMS EXCEPT:

A) Physical symptoms of bloating, swelling, and/or fatigue.
B) Elevated luteinizing hormone to follicle stimulation hormone (LH:FSH) ratio.
C) Restriction of symptoms to the luteal phase of the menstrual cycle.
D) Exclusion of other diagnoses that may better explain the symptoms.

Discussion

The correct answer is "B." PMS is a clinical entity and no laboratory data exist to aid in diagnosis. All other options described above are correct. An elevated LH:FSH ratio of 3:1 in the face of appropriate symptoms is suggestive of PCOS.

Each of the following is a possible treatment option for PMS and PMDD EXCEPT:

A) Supportive therapy/counseling.
B) Aerobic exercise.
C) Selective serotonin reuptake inhibitors.
D) Thiazide diuretics.
E) Calcium.

Discussion

The correct answer is "D." Thiazide diuretics are not helpful in PMS or PMDD, but all of the other options are potentially useful. Treatment options that have been shown to help with PMS are listed in Table 15–5.

Objectives: Did you learn to . . .

- Evaluate concerns about menarche and describe normal early menstrual patterns?
- Evaluate and manage dysmenorrhea?
- Diagnose and treat PMS?

Table 15–5 TREATMENT OPTIONS FOR PREMENSTRUAL SYNDROME

Nonpharmacologic
Aerobic exercise
Increased intake of complex carbohydrates and fiber
Reduction in sodium, caffeine, and alcohol intake
Supportive therapy
Pharmacologic
Anxiolytics such as buspirone and benzodiazepines
Bromocriptine
Calcium, magnesium
Danazol
Hormonal treatment (OCPs, GnRH agonists, progesterones)
NSAIDs
Serotonergic antidepressants such as SSRIs and venlafaxine
Spironolactone (NOT thiazide diuretics)
Vitamin B_6 (pyridoxine)
Vitamin E

CASE 17

A frantic 25-year-old patient calls you. She and her boyfriend were having intercourse and the condom broke at the time of ejaculation about 16 hours ago. She does not use any other form of contraception. Her last menstrual period was about 2 weeks ago. You tell her that 8% of women become pregnant after a single act of coitus. She is mortified, exclaiming, "I've always been in the top 8% of everything!"

Appropriate methods of "emergency contraception" for this patient include:

A) Levonorgestrel (Plan B).
B) Ethinyl estradiol plus levonorgestrel (Yuzpe regimen).
C) High-dose ethinyl estradiol (Ivanapyuk method).
D) A and B only.
E) A, B, and C.

Discussion

The correct answer is "D." Many OCPs are also effective if used at the right doses and within 72 hours (the Yuzpe method). However, as of 2011, only Plan B and ulipristal (an antiprogestin, brand name Ella) are the only FDA-approved drugs for postcoital contraception. Plan B uses a high dose of levonorgestrel and is more effective than the combined OCPs for postcoital contraception. Plan B is available over the counter (in the United States in 2011). Ulipristal appears to be more effective than Plan B and may be taken up to 120 hours after unprotected intercourse but is only available by prescription. Copper IUD is another option and may be used up to 8 days after unprotected intercourse. "C" is incorrect as estrogen alone is not known to be effective as emergency contraception, and "Ivanapyuk" is a made-up name anyway.

HELPFUL TIP: Prescribe an antiemetic with postcoital OCPs as nausea and vomiting are common side effects. Plan B has fewer GI side effects. About the only contraindication to postcoital treatment is active pregnancy. Use a progestin-only regimen in women with a history of thromboembolism.

HELPFUL TIP: Mifepristone (RU486) is not available in the United States for postcoital pregnancy prophylaxis but is very effective (99–100%) and has a more favorable side effect profile when compared with other regimens. As of February 2012 it is available for treating DM II in those with Cushing syndrome. What you prescribe it for is up to you.

* *

You recommend Plan B. Since she now trusts you, she schedules an appointment with you for evaluation of intermittent abdominal and pelvic pain. Her pain has gradually worsened over the last 2 years and is almost omnipresent. Now she complains of severe abdominal cramping and stabbing in the right lower quadrant. The pain radiates to the left lower quadrant at times and is worse during her menstrual periods. Her periods have become heavier and occasionally irregular. She has no bowel or bladder symptoms. She has been missing work 1–2 days each month and is now concerned about her job.

Your examination reveals a well-developed woman who looks depressed and uncomfortable. Her abdomen is soft, nondistended, and diffusely tender to palpation in the lower quadrants. There is no evidence of guarding, rebound tenderness, or palpable masses. She has no back tenderness. The external genital and vaginal examinations show no lesions or erythema. There is a creamy discharge noted at the cervix. Bimanual reveals a retroverted uterus with uterosacral nodularity palpable. Both adnexal areas are tender to examination, but without masses.

You get a pregnancy test (negative), cultures (negative), and UA, all of which are negative.

Based on her symptoms and your physical exam, what is the most likely etiology of the patient's chronic pelvic pain?

A) Irritable bowel syndrome.
B) Myofascial pain disorder.
C) Endometriosis.
D) Cervical dysplasia.
E) Interstitial cystitis.

Discussion

The correct answer is "C." There were no bowel symptoms elicited on the history to suggest irritable bowel syndrome. There were no signs elicited on the examination to suggest a myofascial pain disorder. The patient's history and physical examination, including uterosacral nodularity, is consistent with a diagnosis of endometriosis. Dysplasia is typically asymptomatic. There were no bladder symptoms elicited on the history to suggest interstitial cystitis.

HELPFUL TIP: If after a careful assessment the diagnosis of endometriosis is highly likely, empiric therapy is considered a viable alternative to laparoscopy and preferred by many experts. However, definitive diagnosis relies upon direct visualization of endometrial implants confirmed by histologic examination.

* *

She dose not want laparoscopy. You offer alternatives, and she elects to undergo cycle suppression with a 3-month trial of leuprolide (Lupron) and to complete a pain calendar. You see her in follow-up in 3 months, and she is feeling much better. The pain has been almost completely suppressed, and she has missed only 1 day of work since you last saw her—but that was for a Star Trek convention. She has hot flashes, but they are minor.

What is the most appropriate management at this point?

A) Continue the Lupron for another 3 months (6 months total).
B) Stop the Lupron and monitor.
C) Switch to a trial of cycle suppression using Depo-Provera (medroxyprogesterone acetate) or continuous low-dose OCPs.
D) Switch to a trial of Premarin (conjugated estrogens).
E) A or C.

Discussion

The correct answer is "E." For pain relief, treatment with a GnRH agonist for 3–6 months is effective in most patients. Oral contraceptives and oral or depot progestins are more effective than placebo. Given the marked treatment success with the depot-Lupron, discontinuing treatment would likely result in recurrence of the patient's pain symptoms. Since endometriosis is estrogen dependent, use of estrogen (Premarin) theoretically could worsen symptoms. Another option is treatment with danazol. However, danazol is less well tolerated than GnRH agonists, Provera, or OCPs.

> HELPFUL TIP: NSAIDs are useful monotherapy in patients with mild endometriosis and are useful in combination with hormonal therapy for patients with more severe symptoms.

* *

The patient is concerned about how endometriosis may affect her future fertility. You recall that she is 25 years old and has never attempted pregnancy (at least not intentionally). She has regular menstrual cycles.

What will you tell her?

A) "You are surely infertile. Look into adoption."
B) "You just cannot know for sure until you have tried to conceive."
C) "What are you worried about? There is no association between endometriosis and infertility."
D) "Look at my face. See how tired I am? Do you really want kids?"

Discussion

The correct answer is "B." It is impossible to predict fertility and infertility based on the available information. Early-stage endometriosis is not likely to be associated with alterations in fecundity. If the patient is willing, a diagnostic laparoscopy may aid in visualization of anatomic pathology and allow one to render a guess as to tubal disease.

> HELPFUL TIP: Chronic pelvic pain is a symptom, not a specific disease. By definition, chronic pelvic pain refers to pain that has been present for more than 6 months and for which a thorough investigation has been negative.
> **Is the pain cyclic?** It may be related to endometriosis, dysmenorrhea, adenomyosis, and also other diseases that respond to hormones such as irritable bowel syndrome and interstitial cystitis.
> **Is the pain noncyclic?** It may be urinary, constipation, a myofascial trigger point in the abdominal wall, etc.
> **Always ask about sexual abuse:** There is a high correlation between chronic pelvic pain and a history of sexual abuse. To go by the textbook, the "diagnosis" of chronic pelvic pain requires a negative diagnostic laparoscopy. However, laparoscopy may not be performed in all cases.

Objectives: Did you learn to . . .

- Manage patients who desire emergency oral contraception?
- Define and evaluate chronic pelvic pain?
- Describe the ramifications, evaluation, diagnosis, and management of endometriosis?

QUICK QUIZ: A "TRICHY" ONE

A 19-year-old sexually active female presents to your urgent care center with a foul smelling vaginal discharge. She has noted the discharge for about 3 days. On examination she is in no acute distress, and her vital signs are normal. Her pelvic examination is remarkable for mild vaginal erythema and a frothy gray discharge. You note a malodorous discharge and suspect *Trichomonas* (bacterial vaginosis can also be malodorous, of course, with a fishy smell). A wet prep confirms your diagnosis.

At this point in time, you recommend that she also be tested for:

A) Chlamydia and gonorrhea.
B) Herpes simplex.
C) Hepatitis A.
D) All of the above.

Discussion

The correct answer is "A." Routine screening for chlamydia and gonorrhea infection is recommended for all sexually active adolescents. Given the presence of one STI, it is appropriate to offer testing for other STIs at this visit. Currently, herpes simplex virus (HSV) is not routinely tested for in asymptomatic persons, and the USPSTF recommends against serologic screening for HSV. Hepatitis A is not a sexually transmitted disease. It may be appropriate to offer testing for hepatitis B, HIV, syphilis, etc., as individual cases dictate.

QUICK QUIZ: PROLAPSE

An 80-year-old woman presents for evaluation of a "bulge" she noted after gardening over the weekend . . . or maybe it's been there for years—she's not sure. She has no discomfort and no difficulty with bowel or bladder elimination. On examination, you note her cervix extends 1 cm beyond the vestibule (vaginal opening) with straining. There are no lesions or excoriations noted.

Of the following, what is the best initial treatment option?

A) Hysterectomy.
B) Trachelectomy.
C) Pessary trial.
D) Bed rest.
E) Hormone therapy.

Discussion

The correct answer is "C." Seventy percent of women who are fitted with a pessary are satisfied at 5-year follow-up. Hysterectomy and trachelectomy (removal of the cervix) are both unnecessarily invasive without trying a conservative strategy.

QUICK QUIZ: OVARIAN MASS

What is the best way to manage an *asymptomatic* 4-cm ovarian mass found on routine pelvic exam in a 22-year-old female who is otherwise healthy?

A) Referral to a gynecologist.
B) Start hormonal therapy to reduce ovulation.
C) Expectant management with repeat examination in 2 months.
D) Serum CA-125 level.

Discussion

The correct answer is "C." A 4-cm ovarian mass likely represents a functional cyst in a woman who is cycling (reproductive age). Since it is asymptomatic and easily palpable, expectant management is the best option. No further evaluation is warranted at this time. **If you are not sure of your exam, ultrasound is a good option.** CA-125 is a tumor marker for epithelial ovarian cancer, but it is not useful as a screening test.

QUICK QUIZ: OVARIAN MASS

What is the best first step in managing an asymptomatic 4-cm ovarian mass in a 76-year-old postmenopausal woman?

A) Referral to a gynecologist.
B) Start hormonal therapy to suppress FSH and LH.
C) Expectant management with repeat exam in 2 months.
D) Serum CA-125 level.
E) Pelvic ultrasound.

Discussion

The correct answer is "E." Unlike a relatively small palpable ovarian mass in a reproductive-age woman, a palpable ovarian mass in a postmenopausal woman represents ovarian malignancy until proven otherwise. The best initial imaging study for evaluation of a pelvic mass is ultrasound. Ultrasound will not only identify the location of the mass but will also identify its internal consistency. Characteristics suggestive of cancer include bilaterality, solid and cystic components, thick septations, and the presence of ascites. CA-125 is a marker for epithelial ovarian cancer and may assist in evaluation, but it cannot be relied upon to rule in or to rule out cancer as a diagnosis. CA-125 levels greater than 65 U/mL in postmenopausal women with pelvic masses are predictive of malignancy in 75% of cases. CA-125 is useful in follow-up of patients with a history of ovarian cancer.

QUICK QUIZ: GYNECOLOGIC CANCERS

What is the leading cause of death from a gynecologic malignancy in American women?

A) Ovarian cancer.
B) Uterine cancer.
C) Cervical cancer.
D) Fallopian tube cancer.
E) Vaginal cancer.

Discussion

The correct answer is "A." Ovarian cancer is the leading cause of death from gynecologic malignancy, is the second most common gynecologic malignancy, and is the fourth leading cause of cancer death in women. Endometrial cancer is the most common gynecologic malignancy but also one of the most treatable. Cervical cancer is the third most common gynecologic malignancy. Both fallopian tube and vaginal malignancy are relatively rare.

QUICK QUIZ: OVARIAN CANCER

How does ovarian cancer typically present?

A) Early satiety.
B) Abdominal fullness and pain.
C) Urinary obstruction.
D) Asymptomatic mass noted on routine exam.
E) A and B.

Discussion

The correct answer is "E." There are no specific early symptoms of ovarian cancer. Thus, most patients present with symptoms associated with increasing tumor mass: early satiety, abdominal fullness, and abdominal pain. Unfortunately, ovarian cancer is rarely identified at an early stage on routine annual exam.

> HELPFUL TIP: An ovarian mass is more likely to be malignant if the patient is premenarcheal or postmenopausal and the mass greater than 10 cm in diameter and solid on ultrasound.

CASE 18

While covering the emergency department on the graveyard shift (so-called because of the time of day, not because of the number of patients who die), a 21-year-old college student presents sobbing with a friend. Her friend says, "She's been raped."

Relevant history includes all of the following EXCEPT:

A) Whether force was used and what type.
B) Physical characteristics of the assailant.
C) Details regarding penetration (vaginal, anal, oral).
D) Number of sexual partners the victim has had in her lifetime.
E) Condom use.

Discussion

The correct answer is "D." The patient's past sexual history is not relevant in the evaluation of sexual assault. The other issues are pertinent to the case. Although it may be difficult for the patient to relive the experience, you should try to obtain a detailed history of the assault. In order to assess her risk for pregnancy and infection, you need to ask about the area penetrated (e.g., vaginal, oral, or anal penetration), whether the assailant ejaculated, and if a condom was used. In a sexual assault case, your job is also to collect evidence, including pertinent historical elements (e.g., number of assailants, names, physical appearance, whether force was used, and what type—threat, restraints, weapons, etc.).

> HELPFUL TIP: Sexual assault includes genital, anal, or oral penetration by a part of the accused's body or by an object. By definition, it occurs without the victim's consent and need not involve direct force or violence.

Which of the following are important physical elements to collect for the forensic evaluation in this case?

A) Combed specimens from the scalp and pubic hair.
B) Swabs of the oral, vaginal, and rectal mucosa.
C) The patient's clothing.
D) Fingernail scrapings.
E) All of the above.

Discussion

The correct answer is "E." All of the items listed will be important to the investigation. Evidence collection kits for sexual assault cases ("rape kits") should be available in your emergency department.

* *

Although apparently inebriated, the patient is able to give a coherent history. When you broach the subject of physical examination, her friend says, "Look, she was raped an hour ago. Can't you let her just recover a bit before you violate her all over again?"

Which of the following is the most appropriate response?

A) "Of course. Come back tomorrow after you have sobered up and taken a shower."
B) "An examination is important for your health and in the event that this becomes a criminal case. The yield of the exam declines with time. Even if you don't feel like prosecuting now, you may decide to do so in the future, and the best evidence is gathered early."
C) "The exam has a fairly high yield even a week after the assault, so take your time on this."
D) "Under federal law I am required to perform this exam."

Discussion

The correct answer is "B." The yield of a forensic exam declines with time. Even if a patient states that she does not want to prosecute the assailant, she should be encouraged to have the exam done in case she changes her mind. Also, you are concerned about her health, and she may be at risk for sexually transmitted diseases, pregnancy, and traumatic injury. Despite the fact that yield does decline with time, reliable evidence may still be gathered up to 5 days after the assault.

HELPFUL TIP: "Rape trauma syndrome" generally occurs in three stages. The first includes anger, anxiety, guilt, shame, sleep disturbance, etc. The second stage includes somatic complaints (pelvic pain, other pain) and psychiatric complaints (depression, phobias, etc.). Some patients will resolve these issues while others will develop posttraumatic stress syndrome. The third stage is renormalization.

Further discussion of this topic is beyond the scope of this book but is available in other resources.

Which of the following is the LEAST appropriate to offer this patient at this point in time?

A) HIV antigen/antibody testing.
B) HSV antibody testing.
C) Prophylactic treatment for gonorrhea and Chlamydia.
D) Mental health services referral.
E) Emergency contraception.

Discussion

The correct answer is "B." Herpes virus antibody testing will only tell you if she has been exposed to HSV in the past. Further recommendations include syphilis testing, hepatitis B antibody testing, HIV testing, performing a wet prep of a vaginal sample, and checking a urine pregnancy test.

Objectives: Did you learn to . . .

- Evaluate a patient for sexual assault?
- Manage a patient who has been the victim of sexual assault?

CASE 19

A 21-year-old woman presents to your office complaining of pelvic pain with intercourse, worse over the last 2 weeks. She also complains of not getting pregnant, even though she's had several partners over her last 3 years of sexual activity and has been trying to get pregnant with the same partner for the past 6 months. She states she never has used birth control of any type—not even once. You commend her on commitment to her principles. She started her periods around age 14 but has only had a couple of periods since then. Apparently, this pattern of menstruation is normal for her family, as her mother was the same way.

On physical exam, you notice the patient is a centrally obese young woman, afebrile, with (culturally defined) excess hair noted down the side of her face and under her chin. She also has some erythematous pustules on her cheeks.

Which of the following lab results would be most consistent with the history and exam findings?

A) Positive urine pregnancy test.
B) Low TSH level.
C) Elevated CA-125 level.
D) LH:FSH ratio greater than 3:1.
E) Prolactin level more than three times normal.

Discussion

The correct answer is "D." This patient gives a history and has an appearance consistent with PCOS. The clinical features of PCOS include oligomenorrhea (90%), hirsutism (80%), obesity (50%), amenorrhea (40%), and infertility (40%). Early symptoms in an adolescent may consist only of irregular periods, acne, and central obesity. An LH:FSH ratio greater than 3:1 adds further support to the diagnosis. You should certainly do a pregnancy test, a TSH, and a prolactin level. However, this patient most likely has PCOS.

HELPFUL TIP: The most recent evidence points to insulin resistance as the underlying cause of PCOS and these patients may have acanthosis nigricans. Insulin resistance can be quantified by calculating the ratio of fasting glucose to insulin. A ratio of less than 4.5 indicates insulin resistance. Insulin resistance stimulates ovarian androgen production, which leads to anovulation.

* *

You proceed with the pelvic portion of the exam, noting the patient also has a diamond-shaped, rather than triangular-shaped, pubic hair pattern. You find no lesions on the vulva or in the vagina. However, the cervix appears reddened, with an almost strawberry texture. And, even though there is a generous amount of yellowish, malodorous leukorrhea in the vaginal vault, there is no notable pus at the cervical os. Bimanual exam is limited due to the patient's obesity.

Of the following, which is the most likely cause of her cervicitis?

A) HSV infection.
B) *Trichomonas vaginalis* infection.
C) *Candida albicans* infection.
D) PID.
E) Bacterial vaginosis.

Discussion

The correct answer is "B." *Trichomonas* is a protozoan that is sexually transmitted and can cause urethritis in both sexes. However, in women, it most commonly causes ulceration of the cervical mucosa with punctuate hemorrhages known as a "strawberry cervix." Signs and symptoms also include a malodorous discharge and occasional vulvar and vaginal irritation. The cervix can be somewhat tender to touch, either during exam or intercourse, and patients often complain of a nonspecific pelvic pain. Males are often asymptomatic.

* *

The wet mount demonstrates *Trichomonas*; there is no evidence of yeast or clue cells. You send samples for Chlamydia and gonorrhea tests as well as a Pap smear. You recommend testing for HIV, syphilis, and hepatitis, and she agrees.

For her *Trichomonas* vaginal infection, you prescribe:

A) Flagyl (metronidazole) 2 g orally in a single dose.
B) MetroGel-Vaginal (topical vaginal metronidazole) 5 g applied nightly for 5 days.
C) Diflucan (fluconazole) 150 mg orally in a single dose.
D) Zithromax (azithromycin) 1 g orally in a single dose.
E) Levaquin (levofloxacin) 250 mg orally in a single dose.

Discussion

The correct answer is "A." The best choice is oral metronidazole. Topical antibiotic gels, creams, or ovules—either metronidazole or clindamycin (Cleocin)—only treat bacterial vaginosis, as the concentration is insufficient to reach the protozoa in the glands and urethral areas. The rest options are all incorrect for treating *Trichomonas*. See Table 15–6 for more on diagnosis and treatment of infectious vaginitis.

HELPFUL TIP: As with other STIs, a patient with *Trichomonas* should have her partner tested and treated (or just treated).

HELPFUL TIP: While it makes sense that single-dose azithromycin would work better in treating Chlamydia because of compliance

Table 15–6 VAGINITIS DIAGNOSIS AND TREATMENT

Organism	Discharge	Odor	Microscopic	pH	Treatment
Bacterial vaginosis	Thin, gray, homogeneous	Fishy with positive "wiff test"	Clue cells	>4.5	Metronidazole 500 mg BID × 7 days or clindamycin 300 mg BID × 7 days or topical metronidazole (lower success rate)
Candida	Adherent, white, "cottage cheese" like	Neutral	Pseudohyphae but only 65–85% sensitive	<4.5	Fluconazole oral, topical clotrimazole, miconazole, etc.
Trichomonas	Copious yellow, gray, green, foamy. Friable "strawberry" cervix	Malodorous	See trichomonads on microscopic	>4.5	Metronidazole 2 g × 1 (recommended), or 500 mg BID × 7 days (alternative)

issues, the cure rate is the same whether azithromycin or the doxycycline is used.

* *

You now return your attention to her PCOS (remember, way back then, the reason she came in?). Her lab results demonstrated a LH:FSH ratio >3; normal TSH and prolactin; slightly elevated testosterone, but still well below the normal male range; fasting glucose : Insulin <4.5; and slightly elevated total cholesterol and triglycerides. Her LH:FSH ratio was consistent with the diagnosis of PCOS. She has not menstruated for 12 months. A urine hCG is negative, and a repeat fasting glucose is 120 mg/dL.

Which of the following recommendations should you make now?

A) Initiate metformin.
B) Attempt weight loss through a nutritious diet and increased exercise.
C) Initiate oral contraceptives to regulate menses.
D) A and C.
E) All of the above.

Discussion

The correct answer is "E." This patient has glucose intolerance (elevated fasting glucose and ratio of glucose: insulin <4.5), and it is reasonable to initiate dietary and medical therapy at this point in time. Another option is to start with lifestyle modifications and check fasting glucose again 3–6 months later. Due to increased risk of endometrial carcinoma in patients who have rare menses, it is important to regulate her cycles. OCPs ("C") can accomplish menstrual regulation.

HELPFUL TIP: For hirsutism of PCOS, spironolactone is usually first-line therapy, unless the patient has a contraindication; traditional hair removal techniques will still be required for the existing hair growth. Since spironolactone can result in feminization of a male fetus, patients taking spironolactone must be using reliable birth control.

HELPFUL TIP: Not all women with PCOS are obese and hirsute. Many patients may be thin with sparse body hair and present with menstrual irregularities and fertility concerns.

Objectives: Did you learn to . . .

- Identify the clinical presentation of polycystic ovarian syndrome?
- Diagnose and treat *Trichomonas* infection?
- Treat gonorrhea?
- Diagnose and manage polycystic ovarian syndrome?

QUICK QUIZ: SCREENING

A 16-year-old female presents with her mother. They don't look happy. Her mother says, "She needs a Pap smear because she's been having sex with a couple of boys—in my house, I will have you know—for a year!" The patient rolls her eyes.

Consistent with published guidelines, you recommend:

A) Pap smear.
B) Gonorrhea and chlamydia testing.
C) Pap smear and gonorrhea and chlamydia testing.
D) Return for a Pap after sexually active for 3 years (age 18 for this patient).
E) A chastity belt.

Discussion

The correct answer is "B." Most major medical group guidelines (ACOG, ACS, USPSTF, etc.) now recommend delaying cervical cancer screening until age 21, even if the woman has been sexually active. The reasoning: although adolescent females are frequently infected with HPV, they also easily clear these infections, with 95% of lesions spontaneously regressing. Exceptions to this rule include patients who are immunocompromised (e.g., organ transplant, HIV infection).

QUICK QUIZ: AN ITCHY VULVA

A 65-year-old female presents for a health maintenance examination. She complains of a vulvar itching due to what she calls "recurrent yeast infections," and her symptoms have worsened over the last few months. She is sexually active with her husband and has experienced dyspareunia with penetration lately. She always uses a water-based lubricant with intercourse. On examination, you find complete loss of the borders of the labia minora, constriction of the vaginal outlet, and several thin white plaques (like parchment paper) on the vulva. There is no other skin or mucosal involvement.

What is the most likely diagnosis?

A) Lichen planus.
B) Lichen simplex.
C) Lichen sclerosus.
D) Vulvovaginal candidiasis.
E) Squamous carcinoma.

Discussion

The correct answer is "C." The clinical description above is characteristic of lichen sclerosus, which occurs more commonly in older women but also has a peak in young girls. Almost all lichen sclerosus is intensely pruritic. As lichen sclerosus progresses, there may be loss of labial architecture, stenosis of the introitus, and obliteration of the clitoris. The lesions are usually multiple and appear as thin, shiny, white, wrinkled patches or plaques. The rest are incorrect. However, "E," squamous carcinoma, occasionally can be confused for lichen sclerosus but is more likely to present with ulceration and induration and is less common (though if you are suspicious of cancer, a biopsy is indicated). Patients with lichen sclerosis have a squamous cell cancer risk of 3–7% and should have an exam every 6–12 months and biopsies as indicated for persistent and nonhealing lesions, etc.

HELPFUL TIP: Initial treatment for lichen sclerosus involves local steroid ointment application. High-potency steroids are initiated and then tapered to the lowest effective potency and frequency that maintain symptom control. Testosterone creams have fallen out of favor due to lesser efficacy and secondary virilization. Vaginal dilators can be used if there is constriction of the vaginal opening that causes dyspareunia, etc.

QUICK QUIZ: VULVOVAGINAL CANDIDIASIS

A 48-year-old perimenopausal female presents with a 3-day history of vulvar pruritus. Her history is significant for mitral valve replacement and she is on warfarin with INR 2–3. A limited vulvar and vaginal exam reveals significant erythema with satellite lesions on the labia majora. Wet prep microscopy reveals abundant pseudo-hyphae and inflammatory cells. You somehow assemble all these clues into a diagnosis of candidal vulvovaginitis (and you can tell the patient is impressed when she says, "That's right, genius. I've got a yeast infection."). She inquires about use of oral therapy, as vaginal creams are "messy."

How will you counsel this patient regarding use of oral fluconazole (Diflucan)?

A) "You have no contraindications to oral fluconazole."
B) "Given your use of warfarin, you should not use oral fluconazole."

C) "You will need to stop warfarin while taking oral fluconazole."
D) "You should take extra warfarin if you take oral fluconazole."

Discussion

The correct answer is "B." There are numerous drug interactions with oral fluconazole, including warfarin (both inhibit CYP3A4). The INR will increase after even one dose of fluconazole therapy. Similarly, the ubiquitous statins are affected by oral fluconazole with several case reports of rhabdomyolysis in the literature.

CASE 20

A 27-year-old female presents with her husband seeking advice regarding pregnancy loss. She recently had a miscarriage. Your patient states that this was her third miscarriage in the last 2 years. Both occurred at about 9 weeks of gestation.

Possible explanations for recurrent pregnancy loss in this patient include each of the following EXCEPT:

A) Parental structural chromosome abnormalities.
B) Uterine anatomic abnormalities.
C) Anticardiolipin antibody syndrome.
D) Unexplained etiology.
E) Conception while on oral contraceptives.

Discussion

The correct answer is "E." Conception while on oral contraceptives will not increase the risk of **recurrent** spontaneous miscarriages. Parental structural chromosome abnormalities (balanced structural chromosome rearrangement in one partner) are responsible for pregnancy loss in 2–4% of couples. "B," uterine anatomic abnormalities, have been associated with 10–15% of pregnancy loss. "D" is true. The majority of couples with recurrent pregnancy loss will have an uncertain etiology despite extensive evaluation (>50%).

HELPFUL TIP: Recurrent pregnancy loss is classically defined as loss of three or more consecutive pregnancies.

* *

The couple desires testing for possible causes of the pregnancy losses.

Of the following, which test(s) should be included in the evaluation?

A) Cultures for bacteria.
B) Test for glucose intolerance.
C) Maternal antipaternal antibodies.
D) Lupus anticoagulant and anticardiolipin antibody.
E) All of the above.

Discussion

The correct answer is "D." Antiphospholipid syndrome is associated with pregnancy loss in 3–15% of women with recurrent pregnancy loss. The others are not useful. However, chromosomal testing of the parents may be useful.

* *

Evaluation of the recurrent pregnancy loss fails to identify a cause. Thus, like most couples with recurrent pregnancy loss, the etiology remains unexplained.

What is the likelihood that this couple will have a successful pregnancy outcome in the next pregnancy?

A) Highly unlikely, they should consider adoption.
B) Less than one in four chances of successful pregnancy.
C) 60–70% chance of successful next pregnancy.
D) You cannot hazard a guess. Amazingly, this has not been studied.

Discussion

The correct answer is "C." Studies suggest that 60–70% of couples with unexplained recurrent pregnancy loss will have a successful next pregnancy.

Objectives: Did you learn to . . .

- Define recurrent pregnancy loss and discuss some of its epidemiologic aspects?

- Enumerate potential causes of recurrent pregnancy loss?
- Identify etiologies and the workup of recurrent pregnancy loss?

QUICK QUIZ: WEIGHT GAIN IN PREGNANCY

A 28-year-old primigravida female presents for an initial obstetric visit. Pelvic examination is consistent with a 6–8-week gestation uterus, and the remainder of the exam is unremarkable. As this is her first pregnancy, she has a number of questions. She wants to know how much weight gain is expected and whether she should "watch her weight."

You calculate her BMI as 24 kg/m^2 and recommend the following:

A) "Eat anything you want. You're eating for two!"
B) "Your BMI is normal. Your goal is to gain no more than 20 pounds."
C) "Your BMI is low. Your goal is to gain 40 pounds."
D) "Your BMI is high. Your goal is to gain no more than 15 pounds."
E) "Your BMI is normal. Your goal is to gain 30 pounds."

Discussion

The correct answer is "E." The Institute of Medicine recommends weight gain in pregnancy based on pregravid BMI (see Table 15–7). In this patient, her BMI is in the normal range, so her goal for weight gain in pregnancy is 25–35 pounds. Women with a normal pre-pregnancy BMI should gain about one pound per week during their second and third trimesters.

Table 15–7 PREGNANCY WEIGHT GAIN GUIDELINES

BMI (kg/m^2)	Goal weight gain (kg)	Goal weight gain (lb)
<18.5	12.5–18.0	28–40
18.5–24.9	11.5–16.0	25–35
25.0–29.9	7.0–11.5	15–25
>30	5–9	11–20

Adapted from Institute of Medicine, Resource Sheet, May 2009: Weight Gain During Pregnancy: Reexamining the Guidelines: http://www.iom.edu/Reports/2009/Weight-Gain-During-Pregnancy-Reexamining-the-Guidelines.aspx

QUICK QUIZ: AMENORRHEA

A 32-year-old female is coming to see you for amenorrhea. She had regular menses until the last year when they became irregular. She has not had any menses for the past 6 months. She is somewhat distraught because she wants to have a family. Being the smart doctor that you are, you know that a pregnancy test is the first thing to do: it is negative. Being the smart doctor that you are, you also think about the female athlete triad: amenorrhea, an eating disorder, and osteoporosis. She does not meet this profile.

You take more of a history.

- There is no additional stress (such as starting college or a new job), weight loss, or illness, etc., in her life that might lead to hypothalamic amenorrhea.
- She has no galactorrhea (prolactinoma).
- She has no flashes, vaginal dryness, etc. (premature menopause).
- She denies headaches, visual changes, fatigue, polydipsia, or polyuria (pituitary problems).
- She has no acne, hirsutism, etc., suggestive of PCOS.
- Hey, did you notice how we are cleverly giving you the workup of secondary amenorrhea in the question?

As recommended, you check a TSH and prolactin; they are normal.

The next step in the evaluation of this patient's amenorrhea is:

A) A progestin challenge.
B) Hysterosalpingogram to prove cervical patency.
C) A trial of oral contraceptives to prove cervical patency.
D) An LH to rule out menopause.
E) All of the above.

Discussion

The correct answer is "A." A progestin challenge should cause a withdrawal bleed if there is still adequate estrogen (thus ruling out premature ovarian failure). The step following this would be oral contraceptives. Failure of induce menses with OCPs suggests a mechanical blockage such as Asherman syndrome (scaring of the endometrial lining with intrauterine adhesions). This can be followed by a hysterosalpingogram or hysteroscopy to identify any mechanical problems.

* *

You did it! You successfully worked up secondary amenorrhea.

> HELPFUL TIP: But wait, there is more! Check an FSH as well. If this is high, it might indicate ovarian failure. If it is normal or low in the absence of circulating estrogen (remember the progestin challenge?), consider a pituitary cause of amenorrhea including possible hypothalamic–pituitary axis dysfunction from weight loss, stress, etc.

BIBLIOGRAPHY

American College of Obstetricians and Gynecologists. ACOG Practice Bulletin no. 106: Intrapartum fetal heart rate monitoring, nomenclature, interpretation and general management principles. *Obstet Gynecol.* 2009;114(1):192-202.

American College of Obstetricians and Gynecologists. ACOG Practice Bulletin no. 109: Cervical cytology screening. *Obstet Gynecol.* 2009;114(6):1409-1420.

American College of Obstetricians and Gynecologists. ACOG Practice Bulletin No. 112: Emergency contraception. *Obstet Gynecol.* 2010;115:1100-1109.

Allen RH, Goldberg AB. Emergency contraception: A clinical review. *Clin Obstet Gynecol.* 2007;50(4):927-936.

Briscoe D, et al. Management of pregnancy beyond 40 weeks' gestation. *Am Fam Physician.* 2005;71:1935-1941.

Crossman SH. The challenge of pelvic inflammatory disease. *Am Fam Physician.* 2006;73:859-864.

Frey KA, Patel KS. Initial evaluation and management of infertility by the primary care physician. *Mayo Clin Proc.* 2004;79(11):1439-1443.

Hatcher RA, et al. *A Pocket Guide to Managing Contraception.* 6th ed. New York: Ardent Media, Inc; 2005.

Kirkham C, et al. Evidence-based prenatal care: Part I. General prenatal care and counseling issues. *Am Fam Physician.* 2005;71:1307-1316.

Kirkham C, et al. Evidence-based prenatal care: Part I. Third-trimester care and prevention of infectious diseases. *Am Fam Physician.* 2005;71:1555-1562.

Magnotti M, Futterweit W. Obesity and the polycystic ovary syndrome. *Med Clin North Am.* 2007;91(6):1151-1168.

Raina R, et al. Female sexual dysfunction: classification, pathophysiology, and management. *Fertil Steril.* 2007;88(5):1273-1284.

Scott A, Glasier A. Evidence based contraceptive choices. *Best Pract Res Clin Obstet Gynaecol.* 2006;20(5):665-680.

Tan PC, et al., Obstet Gynecol. 2006;108(1):134-40.

Workowski KA, Berman S; Centers for Disease Control and Prevention. Sexually transmitted diseases treatment guidelines, *MMWR Recomp Rep.* 2010;59(RR-12):1-110.

Wright TC, et al. 2006 consensus guidelines for the management of women with abnormal cervical cancer screening tests. *Am J Obstet Gynecol.* 2007;197(4):346-355.

16

Men's Health

Jason K. Wilbur

CASE 1

A 58-year-old black male presents to your clinic complaining of hesitancy, frequency, and nocturia three to four times per night, which has been steadily worsening over the past few years. His urinary stream is weaker than it was a few years ago. He feels like he does not empty his bladder completely, but he denies a history of urinary tract infections (UTIs) or painful urination. He is otherwise well with no significant past medical or surgical history. Currently, he takes no medications and has no allergies. On reviewing his family history, you find that his father and older brother died of prostate cancer in their 50s. General physical exam is normal. Genital exam is unremarkable. Rectal exam reveals a smooth prostate with no nodules or tenderness.

Based on this patient's history and physical exam, all of the following would be appropriate at this stage EXCEPT:

A) Screening prostate-specific antigen (PSA) blood test.
B) American Urological Association (AUA) symptom score.
C) Postvoid residual urine volume.
D) Transrectal ultrasound with prostate biopsies.
E) Urinalysis.

Discussion

The correct answer is "D." Although your patient has an increased risk of prostate cancer, transrectal ultrasound with prostate biopsies is not indicated at this stage. This diagnostic test should be reserved for suspicion of prostate cancer. Based on this patient's family history and the fact that he is black (blacks have a 50% higher incidence of and mortality from prostate cancer compared with whites), PSA screening is very appropriate. A rectal exam, while classically taught to be important, adds no additional information in most cases and is not recommended by the US Preventive Services Task Force (but . . . force of habit, so you did it). Since your patient may not empty his bladder well, a postvoid residual urine volume and urinalysis will help determine if he is likely to get a UTI from urine retention and if he already has an infection. The AUA symptom score is a seven-item questionnaire about symptoms of urinary outlet obstruction, and it can be used in the diagnosis and management of benign prostatic disease.

When considering benign prostatic hyperplasia (BPH), you reflect on the common symptoms of this syndrome, which include all of the following EXCEPT:

A) Urinary retention.
B) Postvoid dribbling.
C) Frequency.
D) Nocturia.
E) Hematuria.

Discussion

The correct answer is "E." Hematuria is not usually associated with BPH. However, it can occur if a man's prostatic urethra is very enlarged and friable. Enlargement of the prostate often results in obstructive flow symptoms (e.g., hesitancy and slow, weak stream), which in turn can lead to irritative symptoms (e.g., frequency, urgency, and nocturia). Obstruction from an enlarged prostate alone can cause hypertrophy of the detrusor, or it can lead to an infection that results in detrusor instability—the cause of irritative symptoms. **If irritative symptoms are present without obstructive symptoms, other diagnoses should be considered, including bladder cancer, urolithiasis, infection, or neurogenic bladder.**

* *

Your patient's urinalysis and PSA are normal. After emptying 250 mL of urine, the postvoid residual urine volume is 50 mL.

With this information, you recommend which of the following strategies?

A) Urodynamic studies.
B) Medical therapy.
C) Surgical therapy.
D) Scheduled bladder catheterization.
E) Biofeedback.

Discussion

The correct answer is "B." You have enough information to diagnose symptomatic BPH, and further studies are not necessary. Depending on the patient's preferences, the next step is to begin treatment, and in most cases, medical therapy is initiated first. If medical therapy fails or if a patient has severe BPH with ongoing obstruction, retention of large volumes of urine, or recurrent UTIs, surgical therapy should be considered. The most commonly performed surgery is transurethral resection of the prostate (TURP), but other techniques are employed as well, including transurethral incision of the prostate, minimally invasive procedures, and open surgery for very enlarged glands. Answer "D" is incorrect. Scheduled bladder catheterization is unlikely to benefit your patient since his postvoid residual is not very large. A postvoid residual greater than 200 mL is associated with an increased risk of UTIs, and such patients may benefit from scheduled catheterizations if medical or surgical interventions do not correct the problem or are contraindicated. Biofeedback (answer "E") may be used to treat urge incontinence but is not used in BPH.

* *

You are satisfied that the patient's urinary symptoms are due to BPH. Your patient desires treatment.

To give him the most immediate relief, you prescribe which of the following?

A) Finasteride.
B) Oxybutynin.
C) Terazosin.
D) Imipramine.
E) Furosemide.

Discussion

The correct answer is "C." Timing and type of intervention should depend on how much the patient is bothered by his symptoms and whether complications of BPH are present. If the symptoms do not significantly interfere with your patient's life, he may choose to wait and take no treatment once he is reassured that he does not have a life-threatening illness. In general, medical management begins with a selective alpha-1 receptor blocker, such as doxazosin or terazosin. A medication specific for the alpha-1a receptor subtype (e.g., tamsulosin) may be used in patients who cannot tolerate traditional alpha-1 receptor blockers. If the patient does not receive sufficient relief from maximum doses of an alpha-1 blocker, a 5-alpha reductase inhibitor (e.g., finasteride or dutasteride 0.5 mg) may be added. However, it may take up to 6 months for a 5-alpha reductase inhibitor to result in a noticeable difference in symptoms (thus, answer "A" should not be the first treatment), whereas the full benefit of an alpha-blocker will be apparent within 4–6 weeks. Answers "B" and "D" are incorrect because these anticholinergic drugs are used for incontinence due to detrusor instability and may make urinary retention worse in patients with outlet obstruction. Answer "E," furosemide, is a potent diuretic and would be a cruel joke to play on this patient.

As you write the prescription for terazosin, you review the side effects. Potential side effects of alpha-blockers include all the following EXCEPT:

A) Retrograde ejaculation.
B) Hypertension.
C) Intraoperative floppy iris syndrome.
D) Priapism.

Discussion

The correct answer is "B." Hypotension (not hypertension) is the most commonly encountered problem with terazosin and other alpha-blockers. In elderly males, the hypotension can be particularly problematic as the propensity for falling may increase. Additionally, alpha-blockers in combination with phosphodiesterase inhibitors (e.g., sildenafil) can cause dangerously low blood pressures. Retrograde ejaculation ("A") and priapism ("D") are not common but have been reported. And, as if we needed it, here is more evidence for a direct link between the male ocular and genital systems: intraoperative floppy iris syndrome has been observed in men taking alpha-blockers and undergoing cataract surgery; causality has not been proven. Yes, you may have thought we made this up but we didn't.

* *

You start terazosin, slowly increasing the dose and administering the medication at night. Unfortunately, the patient is not able to tolerate terazosin due to dizziness. His symptoms are bothersome enough that he wishes to try something else, and you prescribe tamsulosin. He tolerates this medication well, but his symptoms are not relieved to his satisfaction. You consider finasteride.

Which of the following is true of finasteride?

A) It permanently reduces prostate volume, even after the drug is stopped.
B) It is approved by the Food and Drug Administration (FDA) for abnormal hair growth in women.
C) It may reduce the overall risk of developing prostate cancer but increase the risk of developing high-grade prostate cancers.
D) It improves symptoms within 1 week of starting the drug.
E) None of the above.

Discussion

The correct answer is "C." This is important: **5-alpha-reductase inhibitors lower the overall risk of cancer but increase the risk of those cancers being high grade.** Finasteride (and dutasteride) works by inhibiting 5-alpha-reductase, which is the enzyme that converts testosterone to dihydrotestosterone. Dihydrotestosterone stimulates hyperplasia of the prostate gland, and removing this stimulus results in decreased prostate volume. However, removal of finasteride allows hyperplasia to continue, and thus answer "A" is incorrect. Answer "B" is also incorrect because finasteride for hirsutism in women is not approved by the FDA. Additionally, finasteride is category X in pregnancy, with potential teratogenic effects on the fetus. Answer "D" is incorrect because finasteride takes time to work—a lot of time. As previously mentioned, its peak effectiveness is not seen for 3–6 months after starting the medication.

HELPFUL TIP: In comparison trials with alpha-blockers, 5-alpha reductase inhibitors have shown variable results. The addition of a 5-alpha reductase inhibitor to an alpha-blocker does not seem to have additional benefit over alpha-blocker therapy alone in the *near term*, but combination therapy has shown educed incidence of clinical progression of BPH in *longer trials*.

* *

You decide to add finasteride. You see him again 2 months later when he presents with a febrile illness. He thinks that he might have the flu, but his BPH symptoms worsened at the same time. For the last 2 days, he has felt feverish with back pain, perineal pain, and generalized malaise. He complains of dysuria and worsening urinary frequency and urgency.

During your exam, you make sure NOT to:

A) Perform a rectal exam.
B) Massage the prostate.
C) Swab the urethra for chlamydia.
D) Perform urinalysis and microscopic exam of the urinary sediment.

Discussion

The correct answer is "B." There is a risk of seeding bacteria into the bloodstream when an infected prostate is massaged. This patient has symptoms of prostatitis; thus, you should **avoid prostatic massage**. Nonetheless, you should perform a prostate exam. The following physical findings are associated with prostatitis: tenderness, warmth, enlargement, and bogginess.

* *

You suspect prostatitis and obtain urine for analysis.

All of the following laboratory abnormalities are consistent with the diagnosis of acute prostatitis EXCEPT:

A) Leukocytosis.
B) Hematuria.
C) Bacteriuria.
D) Elevated creatinine.
E) Elevated PSA.

Discussion

The correct answer is "D." Tests of renal function should not be abnormal in simple, acute prostatitis. Chronic partial or complete urinary outlet obstruction may cause abnormal renal function but not acute prostatitis. Abnormal serum BUN and/or creatinine in the setting of prostatitis should prompt further investigation. The urine often shows bacteriuria, pyuria, and hematuria. However, the urine may also be negative. Urine should be sent for culture and sensitivity to definitively determine the pathogen and direct further treatment. Answer "E" is true: the PSA is often elevated in prostatitis. However, it is not necessary nor is it recommended to obtain a PSA in order to diagnose prostatitis. When the PSA is elevated due to acute prostatitis, it may not return to normal levels for 1 month or more after the resolution of inflammation.

HELPFUL TIP: Obtaining urine is important in the diagnosis of prostatitis, but you should avoid bladder catheterization due to the potential to spread infection. Besides, you want urine that has been in contact with the prostate.

* *

On exam, you find an uncomfortable appearing male in no distress. His temperature is 38.4°C, and the rest of his vital signs are normal. The prostate is tender, enlarged, warm, and boggy. The remainder of the exam is unremarkable. Urinalysis is consistent with an infection. He has a **sulfa allergy**.

Which of the following is the most appropriate treatment plan for this patient?

A) Amoxicillin 500 mg TID for 10 days.
B) Ciprofloxacin 500 mg BID for 28 days.
C) Admit for IV levofloxacin 500 mg daily for 14 days.
D) Admit for IV levofloxacin 500 mg daily, followed by completion of therapy with oral levofloxacin 500 mg daily for 14 days when the patient is stable.
E) Unable to determine at this time because a transrectal ultrasound must be performed to rule out prostatic abscess.

Discussion

The correct answer is "B." The most appropriate treatment for this patient is a fluoroquinolone, such as ciprofloxacin, for at least 28 days. Some authorities recommend longer treatment (up to 6 weeks) to reduce the risk of chronic prostatitis. In patients who are not allergic, a sulfa antibiotic could be considered as an alternative to a fluoroquinolone. In this case, answers "C" and "D" are overkill. Admission is appropriate for patients who appear septic, have not responded to oral antibiotics, or who have significant comorbidities. However, fluoroquinolones have 100% bioavailability PO. Thus, there is no indication for giving these drugs IV unless the oral route is unavailable (e.g., vomiting). Answer "E" is incorrect because abscesses are rare and imaging for an abscess is only undertaken if the patient does not respond to appropriate antibiotics.

HELPFUL TIP: The most common cause of acute prostatitis is *Escherichia coli*.

* *

When you see this patient again, his symptoms of prostatitis have cleared, but he does not think that finasteride is really helping. His AUA symptoms score is 21 (severe). He is wondering if a TURP might help him, and he wants to discuss the downsides of the operation.

Compared with watchful waiting, all of the following are observed at greater rates in men who undergo TURP EXCEPT:

A) Erectile dysfunction.
B) Urinary incontinence.
C) Urethral stenosis.
D) Increased urine flow.
E) Decreased postvoid residual urine volume.

Discussion

The correct answer is "A." TURP is a commonly performed procedure for BPH. Indications for TURP include failure of medical therapy, recurrent infections, bladder calculi, renal insufficiency, and patient preference. Patients who undergo TURP typically experience decreased AUA symptom scores, increased urine flow rates, and decreased postvoid residual volumes. There are downsides to TURP, including urinary incontinence, urethral stenosis, and the need to repeat the surgery. Strange as it may seem, several studies have shown that erectile dysfunction does NOT occur at increased rates in patients undergoing TURP compared with watchful waiting. However, men can have retrograde ejaculation status post-TURP.

> HELPFUL TIP: Cialis (taladafil) has been approved for treating BPH. But, the benefit over placebo is only 2.3 points on a 35-point scale . . . don't expect miracles.

Objectives: Did you learn to . . .

- Recognize the pattern of voiding dysfunction seen in BPH?
- Manage a patient with BPH and understand the potential adverse effects of medications used to treat BPH?
- Diagnose and treat acute prostatitis?
- Describe indications for and complications of TURP?

QUICK QUIZ: SEXUALLY TRANSMITTED INFECTIONS

A 21-year-old college student, self-described as a "ladies' man," (interpret: jerk) presents because of a concerning spot that developed on his penis. He complains of pain at the spot but denies itching. He reports no fever. When asked further about his sexual practices, he reports no condom use because his partners are all "on the pill." He had chlamydia in high school but is otherwise healthy. His review of systems is negative. On examination of the penis, you find a 1-cm tender, erythematous papule with a deep central ulceration at the glans penis. There is some mild, tender lymphadenopathy in the inguinal area. The rest of the exam is unremarkable.

This lesion is most likely caused by:

A) *Haemophilus ducreyi.*
B) *Neisseria gonorrhoeae.*
C) *Staphylococcus aureus.*
D) *Treponema pallidum.*
E) None of the above.

Discussion

The correct answer is "A." This is the lesion of *H. ducreyi*, otherwise known as chancroid. It can be confused with the chancre of primary syphilis, caused by *T. pallidum*, but the syphilis chancre is painless. Gram stain (gram-negative rods in chains), culture, or biopsy (which this guy deserves) may confirm the diagnosis. A few more notes: chancroid is rarely diagnosed in the United States and is probably underdiagnosed; it frequently coinfects with syphilis and tends to occur in clusters. A number of treatments are available, including ceftriaxone (250 mg IM once), azithromycin (1 g PO once), ciprofloxacin (500 mg PO BID for 3 days), and others.

CASE 2

A 22-year-old male presents complaining of a painless lump on his left testicle. He denies penile discharge, dysuria, or other urinary complaints. He underwent a left orchidopexy for an undescended testicle at age 6. Otherwise, his past medical history is unremarkable. On exam, the penis is circumcised with no lesion or discharge. There is adenopathy in the left inguinal area. His testicles are descended bilaterally with a 1-cm palpable, irregular mass on the midlateral portion of the left testicle. His exam is otherwise unremarkable. Your patient is worried about testicular cancer and wants to know if he is at risk.

All of the following are associated with an increased risk of testicular cancer EXCEPT:

A) Vasectomy.
B) HIV infection.
C) Cryptorchidism.
D) Klinefelter syndrome.
E) Family history.

Discussion

The correct answer is "A." Epidemiologic data do not support an association between testicular cancer and vasectomy. As is true of some other malignancies, males with HIV infection have an increased risk of testicular cancer. Also, males with cryptorchidism (failure of one or both testicles to descend into the scrotum) and Klinefelter syndrome are at increased risk of testicular cancer. About 25% of testicular cancers occurring in patients with cryptorchidism arise in the contralateral (normally descended) testicle. While testicular cancer does not have as strong of a hereditary component, a positive family history is a risk factor for testicular cancer. Of note, black males have a much **lower** incidence of testicular cancer than do white males.

If your patient had not had an orchidopexy to repair the undescended testicle, he would be at risk for developing all of the following problems EXCEPT:

A) Infertility.
B) Inguinal hernia.
C) Testicular torsion.
D) Testicular malignancy.
E) Impotence.

Discussion
The correct answer is "E." Organic impotence is not a consequence of cryptorchidism. All of the other problems listed occur at an increased frequency in males with an undescended testicle. The best time to begin treatment for an undescended testicle to minimize future sequelae is between 6 and 18 months of age and preferably by the end of the first year. The consequence of not treating an undescended testicle is a 20–40% increase in risk of developing a testicular malignancy, which often presents as a painless mass (although it is not clear that fixing the undescended testicle lowers the cancer risk). Therefore, the reasons to treat cryptorchidism are (1) to better palpate the testicle to assess for potential malignant transformation; (2) to decrease the risk of malignant transformation (maybe); (3) to improve chances of fertility; (4) to decrease risk of testicular torsion; (5) to decrease psychological effects from having an empty scrotum; and (6) to repair an inguinal hernia at the same time, if it is present.

> HELPFUL TIP: In patients with hypospadias and unilateral or bilateral empty scrotum, there is a higher rate of chromosomal anomalies.

After an appropriate history and physical examination, which of the following tests is the initial diagnostic study of choice in your patient?

A) CT scan.
B) Ultrasound.
C) CBC.
D) Alpha fetoprotein (AFP).
E) Pelvic x-ray.

Discussion
The correct answer is "B." The best initial diagnostic test would be a scrotal ultrasound to determine if this mass is cystic or solid. If it is determined to be a solid mass suspicious for malignancy, then other diagnostic studies would be warranted, such as beta-hCG and AFP. Answer "A" is incorrect, as ultrasound is considered the test of choice. In conjunction with a radical inguinal orchiectomy for testicular cancer, a CT scan would be indicated to evaluate for metastatic disease. Answer "C," CBC, would have a role in suspected infection. Answer "E," x-ray, really has no role in the evaluation of this patient.

> HELPFUL TIP: If the ultrasound of a scrotal mass is equivocal, MRI or urological referral should be considered next.

In taking this patient's history, if he had described a *painful* lump in his scrotum, the LEAST likely cause would be:

A) Chlamydia.
B) Inguinal hernia.
C) Hydrocele.
D) Testicular torsion.

Discussion
The correct answer is "C." Spermatoceles and hydroceles are usually not painful. When a young, sexually active male presents with a painful scrotal mass or swelling, epididymitis from chlamydia or gonorrhea should be considered. Testicular torsion often has a very abrupt onset of pain and is a surgical emergency. Inguinal hernias can be intermittently painful if moving freely in the inguinal canal. However, if one becomes incarcerated, intense pain occurs. Of note, varicoceles are usually an incidental finding; however, large varicoceles may occasionally be painful. Likewise, testicular cancers are usually not painful but can become so if the tumor growth is rapid.

* *

Your patient's ultrasound is concerning for testicular cancer, and you refer him to a urologist.

The next day the patient's 15-year-old brother presents with scrotal pain. You wonder if you are on the cusp of discovering an infectious cause of testicular cancer, but alas, it appears to be coincidence or God's sense of humor at work.

This patient's pain is on the right and he can localize it well to the front of the testicle. It has been present for 3 days and seemed to occur gradually over a few hours. There is no radiation of the pain. Running makes it worse, and cool packs seem to help. Yesterday he noticed a slight swelling of the scrotum on the same side. He denies trauma to the area, any history of sexual activity, other genitourinary complaints, fever, nausea, or vomiting. On exam, you find normal vitals. He has a well-localized tender spot at the anterior superior right scrotum with a bluish discoloration under the skin.

Which of the following is the most likely diagnosis?

A) Torsion of the appendix testis.
B) Torsion of the testicle.
C) Varicocele.
D) Abscess.
E) Spermatocele.

Discussion

The correct answer is "A." This is the classic presentation of torsed appendix testis. The appendix testis is a pedunculated, vestigial structure at the anterior superior testicle. Torsion of the appendix testis is one of the most common causes of scrotal pain in children. The pain is usually well localized. There may be a reactive hydrocele. Diagnosis is confirmed by ultrasound. Unlike a torsed testicle, a torsed appendix testis is not an emergency. It may be treated by conservative therapy (rest, NSAIDs, ice) or surgical excision.

Objectives: Did you learn to . . .

- Recognize potential causes of a painless scrotal mass?
- Evaluate a testicular mass?
- Recognize the significance of cryptorchidism?
- Identify torsion of the appendix testis?

QUICK QUIZ: HEMATOSPERMIA

A 28-year-old male presents to your office looking quite concerned. Several days ago after sexual intercourse with his girlfriend, he noticed bloody ejaculate in the condom. Since then he has avoided sex and masturbation. He denies pain, hematuria, dysuria, fevers, night sweats, and weight loss. He reports that he is otherwise healthy. His examination, including genitourinary and rectal exam, is normal, and a urinalysis shows 1–2 RBCs/hpf.

What is your next step in the evaluation and management of this patient?

A) Reassurance and follow-up.
B) Scrotal ultrasound.
C) Pelvic CT scan.
D) Transrectal ultrasound.
E) PSA.

Discussion

The correct answer is "A." Hematospermia, the name given to bloody penile ejaculate, is fairly uncommon. It can occur in men of any age and is perhaps most common after prostate biopsy or prostate surgery. In otherwise healthy young men, the cause is most often idiopathic and is almost always benign. History should focus on traumatic causes (e.g., long bicycle ride), symptoms of prostate disease, and symptoms of infection. A genital and prostate examination should be performed. Urinalysis is helpful to exclude infection. Consider gonorrhea and chlamydia cultures in the appropriate patients. In this patient, reassurance is adequate. In an older male (>40 years old) with the same complaint, PSA and transrectal ultrasound may be indicated. Other studies (e.g., MRI and cystoscopy) may be indicated depending on the findings on history, physical exam, and initial lab studies. Of note, in other parts of the world, schistosomiasis is a frequent cause of hematospermia and hematuria. In most cases of hematospermia, semen analysis is not warranted, but it can be diagnostic in patients with schistosomiasis. Finally, otherwise healthy patients with **persistent hematospermia** (>1 month) should be treated with a month trial of antibiotics (although there is no evidence for benefit) to treat possible prostatitis and then should be referred to a urologist if hematospermia persists.

CASE 3

A couple you have known for a few years comes to your office to announce that they are expecting and that they want you to be the baby's doctor (strange that they didn't ask you to be the mother's doctor, but you let it slide). According to an ultrasound, the fetus is male. The couple is ambivalent about neonatal circumcision and wants your advice.

You start the conversation by saying:

A) "Circumcision is a relic of history and should be illegal."
B) "All major medical organizations (e.g., AAFP, AAP, AMA) recommend routine neonatal circumcision."
C) "The decision to perform circumcision is a personal one, influenced by a number of factors—but primarily by cultural, religious, and familial issues."
D) "Do whatever you want. I don't really care what you do with a tiny piece of skin."

Discussion

The correct answer is "C." One of the strongest predictors of whether a newborn in the United States will be circumcised is the circumcision status of the father. There are other reasons cited by parents as well (discussed later in the case). "A" is incorrect simply because the statement is effused with emotion and lacks logic. "B" is incorrect. The AAFP has no policy statement on circumcision. In 2012 the American Academy of Pediatrics changed its statement on circumcision (since 1999 the AAP did not find the data sufficient to recommend routine neonatal circumcision) to the following: the health benefits outweigh the risks, and circumcision should be made available to all families who choose it. However, 'routine' universal circumcision is still not recommended. If you chose "D," you need to work on your bedside manner!

Consequences of circumcision include which of the following?

A) Overall reduction in mortality of circumcised infants compared with uncircumcised infants.
B) Reduction in UTIs in the first year of life.
C) Reduction in the number of sexual partners.
D) All of the above.

Discussion

The correct answer is "B." The rate of UTIs in uncircumcised males in the first year of life is about 10 times greater than the rate for circumcised males. In order to prevent one UTI in the first year of life, about 100 circumcisions need to be performed. The effect of circumcision on rates of UTI later in life is not well studied. The rate of UTI may be higher shortly after circumcision (within the first 2 weeks). "A" is incorrect because there is no data showing any difference in mortality between circumcised and uncircumcised infants. "C" is incorrect; some surveys have shown increased frequency and variety of sexual practices in circumcised males compared with uncircumcised (note that this is an association, not a causal relationship).

> **HELPFUL TIP:** Circumcision reduces the rate of cervical cancer in the female partners of males who were circumcised and previously had six or more sexual partners.

> **HELPFUL TIP:** It is abundantly clear that circumcision reduces the transmission of HIV. This has led to a call for routine circumcision in high-risk populations (e.g., some parts of sub-Saharan Africa, etc.).

Neonatal circumcision is associated with all of the following EXCEPT:

A) Risk of hemorrhage with the procedure.
B) Psychological trauma and decreased sexual satisfaction later in life.
C) Reduced risk of infection with human papillomavirus (HPV).
D) Reduced risk of penile cancer.

Discussion

The correct answer is "B." Despite what some anti-circumcision web sites maintain, circumcision does not appear to result in any significant psychological trauma or decreased sexual satisfaction for most men later in life. "A" is true. There is a small but real risk of hemorrhage with the procedure, and this occurs mostly in patients who have an unknown or unrealized coagulopathy. In fact, abnormal bleeding after circumcision is a common way in which sporadic cases of hemophilia are discovered (including one case discovered this way by one of the editors—and he still feels bad!). "D" is true. Several studies have demonstrated that circumcised men are less likely to have HPV infection. The data for the risk of other sexually transmitted infections (STIs) are somewhat contradictory, but generally favor a reduced risk of STIs in circumcised males. "D" appears to be true—at least in the United States. Retrospective studies have shown that the rate of squamous cell carcinoma of the penis is about threefold higher in uncircumcised men. However, the American Cancer Society does **not** recommend routine neonatal circumcision for the prevention of penile cancer but does recommend that all risk factors be addressed.

HELPFUL TIP: Penile cancer is exceedingly rare (incidence about 1/100,000 in the United States). In addition to uncircumcised status, risk factors associated with penile cancer include smoking, risky sexual behavior, poor hygiene, and genital warts.

* *

You have a nice, long conversation with the couple, discussing the potential benefits and risks, and they decide to have their son circumcised. After the birth, you are performing a thorough examination when you find something slightly abnormal with the penis.

Routine circumcision is absolutely or relatively contraindicated in all of the following situations EXCEPT:

A) Congenital phimosis.
B) Micropenis.
C) Hypospadias.
D) Ambiguous genitalia.
E) Religious beliefs of the parents that circumcision is wrong.

Discussion

The correct answer is "A." Significant congenital phimosis rarely occurs and is an **indication** for circumcision. Phimosis is defined as the inability to retract the foreskin (prepuce) over the glans. This is a **normal** finding in uncircumcised infants. However, **significant** congenital phimosis may completely cover the urethra and not allow the normal passage of urine. "B," "C," and "D" are reasons to avoid routine circumcision and to call on the aid of a urologist. If you chose "E," you need a coffee break. If the parents have a religious or cultural objection to circumcision, it should be avoided.

HELPFUL TIP: When performing circumcision, local anesthetic is recommended, and either dorsal penile nerve block or subcutaneous ring block is preferred. Other pain control modalities may be used as well, including preprocedure acetaminophen, sucrose-coated pacifier, etc.

Objectives: Did you learn to . . .

- Discuss the benefits and risks of circumcision with parents?
- Identify indications and contraindications for neonatal circumcision?
- Employ pain control measures for the procedure of circumcision?

CASE 4

A 32-year-old male presents to discuss permanent sterilization. He clearly states that he wants a vasectomy, and sooner is better than later. He is married and has three children at home. His wife just gave birth to twins. He is healthy and takes no medications. He looks tired and anxious. You examine him and find no abnormalities. The vas deferens is easily isolated bilaterally.

What is your next step?

A) Refer him for psychological counseling as he is clearly under a great deal of stress.
B) Provide him with detailed counseling on vasectomy, give him written material on the procedure, and ask him to discuss it with his wife.
C) Schedule the procedure as soon as possible.
D) Tell him that he is not an appropriate candidate for vasectomy.

Discussion

The correct answer is "B." Patient education, counseling, and selection are very important aspects of vasectomy. When you counsel him on vasectomy, you should explore his reasons for wanting the procedure. You should not schedule a vasectomy without providing counseling and assuring that he understands the procedure in detail. This patient appears to be fatigued—an issue that should be explored further . . . and he has newborn twins at home. Who the heck wouldn't be tired! So, immediate referral for psychological counseling without investigating the underlying cause is not appropriate.

While counseling this patient, you discuss which of the following issues?

A) Partner's desire for permanent sterility.
B) Effect of the procedure on sexual function.
C) Reversibility of the procedure.
D) Complications.
E) All of the above.

Discussion

The correct answer is "E." All of these issues are important to discuss prior to scheduling the procedure. It is important that the couple agree on this procedure because it is the couple—not just your patient—who will be sterile. Aside from psychological effects of vasectomy, the procedure should not directly affect sexual function, orgasm, or ejaculation. Patients should be aware that vasectomy results in permanent sterility and that reversal procedure are only successful about half of the time. Potential complications include failure and unwanted pregnancy, infection, pain, bleeding, hematoma, etc.

* *

After discussing the situation with his wife, the patient calls to ask your opinion on another option that they are considering. Although he is ready to have the vasectomy, his wife recently thought that maybe she should have a tubal ligation instead.

All of the following are advantages of vasectomy over tubal ligation EXCEPT:

A) Effectiveness of the procedure.
B) Risks of anesthesia.
C) Risks of procedural complications.
D) Cost.
E) Verification of sterility.

Discussion

The correct answer is "A." The failure rates of vasectomy and tubal ligation are fairly similar and are under 1% (although the failure rate of laparoscopic tubal ligation is up to 3% over 10 years). All the rest are true. In general, local anesthesia is used for vasectomy, compared with spinal or epidural anesthesia for tubal ligation. Vasectomy is safer and less expensive. Men usually leave the office shortly after the vasectomy is completed, whereas tubal ligation is typically performed in a surgical suite and requires several hours of postoperative observation. Abdominal organs can be injured during tubal ligation (e.g., bowel perforation). If you injure abdominal organs during a vasectomy, you need to go to remedial anatomy class. Another advantage of vasectomy is the ability to verify sterility with a semen analysis after the vasectomy.

* *

Your patient decides to "get snipped" as he puts it. You perform the vasectomy using a no-scalpel technique. The procedure was fairly easy, and the patient tolerated it well. One month after the procedure, the patient calls to complain about a painful swelling that has developed superior and slightly posterior to the left testis. He has no other symptoms.

Which of the following is the most likely diagnosis?

A) Hematoma.
B) Varicocele.
C) Congestive epididymitis.
D) Abscess.

Discussion

The correct answer is "C." Without any further information, congestive epididymitis is the most likely cause of this patient's current complaint. Congestive epididymitis occurs in about 3% of patients postvasectomy, and the onset is usually within weeks to months after the procedure. "A," hematoma, can be avoided in most cases if hemostasis is achieved during the procedure and the patient does not overexert himself immediately postop. A hematoma is more likely to develop early rather than a month later. Likewise, an infection ("D") would be unlikely so far out from the procedure. "B" is incorrect because varicoceles do not develop after vasectomy (unless you are operating far away from where you are supposed to be). Overall, the most common scrotal pathology after vasectomy is sperm granuloma, which occurs in up to 40% of patients but is generally asymptomatic.

HELPFUL TIP: The treatment of congestive epididymitis can be frustrating. Most men who have a vasectomy will have some element of congestive epididymitis, but most will have minor swelling without pain. For patients with painful congestive epididymitis, a trial of NSAIDs and sitz baths for several months is indicated. Failing conservative therapy, steroid injection or surgery may be indicated.

* *

Two months after the vasectomy, your patient returns with a semen sample, showing no sperm. His surgery was successful, but failures do occasionally occur.

Vasectomy failure is usually due to:

A) Failure to identify and transect the vas at the time of surgery.
B) Recanalization.
C) Left-handed doctors.
D) Infection.
E) Immaculate conception.

Discussion

The correct answer is "B." Although "redundant systems" (removing a segment of the vas deferens, clipping or suturing the free ends, cauterizing the transected vas, suturing fascia around one free end while leaving the other outside the fascia) are employed to avoid this complication, recanalization can occur. A new pathway can form between the free ends of the transected vas deferens, allowing sperm into the ejaculated semen. Therefore, all patients should return postvasectomy for semen analysis. "A" and "D" are potential, but infrequent, causes of failure. "C" is incorrect. What have you got against lefties? As to "E," only God knows.

* *

Your patient is ultimately pleased with his vasectomy results. He returns to see you several years later because of concerns that he is balding. On exam, you find nonscarring hair loss at the vertex. The scalp appears normal otherwise.

You should entertain all of the following diagnoses EXCEPT:

A) Androgenetic alopecia (yes, it is "androgenetic" and not "androgenic").
B) Telogen effluvium.
C) Alopecia areata.
D) Hypothyroidism.
E) Tinea capitis.

Discussion

The correct answer is "E." Hair loss is common in males, affecting up to two-thirds of all men. Alopecia is often divided in scarring and nonscarring forms. Most infectious causes of hair loss (e.g., tinea capitis and folliculitis) are scarring if not treated, whereas the other causes listed ("A" through "D") are nonscarring. Without any signs of inflammation or hyperkeratosis, tinea capitis is unlikely. "A," androgenetic alopecia, is quite common in adult males (male balding). "B," telogen effluvium, presents with diffuse hair loss usually secondary to metabolic (including dieting) or emotional stress. This occurs as an abnormal percentage of hair enters the telogen phase during which they are shed. Grab some hair: if more than 5 hairs in telogen phase come out, you have your diagnosis. "C," alopecia areata, results in patchy hair loss in round or oval shapes. Metabolic conditions should also be in the differential diagnosis of hair loss, and these might include hypothyroidism ("D"), hyperthyroidism, and iron deficiency.

HELPFUL TIP: Secondary syphilis causes a noninflammatory, nonscarring hair loss that may be patchy or diffuse. Consider testing for syphilis in appropriate patients.

* *

The patient reports a strong family history of baldness. On your exam, the patient has thin hair at the vertex and recession of the hairline in an "M" shape at the frontotemporal area. On the basis of the history and exam, you diagnose androgenetic alopecia. He would like to do something about his hair loss.

Regarding androgenetic alopecia, which of the following statements is true?

A) Minoxidil must be used for at least 2 years to achieve permanent hair regrowth.
B) Lower doses of 5-alpha reductase inhibitors (e.g., finasteride) are used in treating androgenetic alopecia compared with BPH.
C) Hair transplant should be avoided unless all other therapeutic attempts have failed.
D) Topical steroids are an effective therapy for androgenetic alopecia.
E) A toupee looks great on anyone.

Discussion

The correct answer is "B." Finasteride (Propecia) is FDA approved for androgenetic alopecia, and the dose is 1 mg/day rather than the 5 mg/day dose used to treat BPH symptoms. Minoxidil applied to the scalp is also an effective therapy for androgenetic alopecia. Both minoxidil and finasteride must be continued indefinitely to be effective. Hair transplant is a viable option for men and women with androgenetic alopecia, and it is sometimes used as a first-line therapy. Thus, "C" is incorrect. Topical steroids are not effective for this type of hair loss. "E" is clearly wrong; there are a lot of bad toupees out there.

Objectives: Did you learn to . . .

- Provide pre-vasectomy counseling?
- Recognize complications of vasectomy?
- Identify causes of hair loss in men?
- Describe current treatment options for androgenetic alopecia?

QUICK QUIZ: DEATH RATES IN MEN

For all of the following causes of death, the age-adjusted death rate is higher for males than for females EXCEPT:

A) Liver disease.
B) Alzheimer disease.
C) Coronary artery disease.
D) Suicide.
E) Cancer.

Discussion

The correct answer is "B." When it comes to Alzheimer disease, men get a break; the death rate is higher for females. All of the other causes of death listed have greater death rates in males. For example, compared with women with liver disease, same age men with liver disease are twice as likely to die of their liver disease.

QUICK QUIZ: DEATH RATES IN MEN

The relative risk of death for males is greater throughout the life span.

Compared with same age females, at what age range is the relative risk of death greatest for males?

A) <1 year.
B) 5–14 years.
C) 15–24 years.
D) 25–34 years.
E) >85 years.

Discussion

The correct answer is "C." Unfortunately, males aged 15–24 years have a relative risk of death of greater than 2.5 compared with same age females (usually preceded by a cry of "Hey, look what I can do!"). Mother nature has a way of making up for boys and young men dying: more male fetuses are conceived than female. However, the miscarriage rate is also greater for male fetuses. Nonetheless, about 105 males are born in the United States for every 100 females. By age 35, enough males have died off that the number of males and females that age is about equal, and thereafter the number of females exceeds the number of males (in other words, the singles scene improves markedly for the remaining males).

CASE 5

A 14-year-old male presents with his mother, who is worried that he has growing breasts. Over the last 2 or 3 months, the patient has developed swellings beneath both nipples. He denies discharge or pain, but the nipples are tender at times.

You can tell this patient that physiologic gynecomastia (subareolar breast tissue) is a condition that affects:

A) Newborns.
B) Adolescents.
C) Elderly males.
D) All of the above.

Discussion

The correct answer is "D." The incidence of physiologic gynecomastia is trimodal, with peaks in the neonatal period, adolescence, and old age. Data can be contradictory at times, but clinically palpable breast tissue (either fat or true breast tissue) may be present in more than 50% of males in each of these three age groups.

Which of the following hormones is responsible for the proliferation of breast tissue?

A) Testosterone.
B) Estrogen.
C) Androstenedione.
D) Growth hormone.
E) Progesterone.

Discussion

The correct answer is "B." Estrogens induce ductal hyperplasia and growth of glandular tissue. Testosterone and androstenedione inhibit the actions of estrogens on the breast tissue. Some men with gynecomastia have increased sensitivity of breast tissue to circulating estrogens; others may have an increased proportion of estrogens compared with androgens; yet, others may have a mixture of both processes or another process altogether.

Potential causes of gynecomastia include all of the following EXCEPT:

A) Renal failure.
B) Marijuana use.
C) Testicular cancer.
D) Hypothyroidism.
E) Phenothiazines.

Discussion

The correct answer is "D." **Hyper**thyroidism, not **hypo**thyroidism, can cause gynecomastia through increased aromatization of testosterone to estradiol and androstenedione to estrone. A number of drugs are associated with gynecomastia, including marijuana, alcohol, 5-alpha reductase inhibitors, phenothiazines, tricyclic antidepressants, androgens, estrogens, growth hormone, calcium channel blockers, and spironolactone. Other causes of gynecomastia include hypogonadism, hyperprolactinemia, testicular tumors (some secrete estrogens), renal failure, and liver diseases (cirrhosis).

HELPFUL TIP: Obesity causes "pseudogynecomastia." It is the deposition of fat in the breast region and not of breast tissue itself.

* *

A thorough drug history is negative. On physical examination, you find palpable, nontender tissue beneath the nipples, with slightly more prominent tissue mass on the right. The tissue is about 2–3 cm in diameter, and no discrete masses are palpable. There is no nipple discharge. An adult male's hair growth pattern is evident in the axillary and inguinal areas. The testicles are normal size without masses.

At this point in time, you recommend which of the following?

A) Observation.
B) Referral to a surgeon.
C) Limited laboratory studies, including thyroid-stimulating hormone (TSH), testosterone, and liver enzymes.
D) Biopsy of the tissue.
E) Mammogram and/or ultrasound.

Discussion

The correct answer is "A." As previously mentioned, physiologic gynecomastia is quite common in adolescent males. The findings on exam are reassuring. This patient does not display any other signs of testosterone deficiency, and further workup is not indicated at this time. If there are no discrete masses on exam, a mammogram, ultrasound, or biopsy is not likely to be helpful. Referral to a surgeon is premature, as 90% of these patients experience spontaneous involution of the breast tissue over 3 years.

HELPFUL TIP: In adolescent males with gynecomastia, further evaluation with laboratory studies and imaging is indicated if the breast tissue is rapidly enlarging or is greater than 5 cm in diameter, a mass (not normal breast tissue) is palpable, or other signs of under androgenization are present.

* *

You provide the patient and his mother with reassurance and have them return in a year. At follow-up, there is no palpable tissue. When you see the patient again, he is 17 years old. He told his mother that he was having abdominal pain, but really he is worried that he may have contracted a STI. He has become fairly promiscuous and does not use condoms. In the last week, he has developed dysuria and a yellowish urethral discharge. He has no other symptoms.

Which of the following is the most likely diagnosis?

A) HPV.
B) Syphilis.
C) Gonorrhea.
D) Trichomonas.
E) Herpes simplex.

Discussion

The correct answer is "C." This patient's symptoms are typical of gonococcal urethritis. However, ***N. gonorrhoeae*** **may be present in the urethra without any symptoms and *Chlamydia trachomatis* can present with a purulent discharge that is classically thought of as gonorrhea;** gonorrhea and chlamydia cannot be reliably distinguished on clinical grounds. "A" is incorrect as HPV causes genital warts, not urethritis. "B," syphilis, may present as a painless ulcer (primary syphilis). "D" is incorrect because most men infected with *Trichomonas vaginalis* are asymptomatic, although some will have mild urethritis. Finally, "E," herpes simplex, presents with painful vesicles at the area of inoculation.

* *

You take urethral samples for gonorrhea and chlamydia (you could use a PCR but are feeling contrary). You discuss other STIs and decide to perform some other tests (e.g., HIV, hepatitis B, RPR/VDRL).

At this point in time, you are compelled to do all of the following EXCEPT:

A) Recommend safe sexual practices.
B) Inform the public health services if he tests positive.
C) Treat him with antibiotics now.
D) Encourage him to contact his partners and tell them to get tested.
E) Inform his mother of your findings.

Discussion

The correct answer is "E." In general, adolescents can seek care for STIs and be treated without parental consent. However, clinicians should refer to the laws of the state in which they practice for ultimate legal authority in this matter. Of course, the time of diagnosis and treatment should be used as an opportunity to educate the patient regarding safe sexual practices. "B" is true. Gonorrhea and chlamydia are reportable diseases in every state. Again, clinicians should refer to the laws of their state and the reporting protocols of the clinic in which they practice. Empiric treatment is the rule here, so "C" is correct. "D" is also correct since all of this patient's partners should be contacted, tested, and treated. There are several ways to contact the partners, and allowing the patient to do so is only one way. The clinician or the public health authorities could contact the partners as well.

> HELPFUL TIP: Expedited partner treatment in which the patient being treated for an STI is also given medication for his/her partner(s) is recommended by the Centers for Disease Control and Prevention (CDC) and others. See http://www.cdc.gov/std/ept/ for more information and the legality of the practice in your state.

Which of the following methods maintains a high degree of sensitivity and is also the quickest and least expensive way to diagnose gonococcal urethritis in a symptomatic male?

A) Culture.
B) Gram stain.
C) Serologic antibody assay.
D) PCR.
E) DNA probe.

Discussion

The correct answer is "B." In **symptomatic** males, Gram stain of a urethral sample can identify gram-negative diplococci (*N. gonorrhoeae*) with a sensitivity of about 90–95%. The sensitivity drops to about 70% in asymptomatic males. If the materials and expertise are readily available, a Gram stain is quick and inexpensive. Culture of a urethral specimen on Thayer-Martin agar takes longer and false-negative tests can occur with high frequency (due to the need to have a CO_2-rich environment and to keep the culture in a narrow temperature range). However, culture is still the "gold standard." PCR and other nucleic acid testing are more sensitive than cultures but still not 100%. PCR is particularly attractive as a screening test, as it can be performed on urine specimens instead of urethral swab specimens. Serologic assays for gonorrhea would not be helpful in diagnosing urethritis.

Your clinical suspicion of gonorrhea is high. What is your next step?

A) Single doses of ceftriaxone 125 mg IM.
B) A single dose of penicillin G 1.2 million units IM and erythromycin 500 mg PO QID for 7 days.
C) Tetracycline 500 mg PO QID for 10 days.
D) Single doses of ciprofloxacin 500 mg PO and cefixime 400 mg PO.
E) Single dose of ceftriaxone 250 mg IM and azithromycin 1 g PO.

Discussion

The correct answer is "E." If there is any concern for compliance, it is best to treat the patient in the office if you have access to the appropriate antibiotics. When you are treating for gonorrhea either empirically or on the basis of a positive test result, **you should also treat for chlamydia**. Therefore, of the options listed, "E" is most appropriate. As of 2011, the CDC recommends ceftriaxone 250 mg IM as a single dose (rather than 125 mg, due to increasing resistance) for uncomplicated gonococcal urethritis, **and** azithromycin 1 g PO as a single dose for chlamydia urethritis. The first-line treatments for gonorrhea are third-generation cephalosporins. **Fluoroquinolones are no longer recommended for gonorrhea due to high rates of resistance in some communities.** "A" is incorrect because ceftriaxone alone will not provide empiric coverage for chlamydia, and the dose is too low anyway. "B" is incorrect because penicillin should never be used to treat gonorrhea (due to the prevalence of penicillinase-producing strains of the bacteria). "C" is incorrect. Tetracycline antibiotics provide adequate coverage for chlamydia and some strains of *N. gonorrhoeae*, but other strains of *N. gonorrhoeae* are resistant to tetracyclines, so these drugs are not used as first-line agents in treating gonorrhea. "D" is incorrect because it gives two medications that are used for the treatment of gonorrhea and none for the treatment of chlamydia.

HELPFUL TIP: Another equally effective regimen for chlamydia is doxycycline 100 mg BID for 7 days. This is equal in efficacy to azithromycin regardless of the fact that some doses may be missed. But then again, there is something satisfying about watching your patient swallow his medicine.

* *

You treat this patient with ceftriaxone and azithromycin and tell him to contact his partners so that they can get treated. When your patient returns to discuss his lab tests, he is feeling much better. You tell him that he was infected with both gonorrhea and chlamydia but that the rest of his tests were negative. He is relieved that he does not have HIV, but he wonders what problems chlamydia can cause.

***C. trachomatis* has been implicated in which of the following?**

A) Reiter syndrome.
B) Lymphogranuloma venereum.
C) Proctitis.
D) Epididymitis.
E) All of the above.

Discussion

The correct answer is "E." A small percentage of men with chlamydia urethritis develop reactive arthritis, and a subset of these will go on to have the triad of Reiter syndrome (urethritis, arthritis, and uveitis). Lymphogranuloma venereum is also due to a particularly virulent strain of *C. trachomatis*, but it produces genital ulcers and lymphadenitis and is generally seen in tropical areas. Lymphogranuloma venereum is treated with extended courses of doxycycline (100 mg PO BID for 21 days) or azithromycin (1 g PO weekly for 3 weeks). Chlamydia proctitis occurs almost exclusively in homosexual men and presents with rectal pain, bleeding, and discharge. Diagnosis is confirmed by rectal swab, and the treatment is the same as for chlamydia urethritis. "D," epididymitis is most often the result of infection with *C. trachomatis* or *N. gonorrhoeae*. CDC guidelines recommend treatment with a single injection of ceftriaxone 250 mg IM and doxycycline 100 mg PO BID for 10 days.

HELPFUL TIP: The majority of males (and females) who are infected with chlamydia and/or gonorrhea **do not have symptoms**. Therefore, there is a good argument to be made for screening asymptomatic males in high-risk populations (e.g., adolescents, young adults, and those with multiple sexual partners). For females, see Chapter 15.

Objectives: Did you learn to . . .

- Define gynecomastia and understand its causes?
- Identify when to initiate further evaluation in a patient with gynecomastia?
- Recognize symptoms of gonorrhea and chlamydia?
- Initiate treatment in a male with urethritis?
- Recognize manifestations of chlamydia infection in men?

QUICK QUIZ: AN INFLAMED GLANS

A 36-year-old male diabetic patient presents with a 3-day history of irritation, itching, dysuria, and redness at the tip of his penis. He is monogamous with his wife, and he denies any history of high-risk sexual behavior or STIs. On exam, you find an afebrile patient in no acute distress. The penis is circumcised, and the glans penis is red, tender, and edematous. There are numerous small, white papules on the glans.

Which of the following is the most appropriate treatment?

A) Sitz baths and improved hygiene.
B) Oral doxycycline.
C) Topical bacitracin.
D) Topical miconazole.
E) Topical steroids.

Discussion

The correct answer is "D." This patient has balanitis, which is defined as an inflammatory condition of the glans penis (balanoposthitis is the name applied to inflammation of the glans and foreskin). Some authors believe that balanitis is a noninfectious, inflammatory condition. Others implicate infectious causes. Of infectious causes, the most common is *Candida albicans*, especially in diabetic patients. This patient has classic findings of candidal balanitis and is diabetic. Therefore, the most appropriate therapy is a topical antifungal agent, such as miconazole. Fluconazole is an option. Topical and oral antibiotics will not help, and topical steroids should be avoided. Sitz baths and improved hygiene should be encouraged, but they should not be employed without an antifungal agent.

CASE 6

While covering the emergency department (ED), a 40-year-old male presents with a painful erection that began 4 hours ago "out of the blue."

Which of the following is true regarding priapism and normal erections?

A) Normal erections can last up to 12 hours, so this is not priapism.
B) Abnormally prolonged sexual desire can "convert" a normal erection into priapism.
C) The corpus spongiosum and glans penis are not involved in priapism.
D) Acute urinary retention may lead to priapism and vice versa.
E) All of the above are true statements.

Discussion

The correct answer is "C." Priapism is defined as the prolonged engorgement of the penis (or—rarely—the clitoris in females), unrelated to sexual desire or stimulation. The word priapism comes from the Greek god Priapus, apparently well known for his lasciviousness and generous genital endowment. In most cases of priapism, the corpus spongiosum and glans penis are not involved. Only the corpora cavernosa are engorged and rigid. Priapism typically lasts longer than 6 hours, whereas normal erections last minutes to hours. With normal erections, detumescence occurs after ejaculation or after the stimulus is removed. This is not the case with priapism, and sexual desire does not play a role in the development of priapism; thus, "B" is incorrect. "D" is also incorrect. Urinary retention is not thought to cause priapism, and priapism does not lead to urinary retention.

Priapism may be secondary to all of the following EXCEPT:

A) Sickle cell disease.
B) Penile trauma.
C) Leukemia.
D) Iron deficiency anemia.
E) Trazodone use.

Discussion

The correct answer is "D." A number of different disease states and drugs have been implicated in the etiology of priapism. In one way or another, these diseases and drugs affect the balance of blood flow into the penis, leading to increased arterial blood flow and/or decreased venous outflow. Local malignancies, such as bladder and prostate cancers, can cause obstruction. Likewise, any condition that increases blood viscosity (e.g., sickle cell disease, polycythemia, leukemia) or results in thromboembolic phenomena (e.g.,

Table 16–1 DRUGS ASSOCIATED WITH PRIAPISM

Psychotropics
- Trazodone
- Chlorpromazine

Agents used to treat erectile dysfunction
- Intracavernosal injections (e.g., papaverine)
- Phosphodiesterase inhibitors (e.g., sildenafil)

Antihypertensives
- Hydralazine
- Prazosin

Anticoagulants
- Heparin

Drugs of abuse
- Alcohol
- Cocaine
- Marijuana

vasculitis) can cause priapism. Penile trauma that results in laceration of penile arteries can cause priapism. Numerous drugs have also been implicated (see Table 16–1), but in most cases, the cause is not identified.

What is your next step in management of this patient?

A) Reassurance.
B) Call for emergent urologic consultation.
C) Give oral alpha-blockers.
D) Engage patient in guided imagery to lead his thoughts away from sex.

Discussion

The correct answer is "B." Priapism is a urologic emergency and needs to be treated ASAP. All the other answers could result in your undesired new title of "defendant."

> HELPFUL TIP: After recovery, about 50% of men with priapism suffer erectile dysfunction. Penile implants are an option.

* *

The urologist will be in the ED in 30 minutes.

What should you do while you wait?

A) Administer intracavernosal metoprolol.
B) Administer supplemental oxygen, IV hydration, and analgesics.
C) Insert a needle into the glans penis and withdraw blood.
D) See the next patient waiting... or "take 5" and get a cup of coffee.

Discussion

The correct answer is "B." Until the urologist arrives, conservative measures are probably best, and you should try to make the patient comfortable using analgesics, oxygen, and hydration. Check a CBC since leukemia can rarely present with priapism. Some patients will respond to analgesics and ice packs. Oral or subcutaneous terbutaline may be helpful. Some authors recommend sedatives, such as benzodiazepines. "A," giving metoprolol, is the exact opposite of what you should be doing. "C" is incorrect because any attempt to withdraw blood from the penis should be directed at the corpora cavernosa, not the glans. Maybe "E" is tempting, but you can get your coffee after you do "B."

> HELPFUL TIP: If a urologist is not available and/or you are comfortable performing the procedure (and you have a good lawyer), you can attempt detumescence. A needle is inserted into the corpora cavernosa and blood is withdrawn. Then a vasoactive agent (e.g., phenylephrine) is injected. This procedure is repeated every 5 minutes until detumescence occurs. It should go without saying that the patient's vital signs must be closely monitored during this intervention because they will likely need sedation.

Objectives: Did you learn to . . .

- Recognize priapism and its causes?
- Manage a patient with priapism?

QUICK QUIZ: DEPRESSION AND SUICIDE

Which of the following groups has the highest rate of death by suicide?

A) Black males.
B) White males.
C) Black females.
D) White females.
E) Hispanic males.

Discussion

The correct answer is "B." In the United States, white males make up about 70% of all deaths due to suicide. Although females account for more suicide attempts, males are at greater risk of death from suicide. Men tend to use deadlier means, such as guns, hanging, and car collisions. In other words, men are very efficient at suicide. White men older than 85 years have one of the highest rates of death due to suicide: 59/100,000 (with the rate in the general public being 10.6/100,000). As a group, black males have the second highest rate of suicide. Of those groups listed above, black females have the lowest risk of death from suicide.

CASE 7

A 78-year-old male presents to your office after sustaining a backward fall last night. He went to the bathroom and slipped on a throw rug. He complains of mid back pain. He smokes cigarettes, considers himself healthy, and takes no medication. On examination, you find a pleasant male in some discomfort. His vital signs are normal. Radiographs of the thoracic spine show an acute wedge compression fracture of the T11 vertebral body.

Which of the following is the most appropriate next step in the evaluation of this patient?

A) Bone scan.
B) Dual energy x-ray absorptiometry (DEXA) scan.
C) Chest x-ray.
D) PSA.

Discussion

The correct answer is "B." Normal, healthy vertebral bodies should not break from low impact trauma, such as falling from a standing height. This patient almost certainly has diseased bone, most likely osteoporosis. The next step is to confirm your suspicion by obtaining a bone mineral density test, and DEXA is the most well-standardized test currently available. The other radiologic studies are less likely to be useful. Fracture due to metastatic prostate cancer is a reasonable concern, and a PSA and rectal exam can help rule out or rule in prostate disease. However, prostate cancer metastatic to bone typically causes lytic lesions, which should be seen on x-ray. Therefore, a PSA would be expected to have lower yield than a DEXA scan.

HELPFUL TIP: Regarding bone mineral density, the numbers to watch do not change for men. Use T-scores. If the T-score is between −1 and −2.5, the diagnosis is osteopenia. If the T-score is −2.5 or less, the diagnosis is osteoporosis.

* *

The DEXA scan results show that this patient has osteoporosis.

What further tests are indicated in this patient at this point in time?

A) TSH.
B) Calcium.
C) Skeletal survey.
D) A and B.
E) All of the above.

Discussion

The correct answer is "D." Secondary causes of osteoporosis are found more commonly in men when compared with women. You should not assume that this patient's osteoporosis is idiopathic as 50% or more of males with symptomatic vertebral fractures due to osteoporosis have a secondary cause of osteoporosis. Common causes of osteoporosis in males include long-term corticosteroid use, thyroid and parathyroid disorders, gastrointestinal disease (adversely affecting calcium and vitamin D absorption), testosterone deficiency, alcoholism, and renal disease. While multiple myeloma may result in decreased bone mineral density, it is less common, and a skeletal survey ("C") is not the preferred screening test. Instead, you would want to order serum and urine protein electrophoresis, looking for a monoclonal band.

* *

Your patient's laboratory tests are normal. In addition to calcium and vitamin D, you want to start him on a medication for osteoporosis.

Which of the following medications has the best evidence for use in men with primary osteoporosis?

A) Alendronate.
B) Estrogen.
C) Testosterone.

D) Calcitonin.
E) Fluoride.

Discussion

The correct answer is "A." Bisphosphonates, like alendronate, have the best evidence for treatment of primary osteoporosis in men. In addition to stabilizing bone density, alendronate and risedronate have been shown to decrease the incidence of osteoporotic fractures in men. If you choose to treat with bisphosphonates, the doses are the same for men and women. The other medications listed simply do not have the efficacy data published for bisphosphonates. If a patient cannot tolerate oral bisphosphonates, an IV bisphosphonate preparation should be considered. Estrogen ("B") may be effective, but the side effect profile would prohibit its use. "C" (testosterone) and "D" (calcitonin) are incorrect, as both have been shown to improve bone mineral density but have not shown reduced hip fracture risk. Finally, "E" is incorrect, as fluoride does not appear to be effective.

HELPFUL TIP: If a male patient with osteoporosis has testosterone deficiency, testosterone supplementation may be a reasonable treatment option, but the efficacy of testosterone in this scenario is **not** well studied. Although testosterone contributes to peak bone mass in young men and low testosterone is associated with an increased fracture risk in older men, testosterone for the treatment of osteoporosis has been **disappointing**.

HELPFUL TIP: Teriparatide (recombinant parathyroid hormone 1–34) is FDA approved for treatment of men at high risk for osteoporotic fractures (severe osteoporosis, failed other therapies, previous osteoporotic fractures). However, its use is limited by cost, need for daily injection, and the finding of increased osteosarcoma incidence in lab rats.

* *

Just to be on the safe side, you order a bunch of laboratory tests, all of which are normal except for serum testosterone. Lo and behold, his testosterone level is low. You are considering starting testosterone supplementation.

Which of the following testosterone supplementation products would you AVOID?

A) Transdermal testosterone.
B) Buccal testosterone.
C) Oral testosterone.
D) Intramuscular testosterone.
E) None of the above.

Discussion

The correct answer is "C." Oral testosterone should be avoided due to significant first-pass metabolism and potential liver toxicity. The other choices listed are viable options for testosterone replacement (see Table 16–2).

Which of the following is true regarding testosterone supplementation in older men with testosterone deficiency?

A) Testosterone supplementation has markedly beneficial effects on depression.
B) The effects of testosterone supplementation in young hypogonadal males and older testosterone-deficient males are the same.
C) In testosterone-deficient older males with erectile dysfunction, testosterone supplementation dramatically improves erections.
D) In testosterone-deficient older males with poor libido, testosterone supplementation improves libido.
E) Testosterone supplementation has no effect on lean muscle mass or grip strength.

Discussion

The correct answer is "D." In testosterone-deficient older males, testosterone supplementation does improve libido. Unfortunately, "C" is incorrect: its effects on erectile dysfunction are not impressive. Even in testosterone-deficient men with erectile dysfunction, a phosphodiesterase inhibitor (e.g., sildenafil) is more likely to be successful. In terms of the neuropsychiatric effects of testosterone, many questions are as yet unanswered. However, testosterone supplementation does not appear to significantly affect depression, so "A" is incorrect. "B" is not true. Young hypogonadal males who are treated with testosterone have increased peak bone mass and virilization. But the effects on older males are different: older males have improved strength, libido, and sense of well-being without some of the effects seen in the young hypogonadal males. "E" is incorrect because testosterone has

Table 16–2 TESTOSTERONE SUPPLEMENTATION PRODUCTS

Agents	Dosages	Comments
Striant (buccal tablet)	Dosed 30 mg BID and must be kept beside buccal mucosa	The product does not dissolve completely
Androgel, Testim (transdermal gels)	Dosed daily	Cover the application area to reduce risk of spreading by contact with others
Androderm (transdermal patch)	Applied daily	Rotate sites to reduce skin irritation
Scrotal patches (Testoderm)		Now rarely used due to scrotal irritation and more acceptable alternatives
Itramuscular injections (Depo-testosterone, Delatestryl)	Dosed every 2–4 weeks	Serum testosterone levels fluctuate significantly between doses
Subcutaneous pellets (Testopel)		These are implanted (like Norplant) and are rarely used for supplementation
Oral agents (methyltestosterone)		AVOID due to significant first-pass metabolism, fluctuating serum levels, and risk of liver toxicity

been shown to consistently improve lean muscle mass and grip strength.

HELPFUL TIP: Hypogonadal males should **not** take testosterone replacement while trying to impregnate their partners because it will further decrease their sperm counts (due to the effect of exogenous testosterone feeding back on the hypothalamic–pituitary–gonadal axis). To improve fertility in these patients, unproven empiric therapy is often used, including clomiphene, human chorionic gonadotropin, and gonadotropin-releasing hormone.

HELPFUL TIP: Topical testosterone can have an androgenizing effects on women and children if they come in contact with the gel on a male's skin.

* *

You have a conversation with your patient about starting testosterone therapy. He would like to try it.

You tell him about adverse effects and monitoring and tell him it is important to periodically check:

A) Hematocrit.
B) Potassium.
C) Alanine aminotransferase.
D) A and B.
E) A and C.

Discussion

The correct answer is "E." There are good reasons behind the recommendation for periodic monitoring with certain serum tests. Testosterone increases erythropoietin production and can cause erythrocytosis. In fact, testosterone should not be started in a patient with a hematocrit greater than 50% (or severe heart failure or untreated sleep apnea). Testosterone can cause elevated liver enzymes, increased cholesterol, and growth of prostate and breast tissue, including prostate and breast cancers. Prostate exam and PSA are recommended prior to starting therapy and periodically while on testosterone. Of course, it makes sense to periodically monitor serum testosterone levels to assure that the patient is in the normal range and not sub- or supratherapeutic. Potassium ("B") is not directly affected and no monitoring is recommended.

Objectives: Did you learn to . . .

- Recognize the importance of osteoporosis in older males?
- Evaluate a patient with an osteoporotic fracture?
- Discuss management strategies for osteoporosis in males?

- Identify testosterone replacement products and discuss how older males might benefit from them?
- Recognize some of the risks associated with testosterone supplementation?

CASE 8

A 50-year-old male presents for a "get acquainted" visit. He has a history of hyperlipidemia treated with lovastatin. He takes no other medications and states that he is otherwise healthy. After watching a television feature on prostate cancer, he thought he should be screened.

In order to assess his risk for prostate cancer, you should take into account all of the following factors EXCEPT:

A) Age.
B) Race.
C) Family history.
D) Diet.
E) Ultraviolet light exposure.

Discussion

The correct answer is "E." Ultraviolet light exposure increases the risk of skin cancer but not prostate cancer (it is where "the sun don't shine"). Advancing age is strongly and directly associated with the development of prostate cancer. Between ages 50 and 70 years, the incidence of prostate cancer more than quadruples, and it continues to increase thereafter. Black ancestry and positive family history are associated with an increased risk. Interestingly, dietary factors may have a role in the development of prostate cancer, although the associations are not strong. A diet rich in fish and vegetables and low in red meat may reduce the risk of prostate cancer.

* *

Your patient is Caucasian and denies any family history of prostate cancer. He has no urinary symptoms and denies sexual dysfunction.

If he did have urinary symptoms, which of the following could be used to reliably distinguish BPH from prostate cancer?

A) Urgency.
B) Nocturia.
C) Frequency.
D) Hesitancy.
E) None of the above.

Discussion

The correct answer is "E." A male who presents with urinary symptoms of urgency, nocturia, frequency, and/or hesitancy most likely has BPH and not prostate cancer. However, urinary tract cancers (including prostate and bladder cancers) can present with these symptoms and must be considered. The point is that we cannot always attribute urinary symptoms in an older male to BPH. In fact, similar symptoms are found in high rates in older *women* and are often attributable to bladder problems rather than prostate problems. Urinary outlet obstruction is being increasingly recognized in women.

* *

You discuss prostate cancer screening with him, and he chooses to undergo digital rectal exam and PSA testing. The exam is remarkable for a slightly enlarged, smooth, nontender prostate with no nodules. The PSA level is 16 ng/mL (normal 0–4 ng/mL).

The most appropriate next step is to:

A) Repeat the PSA in 3–6 months.
B) Order a transrectal ultrasound of the prostate.
C) Refer to urology for further evaluation and prostate biopsy.
D) Repeat the rectal exam and try to find the nodule that you missed.
E) Order a free PSA.

Discussion

The correct answer is "C." This patient is at relatively high risk of having prostate cancer based on his PSA level and age at presentation. Sending him to a urologist for prostate biopsy is the most prudent step. Follow-up PSA alone ("A") would be more defensible if the PSA level were <10 ng/mL and/or the patient were much older. "B," a transrectal ultrasound, is likely to miss more than it would find in this case. With this patient's PSA and current life expectancy, ultrasound should only be used as part of a larger urologic evaluation, including biopsy. "D," repeating the rectal exam, is just nuts. There is no need for this. Did you miss a nodule? Maybe. If so, you will eventually get over it. More likely, there was no palpable nodule. This patient could have stage T1 prostate cancer in which, by definition, no nodules are palpable. He could have a nodule located anteriorly in the prostate—a location you cannot palpate. He also may have a PSA elevation for reasons other than prostate cancer. Finally, "E" is incorrect. The free PSA is most helpful when the total PSA is in the intermediate risk zone (4.1–10 ng/mL). When the PSA is higher (>10 ng/mL), the risk of cancer is too great to make the free PSA useful. The fraction of PSA that is "free" (not bound to plasma proteins) is inversely proportional to risk of prostate cancer: the lower the free PSA compared with total PSA, the greater the risk of prostate cancer (cutoff percentages vary from 10% to 25%).

* *

Thankfully, this patient has only one medication and you don't have to think too hard.

If he were taking _____, you would need to interpret his PSA differently.

A) Finasteride.
B) Hydrochlorothiazide.
C) Sildenafil.
D) Testosterone.
E) Tamsulosin.

Discussion

The correct answer is "A." With chronic use, 5-alpha reductase inhibitors (finasteride, dutasteride) are known to lower PSA values by about 50%. Therefore, many experts recommend doubling the measured PSA when a patient is taking a 5-alpha reductase inhibitor in order to reduce the risk of a false-negative result. Brief interruption in 5-alpha reductase inhibitor therapy is not a viable approach, as the PSA measure only returns to baseline after therapy has been stopped for at least 6 months. The other options are incorrect, as they do not affect PSA levels.

HELPFUL (OR NOT SO HELPFUL) TIP: The determination of when to send a patient for prostate biopsy is made on clinical grounds and must take into account the patient's risk, comorbidities, exam findings, PSA level, possibility of false-positive or negative tests, patient's preference, etc. This decision cannot be made based on an arbitrary PSA value.

Which of the following is true of the PSA test when used for screening purposes?

A) The positive predictive value approaches 100%.
B) Since PSA testing has become widespread, prostate cancer incidence and mortality have increased.
C) The false-negative rate is 20–25%.
D) Age-specific cutoff values for PSA have proven to increase positive predictive value and specificity.
E) Race-specific cutoff values for PSA have proven to increase positive predictive value and specificity.

Discussion

The correct answer is "C." There is a substantial false-negative rate—from 20% to 25%—limiting the use of PSA for screening purposes. "A" is incorrect by a long shot. The positive predictive value (likelihood of a positive test indicating true prostate cancer) ranges from about 20% to 60%, depending on the PSA level. The positive predictive value increases with increasing PSA level. "B" is incorrect. Since the PSA test has come into widespread use, the incidence of prostate cancer has increased, but mortality due to the disease has decreased. The reason for these trends has not been completely explained, and the role of the PSA test in these trends is not known. "D" and "E" are incorrect. Since older males seem to have higher PSA values in the absence of prostate cancer and black males tend to have prostate cancer found at lower PSA levels, age-specific and race-specific cutoff values have been proposed and investigated. However, the use of age-specific and race-specific PSA cutoff values is of questionable value.

HELPFUL TIP: It is important to realize that there is great controversy over the role of digital rectal exam and PSA in screening for prostate cancer. Neither is considered a "good" screening test (high rate of false positives and false negatives), but there is nothing else to offer at this time. The AUA and American Cancer Society recommend routine prostate cancer screening with DRE and PSA, and in 2009, they lowered the screening age to 40. However, the US Preventive Services Task Force now (as of 2012) recommends AGAINST using PSA for prostate cancer screening. The two large studies (the Prostate, Lung, Colon, and Ovarian Cancer Screening Trial [PLCO] and the European Randomized Study of Screening for Prostate Cancer [ERSPC]) done to answer the question of how PSA screening affects mortality arrived at opposite conclusions (PLCO showed no mortality effect with screening, while the ERSPC showed a prostate cancer-specific mortality reduction with PSA screening). However you approach this issue, you're not alone, and the company you keep is just as confused. Everyone agrees that screening for men older than 75 years or with less than 10 years to live is not useful.

HELPFUL TIP: The results of a randomized trial suggest that vitamin E supplementation may increase the rate of prostate cancer. Don't do it (*JAMA* 2011;306(14):1549-1556; doi: 10.1001/jama.2011.1437.)

Objectives: Did you learn to . . .

- Identify risk factors for prostate cancer?
- Discuss prostate cancer screening with a patient?
- Interpret an elevated PSA?
- Recognize the limitations of prostate cancer screening?

CASE 9

A 32-year-old male accompanied by his wife presents for evaluation of infertility. They have been married for 5 years and have been attempting conception for 3 years without success. The patient's wife has a 7-year-old daughter from a previous marriage. The patient has no significant past medical or surgical history. He does not smoke but drinks a six pack of beer and one cup of coffee daily—not necessarily in that order. He relaxes after work and on weekends by sitting in their hot tub. His BMI is 32 kg/m^2. He has normal facial and body hair and his testicles are descended bilaterally. You estimate the testicular volume to be 13 cc on the left and 18 cc on the right. You note a moderate sized varicocele on the left.

Which of the following is *not* a modifiable risk factor for male subfertility?

A) Alcohol intake.
B) Hot tub usage.
C) Varicocele.
D) Tobacco use.
E) Obesity.

Discussion

The correct answer is "D." We should note that the study of infertility risk factors and treatments is complicated by inconsistent outcome measures (e.g., sperm count, sperm motility, conception, pregnancy resulting in live birth). However, there are no conclusive studies correlating tobacco use with male subfertility. The other answers are modifiable risk factors and have been directly linked to subfertility, either in decreased sperm count or decreased sperm motility. It is important to ask about alcohol use ("A"). Other drug use, such as marijuana, should be investigated as well. "B" is true. Hot tub usage, febrile illnesses, and the presence of a varicocele raise the temperature of the testicles, thereby decreasing the optimal environment for the maturation of sperm. But how about the boxers or briefs controversy? Type of underwear does not seem to affect scrotal temperature significantly, and more to the point, tight underwear is not associated with decreased fertility. "C," the presence of a varicocele, is an interesting issue. It certainly is modifiable in that the patient could undergo a varicocelectomy, which might help if the varicocele is moderate to large in size. However, the degree to which a varicocele contributes to infertility is not well known. Varicoceles are noted to occur more commonly in infertile men, but they also occur in 10–15% of the normal, fertile male population. "E," obesity, contributes to the increased peripheral aromatization of testosterone into estradiol in fatty tissue.

Other factors that contribute to subfertility/infertility include a history of cryptorchidism, hypospadias, viral orchitis after puberty, prior chemotherapy or radiation, intake of calcium channel blockers, and retrograde ejaculation associated with diabetes and multiple sclerosis. It has been noted that roughly one-third of men with a history of unilateral cryptorchidism and two-thirds of men with bilateral cryptorchidism are infertile.

HELPFUL TIP: Infertility in a couple is defined as inability to conceive despite 1 year of frequent (how frequent is not defined), unprotected sexual intercourse. In the United States, the prevalence of infertility is 7–15% depending on how the statistic is measured.

Which of the following laboratory tests would you order first?

A) Seminal fluid analysis (SFA) including sperm count.
B) Testosterone.
C) Karyotype.
D) FSH.
E) Y chromosome analysis for microdeletion.

Discussion

The correct answer is "A." If the main concern is infertility, the initial step in evaluation beyond the history and physical exam is an SFA. Depending on the results of the SFA, additional laboratory studies may need to be ordered. If the sperm count is abnormal, then hormonal studies (e.g., testosterone, FSH, LH) should be ordered. If the patient is obese, an estradiol level may also be appropriate since obesity contributes to the increased peripheral aromatization of testosterone into estradiol in fatty tissue. Karyotype and Y chromosome analysis are important tools in the right patient population, but should not be employed in the early stages of the evaluation unless a chromosomal disorder is strongly suspected.

This patient's sperm density is 12 million/mL with a motility of 35%. This finding is:

A) Normal for both sperm count and motility.
B) Normal for sperm count but abnormal for motility.
C) Abnormal for sperm count but normal for motility.
D) Abnormal for both sperm count and motility.

Discussion

The correct answer is "D." As a general rule, normal sperm concentration for fertility is considered to be 15 million/mL or greater. However, as they say, it only takes one sperm to make a baby, so men with lower sperm counts can be fertile. At least 40% or more should be motile. Another finding of importance on SFA is the sperm morphology. Using strict criteria, normal morphology should be 4% or more (yes, unfortunately for men, only 4%).

* *

You repeat the SFA 2 weeks later, and again it is abnormal. His testosterone level is low for his age, and his FSH and LH are high.

Which of the following is most likely to be the cause of his decreased fertility?

Table 16–3 A PARTIAL LIST OF CAUSES OF MALE INFERTILITY

Mechanism	Specific examples
Hypothalamic-pituitary disorders	Congenital disorders (Kallmann syndrome), pituitary tumors, pituitary infarction, hormonal or psychotropic drug use.
Primary hypogonadism	Klinefelter syndrome, cryptorchidism, alcohol use, chemotherapeutic agents, testicular torsion, hyperthermia.
Disorders of sperm transport	Congenital absence of the vas deferens, epididymal dysfunction, spinal cord injury.
Idiopathic infertility	Unexplained satisfactorily by history, exam, and laboratory evaluation.

A) Congenital absence of the prostate gland.
B) Primary hypogonadism.
C) Bilateral complete vas deferens obstruction.
D) Androgen resistance.

Discussion

The correct answer is "B." A low testosterone level accompanied by elevated LH and FSH could indicate testicular failure, or primary hypogonadism. "A" is not a known cause of infertility, and in fact it is not a known disorder as far as the editors can determine. The prostate gland's only important function is to provide a subject for an endless debate over screening so that epidemiologists have something to do. Just kidding... The prostate gland actually has a role in producing important substances that are part of the seminal fluid and assist sperm in their migration through the female genital tract. However, prostate problems do not seem to cause infertility. "C," an obstruction of the vas deferens, would most likely result in azoospermia with normal or high testosterone levels. "D" is incorrect. You would expect to see elevated testosterone levels in patients with androgen resistance. See Table 16–3 for a list of causes of infertility in males.

How can you now best help this patient achieve fertility, assuming that there are no problems with his partner?

A) Empiric treatment for gonorrhea and chlamydia.
B) Empiric treatment with testosterone injections.

C) Empiric treatment with gonadotropin-releasing hormone.
D) Referral to an infertility treatment center.

Discussion

The correct answer is "D." At this point in time, you have performed a reasonably complete evaluation and even arrived at a potential cause of infertility. However, treatments for male infertility are the subject of much debate, and the patient is probably best served by referral to an infertility treatment specialist. "A" is incorrect. Genital infections are not thought to play a major role in male subfertility/infertility, so without clear evidence of gonorrhea and/or chlamydia, treating for these diseases is not recommended. "C" is incorrect because this patient does not appear to have a hypothalamic source for his infertility. "B," testosterone injection, can actually make the problem worse. The most effective therapy for patients with infertility and primary hypogonadism (i.e., this patient) may be sperm retrieval for intracytoplasmic sperm injection (not typically thought of as an office procedure for the family physician).

* *

You refer this gentleman to an infertility treatment center in your neck of the woods. He is so pleased with your attention to detail and well-reasoned approach that he refers his best friend to you for the same problem—infertility. This new patient reports never conceiving, although his wife has had one child from a previous marriage. On physical exam, you note a thin frame, mild symmetric gynecomastia, and small, firm testicles. He has complete azoospermia on two semen analyses.

His most likely diagnosis is:

A) Cystic fibrosis.
B) History of vasectomy.
C) Klinefelter syndrome.
D) Testicular cancer.
E) Turner syndrome

Discussion

The correct answer is "C." The triad of small firm testicles, gynecomastia, and azoospermia are classic findings in patients with Klinefelter syndrome. Klinefelter syndrome occurs in 1 in 1000 live male births and is responsible for 14% of cases of azoospermia. The most common (90%) chromosomal abnormality in Klinefelter syndrome is 47,XXY. "A" is incorrect. Although males with cystic fibrosis can have congenital absence of the vas deferens, these patients usually have normal-sized testicles and no gynecomastia. The same would be true for a patient status postvasectomy (no sperm, no gynecomastia, normal testicles), so "B" is incorrect. "D" is incorrect. Patients with testicular cancer usually have an enlarged testicle with a mass on the surface or inside the testicle. Although the treatments for testicular cancer may result in infertility, patients with testicular cancer do not typically present with infertility. "E" is incorrect. Turner syndrome (45,X) is associated with unambiguously female genitalia with no breast development.

Objectives: Did you learn to . . .

- Define modifiable risk factors for male subfertility/infertility?
- Recognize the significance (or lack of significance) of a varicocele?
- Identify the appropriate indications for obtaining laboratory studies in male patients with infertility concerns?
- Recognize some important causes of infertility?

CASE 10

A 63-year-old male with a history of insulin-dependent diabetes complains of decreased libido and difficulty maintaining an erection which has been worsening over the past few years. He had a similar problem at age 30 when he was experiencing a "deep depression." He does have occasional erections sufficient for penetration and awakens with an erection at times. His medical history is also significant for hypertension and an appendectomy. His medications include insulin, lisinopril, and hydrochlorothiazide. He has been married for 30 years and has two grown children, ages 24 and 26.

Which of the following historical elements is NOT likely to contribute to this patient's erectile dysfunction?

A) Diabetes.
B) Depression.
C) Hypertension.
D) History of appendectomy.
E) Antihypertensive medications.

Discussion

The correct answer is "D." We're checking to see if you're still awake. All the other options could cause some degree of erectile dysfunction. Any disease process that affects the nervous, vascular, endocrine, or smooth-muscle systems can result in erectile dysfunction. A partial list of other risk factors for erectile dysfunction includes advancing age, prostate disease or surgery (if the nerves are cut... not an issue with TURP), pelvic fracture, alcohol or other substance abuse, medications (addressed later), spinal radiculopathy or spinal cord injury, multiple sclerosis, endocrine disorders (e.g., hypothyroidism, hyperthyroidism), smoking, cardiovascular disease, chronic renal failure, and Peyronie disease (a localized plaque-like fibrosis leading to possible erectile dysfunction, penis curvature, shortening of the penis.

HELPFUL TIP: There are two categories of erectile dysfunction—psychogenic and organic. In men younger than 35 years, psychogenic erectile dysfunction is more common. In contrast, men older than 50 years are more likely to have an organic cause for their erectile dysfunction.

What further historical element(s) is/are useful in the evaluation of erectile dysfunction?

A) Rapidity of onset of sexual dysfunction.
B) Presence of nocturnal erections.
C) Status of relationship with the sexual partner.
D) Partner's interest in sex.
E) All of the above.

Discussion

The correct answer is "E." Further history should involve all of the elements listed. Patients with a sudden onset of erectile dysfunction often have a primary psychogenic erectile dysfunction. The presence of nocturnal erections establishes that the patient's neurologic and vascular mechanisms work to produce an erection. An organic disorder may still be playing a role, but the circuit is working. The status of the relationship with the patient's partner, his attraction to that partner, and the partner's interest in sex are important. If the patient and his partner are having relationship problems outside of the sexual arena, counseling may be the best first step in trying to address the erectile dysfunction.

All of the following drugs or classes of drugs can adversely affect male sexual function EXCEPT:

A) Cimetidine.
B) Chlorthalidone.
C) Prednisone.
D) Clonidine.

Discussion

The correct answer is "C." There are many drugs, prescription and recreational, that affect sexual function, and some of these include antihypertensives, antidepressants, antipsychotics, anxiolytics, hormonal agents (e.g., antiandrogens, estrogens, progestational agents, and anabolic steroids), and the H_2 blocker cimetidine (apparently not ranitidine or famotidine). The effects range from decreased libido to impotence and/or ejaculatory dysfunction. Various recreational drugs such as alcohol, marijuana, heroin, and cocaine may initially cause a state of disinhibition and enhanced libido. However, excessive or chronic use leads to erectile dysfunction. Prednisone is not known to cause significant erectile dysfunction.

* *

On physical examination, you find normal genitalia, normal femoral and dorsalis pedis pulses, appropriate virilization, and slightly diminished sensation at the plantar aspects of the feet with an otherwise intact neurological exam.

Which of the following will be most useful in evaluating a cause for his erectile dysfunction and directing further therapy?

A) BUN and creatinine.
B) TSH.
C) PSA.
D) Nocturnal penile tumescence study.
E) Arterial and venous Doppler studies.

Discussion

The correct answer is "B." With the advent of safe and efficacious therapy for erectile dysfunction, many clinicians proceed directly to a medication trial without laboratory studies. In many patients, this approach is acceptable. Other patients may benefit from a limited laboratory evaluation—especially those men with other symptoms and/or comorbidities. Initial labs might include TSH, testosterone, and prolactin. If not done already, screening for diabetes and vascular risk (e.g., lipids) is appropriate. The role of nocturnal penile tumescence is debated, but it is not necessary prior to a therapeutic trial and this patient reported having nocturnal erections anyway. BUN, creatinine, and PSA are not likely to be helpful. Doppler flow studies of femoral vessels are unlikely to change therapy as long as the physical exam demonstrates normal distal blood flow. In this patient, you know that he has vascular disease (diabetes, hypertension, and now erectile dysfunction), so his treatment should already involve lowering his vascular risk factors.

Concurrent use of which of the following drugs is an absolute contraindication to taking a phosphodiesterase type 5 inhibitor (e.g., tadalafil, vardenafil, sildenafil)?

A) Hydrochlorothiazide.
B) Isosorbide dinitrate.
C) Testosterone.
D) Finasteride.
E) Saw palmetto.

Discussion

The correct answer is "B." In patients who take nitrates for coronary heart disease, phosphodiesterase inhibitors are contraindicated. The combination has been shown to cause hypotension, in rare cases severe enough to result in stroke. While concurrent use of finasteride is safe, the alpha-blockers used to treat BPH are another story (see below). Drugs that inhibit cytochrome P450 isoenzyme, such as cimetidine, erythromycin, clarithromycin, itraconazole, ketoconazole, and HIV protease inhibitors, may warrant phosphodiesterase type 5 inhibitor dosage reductions. Caution with phosphodiesterase inhibitors is advised in patients with uncontrolled hypertension, recent stroke or myocardial infarction, life-threatening arrhythmias, unstable angina, or heart failure. Other potential medical therapies for erectile dysfunction include testosterone supplementation and yohimbine. There are even more treatment modalities: sex therapy, vacuum erection devices, intracavernosal injection therapy, intraurethral pharmacotherapy, arterial revascularization, penile prosthesis implantation, and combined therapy.

An important difference between the phosphodiesterase inhibitors is:

A) Tadalafil and vardenafil have a shorter half-life than sildenafil.
B) Tadalafil and vardenafil are contraindicated with alpha-blockers, but sildenafil is safe.
C) Tadalafil and vardenafil must be taken at least 6 hours before intercourse, whereas sildenafil acts much faster.
D) Tadalafil and vardenafil affect color vision changes, whereas sildenafil does not.
E) None of the above.

Discussion

The correct answer is "E." Tadalafil (Cialis) and vardenafil (Levitra) both have a longer half-life than sildenafil (Viagra), and tadalafil has a duration of action of 24–36 hours, thus earning it the title "the weekender." Tadalafil, vardenafil, and sildenafil all have precaution warnings for use with alpha-blockers (alpha-blocker + phosphodiesterase inhibitors = hypotension). Sildenafil can cause some changes in color vision (everything looks a little blue) because it affects phosphodiesterase in the retina. All of the phosphodiesterase inhibitors have about the same time to onset of action and should be taken 30–60 minutes before sexual activity. Tadalafil and vardenafil are allegedly more specific for phosphodiesterase in the penis, but this claim has yet to be proven in clinical practice.

* *

You start the patient on sildenafil. He discovers love again, but his wife finds out. Now you're in trouble!

Objectives: Did you learn to . . .

- Evaluate a patient with erectile dysfunction?
- Describe various etiologies of erectile dysfunction?
- Identify medications that affect erectile function?
- Recognize indications, contraindications, and side effects of therapeutic modalities for erectile dysfunction?

BIBLIOGRAPHY

Bremner WJ. Testosterone deficiency in older men. *N Engl J Med.* 2010;363:189.

Centers for Disease Control and Prevention. Sexually transmitted diseases guidelines, 2010. *MMWR.* 2010; 59(RR-12):1-110.

Ebeling PR. Osteoporosis in men. *N Engl J Med.* 2008; 358:1474.

Edwards JL. Diagnosis and management of benign prostatic hyperplasia. *Am Fam Physician*. 2008;77(10):1403.

Green KL, et al. Prostate specific antigen best practice statement: 2009 update. *J Urol*. 2009;182(5):2232.

Heidelbaugh JJ. Management of erectile dysfunction. *Am Fam Physician*. 2010;81(3):305.

Kolletis PN. Evaluation of the subfertile male. *Am Fam Physician*. 2003;67(10):2165.

Teichman, Joel MH. Urology: 20 Common Problems. New York, NY: McGraw-Hill, 2001.

U.S. Preventive Services Task Force. Screening for prostate cancer: Recommendation and rationale. *Ann Intern Med*. 2002;137(11):915.

17

Dermatology

Jason K. Wilbur

Since dermatology is a visual science, take a look at pictures at www.dermnet.org.nz/sitemap.html, or www.dermnet.com. See Table 17–1 for commonly used dermatology terms.

Table 17–1 DERMATOLOGY TERMS

Crust: Dried exudate on the skin surface (e.g., impetigo)
Desquamation: Heaped up scales and flakes, representing malformed stratum corneum (e.g., psoriasis)
Macule/Patch: A circumscribed area of change without elevation or depression; depending on the text, the size varies, but generally "macule" if <0.5–1 cm and "patch" if larger
Nodule: A solid, firm, round lesion of varying depths
Papule/Plaque: A palpable, superficial, elevated, solid lesion; text definitions vary, but generally "papule" if <0.5–1 cm and "plaque" if larger
Pustule: A well-circumscribed cavity in the skin filled with purulent exudate
Ulcer: A crater-like lesion with loss of epidermis
Vesicle/Bulla: A well-circumscribed cavity in the skin filled with fluid; text definitions vary, but generally "vesicle" if <0.5–1 cm and "bulla" if larger
Wheal: A round or irregular, light red patch that is typically evanescent

CASE 1

A 37-year-old white female presents to clinic for her annual well adult physical exam. After a complete skin examination, you find a suspicious lesion on her back (see Figure 17–1; see also color section). It measures 16 mm × 8 mm. She has approximately 20 nevi that appear normal. The patient reports never performing self-skin exams and does not know if the lesion in question is new. She denies any symptomatic lesions. Her family history is remarkable for "skin cancer" on her father's side. Many family members have "tons of moles." She frequented a tanning parlor in college (too much free time) and occasionally still does so before social events (didn't learn much about skin health in college).

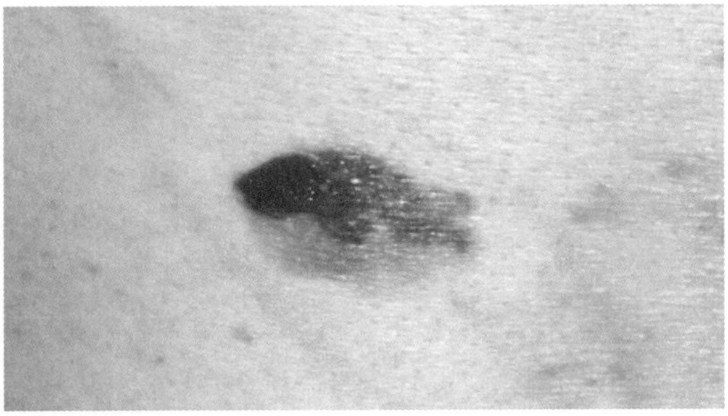

Figure 17–1

How do you evaluate the lesion?

A) Take a photograph and see her back in 2 months.
B) Take a shallow shave biopsy of the lesion.
C) Excise the entire lesion with 1–2 mm margins.
D) Excise the entire lesion with 3 cm margins.
E) All of the above are equally valid approaches.

Discussion

The correct answer is "C." This lesion is worrisome for malignant melanoma. Any time you suspect melanoma, you are obligated to perform at minimum a punch biopsy or preferably complete excision of the lesion and send it for pathology. Do not throw away the specimen; do not perform a pathologic exam yourself. These cases end badly in court. "A" is not an option; if you suspect melanoma, the sooner you make the diagnosis the better. A shave biopsy ("B") is also not recommended because the biopsy is often too shallow and the deep margins are not visible. The depth of the lesion is necessary to stage the melanoma. There is some evidence that deep shave biopsies may be acceptable, but the standard of care for evaluating a lesion suspicious for melanoma is excision. Since a punch biopsy will only get a portion of this lesion, sampling error is a possibility, which is why excisional biopsy with narrow (e.g., 2 mm) margins is preferred. "D" is preferable to "A" and "B"; however, it would be unnecessary to remove the lesion with such large margins when the histopathology is not yet known.

* *

You excise the entire lesion with a small border. The pathology report reveals a malignant melanoma (Table 17–1).

Which of the following lesion characteristics will determine your patient's prognosis?

A) The depth and ulceration.
B) The histologic level of invasion (Clark level).
C) The number of colors in the lesion.
D) Whether or not it arose in a preexisting mole.
E) Number of mitoses per high power field on microscopy.

Discussion

The correct answer is "A." As alluded to previously, the depth of the melanoma is the most important prognostic indicator. Breslow tumor thickness is most commonly used to arrive at a prognosis. Breslow tumor thickness measures the depth of the melanoma from the granular layer in the epidermis to the base of the melanoma in millimeters. The best prognosis is achieved with a Breslow depth $\leq$0.75 mm. Ulceration is associated with more aggressive cancers and a poorer prognosis. Clark's level of invasion ("B") is still reported by many pathologists, but it has less bearing on prognosis than the Breslow depth. The diameter of the lesion has not been associated with prognosis. A very large, clinically atypical pigmented lesion can often be benign. Melanomas can also be one color, many colors, or nonpigmented; color does not correlate with prognosis. Up to two-thirds of melanomas arise in normal skin. They can be just as aggressive as those arising from moles. The number of mitoses in a lesion can be a clue of more aggressive melanomas in some instances but does not possess the same prognostic value as the Breslow depth.

> HELPFUL TIP: For a patient with no metastasis and a melanoma completely excised, Breslow depth is the most important prognostic factor. However, the worst prognostic factor overall is regional or distant spread of disease, with the overall survival dropping to less than 50% for regional metastases and less than 10% for distant metastases.

In the United States in 2011, the lifetime risk of developing melanoma in a Caucasian female is approximately:

A) 1/10.
B) 1/55.
C) 1/105.
D) 1/1500.

Discussion

The correct answer is "B." The lifetime probability of melanoma in the year 2011 for Caucasian females was approximately 1 in 55. Caucasian males in the United States fare worse, with a lifetime probability of 1/37.

* *

Your biopsy reveals a malignant melanoma in situ. You excise the entire lesion with 0.5 cm margins. **There is no penetration of the epidermis.**

What additional evaluation is necessary?

A) Chest x-ray.
B) CT scan of the chest.
C) Serum lactic acid dehydrogenase (LDH).
D) All of the above.
E) None of the above.

Discussion

The correct answer is "E." If the melanoma has not penetrated the epidermis, it is referred to as a melanoma in situ. If excised with 0.5–1 cm margins, the long-term survival at 5 and 10 years approaches

100%. Therefore, any additional workup is not necessary according to the 2010 report from the American Joint Commission on Cancer. When the melanoma depth is greater than 1 mm, there is wide variation in clinical practice regarding imaging and serologic evaluation. In general, chest radiography and a serum LDH level are recommended for malignant melanomas greater than 1 mm in depth, mostly to obtain a "baseline." Serum LDH levels are usually positive in very advanced cases that have metastasized to bone or liver. A CT scan of the chest and pelvis and MRI of the brain can be ordered if metastatic disease is suspected, but these studies are not recommended routinely. Metastatic disease has not been reported with malignant melanoma in situ.

HELPFUL TIP: Sentinel lymph node biopsy is often undertaken in patients at risk for metastatic melanoma (based on ulceration and tumor thickness) who have no clinically evident lymphadenopathy. However, there is no proven survival benefit to this approach.

Which of the following has NOT been associated with an increased risk of the development of melanoma?

A) Blistering sunburns in childhood.
B) Sister with melanoma.
C) Fair hair color.
D) More than 50 moles on a person's body.
E) Smoking.

Discussion

The correct answer is "E." A history of blistering sunburns, melanoma in first-degree relatives, fair hair, and more than 50 moles are all associated with an increased risk of developing melanoma. Also, high socioeconomic class and immunosuppression appear to be risk factors. Smoking has not been linked to malignant melanoma—unlike many other malignancies.

The most common subtype of melanoma in people of African descent is:

A) Superficial spreading melanoma.
B) Lentigo maligna melanoma.
C) Nodular melanoma.
D) Acral lentiginous melanoma.
E) Amelanotic melanoma.

Discussion

The correct answer is "D." There are four classical subtypes of malignant melanoma. The subtype does not predict prognosis. **Superficial spreading melanoma** is the most common type in fair skin populations. It can occur at any site and clinically presents as a brown macule with irregular, notched borders. It grows radially (outward) initially. **Nodular melanoma** is the second most common type in fair skin individuals and, as the name suggests, is an exophytic nodule. **Lentigo maligna melanoma** is usually a brown macule with hue variations that spreads outward slowly. It occurs in the elderly on sun-exposed areas, such as the face and hands. When there is dermal invasion, lentigo maligna is referred to as lentigo maligna melanoma. **Acral lentiginous melanoma** is the least common type in Caucasian populations but is the most common type in races with pigmented skin, such as people of African descent. Acral lentiginous melanoma occurs on the palms, soles, or near the nails. **Amelanotic melanoma** is a subtype of nodular melanoma.

Objectives: Did you learn to . . .

- Evaluate a patient with suspected melanoma?
- Describe how the prognosis of melanoma is determined?
- Recognize the lifetime risk of malignant melanoma in the United States?
- Identify risk factors for the development of melanoma?
- Recognize the four classic subtypes of melanoma and which are the most common in African and Caucasian populations?

QUICK QUIZ: ITCHY ELBOWS

A 22-year-old female presents with a pruritic rash on her elbows and extensor forearms. She's studying for finals, so she's been indoors for days eating Wheat Thins and drinking Mountain Dew. She has a history of celiac disease, but is otherwise healthy and takes no medications. On exam, she is afebrile and has 2–4-mm diameter vesicular lesions in a bilaterally symmetric pattern on her extensor forearms with numerous excoriations.

The most likely diagnosis is:

A) Dermatitis herpetiformis.
B) Poison ivy (contact dermatitis).
C) Herpes simplex.
D) Neurotic excoriations.
E) Nerd elbow.

Discussion

The correct answer is "A." Dermatitis herpetiformis is the most common skin condition to occur in association with celiac disease (gluten enteropathy). This patient seems to have lapsed in her gluten-free diet, and the skin eruption may be the result. Dermatitis herpetiformis, as the name suggests, presents with vesicles similar in appearance to HSV. However, dermatitis herpetiformis is pruritic rather than painful. In fact, it can be intensely pruritic and confused with scabies. Often, only excoriations are seen on exam. Dermatitis herpetiformis is also commonly symmetrical (as opposed to HSV) and may involve several body areas, most commonly extensor surfaces of the extremities. The cornerstone of treatment is a gluten-free diet. Dapsone will speed up resolution of the rash, but the benefits must be weighed against the risks. In this case, "B" is unlikely as there is no reported exposure. "C" is unlikely for the reasons already stated, and neurotic excoriations ("D") do not present with vesicles. If "E" were a real entity, the editors believe it would be an orthopedic disorder—some underuse atrophy of the joint maybe.

CASE 2

A 7-month-old male is brought to clinic for a "rash all over." Six weeks ago, his parents noticed him rubbing his legs against his crib and scratching his head frequently. They are concerned because they find blood on his sheets in the morning, and he has become increasingly irritable. He is eating and drinking normally. His past medical history is unremarkable. His father has sensitive skin and hay fever, but no one else in the family currently has a rash. He does not attend a daycare. On skin exam, you find lichenified and erythematous patches of skin with fissures and bleeding on the ventral heels, dorsal feet, hands, and a few areas on the scalp. His cheeks are bright red with scale. His diaper area is uninvolved and there are no lesions in the web spaces of the hands and feet.

Based on the description, which of the following is the most likely diagnosis?

A) Seborrheic dermatitis.
B) Atopic dermatitis (AD).
C) Scabies.
D) Tinea corpora.
E) Tinea versicolor.

Discussion

The correct answer is "B." The most likely diagnosis is AD, also known by the moniker eczema. AD is characterized by dryness of the skin that is intensely pruritic. A red rash subsequently develops. AD is often referred to as the "itch that rashes." It occurs in characteristic locations. In younger infants, the cheeks and neck are involved. As they begin to crawl, their extensor surfaces are involved. The diaper area, because it is moist, is not usually involved. In older children, the flexural areas, such as the antecubital and popliteal fossae, are involved. Seborrheic dermatitis ("A") is common in infants and usually is seen on the scalp and face, although it can involve the whole body. Seborrheic dermatitis is typically not hyperkeratotic and is less erythematous than AD. Scabies ("C") rarely involves the scalp, but it can do so in infants and the immunocompromised. However, other more typical locations (web spaces, wrists, waist, etc.) should be involved in scabies. Also, he does not appear to have any exposure to scabies. Tinea corpora ("D") is not usually widespread or brightly erythematous. Often, tinea corpora presents with a ring of advancing erythema and a central clearing ("ringworm"). Finally, tinea versicolor ("E") typically involves the trunk and extremities, not the scalp, and is not very pruritic.

* *

You diagnose the patient with AD.

Which of the following is NOT true about AD?

A) The prevalence of AD appears to be increasing worldwide.
B) AD tends to worsen in the winter months.
C) In some patients, food allergies can exacerbate AD.
D) Positive skin prick tests and RAST testing correlate highly with food challenges (e.g., those with

positive tests will have worsening of their rash when given a food challenge).

E) In most infants, AD will significantly improve or resolve by school age.

Discussion

The correct answer is "D." Sixty percent of AD appears in the first year of life, usually after 2 months of age. The cause of AD is not yet known. The role of specific allergens is controversial. In some patients, a food allergy can worsen the disease but is not thought to be the cause. However, in severe, unresponsive AD, food allergens should be evaluated. Most patients who have positive allergy testing to foods do not have improvement in their skin with removal of the allergen. Therefore, "D" is an incorrect statement. AD does tend to improve as the affected child ages.

HELPFUL TIP (OR NOT): The link between allergies of any kind, including food and environmental, and AD has been called into question. It does seem that a subset of patients have AD that flares in response to exposure to certain food and environmental triggers, but these patients are the minority. Random elimination diets are to be discouraged. Only patients with proven food allergy **and** an immediate worsening of symptoms when exposed to that food should eliminate that particular food from their diet.

The *hallmark* of AD is:

A) Lichenification of the skin.
B) Pruritus and relapsing nature.
C) Associated asthma or allergic rhinitis.
D) Elevated IgE serum levels.
E) Redness of the skin with honey crusting.

Discussion

The correct answer is "B." Although all of the above can be associated with AD, waxing and waning pruritus is what defines this common skin condition. Chronic scratching often leads to thickened skin with accentuation of skin lines (lichenification). Early lesions will not have lichenification, however. Asthma and allergic rhinitis can be associated with AD. This common hypersensitivity triad is referred to as atopy (although AD is not allergic in nature). "D," elevated IgE, does occur in patients with AD, and higher levels of serum IgE are associated with more extensive disease of greater chronicity. However, an elevated IgE level is merely an association and is not pathognomonic of AD. "E" is not diagnostic of AD. Erythema of the skin is a nonspecific sign of inflammation and is seen in many skin disorders. Honey crusting implies a secondary bacterial infection (impetigo), which is common in AD but does not define the disease.

Your initial recommendation should include the mainstay of long-term management of AD, which is:

A) Daily use of thick emollients such as white petrolatum.
B) Decreasing the bathing frequency to twice per week.
C) Topical corticosteroids or topical immunomodulators.
D) Oral antihistamines.
E) Oral antibiotics.

Discussion

The correct answer is "A." The protective barrier of the skin is broken down in patients with AD. By adding a protective barrier, such as petrolatum, frequently, the skin becomes less pruritic resulting in less itching-induced skin trauma and rash, thus decreasing the "itch-scratch cycle." This is the most important aspect of long-term management. Topical steroids and immunomodulators work well to decrease the inflammation in the skin and are first-line anti-inflammatory treatment; however, the goal is to protect the skin with thick emollients so that the skin does not dry out and itch, leading to scratching and subsequent inflammation. Daily bathing with mild cleansers and cool water followed by the application of emollients, is recommended. Patients with AD have a higher bacterial count of *Staphylococcus aureus* on their skin. By bathing for short periods daily, the bacterial count is decreased thus decreasing the risk of secondary infection. Oral antihistamines cause some level of sedation, which is often helpful at night when the child is awake and itching. Interestingly, there is almost no evidence to support the use of antihistamines in the treatment of AD, except small studies that have shown nonsedating antihistamines to be no better than placebo. If you choose to recommend an antihistamine, use an older drug (e.g., diphenhydramine). "E" is incorrect. However, oral antibiotics may be necessary if there is extensive impetigo. Finally, bacteria can lead to a flare of atopic dermatitis. Occasionally, treatment with antibiotics may be of benefit (more below).

HELPFUL TIP: Mid-potency steroid (e.g., triamcinolone) ointments are the mainstay of pharmacotherapy for AD flares. For the face, low-potency steroid (e.g., hydrocortisone) creams can be used for a maximum of 2–3 weeks at a time. For severe, acute flares, systemic steroids can be employed for 10–14 days.

HELPFUL TIP: Topical calcineurin inhibitors (e.g., tacrolimus, pimecrolimus) are second-line therapies in the treatment of AD. Although they are generally safe and well tolerated, they are expensive and carry a "black box warning" related to possible cancer risk. There are a few reported cases of lymphoma and cutaneous cancers developing in humans using topical calcineurin inhibitors. Animal studies support this association. They are contraindicated in patients younger than 2 years.

* *

A recent ear infection has caused your patient's skin to worsen. He returns to clinic and your physical exam reveals the skin lesion seen in Figure 17–2 (see also color section). He has appreciably enlarged cervical lymph nodes. The patient has no known drug allergies.

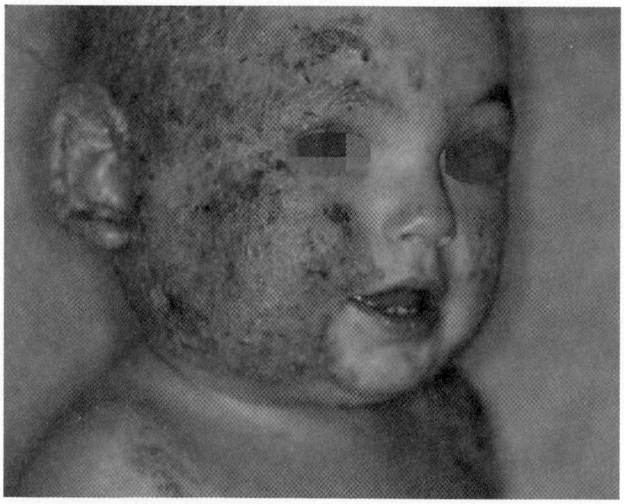

Figure 17–2

Which of the following oral antibiotics would be the best initial choice while you wait for culture and antimicrobial sensitivities?

A) Ciprofloxacin.
B) Trimethoprim/sulfamethoxazole.
C) Amoxicillin/clavulanic acid.
D) Tetracycline.
E) Metronidazole.

Discussion

The correct answer is "B." Patients with AD are prone to certain skin infections that may exacerbate their disease. Ninety percent of patients with AD will grow *S. aureus* on swab cultures of their crusted lesions. By decreasing the bacterial count, inflamed lesions often heal faster. With the rapid spread of community-acquired methicillin-resistant *S. aureus* (CA-MRSA), it is safe to assume that many, or in some communities most, skin infections are due to CA-MRSA. Therefore, trimethoprim/sulfamethoxazole (Bactrim or Septra) is the most appropriate choice. Tetracycline is another option. However, this should be avoided in young children, as should fluoroquinolones (except in rare cases such as cystic fibrosis). Although not an option, cephalexin, a first-generation cephalosporin, would also be a reasonable initial choice as it has good skin penetration with good coverage of gram-positive cocci. However, neither cephalexin nor amoxicillin/clavulanate will cover CA-MRSA.

HELPFUL TIP: Patients with head and neck AD may benefit from systemic antifungal therapy (itraconazole or ketoconazole) for a month. Malassezia yeast is a common skin flora found to cause an inflammatory reaction in patients with head/neck AD, and its eradication may improve AD symptoms in these patients. The evidence is pretty weak, so save it for third-line treatment in patients with more severe symptoms.

Which of the following vaccinations is contraindicated in patients with AD?

A) Smallpox (Vaccinia).
B) Varicella.
C) Measles/Mumps/Rubella.
D) Hepatitis B.
E) Pneumococcus.

Discussion

The correct answer is "A." Vaccination against smallpox (Vaccinia), a live virus vaccine, is contraindicated in people with AD even when the condition is in remission. Vaccination may result in eczema vaccinatum, a severe and potentially fatal reaction. Vaccinia vaccine is also contraindicated in all household contacts (e.g., parents of children with AD). A family history of AD is not a contraindication. Patients with eczema may also develop **eczema herpeticum,** a particularly severe form of disseminated herpes simplex with generalized sever ulcerations. These patients should be treated immediately with antivirals as the disease may be fatal.

* *

As the patient grows, he improves significantly. However, his skin continues to be sensitive to many products. As a teenager, he presents with a recurring rash near his wrist that is intensely pruritic. He has recently started wearing a bracelet... and he won't take it off despite the rash... because he's too cool... even though it seems to be a girl's bracelet (see Figure 17–3; see also color section).

The test most likely to confirm your presumptive diagnosis is:

A) Potassium hydroxide of a skin scraping.
B) Tzanck preparation.
C) Patch testing.
D) Serum thyroid-stimulating hormone level.
E) Serum IgE levels.

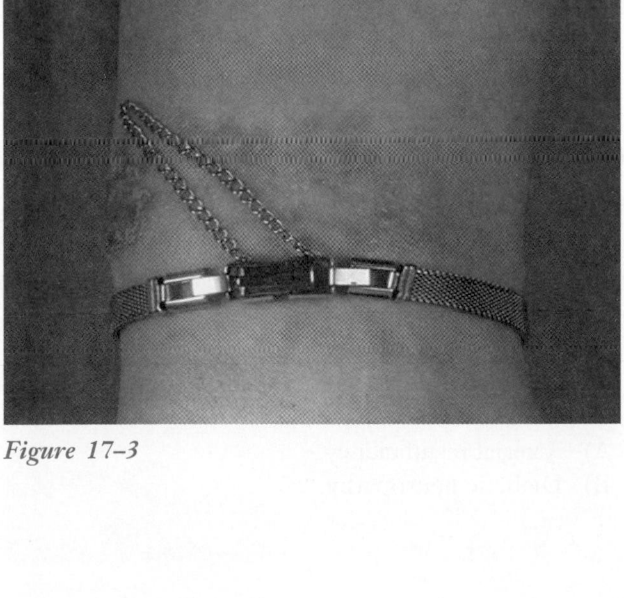

Figure 17–3

Discussion

The correct answer is "C." The patient most likely has an allergic contact dermatitis to the nickel in the metal bracelet on his wrist. Patients with a history of AD are more likely to have contact hypersensitivities. Nickel is a common contact allergen and can also be seen with contact to earrings, optical glasses, and buttons on jeans. Patch testing identifies many of the common contact allergens in the skin. KOH (potassium hydroxide) application to a skin scraping is used to identify fungal elements. KOH dissolves keratin, the protein in skin, to better identify the fungal elements. Tzanck preparations stain blister scrapings to evaluate lesions suspicious for herpes or varicella viruses. Thyroid disease can cause many skin conditions but is not a known cause of allergic contact dermatitis. An abnormality in the TSH level is the least likely to yield a diagnosis in this case. Serum IgE levels may be elevated in atopic patients, but this is not diagnostic as IgE can be elevated in many states.

Objectives: Did you learn to...

- Recognize AD by its classic presentations?
- Identify the hallmarks of AD?
- Manage a patient with AD and its complications?
- Recognize that smallpox vaccination is contraindicated in AD?

CASE 3

A 49-year-old obese white male with poorly controlled diabetes mellitus, hypertension, and hyperlipidemia presents to clinic for a regularly scheduled visit. He complains that his left leg is red. He denies constitutional symptoms or pain. His vital signs are within normal limits. He has a warm leg with circumferential erythema extending from the ankle to the mid-calf. He has 2+ pitting edema bilaterally with hemosiderin staining (brownish macular lesions) of the ankles. There are no open sores or minor trauma noted (see Figure 17–4; see also color section). His complete blood count with differential is within normal limits. You send him for Doppler studies that fail to reveal venous thromboses. You prescribe 7 days of oral antibiotics and send him home, confident that your therapy will not fail.

He returns 3 days later with modest improvement in the redness. After completing the antibiotic course, he presents to clinic 3 weeks later complaining of

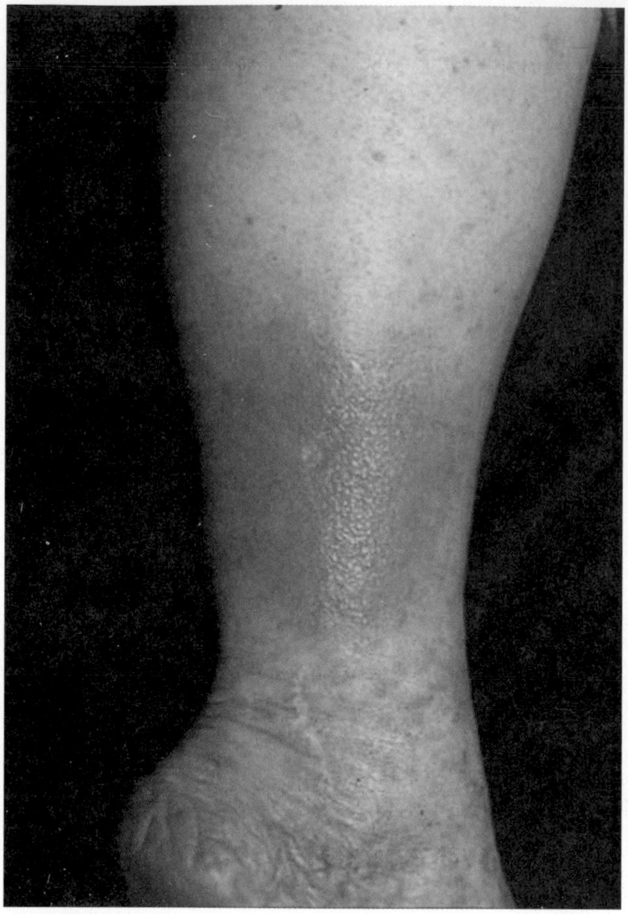

Figure 17–4

return of the redness. (Why don't patients just get better with a pill like they are supposed to?)

The most appropriate next step in the care of this patient is to:

A) Prescribe another course of oral antibiotics for 14 days.
B) Admit the patient to the hospital for intravenous antibiotics.
C) Send a punch biopsy of skin for bacterial culture.
D) Recommend daily leg elevation and compression hose use.
E) Prescribe a diuretic (e.g., furosemide).

Discussion

The correct answer is "D." This patient has a classic history of stasis dermatitis, a condition that is often misdiagnosed as recurrent or chronic cellulitis. Stasis dermatitis is a chronic dermatitis of the lower extremities that results from chronic edema. It can start relatively abruptly and be unilateral or bilateral. The pitting edema with hemosiderin staining is a clue that there is chronic fluid extravasation from the vessels of the lower extremities. Ectatic veins may also be present. The goal of therapy is directed at resolution of the edema. Patients must lose weight and employ a strict routine of compression hose and leg elevation. In the short term, topical corticosteroids can improve the inflammation. In general, diuretics should not be used simply to treat edema, as these drugs have numerous systemic effects. Paradoxically, diuretics can actually make edema worse in the long term by causing low circulating volume and renal retention of sodium and water to make up for the diuretic-induced hypovolemia. Chronic lower extremity edema can lead to local tissue necrosis, resulting in ulceration.

* *

From years of diabetic nephropathy, the patient's kidneys eventually fail leading to transplantation (and use of immunosuppressants). After 5 years of stable renal function and improved control of his diabetes, he develops a new nonhealing lesion on the left forearm.

What cutaneous malignancy is he at the highest risk of developing?

A) Basal cell carcinoma.
B) Malignant melanoma.
C) Squamous cell carcinoma.
D) Metastases from an undiagnosed internal malignancy.
E) Kaposi sarcoma.

Discussion

The correct answer is "C." All primary cutaneous malignancies are increased in immunosuppressed patients. However, squamous cell carcinoma is the most common in transplanted, immunosuppressed patients, surpassing basal cell carcinoma, which is most common in the general population. Depending on sun exposure and length of immunosuppression, the incidence of squamous cell carcinoma in transplant populations is as high as 45%. Any nonhealing lesion should be further investigated with a biopsy.

* *

You removed the lesion, which was indeed squamous cell carcinoma. Good job! The patient develops a shallow ulcer superior to the medial malleolus. "Is that another one of them cancers, Doc?" your patient asks.

The most common cause of an ulceration at this location is?

A) Arterial insufficiency.
B) Diabetic neuropathy.

C) Chronic venous stasis.
D) Pyoderma gangrenosum.
E) Prolonged pressure (e.g., "decubitus" ulcer).

Discussion
The correct answer is "C." Your patient is at risk for many of the above diagnoses; however, venous ulcerations classically occur over the medial lower leg. In contrast to this patient's venous ulceration, arterial insufficiency ulcers classically have a punched out appearance and occur over bony prominences (e.g., malleoli) or distal aspects (e.g., tips of toes) and are extremely painful (in the absence of neuropathy). Poor peripheral pulses, cool extremities, and hairlessness are clues to arterial insufficiency. Abnormal ankle–brachial indices help to confirm peripheral artery disease. Neuropathic ulcers, such as those associated with diabetic neuropathy, also occur over pressure points including on the plantar surface of the foot. The patient may complain of burning or tingling of the foot, but the ulcer is asymptomatic (because of lack of pain sensation from diabetic neuropathy). Pyoderma gangrenosum is a rare cause of ulceration associated with systemic problems such as Crohn disease and ulcerative colitis. Pressure ulceration is common and results from tissue ischemia from prolonged pressure, usually over bony prominences, such as the sacrum, coccyx, and heels.

* *

As you start to exit the exam room, the patient states "Oh by the way, Doc, can you do anything for my toenails?" Your exam reveals three, yellow heaped-up nails on the left foot. You suspect a dermatophyte infection.

What do you do next?

A) Perform a KOH exam of toenail scrapings.
B) Send toenail clippings for culture.
C) Empirically treat with an oral antifungal.
D) Empirically treat with a topical antifungal.
E) Tell the patient that his nails are the least of his worries.

Discussion
The correct answer is "A." The cost of antifungal therapy has declined substantially over the last few years with generic options becoming available. Some experts now argue that "C," empiric therapy, is reasonable in otherwise healthy patients without contraindications. However, a board exam is not real life, and "A" would be the best choice. Here's the argument for testing prior to treating: all that looks fungal is not necessarily fungal. Dystrophic nails can mimic onychomycosis and may be the result of psoriasis, eczema, trauma, etc. Potassium hydroxide (KOH) is an inexpensive and easy test to perform in the clinic setting. If it is negative, then a toenail clipping can be sent for fungal culture or pathologic study with periodic acid-Schiff staining if desired.

* *

The KOH is negative, so you send a toenail clipping for culture. It grows a *Candida* species.

Which of the following would be the LEAST efficacious medication?

A) Amphotericin.
B) Fluconazole.
C) Nystatin.
D) Terbinafine.
E) Voriconazole.

Discussion
The correct answer is "D." All the above medications have some *Candida* species coverage, but terbinafine (Lamisil) has the least yeast coverage. Of note, amphotericin would be the most toxic (but still would work well) and should be avoided.

> HELPFUL TIP: Terbinafine (Lamisil) **is** effective against most dermatophyte infections of the nails. Most cases of onychomycosis are caused by various *Tinea* species, which are sensitive to terbinafine.

* *

The patient wants to know why he has this problem with his toenails.

You tell him that it is related to:

A) Occlusive footwear.
B) Cotton socks.
C) Poor peripheral arterial circulation.
D) Eating mushrooms that are black and slimy.
E) A and C.

Discussion
The correct answer is "E." Patients with peripheral artery disease are more likely to develop onychomycosis. Likewise, occlusive footwear is thought to play a role. Cotton socks are more breathable than

nylon or other materials and do not increase the risk of onychomycosis as much as other materials. As to "D," there is a great restaurant in Jogjakarta, Indonesia, where everything is made out of various types of mushrooms (shelf fungus, etc.). It is pretty yummy.

> HELPFUL TIP: "Cold," nontender nodules and abscesses at injection sites are often caused by *Mycobacterium chelonei*. These are mostly found in immunocompromised patients, such as those with diabetes and organ transplantation.

Objectives: Did you learn to . . .

- Recognize the presentation of stasis dermatitis and describe its etiology?
- Treat stasis dermatitis?
- Recognize the cutaneous malignancies seen in transplanted, immunosuppressed patients?
- Differentiate between common causes and sites of lower extremity ulcerations?
- Diagnose and treat onychomycosis?

CASE 4

You are working in the student health clinic at the local university when a previously healthy 19-year-old female presents with malaise for 3 weeks and a severe sore throat for 3 days. Yesterday, she took some old amoxicillin that her roommate gave her. Today, she developed a diffuse macular, red skin eruption, starting on her chest and spreading to involve her extremities. Her mucous membranes, palms, and soles are free of lesions, but she has enlarged tonsils with exudates and large cervical lymph nodes, including prominent posterior nodes. A rapid *Strep* test is negative.

You suspect:

A) An allergic reaction to the amoxicillin.
B) An Epstein–Barr virus infection (mononucleosis).
C) An enterovirus infection.
D) A gonococcal infection.
E) Scarlet fever.

Discussion

The correct answer is "B." All of the above infections except for enterovirus can present with an exudative pharyngitis; enterovirus presents with gastrointestinal or meningeal symptoms. The clinical scenario describes the usual course of infectious mononucleosis: a college-age student, a few week prodrome of malaise, and posterior cervical lymphadenopathy. Amoxicillin or ampicillin given to patients with infectious mononucleosis can result in a macular, diffuse rash. This is not an allergy but can be mistaken for one. Scarlet fever, which this patient does not have, is a complication of group A streptococcal infection which presents with an erythematous, coarse ("sandpaper") rash, strawberry tongue, and skin desquamation.

* *

Later that same day, a 20-year-old male presents with a mildly pruritic rash on his trunk. He had a cold a few weeks earlier but is otherwise healthy. He denies high-risk sexual behavior (of course, your definition of "high-risk" and his may not be the same!) or intravenous drug use. Your exam reveals the findings in Figures 17–5 and 17–6 (for both figures, see also color section).

You tell the patient:

A) This skin condition is usually chronic and relapsing.
B) That although you trust his history, you suspect a sexually transmitted disease is the cause.
C) That topical corticosteroids are needed to speed up the healing.
D) That the rash usually resolves within 6–8 weeks without treatment.
E) That the rash is likely to be fatal.

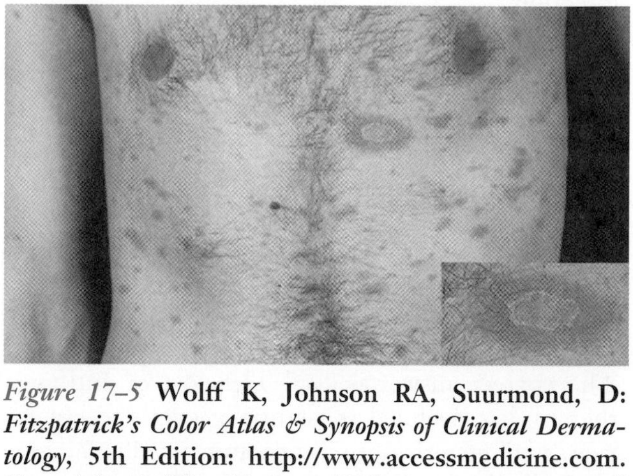

Figure 17–5 **Wolff K, Johnson RA, Suurmond, D: *Fitzpatrick's Color Atlas & Synopsis of Clinical Dermatology*, 5th Edition: http://www.accessmedicine.com. Copyright © The McGraw-Hill Companies, Inc. All rights reserved.**

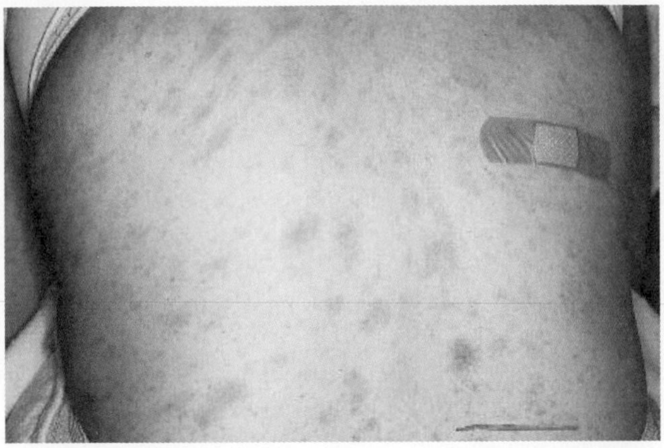

Figure 17–6 **Knoop KJ, Stack LB, Stack LB, Storrow AB: *Atlas of Emergency Medicine*, 2nd Edition: http://www.accessemergencymedicine.com. Copyright © The McGraw-Hill Companies, Inc. All rights reserved.**

Discussion

The correct answer is "D." The rash is consistent with pityriasis rosea (PR), which is an acute, often asymptomatic, eruption on the trunk and proximal extremities. The etiology is (still) unknown. Secondary syphilis, which is on the rise in some areas of the United States, can mimic PR. A sexual history is necessary, and appropriate laboratory studies should be undertaken if high-risk behaviors have occurred or if local syphilis rates are high. PR, unlike syphilis, often resolves within 8 weeks without treatment and does not usually recur. Topical steroids are not necessary for healing but may be helpful in the minority of patients who experience itching. "E" is incorrect. This rash just isn't that serious.

HELPFUL TIP: PR starts with a "herald patch," a salmon colored 2–5 cm oval-shaped lesion on the back, neck, or chest (see inset in Figure 17–5). The herald patch may clear a bit and scale and is then followed by numerous smaller lesions that crop up mostly on the trunk. These lesions tend to be oval in shape and are oriented along skin lines, giving a "Christmas tree" appearance.

* *

Your next patient is a 20-year-old female complaining of "a rash down there." You confirm that she is talking about a vulvar rash and ask about her sexual history.

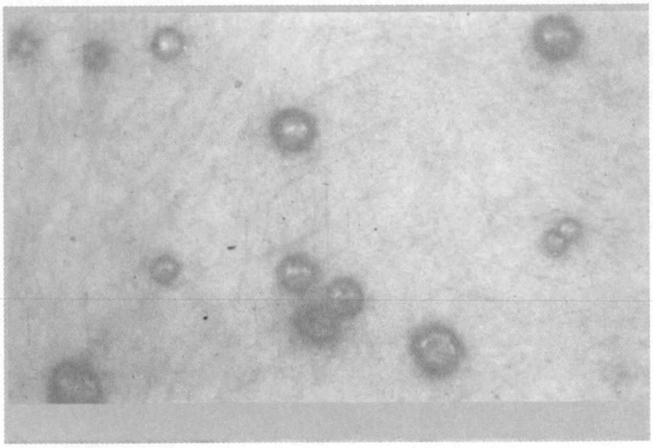

Figure 17–7

She says that she had not been sexually active with anyone for about 1 year until a recent spring break liaison in Florida. On exam, you find a rash over the pubic region and extending into the inguinal areas and medial thighs. There is no pain or pruritus (see Figure 17–7; see also color section).

Which of the following is FALSE?

A) These lesions are transmitted in adults only by sexual contact.
B) If not treated, the lesions may resolve on their own.
C) Topical corticosteroids **do not** improve this skin condition.
D) The lesions are contagious and can spread readily and rapidly.
E) The skin lesions are a result of a viral infection.

Discussion

The correct answer is "A." These lesions, referred to as molluscum contagiosum, result from a pox virus. Molluscum is commonly spread via sexual contact in adults; however, **any** physical human contact (not necessarily sexual) can also spread it. Molluscum is extremely common in children in day care settings. The lesions generally resolve in time without treatment. Because they can be autoinoculated, the molluscum lesions can rapidly increase in number, and it is for this reason that treatment is recommended. Treatment consists of destructive methods, such as cryotherapy or curetting. The immune modulator imiquimod has been used, but is not approved by the Food and Drug Administration (FDA) for molluscum, and only small trials have been undertaken. Topical steroids are not indicated. In immunocompromised patients, molluscum lesions can be widespread and persist much longer.

> HELPFUL TIP: Other molluscum therapies appear effective in small trials but are not FDA approved, including podofilox 0.5%, potassium hydroxide 5–10%, and cantharidin.

* *

A healthy 18-year-old male presents for treatment of plantar warts. He has tried topical salicylic acid 17% at home. He used it for a few weeks without significant improvement.

What is the single best therapy for plantar warts?

A) Cryotherapy (liquid nitrogen).
B) Duct tape occlusion.
C) Imiquimod.
D) Candida antigen injection.
E) None of the above is best.

Discussion

The correct answer is "E." No therapy for cutaneous warts (plantar or otherwise) has been proven superior. All of the options given have their pros and cons. "A," cryotherapy, is easily performed in the office and is quick but may be too painful for children to tolerate. Also, cryotherapy may result in hypopigmented scarring in dark-skinned patients. As we all know, duct tape can be used for anything (e.g., holding your muffler together and protecting you from terrorist attacks) and has been used to treat warts, but the evidence is conflicting. "C," imiquimod, is painless and unlikely to cause scarring, so it's a good choice for facial warts or dark-skinned patients. However, it is the most expensive option. "D," candida antigen injection, is a therapy that aims at stimulating an immune response to the warts. Mumps antigen has been used as well. In the antigen injection studies, only one wart was injected to achieve treatment for all of a patient's warts. Destructive methods are all approximately 70% effective at eradicating warts. It is important to remind patients that one method is no more likely to work than another. In immunocompetent patients, most warts resolve in time without treatment. For young children, this is an important issue, since they cannot understand the pain associated with most treatment modalities.

> HELPFUL TIP: To use duct tape for warts, the patient should put a piece of duct tape on the wart and leave it on for 6 days. On day 7, remove the duct tape, soak, and abrade the wart with a "pumice stone." Reapply the duct tape the next day.

Objectives: Did you learn to . . .

- Recognize that ampicillin/amoxicillin given to patients with mononucleosis will often result in a macular rash?
- Diagnose PR and recognize secondary syphilis as a mimic?
- Recognize and treat molluscum contagiosum?
- Describe the treatment modalities for verruca plantaris?

QUICK QUIZ: ID REACTIONS

Which of the following represents an id reaction?

A) Granuloma annulare
B) Dyshidrotic eczema
C) Sézary syndrome
D) Tinea versicolor
E) Acanthosis nigricans

Discussion

The correct answer is "B." Dyshidrotic eczema does not have a well-characterized etiology and several causes have been implicated. Some cases are "id" reactions, which occur as a result of a dermatophyte infection. Dyshidrotic eczema is characterized by pruritic, small, fluid-filled blisters ("tapioca-like") generally on the sides of the fingers and toes. You should look for a dermatophyte infection and treat it if present. Otherwise, if no dermatophyte is found, topical steroids of medium-to-high potency are useful.

CASE 5

You are rounding in the newborn nursery. A healthy 2-day-old term infant has a new rash characterized by yellow pustules on an erythematous base

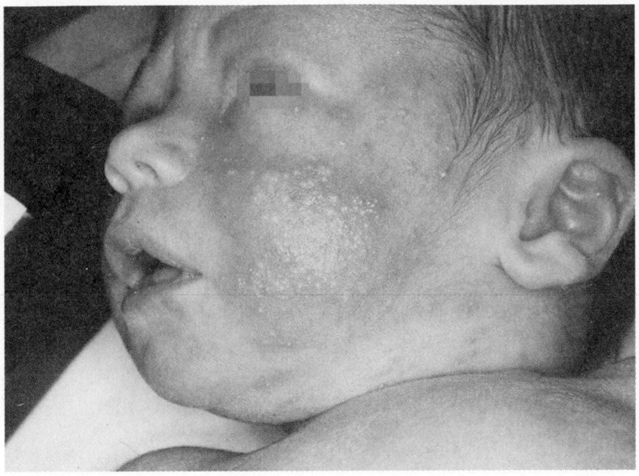

Figure 17–8

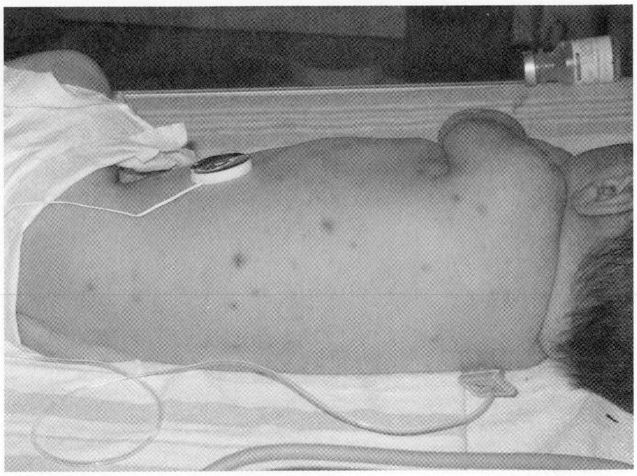

Figure 17–9

(Figure 17–8; see also color section) involving the trunk and extremities but sparing the palms and soles.

What is the diagnosis?

A) Transient neonatal pustular melanosis.
B) Herpes simplex.
C) Miliaria.
D) Erythema toxicum neonatorum.
E) Epidermolysis bullosa.

Discussion

The correct answer is "D." Erythema toxicum neonatorum is a common, benign, self-limited rash seen in term infants. Lesions usually appear after 24 hours of age. Lesions may begin as erythematous macules that progress to yellow pustules on an erythematous base, may be sparse or numerous and involve the trunk and extremities, sparing the palms and soles. The etiology is unknown and the diagnosis is clinical. Transient neonatal pustular melanosis usually affects term African American infants presenting at birth with pustules on a hyperpigmented macule that may involve the palms and soles. Neonatal herpes presents with blisters or erosions and an ill-appearing child. Diagnosis is made via a Tzanck preparation demonstrating multinucleated giant cells, viral culture, or direct fluorescent antibody for HSV 1 or 2. Commonly seen in warm climates, miliaria or "prickly heat" is due to blocked sweat ducts presenting as noninflamed pinpoint clear diffuse vesicles. Epidermolysis bullosa is a chronic blistering disease presenting as blisters at sites of mild trauma.

HELPFUL TIP: Neonatal acne presents as a pustular, facial eruption with a mean onset at 2–3 weeks of life. It is asymptomatic and diagnosed clinically. Fungal organisms have been found in some pustules. Treatment for acne is not necessary as most lesions resolve in several weeks. Besides, we doubt neonatal acne will affect the child's chance of landing a prom date.

* *

While taking care of the neonate in the newborn nursery, you notice a child in isolation. His skin catches your eye (see Figure 17–9; see also color section).

The most common cause of this rash in newborns in the United States is:

A) Cytomegalovirus (CMV).
B) Rubella.
C) Langerhan cell histiocytosis.
D) Rh incompatibility.
E) Parvovirus B19.

Discussion

The correct answer is "A." All the above can present as a "blueberry muffin baby"; however, CMV is the most common cause in the United States. CMV is the most common congenital viral infection, affecting about 1–2% of all births. Rubella was the most common cause in the prevaccination era. In most cases, the purple plaques represent extramedullary hematopoeisis.

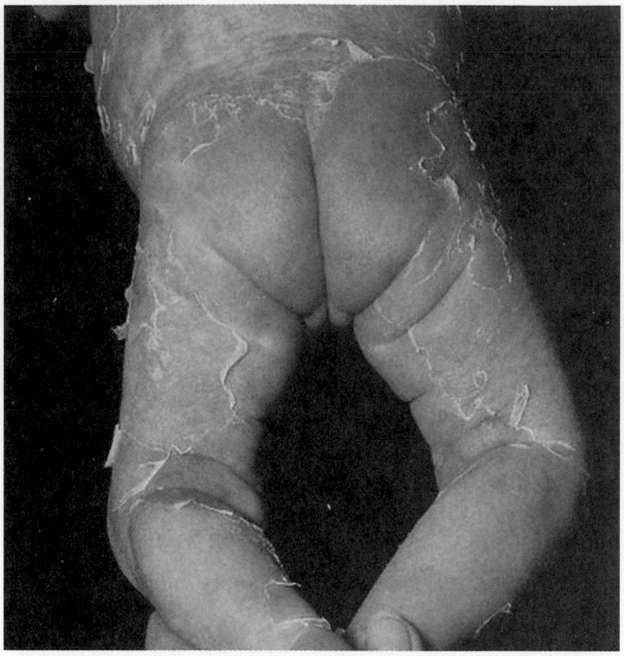

Figure 17–10 **Wolff K, Johnson RA, Suurmond, D: *Fitzpatrick's Color Atlas & Synopsis of Clinical Dermatology*, 5th Edition: http://www.accessmedicine.com.**

* *

Later that same morning, a previously healthy neonate age 3 weeks presents to your clinic with peeling of the skin and a fever (Figure 17–10; see also color section). She had appeared well until 2 days ago when she became more irritable. Her mother noted a decrease in her urine output. The child was born vaginally without complications and has no known medical conditions. On physical exam, you notice a well nourished, crying infant with large sheets of desquamating skin on her extremities. **Her mucus membranes appear normal.** You order complete blood count and urine analysis.

The most likely diagnosis is:

A) Toxic epidermal necrolysis (TEN).
B) Bullous impetigo.
C) Staphylococcal scalded skin syndrome (SSSS).
D) Diffuse cutaneous mastocytosis.

Discussion

The correct answer is "C." This is staphylococcal scaled skin syndrome. So what differentiates "C" from "A?" TEN presents with shedding of sheets of skin **and often has mucosal involvement that separates it clinically from SSSS.** Usually, TEN is a result of drug hypersensitivity, or bacterial sepsis, in the case of the neonate children are quite ill compared with children with SSSS. In TEN, a biopsy would show full-thickness necrosis of the epidermis versus an intraepidermal split in SSSS. "B," bullous impetigo, is a result of *S. aureus* skin infection in 85% of the cases. The erosions and blisters result from the local production of epidermolytic toxins. "D," diffuse cutaneous mastocytosis, can present with hemorrhagic blisters and erosions, but these are usually focal areas, not sheets of skin loss. See below for further discussion of SSSS.

In this case of SSSS, peeling of the skin is a result of:

A) Necrosis of the entire epidermis from lymphocyte attack.
B) A widespread bacterial skin infection.
C) Histamine released in the skin with edema and blistering.
D) Toxin-mediated skin blistering from nonskin source of infection.

Discussion

The correct answer is "D." This clinical scenario describes SSSS, which is an epidermolytic toxin-driven disease. Extreme tenderness of the skin precedes superficial, widespread desquamation. The skin is usually bright red with areas of flakiness. Radial wrinkling of the mouth, giving an "old man" appearance, is common. The source of infection is not the skin but rather an occult site such as nasopharynx or urinary tract; therefore, investigation for a causative infection should be undertaken (e.g., blood and urine cultures).

Objectives: Did you learn to . . .

- Recognize neonatal benign cutaneous eruptions?
- Identify a blueberry muffin neonate and know the common causes?
- Recognize SSSS and consider its differential diagnosis?

QUICK QUIZ: NAILS

Which of the following nail findings–systemic disease pairing is INCORRECT?

A) Muehrcke nails—nephrotic syndrome.
B) Plummer nail—hyperthyroidism.

C) Periungual fibroma—tuberous sclerosis.
D) Splinter hemorrhages—infective endocarditis.
E) Koilonychia—systemic lupus erythematosus.

Discussion

The correct answer is "E." Koilonychia, otherwise known as "spoon nail," is a result of softening and thinning of the nail plate and is found in patients with long-standing iron deficiency anemia, Plumer–Vinson syndrome, Raynaud disease, hemochromatosis, and trauma. It can also be inherited as an autosomal-dominant trait. Connective tissues diseases, such as lupus, are more commonly characterized by nail fold abnormalities, such as nail fold telangiectasias, rather than koilonychia. Muehrcke nails ("A") have paired narrow horizontal white bands, separated by normal nail, that remain static as the nail grows. They are most often seen in patients with nephrotic syndrome, and their presence reflects the degree of hypoalbuminemia. When you see onycholysis (separation of the nail plate from the nail bed that appears opaque), consider trauma, onychomycosis, psoriasis, and other systemic disease. When onycholysis is present in hyperthyroidism, it is called Plummer nail and often affects the ring finger only for unclear reasons. A periungual fibroma ("C") should prompt evaluation for tuberous sclerosis with brain imaging for tuberous lesions. Splinter hemorrhages ("D") are usually a result of trauma but can be a sign of infectious endocarditis.

HELPFUL TIP: Paronychia, inflammation around the nail, may be acute or chronic. Acute paronychia is often due to bacterial infection and is treated with oral antibiotics, drainage, warm compresses, and soaks. Chronic paronychia is related to eczema and may have secondary *Candida* infection. Treatment is with topical steroids, topical antifungals, and oral antifungals.

QUICK QUIZ: DERM PHOTO

A 52-year-old white male presents to clinic with a nonhealing, asymptomatic "pimple" on the cheek. It has been present for 6 months and has recently started to bleed when he shaves. On exam, you note his fair skin, blue eyes, and ruddy complexion. You find the lesion in Figure 17–11 (see also color section).

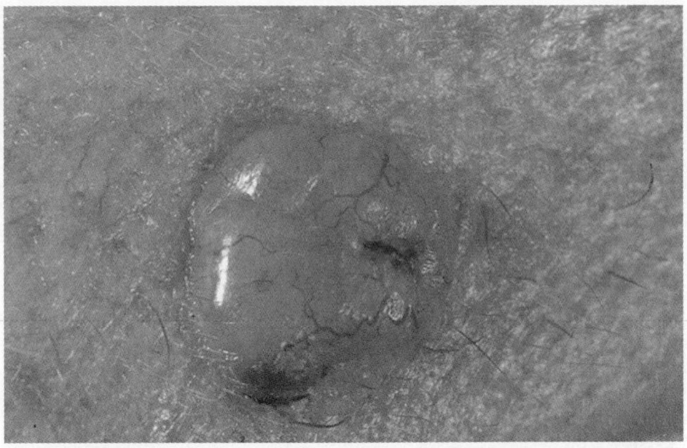

Figure 17–11

Your preliminary diagnosis is:

A) Sebaceous hyperplasia.
B) Squamous cell carcinoma.
C) Basal cell carcinoma.
D) Metastases from internal malignancy.
E) Merkel cell carcinoma.

Discussion

The correct answer is "C." The photograph is a classic picture of a basal cell carcinoma with its rolled, pearly pink borders, and telangiectasias. It is found commonly on the head and neck. People with fair skin and light hair and eyes are at particular risk. Sebaceous hyperplasia can look similar but is ivory or yellow in appearance and has a central pore. Squamous cell carcinoma is usually a hyperkeratotic or ulcerated papule or plaque. Metastases from solid organ malignancies are subcutaneous, firm nodules, although they may ulcerate. Merkel cell carcinoma is a rare tumor on the head and neck that usually appears as an ill-defined, violaceous nodule or plaque.

CASE 6

While working in the emergency department, a 6-month-old healthy female infant is brought in by her grandmother. She is bleeding from her birthmark on her buttocks (see Figure 17–12; see also color section). Her grandmother watches her during the day while her mother is at work and has noticed the lesion getting larger recently. After holding pressure on the lesion for about 20 minutes, the bleeding stops. You

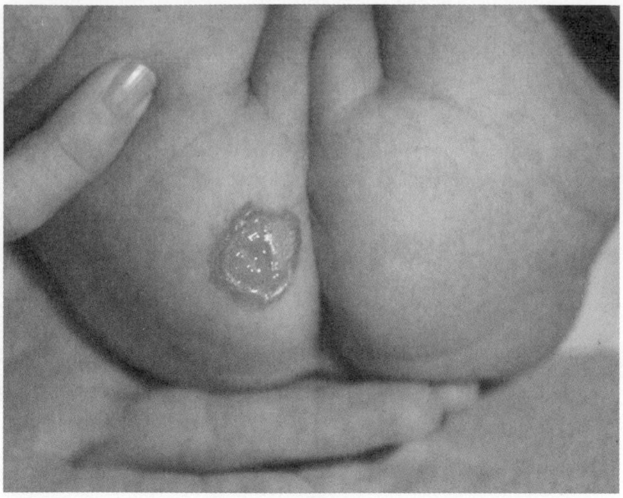

Figure 17–12

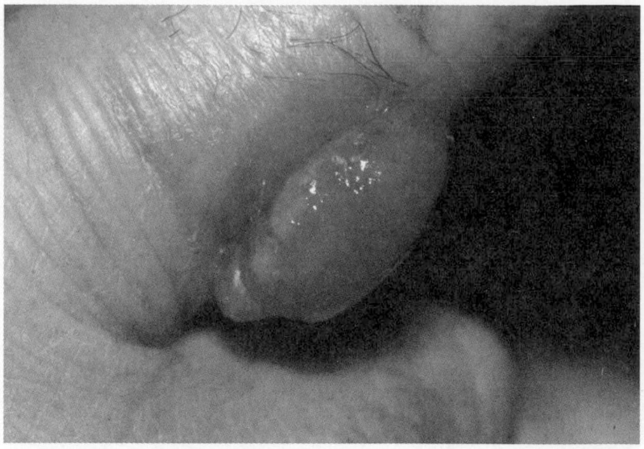

Figure 17–13

educate the grandmother about the natural history of the "birthmark."

Which of the following is NOT a true statement about this type of birthmark?

A) This is the most common type of soft-tissue tumor of infancy.
B) Most of these birthmarks undergo complete or partial resolution.
C) Treatment is indicated in all lesions lest they become malignant.
D) Pulse dye laser therapy is used primarily for ulcerated lesions.
E) Many are not present at birth but develop shortly thereafter.

Discussion

The correct answer is "C." The child has an ulcerated hemangioma of infancy. Infantile hemangiomas are benign proliferations of endothelial cell lineage that are usually present at birth or soon thereafter. They are characterized by rapid growth in the first several months of life and then stop growing about 1 year of age. They spontaneously involute over years. Treatment options must be individually tailored. Most are treated if they ulcerate or if they are impairing a normal function, such as vision. Pulse dye laser therapy can heal ulcerated hemangiomas but does not significantly change the size of lesions. Most ulcerated lesions are successfully treated with topical antibacterial agents and nonadhesive dressings. Hemangiomas on the head and neck or multiple hemangiomas should be further evaluated with imaging studies.

* *

The same patient returns, this time with mom, at age 5. The hemangioma has healed. About 2 months ago, the mother noticed a spot on the patient's left index finger, and now she is concerned that it is not resolving. The patient is not bothered by the lesion, except that it occasionally bleeds when she bumps it on something. On exam, you find a 3-mm dome-shaped, bright red nodule on the palmar aspect of the left index finger. It is nontender and smooth (see Figure 17–13; see also color section).

The most likely diagnosis is:

A) Basal cell carcinoma.
B) Squamous cell carcinoma.
C) Acne.
D) Pyogenic granuloma.
E) Nodular melanoma.

Discussion

The correct answer is "D." This patient most likely has a pyogenic granuloma, which is essentially a nodular hemangioma arising at sites of trauma, especially the fingers and toes. Although pyogenic granuloma is not cancerous, it can be confused with basal and squamous cell carcinomas as well as melanoma. For this reason, it is prudent to perform excision and histologic examination. After excision, the base of the lesion should be ablated (electrocautery or laser), or the pyogenic granuloma may return. "C," acne, should not be a consideration, as sebaceous glands are not found on the palms. By the way, did you notice that this poor child has developed coarse, dark hair growth on her knuckles? Now that seems to be a serious skin condition, but you'll just have to wait until the next edition to find out.

Objectives: Did you learn to . . .

- Describe the natural history of infantile hemangiomas?
- Identify options for treating ulcerated hemangiomas?
- Describe the features and management of pyogenic granuloma?

CASE 7

A 78-year-old female presents with a rash on her legs. It started 1 week ago and was preceded by itching of the legs without any visible changes. Then red blotches developed that quickly became blisters. She denies pain or drainage. She also has some sores in her mouth. She reports overall good health and takes no medications. On exam, you find an afebrile, comfortable looking female. There are several small ulcers on her hard palate. She has 1+ pitting edema at her ankles. You notice round, tense bullae erupting on erythematous patches on the lower extremities bilaterally. The bullae break open with slight pressure applied to the edge, and several are draining clear fluid. There is no purulence or bleeding (see Figure 17–14; see also color section).

Which of the following is the most likely diagnosis?

A) Pemphigus vulgaris.
B) Bullous pemphigoid.

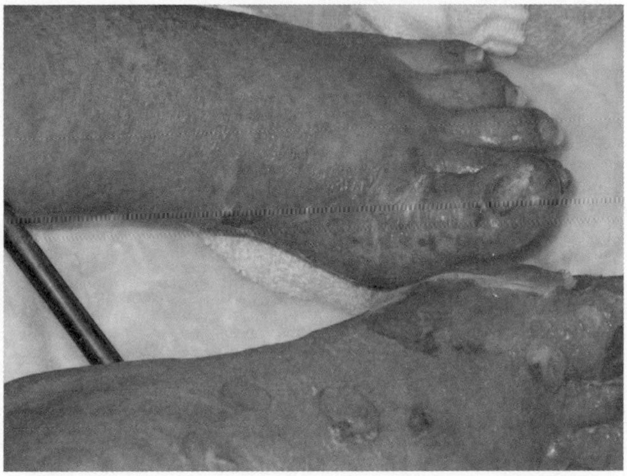

Figure 17–14

C) Varicella zoster.
D) Dermatitis herpetiformis.
E) Stevens–Johnson syndrome (SJS).

Discussion

The correct answer is "B." Bullous pemphigoid is an autoimmune disorder and is primarily a disease of the elderly. Often patients will have some sort of prodrome prior to the eruption of typical bullous lesions. Prodromal symptoms can include pruritus, erythema, and urticaria. When the bullae form, they are frequently asymptomatic but can be intensely pruritic and mildly tender. In contradistinction to pemphigus vulgaris and SJS, systemic symptoms are not part of bullous pemphigoid. Additionally, pemphigus vulgaris lesions are painful, and classically the bullae are flaccid rather than tense. SJS generally occurs in response to medications, and this patient is taking none. Varicella zoster should follow a dermatomal pattern rather than appear bilaterally; zoster is usually associated with pain and paresthesia. Dermatitis herpetiformis presents with crops of vesicles and excoriations rather than bullae.

* *

Although she feels well, the lesions are dramatic, and the patient is very concerned that she might have cancer. To confirm your diagnosis, you decide to biopsy the skin.

The most appropriate way to perform a biopsy in this situation is:

A) 4-mm punch biopsy of the margin of an intact bulla for light microscopy.
B) 4-mm punch biopsy of normal skin for light microscopy.
C) 4-mm punch biopsy of normal skin for immunofluorescence.
D) A and B.
E) A and C.

Discussion

The correct answer is "E." Bullous pemphigoid is diagnosed definitively by demonstration of autoantibodies deposited along the basement membrane of **normal** skin. Immunofluorescent exam of normal-appearing skin can demonstrate IgG and complement deposits. A biopsy of the edge of an intact bulla will show the characteristic pathology of separation at the basement membrane and subepidermal blister. For a definitive diagnosis, both "A" and "C" should be done.

* *

You assure her that the lesions are not cancerous.

What else can you tell her about the prognosis of bullous pemphigoid?

A) There is a 50% chance that it will resolve in 3 years.
B) It is associated with an increased risk of all forms of skin cancer.
C) It is associated with a high mortality rate.
D) It will likely spread to cover her entire body until she's one big blister, and her hair will fall out.

Discussion

The correct answer is "A." Bullous pemphigoid may undergo complete resolution and never recur. Alternatively, the disease may have resolutions and exacerbations over time. It is not associated with an increased risk of cancer or a high mortality rate. Very extensive involvement may lead to skin infections and bacteremia, but diffuse disease is not common.

* *

She seems miserable. You want to offer her the safest, most effective therapy to treat this condition.

What is the FIRST therapy that you want to offer her?

A) Oral azathioprine.
B) Oral cephalexin.
C) Oral prednisone.
D) Topical antimicrobials.
E) Topical clobetasol.

Discussion

The correct answer is "E." Bullous pemphigoid is an autoimmune disease, so anti-inflammatory medications and immunosuppressive agents are used to treat it. There is some concern about increased mortality in elderly patients treated with systemic steroids, and there is good evidence that even moderate-to-severe cases will respond to topical steroids. Therefore, potent topical steroids (e.g., clobetasol) are currently the preferred therapy. However, topical clobetasol may be impractical and is much more expensive than oral prednisone. Thus, many cases are still treated with oral steroids, sometimes in combination with another immunosuppressive agent such as azathioprine or methotrexate. Dapsone may be used as well. When using oral steroids, it is prudent to taper the medication to achieve the lowest effective dose. Topical antimicrobials are used when treating infected, open bullae but are not effective for the treatment of the disease itself.

Objectives: Did you learn to . . .

- Distinguish bullous diseases from one another?
- Diagnose and treat bullous pemphigoid?

QUICK QUIZ: PAPULAR ERUPTION

A 30-year-old female presents with a several month history of bumps on her chin and around her mouth. Although she has never had problems with acne, she thought that she was developing acne and tried benzoyl peroxide. A month ago, she stopped the benzoyl peroxide because it did not seem to work, and she switched to hydrocortisone cream, which has worsened the outbreak if it has done anything. The rash is neither itchy nor painful. She works in an office and cannot recall any contact irritants. On exam, you find erythematous papules with small pustules on the chin and laterally around her mouth (see Figure 17–15; see also color section). The neck and the remainder of the face are not involved.

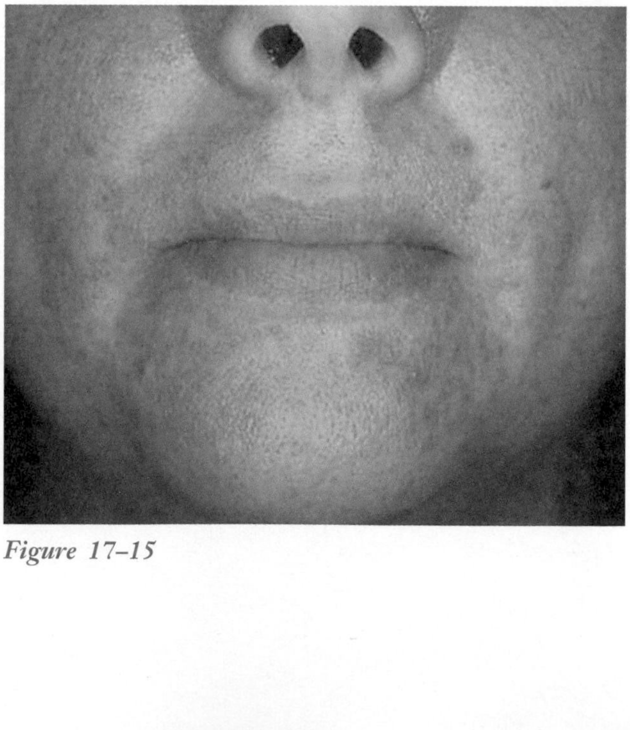

Figure 17–15

* *

You decide that this patient probably has cold urticaria (the fact that it is summer does not dissuade you).

The next drug you might want to try on this patient is:

A) Cyproheptadine (Periactin).
B) Prednisone.
C) Montelukast.
D) Nifedipine.
E) Aspirin.

Discussion

The correct answer is "A." The physical urticarias (cold and pressure especially) may respond better to cyproheptadine than other modalities. If this patient had a "typical" urticaria, you might want to try prednisone, one of the leukotriene inhibitors or nifedipine (which interferes with mast cell degranulation). **Remember that leukotriene inhibitors, steroids, etc., are second line and should be used only when first-line drugs have failed or are not tolerated** (cyproheptadine for physical urticaria; doxepin, antihistamines, etc., for "typical" urticaria). There are no good studies on the effectiveness of leukotriene inhibitors (anecdotal evidence only), but they might be worth trying when all else fails.

HELPFUL TIP: Any number of drugs can cause urticaria. Look at the med list!

Objectives: Did you learn to . . .

- Recognize urticaria?
- Identify potential causes of urticaria?
- Develop a treatment strategy for patients with urticaria?

QUICK QUIZ: DERMATOLOGY

Actinic keratoses (AKs) are precursors to what?

A) Nothing.
B) Melanoma.
C) Basal cell carcinoma.
D) Squamous cell carcinoma.
E) Granuloma annulare.

Discussion

The correct answer is "D." AKs are precursors to squamous cell carcinomas. As such, they should be treated. Options include cryotherapy, laser therapy, or 5-fluorouracil topically.

HELPFUL TIP: Less than 1% of AKs progress to squamous cell carcinoma per year. Some spontaneously involute and some remain as AKs. However, in an individual, the risk of an AK developing into a squamous cell carcinoma increases with the number of AKs present.

QUICK QUIZ: DERMATOLOGY

Seborrheic keratoses are precursors to what?

A) Nothing.
B) Melanoma.
C) Basal cell carcinoma.
D) Squamous cell carcinoma.
E) Granuloma annulare.

Discussion

The correct answer is "A." Seborrheic keratoses are precursors to nothing. They are the greasy looking, stuck on, growths that occur with age. They can be treated, if necessary, with freezing and curetting. They look ugly, patients hate them, but they are harmless.

CASE 11

A 50-year-old female with type 2 diabetes controlled with insulin complains of a rash that has developed on her legs over the past year. It started as a small patch on her left leg and then "spread" to her right leg. It is neither painful nor pruritic. You are impressed by the rash she shows you in Figure 17–17 (see also color section).

The most appropriate next step in the management of these lesions is which of the following?

A) A topical mid-potency steroid under occlusion or intralesional steroids.
B) Discontinue insulin.
C) Increase her insulin dose.
D) Liberal use of emollients (e.g., petrolatum).

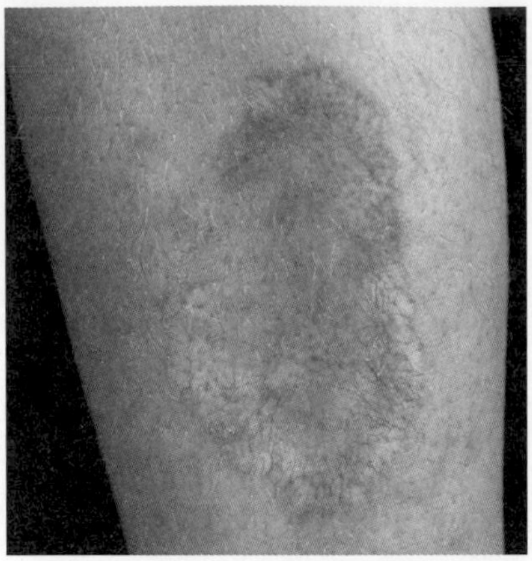

Figure 17–17 **Wolff K, Johnson RA: *Fitzpatrick's Color Atlas & Synopsis of Clinical Dermatology*, 6th Edition: http://www.accessmedicine.com. Copyright © The McGraw-Hill Companies, Inc. All rights reserved.**

E) Leg elevation and application of compressive stockings.

Discussion

The correct answer is "A." This patient has developed necrobiosis lipoidica, a benign condition of the skin affecting a small percent of diabetics, usually those on insulin. Look for brownish red patches or plaques with yellowish areas through the center. The center is often shiny with telangiectasias. The legs are most often involved and the lesions may be painful. The name describes the pathology: necrobiosis refers to the inflammation around destroyed collagen, and lipoidica refers to the yellowish color associated with lipid deposits. It does not seem to be caused by insulin or affected by glucose control, so "B" and "C" are not appropriate choices. These lesions can be confused for eczema, and in fact may respond to topical steroids ("A"); however, emollients are not useful. Finally, necrobiosis lipoidica might be confused with the skin changes associated with venous stasis and chronic edema, which would be treated as in "E." Patients should know that necrobiosis lipoidica is often chronic and difficult to treat but benign. The diagnosis is clinical but can be confirmed by biopsy, and treatment is not always necessary.

* *

Your patient also complains of thick, dark, velvety patches under her arms (Figure 17–18; see also color section). She's unsure of the duration, but states, "They've been with me a while. I just wondered if my medication might cause these." She gives you an accusing look, and you have to admit that she takes more than a few medicines related to her diabetes.

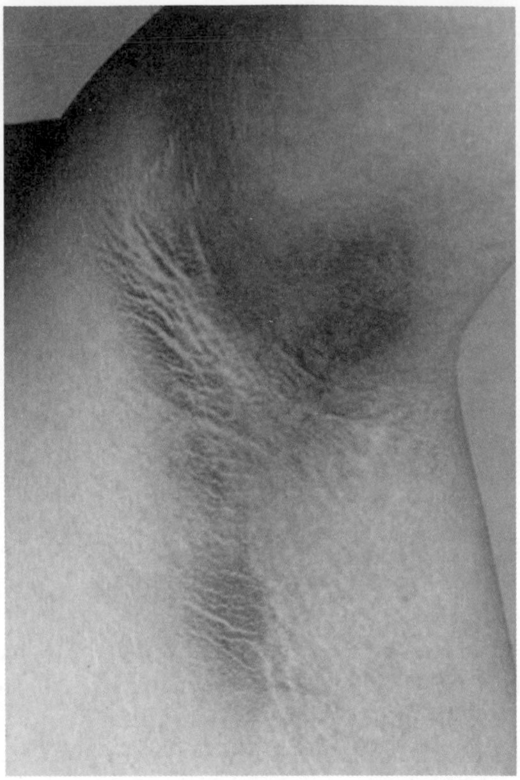

Figure 17–18 **Wolff K, Johnson RA, Suurmond, D: *Fitzpatrick's Color Atlas & Synopsis of Clinical Dermatology*, 5th Edition: http://www.accessmedicine.com. Copyright © The McGraw-Hill Companies, Inc. All rights reserved.**

The most likely culprit is:

A) Aspirin.
B) Lisinopril.
C) Insulin.
D) Simvastatin.

Discussion

The correct answer is "C." The lesions are typical of acanthosis nigricans, a hyperkeratotic, hyperpigmented condition affecting skin folds (neck, inguinal area, axilla, etc.). The common causes of acanthosis nigricans are obesity, insulin resistance, and diabetes. Some drugs have been known to cause it, including insulin, corticosteroids, and nicotinic acid. From med school, we all remember acanthosis nigricans as a cutaneous manifestation of internal malignancy. But such a presentation is rare. Cancer is more likely in patients with extensive and quickly progressing lesions, and as you might expect, it's not a good sign.

HELPFUL (ISH) TIP: Another cutaneous manifestation of internal malignancy is the sign of Leser–Trelat: a large crop of seborrheic keratoses that erupt quickly. Note that seborrheic keratoses themselves are benign and that knowing about Leser–Trelat is mostly good for looking smart.

* *

Your patient returns a year later and the lesions on her legs have essentially disappeared. Now she has a new concern. She reports a sore on the bottom of her great toe. She's uncertain how it occurred and thinks it has only been present for a few days. You find a 1-cm circular ulcer at the plantar aspect of her great toe.

Of the following options, the most important next step is to:

A) Culture the wound.
B) Assess for adequate vascular supply to the foot.
C) Perform MRI of the foot.
D) Perform monofilament testing to check sensation in the foot.
E) Debride the wound.

Discussion

The correct answer is "B." The described wound is most likely a diabetic foot ulcer, but the location and the patient's history of diabetes do elicit concern for an ulcer related to vascular disease. Additionally, good vascular supply to the foot is necessary for wound healing. Therefore, you need to know the status of blood flow to the foot. This may be accomplished by physical exam. For patients at high risk for peripheral vascular disease or without strong pulses, ankle–brachial indices would be the next step. As to the other answers: culture of an open foot ulcer is pretty much worthless; x-ray may be warranted to evaluate for osteomyelitis, but MRI is jumping the gun; sensation is important, but not as urgent to wound healing as vascular supply (although we are confident, you will assess her sensation); wound debridement may be needed, but you would want to know that the debrided area will have good blood flow first.

* *

Her pulses are good, her feet are warm, and the rest of her skin is in good condition. Through her diligent care and control of her diabetes, the ulcer heals. She returns 3 months later with a new skin concern. On her forearm, she has developed a clear fluid-filled blister about 1 cm in diameter and irregular in shape. There is no erythema, no pruritus, and no pain. She denies trauma and new environmental contacts.

Which of the following is the most likely diagnosis?

A) Dyshidrotic eczema.
B) Contact dermatitis.
C) SSSS.
D) Bullosis diabeticorum.
E) Drug eruption.

Discussion

The correct answer is "D." Bullosis diabeticorum, or bullous disease of diabetes, occurs in less than 1% of diabetic patients. However, patients may be alarmed by it and seek treatment. The cause is unknown, but it typically follows a benign course and resolves spontaneously over a few weeks or months. Because it requires no intervention, it is useful to distinguish bullosis diabeticorum from dyshidrotic eczema and contact dermatitis, both of which may mimic the disease except for pruritus and inflammation.

Objectives: Did you learn to . . .

- Identify necrobiosis lipoidica, acanthosis nigricans, and bullosis diabeticorum?
- Treat these conditions (if necessary)?
- Evaluate a diabetic foot ulcer?

QUICK QUIZ: DERMATOLOGY

The pruritic lesion in Figure 17–19 (see also color section) is most likely:

A) Grover disease.
B) Lichen planus.
C) Contact dermatitis.
D) Atopic dermatitis.
E) Pyoderma gangrenosum.

Discussion

The correct answer is "C." This is contact dermatitis, which may be acute, subacute, or chronic. It is an erythematous, pruritic eruption that usually blisters and leaves a crust. More chronic forms of contact dermatitis present with lichenification and scaling. The rash

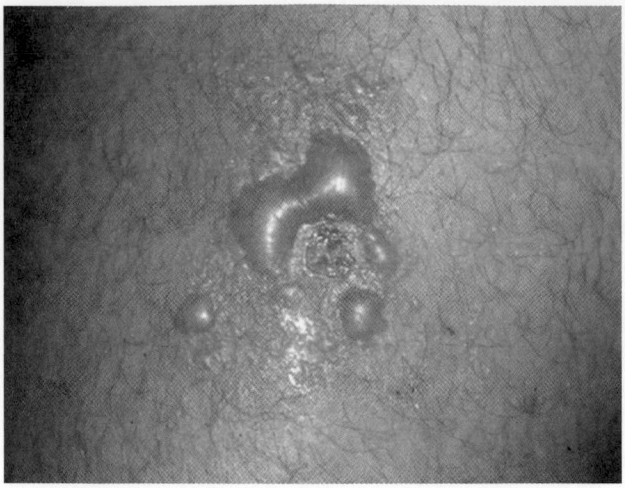

Figure 17–19

in Figure 17–19 does not look like any of the other choices. Grover disease, or transient acantholytic dermatosis, presents with small, sometimes pruritic, erythematous papules on the back and chest which may blister. Lichen planus presents with pruritic, red to purple, flat-topped papules. AD is discussed earlier in the chapter. Pyoderma gangrenosum presents with painful, red nodules and pustules that ulcerate. Again, since we cannot print pictures of all diseases mentioned, please look at one of the Web sites included at the beginning of this chapter.

> HELPFUL TIP: Pyoderma gangrenosum is often associated with underlying systemic illness, most commonly ulcerative colitis and Crohn disease.

QUICK QUIZ: MR. SCRATCHER

A 76-year-old male comes to your clinic with a 1-year history of pruritic, eczematous rash on his chest and back. He has no atopic history or eczema as a child. He has no other active medical issues. He has tried moisturizers and over-the-counter hydrocortisone cream, which have provided minimal relief.

Which of the following is the most appropriate next step in his management?

A) Tacrolimus ointment.
B) Skin scraping for KOH preparation.
C) High-dose topical steroids.
D) Skin biopsy.
E) Oral antihistamines.

Discussion

The correct answer is "D." The development of a new, eczematous rash in an adult patient should raise the concern for a more serious condition. It is rare for an elderly person to develop AD de novo. This may be indicative of an underlying lymphoproliferative malignancy such as cutaneous T-cell lymphoma. Bowen disease (squamous cell carcinoma in situ) is another possibility. The most appropriate next step in this patient's management would be skin biopsy.

QUICK QUIZ: ALLERGY

A 4-year-old girl comes to clinic accompanied by her mother for her yearly checkup. Her mother requests that you examine her daughter's skin because of a rash. Upon examination, you identify scattered reddish-brown macules on the back and chest. When stroked, the lesions urticate. There are no other complaints or abnormalities on physical examination.

What is the most likely diagnosis?

A) Atopic dermatitis.
B) Contact dermatitis.
C) Congenital nevi.
D) Cutaneous lupus.
E) Urticaria pigmentosa.

Discussion

The correct answer is "E." This child's rash is most likely secondary to urticaria pigmentosa, which is a cutaneous form of mastocytosis. Clinical findings include reddish-brown macules or slightly raised papules, which represent cutaneous accumulations of mast cells. These occur most commonly on extensor surfaces, thorax, and abdomen. When stroked, these lesions can urticate (Darier sign). Urticaria pigmentosa is the most common skin manifestation of mastocytosis in children and adults. Eighty percent of cases appear during the first year of life. Lesions resolve in >50% of patients by adolescence. The diagnosis is confirmed by skin biopsy. In children, urticaria pigmentosa is rarely associated with systemic disease.

BIBLIOGRAPHY

Bruckner AL, Frieden IJ. Hemangiomas of infancy. *J Am Acad Derm*. 2003;48:477-493.

Di Lorenzo G, et al. Leukotriene receptor antagonists in monotherapy or in combination with antihistamines in the treatment of chronic urticaria: A systematic review. *J Asthma Allergy*. 2008;2:9-16.

Gershenwald JE, et al. 2010 TNM staging system for cutaneous melanoma . . . and beyond. *Ann Surg Oncol*. 2010;17:1475-1477.

Hurwitz S, eds. Eczemetous eruptions in childhood. In: *Clinical Pediatric Dermatology*. 3rd ed. Philadelphia, PA: W.B. Saunders Co; 2005.

Khumalo N, et al. Interventions for bullous pemphigoid. *Cochrane Database Syst Rev*. 2003;(3):CD002292.

O'Connor NR, McLaughlin MR. Neonatal skin: Parts I and II. *Am Fam Physician*. 2008;77:47-60.

Rager EL. Cutaneous melanoma. *Am Fam Physician*. 2005; 72:269-276.

Ramsey HM, et al. Factors associated with nonmelanoma skin cancer following renal transplantation. *J Am Acad Dermatol*. 2003;49(3):397-406.

Smallpox Vaccination: Contraindications. Reviewed December 12, 2011, from http://www.CDC.gov

Usatine RP, et al. *The Color Atlas of Family Medicine. Part 13: Dermatology*. New York: McGraw-Hill; 2009.

Wolff K, Johnson RA. *Fitzpatrick's Color Atlas and Synopsis of Clinical Dermatology*. 6th ed. New York: McGraw-Hill; 2009.

18 Neurology

Jason Maxfield and Alex Ellison

CASE 1

A 75-year-old right-handed man presents to the emergency department (ED) with dizziness that started 1 hour ago. His dizziness consists of a spinning sensation and he feels off balance as he walks. He reports coughing when trying to drink water earlier, but otherwise notes no symptoms. He has an unremarkable past medical history and is taking no medications. On exam, he is found to have left-sided ptosis and left facial numbness to pinprick. Gag reflex is absent. Motor examination is otherwise unremarkable. Sensory examination revealed decreased pinprick sensation of the right arm and leg. He is unsteady while walking, tending to lean leftward.

What is the most likely diagnosis in this patient?

A) Acute vestibulitis/labyrinthitis.
B) Benign paroxysmal positional vertigo (BPPV).
C) Cerebellar stroke.
D) Brain stem stroke.
E) Ménière attack.

Discussion

The correct answer is "D." Although dizziness can be associated with all of the above disorders, a brain stem stroke is the most likely answer. The associated symptoms of ptosis (suggestive of Horner syndrome), absent gag with patient report of possible dysphagia, and crossed sensory findings (left side face, right side body) are most consistent with brain stem localization. In peripheral etiologies of vertigo ("A," "B," and "E"), one would not expect sensory phenomena, ptosis, or swallowing difficulties. In BPPV, one would expect brief attacks, lasting seconds to minutes, and not a prolonged attack. In Ménière's, there should be some history of tinnitus and/or hearing loss (low frequency initially). A pure cerebellar stroke would not be expected to have sensory findings.

> HELPFUL TIP: When a patient complains of dizziness, ask what the patient means by "dizziness." Dizziness is defined differently by different patients. The report of "dizziness" may represent vertigo, lightheadedness, presyncope, disequilibrium when walking (e.g., falling to one side), anxiety, etc.

* *

In considering the management of this patient, tissue plasminogen activator (tPA) was discussed.

Which one of the following is NOT a contraindication to intravenous (IV) tPA?

A) Age >75.
B) INR >1.7.
C) Platelets <100,000.
D) Stroke within last 3 months.
E) Glucose <50.
F) Hemorrhage seen on head CT.

Discussion

The correct answer is "A." Acute stroke treatment with thrombolytics **may be** of benefit if administered

Table 18–1 ELIGIBILITY AND CONTRAINDICATIONS FOR tPA, SYMPTOM ONSET 0–3 HOURS

Eligibility

- Age >18 years
- Clinical diagnosis of ischemic stroke causing measurable neurological deficit

Contraindications

- Symptoms minor or rapidly improving
- Seizure with postictal residual neurological impairments
- Stroke or serious head trauma within 3 months
- Major surgery within 14 days
- Known history of intracranial hemorrhage
- Symptoms suggestive of subarachnoid hemorrhage
- Sustained blood pressure of SBP >185 or DBP >110
- GI or urinary hemorrhage within 21 days
- Arterial puncture at noncompressible site within 7 days
- Platelet count of <100,000
- Heparin within last 48 hours with elevated PTT or anticoagulation with an INR of >1.7 or PT >15

to carefully selected patients within **3 hours** of symptom onset or **4.5 hours** of symptom onset if certain criteria are met (see Tables 18–1 and 18–2). When administered properly, the number needed to treat for improvement at 3 months is **6**. However, there is no survival benefit. The risk of hemorrhage is 6% (1 in 16). Of those with symptomatic hemorrhagic transformation, 60% are fatal. There is no upper age cutoff for administration of tPA. Strong contraindications include minor or rapidly improving symptoms as well as those listed above. In selected patients, there is a role for neurointerventional procedures including intra-arterial tPA. Unlike IV tPA, there are not clearly defined criteria for inclusion/exclusion. In general, patients should be within 6 hours of onset of symptoms and have well-localized symptoms for treatment with intra-arterial, intracranial tPA.

Table 18–2 ELIGIBILITY AND CONTRAINDICATIONS FOR tPA, SYMPTOM ONSET 3–4.5 HOURS

Eligibility

- Age >18 years but <80 years
- Clinical diagnosis of ischemic stroke causing measurable neurological deficit
- NIH stroke scale must be <25

Contraindications include all of the 0–3-hour criteria plus:

- History of prior stroke AND diabetes
- Taking oral anticoagulation therapy

HELPFUL TIP: Make sure you are compulsive about inclusion and exclusion criteria!! When in doubt, call the nearest stroke accredited hospital to speak to the on-call neurologist.

* *

The patient is outside of the 4.5-hour window for thrombolysis and has a blood pressure of 200/100.

The best next step in treatment at this point is to:

A) Administer IV labetalol with a blood pressure goal of 140/90.
B) Administer IV labetalol with a blood pressure goal of 130/85.
C) Administer IV nitroglycerin with a blood pressure goal of 150/90.
D) Administer sublingual nifedipine with a blood pressure goal of 160/95.
E) Monitor the patient's blood pressure and avoid antihypertensives.

Discussion

The correct answer is "E." Do not treat this patient's blood pressure unless the blood pressure is >220 mm Hg systolic or 120 mm Hg diastolic. Treating the blood pressure reduces central nervous system (CNS) perfusion and puts ischemic brain at risk. Obviously, this does not apply if the patient has a hypertensive urgency or hypertensive crisis (CHF or other end-organ dysfunction—renal, CNS, optic, etc.). **Note that this is for ischemic stroke and not hemorrhagic stroke. Lowering the blood pressure to a systolic of around 160 mm Hg is indicated in hemorrhagic stroke.** In this scenario, if you use an antihypertensive, labetalol is preferred. Why labetalol and not nitrates? Nitrates cause intracranial vasodilatation increasing CNS pressure.

After admission to a monitored bed, which of the following diagnostic evaluations is LEAST likely to be of further benefit in this patient?

A) Fasting lipid profile.
B) Magnetic resonance angiography (MRA) of the head and neck.
C) Fasting glucose.
D) Hypercoagulable testing.
E) Transesophageal echocardiogram.

Discussion

The correct answer is "D." Hypercoagulable states are an uncommon cause of stroke and evaluation of such should be done in a situation where another etiology is not found, especially in a low-risk patient. In addition to monitoring the patient for signs of neurologic decline or complications, evaluation of potential risk factors for recurrent stroke is an integral part of stroke care. Hypertension, hyperlipidemia, cardiac arrhythmia or structural defects, illicit drug use (IV drugs and stimulants), smoking, and diabetes mellitus are risk factors for recurrent stroke and should be evaluated. MRA allows noninvasive evaluation of intracranial and cervical blood vessels in both the anterior and posterior circulation. Echocardiography is also an important part in the evaluation of stroke, and **transesophageal** echocardiography is more sensitive for identifying thrombotic sources for stroke when compared with transthoracic echo.

* *

The patient is found to have a lateral medullary stoke on MRI and has heavy atherosclerotic burden in their vertebral arteries. Echocardiogram and telemetry are normal.

What would be the optimal antithrombotic medication in this patient for prevention of recurrent stroke?

A) Coumadin (warfarin).
B) Aspirin.
C) Plavix (clopidogrel).
D) Aggrenox (aspirin/dipyridamole).
E) Pletal (cilostazol).

Discussion

The correct answer is "B." In patients with a noncardiogenic source for their stroke, there is no data to support the use of anticoagulation (warfarin) for stroke prevention. Similarly, there is no prospective data to support a role for cilostazol or pentoxifylline in the prevention of stroke.

With regard to antiplatelet agents, aspirin is the first-line choice. There is no benefit to dual therapy (i.e., clopidogrel [Plavix] and aspirin). There is also no benefit in increasing the dose of aspirin to more than 81 mg every day. If a patient fails aspirin (recurrent stroke of same mechanism), either change to clopidogrel or Aggrenox (combination aspirin/dipyridamole); both are equally effective in stroke prevention. Because of cost, most authors recommend aspirin as a primary preventive agent in those who have had a transient ischemic attack (TIA).

HELPFUL TIP: Patients on a "stroke service" have better outcomes than those taken care of by other services. **This is because stroke services are compulsive about evaluation and treatment** (e.g., swallow studies, early physical therapy, and secondary prevention). You can be compulsive too!

* *

It seems that there's a 2-for-1 special on neurologic symptoms in your ED this evening. Your next patient is a 59-year-old male who appears to have had a simple TIA with left-sided focal weakness. The TIA lasted <10 minutes and the patient has a normal blood pressure and is nondiabetic.

His risk of having a stroke in the 48 hours after a simple TIA is:

A) 1%.
B) 5%.
C) 10%.
D) 20%.
E) 30%.

Discussion

The correct answer is "A." The overall risk of stroke ranges from 4% to 20% in the 90 days after a TIA. This is a pretty wide range. To narrow down the range a bit, the ABCD^2 has been developed and takes into account age, duration of symptoms, blood pressure, and diabetes. This can be used to predict the 48-hour risk of stroke.

ABCD²
Age: 1 point for age ≥60 years
Blood pressure: 1 point for systolic >140 or diastolic >90
Clinical features: Focal weakness (2 points) or only speech difficulty (1 point)
Duration of symptoms: >60 minutes (2 points), ≤59 minutes (1 point)
Diabetes: 1 point

The 2-day risk of stroke is **0–3 points**: 1%; **4–5 points:** 4.1%: **6–7 points:** 8.1%.

Rapid evaluation of the at-risk patient is warranted, although it is unclear if earlier interventions make a difference (beyond starting antiplatelet agents, etc.).

Objectives: Did you learn to . . .

- Identify signs/symptoms suggestive of acute ischemic stroke (cerebral infarction)?
- Initiate a diagnostic evaluation for a patient with a possible stroke?
- Describe the role of intravenous and/or intra-arterial tPA in the treatment of acute ischemic stroke?
- Evaluate options for secondary prevention of stroke?
- Assess stroke risk after TIA?

QUICK QUIZ: WHEN TO CUT?

Which of the following referrals for carotid endarterectomy is most likely to result in a benefit to the patient?

A) A symptomatic **woman** with 70% or greater stenosis to a surgeon who has a 5% complication rate.
B) An asymptomatic **man** with 60% stenosis to a surgeon who has a 7% complication rate.
C) A symptomatic **woman** with a 50–69% stenosis and a life expectancy of >5 years to a surgeon who has a 5% complication rate.
D) None of the above.

Discussion

The correct answer is "A." All sources agree that a symptomatic patient who has ≥70% stenosis of the carotid will benefit from surgery provided that the surgeon's complication rate is sufficiently low. Men, but not women, seem to have a benefit with symptomatic stenosis of 50–69% if there is >5-year life expectancy **and** the surgeon's complication rate is <6% (NNT 22). In asymptomatic patients, those with >60% stenosis will benefit from carotid endarterectomy, but NNT is 33 and the benefit is less than those with symptomatic disease.

CASE 2

A 24-year-old right-handed woman presents to you in the ED after her second episode of loss of consciousness. The first spell occurred 6 months ago and was associated with a 60-second loss of consciousness and jerking movements of her arms and legs. Following the spell, she was confused for about 15 minutes. At that time, her initial ED evaluation was unremarkable. She presents today following a spell that occurred about 45 minutes ago. Her friends observed her to fall to the ground and shake her arms and legs for about 2 minutes. They could not get her to respond during this time. Afterward, she was confused and they brought her to the ED. Upon arrival in the ED, she is mildly drowsy but otherwise oriented. She has no memory of the earlier events. Her general medical examination and neurological examination are unremarkable.

Which of these tests would be LEAST helpful in determining the etiology of this spell?

A) Urine toxicology screen.
B) Electrolytes.
C) Neuroimaging (head CT or MRI).
D) Electrocardiogram (ECG).

Discussion

The correct answer is "D." In this case, ECG would be the lowest yield, as this spell is most suggestive of seizure. Syncopal episodes, which can be caused by cardiac disease, are generally of shorter duration without postictal confusion. Although a few tonic–clonic movements can be seen with syncope (convulsive syncope), it would be atypical for those movements to continue throughout the entire period of loss of consciousness.

All of the other tests would be useful. Evaluation of a first-time seizure should include assessment for alcohol or other drug withdrawal (especially benzodiazepines and barbiturates) as well as drug intoxication (cocaine, methamphetamine, and other sympathomimetics). Infection, including meningitis and encephalitis, can provoke a seizure. Hyponatremia, hypernatremia, hypocalcemia, hypoglycemia, hyperglycemia, hypomagnesemia, hypophosphatemia, and uremia are all associated with seizures. To rule out structural lesions (e.g., tumor and AV malformation) and hemorrhage, neuroimaging should be performed. Although MRI has greater sensitivity, it is often not available in a timely manner, and thus, CT is the modality of choice.

HELPFUL TIP: All patients with syncope, including children, deserve at least one ECG in order to rule out prolonged QT interval, Brugada syndrome, etc. If the spell is not clearly a seizure and could be syncope, get an ECG.

HELPFUL TIP: The most common cause of status epilepticus in a patient with seizure disorder is noncompliance! One of the most common causes of breakthrough seizures in those with a known seizure disorder is sleep deprivation.

* *

Evaluation in the ED, including electrolytes, CBC, brain CT scan, and urine toxicology, is unremarkable. An electroencephalogram (EEG) is obtained in the ED and read as normal. The patient is feeling well and does not wish to remain in the hospital. Her friends assure you that they will be with her over the next 24 hours. She returns to your clinic in 2 days.

After reviewing her test results with her, what do you recommend for further management?

A) Continued follow-up with no further workup or treatment.
B) Video/EEG monitoring.
C) Initiate treatment with antiepileptic drug(s).
D) Tilt table testing.

Discussion

The correct answer is "C." This is this patient's second seizure. In adults with a first seizure, only 30–60% will go on to have a second seizure. In patients who have a second seizure, the likelihood of going on to have a third is 80–90%; therefore, after a second unprovoked seizure, treatment is recommended. Video/EEG monitoring is appropriate for classifying spells of unclear etiology. In order for video/EEG to be an effective tool, the patient should have spells frequently enough to capture them during a reasonable inpatient stay (3 days average). Tilt table testing would not be of value, as syncope is unlikely to be the cause of these spells.

* *

You discuss her case with the neurologist, Dr. Lotta Branes, who recommends that she start an antiepileptic drug (AED) since this is her second unprovoked seizure. "Huh? What?" you say. "Start her on an antiepileptic drug? Didn't she have a negative EEG?"

What is the sensitivity of a single interictal EEG for seizure focus?

A) 20%.
B) 30%.
C) 50%.
D) 60%.
E) 90%.

Discussion

The correct answer is "D." A single interictal EEG has only a 60% sensitivity for picking up a seizure focus. The sensitivity goes up to 90% after three interictal EEGs. However, this still means that an EEG will be negative in 10% of those with seizures after three EEGs.

* *

She has multiple questions about AEDs... and so do you... hold on!

Which of the following AEDs is *NOT* typically associated with weight gain?

A) Depakote (valproic acid).
B) Lamictal (lamotrigine).
C) Tegretol (carbamazepine).
D) Neurontin (gabapentin).

Discussion

The correct answer is "B." Depakote, Tegretol, and Neurontin are all associated with weight gain. Gabitril (tiagabine) is also associated with weight gain. Lamictal is typically weight neutral. Felbatol (felbamate) and Topamax (topiramate) are associated with weight loss.

Which of the following adverse effects is NOT typically associated with phenytoin (Dilantin)?

A) Cerebellar atrophy.
B) Gingival hyperplasia.
C) Stevens–Johnson syndrome.
D) Hypertension.
E) Bone demineralization.

Discussion

The correct answer is "D." Phenytoin (Dilantin) is associated with a number of idiosyncratic effects including cerebellar atrophy, hirsutism, Stevens–Johnson syndrome, and gingival hyperplasia. Diplopia and nystagmus can be prominent side effects, particularly with supratherapeutic doses. Dizziness, drowsiness, fatigue, headache, nausea, vomiting, weight loss, and urine discoloration (pink, red, or reddish-brown) are among some of the side effects seen with phenytoin. Many AEDs cause increased metabolism of vitamin D via the liver. Long-term use of AEDs may lead to osteoporosis, so vitamin D supplementation with calcium is routine. Phenytoin is associated with hypotension and cardiac dysrhythmia (particularly with IV administration) and can cause "purple glove syndrome" if their peripheral IV infiltrates. This is due to the solution/carrier for the drug. Fosphenytoin (Cerebyx) does not have risk of "purple glove syndrome" and has much lower incidences of hypotension and arrhythmias, so is the formulation of choice when giving IV.

Which of the following is NOT Class D for pregnancy?

A) Valproic acid (Depakote).
B) Phenytoin (Dilantin).
C) Topiramate (Topamax).
D) Phenobarbital.
E) Primidone.

Discussion

The correct answer is "C." Valproic acid, phenytoin, phenobarbital, primidone, and carbamazepine are all Class D drugs in pregnancy. The newer AEDs including Neurontin (gabapentin), Lamictal (lamotrigine), Keppra (levetiracetam), Trileptal (oxcarbazepine), Gabitril (tiagabine), Topamax, and Zonegran (zonisamide) are currently Class C in pregnancy. In particular, valproic acid has a known association with neural tube defects. As a result, it is recommended that **all** women of childbearing age be on folate and a prenatal vitamin while on AEDs. It is **not** recommended that women discontinue AEDs when pregnant, but simplifying to monotherapy is recommended if possible.

HELPFUL TIP: In the third trimester, vitamin K 10 mg PO daily is recommended by some experts due to depression of clotting factor levels with many antiepileptics. This lowering of clotting factors has been associated with neonatal bleeding.

Which of the following drugs does *NOT* have potential interactions with oral contraceptives?

A) Depakote (valproic acid).
B) Tegretol (carbamazepine).
C) Trileptal (oxcarbazepine).
D) Dilantin (phenytoin).
E) Topamax (topiramate).

Discussion

The correct answer is "A." Interactions with oral contraceptives, decreasing the efficacy of the OCP **not** the anticonvulsant, have been reported with oxcarbazepine, phenobarbital, phenytoin, lamotrigine, and topiramate.

Zonisamide, (zongran), valproic acid (Depakote), tiagabine (Gabitril), levetiracetam (Keppra), gabapentin (Neurontin), and felbamate (Felbatol) do not interfere with oral contraceptives. A barrier method of contraception, in addition to oral contraceptives, is recommended in women on AEDs, particularly those with known interactions with oral contraceptives.

Which of the following is NOT part of routine counseling with epilepsy and *initiation of therapy with an antiepileptic drug?*

A) Work safety.
B) Calcium and vitamin D supplementation.
C) Driving.
D) Alcohol consumption.
E) Epilepsy surgery.

Discussion

The correct answer is "E." Epilepsy surgery is reserved for patients who are intractable to medical management and have failed at least two AEDs. Exceptions would include patients with focal pathology (e.g., malignancy or vascular malformation). "B," calcium and vitamin D supplementation, should be initiated in patients on AEDs due to increased risk of osteoporosis. "A" and "C," work and driving safety issues, should be discussed. Most states have specific laws regarding driving and seizures and the time before resumption of driving privileges varies greatly; check the laws in your state(s) of practice. Epileptic patients should be warned of potentially dangerous activities at work and home (e.g., working on ladders, with heavy equipment, bathing, and swimming). "D," alcohol use, should be discussed with patients. Patients should also be warned of potential factors that could lower their seizure threshold, including alcohol consumption, herbal ephedra supplements, sleep deprivation, infection, and medication noncompliance.

Objectives: Did you learn to . . .

- Evaluate a patient with a potential new diagnosis of epilepsy?
- Identify some areas of specific concern regarding women's issues in epilepsy?
- Recognize commonly encountered or serious side effects with antiepileptic drugs?
- Counsel of patients with epilepsy for daily activities and regarding medication management?

QUICK QUIZ: SEIZURE DISORDERS

All of the following are indicated in the treatment of petit mal seizures (aka absence seizures, aka generalized nonconvulsive epilepsy) EXCEPT:

A) Ethosuximide.
B) Acetazolamide.
C) Valproic acid.
D) Clonazepam.
E) Phenytoin.

Discussion

The correct answer is "E." Phenytoin is not indicated in the treatment of petit mal seizures. The other options are indicated. Other drugs known to be useful in petit mal seizures include lamotrigine, phenobarbital, and topiramate.

> HELPFUL TIP: For grand mal seizures, valproic acid seems to be the drug that is most effective and thus the best drug to start with. For partial seizures (e.g., temporal lobe epilepsy), lamotrigine seems to be the best drug to start with.

CASE 3

A 60-year-old left-handed man comes in with a complaint of numbness and tingling in his lower extremities for about 10 months. He notes no weakness. He has had type 2 diabetes mellitus for 6 years and has a 30-pack-year smoking history. Examination reveals decreased sensation to light touch, pin prick, and vibratory sensation in the feet extending to 7 cm below the knees symmetrically. You also notice lack of hair on his leg to the same level. Chest, abdomen, and upper extremities have normal sensation. His reflexes are 1+ in the upper extremities and quadriceps with absent Achilles bilaterally. The remainder of his neurological and general medical examination is unremarkable. He says his diet is good but always brings you a dozen doughnuts when he visits . . . with one or two missing.

This history is most consistent with:

A) Stroke.
B) Early mononeuritis multiplex.
C) Guillain–Barré syndrome (GBS).
D) Brown–Sequard syndrome.
E) Peripheral neuropathy.

Discussion

The correct answer is "E." This is the quintessential presentation of a patient with diabetic peripheral neuropathy. "A" is incorrect because of the distribution. Bilateral distal lower extremity sensory changes are not likely from a stroke. "B," mononeuritis multiplex, is—at least initially—not in a stocking-glove distribution. Patients with mononeuritis multiplex will notice a stepwise loss of sensation and motor ability in discrete peripheral nerve distributions. Eventually, these may become confluent and resemble a stocking-glove neuropathy. However, this is found late in the disease. Additionally, there is usually motor involvement. "C" is unlikely because GBS has a relatively rapid onset and is associated with motor findings. "D," Brown–Sequard syndrome, is the result of a lesion in one side of the spinal cord. Patients have diminished proprioception, vibration sense and strength on the side of the lesion, decreased sharp sensation, and loss of temperature sense on the other side. Since our patient's findings are symmetrical in both distribution and manifestation, it is not Brown–Sequard syndrome.

Which of the following lab tests would NOT be useful in helping to determine a particular cause of this patient's neuropathy?

A) Serum immunofluorescence electrophoresis.
B) TSH/free T4.
C) Hemoglobin A_{1C}.
D) Electrolytes (Na, K, Cl, CO_2).
E) Vitamin B_{12}.

Discussion

The correct answer is "D." Electrolytes are not likely to give us a diagnosis in this patient. The initial evaluation of a patient with "stocking-glove" sensory loss should focus on finding potentially treatable causes of neuropathy. These would include hypothyroidism and vitamin B_{12} deficiency. In addition, serum immunofluorescence electrophoresis can help to identify monoclonal gammopathy, which is associated with neuropathy. Hemoglobin A_{1C} is a marker of glycemic control in diabetes and would be associated with diabetic polyneuropathy.

HELPFUL TIP: A history of alcohol use is important, as chronic alcohol abuse is commonly associated with polyneuropathy, even in the absence of vitamin B_{12} or other nutritional deficiencies.

* *

Your patient is on a number of medications.

Which of the following medications is known to cause a peripheral neuropathy?

A) Metronidazole.
B) HMG-CoA reductase inhibitors.
C) Amiodarone.
D) Disulfiram.
E) All of the above.

Discussion

The correct answer is "E." All of the above can cause a peripheral neuropathy. Some of the other drugs that can cause neuropathy include phenytoin, gold, isoniazid, several chemotherapeutic agents, nitrofurantoin, ddC, and D4T. See Table 18–3 for more causes of peripheral neuropathy.

Table 18–3 VERY PARTIAL LIST OF CAUSES OF PERIPHERAL SENSORY NEUROPATHY

Infectious	
	Syphilis
	Lyme disease
	Mycoplasma
	West Nile virus
	Leprosy
Nutritional	
	Vitamin B_{12} deficiency
	Thiamine (vitamin B_1) deficiency
	Folic acid deficiency
	Vitamin B_6 toxicity
	Celiac disease
Drugs	
	Metronidazole
	Isoniazid
	Phenytoin
	Thalidomide
Metabolic	
	Diabetes
	Hypothyroidism
Toxic	
	Mercury
	Thallium
	Other heavy metals
	Alcohol
Miscellaneous	
	Amyloid
	Paraneoplastic syndromes
	Mitochondrial disease
	Chronic inflammatory demyelinating polyneuropathy (motor > sensory)

Electrophysiological testing (electromyography/nerve conduction studies, EMG/NCV) can be helpful for all of the following EXCEPT:

A) Confirming the presence of sensory deficits.
B) Identifying subclinical motor deficits.
C) Identifying a specific etiology of the neuropathy (e.g., diabetic vs. B_{12} deficiency).
D) Determining axonal damage versus demyelination as the primary pathologic process.
E) Differentiating between primarily myopathic and neuropathic processes.

Discussion

The correct answer is "C." EMG and NCV are not capable of yielding results specific to the etiology of neuropathy (e.g., identifying diabetic neuropathy vs. B_{12} vs. syphilis); however, they can yield a pattern suggestive of a particular etiology. For example, increasing motor reaction to repeated stimulation is classic Eaton–Lambert syndrome (a paraneoplastic syndrome), while a decreasing motor response with repeated stimulation is suggestive of myasthenia gravis. EMG and NCV can be helpful in confirming the presence of a radiculopathy in the proper clinical setting. They can also determine if the process is primarily axonal (damage directly to the axons/reduction in the number of axons) versus demyelinating (damage to the myelin sheath). NCV can confirm the presence of sensory deficits (although NCV is looking at large fibers and may not identify small fiber, painful neuropathies) as well as identifying subclinical motor involvement. EMG and NCV can be used to differentiate between myopathic and neuropathic processes.

HELPFUL TIP: If electrophysiological testing shows a primary demyelinating neuropathy, a neurologic consult is recommended. These may respond to intravenous immunoglobulin (IVIG), steroids or other immunosuppressives, and plasma exchange, among others.

* *

After being followed in clinic for several years, the patient begins to complain of a painful, burning sensation developing in his feet and ankles. This pain developed gradually over the last few years in the areas that previously were numb. He has a friend who was started on gabapentin (Neurontin) for a similar problem and is wondering if this would be a good drug for him.

Which of the following is NOT an adverse reaction or contraindication to gabapentin?

A) Dizziness.
B) Peripheral edema.
C) Fatigue and drowsiness.
D) Hepatic failure.
E) Paresthesias.

Discussion

The correct answer is "D." Gabapentin (Neurontin) is not hepatically metabolized or cleared. In the setting of renal dysfunction, reduced dosing is necessary. Although gabapentin is generally well tolerated, numerous side effects have been reported. Among the most prominent complaints are those of dizziness, vertigo, and ataxia. Fatigue and drowsiness are also relatively common adverse effects; paresthesias, myalgias, and weakness have also been reported. Peripheral edema (particularly lower extremities) and facial edema are also seen as a result of therapy with gabapentin. Titrating slowly to the target dose over several weeks can improve tolerance.

* *

Your patient is concerned about swelling in his legs, as he has had problems with this in the past and does not want to try gabapentin at this time.

Which of the following medications would NOT be a reasonable FIRST choice for treatment of painful neuropathy (not specifically in this patient but in general)?

A) Amitriptyline.
B) Topical lidocaine patch.
C) Oxycodone.
D) Capsaicin cream.
E) Valproic acid.

Discussion

The correct answer is "C." Narcotics are not the treatment of choice for peripheral neuropathy and tend not to be as effective in this setting as in other types of pain. **Tricyclic antidepressants are commonly used in the setting of neuropathic pain and remain the first-line therapy.** The evidence for TCAs suggests they are superior to other classes of drugs. If pain is confined to a small area, a topical treatment such as capsaicin cream or a Lidoderm patch may be effective. The use of Lidoderm patches outside the setting of postherpetic neuralgia is an off-label use.

> **HELPFUL TIP:** Other treatments for neuropathic pain once the patient has failed a TCA include anticonvulsant drugs such as gabapentin, pregabalin, valproic acid, and carbamazepine. Finally, methadone is more effective than other opiates for neuropathic pain.

What is the most common infectious cause of peripheral neuropathy in the world (not just in the United States)?

A) HIV.
B) Lyme.
C) Leprosy.
D) Hepatitis C.
E) Tuberculosis.

Discussion

The correct answer is "C." The most common infectious cause of peripheral neuropathy in the world is leprosy. Leprosy (Hansen disease) is caused by *Mycobacterium leprae*, an acid-fast bacillus. It usually presents with a hypopigmented anesthetic patch. The sensory deficits start with loss of temperature sensation followed by loss of pain and then tactile sensations. Modalities carried by the posterior columns (proprioception and vibration) are spared. Sensation in the palms, soles, mid-chest, and mid-back is preserved until late in the disease.

HIV can cause peripheral neuropathy, most commonly being a symmetric, distal polyneuropathy. Autonomic dysfunction and mild weakness accompany distal paresthesias and burning sensations with sensory loss. Keep in mind that many of the medications used in HIV therapy are also associated with peripheral neuropathies.

Early neurologic manifestations of Lyme disease include lymphocytic meningitis, cranial neuropathy (a Bell palsy-like picture), or painful radiculoneuritis. GBS and mononeuritis multiplex can be seen early in the course of Lyme disease. Advanced (late) neurologic complications of Lyme disease include peripheral neuropathy and encephalomyelitis.

Hepatitis B and C can cause peripheral nerve manifestations. Hepatitis B has been associated with GBS (demyelinating) and mononeuritis multiplex. Hepatitis C is also associated with multiple mononeuropathies.

Tuberculosis has rarely been associated with neuropathy, but isoniazid is well known to cause peripheral neuropathy (that's why we prescribe pyridoxine with it).

> **HELPFUL TIP:** In the United States, diabetes and alcohol use disorders are the most common causes of peripheral neuropathy.

Objectives: Did you learn to . . .

- Recognize common etiologies of peripheral neuropathy?
- Identify appropriate uses of electrophysiological testing?
- Identify types of neuropathy that are potentially treatable?
- Prescribe medical therapy for painful peripheral neuropathy?

QUICK QUIZ: WRIST DROP

Which of the following is most likely to cause an isolated wrist drop?

A) C-3 disk lesion.
B) Ulnar nerve compression.
C) Radial nerve compression.
D) C-4 disk lesion.
E) Median nerve compression.

Discussion

The correct answer is "C." Compression of the radial nerve (such as sleeping with someone's head on your arm) can cause an isolated wrist drop, the so-called Saturday Night Palsy. Suspect alcohol or other drug abuse in patients with this lesion. It is pretty hard to get this type of compressive lesion if you are not passed out or very sedated. "B," ulnar nerve compression (cubital tunnel syndrome), presents with pain and numbness in the elbow and fourth and fifth fingers and weakness of the intraosseous muscles (weakness with spreading fingers). "E," median nerve compression (including carpal tunnel syndrome), leads to numbness on the palmar surface of the thumb and fingers two, three, and the radial half of four. There is weakness and perhaps atrophy of the thenar muscles (unable to maintain opposition of thumb to fifth finger against resistance).

CASE 4

A 25-year-old woman presents to your clinic complaining of a bifrontal headache that started this morning. She describes the pain as throbbing and 8/10 in severity. She is complaining of photophobia and nausea. She has had similar headaches in the past, lasting a few hours to all day. She is unable to work during these headaches and prefers a dark, quiet room. The physical examination, including neurological exam, is unremarkable.

Which of the following statements is most accurate?

A) She likely does not have migraine headaches because her headache is bilateral.
B) She likely dose not have migraine headaches because they most commonly present in the fourth to fifth decade of life.
C) She likely does not have migraine headaches because they rarely occur in the morning.
D) She likely has migraine headaches.

Discussion

The correct answer is "D." She likely has migraine headaches. Migraine headaches may vary considerably in severity, time of day, and characteristics. The International Headache Society (IHS) has a useful classification system with criteria for the diagnosis of migraine headaches (Table 18–4). "B" is incorrect because migraine headaches typically present in the first three decades of life. Attacks typically last less than 1 day although they may occasionally last longer. Migraine headaches are typically moderate to severe in intensity, may occur at any time during the day, and occur with or without aura. Most migraine headaches are unilateral, preceded by aura, and accompanied by nausea and vomiting. They are more prevalent among women, with a 1-year prevalence rate of approximately 18% in women, 6% in men, and 4% in children. Family history is important as 80% of patients with migraine headache have a first-degree relative with migraines.

Migraine headaches were formerly classified as classic type (migraine with aura) and common type (migraine without aura.) Typical auras develop over several minutes and last for less than 60 minutes. Auras may involve visual, language, sensory, or motor deficits. The visual auras are by far the most common and may appear as photopsias (flashes of light), scotomas (blind spots), or complex shapes that build or move across the visual field. The IHS criteria for migraine with aura are listed in Table 18–5.

Table 18–4 CRITERIA FOR THE DIAGNOSIS OF MIGRAINE WITHOUT AURA

At least five attacks fulfilling the following criteria:

Headache lasting 4–72 hours (untreated or unsuccessfully treated)

Headache has at least two of the following characteristics:
1. Unilateral location
2. Pulsating quality
3. Moderate or severe intensity (inhibits or prohibits daily activities)
4. Aggravation by walking stairs or similar routine physical activity

During headache at least one of the following:
1. Nausea and/or vomiting
2. Photophobia and phonophobia

No evidence of organic disease

Table 18–5 CRITERIA FOR THE DIAGNOSIS OF MIGRAINE WITH AURA

At least two migraines (see Table 18–4) fulfilling at least three of the following characteristics:
1. One or more fully reversible aura[a] symptoms indicating brain dysfunction
2. At least one aura symptom develops gradually over 5 minutes (or longer) or two or more symptoms occur in succession.
3. No single aura symptom lasts more than 60 minutes.
4. Headache begins during aura or within 60 minutes of the end of the aura.

History, physical, and appropriate diagnostic tests exclude a secondary cause

[a]An aura should have symptoms from two neurologic domains—visual and/or sensory and/or speech. The symptoms may be positive (e.g., flickering lights, pins/needles sensation) or negative (e.g., scotoma, numbness).

HELPFUL TIP: The IHS criteria are meant as research criteria rather than strict clinical criteria. While patients with a certain type of migraine headache will ideally meet all criteria, it is not necessary to meet all criteria to make a clinical diagnosis of migraine headache.

* *

You have decided to treat this woman's migraine headache.

Which medication would be LEAST appropriate for acute management of her headache?

A) Oral ibuprofen.
B) Intranasal sumatriptan.
C) IV meperidine (Demerol).
D) Intranasal DHE.

Discussion

The correct answer is "C." The least appropriate treatment from the above list would be Demerol (meperidine). The long-term use of opiates for rescue therapy has not been found to improve the quality of life in patients with migraines. Oral NSAIDs ("A"), including aspirin and combination analgesics containing caffeine, are a first-line choice for mild-to-moderate migraine attacks or severe attacks that have been NSAID responsive in the past. "B," the "migraine-specific" treatments, commonly called the "triptans" (e.g., sumatriptan, zolmitriptan, naratriptan, rizatriptan, almotriptan, eletriptan, and frovatriptan—wow, talk about "me too" drugs...), are effective and relatively safe for the acute treatment of migraine headaches. Triptans are an appropriate initial treatment choice in patients with moderate-to-severe migraines who have no contraindications to their use (see below). Alternative vasoconstrictive agents, including DHE nasal spray (dihydroergotamine, answer "D"), can provide a safe and effective treatment of acute migraine attacks. DHE can be administered IV as well. Vasoconstrictive side effects, including the risk of coronary artery spasm, should specifically be discussed with patients prior to initiation of therapy.

> HELPFUL TIP: Adding oral metoclopramide to aspirin or NSAIDs will improve their rate of success. Part of the nausea and vomiting from migraines (and the reason that oral medications often do not work) is from gastric paresis. Metoclopramide overcomes this problem and treats nausea as well.

Which of the following statements is correct?

A) If a patient doesn't respond to sumatriptan, there is no point in trying another triptan because the patient will not respond.
B) DHE and sumatriptan may be safely used within the same 24-hour time period.
C) Sumatriptan use is contraindicated in patients with known coronary artery disease, regardless of age.
D) Flushing, sweating, and paresthesias after a dose of sumatriptan is an indication of a severe reaction and continued use of this medication is contraindicated.

Discussion

The correct answer is "C." The triptans should not be used in patients with known coronary disease. Patients who do not respond to one triptan may respond to other triptans, and a trial of other triptans is appropriate. Also, a patient may respond initially to a triptan but not respond on other occasions. Each triptan has a maximum recommended dose, and a good rule of thumb is that the initial dose may be repeated once in a 24-hour period of time. However, avoid the use of DHE within 24 hours after a triptan has been given due to increased vasoconstriction and the possibility of vasospasm.

Contraindications to the use of "triptans" include all of the following EXCEPT:

A) Lung cancer.
B) Coronary artery disease.
C) Uncontrolled hypertension.
D) Use of an MAO inhibitor within the last 2 weeks.
E) Use of an ergot preparation within the last 24 hours.

Discussion

The correct answer is "A." Lung cancer is not a contraindication to the use of triptans. In addition to "B"–"D," caution should be used in patients with history of stroke, known cardiac risk factors, and impaired liver function.

> HELPFUL TIP: Common reactions to triptans include jaw tightness, flushing, anxiety, dizziness, and sweating. These are uncomfortable but not dangerous. Serious reactions to triptans include coronary vasospasm, anaphylaxis, or hypertensive crisis in patients with known CAD, hypersensitivity to triptans, or uncontrolled hypertension. See Table 18–6 for acute treatment of migraine headaches.

Table 18–6 US HEADACHE CONSORTIUM GUIDELINES FOR TREATMENT OF HEADACHE

Group 1: Proven, pronounced statistical and clinical benefit (at least two double-blind, placebo-controlled studies and clinical impression of effect)	• Sumatriptan SC/IN • DHE (IV/IM/SC/IN) • Prochlorperazine IV • Butorphanol IN
Group 2: Moderate statistical and clinical benefit (one double-blind, placebo-controlled studies and clinical impression of effect)	• Prochlorperazine IM/PR • Chlorpromazine IV/IM • Metoclopramide IV • Ketorolac IM • Lidocaine IN • Meperidine IM/IV • Butorphanol IM • Methadone IM
Group 3: Conflicting or inconsistent evidence.	• Metoclopramide IM/PR
Group 4: Proven to be statistically or clinically ineffective (failed efficacy vs. placebo)	• Chlorpromazine IM • Granisetron IV • Lidocaine IV
Group 5: Clinical and statistical benefits unknown (insufficient evidence available)	• Dexamethasone IV • Hydrocortisone IV

Data from US Headache Consortium: http://www.americanheadachesociety.org/professional_resources/us_headache_consortium_guidelines/

HELPFUL TIP: Consider dexamethasone as an adjunct therapy in severe headache. A single dose of dexamethasone 10 mg PO, IV, or IM after abortive therapy in the ED may prevent headache recurrence in patients who have had a headache for more than 24 hours (NNT 9).

* *

Your patient has decided to take ibuprofen for her headaches. This medication seemed to be effective at first, but she notes for the last several weeks that she is taking two to three doses of ibuprofen per day without significant headache relief. She has had a dull bilateral headache that is moderate in severity for the last 2 weeks. She has no personal or family history of coronary artery disease.

Which of the following statements is correct?

A) She likely has a tension headache and should increase her frequency of ibuprofen and continue to take it on a daily basis.
B) She likely has a medication-overuse headache in addition to chronic migraine headache (status migrainous) and should taper and then discontinue ibuprofen.
C) A medication such as sumatriptan used on a daily basis does not increase the risk of rebound headache.
D) She likely does not have medication-overuse headache because opiates are the only medications that increase the risk of these headaches.

Discussion

The correct answer is "B." See below for a discussion.

Which of the following medications taken on a frequent basis is LEAST likely to cause medication-overuse or rebound headache?

A) Sumatriptan.
B) Morphine.
C) Ibuprofen.
D) Amitriptyline.
E) All of the above are equally likely to cause rebound headache.

Discussion

The correct answer is "D." Frequent use of opiates, ergotamine, triptans, and any other analgesics may put a patient at risk for medication-overuse or rebound headache. Although analgesic rebound headache characteristics can vary significantly, the patient typically reports a pattern of headache that decreases modestly in severity with the use of their analgesic of choice, and then in 2–4 hours (depending on the medication), the headache returns to its previous severity or worsens further. Failure to repeat analgesic use results in a withdrawal headache (similar to the caffeine withdrawal headaches physicians often experience when they miss their morning coffee). In the case of triptans, the headache may not worsen for many hours or even until the next day, but a cycle of regular use of the medication is still established. At this time, no clear consensus on the duration of therapy necessary to produce analgesic rebound is reported. As a general rule, it is best to limit the use of analgesic medications to no more than 2–3-headache days per week. In addition, limit the patient's analgesic use to no more than 2–3 weeks per month. Patient education is the most important part of therapy in treating analgesic rebound or medication-overuse headaches.

HELPFUL TIP: Treatment of rebound headaches consists of discontinuing the medication. Several approaches have been tried to reduce headaches after the analgesic has been withdrawn. These include IV or oral steroids, long-acting NSAIDs (naproxen), and elective admission and therapy with IV DHE (dihydroergotamine) or Thorazine (chlorpromazine). These should be combined with a prophylactic medication such as amitriptyline (or other tricyclic) used on a daily basis. Patients can also take hydroxyzine and prochlorperazine when they have a breakthrough headache; these medications do not cause rebound headaches.

Which of the following medications would be the LEAST appropriate for the preventative treatment of your patient's migraine headaches?

A) Verapamil.
B) Propranolol.
C) Amitriptyline.
D) Clonazepam.

Discussion

The correct answer is "D." Clonazepam is not used as a preventive treatment for migraine headaches. Keep in mind the common side effects of these medications and the appropriateness in your specific patient. For example, valproate would be a bad choice for many patients secondary to weight gain or teratogenicity. Propranolol may cause hypotension. Amitriptyline may cause cardiac arrhythmia in certain patients, while constipation and urinary retention are relatively common in elderly patients. Topiramate (Topamax) may actually cause weight loss, and impaired cognition is common.

HELPFUL TIP: A number of medications are useful in the prevention of migraine headaches.

- Medications that have been found to have medium-to-high efficacy, good strength of evidence, and mild-to-moderate side effects include amitriptyline, divalproex sodium, and propranolol/timolol.
- Medications of lower efficacy include atenolol/metoprolol/nadolol, nimodipine/verapamil, aspirin/naproxen/ketoprofen, fluoxetine, ACE inhibitors, gabapentin, feverfew, magnesium, and vitamin B_2.
- Antidepressants such as fluvoxamine, paroxetine, nortriptyline, sertraline, trazodone, and venlafaxine have also been found to be clinically efficacious based on consensus and clinical experience, but no scientific evidence of efficacy has been established. Efficacy has also been demonstrated for the antiepileptic drugs Depakote (valproic acid) and Topamax (topiramate); other antiepileptic drugs have been tried as well, although there is little to no evidence to support their use at this time.

HELPFUL TIP: Combination products such as butalbital/caffeine/acetaminophen/codeine (e.g., Fiorinal with codeine) have no role in the treatment of migraine or other headaches. Addiction, abuse, and diversion are potential issues with these drugs.

Which one of the following medications is rated Class B or better in pregnancy?

A) Phenergan (promethazine).
B) Imitrex (sumatriptan).
C) Codeine.
D) Amitriptyline.
E) None of the above.

Discussion

The correct answer is "E." Headache treatment in pregnancy remains a difficult problem. Although numerous medications are available for headache treatment, their safety in pregnancy has not been established. Amitriptyline and valproic acid are class D in pregnancy. Other commonly used tricyclics include imipramine (Class C) and nortriptyline (Class D); venlafaxine is Class C. Promethazine, prochlorperazine, codeine, hydrocodone, and meperidine are all Class C. Ergotamine (DHE 45) is Class X. The triptan class of medications, including sumatriptan, remains Class C, though pregnancy registries, retrospective and observational studies suggest that sumatriptan is safe (Duong, *Can Fam Physician* 2010) (Evans, *Ann Pharmacother* 2008).

In which of the following patients is neuroimaging LEAST likely to be useful?

A) A 30-year-old woman with a headache typical of a migraine.
B) A 23-year-old woman with a history of migraine headaches that is very concerned because her current headache of 1-week duration is more severe than her typical migraine headaches.
C) A 60-year-old man with new headache, worse in the morning and of 6 weeks duration.
D) A 40-year-old man with a headache and right arm weakness.

Discussion

The correct answer is "A." According to the U.S. Headache Consortium, neuroimaging is not typically recommended in **migraine** patients with a normal neurologic examination. Imaging may be considered in patients who are disabled by their fear of serious pathology or if the provider is suspicious about underlying pathology. Factors that may lead one to consider neuroimaging include a nonacute, atypical headache or unexplained abnormal neurologic examination.

HELPFUL TIP: Not all unilateral headaches are migraines. Think of occipital neuralgia, temporal arteritis, jolts and jabs (icepick) headache, temporalis muscle overuse/TMJ syndrome, chronic paroxysmal hemicrania, SUNCT syndrome, and cluster headaches, among others.

Objectives: Did you learn to . . .

- Recognize and diagnose migraine headaches?
- Initiate appropriate acute therapy for migraine headaches?
- Identify contraindications and adverse reactions of the triptan medications?
- Recognize and treat analgesic-related headaches?
- Identify appropriate preventive therapy for chronic headaches?

CASE 5

A 30-year-old woman presents to your office with a 2-day history of progressive, **unilateral** arm (proximal and distal) numbness without weakness. She has been diagnosed with fibromyalgia in the past. She is taking fluoxetine for depression and has a history of previous hospitalizations for depression.

Which of the following is the most appropriate next step?

A) Monitor her symptoms and reassure that her numbness is likely related to her fibromyalgia.
B) Order nerve conduction (NCV) studies.
C) Order a head CT.
D) Get additional history; ask about previous similar episodes or other neurological concerns.
E) Order a chest radiograph (CXR) and complete blood cell count (CBC).

Discussion

The correct answer is "D." Of course, the answer is "more history." With a progressive neurological deficit, the first step in the workup is to further explore the history. Frequently, patients will not mention previous neurological symptoms because they—the symptoms, not the patients—are vague.

* *

When you ask about previous spells, she notes that she had an episode of left leg numbness that lasted about 1-week several years ago, but she thought nothing of it as it was mild. Six months ago, she had a 3-day visual disturbance in her right eye, during which she found it difficult to read and focus on objects; no blind spot was noticed. However, she had pain in the eye, especially when moving it.

What is the most likely diagnosis based on the history given?

A) Multiple sclerosis (MS).
B) Fibromyalgia.
C) Conversion disorder.
D) Migraine.
E) TIAs.

Discussion

The correct answer is "A." MS would be the most likely diagnosis based on the history related above. MS most commonly presents in women 20–35 years old and in men 35–45 years old. It is almost five times more prevalent among women than among men and is more common in the Caucasian population. MS is a central nervous system demyelinating disease that is thought to occur by an immune-mediated process. The demyelinating lesions of MS can occur anywhere in the CNS including the brain stem and spinal cord. The presenting symptoms of MS vary, but common symptoms are visual complaints, weakness, and sensory deficits. Although migraine can be associated with neurologic symptoms, one would expect more stereotypic events and a history of previous headaches. Fibromyalgia is associated with numerous somatic complaints, but is not typically associated with sensory deficits or visual problems. Conversion disorder can produce all of the symptoms described earlier but is a diagnosis of exclusion. TIAs would be unusual in a patient of this age, though not impossible by any means, and would typically present with stroke-like symptoms (dysarthria, vertigo, hemiparesis, etc.).

HELPFUL TIP: MS has a geographic predilection. The incidence of MS increases with increasing distance from the equator. Various theories have suggested an association with sunlight exposure, vitamin D, virus exposure, or ethnicity.

If your patient indeed does have MS, which type is most likely?

A) Devic disease.
B) Relapsing–remitting.
C) Primary progressive.
D) None of the above.

Discussion

The correct answer is "B." The two common forms of MS are primary progressive and relapsing–remitting. The diagnosis of relapsing–remitting MS is based on clinical grounds and laboratory data. Clinically, symptoms of CNS dysfunction develop over hours to days, stabilize, and then improve. It is important to identify clinical events disseminated in space and time. In this case, your patient had a prior history of optic neuritis and lower extremity numbness and now has arm numbness. "A," Devic disease (neuromyelitis optica), is a central nervous system demyelinating illness that is characterized by **bilateral** optic neuritis (simultaneous or occurring at different times) and spinal cord demyelination.

Which of the following tests would NOT be helpful in further diagnosing MS?

A) MRI brain.
B) Lumbar puncture.
C) Nerve conduction studies.
D) Visual evoked potentials.

Discussion

The correct answer is "C." MS is a central demyelinating process and does not produce abnormalities that would be seen on nerve conduction studies. "A," an MRI, would be helpful. Brain MRI is 85–97% sensitive in detecting MS plaques. Multiple areas of increased signal in the periventricular area are suggestive of, but not specific for, MS. Gadolinium-enhancing lesions suggest active disease. "B," lumbar puncture, can also be useful. Cerebrospinal fluid (CSF) abnormalities suggestive of MS include oligoclonal bands and increased synthesis of IgG. A spinal fluid examination may be considered if the clinical diagnosis of MS is suspected but is not definite. However, the positive and negative predictive value of CSF oligoclonal bands is inadequate to do more than support the clinical diagnosis. Recent evidence for serum antibody testing to other myelin components has yielded promising initial results as a supportive diagnostic tool. Finally, "D," visual evoked potentials, may be helpful. Evoked potential may be used to aid in the diagnosis of MS by indicating prior demyelination of the optic tract (optic neuritis) if the clinical history is vague (e.g., eye pain without vision loss or no recollection of symptoms). This will aid in proving the occurrence of different events separated by space and time.

Which of the following is not a recognized therapy for MS?

A) Corticosteroids.
B) Interferon-beta.
C) Glatiramer acetate.
D) Sulfasalazine.
E) Amantadine.

Discussion

The correct answer is "D." Sulfasalazine is not useful in the treatment of MS. Immune-modulating therapy reduces the number of exacerbations and active lesions on MRI. These include interferon-beta-1a (Avonex and Rebif) and interferon-beta-1b (Betaseron), as well as glatiramer acetate (Copaxone). These medications are more efficacious if started early in the course of the disease. Common adverse effects of interferon include fatigue, depression, and myalgias. Amantadine is given commonly as monotherapy and in combination with immunomodulatory therapy to treat fatigue associated with MS. Corticosteroids have a role in treating severe acute exacerbations (e.g., optic neuritis, severe neurological impairments limiting activities of daily living) in the form of a short burst and taper (typically methylprednisolone, 1 g/day often followed by an oral prednisone taper). Oral steroid use does not appear to offer long-term functional benefit, excluding the possible exception of IV pulsed steroid dosing. Currently, oral immunosuppressive therapies (mycophenolate mofetil, azathioprine, and cyclosporin) are being considered in treating refractory MS, but their long-term efficacy and safety are not known. Similarly, the value of IVIG and plasma exchange has not been conclusively demonstrated and use of these treatment modalities is reserved for refractory patients.

Which of the following treatments would you most likely choose for this patient, given her history of depression?

A) Avonex (interferon-beta-1a).
B) Amantadine.
C) Copaxone (glatiramer acetate).
D) Betaseron (interferon-beta-1b).

Discussion

The correct answer is "C." The interferon agents (Avonex, Rebif, and Betaseron) and amantadine are associated with worsening of depression. Given this patient's history of severe depression requiring hospitalization, one would favor Copaxone as an initial therapy, although treatment with interferon is not absolutely contraindicated.

* *

The patient is wondering what she can do to prevent exacerbations.

Which of the following is associated with exacerbation of MS symptoms?

A) Cold temperatures (you could recommend she move to Florida).
B) Urinary tract infection.
C) Influenza vaccination.
D) Trauma.

Discussion

The correct answer is "B." Urinary tract infections can exacerbate MS. Unfortunately, urinary tract infections are particularly common in those with MS because of the frequent occurrence of neurogenic bladder. Systemic infection has also been reported to provoke MS exacerbations. "A" is of special note. Cold is not associated with exacerbations, **but heat is** notorious, and this phenomenon actually has a name—Uhthoff phenomenon. Patients with MS should be instructed to avoid hot tubs, saunas, steam rooms, etc. "C," vaccinations, including influenza vaccine, had been posited as a cause of exacerbations. However, a review of multiple clinical trials showed no increased risk of exacerbations in patients with MS receiving the influenza, hepatitis B, or tetanus vaccinations. **Note that we do not have experience with nasal influenza vaccine and MS. Since the nasal vaccine contains live virus, it should probably be avoided in patients with MS.** "D," trauma, has been suggested as a possible exacerbation trigger, but the American Academy of Neurology clinical practice guidelines state that the majority of class II evidence available on this issue supports no connection.

HELPFUL TIP: There are several new drugs for MS. The first, Ampyra (dalfampridine), is supposed to increase walking distance. The second, Zenvia (dextromethorphane + quinidine), is designed to reduce pseudobulbar symptoms (emotional lability with spontaneous laughing, crying). Both are of marginal benefit.

Objectives: Did you learn to . . .

- Identify epidemiologic characteristics of MS?
- Identify appropriate workup for patients with possible MS?

- Diagnose MS?
- Discuss potential treatment options available for long-term disease modification as well as acute exacerbations?
- Recognize factors that might result in exacerbations of MS?

CASE 6

A 43-year-old woman with a history of myasthenia gravis presents to the ED while on vacation. She reports she is feeling tired and rundown and endorses flu-like symptoms in addition to some worsening of her proximal lower extremity weakness. On examination, she is afebrile with a respiratory rate of 18. She has mild diplopia with lateral gaze. Her strength is 4/5 proximally and 4+/5 distally bilaterally. Her sensory examination is normal. Plantar responses are down-going bilaterally.

In determining this patient's further disposition, what is the most important test?

A) Arterial blood gas.
B) CXR.
C) Head CT.
D) Spirometry (forced vital capacity [FVC] and negative inspiratory force [NIF]).
E) CBC.

Discussion

The correct answer is "D." This patient is experiencing an exacerbation of myasthenia gravis. This could be occurring for any number of reasons including concurrent illness or possibly noncompliance with her regimen. The greatest morbidity and mortality for this patient lies in the potential for respiratory failure and arrest. In primary neuromuscular respiratory failure (e.g., myasthenia gravis, acute inflammatory demyelinating polyradiculoneuropathy, GBS), the arterial blood gas may remain normal despite impending respiratory collapse. The best way to evaluate respiratory status is with the FVC and NIF. If the FVC is less than 15 mL/kg or NIF less than −20 cm H_2O, elective intubation is recommended, although some centers will choose to monitor these patients closely in an intensive care setting. Once a myasthenic patient has been intubated, you should stop their pyridostigmine as it will increase respiratory secretions and GI motility leading to diarrhea. Neither of these is desirable in an intubated ICU patient (the nurses will love you for this one) and the pyridostigmine will not liberate them from the ventilator. Monitoring the FVC/NIF should be done regularly throughout the hospital course until the patient is clinically improved and stable.

* *

You decide to give this patient a dose of edrophonium trying to reverse her symptoms. When you do this, she becomes increasingly weak, requiring intubation.

The BEST explanation of this is:

A) Since she has missed multiple doses of her pyridostigmine, she has become desensitized and will have an overwhelming response to small doses of IV edrophonium.
B) Influenza has made her particularly susceptible to edrophonium.
C) The patient has taken too much pyridostigmine by accident.
D) The alcohol that she has had on vacation has changed her pyridostigmine requirement.

Discussion

The correct answer is "C." Myasthenic crisis can be due to two causes. First, the patient may have not taken enough medication or may have missed doses. In this case, edrophonium will improve symptoms. The second cause is **too much** pyridostigmine. This will also cause weakness. In this case, the edrophonium will worsen the patient's symptoms. Here's how it works. Pyridostigmine and edrophonium are both cholinesterase inhibitors similar to organophosphates. They act by binding to acetylcholinesterase and preventing the breakdown of acetylcholine. Too much of either drug (or a combination of the drugs) will cause weakness and an organophosphate toxicity-like syndrome (salivation, lacrimation, defecation, urination, weakness, etc.).

Which of the following IS NOT likely to contribute to the diagnosis of myasthenia gravis?

A) Tensilon (edrophonium) test.
B) Nerve conduction studies.
C) Antithymocyte antibodies.
D) Antiacetylcholine receptor antibodies.

Discussion

The correct answer is "C." Antithymocyte antibodies are used to treat renal rejection and have also been used in aplastic anemia, red cell aplasia, and other disorders. They have no relationship at all to myasthenia gravis. All of the others can be used in the diagnosis of myasthenia gravis. The edrophonium test is a functional test. One must be ready to intubate the patient when performing an edrophonium test. Nerve conduction studies show a reduction in the amplitude of the response to repeated stimulation (thus, patients get weaker with repeated muscle use). Antiacetylcholine receptor antibodies are found in the majority (80–90%) of patients with myasthenia gravis. In fact, when an ultrasensitive test is done, it is found in 70% of "antibody negative" cases of myasthenia gravis.

HELPFUL TIP: Myasthenia gravis can be systemic or limited to the ocular muscles. It is often associated with a thymoma (or thymus hyperplasia), and patients with myasthenia gravis should have a chest CT scan to rule out thymoma or thymus hyperplasia. If present, removal of the thymoma will often "cure" the patient's disease.

Which of the following is LEAST likely to be confused with myasthenia gravis on the basis of its neurologic symptoms?

A) Eaton–Lambert syndrome.
B) Guillian-Barre syndrome (GBS).
C) Amyotrophic lateral sclerosis.
D) Botulism toxicity.
E) Penicillamine-induced myasthenia gravis.

Discussion

The correct answer is "B." GBS includes sensory findings of pain, paresthesias, numbness, etc., that are generally absent in the other syndromes. "A," Eaton–Lambert syndrome, is a paraneoplastic process, which consists of weakness **that gets better with repetitive movement.** This is the exact opposite of what is seen with myasthenia gravis where repetitive tasks lead to increased weakness. Thus, Eaton–Lambert syndrome is often worse in the morning and better toward the afternoon—the reverse of what is seen with myasthenia gravis. Patients with amyotrophic lateral sclerosis, botulism, and penicillamine-induced myasthenia gravis do not have sensory symptoms. Thus, these can be confused with myasthenia gravis.

* *

The patient and her husband have some questions about myasthenia gravis and are wondering if there are any medications that might exacerbate this patient's weakness.

Which of the following can worsen myasthenia gravis?

A) Fluoroquinolones.
B) Verapamil.
C) Beta-blockers.
D) Oral contraceptives.
E) All of the above.

Discussion

The correct answer is "E." All of the above can worsen myasthenia gravis. Other drugs of note include aminoglycosides, anesthetic and paralytic agents, diuretics, tetracyclines, and magnesium, among many others.

* *

You decide to add to the treatment of this patient.

Which of the following is considered a standard therapy for myasthenia gravis?

A) Plasmaphoresis for an acute myasthenic crisis.
B) IVIG.
C) Prednisone.
D) Azathioprine.
E) All of the above are used for myasthenia gravis.

Discussion

The correct answer is "E." Do you see a pattern here? All of the treatments are immunomodulators. Most people will start with prednisone and azathioprine. Other options are cyclosporin and mycophenolate. The idea here is to reduce anti-endplate antibodies (although nobody is quite sure how IVIG works). Prednisone is generally considered first-line therapy for an exacerbation. It may be that immunomodulators will become first line (and many neurologists are already using them as first line and using pyridostigmine only as a bridge until the immunomodulator kicks in). Remember thymectomy.

Objectives: Did you learn to . . .

- Manage a patient with an exacerbation of myasthenia gravis?
- Understand the use of diagnostic tests in myasthenia gravis?

- Recognize diagnoses that can be confused with myasthenia gravis?

CASE 7

A 29-year-old woman presents to the ED with sudden onset of a severe headache involving **bilateral occipital** pain associated with nausea. The headache has not responded to her sumatriptan (Imitrex) injection. She has a history of migraine headaches consisting of **right-sided throbbing** pain that typically respond to sumatriptan but occasionally require IM hydroxyzine and morphine. She appears to be in moderate pain but otherwise has a normal general and neurological examination. This is the worst headache of her life.

What is the next step in the management of this patient?

A) Ketorolac (Toradol) IM or IV.
B) Aspirin plus metoclopramide.
C) IV dihydroergotamine (DHE).
D) Head CT.
E) Lumbar puncture.

Discussion

The correct answer is "D." Although this patient has a history of migraines, she is reporting a sudden onset headache that is markedly changed from her typical pattern of headache. In this setting—especially with the "worst headache of her life"—the diagnosis of subarachnoid hemorrhage (SAH) must be ruled out. Requiring a CT before LP is dogma, which is unsupported in the literature unless the patient has a focal neurological exam. None of the other answers are correct. While pain management can be given before CT (e.g., IV morphine or fentanyl), ketorolac, aspirin, and DHE are inappropriate if there is a question of SAH. Ketorolac and aspirin have antiplatelet effects, which can increase bleeding. DHE can cause vasospasm and worsen brain ischemia. Finally, if you recall, this patient tried her sumatriptan. One should not use DHE within 24 hours of a triptan.

HELPFUL TIP: Did you notice that the patient usually gets hydroxyzine and morphine IM? IM hydroxyzine has been known to cause severe muscle necrosis and should be avoided.

* *

The patient's head CT is negative.

What next?

A) Lumbar puncture.
B) IV hydroxyzine and meperidine and discharge when the patient is comfortable.
C) IV hydroxyzine and promethazine (Phenergan) and discharge when the patient is comfortable.
D) Discharge home with prescription for acetaminophen and oxycodone (Percocet).
E) Discharge home with prescription for rizatriptan (Maxalt).

Discussion

The correct answer is "A." In the setting of a "worst headache of life," a CT scan to rule out SAH is required. The sensitivity of CT scan of the brain for hemorrhage in the setting of SAH is 90–95% within 24 hours of the event (decreases to 80% at 72 hours). As a result, **a negative head CT does not adequately rule out SAH** and should be followed with a lumbar puncture. The CSF from the lumbar puncture must be spun down immediately to examine for xanthochromia; delay in examining the CSF may result in false-positive results. Xanthochromia is a yellow discoloration of the normally clear CSF resulting from degradation of hemoglobin. In addition to xanthochromia, markedly elevated RBC counts are indicative of SAH. If either the CT or LP is positive for SAH, an emergent 4-vessel cerebral angiogram (or MR angiogram or CT angiogram) is indicated.

HELPFUL TIP: Thirty-nine percent of patients with an SAH have no neurologic signs or symptoms. Only 10% of patients with SAH have an initially focal exam. Patients with SAH may have a fever and leukocytosis. While looking at the patient's fundi is important, the absence of papilledema does not rule out SAH. SAH can present as back pain. Since each bleed carries a 50% mortality, this is one diagnosis you do not want to miss. Use LP liberally in appropriate patients.

Objective: Did you learn to . . .

- Identify a patient presenting with symptoms of SAH?

CASE 8

A 40-year-old man presents with a complaint of low back pain that is dull in nature, which started 2 days ago. This morning he woke up with a feeling of numbness and tingling in his feet, which gradually seemed to worsen. By noon, he noted difficulty walking and decided to come to the ED. He denies bowel or bladder incontinence. On exam, he is in no acute distress and has a respiratory rate of 12. He has strength of 5/5 in his upper extremities, and in his lower extremities, strength is 4/5 proximally and 3/5 distally. Sensory examination reveals a mild decrease in pinprick and light touch in a stocking distribution to the mid-calf. Reflexes in the upper extremities are 2+/4 and in the lower extremities are trace at the knees and absent at the Achilles. Plantar response is down going bilaterally.

What is the most likely diagnosis?

A) Diabetic polyneuropathy.
B) Gullian-Barre syndrome (GBS).
C) Diabetic amyotrophy.
D) Stroke.
E) Conversion reaction.

Discussion

The correct answer is "B." Of the choices given above, the most likely diagnosis is acute inflammatory demyelinating polyradiculoneuropathy (GBS). With an acute onset of bilateral lower extremity weakness and sensory deficits, the diagnosis of an acute cord-compressing lesion (e.g., tumor and epidural abscess) should also be considered and ruled out, especially with back pain. The time course described above is not consistent with diabetic polyneuropathy nor would one expect to see weakness as a prominent symptom. Diabetic amyotrophy is characterized by painful **proximal** muscle weakness with minor sensory loss. The onset of diabetic amyotrophy can be subacute or acute. The time course described above of gradually progressing deficits is not consistent with stroke. Additionally, the findings of a stroke should not be bilateral.

Which of the following is/are associated with GBS?

A) *Campylobacter jejuni* infection.
B) Lyme disease.
C) Epstein–Barr virus.
D) CMV virus.
E) All of the above.

Discussion

The correct answer is "E." All of these infectious agents are associated with GBS. Other associations include URIs, HIV, immunizations (rare), mycoplasma, epidural anesthesia, sarcoid, lupus, etc. The point here is that one should look for an underlying illness in patients with GBS.

> HELPFUL (AND INTERESTING) TIP:
> Antibodies to *Campylobacter* have recently been shown to cross-react with nerve tissue, thus the association of *Campylobacter* with GBS.

Which of the following actions would NOT be appropriate for additional diagnosis and/or management of this patient with progressive weakness?

A) Cardiac monitoring.
B) FVC.
C) Discharge to home on steroids with a follow-up in the morning.
D) EMG/NCV.

Discussion

The correct answer is "C." This patient should not be sent home. Did you even consider it? Discharge is a particularly bad idea because his disease has worsened rapidly over the last 12 hours. As with other potential causes of neuromuscular respiratory failure, an FVC and NIF are necessary to determine adequate respiratory reserve. The FVC and NIF should be monitored closely during the acute illness. GBS can have a rapid and catastrophic worsening that necessitates monitoring during the acute phase of illness. Typically, patients reach the peak of severity about 2 weeks into the illness. Autonomic dysfunction is associated with GBS, and close cardiovascular monitoring is important. EMG/NCV can be of value in diagnosing GBS—although early on in the course of the disease, these tests may be normal.

* *

A diagnosis of GBS is made.

Which of the following is NOT an appropriate treatment modality?

A) IVIG.
B) Plasma exchange.
C) Elective intubation if FVC is <15 cc/kg.
D) Corticosteroids.

Discussion

The correct answer is "D." Treatment options for GBS include careful monitoring of disease with no intervention, IVIG, or plasma exchange. Corticosteroids are not used in the treatment of GBS. Multiple studies have shown no benefit to corticosteroids in this disease. If a patient requires ventilatory support or has weakness that precludes ambulation, treatment should be started immediately. Elective intubation is appropriate if the FVC is less than 15 cc/kg. As discussed in regard to neuromuscular respiratory failure with myasthenia gravis, arterial blood gases are not reliable markers of impending failure, and the FVC must be closely monitored.

* *

The family would like to know what the outcome in this patient with GBS will be, so you pull out your crystal ball.

Well, instead of sarcasm, you actually opt for compassion and tell them that FULL RECOVERY can be expected in__________percent of patients.

A) 15%.
B) 50%.
C) 80%.
D) Greater than 95%.

Discussion

The correct answer is "A." Fifteen percent of all patients with GBS will have **complete** resolution of their symptoms. Sixty-five percent will be left with minor deficits, and about 10% will become disabled. Despite excellent care, some patients still die.

HELPFUL TIP: West Nile virus infection can present as either a GBS (symmetrical neurological symptoms with loss of reflexes) or a poliomyelitis syndrome (generally asymmetrical weakness with worse weakness proximally, loss of reflexes, fasciculations).

Objectives: Did you learn to . . .

- Recognize the clinical presentation of GBS?
- Identify underlying illnesses that are associated with GBS?
- Manage a patient with GBS?

CASE 9

A 38-year-old woman is brought to the ED by her husband who expresses concerns over changes in her mental status over the past 2 days. She has become confused, forgetting the names of persons well known to her and forgetting what she is doing. Her conversations have become increasingly more difficult to follow, and over the past 12 hours, she has gradually become sleepier. On examination, she has a temperature of 38.0°C. She is drowsy but can be aroused. She has no meningismus. She is oriented only to person. She responds to questions slowly and incorrectly and follows only simple commands (stick out your tongue). The remainder of her neurological examination is essentially normal, given her limited ability to cooperate. CBC, coagulation studies, and electrolytes (including calcium, magnesium, and phosphorous) are normal.

What is the best next step in evaluating this patient?

A) Lumbar puncture.
B) Head CT.
C) EEG.
D) CXR.

Discussion

The correct answer is "B." Although performing all of the above tests will be helpful in evaluating this patient, the most important test to do at this time is a head CT to rule out any mass lesion or hemorrhage. You could argue that "A," an LP, could be done first, and you would technically be correct. However, the standard in the United States is to do the CT scan first if there is any possibility of a mass lesion. There is a possibility that nonconvulsive status epilepticus is causing these mental status changes. However, even if the EEG showed nonconvulsive status epilepticus, a head CT and lumbar puncture would remain necessary. Although pneumonia could cause confusion, a CXR is unlikely to be of high yield in this setting.

* *

Her head CT is normal. Lumbar puncture revealed 18 WBCs (all lymphocytes), 12 RBCs, CSF protein 67 mg/dL (elevated), and CSF glucose 70 mg/dL (normal). An EEG is normal.

What is the next step in managing this patient?

A) Admit for viral encephalitis with close monitoring.

B) Admit for viral encephalitis and start acyclovir and antibiotics.
C) Admit for bacterial meningitis and start antibiotics.
D) Discharge to home with close follow-up tomorrow at 8 am.

Discussion

The correct answer is "B." The probable diagnosis in this setting is herpes simplex encephalitis. Her CSF results are consistent with a viral process and are not consistent with bacterial meningitis (due to the normal glucose and only lymphocytes in the differential). Given the mortality of herpes simplex encephalitis (30–70%), all patients in whom the diagnosis is suspected should be started on acyclovir 10 mg/kg every 8 hours IV empirically (with appropriate dosage adjustments for renal failure), while further confirmatory testing is pending (CSF PCR for the herpes simplex virus). Treatment should be for a minimum of 10 days and has been advocated (with little evidence to support it) to be as long as 21 days. It is important to recognize that the EEG and CT may be normal in herpes simplex encephalitis, particularly early in the disease. On CT, one may see evidence of temporal lobe hemorrhage and/or hypodensity in the temporal lobes. EEG can show either periodic lateralized epileptiform discharges or focal slowing in the temporal lobes. Temporal lobe changes may be even more prominently visualized on MRI, and this may be of benefit in cases in which the diagnosis remains unclear. Even with prompt, appropriate treatment, only 38% of patients returned to normal or near-normal neurologic functioning at 2 years. "B" includes antibiotics because most clinicians would cover for bacterial meningitis until the CSF cultures come back negative.

Objectives: Did you learn to . . .

- Recognize the clinical presentation of and the laboratory findings in viral encephalitis?
- Initiate appropriate treatment in a patient with a presumptive diagnosis of herpes encephalitis?

CASE 10

A 70-year-old male presents to your office as a new patient. He is with his wife, who assists in providing the history. His appetite is reduced, and he has lost 10 pounds in the past 6 months. His only medication is aspirin, and he has no significant past medical history. On exam, his vital signs are normal, and he is in no acute distress. His gait is slow, and he takes eight steps to turn. He has retropulsion (takes two steps backward when you pull him from behind). There is a resting tremor in both hands but more prominently in the right. You find cogwheel rigidity in both arms as well. His cognitive screening tests are normal.

The most likely diagnosis is:

A) Essential tremor.
B) Parkinson disease.
C) Normal pressure hydrocephalus (NPH).
D) Progressive supranuclear palsy.
E) Stroke.

Discussion

The correct answer is "B." This patient most likely has Parkinson disease. "A" is incorrect because essential tremor is typically worsened by activity and is not associated with the other neurologic findings seen in this patient. "C" is incorrect. The classic triad of NPH includes urinary incontinence, gait ataxia, and dementia. "D" might be a consideration, but there is no specific finding of progressive supranuclear palsy here (e.g., aggressive course, more severe axial rigidity, dysarthria, dysphagia, and downward gaze paresis). Stroke is quite unlikely to present in this insidious fashion with generalized findings. However, there is a controversial entity called "vascular parkinsonism" in which lacunar infarcts of the basal ganglia are thought to cause parkinsonism.

Which of the following is NOT a common feature of idiopathic Parkinson disease?

A) Rigidity.
B) Extraocular movement paresis.
C) Bradykinesia.
D) Loss of postural reflexes or gait disturbance.

Discussion

The correct answer is "B." There are four cardinal features of Parkinson disease: tremor, bradykinesia, rigidity, and postural instability. Two or more of these features should be present to make the diagnosis. The tremor of parkinsonism is a resting tremor (as opposed to the postural, intention, or action tremor) and is most common in the hands. Rigidity ("A") is described as increased resistance to passive movement and may be reinforced by having the patient open and close the fist on the opposite hand. Cogwheel rigidity is a ratchet-like sensation noted when testing a limb with concurrent tremor. Bradykinesia ("C") may be observed by monitoring the speed and amplitude of movements. Gait disturbance ("D") with reduced stride length and stooped posture is a common finding but generally occurs later in the course of the disease. Postural reflexes and ability to rise from a chair are also impaired. Postural reflexes may be tested by retropulsion.

* *

You are fairly certain that your patient has Parkinson disease.

What else might you find with idiopathic Parkinson disease?

A) Micrographia.
B) Urinary incontinence.
C) Apraxia.
D) Autonomic dysfunctions.
E) Alien limb phenomenon.

Discussion
The correct answer is "A." Micrographia, writing in small letters, is associated with Parkinson disease. The others are not. This is important because there are a number of neurologic syndromes that can mimic Parkinson disease. Decreased facial expression (hypomimia) with decreased rate of eye blink and diminished vocal volume (hypophonia) is also common with Parkinson disease. Other conditions that occur in patients with Parkinson disease include depression, cognitive impairment, and REM sleep behavioral disorder (for example kicking and screaming during REM sleep in response to vivid, disturbing, dreams).

HELPFUL TIP: There are "Parkinson plus" syndromes, so-called because they present with parkinsonian features with another characteristic. Look for these syndromes in those that you believe may have Parkinson disease:

(1) Progressive supranuclear palsy, which is associated with supranuclear gaze palsy, dysarthria, dysphagia, postural instability, and axial rigidity.
(2) Shy–Drager syndrome, which is notable for autonomic dysfunction, including marked orthostatic hypotension.
(3) Cortico-basal ganglionic degeneration, which is associated with apraxia, cortical sensory dysfunction, and the "alien limb phenomenon." Alien limb phenomenon occurs when the patient's arm moves by itself (e.g., will reach up to touch the patient's face). The patients do not believe that the limb belongs to them. Spontaneous limb movements also occur when the patient is startled or the limb is touched (anyone see Dr. Strangelove?).

The diagnosis of Parkinson disease is most appropriately made:

A) With a brain MRI.
B) By CSF analysis.
C) Clinically.
D) By a neurologist.

Discussion
The correct answer is "C." The diagnosis is based on a history and physical examination that are consistent with Parkinson disease. Additionally, a response to dopaminergic agents is virtually diagnostic of Parkinson disease. If the patient does not have some response to a dopaminergic agent, reconsider you diagnosis. "A" is incorrect because there are no findings on neuroimaging that are specific for the diagnosis of Parkinson disease. Likewise, "B" is wrong because CSF analysis cannot provide the diagnosis. "D" is clearly wrong—do you really need a neurologist for this? The "gold standard" for diagnosis is neuropathologic exam, but you would rather not wait for the autopsy to diagnose Parkinson disease.

HELPFUL TIP: Up to 10% of patients with Parkinson's disease will have some degree of intention tremor in addition to their rest tremor.

* *

Your patient takes only aspirin, which you know is not a cause of parkinsonism.

Which of the following medications is frequently associated with a Parkinson-like syndrome in the elderly?

A) ACE inhibitors.
B) HMG-CoA reductase inhibitors.

C) Calcium channel blockers.
D) Metoclopramide.
E) All of the above.

Discussion
The correct answer is "D." Metoclopramide is a frequent cause of the misdiagnosis of Parkinson's disease in the elderly. Additional medications, such as SSRIs, antipsychotics, and others, can mimic Parkinson disease. Importantly, **drug-induced parkinsonism may last for up to 6 months after discontinuation of the offending agent**.

* *

You think it is best to initiate treatment in this patient.

Possible treatments of Parkinson disease include all of the following EXCEPT:

A) Levodopa.
B) Pallidotomy.
C) Pramipexole.
D) Donepezil.
E) Selegiline

Discussion
The correct answer is "D." Donepezil is used to treat Alzheimer disease. The initial symptoms of Parkinson disease typically respond well to levodopa and the dopamine agonists. Selegiline is a monamine oxidase B inhibitor and yields modest symptomatic benefits. Dopamine receptor agonists, such as pramipexole (Mirapex), ropinirole (Requip), and bromocriptine, are important medications that may be used in the initial treatment of Parkinson disease.

> HELPFUL TIP: Surgical options for advanced Parkinson disease include pallidotomy and deep brain stimulation. In general, stimulation of the thalamus is used to treat tremor but has little impact on the other symptoms of Parkinson disease (bradykinesia, etc.). Subthalamic nucleus stimulation is more beneficial for ameliorating the other features of Parkinson disease, but may have a less profound impact on tremor.

Which of the following is *NOT* a common side effect of levodopa?

A) Nausea.
B) Paresthesias.
C) Dyskinesia/dystonia.
D) Hallucinations.

Discussion
The correct answer is "B." Paresthesias are not associated with the use of carbidopa/levodopa. The use of carbidopa with levodopa allows the dose of levodopa to be optimized. Carbidopa helps to prevent levodopa-induced nausea ("A"). Dystonia and dyskinesia ("C") are common with therapy more than 2 years or at peak dose responses and may necessitate lowering the doses. Psychiatric problems ("D"), including hallucinations and psychosis, can be seen with dopaminergic agonists and levodopa. Other common side effects of levodopa include hypotension, confusion, and other psychiatric disturbances.

> HELPFUL TIP: Levodopa is a dopamine precursor, and carbidopa is a peripheral dopadecarboxylase inhibitor that does not cross the blood–brain barrier. The symptoms of tremor, rigidity, and bradykinesia are initially relieved by levodopa. However, with time, larger doses are required to maintain control of symptoms.

> HELPFUL TIP: One of the dopamine agonists (pramipexole, ropinirole, and bromocriptine) can be used to help minimize the dose of levodopa needed, thus minimize the side effects of levodopa.

* *

You decide to start levodopa/carbidopa (Sinemet) and bromocriptine. At the follow-up visit, the patient is doing relatively well on this combination. However, he notices that in the mornings and evenings, he tends to be stiff and has difficulty ambulating.

The most appropriate next step is to:

A) Initiate a "drug holiday" to restore the patient's sensitivity to the drug.
B) Add another dopaminergic agent such as ropinirole (Requip).
C) Add a catechol-*O*-methyl-transferase (COMT) inhibitor such as entacapone (Comtan).
D) Add an anticholinergic agent such as benztropine (Cogentin).

Discussion

The correct answer is "C." The patient is experiencing the "wearing-off" phenomenon. There are several ways to address this. One option is to add a COMT inhibitor (like tolcapone [Tasmar] or entacapone [Comtan]) in order to slow down the metabolism of levodopa. COMT inhibitors have no effect on their own and should only be used with levodopa. Another option is to switch the patient from immediate release carbidopa/levodopa to a sustained release product (e.g., Sinemet CR). The effectiveness of this strategy is not conclusively proven, and there is no benefit from using controlled-release carbidopa/levodopa as the initial agent in Parkinson disease. Another common approach to the "wearing-off" phenomenon is altering the dosing of carbidopa/levodopa—either increasing the dose or shortening the interval between doses.

HELPFUL TIP: Tolcapone (Tasmar) is associated with fatal hepatic necrosis and requires monitoring of liver function tests (LFTs). Thus, entacapone (Comtan) is the preferred drug.

* *

When you counsel your patient regarding medication use, you urge him not to stop taking his medication all at once.

Which of the following is NOT a potential adverse effect of abrupt discontinuation of dopaminergic agonists and/or levodopa?

A) Neuroleptic malignant syndrome (NMS).
B) Severe rigidity.
C) Confusional state.
D) Severe dyskinesias.

Discussion

The correct answer is "D." Levodopa and dopamine agonists should be tapered. Abrupt discontinuation of these medications may precipitate NMS. In addition, abrupt withdrawal is also associated with an acute confusional state separate from the mental status changes seen in NMS. Severe worsening of the patient's parkinsonism is expected, which can result in prominent rigidity. Dyskinesias are frequently seen with dopaminergic agonist/levodopa **therapy**, but are not exacerbated or triggered by **withdrawal** of these agents.

HELPFUL TIP: Diagnostic criteria for definite NMS include hyperthermia, muscle rigidity, and five of the following: mental status changes, tremor, tachycardia, incontinence, labile blood pressure, metabolic acidosis, tachypnea/hypoxia, elevation of creatine kinase, diaphoresis/sialorrhea, and leukocytosis. Treatment includes supportive care as well as the use of bromocriptine and propranolol, although there is limited data to support the use of either agent. **Dantrolene is ineffective.**

* *

A year later your patient returns and seems to be doing well. You ask him about symptoms of Parkinson disease, if he is having any adverse effects of medications, and if he is experiencing any of the Parkinson-associated diseases.

Which of the following is NOT associated with Parkinson disease?

A) Depression.
B) Dementia.
C) REM sleep disorder.
D) Narcolepsy.
E) Decreased visual contrast sensitivity.

Discussion

The correct answer is "D." Narcolepsy has not been associated with Parkinson disease. However, excess daytime sleepiness has been associated. This is likely due to a combination of factors, such as sleep disturbance, depression, dopaminergic drugs, and Parkinson disease itself. Depression is commonly seen in Parkinson disease and is reported to occur in up to 41% of patients. Dementia, typically with Lewy bodies present on pathological analysis, is seen and can affect the decision to proceed with surgical treatment of Parkinson disease, as patients with advanced dementia get less benefit from surgery. Also, REM sleep behavior disorders are seen in Parkinson disease and can be a source of stress for families and caretakers. REM sleep behavior disorder is characterized by acting out of dreams that can consist of vocalizations as well as active and even violent movements. Typically, REM sleep behavior disorder responds to clonazepam. Finally, decreased visual contrast sensitivity can occur with Parkinson disease as well.

HELPFUL (AND COOL) TIP: The dopamine agonists (pramipexole, ropinirole, etc.) have been associated with compulsive behavior (sexual compulsion, compulsive gambling, etc.). This may explain why our elderly patients like to go to Las Vegas and Atlantic City...

Objectives: Did you learn to...

- Identify common features of Parkinson disease?
- Diagnose Parkinson disease?
- Manage a patient with Parkinson disease?
- Understand pharmacotherapy available for Parkinson disease and some of the potential adverse effects of drug therapy?

CASE 11

A 45-year-old left-handed woman who is a busy executive for a Fortune 500 company presents with excessive daytime sleepiness. She is otherwise healthy and takes no medications.

How do you approach this problem?

A) Reassure her that it is normal for people to be drowsy under stressful work conditions.
B) Begin zolpidem at night for sleep.
C) Schedule the patient for polysomnography.
D) Discuss the patient's sleep hygiene.
E) Administer modafinil (Provigil) prior to important board meetings.

Discussion

The correct answer is "D." It is essential that all patients with complaints of either insomnia or excessive daytime sleepiness have a thorough sleep history taken. Polysomnography may be necessary, but this test—like all diagnostic tests—should be driven by a hypothesis. A history is necessary to develop a hypothesis and determine a test's utility. Starting hypnotic agents ("B") or stimulants ("E") without thoroughly investigating the underlying problem may cover up a significant, treatable problem and is considered bad form.

Which of the following is NOT an important aspect of a sleep history?

A) Sleeping and waking times.
B) Use of stimulants and alcohol.
C) Sleep interruptions (children, pagers, etc.).
D) Work schedule.
E) Listening to "soft rock" ("easy listening" or "adult contemporary").

Discussion

The correct answer is "E." Okay, maybe this one was too easy, but we hate "easy listening" music. The Geneva Convention prohibits its use on prisoners of war... we've been told. All ranting aside, this tidbit of her history has no bearing on her sleep. Important parts of the sleep history include the sleeping environment (alone, with spouse or other individual, in the daylight hours, etc.), nap history, family history of sleep problems, and symptoms of specific sleep disorders (snoring, hypnagogic hallucinations, etc.). A medication history is important as well as a history of watching TV in bed, eating in bed, etc., which indicate poor sleep hygiene.

HELPFUL TIP: One of the favorite parasomnias of the editors is "exploding head syndrome" (this is actually real, not a joke). Patients have the feeling of popping or explosions occurring in their head as they fall asleep. Another great diagnosis is "moss brain," an archaic term for a type of CNS disease.

Which of the following is NOT part of a typical sleep study?

A) Monitoring of EEG.
B) Monitoring respirations and oxygen desaturations.
C) Evaluating the sleep latency in response to sleep aids, such as zolpidem and trazodone, to maximize effective pharmacologic therapy.
D) Monitoring EMG.
E) Video monitoring of sleep.

Discussion

The correct answer is "C." Sleep studies are generally done in the naïve state without the use of medications. All of the rest are true. "D" and "E" deserve more attention. "D," monitoring EMG, allows informing the physician about muscle activity during sleep (e.g., restless limbs). "E," video monitoring and taping, allows the physician to look for problems, such as awakening, evidence of restless leg syndrome, and sleep apnea.

In considering a diagnosis of narcolepsy, which of the following is NOT part of the diagnosis?

A) Cataplexy.
B) Sleep paralysis.
C) Hypnagogic hallucinations.
D) Sleep myoclonus.
E) Excessive daytime sleepiness.

Discussion

The correct answer is "D." Sleep myoclonus (hypnagogic jerks) is commonly seen in normal people as they begin to fall asleep (witness colleagues at grand rounds with sudden tossing of the head) and is not a part of narcolepsy. Narcolepsy is a disorder characterized by four cardinal traits, although not all need be present to make the diagnosis: cataplexy, excessive daytime sleepiness, sleep paralysis, and hypnagogic hallucinations. "A," cataplexy, is a sudden loss of voluntary muscle control during which the patient may appear to be asleep; however, cataplexy does not have to be accompanied by sleep attacks, and the patient may be aware throughout the attack. "B," sleep paralysis, can occur either at the onset of sleep or upon awakening and can be quite frightening to the patient. "C," hypnagogic hallucinations, are vivid and typically fearful dreams that occur at the onset of sleep but can also occur upon awakening (hypnopompic hallucinations). "E," excessive daytime sleepiness, is a hallmark of narcolepsy and can include sleep attacks as well as persistent drowsiness and "micro sleep" (brief intrusions of sleep during a waking state). The complete tetrad of symptoms is seen in only 10% of patients with narcolepsy.

Which of the following is NOT a treatment for narcolepsy?

A) Amitriptyline.
B) Clonazepam.
C) Fluoxetine.
D) Modafinil (Provigil).
E) Sodium oxybate.

Discussion

The correct answer is "B." Clonazepam is not a treatment for narcolepsy. Treatment of narcolepsy can be divided into two primary goals. The first goal is to address daytime sleepiness, which is primarily done with stimulants such as modafinil or methylphenidate. The second goal is to reduce the symptoms of cataplexy. This can be accomplished with agents such as tricyclic antidepressants, and to a lesser extent, SSRIs. Sodium oxybate (also known as gamma hydroxybutyrate) can be used for treatment of cataplexy as well as sleep hallucinations and sleep paralysis. Some evidence suggests it may also help with excessive daytime sleepiness. Given its street popularity and abuse potential (including date rape), prescriptions are centrally controlled nationally for this medication at the time of this publication.

* *

After a thorough history, you find nothing to suggest narcolepsy besides daytime sleepiness. Of course, you are considering other diagnoses simultaneously—unless you are experiencing a sleep attack yourself.

Which of the following would *NOT* suggest a possible diagnosis of obstructive sleep apnea?

A) Difficulty falling asleep.
B) Frequent nighttime arousals.
C) Obesity.
D) Paroxysmal nocturnal dyspnea.
E) Snoring.

Discussion

The correct answer is "A." Difficulty falling asleep is not one of the components of obstructive sleep apnea. Snoring, obesity, excessive daytime sleepiness, and paroxysmal nocturnal dyspnea are all associated with obstructive sleep apnea. Some patients will note frequent arousals from sleep with or without accompanied shortness of breath.

> HELPFUL TIP: It is important to note that not all patients with sleep apnea are overweight, and this diagnosis must be considered in all patients with excessive daytime sleepiness or other suggestive symptoms. Small oropharyngeal airway (especially in **thin** women) and gastroesophageal reflux are associated with sleep apnea.

What treatment options would NOT be appropriate to consider in your patient if she has obstructive sleep apnea?

A) Bilevel positive airway pressure (BiPAP).

B) Continuous positive airway pressure (CPAP).
C) Positional therapy.
D) Uvulopalatopharyngoplasty (UPPP).
E) Zolpidem.

Discussion

The correct answer is "E." Sleep aids, including benzodiazepines, do not have a role in the treatment of obstructive sleep apnea and may actually worsen symptoms. CPAP and BiPAP are both potential treatments. Polysomnography (sleep testing) with titration of CPAP or BiPAP should determine which modality to use and the pressure settings. These should not be arbitrarily set to the "normal settings" for a patient. Positional therapy, avoiding sleeping on one's back, may be effective in some patients. Some techniques for achieving this goal include sewing an object on the back of the pajama shirt that will irritate the patient when they roll onto it. Weight loss, although not mentioned above, can provide improvement in symptoms as well. Surgical therapies including UPPP can also be considered based on the patient's symptoms and preferences.

* *

Further history leads you to suspect that she has restless legs syndrome, and you confirm the diagnosis with a sleep study.

Which would be a *first-line* agent for treatment of restless legs syndrome?

A) Clonazepam.
B) Codeine.
C) Methadone.
D) Pramipexole
E) Tramadol.

Discussion

The correct answer is "D." Restless legs syndrome is characterized by an urge to move the lower extremities due most often to an uncomfortable sensation. This sensation usually occurs during rest and is typically relieved by moving the legs. Dopaminergic agents, either levodopa (e.g., Sinemet) or agonists, such as ropinirole (Requip) and pramipexole (Mirapex), are the first-line treatments for restless legs syndrome. Benzodiazepines ("A") and narcotic medications ("B" and "C") as well as the nonnarcotics tramadol and gabapentin have all been reported to be successful alternative therapies for restless leg syndrome.

What other workup would you suggest for this patient once the diagnosis of restless legs syndrome is made?

A) No further workup is indicated, initiate treatment as above.
B) Serum calcium.
C) Serum iron studies, including ferritin.
D) Serum vitamin B_{12}.
E) Serum vitamin B_6.

Discussion

The correct answer is "C." Recent studies have shown a link between low iron stores and restless legs syndrome. All patients with restless legs syndrome should have an iron profile performed, and low iron or ferritin levels merit iron supplementation (and workup for underlying cause, of course). Other associations are diabetes, pregnancy, end-stage renal disease, Parkinson disease, venous insufficiency, folate deficiency, and caffeine intake (dump that fourth cup of coffee . . .).

Objectives: Did you learn to . . .

- Take an appropriate sleep history?
- Generate a differential diagnosis for daytime sleepiness?
- Gain familiarity with the diagnostic testing used in a sleep laboratory?
- Identify the presentations of and treatments for common sleep disorders, including narcolepsy, obstructive sleep apnea, and restless legs syndrome?

CASE 12

A 60-year-old right-handed gentleman presents with the complaint of head pain.

Which of the following historical descriptions is of the LEAST VALUE in identifying a specific diagnostic classification for head/face pain?

A) Right-sided, electric, stabbing pain involving primarily the cheek, occurring for seconds to minutes repeatedly throughout the day.
B) Right-sided, electric, stabbing pain involving primarily the throat, tongue, and right ear.

C) Right-sided severe headache involving the orbit and associated with lacrimation and rhinorrhea typically occurring in groups.
D) "Sinus pressure" with a history of sinus headaches responsive to antibiotics in the past.
E) Pattern of severe right-sided "stabbing and boring" headaches around the age of 30 that went away with scheduled indomethacin.

Discussion

The correct answer is "D." Sinus headaches are typically a diagnosis of exclusion. Acute sinusitis can cause severe head and face discomfort, but **sinusitis remains a relatively uncommon etiology for recurrent head and face pain.** The specific headache syndromes described in "A," "B," "C," and "E" are described in more detail in the following questions.

If this patient gives you the history of right-sided severe headache involving the orbit associated with lacrimation and rhinorrhea typically occurring in groups, which of the following would you use for initial acute treatment of this headache syndrome?

A) Naproxen.
B) Oxygen.
C) Tylenol.
D) Verapamil.

Discussion

The correct answer is "B." The type of headache syndrome described is most consistent with cluster headaches. These are most commonly seen in men and are characterized by exquisite pain, typically centered at the orbit. Conjunctival injection, rhinorrhea, and lacrimation frequently accompany the headache. Pain is often disabling. As the name suggests, the patient tends to have headaches in groups (or clusters). These headaches are more common at night, and REM sleep is thought to be a triggering factor. For acute treatment, conventional headache medications such as DHE and the triptans can be effective. Treatment with high-flow oxygen has also shown significant efficacy as an abortive treatment: typical protocol would be 8 L oxygen on non-rebreather for 15 minutes, with reports of 70% of patients achieving headache relief. Verapamil can be effective for prophylaxis but is not effective as an abortive. Other, more typical migraine prophylactic agents (propranolol, topiramate, indomethacin, valproic acid) have been tried, but no systematic studies have been done to evaluate their efficacy in cluster headaches.

If your patient describes a history of severe right-sided "stabbing and boring" headaches around the age of 30 that went away with scheduled indomethacin, this would be most consistent with which of the following headache syndromes?

A) Tension headache.
B) Paroxysmal hemicrania.
C) Migraine without aura.
D) Chronic daily headache.
E) Analgesic rebound headache.

Discussion

The correct answer is "B." Paroxysmal hemicrania is classically described as a unilateral headache with a stabbing/boring character. Although age of onset can vary greatly, it classically occurs in women in their 30s (although it can be seen in men as well). Patients will have between 2 and 40 episodes during a given day, although they do not cluster together as is typical in cluster headaches. Although autonomic symptoms (rhinorrhea, lacrimation, conjunctival injection, and ptosis) can be seen in a majority of patients, these headaches can be differentiated from clusters by the pattern of recurrence (sporadic throughout the day versus in clusters); significant overlap between the two headache syndromes does exist and differentiation can be difficult. Paroxysmal hemicrania typically is exquisitely sensitive to indomethacin, and response to indomethacin is highly correlated with this diagnosis. Migraine headaches typically do not occur multiple times in one day and are usually described as a throbbing pain. Chronic daily headaches as well as analgesic rebound headaches generally are continuous in nature with limited, if any, periods of time without some degree of headache. Chronic daily headache in the setting of prolonged analgesic use is highly suggestive of analgesic rebound headache. The duration of analgesic therapy necessary to trigger and propagate these headaches remains uncertain. However, it can be as little as three times per week.

* *

With further history, your patient describes right-sided, electric, stabbing pain involving primarily the cheek and occurring for seconds to minutes repeatedly throughout the day.

What would be the first-line choice for therapy of this entity?

A) Carbamazepine.
B) Amitriptyline.
C) Ibuprofen.
D) Morphine.
E) Microvascular decompression (Janetta procedure).

Discussion

The correct answer is "A." This description is typical of trigeminal neuralgia. Carbamazepine has been shown to be effective in treating trigeminal neuralgia and was used for treatment of this disorder prior to being used for seizures. Tricyclic antidepressants, opioids, and nonsteroidal anti-inflammatory agents are not first-line agents for treatment. Typically, NSAIDs are of limited, if any, benefit in this setting. Other agents that have been used for treatment with at least anecdotal reports of benefit include gabapentin, oxcarbazepine, clonazepam, baclofen, phenytoin, and topiramate. Microvascular decompression (the Janetta procedure) can be effective in alleviating pain from trigeminal neuralgia (tic douloureux), which is described in the question. However, medical therapy remains the first-line treatment.

> HELPFUL TIP: A unilateral electric, stabbing pain occurring in the tongue, oropharynx, and occasionally extending to the ipsilateral ear has been described; this is known as **glossopharyngeal neuralgia**. Treatment of glossopharyngeal neuralgia is similar to the pharmacologic treatment of trigeminal neuralgia described above. If the patient complains of stabbing eye or temporal headaches lasting seconds, consider the diagnosis of "jolts and jabs" headaches (aka "ice pick" headache). They occur 40–50 times a day or more and are likely a migraine variant.

Objectives: Did you learn to . . .

- Describe the features of various headache syndromes?
- Initiate treatment for cluster headaches, paroxysmal hemicrania, and trigeminal neuralgia?

CASE 13

A 55-year-old male with a history of diabetes and prostate carcinoma presents to your office complaining of back pain, groin numbness, and an inability to initiate voiding.

The most likely explanation for these symptoms is:

A) Cauda equina syndrome.
B) Urinary outlet obstruction secondary to prostate carcinoma.
C) Hydroureter and hydronephrosis secondary to urolithiasis.
D) Neurogenic bladder from long-standing diabetes.
E) All of the above are equally likely.

Discussion

The correct answer is "A." This is a presentation of cauda equina syndrome. Cauda equina syndrome is caused by compression of the cauda equina at the level of L4 or L5 by a protruding disk, tumor, etc. Symptoms include progressive fecal or urinary incontinence (secondary to inability to initiate voiding), impotence, distal motor weakness, and sensory loss in a saddle distribution. This patient's symptoms are not likely to be due to urinary outlet obstruction ("B"). Urinary outlet obstruction should not be associated with sensory changes in a saddle distribution. The same is true of "C." "D," neurogenic bladder from diabetes, could be a possibility. However, this should not include back pain or perineal numbness.

On examination of this patient, you would expect to find:

A) Increased rectal tone.
B) Decreased rectal tone.
C) Normal rectal tone.
D) No rectum.

Discussion

The correct answer is "B." Patients with cauda equina syndrome should have decreased rectal tone. If you chose "D" . . . well, there are a lot of things we could say but won't.

The INITIAL treatment of this patient should include all of the following EXCEPT:

A) Pain management with narcotics.
B) Dexamethasone administered IV.

C) Placement of a Foley catheter.
D) Urgent neurosurgical consultation.
E) Methylprednisolone 30 mg/kg over 1 hour then 5.4 mg/kg/hr for 24 hours.

Discussion

The correct answer is "E." This dose of methylprednisolone is indicated for spinal cord injury (e.g., from trauma) and not for epidural compression by tumor. **High-dose** steroids have been found to be of no additional benefit in cord compression from tumor when compared with lower dose steroids. All of the remaining options are correct. Pain management is critical in any patient. Dexamethasone may reduce tumor-related edema leading to a reduction in cord compression. A Foley catheter is indicated to treat the patient's urinary retention. Since this is a neurosurgical emergency, urgent neurosurgical consultation should be obtained (although there is contradictory data about whether early surgical intervention makes any difference). Local radiation may also be used acutely depending on your surgeon, oncologist, etc.

HELPFUL TIP: The diagnosis of cauda equina syndrome is often delayed for months since many patients initially have incomplete syndromes, including only pain and mild neurologic symptoms. This is unfortunate since outcome depends on the degree of neurologic dysfunction at the time of diagnosis.

Objectives: Did you learn to . . .

- Recognize the clinical presentation of cauda equina syndrome?
- Identify causes of cauda equina syndrome?
- Initiate treatment of a patient with cauda equina syndrome?

QUICK QUIZ: SEIZURE DISORDERS

Absence seizures are characterized by all of the following EXCEPT:

A) Loss of consciousness.
B) Feeling of déjà vu.
C) Rhythmic lip smacking or eye blinking.
D) Staring spells.
E) Occurrence up to hundreds of times per day.

Discussion

The correct answer is "B." Feelings of déjà vu and other "psychic" phenomenon such as hallucinations are associated with temporal lobe (aka simple partial) seizures.

CASE 14

A 2-year-old female presents to the ED after having a seizure. The parents note that the patient was fine this morning, spiked a temperature to 39.9°C, and then had a 5-minute tonic–clonic seizure that resolved spontaneously. This is her second such episode in 18 months. On arrival, the patient is febrile, lethargic, and looks postictal.

Your next step is to:

A) Reassure the parents that this is a simple febrile seizure.
B) Obtain blood cultures and start ceftriaxone.
C) Perform an LP if the CBC shows leukocytosis and elevated bands.
D) Administer acetaminophen and wait for 2 hours to see if the patient returns to baseline before deciding on further treatment.
E) None of the above.

Discussion

The correct answer is "B." This patient **must** be assumed to have meningitis until proven otherwise. Treatment should be started immediately. "A" is incorrect. This is not a simple febrile seizure by history. The child is postictal and looks ill. While it may end up being a febrile seizure, you cannot make that conclusion at this point. If the child did not look lethargic and was up and running around, no further evaluation or treatment would be needed at this time. "C" is incorrect. First, the CBC may be relatively normal even with meningitis. Second, you do not want to delay antibiotics until the CBC and LP are done. "D" is incorrect for the same reason. The standard of care in meningitis is antibiotics within 30 minutes of hitting the door. Waiting to see the patient's response to acetaminophen for 2 hours will clearly put you out of this time window.

* *

You do the right thing and treat the patient with ceftriaxone. The patient does look better in an hour or so and has returned to baseline. She is alert, attentive, and playing with toys. The parents are concerned about whether or not this patient has a seizure disorder. They would like a further evaluation.

Which of the following is indicated at this point, assuming you decide to evaluate the patient for a seizure disorder?

A) EEG done on the same day.
B) Admission to the hospital and EEG the next day.
C) Serum electrolytes and glucose.
D) Trial of antiepileptic drug.
E) None of the above.

Discussion

The correct answer is "C." The workup of a seizure includes serum electrolytes, calcium, magnesium phosphate, glucose, etc. Note that this need not be done for someone with a known seizure disorder who has his or her typical seizure and returns to baseline. In these cases, only a drug level of their antiepileptic drug need be done unless there is some change in the seizure type, mental status, etc. "A" and "B" are incorrect. The EEG will be positive because of the recent seizure and may not reflect the underlying condition. Thus, waiting a couple of weeks after the seizure will give a better picture of what the brain's innate electrical activity looks like. "D" is incorrect because we haven't yet proven this child has a seizure disorder. Prescribing antiepileptic drugs would be premature.

HELPFUL TIP: A "stat" EEG can be helpful if you are not sure if a patient is having (or had) an active seizure versus a pseudoseizure. A "stat" EEG may also be helpful in a patient with mental status changes who you believe may be having nonconvulsive status.

* *

The parents are wondering what to do about treating this patient to prevent further febrile seizures.

Your recommendation to prevent further seizures is:

A) Acetaminophen at the onset of fever.
B) Ibuprofen at the onset of fever.
C) Phenytoin until the child reaches the age of 5.
D) Buccal midazolam at the onset of any fever.
E) None of the above.

Discussion

The correct answer is "E." None of these choices are optimal in the management of this patient. "A" and "B" seem like a good idea but do nothing to reduce the occurrence of febrile seizures. Neither "C" nor "D" is effective. One study suggests that rectal diazepam at the onset of a fever will reduce the occurrence of febrile seizures. However, it is associated with some morbidity (e.g., sleepiness) and should be reserved for those with frequent febrile seizures.

HELPFUL TIP: Phenobarbital **can** prevent febrile seizures but is associated with behavior and learning problems and is generally not recommended.

* *

The parents have another child at home who has had **one** febrile seizure. He is now 12 months old. The parents want to know what his likelihood of having a seizure disorder.

You can let them know that he has *approximately*:

A) 1–5% chance of developing a seizure disorder.
B) 10–15% chance of developing a seizure disorder.
C) 40–50% chance of developing a seizure disorder.
D) 80–90% chance of developing a seizure disorder.

Discussion

The correct answer is "A." Patients who have a single febrile seizure have approximately a 1–5% chance of developing a seizure disorder. This is essentially the same risk as the general population.

HELPFUL TIP: About 50% of patients who have their first febrile seizure under age 15 months will have a recurrent febrile seizure. This drops to 30% if the first seizure is after 15 months of age. Family history is also involved; 45% of those who have a first-degree relative with febrile seizures will have a second seizure.

Objective: Did you learn to . . .

- Diagnose and manage febrile seizures in children?

BIBLIOGRAPHY

Adams HP Jr., et al. Guidelines for the early management of adults with ischemic stroke: A guideline from the American Heart Association/American stroke

Association stroke council, clinical cardiology council, cardiovascular Radiology and Intervention council, and the atherosclerotic peripheral vascular disease and quality of care outcomes in research interdisciplinary working groups. *Circulation*. 2007;115(20):e478-e534.

Chronicle E, Mulleners W. Anticonvulsant drugs for migraine prophylaxis. *Cochrane Database Syst Rev*. 2004; 3:CD003226.

Confavreux C, et al. Vaccinations and the risk of relapse in multiple sclerosis. *N Engl J Med*. 2001;344:319-326.

Fenstermacher N, et al. Pharmacological prevention of migraine. *BMJ*. 2011;342:d583.

Goodin DS, et al. Disease modifying therapies in multiple sclerosis: Report of the Therapeutics and Technology Assessment Subcommittee of the American Academy of Neurology and the MS Council for Clinical Practice Guidelines. *Neurology*. 2002;58:169-178.

Gronseth GS, Ashman EJ. Practice parameter: The Usefulness of evoked potentials in identifying clinically silent lesions in patient with suspected multiple sclerosis (an evidence-based review). Report of the quality standards subcommittee of the American Academy of Neurology. *Neurology*. 2000;54:1720-1725.

Hassan-Smith G, Douglas MR. Management and prognosis of multiple sclerosis. *Br J Hosp Med (Lond)*. 2011; 72(11):M174-M176.

Hughes RA, et al. Pharmacological treatment other than corticosteroids, intravenous immunoglobulin and plasma exchange for Guillain Barré syndrome. *Cochrane Database Syst Rev*. 2011;16(3):CD008630.

Jankovic J, Stacy M. Medical management of levodopa-associated motor complications in patients with Parkinson's disease. *CNS Drugs*. 2007;21(8):677-692.

Johnston SC, et al. National Stroke Association guidelines for the management of transient ischemic attacks. *Ann Neurol*. 2006;60(3):301-313.

Miller AE, et al. A multicenter, randomized, double-blind, placebo-controlled trial of influenza immunization in multiple sclerosis. *Neurology*. 1997;48:312-314.

Pahwa R. Understanding Parkinson's disease: An update on current diagnostic and treatment strategies. *J Am Med Dir Assoc*. 2006;7(Suppl 2):4-10.

Pringsheim T, et al. Prophylaxis of migraine headache. *CMAJ*. 2010;182:E269-E276.

Silberstein SD, et al. Migraine: Diagnosis and treatment. In: Silberstein SD, ed. *Wolff's Headache and Other Head Pain*. New York, NY: Oxford University Press; 2001:121-211.

Subcommittee on Febrile Seizures; American Academy of Pediatrics. Neurodiagnostic evaluation of the child with a simple febrile seizure. *Pediatrics*. 2011;127(2):389-394.

Warden CR, et al. Evaluation and management of febrile seizures in the out of hospital and emergency department settings. *Ann Emerg Med*. 2003;41(2):215-222.

19

Ophthalmology

Mark A. Graber and Jason K. Wilbur

GLOSSARY OF TERMS

Accommodation: Change in the shape of the lens to compensate for changes in focal length. The term is also used more generally to mean the adjustment of the eye in general to compensate for vision of objects at different distances.

Amblyopia: Unilateral or bilateral loss of vision not attributed to structural abnormality of the eye or visual pathway, but rather the brain is suppressing the signal from the eye. This may be a result of strabismus or visual deprivation.

Esotropia: Inward deviation of the eyes when compared with normal.

Exotropia: Outward deviation of the eyes when compared with normal.

Relative afferent pupillary defect (RAPD): The "swinging flashlight test" **in a darkened room** is used to test for an RAPD. The pupillary response should be equal in both eyes. An RAPD is detected when there is a relative difference in the pupillary response to direct and consensual light between the two eyes. So, the eye with an RAPD will dilate with direct light to the eye but constrict normally in response to light shined in the good eye. This occurs when there is optic nerve damage or significant retinal disease (e.g., large retinal detachment, retinal artery occlusion, optic neuritis). One will **not** get an RAPD in refractive errors, vitreous bleeds, etc.

Strabismus: A general term that refers to a misalignment of the eyes. Esotropia, exotropia, and hypertropia (one eye deviated upward) are all examples of strabismus. The term strabismus says nothing about etiology, which can be congenital, neurologic, or muscular.

CASE 1

A mother presents with her healthy 2-month-old male infant. She reports that for the past week his eyes have been noticeably crossed. He appears to fixate with either the right or left eye. She feels that aside from being cross-eyed, he seems to see well. On examination, his eyes are very crossed. When either eye is covered, he fixes and follows with the contralateral eye and appears to have normal motility.

The most likely diagnosis in this patient is:

A) Pseudoesotropia.
B) Congenital esotropia.
C) Accommodative esotropia.
D) Sixth nerve palsy.

Discussion

The correct answer is "B." Esotropia is more common than exotropia. Congenital esotropia is generally found in children younger than 6 months. "C," accommodative esotropia, is the most common cause of esotropia in childhood and develops between age 6 months and 7 years. It is rare for accommodative esotropia to develop before 4 months or after 8 years of age. Pseudoesotropia is common in infants due to their flat nasal bridges and medial epicanthal folds, giving an appearance of esotropia. The thing to do here is to shine a penlight in their eyes. When you look at where the light hits the eye, it will be in the same location bilaterally for pseudoesotropia but

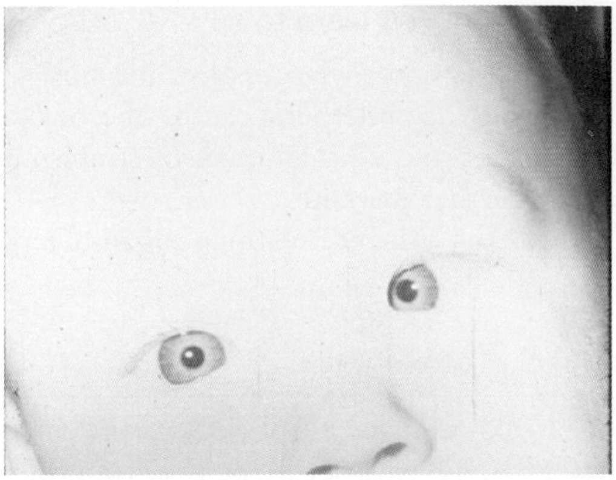

Figure 19–1 **Congenital esotropia. Note the large deviation with abnormal corneal light reflexes. The corneal light reflex of the left eye appears more temporal than that of the right eye. Therefore, the eye is deviated inward.**

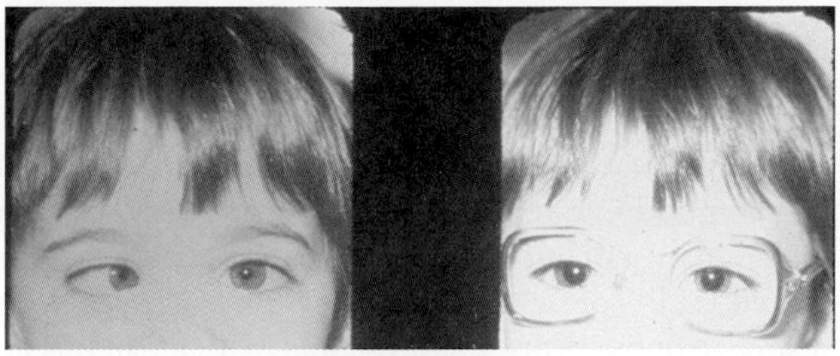

Figure 19–2 **Accommodative esotropia improves when vision is corrected. Adaptation for near vision consists of accommodation (change in lens shape), miosis (constriction of the pupil), and convergence. This can eventually lead to an accommodative esotropia, which can easily be corrected with glasses. After glasses, the patient no longer uses the near response of accommodation and convergence, since the glasses are now providing the correction so the eyes resume normal alignment.**

in different parts of the eye with true esotropia (see Figure 19–1; see also color section).

HELPFUL TIP: It is important to differentiate an esotropia or exotropia from sixth nerve palsy. A sixth nerve palsy affects the lateral rectus muscle and the patient will have limited abduction on the affected side. This is usually the first cranial nerve to go with increased intracranial pressure.

Which of the following statements is FALSE?

A) Congenital esotropia is nearly always present at birth.
B) Alternating fixation (e.g., the ability to fix on an object with either eye) is characteristic of congenital esotropia.
C) Patients with congenital esotropia generally have normal vision with regard to hyperopia (farsightedness).
D) Patients with a high degree of uncorrected hyperopia (farsightedness) can develop an accommodative esotropia.

Discussion

The correct answer (and the false statement) is "A." Congenital esotropia presents by the age of 6 months but is rarely present at birth. If true esotropia is observed at birth, it may be due to another neurologic disorder and further evaluation is indicated. Any form of strabismus may result in vision loss, and for this reason, it is important to treat strabismus early in life. The rest of the answers are true. Answer "B": since patients have two eyes with equal vision, neither is preferred, so they will use both eyes to focus on objects (although not at the same time, of course!). Answer "C": patients with congenital esotropia do have a normal degree of hyperopia for their age. "D" is also correct (see Figure 19–2; see also color section).

Which of the following is NOT an appropriate treatment for strabismus?

A) Surgical correction if correction of refractive errors with full hyperopic spectacle does not resolve the strabismus.
B) Patching the bad eye.
C) Atropine drops or patching the good eye without surgery.
D) Atropine drops or patching the good eye plus surgery

Discussion

The correct answer is "B." The goal of the treatment of strabismus is to prevent amblyopia. Amblyopia is commonly caused by strabismus (ocular misalignment), significant uncorrected refractive error, or disorders that distort images from the eye to the brain (i.e., congenital cataracts). The body basically "turns off" the vision in the bad eye allowing the good eye to work and produce interpretable signals. In addition to surgical treatment (realignment, removal of cataract, etc.), one needs to blur the vision in the **good eye** to strengthen the bad eye. This can be done by patching the good eye (not the bad eye as noted in "B") or by blurring the vision in the good eye using atropine drops if compliance with a patch is an issue (although eye patches remind kids of pirates and pirates are cool).

In which of the following situations would neuroimaging be necessary?

A) A 6-month-old with longstanding esotropia and equal visual acuity bilaterally.
B) A 5-year-old with recent onset esotropia correctable by glasses.
C) A 12-year-old with normal refraction and acute esotropia with diplopia.
D) A newborn with a unilateral congenital cataract and an esotropia.

Discussion

The correct answer is "C." **ANY unexplained new onset strabismus mandates an evaluation.** A 12-year-old with acute esotropia and diplopia and no evidence of hyperopia requires neuroimaging to rule out any underlying neurological disorder. The age of the patient is older than that seen with congenital, acquired, or accommodative esotropia. The refraction is normal, so this does not fit with accommodative esotropia. Diplopia also suggests acute onset. Further workup is therefore necessary. "A" is incorrect because this is a classic history for congenital esotropia. "B" is incorrect because it is consistent with accommodative esotropia. Fixing the nearsightedness would be the first step here. Note that nearsightedness (in this case, high-degree myopia) is a much less common cause of accommodative esotropia compared with farsightedness. "D" is incorrect because we have reason for the esotropia—a congenital cataract.

HELPFUL TIP: Acquired strabismus **always** requires a rapid and complete evaluation. It can be due to tumor, intracranial hemorrhage, botulism, lead poisoning, etc. Any child (or adult, for that matter) with new onset strabismus requires a full ophthalmologic examination.

Objectives: Did you learn to . . .

- Describe the nomenclature of strabismus?
- Determine the underlying causes of esotropia?
- Recognize some unusual cases of strabismus that require further workup?
- Describe the risk and treatment of amblyopia?

CASE 2

A 50-year-old Asian female presents to the emergency department (ED) with severe nausea, vomiting, right eye pain, and blurry vision. She reports the symptoms began only a few hours earlier. She has no significant past medical history. On gross examination, her visual acuity is OD 20/200, her right eye is injected, and her right pupil larger than her left. There does **NOT** appear to be a relative afferent pupillary defect (RAPD) (see glossary at the start of the chapter).

With regard to this patient's presentation, which of the following would NOT be considered in the differential diagnosis?

A) Trauma secondary to blunt injury from a softball.
B) Central retinal artery occlusion.
C) Contact lens-associated bacterial keratitis.
D) Acute angle closure glaucoma.
E) Anterior uveitis.

Discussion

The correct answer is "B." Among these choices, only central retinal artery occlusion would be painless and also associated with an RAPD (from a diffuse retinal ischemia). All of the others will present with pain and WITHOUT an RAPD. "A," blunt injuries, may result in decreased vision secondary to corneal abrasions or edema, intraocular inflammation, hyphema, or retinal injuries. Injury can also cause injection and a traumatic mydriasis (dilation of the pupil). Direct and consensual pupillary reflexes would be normal (no RAPD) unless there was an associated traumatic optic neuropathy or significant retinal damage. "D," acute angle closure glaucoma, would cause diffuse injection with a mid-dilated pupil and no RAPD. "E," anterior uveitis, would also cause injection—but only a ciliary flush—and no RAPD. There is often asymmetry of the pupils in chronic anterior uveitis secondary to central posterior synechiae (adhesions between the iris and lens).

Which of the following is *required* in order to diagnose acute angle closure glaucoma?

A) Slit lamp.
B) Tonometer.
C) Fluorescein and appropriate UV light.
D) Snellen eye chart.
E) A and B.

Discussion

The correct answer is "B." The most important examination technique used to diagnose acute glaucoma is intraocular pressure measurement. This could be a Tonopen, applanation tonometry at the slit lamp, Schiotz tonometer (anyone remember this antique?), etc. "A" is incorrect. A slit lamp is useful for diagnosing structural problems, iritis, etc. "C," fluorescein, is used to diagnose corneal injuries (de-epithelized cornea will take up fluorescein). "D," a Snellen eye chart, is used to determine visual acuity but is not necessary for diagnosing glaucoma. It is always a good idea to check vision in every patient with eye complaints, however (see Figure 19–3; see also color section).

Which of the following is NOT a risk factor for acute angle closure glaucoma?

A) Hyperopia (farsightedness).
B) Asian descent.
C) Male gender.
D) Pharmacologic dilation.
E) Increasing age.

Discussion

The correct answer is "C." Associated risk factors for acute angle closure glaucoma are hyperopia, Asian ancestry, female gender, and older age. Patients with hyperopia have smaller eyes and more crowded anterior chambers. Females also tend to have smaller eyes. As people age, cataracts may develop, become thicker, and crowd the anterior chamber, increasing the likelihood of developing pupillary block leading to glaucoma.

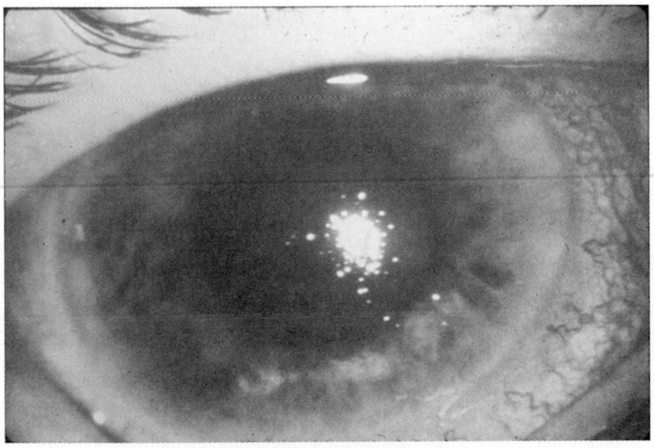

Figure 19–3 **Acute angle closure glaucoma. Note the injection, hazy corneal reflex, and mid-dilated pupil.**

HELPFUL TIP: Pharmacologic dilation may result in an attack of acute angle closure glaucoma. Neovascularization of the eye (such as from diabetes or retinal hypoxia) can lead to "neovascular glaucoma" from neovascularization of the iris and angle. Hyphema can cause glaucoma from clot obstructing the outflow of aqueous humor.

Which of the following is NOT a presentation of acute closed angle glaucoma?

A) Headache.
B) Abdominal pain.
C) Vomiting.
D) Limitation of extraocular motion.
E) Halo's around light.

Discussion

The correct answer is "D." Patients with acute closed angle glaucoma can present with all of the above findings except for the limitation of extraocular motion. Severe eye pain and blurred vision may also be noted.

* *

You call the ophthalmologist to see this patient with acute angle glaucoma. She is going to be delayed because of traffic—it's Iowa, so she's stuck behind a big tractor . . . we don't have "rush hour," only "rush minute."

Which of the following drugs is NOT appropriate to use as a temporizing measure?

A) Topical carbonic anhydrase inhibitors.
B) Topical beta-blockers.
C) Topical glycerin.
D) Topical atropine drops.
E) Oral acetazolamide.

Discussion

The correct answer is "D." Atropine is **contraindicated** in acute glaucoma since it will dilate the eye,

Table 19–1 DRUGS USED FOR ACUTE GLAUCOMA AND HOW THEY WORK

Drug	Mechanism of Action
Topical beta-blockers (e.g., timolol)	Decreases aqueous humor production
Topical alpha-adrenergic agonists (e.g., brimonidine)	Decreases aqueous humor production
Topical carbonic anhydrase inhibitors (e.g., dorzolamide, brinzolamide)	Decreases aqueous humor production
Oral carbonic anhydrase inhibitor (e.g., acetazolamide)	Diuretic and, more importantly, decreases the production of aqueous humor
Mannitol (rarely use now for acute glaucoma, mostly OR cases only)	Osmotic diuretic draws aqueous humor from the eye

exacerbating the problem. Topical beta-blockers and topical or oral carbonic anhydrase inhibitors (e.g., acetazolamide) reduce aqueous production and thereby reduce intraocular pressure. In addition to the medications noted above, a topical alpha-adrenergic agonist (e.g., brimonidine, apraclonidine) should be given to lower intraocular pressure. Topical glycerin is used to clear the corneal edema. Hopefully, this will serve to temporize while the ophthalmologist is on the way. See Table 19–1 for details on glaucoma medications.

HELPFUL TIP: Did you notice that pilocarpine, the classic agent for treating acute glaucoma, is absent from the list? Turns out it doesn't work all that well unless the intraocular pressure is less than 40 mm Hg.

* *

The ophthalmologist makes it to the hospital and wants to take this patient for surgery.

What is the definitive *treatment of choice* for acute angle closure glaucoma?

A) Laser peripheral iridotomy.
B) Tapping of the anterior chamber to lower intraocular pressure.
C) Aqueous suppressant therapy.
D) Surgical iridectomy.
E) Chiropractic manipulation of the iris.

Discussion

The correct answer is "A." The treatment goal is to allow the free flow of aqueous so that it does not accumulate behind the iris to push it forward to obstruct the trabecular meshwork. A laser peripheral iridotomy creates a small hole in the peripheral iris that allows aqueous to enter the anterior chamber. As long as this hole remains patent, the patient is no longer at risk for an attack of angle closure glaucoma, and it is unusual for the hole to close unless there is a history of intraocular inflammation. "B," tapping the anterior chamber, can be used before laser therapy in order to clear the cornea so that visualization is better for the procedure. However, it is adjunctive and not a treatment of choice. Also, topical glycerin works well and can accomplish the same goal without being invasive. "C," aqueous suppressant therapy, is discussed in the previous question. "D," a surgical iridectomy, is performed for patients who are unable to sit still for the laser procedure (i.e., children, mentally incapacitated). As to "E"... nothing against chiropractors, but this might not be the right time.

Which is FALSE regarding closed and open angle glaucoma?

A) The main difference is that the drainage angle (trabecular meshwork) is closed in angle closure glaucoma and open in open angle glaucoma.
B) Scopolamine and other agents with anticholinergic properties are contraindicated in open angle glaucoma but not in closed angle.
C) Acute angle closure glaucoma usually occurs in hyperopic individuals while myopia is associated with open angle glaucoma.
D) The majority of people diagnosed with glaucoma have primary open angle glaucoma.

Discussion

The correct answer (and false statement) is "B." Scopolamine and agents with anticholinergic properties, which would cause dilation of the pupil, are actually **contraindicated** in those with **closed angle glaucoma** (and those with **narrow** angles who may not yet have obstructed). Once peripheral iridotomy is performed, anticholinergics are no longer an issue since the patient is no longer at risk. All of the rest of the statements are correct.

Which of the following does NOT increase a patient's risk for primary *open angle* glaucoma?

A) Family history.
B) Caucasian race.
C) Elevated intraocular pressure (>21 mm Hg).
D) Age >40.

Discussion
The correct answer is "B." Black patients are much more likely to develop open angle glaucoma than whites and are also more likely to suffer vision loss from glaucoma. Family history, high intraocular pressures, and thin corneas are all risk factors for the development of open angle glaucoma. High intraocular pressures lead to optic nerve damage. Minor risk factors include diabetes and myopia (nearsightedness). All patients should be screened for glaucoma as part of their routine eye exam.

Which of the following is typical of early open angle glaucoma?

A) Central vision loss.
B) Peripheral vision loss.
C) Lack of symptoms.
D) Decreased contrast.
E) Blurring of vision.

Discussion
The correct answer is "C." Most people with early open angle glaucoma are asymptomatic. This is why screening is so important. A significant number of axons of the optic nerve may be damaged before this manifests itself as visual field loss. Examination of the optic nerve for abnormalities is the best way to diagnose early glaucoma. Later symptoms involve loss of peripheral or central vision.

Which of the following is necessary to diagnose a patient with *open* angle glaucoma?

A) Optic nerve head cupping with corresponding visual field loss.
B) Thin corneas.
C) Elevated intraocular pressure.
D) Narrow but open drainage angle.

Discussion
The correct answer is "A." Cupping of the optic nerve head is thinning of the neural rim secondary to damage from high intraocular pressure. There should be a corresponding visual field defect consistent with the appearance of optic nerve cupping to diagnose a patient with glaucoma. In open angle glaucoma, the mechanism of injury to the optic nerve is thought to be direct mechanical compression. **Note that elevated intraocular pressure does not diagnose open angle glaucoma. Glaucoma describes the changes secondary to ocular hypertension.** Elevated intraocular pressure by itself is considered a risk factor for glaucoma. When **not** accompanied by cupping or visual field loss, it is considered ocular hypertension. Patients with ocular hypertension still need to be monitored and treated to prevent the development of open angle glaucoma. Thin corneas ("B") increase the risk of glaucoma but are not required for diagnosis (you wouldn't require smoking to diagnose lung cancer, right?). Answer "D" is incorrect. The drainage angle must be widely open—thus the name "open angle glaucoma."

Which of the following statements regarding glaucoma is true?

A) If treated early enough, normalizing the intraocular pressure can reverse the process of glaucoma and restore sight.
B) The funduscopic exam in patients with glaucoma will generally show small retinal hemorrhages in addition to optic nerve cupping.
C) Papilledema is seen with glaucoma as a result of increased pressure on the optic nerve.
D) All of the above.
E) None of the above.

Discussion
The correct answer is "E." So, wrong, wrong, and wrong. Once there is visual loss, it cannot be restored. Papilledema results from increased **intracranial—**not intraocular—pressure. Optic nerve hemorrhages, and not retinal hemorrhages, are seen in glaucoma. See Figure 19–4 (see also color section) for images of normal-appearing optic nerves, and compare these with Figure 19–5 (see also color section), which shows optic nerve findings in patients with glaucoma.

Objectives: Did you learn to . . .

- Recognize the signs and symptoms of acute angle closure glaucoma?
- Identify risk factors associated with acute angle closure glaucoma?

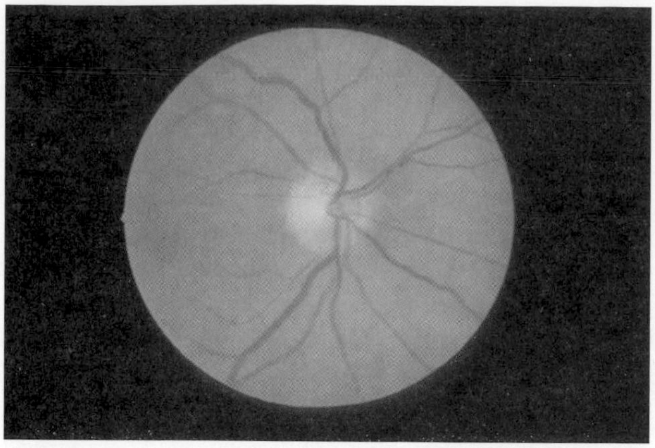

Figure 19–4 **Normal optic nerve.**

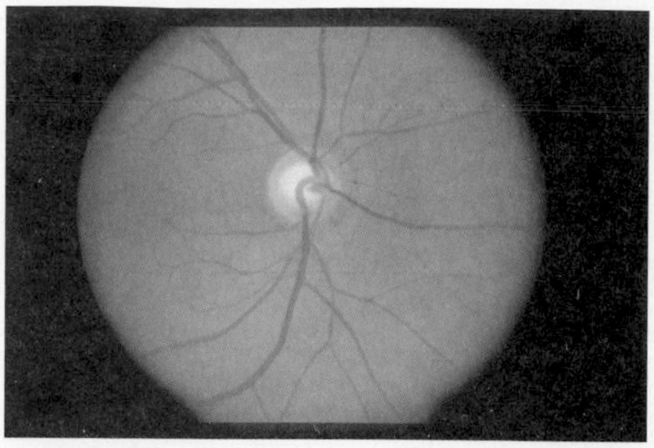

Figure 19–5 **Glaucomatous optic nerve. Observe the cupping of the optic nerve head. The cup (central depression, seen as the bright part of the disc) of the optic nerve, which represents the axons diving down into the optic nerve, is larger compared with normal. A cup >50% of the disc width is indicative of glaucoma. Cupping represents damage to the optic nerve and fewer axons are present.**

- Describe the pathology and basis for treatment for glaucoma?
- Differentiate between angle closure and open angle glaucoma?
- Describe optic nerve findings in glaucoma?

QUICK QUIZ: GLAUCOMA AGENTS

Topical beta-blockers lower intraocular pressure by decreasing aqueous production.

Which of the following is NOT considered a systemic side effect of these medications?

A) Bronchospasm.
B) Bradycardia.
C) Worsening of congestive heart failure.
D) Increased low-density lipoprotein (LDL).

Discussion

The correct answer is "D." Beta-blockers do not increase LDL. The take home message here is that **topical beta-blockers can have systemic effects including congestive heart failure and bradycardia.** Be aware of these, especially in the elderly.

QUICK QUIZ: VISION LOSS

A 70-year-old white female presents with sudden loss of the upper half of her vision in the left eye. **She reports no pain.** Her past medical history is significant for hypertension and type 2 diabetes.

Which of the following is the LEAST likely diagnosis given this history?

A) Retinal detachment.
B) Branch retinal artery/vein occlusion.
C) Optic neuritis.
D) Anterior ischemic optic neuropathy.

Discussion

The correct answer is "C." Retinal detachment, branch retinal artery/vein occlusion, and anterior ischemic optic neuropathy all cause **painless** sectorial loss of vision in this age group. **Optic neuritis** usually occurs in a younger age group and is associated with pain and a central scotoma (blind spot).

> HELPFUL TIP: Many patients complain of pain when they move their eyes. Diagnoses to consider include optic neuritis, intraorbital infection/inflammation, sinusitis, and orbital myositis (e.g., orbital cellulitis, acute Graves disease, orbital pseudotumor, sarcoidosis, polyarteritis nodosum, systemic lupus erythematosus, dermatomyositis, rheumatoid arthritis, and Wegener granulomatosis).

QUICK QUIZ: ANTERIOR ISCHEMIC OPTIC NEUROPATHY

Ischemic optic neuropathy is the most common cause of optic nerve lesions with visual loss in patients older than 50 years. It is referred to as "anterior" when it affects parts of the optic nerve behind the optic disk. It generally results from ischemia of the optic disk (sort of makes sense since it is called "anterior ischemic optic neuropathy").

Which of the following is correct regarding nonarteritic (not related to temporal arteritis) anterior ischemic optic neuropathy (NA-AION)?

A) It is not associated with diabetes.
B) Women are affected five times as often as men.
C) As with giant cell arteritis, it responds quickly and dramatically to systemic corticosteroids.
D) Avoiding nocturnal hypotension is an important aspect of treatment.

Discussion

The correct answer is "D." It is important to ***avoid* nocturnal hypotension.** Occasionally, midodrine needs to be prescribed to support the blood pressure at night. The remaining statements are incorrect. Think of NA-AION as being equivalent to peripheral vascular disease: it is associated with hypertension, smoking, diabetes, etc. Males and females are equally affected. While the age of patients with NA-AION overlaps with that of patients with giant cell arteritis, the patients with NA-AION tend to be younger and NA-AION is painless. Unlike giant cell arteritis, steroids are not the treatment of choice.

HELPFUL TIP: Surgical intervention for NA-AION is not helpful and may lead to worsening blindness. In fact, there is no known effective therapy. Treatment of risk factors is paramount.

CASE 3

A 65-year-old white male complains of "seeing wavy lines" or "window blinds" when looking at the doorway with his right eye. He has no pain or other ocular symptoms. His past medical history is significant for hypertension. He has a 40-pack-year smoking history. On examination, his visual acuity is 20/400 in the right eye. He has no RAPD and slit-lamp exam reveals that his anterior segment examination is normal. Examination of his right fundus reveals a subretinal hemorrhage involving his fovea.

Which of the following is the most likely cause of this patient's vision loss?

A) Age-related macular degeneration (AMD).
B) Acute angle closure glaucoma.
C) Cataract.
D) Diabetic retinopathy.

Discussion

The correct answer is "A." This is a typical presentation for AMD (continue to the next question for more information). "B" is incorrect because acute angle closure glaucoma presents with pain. "C" is incorrect since cataracts cause slowly progressive vision loss. Finally, "D" is incorrect. This would be an unusual presentation for diabetic retinopathy, and the patient has no known history of diabetes.

Which of the following statements is FALSE?

A) AMD is the leading cause of **severe central** vision loss in persons older than 50 years in the United States.
B) Smoking has been shown to be a risk factor in the development of wet AMD.
C) AMD is more common in the black population when compared with other populations.
D) The Age-Related Eye Disease Study has shown a beneficial effect of vitamin E, vitamin C, beta-carotene, copper, and zinc in delaying the progression to wet AMD.
E) The main complaint of wet AMD is metamorphopsia, which is distortion or waviness centrally in the visual field.

Discussion

The correct answer is "C." AMD is more commonly seen in the Caucasian population. "A" and "B" are correct. Smoking is a risk factor in the progression to wet AMD; AMD is the leading cause of **central** vision loss in patients older than 50 years. "D" is correct. The listed micronutrients are beneficial in delaying the progression from dry to wet AMD. "E" is also correct. Patients with AMD complain of distortion and/or waviness in the central visual field.

HELPFUL TIP: Dry AMD is the nonneovascular form of AMD. It is characterized by drusen (yellow lesions in the outer retinal layers of the macula) or atrophy within the macula. Dry AMD may lead to wet (neovascular)

AMD, which is associated with a choroidal neovascular membrane (CNVM). The CNVM is an abnormal growth of blood vessel in the outer layers of the retina, which grows in the macula or fovea and affects vision.

HELPFUL (BUT UNFORTUNATE) TIP: Micronutrients for the general population do not seem to prevent the development of AMD. However, they do seem to work to prevent progression once the patient has AMD.

HELPFUL TIP: There are several treatments available for neovascular AMD. These include laser of the CNVM, intravenous injection of photosensitizing drug (verteporfin) followed by nonthermal red light, intravitreal injection of antivascular endothelial growth factor medications, and surgical removal of CNVM. With regard to photosensitizing drugs, the NNT to **improve** vision is 12, the NNH with vision loss is 100. All treatments are aimed toward preserving existing vision, not improving vision. In addition, patients should be encouraged to cease smoking.

Objectives: Did you learn to . . .

- Recognize the signs and symptoms of AMD?
- Differentiate between dry and wet AMD?
- Recognize treatment modalities for wet AMD?

CASE 4

A 55-year-old white male with a history of newly diagnosed type 2 diabetes mellitus presents for routine evaluation. He has no complaints, including ocular complaints. On nondilated direct ophthalmoscopic examination, both fundi appear to be normal.

When should this patient be referred for formal ophthalmologic examination?

A) Immediately upon diagnosis.
B) Within 3 months.
C) Within 6 months.
D) Within 1 year.
E) When he develops visual symptoms, maybe 2 days before he goes blind.

Discussion

The correct answer is "A." Patient with type 2 diabetes should be referred for a dilated exam immediately upon diagnosis since they may have been undiagnosed for a long time period and may already have a degree of retinopathy. **For type 1 diabetic patients**, the recommendation is to refer within 5 years of diagnosis.

What are the common findings seen on direct ophthalmoscopic examination in nonproliferative diabetic retinopathy?

A) Exudates.
B) Cotton wool spots.
C) Dot-blot hemorrhages.
D) Microaneurysms.
E) All of the above.

Discussion

The correct answer is "E." Direct ophthalmoscopic examination may reveal all of these findings in nonproliferative diabetic retinopathy. These are caused by the increased fragility of capillaries and arterioles of the retina with diabetes.

What is the main cause of vision loss in *nonproliferative* diabetic retinopathy?

A) Dot-blot hemorrhages.
B) Macular edema.
C) Cataract.
D) Neovascularization.

Discussion

The correct answer is "B." Nonproliferative diabetic retinopathy by definition has no neovascularization (new, fragile blood vessel growth secondary to microvascular disease). The main source of decreased vision is macular edema. Treatment of focal macular edema consists of focal laser to leaking microaneurysms. If the patient has diffuse macular edema, a more extensive ("grid laser") pattern is used.

What is the main cause of vision loss in *proliferative* diabetic retinopathy?

A) Cataract.
B) Macular edema.
C) Vitreous hemorrhage.
D) Neovascular glaucoma.

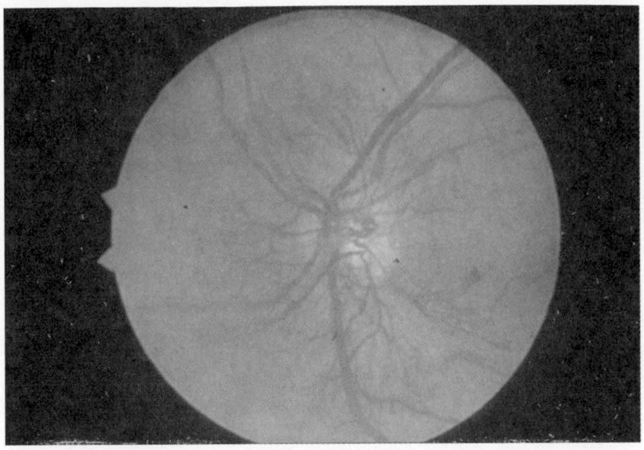

Figure 19–6 **Proliferative diabetic retinopathy. Neovascularization of the optic nerve.**

Discussion

The correct answer is "C." Vision loss in proliferative retinopathy occurs when friable neovascular vessels break open and bleed (vitreous hemorrhage). Vision loss can also occur if the neovascular vessels grow over the drainage angle of the eye, causing glaucoma. This is far less common than vitreous hemorrhage. See Figure 19–6 (see also color section) for an image of neovascularization.

The treatment of proliferative diabetic retinopathy consists of panretinal photocoagulation, which involves lasering the peripheral retina, thereby decreasing the ischemic drive for neovascularization. Treatment of vitreous hemorrhage is observation with the head of bed elevated until the hemorrhage settles out and clears enough for laser treatment. Vitreous hemorrhages may be caused by other things, such as retinal detachments, so ultrasound is usually performed acutely, since one will not be able to see the retina after a significant hemorrhage.

HELPFUL TIP: Aspirin is safe in patients with neovascularization. The risk of bleeding does not increase significantly. The cardiovascular benefit outweighs the risk to the eye.

Objectives: Did you learn to . . .

- Identify when to refer patients for formal ophthalmologic examination in type 1 and type 2 diabetes?
- Recognize the signs of diabetic retinopathy on direct ophthalmoscopic examination?
- Understand the causes of vision loss in those with nonproliferative and proliferative diabetic retinopathy?
- Describe the basis for treatment of both nonproliferative and proliferative diabetic retinopathy?

CASE 5

A 20-year-old male presents to the ED, complaining of a "bloody eye." He was in a fight earlier in the evening and was hit in the eye ("but you should see the other guy!" . . . and with your luck, you probably will . . . .). You examine him and discover the findings in Figure 19–7 (see also color section). His visual acuity in the affected eye is to hand motions only. He also has moderate edema of the lids but is able to open his eyes. On slit-lamp exam, the pupil appears normal. His motility is full and there is no diplopia.

What is the single *most* important first step in evaluation of this patient?

A) Detection of an RAPD.
B) Patching until the heme clears.
C) Evaluation for possible open globe.
D) Immediate CT scanning to evaluate for an orbital fracture.
E) Surgical anterior chamber washout of the heme.

Discussion

The correct answer is "C." This is a hyphema, with blood filling about one-third of the anterior chamber in Figure 19–7. More important is the history of trauma. The first, and most important, step in ocular trauma is to look for evidence of an open or ruptured

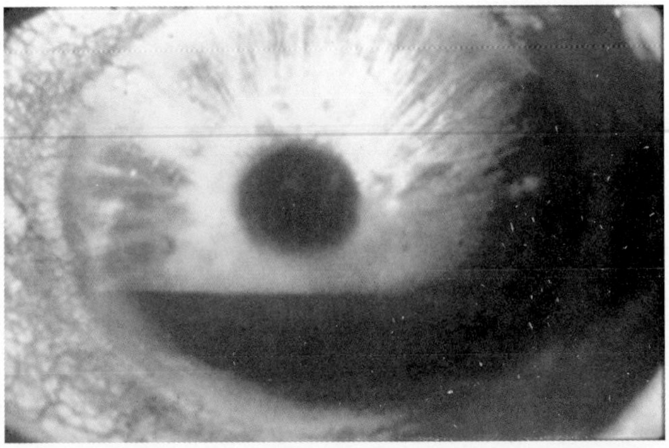

Figure 19–7

globe. **There should be no pressure placed on the eye until an open globe is ruled out.** Signs of ruptured globe would be 360 degrees of conjunctival chemosis (conjunctival swelling), a shallow anterior chamber, an irregular pupil, or low intraocular pressure. **Intraocular pressure measurements should not be taken until an open globe is ruled out. However, a normal globe pressure does not rule out a ruptured globe.** The leak may be small or may be plugged with choroid. If there is any doubt about whether there is an open globe, consult an ophthalmologist. "D" is incorrect and deserves special mention: CT is not sensitive enough to rule out an open globe, even with thin cuts through the globe.

> HELPFUL TIP: When evaluating for a ruptured globe, remember that the most common areas of rupture are the limbus (the margin of the cornea where it meets the sclera) and sclera behind the insertion of rectus muscles. This is where the sclera is thinnest.

> HELPFUL TIP: A "Seidel test" can be used to look for an open globe. A moistened fluorescein strip is gently placed at the site of injury. Slit-lamp exam is done with Cobalt blue light. If a rupture is present, the fluorescein dye will be diluted by the aqueous, which will appear as a dark stream through the green fluorescein.

Which is NOT a complication of hyphema (bleeding into the anterior chamber)?

A) Corneal blood staining.
B) Glaucoma.
C) Rebleeding.
D) Iris heterochromia.

Discussion

The correct answer is "D." Complications of hyphema include rebleeding, which is most common in the first 3–5 days after injury. The hyphema may also stain the cornea; the staining may take months to clear. Glaucoma may also occur because of clogging of the trabecular meshwork by RBCs, leading to a rise in intraocular pressure. Answer "D," iris heterochromia, describes difference in iris coloring (e.g., one blue eye and one brown) and can be caused by a retained foreign body (e.g., iron) but is more often due to an underlying condition.

* *

You rule out ruptured globe and orbital fracture. He's seen by the ophthalmologist on call who recommends treatment.

Which of the following is the most appropriate treatment for this patient?

A) Treat at home with topical steroids.
B) Hospital admission and IV steroids.
C) Hospital admission and IV antibiotics.
D) Hospital admission and topical antibiotics.
E) Treat at home with topical antibiotics.

Discussion

The correct answer is "A." This patient has a hyphema, which is blood in the anterior chamber, usually due to direct trauma. While the party line in the past was that all of these patients require admission, sending a patient home with instructions to avoid further trauma and vigorous activities is sufficient in **reliable** patients with limited disease. However, **an ophthalmologist should be involved in this decision.** In addition to topical steroids, other potential treatments include cycloplegic agents and perhaps antifibrinolytic agents such as aminocaproic acid.

* *

OK. Time for a joke. What is the definition of a double-blind study? Two orthopedic surgeons reading a electrocardiogram.

Objectives: Did you learn to . . .

- Recognize the complications of ocular trauma?
- Identify the complications of hyphema?
- Initiate management of a patient with hyphema?

CASE 6

A 27-year-old male presents with irritation and redness of his right eye after hammering on an old iron fence. He was not wearing safety glasses at the time (they aren't very cool looking and he was hoping his attractive neighbor would be out gardening). He's now 3 days out from his injury. On exam, his visual acuity is 20/200. His right eye is injected, and his pupil is irregularly peaked to one side upon gross inspection. Slit-lamp examination reveals a laceration of his cornea extending to the limbus with a wick of iris occluding the laceration site.

You place a Fox shield on this patient (to prevent any pressure on the globe), update the patient's tetanus and start antibiotics.

What would be the next step in the evaluation and treatment of this patient?

A) Imaging for an intraocular foreign body by orbital CT scanning.
B) Evaluation for an intraocular foreign body by orbital ultrasound.
C) Try to remove the foreign body from the posterior chamber with a magnet.
D) Complete ocular examination, including intraocular pressure and dilated funduscopic examination.

Discussion

The correct answer is "A." Given his history, the patient needs to be evaluated for a possible intraocular foreign body. The best imaging modality is with orbital CT scanning. Orbital ultrasound would also be appropriate, but for surgical planning, CT scanning is preferred. "C" is incorrect because it is likely to cause more damage. This type of foreign body removal is best left to an ophthalmologist in the OR. But, if you are into it... Finally, it would be best to defer intraocular pressure measurements until the extent of the laceration is evaluated since no pressure should ever be placed on a potential open globe.

* *

The patient undergoes an orbital CT. There appears to be a piece of metal within his vitreous cavity.

Which of the following are inert intraocular foreign bodies?

A) Iron.
B) Copper.
C) Glass.
D) Aluminum.
E) C and D.

Discussion

The correct answer is "C." Iron, copper, and aluminum are all reactive species and must be removed from the eye. Glass is inert and may be left in place, depending on the situation and the risk of surgery.

What are signs of a retained *iron* intraocular foreign body?

A) Iris heterochromia.
B) Mydriasis.
C) Glaucoma.
D) Retinal degeneration.
E) All of the above.

Discussion

The correct answer is "E." All of the above are signs of siderosis caused by a retained iron intraocular foreign body. Given the toxicity to the eye, the foreign body must be removed surgically.

> HELPFUL TIP: Corneal foreign bodies may be removed using a needle after the administration of topical anesthetic. Metallic foreign bodies in the cornea may leave a rust ring around the area of the foreign body, which can be removed using an ocular burr. The rust ring may also be left in place if it is out of the visual axis since it does not cause any long-lasting problems.

Objectives: Did you learn to...

- Recognize the signs of a corneoscleral laceration?
- Manage a corneoscleral laceration in the emergency setting?
- Appreciate the effects of intraocular foreign bodies?
- Manage an intraocular foreign body in the emergency setting?

CASE 7

A 55-year-old farmer presents to the ED complaining of ocular pain and irritation. He reports accidentally splashing ammonia in both eyes (in Iowa, this is usually from cooking meth... but not by farmers. Meth cookers drill into tanks of anhydrous ammonia used for fertilizer. They need the ammonia to process the meth). He attempted to rinse his eyes with water prior to coming to the ED. His visual acuity is OD 20/100 and OS 20/80. Both eyes are injected with corneal edema.

What is the immediate first step in the treatment of chemical injuries to the eye?

A) Complete ocular examination, including dilated funduscopic examination.
B) Manual removal of particulate material followed immediately by irrigation with saline until the pH is 7.0.

C) Application of topical glycerin to clear the corneal edema.
D) Topical anesthetic with debridement of surface epithelium.
E) Build rapport by making small talk, asking about his tractor, etc.

Discussion
The correct answer is "B." Immediate irrigation with normal saline (or water or even beer if saline is unavailable) is the initial step even **before** a complete exam. A lid speculum should be placed and topical anesthesia applied. Irrigation may be administered by a handheld bottle or through IV tubing with an irrigation lens. The pH should be checked with a pH strip and irrigation discontinued when the pH reaches 7.0. Any particulate matter should be removed prior to irrigation if it is a reactive substance (e.g., ammonium hydroxide crystals) since fluid may dissolve these causing more injury. The upper lid should be everted to check for any particulate matter. A moistened cotton swab may be used to sweep the superior/inferior fornices to remove any residual debris.

Which of the following is a complication of chemical injuries to the eye?

A) Corneal ulceration.
B) Inflammation.
C) Deepithelialization of the cornea.
D) All of the above.
E) None of the above.

Discussion
The correct answer is "D." All of these are complications of chemical injuries to the eye.

> HELPFUL TIP: Alkali burns tend to be more severe than acid burns. Alkali burns cause ocular surface damage by saponifying fatty acids in cell membranes. Alkaline agents readily penetrate the cornea causing degradation. Acids cause protein denaturation, which creates a barrier to penetration. Therefore, acids cause less tissue destruction. The eye may become insensate from nerve destruction, so absence of burning sensation is not adequate to determine whether further irrigation is needed. **Check the pH as noted above.**

Objectives: Did you learn to . . .

- Describe the difference between acid and alkali injuries to the eye?
- Treat a chemical eye exposure in the emergency setting?
- Recognize the complications of chemical eye injuries?

CASE 8

A 25-year-old college student complains of redness, sensitivity to light, and tearing of her right eye for the past day. She lives in the dorm but reports no exposure to others with a red eye. For the past few days, she has had a sore throat and slight cough. You suspect the dreaded "pink eye" (conjunctivitis).

Regarding conjunctivitis, which of the following is FALSE?

A) Gonococcal conjunctivitis presents with severe hyperacute purulent discharge.
B) Adenoviral conjunctivitis generally begins in one eye and spreads to the contralateral eye.
C) An enlarged preauricular node is a sign of allergic conjunctivitis.
D) Toxic conjunctivitis has been associated with the use of topical antibiotics, antivirals, and preservatives.

Discussion
The correct answer (the FALSE one) is "C." There is no enlargement of preauricular nodes with allergic conjunctivitis. **An enlarged preauricular node is a prominent feature of adenoviral conjunctivitis.** Allergic conjunctivitis tends to itch and affect both eyes. All other statements are true.

* *

Your patient has no purulent drainage. On examination, her visual acuity is 20/40. Her right eye is diffusely injected and tearing; the left eye appears normal to inspection. She has a slightly tender right preauricular lymph node about 1 cm in size.

What do you recommend as the initial treatment of this patient's conjunctivitis?

A) Symptomatic treatment with artificial tears four to eight times per day, cool compresses, and strict hygiene to prevent spread to the contralateral eye or to others.
B) Treatment with topical vasoconstrictors/antihistamines QID for 1–2 weeks.

C) Topical antibiotic treatment for 1 week.
D) Administration of topical steroids, artificial tears, and cool compresses.
E) Lay off the marijuana; she has "toker's eye."

Discussion

The correct answer is "A." This patient appears to have viral conjunctivitis, which is treated symptomatically. There is no need to treat with topical vasoconstrictors and/or antihistamines unless there is a significant itching component. It's not bacterial, so no antibiotics are needed. Additionally, prophylactic antibiotics are not necessary since there is rarely a secondary bacterial infection. Occasionally, corneal subepithelial infiltrates will develop that reduce vision. In these cases, topical steroids may be used for 1 week then tapered to prevent significant scarring. However, this is rare. See Figure 19–8 (see also color section) for an image of viral conjunctivitis.

HELPFUL TIP: Antibiotics have magical powers in viral conjunctivitis. How else can you explain the fact that a single dose of topical antibiotics is enough to get a child back into school or day care? In reality, even with bacterial conjunctivitis, there is little difference between antibiotics and placebo at 6 days . . . and most of the people we treat have viral conjunctivitis anyway making the NNT huge.

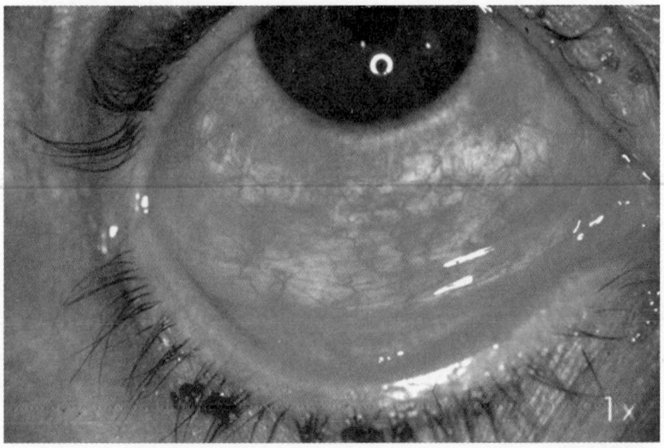

Figure 19–8 **Viral conjunctivitis. Note the follicles that are round collection of lymphocytes in the inferior fornix.**

If your patient is a part-time nursing assistant at a care facility, how long should she stay away from patient care?

A) Two days.
B) Two weeks.
C) Until her eyes are clear.
D) Until she has taken antibiotics for 24 hours.

Discussion

The correct answer is "C." Viral conjunctivitis is highly contagious and is thought to be infectious as long as the eye is red and producing discharge. Promote good hand hygiene and avoidance of contact with others until the eye clears. In many instances, complete removal from school and/or work is not feasible, but patient education regarding the highly contagious nature of viral and bacterial conjunctivitis remains important.

Which of the following is/are appropriate in the treatment of acute gonococcal conjunctivitis?

A) Conjunctival Gram stain and culture.
B) Ceftriaxone IM/IV.
C) Saline irrigation.
D) None of the above.
E) All of the above.

Discussion

The correct answer is "E." The hallmark of acute gonococcal conjunctivitis is severe purulent discharge, which occurs within 12–24 hours of infection. Preauricular adenopathy may also be seen. Management consists of Gram stain of purulent material to document gonococcus, culture, ceftriaxone IM/IV + azithromycin (or spectinomycin if cephalosporin allergic), eye irrigation, and treatment for possible concurrent chlamydia infection. Fluoroquinolones are no longer recommended as initial therapy. See Figure 19–9 (see also color section) for an image of bacterial conjunctivitis and Figure 19–10 (see also color section) for an image of ophthalmia neonatorum.

Which of the following is NOT indicated in the treatment of allergic conjunctivitis?

A) Cool compresses.
B) Artificial tears.
C) Chronic topical vasoconstrictors/antihistamines.
D) Short-term topical steroids.
E) Diphenhydramine.

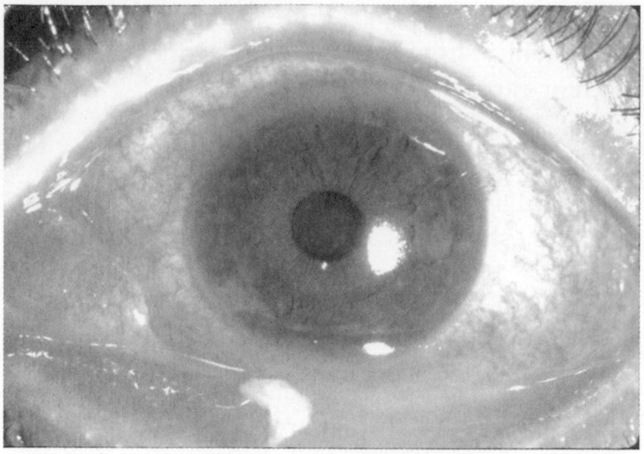

Figure 19–9 **Bacterial conjunctivitis. Note the mucopurulent discharge.**

Discussion

The correct answer is "C." Given the possibility of rebound hyperemia with prolonged use, chronic vasoconstrictors/antihistamines are never indicated. Topical steroids should be reserved for severe cases and tapered over 1–2 weeks. Topical NSAIDs, such as ketorolac, and antihistamines, such as levocabastine and olopatadine, may be used to alleviate intense itching but are very expensive.

Objectives: Did you learn to . . .

- Differentiate among viral, bacterial, and allergic conjunctivitis?
- Choose appropriate treatments modalities for the various causes of conjunctivitis?

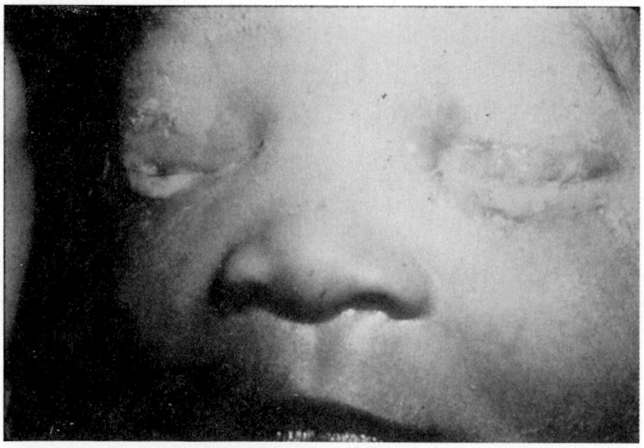

Figure 19–10 **Ophthalmia neonatorum. Note the severe mucopurulent discharge.**

CASE 9

A patient complains of possible foreign body in her eye. She was scraping barnacles off the bottom of her several million-dollar yacht currently dry-docked (Could she be a radiologist? Maybe a plastic surgeon?) when she felt something fly into her eye.

Which of the following is FALSE regarding the use of topical fluorescein, which is used to highlight epithelial defects of the cornea?

A) Fluorescein is a nontoxic, water-soluble dye.
B) It fluoresces under a cobalt blue filter.
C) It exhibits positive staining of epithelial defects.
D) Fluorescein does not penetrate the cornea.

Discussion

The correct answer is "D." Fluorescein **does** diffuse through the corneal stroma and causes a green flare in the anterior chamber. Rapid staining of the anterior chamber after the removal of a corneal foreign body suggests a large, deep corneal injury.

HELPFUL TIP: **Always** evert the upper eyelid to look for additional foreign bodies. These can be removed using a cotton-tipped swab. Irrigation may also be useful.

* *

During your complete exam, you notice a small fleck of what looks like paint on the cornea. After successfully removing the piece of paint, you plan to discharge the patient.

Which of the following is NOT an appropriate treatment for corneal abrasions?

A) Observation alone.
B) Topical antibiotics.
C) Cycloplegics.
D) Topical steroids.
E) Patching.

Discussion

The answer is "D." In uncomplicated corneal abrasions in noncontact lens wearers, observation alone is often adequate. Antibiotics should be used for all contact lens-related abrasions (or in nonwearers if you are particularly worried about the wound). Topical erythromycin or sulfacetamide are good first-line choices in those without contact lenses. A topical fluoroquinolone can be used in contact lens wearers. The patients should also be advised to withhold contact lens use until the abrasion is healed. Patching may also be used for patient comfort but is unnecessary and may actually increase pain and prolong healing time. Topical steroids may inhibit epithelial healing and promote infection and should be avoided. "C" deserves special mention. While cycloplegics are acceptable, there is no data supporting (or refuting) their use in corneal abrasions.

> **HELPFUL TIP:** Multiple vertical corneal abrasions suggest a foreign body under the upper lid. Blinking and closing the eye will leave a vertical abrasion on the cornea. Evert the eyelid and sweep the fornices with a moistened cotton swab to remove any residual foreign body.

* *

As you already know, most corneal abrasion should heal within 24 hours. You ask the patient to follow up the next day to make sure that things are going well. On arrival (the fact that she followed up at all rules out the possibility that she is a physician . . . maybe a stock broker?), she notes increased pain in the eye with increased injection and photosensitivity. You place anesthetic drops in her eye but the pain does not resolve. The corneal abrasion seems to be healed.

What do you expect to see on slit-lamp exam in her anterior chamber?

A) Cells and flare.
B) Opacity of the lens.
C) Foreign bodies of Schlemm.
D) A tear of the anterior lens capsule.
E) None of the above. I am not so good with a slit lamp.

Discussion

The correct answer is "A." This patient is presenting with typical posttraumatic iritis. Findings would be "cell and flare" in the anterior chamber. "B" and "D" are obviously not going to be a result of a superficial corneal abrasion. "C" is something we made up, but "Canal of Schlemm" is one of our favorite names in medicine . . . it is just humorous (. . . humorous, get it . . .). As to "E," well, in real life, "Help me!" is an acceptable answer, but a board exam is not real life.

> **HELPFUL TIP:** Iritis, also called anterior uveitis, characteristically presents with ciliary flush (a red ring around the iris) without tearing or discharge. On slit-lamp exam, the "cell and flare" are due to individual inflammatory cells and foggy-appearing protein leaked from blood vessels.

Appropriate treatment for this patient with posttraumatic iritis includes which of the following?

A) Topical antibiotics.
B) Cycloplegic agents.
C) Topical steroids.
D) A, B, and C.
E) B and C only.

Discussion

The correct answer is "E." Posttraumatic iritis is generally treated with topical steroids and cycloplegic agents. Again, we usually do this in consultation with an ophthalmologist. Of special note is "C." While we all worry about promoting infection with topical steroids, they also increase intraocular pressure. This is generally more of a concern. So, these patients require close follow-up.

* *

Assume that this patient was presenting *de novo* with iritis and it is not posttraumatic.

Which of the following do you NOT have to worry about as an etiology of iritis?

A) Rheumatoid arthritis.
B) Diabetes mellitus.
C) Syphilis.
D) Sarcoid.
E) Lyme disease.

Discussion

The correct answer is "B." Iritis is an inflammatory process that can be caused by multiple underlying illnesses including ankylosing spondylitis, lupus (rarely), Bechet disease, syphilis, sarcoid, TB, Reiter syndrome, toxoplasmosis (common, even in nonimmunosuppressed), juvenile idiopathic arthritis, and many others.

Objectives: Did you learn to . . .

- Remove a corneal foreign body?
- Use topical fluorescein in corneal abrasions?

- Manage uncomplicated corneal abrasions?
- Recognize iritis and its causes?

CASE 10

A 65-year-old white male with a history of hypertension, adult-onset diabetes, rheumatoid arthritis, and rosacea presents with chronic complaints of redness, tearing, and irritation OU. He sometimes also has "a film over his vision" that comes and goes. His ocular examination appears normal. He does, however, have an oily tear film with rapid breakup of his tears over his ocular surface. There is evidence of plugging of his meibomian glands (sebaceous glands along his lid margins), but the eyelids are otherwise normal in appearance.

Which of the following is the most likely diagnosis?

A) Meibomian gland dysfunction.
B) Staphylococcal blepharitis.
C) Hordeolum.
D) Chalazion.
E) Seborrheic blepharitis.

Discussion

The correct answer is "A." Meibomian glands are the sebaceous glands of the upper and lower eyelids, which are located along the posterior lid margin behind the lashes. These are punctate openings along the lid margin, which become inspissated with thick secretions. This eventually leads to an unstable tear film, creating symptoms of burning, redness, foreign body sensation, and filmy vision. It is considered a form of blepharitis (inflammation of the eyelids). "B" and "E" are incorrect. Staphylococcal and seborrheic blepharitis have similar symptoms but involve the anterior eyelid margin at the base of the lashes **(not the meibomian glands as noted in this case)**. Both typically have predominant signs of crusting or mattering. Seborrheic blepharitis often has crusting of an oily or greasy consistency. "C" and "D" are inflammatory processes, commonly but incorrectly grouped together as "styes." A hordeolum affects the anterior lid margin glands, which become acutely plugged. A chalazion affects the posterior lid margin glands, which become plugged and chronically inflamed. "Stye" typically is synonymous with hordeolum; however, both hordeolum and chalazion grossly appear similar on examination.

What part of his past medical history is associated with meibomian gland dysfunction?

A) Hypertension.
B) Diabetes.
C) Rheumatoid arthritis.
D) Rosacea.

Discussion

The correct answer is "D." Meibomian gland dysfunction is associated with rosacea. Typical findings of rosacea include facial papules, pustules, telangiectasia, erythema, and rhinophyma.

What treatment do you prescribe for this patient?

A) Observation and reassurance.
B) Daily warm compresses, lid scrubs with dilute baby shampoo, and oral doxycycline or metronidazole.
C) Erythromycin ophthalmic ointment PRN.
D) Daily warm compresses, topical steroids, and frequent use of artificial tears.

Discussion

The correct answer is "B." The treatment of meibomian gland dysfunction consists of lid hygiene and doxycycline 50–100 mg QD–BID for 3–6 weeks (which will help treat the rosacea). The dosage may then be tapered according to symptoms. Gastrointestinal upset and photosensitivity are common side effects of doxycycline.

Seborrheic blepharitis is often treated with aggressive lid hygiene. Topical steroids are only used for short duration if there is significant inflammation present and should generally be prescribed by an ophthalmologist for this condition.

Which of the following is a common complication of meibomian gland dysfunction?

A) Bacterial keratitis.
B) Preseptal cellulitis.
C) Chalazion.
D) Scleritis.
E) Chronic conjunctivitis.

Discussion

The correct answer is "C." Meibomian gland dysfunction can cause a chronic granuloma to form behind the plugged meibomian gland, which is called a chalazion. The inflammation is sterile—unlike a hordeolum ("stye"), which is a painful purulent abscess. Treatment of a chalazion involves frequent warm compresses and massage. Topical antibiotics are of little value since it is sterile. If these measures fail, an intralesional injection of steroids or incision and drainage is warranted. Hordeola (styes) often resolve spontaneously but warm compresses and massage are often helpful. If there is any evidence of cellulitis, systemic antibiotics are indicated. Drainage using a needle may also be helpful. Topical antibiotics are often not effective.

Objectives: Did you learn to . . .

- Recognize the signs and symptoms of blepharitis and meibomian gland dysfunction?
- Describe the etiologies of blepharitis and meibomian gland dysfunction?
- Differentiate among meibomian gland dysfunction and staphylococcal and seborrheic blepharitis?
- Determine appropriate treatment for blepharitis and meibomian gland dysfunction and the complications of hordeola and chalazion?

CASE 11

A 7-year-old female presents with painful swelling and redness of upper and lower lids of her right eye. She reports having a bug bite near her right eye a week ago, and it's been very itchy. Now, it has become more erythematous and painful (infected, one might say . . .). On examination, her right eyelids are extremely edematous with a well-demarcated area of erythema. Her ocular exam is normal, including normal vision. She has no RAPD, proptosis, or motility deficit.

This presentation is most consistent with:

A) Orbital cellulitis.
B) Preseptal cellulitis.
C) Anaphylactoid reaction to the insect bite.
D) Blepharitis.
E) None of the above.

Discussion

The correct answer is "B." The presentation of this patient is consistent with preseptal cellulitis, which is defined as inflammation/infection anterior to the orbital septum. This is less dangerous than orbital cellulitis, which occurs posterior to the orbital septum and has the risk of spread of infection into adjacent structures. "A" is incorrect. Infection occurring **posterior** to the orbital septum is called orbital cellulitis. This is characterized by fever, proptosis, restriction of orb motility, chemosis, and pain on eye movements. Orbital cellulitis can be complicated by subperiosteal abscess, cavernous sinus thrombosis, meningitis, or intracranial abscesses. "C" is incorrect since an anaphylactoid reaction is systemic.

Which of the following is TRUE?

A) The most common cause of preseptal cellulitis in children is sinusitis.
B) The most common cause of preseptal cellulitis in teens and adults is sinusitis.
C) Orbital cellulitis is most commonly caused by bacteremia from a secondary source, as opposed to direct spread from an adjacent structure.
D) The most common secondary source for orbital cellulitis is otitis media.

Discussion

The correct answer is "A." The most common cause of preseptal cellulitis in children is sinusitis. In contrast, teens and adults usually have preseptal cellulitis from a superficial source, such as skin trauma with inoculation.

HELPFUL TIP: **Both** orbital cellulitis and preseptal cellulitis are commonly secondary to sinusitis. Both preseptal and orbital cellulitis may also occur from direct inoculation or bacteremia from a distant source.

The most common pathogen causing preseptal cellulitis from a skin trauma with inoculation is which of the following?

A) *Staphylococcus epidermidis.*
B) *Haemophilus influenzae.*
C) *Staphylococcus aureus.*
D) *Streptococcus pneumoniae.*

Discussion

The correct answer is "C." *S. aureus* is the most common pathogen of preseptal cellulitis from skin trauma. Some may have chosen "B." Prior to the introduction of the HIB vaccine, children younger than 5 years often had preseptal cellulitis secondary to *H. influenzae*. However, this is no longer the most common pathogen. Most cases of preseptal and orbital cellulitis in children are caused by gram-positive cocci. Orbital cellulitis in children is usually caused by a single organism. In contrast, adults with orbital cellulitis frequently have polymicrobial infections including gram-positive cocci, *H. influenzae*, and anaerobes. Mucormycosis should be suspected in diabetic patients and immunocompromised individuals.

HELPFUL TIP: **Orbital cellulitis** is an ophthalmologic emergency. In addition to spread to other structures (e.g., cavernous sinus thrombosis), orbital cellulitis may cause a tense proptosis leading to blindness. Think about this as a compartment syndrome of the eye. A compartment syndrome (and blindness) can also be seen with trauma and secondary intraorbital (postseptal) bleeding (retrobulbar hematoma) leading to proptosis. The treatment is emergent lateral canthotomy.

Objectives: Did you learn to . . .

- Differentiate between orbital and preseptal cellulitis?
- Recognize conditions that predispose patients to these processes?

CASE 12

A 67-year-old white man with a history of coronary artery disease, hypertension, and peripheral vascular disease presents with the sudden onset of painless loss of vision OD several hours ago. He states he was watching TV when "things went black" in his right eye. He notes that this happened a few times before, but his vision always returned to normal after a couple of minutes. On examination, he has light perception vision, the presence of an RAPD, and a normal anterior segment of the eye. Upon funduscopic exam, the fundus appears diffusely white with a reddish hue within the macula (see Figure 19–11; see also color section).

The patient's history and examination are most consistent with which of the following?

A) Central retinal vein occlusion.
B) Anterior ischemic optic neuropathy.
C) Central retinal artery occlusion.
D) Choroidal ischemia.

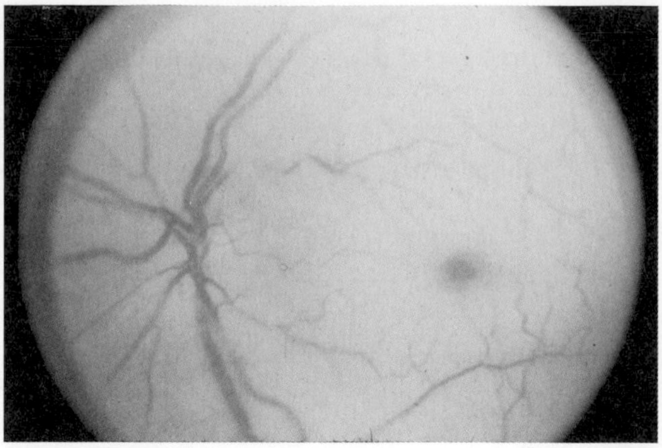

Figure 19–11

Discussion

The correct answer is "C." A central retinal artery occlusion is characterized by acute painless loss of vision. The ischemia and edema of the retina cause diffuse whitening. There is a cherry-red spot in the macula, which is the normal choroidal circulation amidst the ischemic retina (again, see Figure 19–11). The extensive ischemia causes an RAPD and significant visual loss. His previous history of recurrent episodes of loss of vision that returned to normal is consistent with amaurosis fugax.

In a patient with this history, irreversible retinal damage occurs after what time frame?

A) 10 minutes.
B) 30 minutes.
C) 60 minutes.
D) 90 minutes.
E) 6 hours.

Discussion

The correct answer is "D." Amaurosis fugax, or transient monocular blindness, is typically caused by carotid disease. It is often described as a curtain or shade coming over the vision. It lasts from a few seconds to 15 minutes. If occlusion is complete for more than 90 minutes, irreversible retinal damage and visual loss ensue. Patients should seek medical care immediately. Patients with a history of amaurosis fugax should be evaluated for carotid and cardiac disease.

Treatment for central retinal artery occlusion includes all of the following EXCEPT:

A) Thrombolytics.
B) Digital compression/decompression of the globe.

C) Oxygen.
D) Increasing blood carbon dioxide levels (e.g., rebreathing).
E) Acetazolamide.

Discussion
The correct answer is "A." Therapy for central retinal artery occlusion is aimed at dislodging the embolism, maintaining retinal viability, and reducing intraocular pressure (to increase the pressure gradient between the artery and the eye). This can be accomplished by digitally compressing then decompressing the eye with a finger (to dislodge the embolism), oxygen (which will increase oxygen delivery), increasing serum carbon dioxide levels (thus dilating intracranial arteries), and acetazolamide (to reduce intraocular pressure).

Comparing central retinal *artery* occlusion to central retinal vein occlusion, which of the following is TRUE?

A) Central retinal artery occlusion is more likely to be associated with giant cell arteritis.
B) The main feature of both is retinal whitening with a cherry red spot.
C) Central retinal vein occlusion usually results from atherosclerotic thrombosis, while central retinal artery occlusion results from hyperviscosity syndromes and hypercoagulable states.
D) An RAPD is characteristic of central retinal artery occlusion but is not seen with central retinal vein occlusion.

Discussion
The correct answer is "A." Giant cell arteritis is seen in 1–2% of central retinal artery occlusion. However, a more limited anterior ischemic retinopathy is generally seen with giant cell arteritis. If a patient presents with symptoms of central retinal artery occlusion, but no embolus is visualized, he/she should be asked about symptoms of giant cell arteritis. "B" is incorrect because only central retinal artery occlusion is associated with retinal whitening and a cherry red spot. The appearance of a central retinal **vein** occlusion is one of tortuous dilated veins, optic nerve edema, and intraretinal hemorrhages/edema (the so-called blood and thunder appearance of the fundus). Although since thunder is a sound, having something look like thunder makes no sense to us... maybe we are just too literal. "C" is incorrect because central retinal **artery** occlusion is usually caused by atherosclerotic thrombosis or emboli, while central retinal **vein** occlusion is associated more with hyperviscosity syndromes (e.g., polycythemia) and hypercoagulable states (e.g., protein C deficiency). In older patients with central retinal vein occlusion, the main risk factors include vasculopathic states such as hypertension and diabetes. "D" is incorrect because an RAPD can be seen with either syndrome. There is always an RAPD with a central retinal artery occlusion due to the diffuse distribution of ischemia. An RAPD may or may not be seen with a central retinal vein occlusion depending on the level of ischemia.

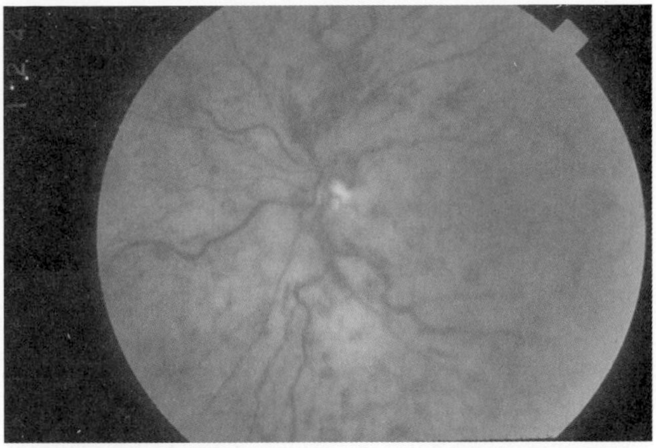

Figure 19–12 **Central retinal vein occlusion. Note the dilated tortuous veins, optic disc edema, and retinal hemorrhage/edema.**

HELPFUL TIP: Other causes of central retinal artery occlusion include vasculitis, such as in giant cell arteritis, or blood dyscrasias. Other causes of central retinal vein occlusions include increased intraorbital or intraocular pressure, glaucoma, blood dyscrasias, lupus anticoagulant, antiphospholipid antibody, and protein C deficiency. See Figure 19–12 (see also color section) for an image of the retina in central retinal vein occlusion.

Further evaluation and treatment of a central retinal artery occlusion include all of the following EXCEPT:

A) Topical timolol.
B) ESR/CRP.
C) Carotid Dopplers.

D) Orbital MRI/MRA.
E) Echocardiogram.

Discussion

The correct answer is "D." There is no need for orbital imaging in the management of a central retinal artery occlusion. All of the other choices are important management steps. In addition, blood pressure, fasting blood sugar or glycosylated hemoglobin, CBC, and PT/PTT should be done. If there is a suspicion of giant cell arteritis, an ESR/CRP should be checked. Other tests might include a rheumatoid factor, syphilis serology, serum protein electrophoresis, and antiphospholipid antibodies. A similar workup is warranted in central retinal vein occlusion, except there is no need to search for an embolic source with a carotid Doppler and echocardiogram.

Objectives: Did you learn to . . .

- Recognize the symptoms of vascular disorders of the eye?
- Differentiate between central retinal artery and vein occlusions?
- Describe some causes of ocular vascular occlusions?
- Determine the appropriate systemic workup for artery and vein occlusions?

CASE 13

A 40-year-old white female presents to your ED complaining of seeing "little floating black spots" in her vision in the left eye. She also notes little sparks of light in the temporal periphery of the left eye. She noted this while shopping today at Walmart. First, you think this may be the revenge of the gods for shopping at Walmart instead of buying locally. But then, you gather your wits about you. On examination, there is no RAPD (she has normal direct and consensual pupillary reflexes). Visual fields to confrontation demonstrate peripheral vision loss in the left eye. Dilated peripheral retinal examination reveals billowing gray folds. The macula appears normal, and her vision is 20/20.

Which of the following is the most appropriate step in the management of this patient?

A) Place a patch over the left eye.
B) Refer to an ophthalmologist immediately.
C) Lower blood pressure acutely with IV labetalol.
D) Apply timolol solution to the affected eye.
E) Offer reassurance.

Discussion

The correct answer is "B." This patient is presenting with urgent ophthalmologic disease. She has classic symptoms of retinal detachment—flashing lights, visual field disruption, and floaters. Also, the majority of her vision is still intact. In her current state, she has a high likelihood of retaining good vision. None of the other treatments offered do anything for retinal detachment. Of note, "C" is treatment for hypertensive retinopathy; "D" is for glaucoma; and "E" is just plain nuts in this case.

Risk factors for retinal detachment include all of the following EXCEPT:

A) Glaucoma.
B) Aphakia (surgical removal of the lens, such as in cataract surgery).
C) Myopia.
D) Trauma.
E) Prior ocular surgery.

Discussion

The correct answer is "A." Glaucoma is not a risk factor for retinal detachment. Both myopia (nearsightedness) and aphakia (surgical removal of lens) are risk factors. Trauma and previous surgery also predispose to retinal detachments. Most persons with retinal detachment are older than 50 years. As patients age, the vitreous detaches from the posterior wall of the eye which can tug on the retina causing a tear.

Objectives: Did you learn to . . .

- Suspect retinal detachment in patients presenting with "floaters" and "flashes?"
- Identify patients who are at risk for retinal detachment?

CASE 14

A 55-year-old white male with type 2 diabetes mellitus complains of a gradual decrease in vision in both eyes. He notes glare with oncoming headlights while night driving. Despite this, he feels that he is able to read better without his bifocals.

20

Otolaryngology

Jason K. Wilbur and Mark A. Graber

CASE 1

A 2-year-old is brought to your office by her mother who is concerned that she has been pulling at her left ear since late last night and has a fever of 101.3°F. She has had recurrent bouts of these symptoms, the last of which was 9 months ago. Each time, the symptoms resolved with one "shot." She is alert and interactive. She has some evidence of mucoid discharge from her nares bilaterally.

Each of the following findings is diagnostic of acute otitis media (AOM) EXCEPT:

A) Profuse, purulent ear discharge without other evidence of otitis externa.
B) Air-fluid level behind the tympanic membrane (TM) with marked redness of the TM and poor movement with pneumatic otoscopy.
C) Bulging, thickened yellow and red TM that does not move well with pneumatic otoscopy.
D) Bubbles in fluid behind the TM with impaired mobility of the TM on pneumatic otoscopy.
E) Yellow, opaque TM, poor movement with pneumatic otoscopy, and substantial ear pain.

Discussion

The correct answer is "D." Suspected ear infections drive many parents to bring their children to a family physician. There may be fluid in the middle ear that is not infected (otitis media with effusion [OME]). In order to diagnose AOM, you need evidence of fluid in the middle ear **and** inflammation. Middle ear effusion is diagnosed by (1) bubbles and/or air-fluid level behind the TM; (2) **two** or more of the following: decreased or absent TM movement with pneumatic otoscopy, opacification of the TM, and discoloration of the TM (yellow, white, blue). These findings get you to OME but not AOM. To diagnose AOM, you will need to have OME with evidence of acute inflammation, such as marked pain, thickened and/or bulging TM, and reddened TM. For these reasons, "B," "C," and "E" are examples of AOM. "A," purulent otorrhea without evidence of otitis externa, would be the one exception where you can diagnose AOM without even seeing the TM. "D" describes OME without inflammation.

> HELPFUL TIP: Don't believe a red eardrum. By itself, redness of the TM has a 15% positive predictive value for diagnosing AOM. In case you're wondering . . . that's terrible! **Use pneumatic otoscopy,** which is the standard of care for diagnosing AOM. **Tympanometry** is an alternative to pneumatic otoscopy. Of course, you still need to look in the ear.

* *

Your patient's left TM is opaque, red, and immobile upon pneumatic otoscopy.

Each of the following factors *increases* her risk for developing otitis media EXCEPT:

A) She attends day care.
B) Her mother smokes inside the house.

C) The patient is a female.
D) Patient still uses a pacifier.

Discussion

The correct answer is "C." The following are known risk factors for the development of AOM: day care attendance, smoking inside the home, **male gender,** pacifier use, children in developing countries, age between 6 and 18 months, and lack of breast feeding.

Which of the following findings is reliably found in patients with AOM?

A) Fever.
B) Ear pulling.
C) Irritability.
D) Rhinitis.
E) None of the above.

Discussion

The correct answer is "E." None of the above is reliably found in patients with AOM. Other unreliable factors include vomiting, diarrhea, and cough. The presence or absence of any of these findings is **not** helpful in making the diagnosis of otitis media. Note that while ear pain is a symptom of inflammation, it is a relatively weak predictor of AOM and must be accompanied by other findings as listed above. However, **pneumatic otoscopy or otoscopy plus tympanometry is the way to make the diagnosis**, but always make sure that you have a good seal or you run the risk of a "false-positive" finding.

> HELPFUL TIP: All children <6 months of age with otitis media should be treated with antibiotics. Patients from 6 months to 2 years should receive antibiotics if the diagnosis is certain **or the diagnosis is suspected and the patient meets high-risk criteria** (moderate-to-severe ear pain, fever >39°C, immunosuppressed). In patients 6 months to 2 years, observation is an option if the diagnosis is uncertain or they meet low-risk criteria (fever <39°C, mild otalgia, immunocompetent, **and** follow-up assured within 48–72 hours). Patients with proven AOM who are older than 2 years may be observed rather than treated with antibiotics as long as they meet low-risk criteria. Analgesics should be given to all patients.

* *

This patient has not had any problems with otitis media for at least 9 months, has not been on antibiotics during that time, is not in day care, and has no allergies. You opt to treat her with an antibiotic.

What is the most appropriate treatment for this patient?

A) Amoxicillin 40 mg/kg/day divided TID.
B) Amoxicillin 80–90 mg/kg/day divided BID.
C) Ceftriaxone 50 mg/kg IM once.
D) Azithromycin 10 mg/kg for 1 day then 5 mg/kg for days 2–5.
E) Amoxicillin/clavulanate 40–80 mg/kg/day divided BID.

Discussion

The correct answer is "B." Amoxicillin is the first-line treatment of AOM. The dose is 80–90 mg/kg/day in all patients whether antibiotic naïve or not. More broad-spectrum (and expensive) drugs such as ceftriaxone and amoxicillin/clavulanate should be reserved for patients who fail initial therapy with a first-line drug or have a penicillin allergy.

> HELPFUL TIP: Remember that you can treat children older than 6 years with a 5-day course of amoxicillin. Amoxicillin/clavulanate should be reserved for treatment failures.

> HELPFUL TIP: **No antibiotic has been proven superior to amoxicillin in the treatment of otitis media. Other antibiotics will work but are more expensive and/or have greater side effects.**

Which of the following statements best characterizes the role of antibiotics in the treatment of AOM?

A) Antibiotics have been shown to reduce suppurative complications of AOM, such as mastoiditis, in developed countries.
B) The majority of patients with AOM benefit from the use of antibiotics.
C) The use of antibiotics for AOM reduces hearing loss and benefits language development.

D) With or without antibiotics, about 75% of children have resolution of AOM symptoms after 7 days.
E) All of the above are true.

Discussion
The correct answer is "D." The benefit of antibiotics for most children with AOM is marginal (number needed to treat [NNT] is about 12); thus, the option exists to observe and not even give antibiotics in children ≥ 2 years old who have mild symptoms, are not immunocompromised, and have good follow-up. The rest of the statements are incorrect. Antibiotics do **not** reduce suppurative complications in **developed** countries, but they do seem to prevent suppurative complications in developing countries where sanitation and health-care access are not optimal. "B" is incorrect. The NNT with antibiotics is up to 12 in order to benefit 1 individual, and this benefit is limited to a 6% absolute reduction in those who have pain at days 2–7 (21% vs. 15%). "C" is incorrect as well, since treating with antibiotics does not impact these outcomes in any way.

HELPFUL TIP: A large (and well publicized) study in the *New England Journal of Medicine* purported to show a benefit to antibiotics in otitis media in children younger than 2 years. For a number of reasons, this study was invalid (and, one might say, absurd). The big "difference" in the groups was that those on antibiotics had a less red TM. Who cares? Clinically, both groups essentially did the same (*NEJM* 2011;364:105-115).

HELPFUL TIP: AOM is usually caused by *Streptococcus pneumoniae*, *Haemophilus influenzae*, *Moraxella catarrhalis*, and various viruses. Most are viral, and the majority of cases—bacterial or viral—will resolve spontaneously.

* *

You prescribe amoxicillin for 10 days and suggest acetaminophen for comfort. A few days later, the patient's mother calls to say that she is no better. You ask her to come in to clinic for evaluation.

When treating AOM, which of these individuals should be considered a treatment failure and switched to another antibiotic?
A) A patient with a fever that continues at 24 hours after starting an oral antibiotic.
B) A child who is still tugging at his ear 5 days into a course of antibiotics.
C) A symptomatic child who still has a bulging, red, immobile TM 3 days after starting antibiotics.
D) A child who continues to have rhinorrhea 1 week after starting antibiotics.
E) All of the above.

Discussion
The correct answer is "C." You should consider switching to a different antibiotic in patients who remain symptomatic at 3 days **and who continue to have positive findings on pneumatic otoscopy.** Symptoms are not enough: they are unreliable. Remember, since most of these are viral infections, you are not doing a whole lot of good with your antibiotics anyway. "A" is incorrect because 24 hours is not sufficient to determine if a particular antibiotic will be effective. "B" is incorrect because patients pull at their ears for a number of reasons besides AOM (such as "Ha! I just discovered I have ears!"). "D" is incorrect. If you chose this one, back to Microbiology 101 for you! Rhinorrhea does not respond to antibiotics and is most likely not bacterial in origin.

HELPFUL TIP: For treatment failures, amoxicillin/clavulanate is recommended by the AAFP and AAP. Other options include cefdinir, cefpodoxime, ceftriaxone, and cefuroxime. Macrolides and TMP/SMX are less effective as second-line therapy because of bacterial resistance (this means azithromycin, folks). Remember the number needed to harm is about 8 with amoxicillin/clavulanate; the diarrhea and resultant diaper rash are often more distressing than the otitis.

* *

She returns with persistent pain and fever after taking amoxicillin for 3 days. On exam, you find evidence of persistent AOM. You switch the patient to your favorite second-line antibiotic. You see her back in 2 weeks for an ear check and find complete resolution.

The mother asks what she could do to avoid these troublesome infections in the future.

All of the following have been shown to reduce the incidence of recurrent otitis media EXCEPT:

A) Antibiotic prophylaxis.
B) Conjugate pneumococcal vaccine **and/or** influenza vaccine.
C) Tympanostomy tubes.
D) Tonsillectomy.

Discussion

The correct answer is "D." Primary tonsillectomy has not been shown to reduce the recurrence of otitis media. However, **adenoidectomy with or without tonsillectomy will reduce the rate of recurrent otitis media in patients who already have tympanostomy tubes.** "A," the use of antibiotic prophylaxis, will reduce recurrent otitis media. **Antibiotic prophylaxis should be considered in the patient who has had $\geq$3 episodes of otitis media in 6 months or $\geq$4 episodes in 12 months.** Reasonable choices for antibiotics include amoxicillin and trimethoprim/sulfamethoxazole. Give half of the usual daily dose. This is generally given at bedtime. Often, antibiotics can be stopped during the summer since an upper respiratory infection (URI) is the precipitant of most cases of otitis media (remember that the great majority are solely viral). Pneumococcal vaccine (e.g., Prevnar) will reduce the risk of recurrence in children with severe and recurrent AOM. The same is true of influenza vaccine. Also recommended to reduce the frequency of AOM: avoid pacifier use, avoid bottle propping at night, avoid smoke exposure, and encourage breast feeding for at least the first 6 months of life.

> HELPFUL TIP: Although it is traditionally done, there is no reason to follow up AOM in patients >15 months of age who are asymptomatic. Clearly, if they are still symptomatic, follow-up is warranted.

> HELPFUL TIP: Adding Cortisporin **suspension** (the solution burns) is appropriate if there is AOM with a ruptured TM (manifested by purulent ear drainage). Other antibiotic drops (ciprofloxacin) can be used as well but are more expensive. No . . . Cortisporin won't cause hearing loss.

* *

The patient returns 4 weeks later with the mother saying, "She is still pulling at her left ear." There are no other complaints. On exam, you find the left TM is without redness or opacity but there is still a fluid level. The right ear exam is unremarkable.

What is your next diagnostic step?

A) Pneumatic otoscopy.
B) Hearing test.
C) Tympanostomy.
D) No further diagnosis needed—treat with antibiotic.

Discussion

The correct answer is "A." Even though we all think we can do it well, the diagnosis of otitis media is fraught with problems. Pneumatic otoscopy should be done in essentially all patients but especially in those in whom long-term therapy is being considered. Remember that fluid can persist for a month or more after an otitis media.

* *

On your exam, the TM does not move with insufflation. The patient's mother asks you if the child should have tubes placed.

Which of the following is NOT a criterion for tympanostomy tubes?

A) Chronic bilateral effusions for more than 3 months with unilateral hearing loss.
B) Failure of antibiotic therapy to prevent recurrent otitis media.
C) Language delay secondary to otitis media.
D) Greater than 20 dB hearing loss bilaterally.

Discussion

The correct answer is "A." Patients should meet the criteria listed above before being considered for tympanostomy tubes. Note that this requires that patients **also** meet the criteria for prophylactic antibiotic therapy ($\geq$3 episodes of AOM in 6 months or $\geq$4 episodes in 12 months). A modification of "A" is also a criterion:

chronic bilateral effusions for more than 3 months with **bilateral** hearing loss. **Although included as a criterion, there is no evidence that tympanostomy tubes improve language development in the short or long term.**

* *

If fluid persists in the middle ear after **AOM**, it is termed OME.

Which of the following interventions has proven benefit in patients with OME?

A) Oral decongestants.
B) Oral antihistamines.
C) Prolonged treatment (≥1 month) with oral antibiotics.
D) Oral corticosteroids.
E) None of the above.

Discussion

The correct answer is "E." For persistent OME, there are no useful medical interventions. Autoinflation ("eustachian tube exercises" or forced exhalation with closed nose and mouth) is often recommended but has not shown a benefit (and try explaining how to do this to a 6-month-old). Patients may benefit from surgical intervention (see the question about tympanostomy tubes above).

Objectives: Did you learn to . . .

- Diagnose otitis media appropriately?
- Initiate treatment in a patient with otitis media?
- Recognize failed antibiotic therapy and choose a new antibiotic for otitis media?
- Describe prevention strategies for recurrent otitis media?
- Recognize indications for tympanostomy tube placement?

QUICK QUIZ: EAR PAIN

Which of the following can cause ear pain?

A) Temporomandibular joint (TMJ) syndrome.
B) Cervical spine degenerative arthritis.
C) Cranial nerve lesions (5, 7, 9, or 10).
D) Bell palsy.
E) All of the above can cause ear pain.

Table 20–1 CAUSES OF EAR PAIN

- Auricular disease
- Canal disease
  - Otitis externa
  - Foreign body
  - Trauma
  - Eczema
  - Ramsay-Hunt syndrome
- Middle ear disease
  - Otitis media
  - Mastoiditis
  - Ménière disease
- Referred pain
  - Dental disease (e.g., abscess)
  - Temporomandibular joint syndrome
  - Carotidynia
  - Pharyngeal disease (e.g., pharyngitis)
  - Cranial nerve lesions (CN V, VII, IX, X)
  - Upper cervical nerve disease, any causes (e.g., disk disease)
  - Bell palsy and other neurologic diseases (e.g., trigeminal neuralgia)

Discussion

The correct answer is "E." All of the above can cause ear pain. A more complete list is given in Table 20–1. The main point here is that not all that hurts in the ear is otitis media.

CASE 2

A 23-year-old female college student presents to your clinic complaining of ear pain. She is on the swimming team and notes that this pain occurs during swimming season. The pain is increased by motion of the pinnae. The external auditory canal is erythematous, edematous, and exquisitely tender when you try to use the otoscope to examine her TM. There is whitish debris in the external auditory canal.

The most likely organism involved in this patient's disease is:

A) *Streptococcus*.
B) *Haemophilus*.
C) *Moraxella*.
D) *Pseudomonas*.
E) *Parainfluenza*.

Discussion

The correct answer is "D." This patient likely has otitis externa. The most common pathogenic organism isolated in cases of otitis externa is *Pseudomonas* followed closely by *Staphylococcus aureus*. However, up to one-third of cases of otitis externa are polymicrobial.

Which of the following is/are considered first-line treatment for otitis externa?

A) Oral ciprofloxacin.
B) Acetic acid ear drops.
C) Polymyxin and neomycin combination ear drops.
D) A and C.
E) B and C.

Discussion

The correct answer is "E." Otitis externa can be treated with a wide array of topical agents. One option is to acidify the external ear canal. Neither *Pseudomonas* nor *Staphylococcus* species can thrive at an acidic pH. Thus, acetic acid drops (VoSol®) can be used: they are cheap and effective. Another approach is to use a topical antibiotic. Polymyxin/neomycin combinations (e.g., Cortisporin) are safe and effective. A number of other antibiotic preparations are available as well. Alcohol-based solutions are another alternative. "A" is incorrect because oral treatment is not indicated for simple otitis externa. However, topical ciprofloxacin may be used.

> HELPFUL TIP: There are a number of much more expensive treatments for otitis externa on the market, including ciprofloxacin otic drops and ofloxacin otic drops. These have no advantage and are very expensive. In fact, **there is no treatment advantage to using antibiotics at all. Topical drying agents, alcohols and acetic acid, have just as good an outcome as do antibiotics.**

This patient is concerned about recurrences of her otitis externa. What advice can you give her?

A) Avoid exposure by putting a petroleum jelly (e.g., Vaseline) impregnated cotton plug in her ear before swimming.
B) Use a blow dryer on her ear after swimming.
C) Instill a 50/50 mixture of alcohol and vinegar in her ears after swimming.
D) Avoid swimming when she has active disease.
E) All of the above.

Discussion

The correct answer is "E." All of the above can be used to minimize disease recurrence. The benefit of "C" is less certain.

> HELPFUL TIP: Remember that **necrotizing (malignant) otitis externa** is a different creature altogether—more a monster compared with an annoying gnat—that occurs primarily in diabetic patients but also in those with HIV. It is an invasive pseudomonal (95%) cellulitis that causes erythema and tenderness around the ear. Complications include osteomyelitis, meningitis, abscess formation, and cranial nerve palsies. It is a true emergency requiring IV antibiotics and surgical consultation.

* *

You treat the patient with neomycin/polymyxin drops, and the symptoms persist and possibly worsen a little after 5 days. The patient has no fever and no signs of cellulitis around the ear.

Of the following possibilities, which is the *LEAST* likely to explain her persistent symptoms?

A) Resistant organisms.
B) Noncompliance with medical recommendations.
C) Misdiagnosis of otomycosis.
D) Development of contact dermatitis.

Discussion

The correct answer is "A." Several things could explain her persistent symptoms. First, the patient should be questioned regarding compliance. Is she still swimming despite advice to the contrary? Is she using the drops at least TID and letting them soak into her ear? Another issue is the development of an allergic reaction, especially in response to neomycin (up to 35% of patients treated chronically with topical neomycin develop a dermatitis). Patients may also "fail" treatment for otitis externa due to misdiagnosis. Otomycosis, a fungal infection of the auditory canal, causes redness, discharge, itching, and sometimes pain. With respect to option "A," treatment failures due to antibiotic resistance are uncommon, and as noted above, antibiotics are not even necessary in the treatment of most cases of otitis externa.

* *

On exam, you notice fine, white, cotton-like fibers filling the ear canal along with the other debris. The exam is otherwise unchanged.

What is your next step?

A) Admit for intravenous (IV) antibiotic and antifungal therapy.
B) Clean the ear canal under direct otoscopy and add oral amoxicillin/clavulanate to her medication regimen.
C) Clean the ear canal under direct otoscopy and add topical clotrimazole 1% to her medication regimen.
D) Order CT or MRI of the head and neck to rule out abscess.
E) Refer to an otolaryngologist.

Discussion

The correct answer is "C." On exam, you have identified signs of otomycosis. It could be that the otomycosis was present initially or developed in the interval with antibiotic administration. Otomycosis is usually due to *Aspergillosis; Candida* only represents 10–20% of cases. Thorough cleaning of the ear canal is an important part of therapy. A topical antifungal that is active against *Aspergillosis* is recommended (e.g., clotrimazole, miconazole, and nystatin).

HELPFUL TIP: Ear wicks are excellent tools for aiding in the delivery of medication deep into the ear canal but **should be changed daily**.

HELPFUL TIP: Cortisporin **suspension** is pH neutral and doesn't burn. The solution causes more pain with instillation.

Objectives: Did you learn to . . .

- Identify bacterial pathogens implicated in otitis externa?
- Diagnose and treat a patient with otitis externa?
- Recommend prevention strategies for otitis externa?
- Determine why treatment for otitis externa may fail?

CASE 3

A 59-year-old male presents with a 3-week history of hoarseness. He denies sore throat or heartburn. He has had no fevers, night sweats, or weight loss. When he initially presented a week ago, your partner treated him empirically for postnasal drainage. He smokes 2 packs of cigarettes per day and drinks alcohol daily. On exam, his vital signs are normal. His voice sounds husky. You find no other abnormalities.

The best next step in the management of this patient is:

A) Empiric antibiotic treatment.
B) Empiric proton pump inhibitor treatment.
C) Direct laryngoscopy.
D) Esophagogastroduodenoscopy (EGD).
E) Neck MRI.

Discussion

The correct answer is "C." The first concern is to rule out malignancy, so the larynx should be visualized. Direct laryngoscopy is a straightforward office procedure and takes only a few minutes. If the equipment and expertise are not available in your office, referral to an otolaryngologist is appropriate. Although there are no firm guidelines, some authors recommend direct laryngoscopy after 2 weeks of hoarseness in patients who are at risk (older patients and those who have a history of tobacco and alcohol use). Since laryngoscopy is such an available, low-cost, low-risk procedure, it is hard to justify postponing it for any patient at risk for malignancy. Therefore, "A" and "B" are incorrect, as further empiric medication trials will only delay laryngoscopy. Besides, antibiotics are not indicated for the lone symptom of hoarseness. In other instances, empiric proton pump inhibitor therapy may be more practical, since gastroesophageal reflux is a common cause of hoarseness. "D" is incorrect. In this case, direct laryngoscopy is preferred to EGD. Finally, "E" is incorrect. Neck MRI is not indicated in the initial evaluation of hoarseness, but it might be used for follow-up after laryngoscopy or to investigate a neck mass.

All of the following are potential causes of hoarseness EXCEPT:

A) Vocal cord mass.
B) Infectious laryngitis.

C) Hypothyroidism.
D) Lung malignancy.
E) A vow of silence.

Discussion

The correct answer is "E." Far from being a cause of hoarseness, voice rest is often recommended for patients with hoarseness due to overuse (e.g., singers). And nobody takes a vow of silence these days except for an occasional monk. All of the other options are known to cause hoarseness. Of particular note is "C": hypothyroidism can result in an accumulation of connective tissue elements, basically myxedema, in the vocal cords. Intrathoracic processes such as lung cancer can present with hoarseness (see "Helpful Tip" below).

Characterizing the nature of the patient's hoarseness can be helpful in narrowing the differential diagnosis. The voice changes may be further characterized as breathy, low-pitched, strained, tremulous, or hoarse. A "breathy" voice may be seen with vocal cord paralysis, abductor spasm, or functional dysphonia. A "low-pitched" hoarseness might be due to edema (seen in smokers), vocal abuse, reflux laryngitis, vocal cord paralysis, or muscle tension dysphonia. A "strained" voice may occur with adductor spasm, muscle tension dysphonia, or reflux laryngitis. A "tremulous" voice occurs in parkinsonism, essential tremor, spasmodic dysphonia, or muscle tension dysphonia. A "hoarse" voice may be due to vocal cord lesions, muscle tension dysphonia, and reflux laryngitis. Vocal fatigue (loss of volume over time) may also be noted and is often caused by muscle tension dysphonia, vocal cord paralysis, reflux laryngitis, or vocal abuse. However, one cannot eliminate a cause of hoarseness based on these characteristics.

HELPFUL TIP: The laryngopharynx is innervated by the recurrent laryngeal nerve, a branch of the vagus nerve (cranial nerve X). In addition to being fun and interesting medical trivia, knowing the innervation is important because chest malignancy, aneurysms, complications of thoracic surgery, etc., can potentially present with hoarseness.

* *

On direct laryngoscopy, you notice a mass lesion on the right vocal cord. You refer the patient to an otolaryngologist. The patient asks if you think that the mass is cancer. Because you are compassionate and also not entirely certain, you avoid saying, "Oh, heck yeah. That's cancer all right. Good thing your life insurance is paid up." You try to be more optimistic.

However, you want to remind him of risk factors for *laryngeal* cancer, which include all of the following EXCEPT:

A) Tobacco smoking.
B) Alcohol use.
C) Epstein–Barr virus (EBV).
D) Family history of head and neck cancers.
E) Male sex.

Discussion

The correct answer is "C." EBV infection is associated with the development of nasopharyngeal cancer, not laryngeal cancer. Additionally, EBV infection has been associated with Burkitt lymphoma (children in Africa), Hodgkin disease, and non-Hodgkin lymphoma. Tobacco and alcohol use are independent risk factors for the development of most types of head and neck cancers (oral, laryngeal, etc.), and the two substances may act synergistically in the promotion of these cancers. A family history of head and neck cancer has a weaker association, but the association is still present. Males are two to four times more likely to have head and neck cancers compared with females.

If this patient is found to have cancer, what pathologic variant is most likely?

A) Adenocarcinoma.
B) Squamous cell carcinoma.
C) Schneiderian papilloma.
D) Neuroblastoma.

Discussion

The correct answer is "B." Upon pathologic examination, the great majority of head and neck cancers are found to be squamous cell carcinomas. Adenocarcinoma may arise from the gastrointestinal tract and could be seen on laryngoscopy but would rarely occur on the vocal cords. Schneiderian papillomas ("C") are polyps that arise from the nasal and sinus mucosae, are associated with HPV, and may transform into carcinomas. Neuroblastomas ("D"), which arise from the sympathetic nervous system, rarely occur in the head and neck region.

* *

During your examination of the oropharynx, you also encountered a small, white, indurated plaque on the underside of the tongue. When you scraped the plaque with a tongue blade, nothing happened.

This lesion is most appropriately described as:

A) Squamous cell carcinoma.
B) *Candida albicans*.
C) Leukoplakia.
D) Geographic tongue.
E) Aphthous ulcer.

Discussion

The correct answer is "C." Leukoplakia is a premalignant lesion of the oropharynx (about 5% will progress to cancer over 10 years). It occurs in response to trauma and/or exposure to irritants and carcinogens, having an especially strong association with smokeless tobacco (e.g., "snuff," "chew") use. In fact, the lesion **could** be squamous cell carcinoma ("A"), and it should be biopsied. However, it would be premature to diagnose the patient with squamous cell carcinoma, and the lesion is more accurately described as leukoplakia. "B," *C. albicans* lesions, may look just like leukoplakia (white plaques on oropharyngeal mucosa), but you should be able to scrape some of the plaques off with a tongue blade (although thrush can be remarkably adherent). "D," geographic tongue, is so named because of the meandering white-bordered patches that occur on the dorsum of the tongue. It is most often asymptomatic, and the lesions vary in shape (or completely resolve) over time. Finally, "E," an aphthous ulcer, is just that—an ulcer, not a plaque. You should not confuse leukoplakia for an aphthous ulcer.

HELPFUL TIP: No interventions have been shown to be useful in promoting the regression of leukoplakia.

* *

You receive a letter from the otolaryngologist stating the patient does indeed have squamous cell carcinoma of the larynx. The patient will be seen in consultation with an oncologist and presented at tumor board. His treatment may consist of surgery, chemotherapy, and/or radiation.

Objectives: Did you learn to . . .

- Generate a differential diagnosis for hoarseness of voice?
- Evaluate a patient with a voice complaint?
- Identify oral lesions, particularly leukoplakia?
- Recognize important issues in the prevention and treatment of head and neck cancers?

CASE 4

A 61-year-old man presents to your office complaining that over the last few months he cannot seem to understand what people are saying when they are standing to his **left** side. He also has episodes of "dizziness," especially when he changes position from sitting to lying and vice versa. He denies nausea and vomiting. He worked for 30 years in a factory and has had bilateral tinnitus for the last 10 years. He has had no previous hearing problems or evaluation. His past medical history is significant for CAD and hypertension. He takes atenolol, chlorthalidone, and aspirin. There is no family history of ear disease. On exam, both ears are normal in appearance. Weber's test is best heard by the patient on his **right** side. Rinne test on both sides was negative (air conduction greater than bone conduction).

These findings are consistent with which type of hearing loss on the *left*?

A) Conductive.
B) Sensorineural.
C) Mixed.
D) Selective.
E) Unable to tell.

Discussion

The correct answer is "B." Hearing can be assessed in the office using the Weber and Rinne tests. The Weber test is performed by putting the tuning fork on the forehead and seeing if the sound lateralizes to one side or the other. In conductive hearing loss ("A"), the sound will be **louder** (i.e., the test will lateralize) to the "bad" side (e.g., the side with wax occluding the canal, otosclerosis). However, in sensorineural hearing loss, the sound will lateralize to the "good" side (e.g., the side not affected by a hearing problem).

The Rinne test is performed by comparing bone conduction (on the mastoid) to air conduction. Patients will notice poor air conduction versus bone conduction if there is a conductive hearing loss.

Normal Rinne tests in both ears suggest that neither ear has **conductive** loss. In our patient, he has decreased hearing on the **left** and the Weber test lateralizes to the **right,** and these findings point to a problem with sensorineural hearing loss in the **left** ear.

Which of the following is LEAST likely to be responsible for this patient's hearing loss?

A) Ménière disease.
B) Acoustic neuroma.
C) Presbycusis.
D) Otosclerosis.
E) Noise exposure.

Discussion

The correct answer is "D." Otosclerosis is a bony overgrowth that involves the stapes and leads to **conductive** loss. Your patient has a sensorineural hearing loss. "A" is correct. Ménière disease presents with the classic triad of hearing loss, tinnitus, and vertigo. These manifestations may be temporally separated with hearing loss, tinnitus, and vertigo occurring at different times. Patients with Ménière disease will note fullness in their ear, which resolves with the onset of vertigo. Typically, the vertigo will last for several hours. "B" is true. Sensorineural hearing loss can also be caused by an acoustic neuroma, a benign tumor that arises from cranial nerve VIII (acoustic nerve), and symptoms include unilateral hearing loss, vertigo, tinnitus, and disequilibrium. "C," presbycusis, is one of the most common causes of sensorineural hearing loss and is often thought of as the "normal" hearing loss that is associated with aging. Presbycusis manifests as an inability to hear high frequencies. This leads to problems with speech discrimination, especially in noisy environments (e.g., parties). It is typically symmetrical and may be associated with tinnitus. However, it may be unilateral, especially in those who have one ear turned toward noisy equipment in their job (e.g., farmers driving tractors and looking behind them—remember, this is being written in Iowa). See Table 20–2 for some causes of conductive and sensorineural hearing loss.

Table 20–2 CAUSES OF CONDUCTIVE AND SENSORINEURAL HEARING LOSS

Conductive Hearing Loss	Sensorineural Hearing Loss
Trauma: ossicle disruption, TM perforation	Presbycusis
Cerumen in the canal	Ménière disease
Otosclerosis	
Barotrauma	Stroke
Otitis media	Tumor (e.g., acoustic neuroma)
Middle ear effusion	Infection (e.g., syphilis, CMV, etc.)

What is the next step in the evaluation of this patient?

A) Audiogram.
B) Brain stem evoked responses.
C) MRI.
D) Tympanogram.

Discussion

The correct answer is "A." An audiogram can further define the air versus bone conductance relationship, check speech discrimination, and define the frequency of hearing loss. Brain stem evoked responses evaluate the neural pathways of hearing and, along with MRI, could be useful if tumor were higher on the differential. A tympanogram, which evaluates movement of the TM, might be useful if conductive hearing loss were suspected.

HELPFUL TIP: Brain stem-evoked potentials measure how long it takes an auditory signal to reach the brain stem. If an acoustic neuroma is present, the brain stem-evoked potential will be prolonged. However, the false-negative rate is up to 30%, and brain stem-evoked potentials have been largely replaced by MRI in the diagnosis of acoustic neuroma.

* *

The audiogram confirms sensorineural hearing loss in the left ear. You order an MRI of the posterior fossa to rule out acoustic neuroma, and the results are negative. The patient continues to have episodes of vertigo, and the hearing loss on his left side persists. When probed further, he does in fact have an increase in tinnitus during his vertiginous episodes.

You should consider all of the following treatments for this condition EXCEPT:

A) Salt, caffeine, and tobacco restriction.
B) Diuretics (e.g., hydrochlorothiazide).

C) Intracochlear injection of gentamicin.
D) Labyrinthectomy or endolymphatic sac shunt.
E) H2-blockers (e.g., cimetidine).

Discussion

The correct answer is "E." The clinical picture now looks most like Ménière disease—a disease for which there is no cure. Luckily not all patients with Ménière disease will experience worsening of their condition over time, and up to 90% are able to maintain normal daily activities with optimal medical management. Few patients progress to debilitating disease. The mainstays of therapy include diet/lifestyle modification and diuretics. Outside the United States, betahistine, an H1-blocker, is commonly used (to theoretically reduce endolymphatic hydrops), but H2-blockers have no role in therapy. A more aggressive approach is indicated in patients with more severe disease, and this might include surgery, intracochlear gentamicin (to kill the nerve and reduce vertigo), labyrinthectomy, or endolymphatic sac shunt.

> HELPFUL TIP: Treating Ménière disease can be problematic. Studies of this condition are frequently of poor quality with a significant placebo effect (including the studies of diuretics and betahistine). This, along with spontaneous remissions and exacerbations, limits the usefulness of data about treatment.

> HELPFUL TIP: Things to remember about tinnitus: It can be caused by a number of medications including NSAIDs, calcium channel blockers, diuretics, etc. It can rarely be caused by a vascular lesion (bruits, A-V shunts, etc.). Other causes include TMJ syndrome, eustachian tube dysfunction, and, most commonly, sensorineural hearing loss (especially presbycusis).

Objectives: Did you learn to . . .

- Evaluate a patient with hearing loss?
- Describe differences between conductive and sensorineural hearing loss?
- Generate a differential diagnosis for hearing loss?
- Diagnose and treat a patient with Ménière disease?

QUICK QUIZ: PERIPHARYNGEAL INFECTION

A 7-year-old female is brought to your office by her concerned parents. Over the last 24 hours, the patient has developed pain in her mouth, drooling, and fever. She refuses to eat. On examination, she is febrile and slightly tachycardic. The sublingual space is swollen and tender bilaterally. The tongue is elevated in the mouth. There are no ulcerations. There is well-demarcated erythema, brawny edema, tenderness, and warmth in the submandibular area. Her respirations are normal, and her lung sounds are clear.

What is the next step in the evaluation and management of this patient?

A) Reassurance, oral rehydration, and analgesics.
B) Oral antibiotics.
C) MRI of the head and neck.
D) IV antibiotics.
E) Intubation and mechanical ventilation.

Discussion

The correct answer is "D." This patient is presenting with classic signs and symptoms of Ludwig angina (related neither to angina nor to Ludwig von Beethoven). The term Ludwig angina is reserved for infection of the submandibular and sublingual areas. The status of the patient's airway must be addressed first. This patient is stable and her airway appears patent; therefore, "E" is incorrect. "A" and "B" are incorrect because patients with Ludwig angina may experience rapid progression of symptoms and should be treated with IV antibiotics and observed in the hospital. Finally, "C" is incorrect because the diagnosis of Ludwig angina is clinical. Also, MRI may delay antibiotic treatment and is unlikely to be of any value, unless you suspect the presence of an abscess. Surgical intervention may be necessary.

> HELPFUL TIP: Trismus is usually absent in Ludwig angina as opposed to peritonsillar abscess, etc.

CASE 5

A 30-year-old man comes to your office complaining of a swollen neck. He noticed it 10 days ago when he was stung by a bee on the right side of his anterior neck. The area has continued to enlarge. It is no longer tender. It was erythematous after the sting, but the redness has resolved. He notes no other symptoms. On exam, you find a 2-cm firm, somewhat tender, enlarged lymph node in the right anterior cervical chain. The node is mobile, nonfluctuant, with no surrounding erythema. There are also shotty anterior and posterior cervical nodes in addition to the larger node described. You find neither supraclavicular, axillary, nor inguinal lymphadenopathy, nor splenomegaly.

What elements of the presentation make malignancy LESS likely?

A) The node is freely mobile.
B) The node is only 2 cm.
C) The node is associated with trauma (bee sting).
D) The node is tender.
E) All of these help to rule out malignancy.

Discussion

The correct answer is "A." Nonmalignant nodes are generally less than 1 cm in size, freely mobile, and rubbery in constancy. Malignant nodes tend to be larger, rock-hard, and fixed. They become immobile secondary to tumor invasion into the surrounding tissues and/or inflammation. Remember that pain in a node is not always indicative of an inflammatory or benign process. Hemorrhage into, or necrosis of, a malignant node can cause capsular distention leading to pain. "C" is of particular note. This patient's bee sting was quite a while ago and is unlikely to be a useful part of the history unless there is ongoing inflammation. Patients will often attribute a physical malady to something in their lives whether or not it makes sense from a biological and medical perspective (one of us had a patient who swore that his purulent sputum was because his lungs were connected to his gallbladder). Of course, lymphadenopathy is not the only source of neck masses. See Table 20–3 for the differential diagnosis of neck masses in adults.

Table 20–3 DIFFERENTIAL DIAGNOSIS OF NECK MASS IN ADULTS

Congenital anomalies
- Lateral neck: brachial cysts and fistulae, cystic hygromas, dermoids
- Central neck: thyroglossal duct cyst, thyroid masses, thymic rests, dermoids

Infection/Inflammation
- Mononucleosis
- Tuberculosis
- Toxoplasmosis
- Cat-scratch disease (*Bartonella henselae*)
- Staphylococcus
- Streptococcus
- Other viral, bacterial, and fungal infections
- Sialadenitis
- Abscess
- Inflammatory or reactive lymphadenopathy

Neoplasm
- Benign masses: lipoma, hemangioma, neuroma, fibroma
- Malignant masses: mucosal head and neck cancers, lymphoma, thyroid cancer, salivary gland cancer, sarcoma, distant metastases

Trauma
- Hematoma (acute or fibrosed)
- Pseudoaneurysm
- AV fistula

Idiopathic and others
- Metabolic: gout, CPPD (pseudogout)
- Inflammatory pseudotumor
- Castleman disease (a benign lymphoproliferative disorder)
- Kimura disease (a chronic subcutaneous inflammatory condition, cause unknown)

What is the most appropriate next step in the management of this patient?

A) Empiric antibiotics.
B) Observation for 4 weeks.
C) Open biopsy of the node.
D) Fine needle aspiration of the node.
E) Incision and drainage.

Discussion

The correct answer is "B." Patients with lymphadenopathy can be observed for 3–4 weeks unless there is a suggestion of malignancy (e.g., fever, night sweats, and weight loss). **Note that a 3–4 week delay makes no difference in patient outcome if the node does turn out to be malignant.** If adenopathy does not resolve, further evaluation including biopsy can be done. Open biopsy and fine needle aspiration each have advantages and disadvantages, but either could be used to obtain tissue. "A," empiric therapy with antibiotics, is possibly correct if you suspect a lymphadenitis or a bacterial infection causing secondary lymphadenopathy. However, in our patient, there is no tenderness or other signs of infection, arguing against lymphadenitis.

Which of the following tests is NOT helpful in arriving at a diagnosis in a patient with GENERALIZED lymphadenopathy?

A) CBC.
B) Chest radiograph.
C) Glucose, BUN, creatinine.
D) HIV.
E) Heterophile antibody.

Discussion

The correct answer is "C." Glucose, BUN, and creatinine are not likely to help you with the diagnosis of generalized lymphadenopathy. Lymphadenopathy in primary care is malignant approximately 1% of the time. After a period of observation, the workup should proceed in stages. First step: CBC, chest radiograph. Second step: PPD, HIV, RPR, ANA, heterophile antibody. Final step: biopsy. Use your clinical judgment to determine the extent of testing necessary in any individual case.

> HELPFUL TIP: Just like in real estate: location, location, location. Supraclavicular nodes are malignant up to 50% of the time in those older than 40 years.

> HELPFUL TIP: Benign lymphadenopathy is common in young children. In patients younger than 5 years presenting for a health maintenance exam, up to 44% have palpable lymph nodes. Occipital and posterior auricular nodes are common in infants but not in children older than 2 years.

Objectives: Did you learn to . . .

- Describe features of malignant and nonmalignant lymph nodes?
- Evaluate a patient with lymphadenopathy?

CASE 6

A 42-year-old businesswoman presents to your office with the chief complaint of 2 days of headache, sore throat, and nasal congestion productive of green mucus. She denies any fever, contact with ill persons, and gastrointestinal symptoms, but she does have a history of seasonal allergies. On exam, she has completely normal vital signs. Her posterior oropharynx has mild erythema and postnasal drainage but no exudates. There is nasal mucosal erythema and swelling with clear rhinorrhea. Her neck is supple with no adenopathy. Respirations are clear.

The most likely agent causing her symptoms and the most common cause of acute rhinosinusitis is:

A) Rhinovirus.
B) *S. pneumoniae*.
C) *H. influenzae*.
D) *M. catarrhalis*.
E) Norwalk virus.

Discussion

The correct answer is "A." Viruses are the most common cause of URIs (or colds or rhinosinusitis). Up to 50% of colds are caused by the 100 different serotypes of rhinoviruses. Other viruses that commonly cause colds include coronaviruses, RSV, parainfluenza, and influenza. Norwalk virus typically causes an intestinal illness. The bacteria listed ("B"–"D") are also associated with infections of the upper respiratory tract, particularly otitis, and sinusitis, but are much less common than viruses.

> HELPFUL TIP: Resident bacteria in the nasopharynx include *S. pneumoniae, H. influenzae*, and *M. catarrhalis*. While most causes of sinusitis are viral, these bacteria make up the great majority of organisms causing bacterial sinusitis. Sinusitis may also result from extension of dental root infection into the sinus cavity, and these infections are caused by microaerophilic and anaerobic bacteria.

Initial treatment for this patient includes:

A) Oral decongestants.
B) NSAIDs.
C) Oral antibiotics.
D) A and B.
E) A and C.

Discussion

The correct answer is "D." Most cases of rhinosinusitis are viral and need only symptomatic treatment. Analgesics and systemic and nasal decongestants are reasonable options. Other treatment options include ipratropium nasal spray (which will also help to decrease mucus production), nasal steroids (at least one well-done randomized trial proved mometasone is superior to placebo), and first-generation antihistamines with anticholinergic activity (e.g., diphenhydramine).

> HELPFUL TIP: Yeah, yeah . . . We know. The party line is that first-generation antihistamines are not useful for rhinorrhea from a URI. However, this is technically incorrect. A Cochrane review showed some benefit of first-generation antihistamines and some effect of combination products. Have you seen someone respond to oral diphenhydramine? Yeah, we thought so—and we have too. (Antihistamines for the common cold. Cochrane Database of Systematic Reviews 2003, Issue 3).

Which of the following does NOT increase the likelihood that a patient has a bacterial sinusitis?

A) Persistence of symptoms for greater than 7 days.
B) Thickened nasal mucosa or effusion on CT scan.
C) Maxillary tooth pain.
D) Unilateral maxillary sinus pain.

Discussion

The correct answer is "B." Radiography is particularly poor at diagnosing bacterial sinusitis. Thickened nasal mucosa is only 40–50% specific for sinusitis (flip a coin, it's cheaper). The other problem with imaging is that essentially all patients with a URI will have fluid in the sinuses. Clinical criteria are more helpful in predicting the presence of bacterial sinusitis; thus, "A," "C," and "D" are correct. Additionally, a biphasic course, sometimes referred to as "double sickening," is a good predictor of bacterial sinusitis: if the patient initially improves and then gets worse, consider a secondary infection. **Thick, green, nasal drainage deserves special mention because green nasal drainage does not necessarily mean that bacteria are present. Secretions will turn green with a viral illness, as with anything else that concentrates protein in the mucous (e.g., anticholinergics).**

> HELPFUL TIP: A viral URI can last up to a month. In fact, 25% of patients with a URI are still symptomatic at 14 days, so duration of symptoms **alone** is not diagnostic of bacterial sinusitis. So, don't tell your patient that she will be better in 4–5 days. Give your patients realistic expectations: 10–14 days.

* *

The patient is initially convinced that only antibiotics will make her better. Through skillful negotiation (and a hefty dose of haloperidol), you manage to avoid prescribing antibiotics for what you strongly suspect is a viral infection. Two weeks later, the patient returns. Initially, she improved, but then she developed subjective fever, face pressure, maxillary tooth pain, and copious green nasal drainage. You now suspect that a bacterial sinusitis has developed. The look on her face says, "I told you so . . . and I am not taking any more of that haloperidol stuff." She has no drug allergies.

Which of the following treatments do you offer as first-line therapy?

A) Azithromycin.
B) Trimethoprim/sulfamethoxazole.
C) Prednisone.
D) Ceftriaxone.
E) None of the above.

Discussion

The correct answer is "B." Most guidelines addressing the treatment of acute bacterial sinusitis recommend narrow-spectrum antibiotics, such as amoxicillin, trimethoprim/sulfamethoxazole, and doxycycline. "C" is incorrect. There is no reason to prescribe steroids here. "D," ceftriaxone, might be considered in cases of treatment failure, but oral antibiotics are generally preferred. Of course, you should continue to recommend that the patient use decongestants and other symptom-oriented therapies.

> HELPFUL TIP: 2012 guidelines now suggest amoxicillin/clavulanate as first line and specifically point out that macrolides (that Z-pack you so love), and TMP/SMX should NOT be used. Doxycycline is considered second line followed by the respiratory quinolones, (http://cid.oxfordjournals.org/). We don't know what the answer on the test will be so we are giving you both the old and new guidelines.

HELPFUL TIP: Even with bacterial sinusitis, the NNT is 9. Most patients are getting no benefit from your careful ministrations.

HELPFUL TIP: Remember that when treating sinusitis you are basically treating an abscess. Draining it is the key: use topical oxymetazoline for limited periods, systemic decongestants, and saline irrigation.

HELPFUL TIP: All noses that run are not infectious. Remember allergic rhinitis, vasomotor rhinitis (now termed idiopathic rhinitis), etc. Vasomotor rhinitis is an exaggerated response to stimuli such as cold, recumbency, and air pollution. It can be differentiated from allergic rhinitis by the absence of other allergic symptoms (itching, eye involvement, perhaps asthma, etc.) and the absence of eosinophils on Hansel stain of mucus (who looks at snot under a microscope anyway?). Other considerations include rhinitis medicamentosum as a result of using topical vasoconstrictors (e.g., oxymetazoline, cocaine).

Objectives: Did you learn to . . .

- Describe the most common pathogens involved in rhinosinusitis?
- Recognize clinical signs and symptoms that are more consistent with bacterial sinusitis than viral rhinosinusitis?
- Prescribe treatment for viral and bacterial sinusitis?

CASE 7

A 65-year-old male presents with dizziness that started a few days ago. He reports that he is otherwise healthy and takes no medications.

Which of the following is the best question to ask him in order to elicit a better characterization of his dizziness complaint?

A) "Is the room spinning round and round?"
B) "Do you feel that you are going to faint?"
C) "Can you describe the dizziness using any other words?"
D) "Do you feel as though you are drunk?"
E) "Are you really just drunk right now?"

Discussion

The correct answer is "C." When exploring a complaint of dizziness, insist that the patient characterizes the nature of the dizziness further without putting words into his mouth. This is a good time for that old technique learned in medical school but rarely used in practice: the open-ended question. There are essentially four types of dizziness: vertigo, presyncope, imbalance (disequilibrium), and undifferentiated dizziness. Patients will usually come up with their own terminology that will allow you to categorize their dizziness into one of these four types.

* *

The patient describes a sensation of the room spinning, usually lasting less than a minute. Further, this sensation comes on in different positions and has led to a fall, which resulted in minor injuries. He denies any upper respiratory symptoms, fevers, hearing loss, or tinnitus. He sometimes feels nauseated with the dizziness but has not vomited. He first noticed the dizziness while in bed and rolling over, but it now occurs more frequently and in various positions. Sudden turning of the head definitely exacerbates his symptoms. It tends to be worse in the morning and better in the evening. You are comfortable calling this type of dizziness vertigo.

Which of the following is LEAST likely to cause vertigo (in a general sense . . . not in this particular patient)?

A) Labyrinthitis.
B) Ménière disease.
C) Migraine aura.
D) Otitis media.
E) Perilymphatic fistula.

Discussion

The correct answer is "D." There are many causes of vertigo, but otitis media should not generally be thought of as one of them (or at least should be a diagnosis of exclusion). Labyrinthitis is usually caused by viral infection and results in severe vertigo that lasts for days. Ménière disease results in episodic vertigo that lasts for minutes to hours. Migraine aura can present with vertigo as well as many other symptoms (e.g., scotoma, diplopia, blindness, and paresthesias). Perilymphatic fistula occurs when perilymph leaks through a tear in the oval window (secondary to a fall or barotrauma—including sneezing). It typically resolves on its own. Although a perilymphatic fistula often results in vertigo, it is a relatively uncommon cause of vertigo.

Which of the following is the best next step in the diagnosis of this patient?

A) Dix–Hallpike maneuvers.
B) Obtain blood for CBC, electrolytes, BUN, and creatinine.
C) MRI brain and brain stem.
D) CT brain.
E) Audiometry.

Discussion

The correct answer is "A." A complete evaluation of the patient with vertigo includes examination of the neurological and cardiovascular systems as well as the ears, eyes, nose, and throat. The Dix–Hallpike maneuver is designed to differentiate central from peripheral vertigo, can be a useful tool (more on this later . . .). In order to perform the maneuver, rapidly move the patient from a seated to a supine position, turning the head to the left or right, and observe for nystagmus. The patient is helped into a seated position, and the maneuver is repeated, turning the head to the other side. If nystagmus occurs within 30 seconds of performing the maneuver, it is considered a positive test. "B" is incorrect. Laboratory tests are rarely helpful. "C" and "D" are not correct because neuroimaging should only be performed if the history and/or exam indicate the need for it. In this case, the exam is not even complete yet! Likewise, audiometry (although helpful in the diagnosis of Ménière disease) is premature.

* *

Dix–Hallpike maneuver is positive with rotation of the head to the left. The rest of the physical exam is unremarkable. The patient gets vertiginous and then it resolves in less than 1 minute.

Given the history and exam, the most likely diagnosis in this patient is:

A) Labyrinthitis.
B) Benign paroxysmal positional vertigo (BPPV).
C) Vertebrobasilar stroke.
D) Motion sickness.
E) None of the above.

Discussion

The correct answer is "B." The history of episodic, positional vertigo and the positive Dix–Hallpike maneuver make BPPV the most likely diagnosis. **Note that the Dix–Hallpike maneuver is not specific for BPPV. The Dix–Hallpike maneuver is designed to differentiate central from peripheral vertigo.** In this case, the history is probably the most important aspect in making the diagnosis. See Table 20–4 for help with interpreting the Dix–Hallpike maneuver. BPPV is more common in older patients but can occur at any age. Women are more commonly affected than men. BPPV is caused by calcium stone deposition in the posterior semicircular canal. BPPV tends to be worse in the morning and better toward evening because, being of peripheral origin, the vertigo response fatigues (see Table 20–4).

Table 20–4 DIX–HALLPIKE MANEUVER

Suggestive of peripheral vertigo
- Delayed onset of nystagmus and symptoms
- Nystagmus always in same direction
- Vertigo reflex fatigable after multiple maneuvers.
- Nystagmus suppressible by patient

Suggestive of central vertigo
- Nystagmus in multiple directions
- No latency to onset of nystagmus
- Reflex not fatigable

The other diagnoses listed are less likely. However, "C" deserves special mention. Stroke should be considered in any patient presenting with sudden onset, persistent vertigo, and risk factors (e.g., hypertension and atrial fibrillation). In general, there should be other findings such as diplopia, dysmetria, and ataxia. However, not every elderly patient with vertigo needs an MRI. If the history is consistent with BPPV, then neuroimaging is not necessary.

HELPFUL TIP: A perilymph leak presents in the opposite manner of BPPV. It is best in the morning and worse in the evening. Gravity is not the patient's friend. As more and more perilymph leaks out during the day, the patient gets progressively more vertiginous.

HELPFUL TIP: "Past pointing" on finger-to-nose testing usually indicates a peripheral lesion. Patients generally fall toward the side of peripheral dysfunction.

For this patient with BPPV, the LEAST appropriate treatment at this time is:

A) Prednisone.
B) Lorazepam.
C) Meclizine (Antivert).
D) Rehabilitation exercises.
E) Dimenhydrinate (Dramamine).

Discussion

The correct answer is "A." Steroids are not likely to improve symptoms in BPPV. Benzodiazepines, anticholinergics, and antihistamines have all been employed in treating the symptoms of BPPV, but **should all be second-line** therapies after rehabilitation and repositioning exercises. Cawthorne rehabilitation exercises (you can find them on the WWW), physical therapy, and physician-directed head positioning (AKA Epley maneuvers to move stones out of the posterior semicircular canal) may be successful. Most patients will improve with time, although many will have relapses.

HELPFUL TIP: Simply treating the patient with medications to suppress the vertigo can actually prolong the course of the disease. The brain needs to learn to adapt to the signal causing vertigo. If your brain was talking (a scary prospect), it would say, "OK, I am not falling. I can ignore that input." Suppressing the vertigo delays this adaptation. However, medications may be necessary for symptom control in some patients.

Objectives: Did you learn to . . .

- Describe types of dizziness?
- Generate a differential diagnosis for vertigo?
- Diagnose and treat a patient with BPPV?

CASE 8

A 15-year-old male wrestler presents to the ED with a nosebleed and a swollen ear. He clearly did not win this round. Prior to coming to the ED, he held pressure to his nose for 30 minutes. He has had nosebleeds before, but none were this bad. When asked how much blood he lost, his father shrugs and says it was "all over the mat." On examination, you see blood oozing slowly from the anterior nasal septum.

Which of the following is/are sources of anterior epistaxis?

A) Ethmoid artery.
B) Sphenopalatine artery.
C) Kiesselbach arterial plexus.
D) Palpatine artery.

Discussion

The correct answer is "C." Kiesselbach plexus is a venous collection system in the anterior nose that contains blood from the ethmoidal, greater palatine and superior labial arteries. It is the most common site of bleeding. The ethmoid and sphenopalatine arteries supply the posterior area of the nose, and bleeding from these sites is more difficult to control. Of special note is "D." Emperor Palpatine, also known as "Darth Sidious," was first seen in the second Star Wars movie. Although evil, he is not known to cause nosebleeds via an eponymous artery.

What is the best next step in managing this patient's nosebleed?

A) Continue to hold pressure against the septum.
B) Pack the anterior naris with gauze.
C) Spray the mucosal surface with phenylephrine.
D) Chemical cautery with silver nitrate.
E) Any of the above can be used.

Discussion

The correct answer is "E." Any of the options listed could be used alone or in combination to try to stop the bleeding. If these methods are not successful, consider electrocautery, laboratory evaluation for signs of bleeding disorders (e.g., CBC, PT/PTT), and otolaryngology consultation. Laboratory studies will rarely be helpful, though.

HELPFUL TIP: If you pack a patient's nose, plan on leaving the packing in place for 24 hours or longer. Also, prescribe antibiotics to prevent sinusitis.

* *

With silver nitrate cautery and direct pressure, you were able to stop the bleeding. You now turn your attention to his left ear. You find a purplish, tender, fluctuant swelling at the left pinna.

The best treatment for this condition is:

A) Analgesics, protection, and observation.
B) Compressive dressing, using a headband (preferably that sweatband in your gym bag).
C) Oral antibiotics.
D) Incision and drainage, leaving the wound open to drain and heal by secondary intention.
E) Needle drainage followed by compressive dressing sutured into the pinna.

Discussion

The correct answer is "E." With traumatic auricular hematoma/seroma, fluid collects between the perichondrium and underlying cartilage, predisposing the cartilage to loss of vascular supply and necrosis. In order to avoid "cauliflower ear" deformity, the hematoma or seroma must be evacuated via incision or needle drainage. However, you cannot stop there: a compressive dressing must then be sutured into the pinna, or the fluid is likely to reaccumulate. "B" is incorrect because compressive dressing alone is insufficient. "D" is incorrect only because it does not include compressive dressing. "A" and "C" are incorrect because taking these actions will delay definitive treatment (and antibiotics are not needed anyway). If the patient were to present late (10 days or more after the injury), he will not benefit from I & D or needle drainage and instead should be referred for otoplasty.

HELPFUL TIP: Repeat after me, "The nose is not the release valve of the cardiovascular system." Most nasal bleeding is venous and not at all related to elevated blood pressure.

Objectives: Did you learn to . . .

- Evaluate and treat a patient with epistaxis?
- Treat a patient with auricular trauma?

QUICK QUIZ: MOUTH SORES

A 20-year-old female presents with three painful ulcerations on her inner lip and tongue. She has no other symptoms. Although she has never had such sores before, everyone else in her family has had similar mouth sores. She only smokes when drinking cheap wine coolers, which occurs about once per week. She is afebrile, and her exam is otherwise unremarkable.

The most likely diagnosis is:

A) Aphthous ulcers.
B) Behçet disease.
C) Crohn disease.
D) Gluten enteropathy.
E) Squamous cell carcinoma.

Discussion

The correct answer is "A." This otherwise healthy young woman with a family history of "similar sores" most likely has aphthous ulcers or "canker sores." The etiology of aphthous ulcers is not well understood, and they are alternatively explained as viral, autoimmune, genetic, traumatic, or due to chemical irritants or other processes (also, karmic retribution, divine punishment for sin, etc.). "B," Behçet disease, is uncommon in the United States. It is thought to be an autoimmune disease, and it presents with recurrent oral and genital ulcerations and skin and eye lesions among other findings. "C" and "D" can both present with isolated oral ulcers but are less common than idiopathic aphthous ulcers. "E" is incorrect because it is highly unlikely that this young, healthy person has developed cancer.

CASE 9

A 34-year-old male dentist presents to your office with a 1-week history of right facial weakness and a bit of tongue numbness. He states that he "just woke up this way one morning." He would have come in sooner, but he was busy with his practice and he has felt fine. He has not noticed any other neurological symptoms. He denies pain, fever, or upper respiratory symptoms. He reports being healthy and taking no medications. On examination, his vital signs are normal. You note that his right eyebrow sags, as does the right corner of his mouth. He cannot close the right eye completely or raise his right eyebrow, and the right nasolabial fold is less prominent than the left. The remainder of the neurological examination is normal.

The neurological finding in this patient that most suggests a cranial nerve process (as opposed to a central brain lesion) is:

A) Normal strength in the upper extremities.
B) Inability to smile on the right.
C) Inability to wrinkle the forehead.
D) Normal blood pressure.
E) Normal speech rate and rhythm.

Discussion

The correct answer is "C." Partial sparing of the forehead muscles suggests a brain lesion because innervation of the forehead contains crossed fibers from both sides of the brain; a bilateral brain lesion is possible but unlikely. Thus, a dense paralysis is more likely to be peripheral (CN7) since all innervation is knocked out when this is involved. This patient's entire right face, including the forehead, is paralyzed, which suggests a lower motor neuron (CN7) process. While "A" and "E" are found in a normal neurologic exam and are reassuring, they are not as helpful in isolating the location of the lesion to a lower motor neuron source. "B," lower facial muscle weakness or paralysis, can occur with upper or lower motor neuron disease. "D," normal blood pressure, is not helpful.

> HELPFUL TIP: Of note, tongue involvement is not unusual in Bell palsy. The seventh nerve is involved in taste sensation on the anterior two-thirds of the tongue.

* *

You tell the patient that you suspect he has Bell palsy. He asks what causes this problem.

Which of the following is the most likely cause of this patient's Bell palsy?

A) Herpes virus.
B) Tick-borne illness.
C) Diabetes.
D) Adenovirus.
E) The dark side of the force.

Discussion

The correct answer is "A." It seems that many cases of Bell palsy are due to reactivation of herpes simplex virus (HSV). Other viral etiologies have been implicated as well, including EBV, CMV, coxsackievirus, and adenovirus ("D"), but all are much less commonly isolated compared with HSV. While "B," tick-borne illnesses such as Lyme disease, cause Bell palsy, these represent a minority of cases. "C," diabetes, may put a patient at increased risk of contracting Bell palsy, but it does not cause the disease.

> HELPFUL TIP: Bell palsy is more likely to occur in pregnancy, especially the last trimester and the first week postpartum.

Which of the following treatments is *most likely* to benefit this patient?

A) Acyclovir.
B) Prednisone.
C) Artificial tears and eye patching at night.
D) A and B.
E) None of the above.

Discussion

The correct answer is "C." In a patient with Bell palsy and weakness to eye closure, good eye care and protection from trauma must be employed to prevent corneal damage (remember that this patient cannot close his right eye). **The evidence for antiviral therapy is negative; acyclovir likely doesn't work, and it is no longer recommended.** There may be some slight benefit to corticosteroid. Steroids are most likely to provide a benefit if started within a few days after the onset of symptoms. Our patient is now a full week out, so steroids won't be of benefit.

* *

You recommend eye care but not medications. Knowing that patients with Bell palsy generally require a lot of reassurance, you discuss the diagnosis in detail, including prognosis.

The patient can expect which of the following?

A) Complete resolution ($\sim$100% likelihood) with nearly zero risk of recurrence.
B) Likely resolution ($>$50% likelihood) with nearly zero risk of recurrence.
C) Likely resolution ($>$50% likelihood) with about 10% risk of recurrence.
D) High probability ($\sim$95% likelihood) of persistent paralysis.

Discussion

The correct answer is "C." Most patients will recover (71% complete, 13% minor impairment with the rest having significant sequelae), but it may take months. If a patient with suspected Bell palsy has no improvement in symptoms after a few months, reconsider the diagnosis. Patients with complete paralysis are more likely to have persistent symptoms, whereas those with partial paralysis usually recover more quickly and completely. Other treatments such as surgical nerve decompression and nerve stimulation have little or no evidence supporting them.

HELPFUL TIP: The Ramsay-Hunt syndrome is the name given to zoster oticus complicated by hemifacial paralysis. If identified early, antivirals may help the patient with Ramsay-Hunt syndrome.

Objectives: Did you learn to . . .

- Differentiate Bell palsy from a central lesion?
- Describe causes of Bell palsy?
- Manage a patient with hemifacial paresis?

QUICK QUIZ: OH, MY ACHING JAW

A 30-year-old female presents with several months of pain and stiffness in her jaw. When asked to localize the pain, she points to the TMJs bilaterally. She notes that the pain is worse with stressful situations, driving, and chewing. Her husband complains that she grinds her teeth at night—and chews him out all day. She is otherwise healthy. On physical examination, you find palpable popping in the TMJs bilaterally, and the remainder of her exam is unremarkable.

You make all of the following recommendations EXCEPT:

A) Start chewing gum daily.
B) Use ibuprofen as needed.
C) Use a bite block at night.
D) Learn relaxation techniques.

Discussion

The correct answer is "A." This patient's history is consistent with TMJ syndrome. In addition to those described in the case, symptoms of TMJ may include ear pain, headache, limited jaw mobility, and crepitus and tenderness on palpation of the joint. TMJ syndrome may occur unilaterally or bilaterally. No one therapy appears to have greater efficacy than any other, and many different interventions have been tried, although poorly studied. "A," increased use of the TMJ by chewing gum, is the exact opposite of what the patient should be doing. Jaw rest is important. All of the other interventions are reasonable. Also, you might recommend a softer diet, hot packs, and TMJ massage.

HELPFUL TIP: The headache of TMJ may be felt in the sinus region, retro-orbitally or as an earache. Check for TMJ when patients present with these types of symptoms.

CASE 10

A 22-year-old female presents to your office complaining of severe facial pain for the past 3 days. She has poor dentition and you find that on exam, there is mandibular swelling and tenderness.

All of the following are causes of mandibular area swelling EXCEPT:

A) Submandibular duct stone.
B) Dental abscess.
C) Retropharyngeal abscess.
D) Ludwig angina.
E) Brachial cleft cyst.

Discussion

The correct answer is "C." Retropharyngeal abscesses are generally not visible but present with fever, throat pain, and symptoms due to swelling of the retropharyngeal space (dysphagia, drooling, odynophagia, and airway obstruction). All of the other options can cause swelling around the mandible.

Which of the following is NOT typical of sialolithiasis (salivary duct stones)?

A) Intermittent swelling of the salivary gland.
B) More than 80% involve the parotid gland.
C) The majority resolve with conservative, nonoperative treatment.
D) Antistaphylococcal antibiotics should be used in their treatment.
E) Sialogogues (e.g., lemon drops) should be used as part of the treatment.

Discussion

The correct answer is "B." **In actuality, more than 80% of cases of sialolithiasis involve the submandibular gland.** "A" is correct. Swelling tends to occur when patients eat and tends to resolve between meals as saliva slowly makes its way through the duct. "C" is correct. Most salivary duct stones pass spontaneously. "D" is correct. Think of this as an abscess. Antistaphylococcal antibiotics should be used until the stone passes. Finally, sialogogues such as lemon drops promote saliva formation. The effectiveness is questionable, but it is worth a try and it gives the patient something to do.

Which of the following is considered good practice with regard to salivary duct stones?

A) Patients should be followed up within 72 hours if the stone does not pass.
B) Stones can be removed using sialolithotomy (using a probe and/or scalpel to nick the outlet).
C) Patients should be referred for lithotripsy if stones do not pass within 4 days.
D) Surgical excision of the duct should be done if the stone does not pass.
E) Tricyclic antidepressant prophylaxis if stones occur frequently.

Discussion

The correct answer is "B." A probe can be used to "dilate" the duct. Occasionally, the outlet needs to be nicked using a scalpel blade to allow the stone to egress. The rest are incorrect. With regard to "A," patients should be followed up in 24 hours if the stone does not pass. "C" is also incorrect. Lithotripsy has actually been used with some good results but is definitely third line. Finally, "D" is incorrect. Excising the duct seems a little dramatic. "E" is very wrong. Anticholinergics reduce salivary flow and thus contribute to stone formation.

* *

You check the patient's mouth and decide that there is likely a dental abscess, not a salivary duct stone. She needs to have her tooth extracted, but the dentist will not be able to see the patient until the morning. She requires antibiotics but is penicillin allergic.

The antibiotic of choice for this patient is:

A) Erythromycin.
B) Clindamycin.
C) Azithromycin.
D) Levofloxacin.
E) Trimethoprim/sulfamethoxazole.

Discussion

The correct answer is "B." Clindamycin is the drug of choice as an alternative to penicillin. The drug used for a dental abscess should cover anaerobes. There is resistance to erythromycin and azithromycin. Neither levofloxacin nor trimethoprim/sulfamethoxazole cover anaerobes.

* *

During your exam, you also noticed a firm nodule in the submental area in the midline. (It is definitely not this patient's day!) It moves up and down when she swallows. She says that it has been there for years—as long as she can remember.

The most likely cause of this midline nodule is:

A) Submandibular gland infection.
B) Thyroglossal duct cyst.
C) Infected frenulum.
D) Brachial cleft cyst.
E) An accumulation of midi-chlorians.

Discussion

The correct answer is "B." This is likely a thyroglossal duct cyst. The rest are not likely. Submandibular glands ("A") and brachial cleft cysts ("D") are lateral to the midline. "C" is incorrect. The frenulum is under the tongue. As for "E," another Star Wars reference. Maybe there will be a Wookie at the end of the chapter. Keep reading.

* *

You start the patient on clindamycin, but she returns in the morning with severe submandibular swelling. **The tongue is elevated in the mouth and there is brawny edema.** You make the diagnosis of Ludwig angina ("Didn't we just do this?" you ask. "Yes, we are going to do it again," we reply.)

At this time, the most appropriate treatment in this patient is:

A) Continue PO clindamycin and add saltwater gargles.
B) Continue PO clindamycin and add PO metronidazole.
C) Incise and drain the swollen area under the tongue.
D) Refer immediately for surgical evaluation for possible tracheostomy.
E) Administer IV fluids and ceftriaxone in the office and follow up tomorrow.

Discussion

The correct answer is "D." This patient's situation has become fairly desperate overnight even while on an appropriate antibiotic. Securing an airway should be your first concern. Unfortunately, these patients do not respond to local incision and drainage, as the swelling is usually diffuse, quickly spreading, and does not result in discreet pus pocket formation until late in the course. She should be admitted for IV fluids, appropriate IV antibiotics (not levofloxacin), and possible tracheostomy. Patients with advancing Ludwig angina do not tolerate endotracheal intubation; thus, an alternative airway is often provided with tracheostomy.

Objectives: Did you learn to . . .

- Diagnose salivary stones?
- Treat salivary stones?
- Recognize the presentation of submandibular masses?

CASE 11

A 21-year-old male presents for a sore throat. His symptoms started 3 days ago. He has had subjective fevers, sweats, fatigue, and mild nausea. He has no cough or rhinorrhea. His temperature is 38.3°C. His vital signs are normal otherwise. He has symmetrically enlarged tonsils with exudates present and tender anterior cervical lymphadenopathy.

At this point, you:

A) Reassure and recommend saltwater gargles.
B) Obtain a routine aerobic culture of the oropharynx.
C) Prescribe penicillin 500 mg BID for 10 days.
D) Prescribe levofloxacin 500 mg daily for 7 days.

Discussion

The correct answer is "C." This patient has 4 of 4 signs/symptoms suggestive of streptococcal (group A strep or *Streptococcus pyogenes*) pharyngitis (the "Centor criteria"): (1) fever, (2) tender cervical adenopathy, (3) exudative pharyngitis, and (4) lack of other URI symptoms. In this case, the most appropriate step would be empiric antimicrobial treatment. "B," performing a culture, will take a few days and does not add much, given the strength of the clinical argument for strep throat. Furthermore, the oropharynx is colonized by many kinds of flora that do not cause disease, and we only really care about group A streptococcus, so a routine aerobic culture is of no value. Alternatively, a rapid assay or a specific "rule out" culture for group A strep could be done rather than treating based on clinical grounds. While saltwater gargles seem to help reduce the pain of pharyngitis, "A" is incorrect because you would want to do more than that for this patient who likely has strep throat. "D" is incorrect because levofloxacin and other fluoroquinolones are not indicated for treatment of strep throat. Here are three strategies for the patient you think might have strep throat:

Strategy 1: No testing (or minimal testing)

In this strategy, one treats based on clinical symptoms. You are looking for four things: fever, exudate, absence of other URI symptoms, and tender anterior cervical adenopathy. Treat patients with 3 or 4 criteria, and do not treat others. Another approach is to treat patients with 4 criteria, do a rapid strep test on those with 3 (and maybe 2) criteria, and avoid treatment and testing of others. This has been recommended by the CDC for nonimmunosuppressed patients in the absence of an outbreak of rheumatic fever in the community.

Strategy 2: Testing

Test all patients and treat those with a positive strep screen. Do not culture others.

Strategy 3: For Children

The majority of group A strep pharyngitis occurs in children between ages 5 and 15 years. In this age group, 15–30% of acute pharyngitis is caused by group A strep. In children, doing a rapid strep test is considered the standard (although many argue convincingly that it is not even necessary here in the older child). Cultures are again optional depending on the reliability of your rapid antigen test. Many would culture **all** rapid strep test negative patients and this is certainly an acceptable strategy as well.

So, now you are quite confused. So is everyone else . . .

Which of the following is true about antibiotic therapy of streptococcal pharyngitis?

A) Azithromycin is the drug of choice because of resistant streptococci.
B) There is no significant resistance seen in Group A beta-hemolytic streptococci, and penicillin is still the drug of choice.
C) Cephalexin is the preferred drug because it covers *H. influenzae*, which is a frequent coinfector with streptococci.
D) Amoxicillin is preferred for strep throat because it does not cause a rash if the patient happens to have mononucleosis.

Discussion

The correct answer is "B." There is no significant resistance among group A beta-hemolytic streptococci to penicillin. Thus, penicillin remains the drug of choice despite drug detailing. There is no reason to use **anything else,** except in the case of allergy where **erythromycin** can be used.

> HELPFUL TIP: Penicillin VK can be used BID in streptococcal pharyngitis, and this administration frequency increases compliance.

Antibiotics should be started within what time period to reduce the risk of rheumatic fever from streptococcal pharyngitis?

A) 2 days after presentation.
B) 2–4 days after presentation.
C) 4–6 days after presentation.
D) 6–8 days after presentation.
E) 8–10 days after presentation.

Discussion

The correct answer is "E." Antibiotics should be started within **9 days after presentation** in order to prevent rheumatic fever, which is really our goal when we treat streptococcal pharyngitis. Thus, there really is no reason to hurry treatment.

* *

Your patient is a student teacher and wants to know how long to stay out of the classroom.

A patient with streptococcal pharyngitis should be considered infectious and kept out of school for what period after beginning antibiotics?

A) 12 hours.
B) 24 hours.
C) 36 hours.
D) 48 hours.

Discussion

The correct answer is "B." Patients should be considered infectious for 24 hours after the initiation of therapy for streptococcal pharyngitis. The risk of transmission goes down markedly after this point. Unfortunately, the patient is actually infectious for the 3–5 days before they become symptomatic, so removing the patient for 24 hours after treatment is closing the barn door after the horses have left. Of course, since this is being written in Iowa, so we are closing the pen after the hogs have left.

* *

You see the same patient 3 weeks later. He took all of his penicillin even though he felt fine a few days after he left your office. (Wow! A compliant patient!) However, he now has the same symptoms, starting 2 days ago. His exam is the same.

Which of the following is the most likely cause for his current symptoms?

A) Gonococcal pharyngitis.
B) Infection with a resistant *streptococcal* organism.
C) Mononucleosis.
D) Recurrent *streptococcal* pharyngitis.

Discussion

The correct answer is "D." Since his symptoms resolved, you either got the diagnosis and treatment right or he had some other self-limited infection. Therefore, it would be unlikely that he had gonococcal pharyngitis or resistant *streptococcal* organisms. Nonetheless, sexual history is important—even when confronted with pharyngitis; if a patient with exudative pharyngitis is not improving, think about gonococcal disease. Remember that gonococcal disease will be missed for two reasons in this scenario: the history is never obtained regarding oral sex and gonococcus requires Thayer-Martin agar to grow, so it will not show up on routine culture. "B," resistant *Streptococcus* organisms causing pharyngitis is non-existent. "C" is unlikely in this case because his symptoms resolved, but mononucleosis can cause prolonged symptoms of sore throat and fatigue and can be confused with strep throat. In this case, recurrent strep throat is most likely and he should be advised appropriately: retreat with penicillin, not a more broad-spectrum antibiotic; consider testing and/or treating cohabitants; have the patient replace his toothbrush.

> HELPFUL TIP: Many causes of throat pain are acute infections (strep throat, other bacterial infections, viral pharyngitis, mononucleosis), but consider other noninfectious causes as well—carotidynia, viral thyroiditis, mouthbreathing, peritonsillar abscess.

* *

The next patient comes in for a sore throat and tender anterior **and** posterior cervical adenopathy. He is febrile and relatively stoic. He has been sick for 2 weeks with significant fatigue and just isn't getting better. In addition to the adenopathy, you notice left-sided abdominal tenderness with minimal guarding but no rebound tenderness. You believe that you feel a spleen edge. However, the patient's heterophile antibody (monospot) is negative. You decide to get anti-EBV antibodies.

* *

The results of the anti-EBV antibody test are as follows (VCA is against the capsid): IgM-VCA positive, IgG-VCA negative, Anti-EBV nuclear antigen antibody negative.

How do you interpret these results?

A) The patient has acute EBV infection.
B) The patient has had EBV at least 6 weeks ago.
C) The absence of anti-EBV nuclear antigen antibody makes acute infection highly unlikely.
D) The patient has never been infected with EBV.

Discussion

The correct answer is "A." The patient has an EBV infection, starting in the last few weeks. Here is why. IgM-VCA is produced acutely and is elevated in the acute infection for 2–4 weeks. Since this patient's IgM-VCA is positive, he has had an acute EBV infection within the past month. IgG-VCA is measurable 3–4 weeks after acute infection and persists for life. Thus, it gives no information about when infection occurred. The absence of IgG-VCA means either (1) the patient has no history of EBV infection or (2) the patient has had a recent EBV infection. Antibodies against the EBV nuclear antigen show up at 6–12 weeks after infection. If this antibody is present in the blood, it suggests that there has not been an acute infection; the infection had to have been at least 6 weeks ago.

Of the following, which DOES NOT cause a mononucleosis-like syndrome?

A) Acute HIV conversion.
B) CMV.
C) Toxoplasmosis.
D) West Nile Virus (WNV).
E) Leptospirosis.

Discussion

The correct answer is "D." WNV is characterized by fever, headache, myalgias, back pain, and anorexia lasting 3–6 days. Much less common manifestations are pharyngitis, nausea, vomiting, diarrhea, encephalitis, etc. Thus, WNV does not cause a mono-like syndrome because it does not last as long and rarely includes pharyngitis. One thing to note is that WNV may include lymphadenopathy. All the other answers can cause a mononucleosis-like syndrome. Other causes of mononucleosis-like syndromes include adenovirus, parvovirus B19 (erythema infectiosum), herpes virus 6 (roseola infantum), and ehrlichiosis (Asian form only). **Remember these diagnoses in heterophile negative mono-like illness.**

HELPFUL TIP: Depending on what population is studied, 1–2% of patients with a mononucleosis-like syndrome who are **heterophile negative** are HIV positive.

If splenomegaly were confirmed in this patient, what would be the generally accepted recommendation with regard to athletic participation (e.g., cage fighting)?

A) No participation until negative acute titers for EBV.
B) No participation for 6 weeks after the diagnosis is made assuming complete resolution of symptoms.
C) No participation until 3 weeks after the diagnosis is made assuming complete resolution of symptoms and then only noncontact training for another week.
D) Full practice and competition allowed immediately unless abdominal pain occurs.

Discussion

The correct answer is "C." It is generally thought that return to practice or **noncontact training** is safe 3 weeks after the diagnosis of mononucleosis, provided that all other symptoms have also resolved. If there are no clinical concerns for splenic enlargement at 4 weeks, then the athlete may be cleared to return to full competition. This recommendation is based on the observation that most cases of splenic rupture in athletes have occurred when those athletes returned to competition in less than 4 weeks from the time of diagnosis.

* *

The patient returns 2 days later and is noting increased pharyngeal swelling and difficulty swallowing. You look into his throat and note "kissing tonsils." There is no stridor, but he feels as though there is something in his throat.

What is the best treatment for this patient at this time?

A) Observation.
B) Amoxicillin.
C) Clindamycin.
D) Prednisone.
E) Tonsillectomy.

Discussion

The correct answer is "A." You may want to give steroids ("D"), but you will find little data to back you up. A Cochrane Collaboration Review updated in 2011 found insufficient evidence for symptom control in patients with mono. However, many physicians still prescribe steroids for patients with significant symptoms. Antibiotics are not indicated for mononucleosis. Tonsillectomy is also not indicated. The patient likely has paratracheal node swelling, as well. In this patient, admission may be indicated if there is enough potential for airway obstruction.

HELPFUL TIP: Amoxicillin is not a good choice for treating patients with streptococcal pharyngitis because if you are wrong and the patient has mononucleosis, he could develop a rash (it occurs but is less common with penicillin). A rash with mononucleosis does not mean that the patient is allergic to amoxicillin.

What is the approximate sensitivity of the heterophile antibody test ("monospot") for mononucleosis within the first 2 weeks of symptoms?

A) 10%.
B) 30%.
C) 50%.
D) 70%.
E) >90%.

Discussion

The correct answer is "D." The sensitivity of the monospot ranges from 60% to 80% 2 weeks into the illness. The point here is not the number per se but the fact that there are heterophile negative mononucleosis syndromes **and** not everyone with EBV mononucleosis will have a positive monospot when tested. However, they should have atypical lymphocytes on WBC differential.

HELPFUL TIP: Remember peritonsillar abscess in a patient with a sore throat. There will generally be a muffled, "hot potato", voice, deviation of the uvula away from the side of the abscess, and protrusion of a tonsil toward midline. This may be an extension of a prior pharyngitis but may also arise de nova. Treatment is antibiotics and drainage (needling it is OK. no need for surgical involvement in all cases). It is also important to pay attention to the airway since there is the possibility of obstruction.

HELPFUL TIP: The monospot is not as sensitive in children. It will become positive in less than 40% of children younger than 5 years when they are infected with EBV. However, anti-EBV antibodies will be positive.

HELPFUL TIP: *Arcanobacterium haemolyticum* is a bacterium that causes pharyngitis especially in young adults (teens–early 20s). It can be confused with strep throat but often has an associated rash especially on the arms (50% only). It does not cause long-term sequelae, so testing for it is not necessarily indicated (but it is cool to identify when the patient comes in with the appropriate rash!).

Objectives: Did you learn to . . .

- Describe different strategies to approaching the patient with symptoms of *streptococcal* pharyngitis?
- Treat a patient with *streptococcal* pharyngitis and recurrent pharyngitis?
- Develop a broad differential for sore throat?
- Diagnose and treat mononucleosis?

QUICK QUIZ

Uh, oh. You have treated a 19-year-old college student for presumed streptococcal pharyngitis with azithromycin (didn't we say not to do this?!). In your defense, he wanted to get better fast because he landed the lead role in the new musical *You Had Me at Arrrgh: A Wookie Love Story*. He returns 1 week later with high fever and a cough, looking quite ill. Chest radiograph shows small pulmonary abscesses and he is tender over the carotid sheath with swelling.

The most likely diagnosis is:

A) Lemierre syndrome.
B) Complication of EBV mononucleosis.
C) Cardiac valvular disease from rheumatic fever.
D) Aspiration pneumonitis from his pharyngitis.
E) Scarlet fever.

Discussion

The correct answer is "A." This is a classic case of Lemierre syndrome, or septic thrombophlebitis of the jugular vein from (generally) *Fusobacterium necrophorum*. This is an anaerobic infection of the posterior pharynx that may be misdiagnosed as streptococcal disease. Generally, patients look ill with a temperature of >39°C, have tenderness in the neck and have septic emboli in the lungs. The basic problem is a septic thrombophlebitis of the jugular vein. It is being increasingly recognized especially in young adults (teens–early 20s). This patient must be admitted for IV antibiotics and may require anticoagulation and/or surgical intervention. In the pharyngitis stage, it is sensitive to penicillin. See, if you would have listened to us and used penicillin in the first place you wouldn't be in this bind! Most causes of throat pain are acute infections (strep throat, other bacterial infections, viral pharyngitis, mononucleosis), but consider other causes as well: carotidynia, viral thyroiditis, mouth-breathing, peritonsillar abscess, etc.

BIBLIOGRAPHY

American Academy of Pediatrics Subcommittee on Management of Acute Otitis Media. Diagnosis and management of acute otitis media. *Pediatrics*. 2004;113(5):1451-1465.

Aring AM, Chan MM. Acute rhinosinusitis in adults. *Am Fam Physician*. 2011;83(9):1057-1063.

Bailey J, Change J. Antibiotics for acute maxillary sinusitis. *Am Fam Physician*. 2009;79(9):757-758.

Buescher JJ. Temporomandibular joint disorders. *Am Fam Physician*. 2007;76(10):1477-1482.

Centor RM, Samlowski R. Avoiding sore throat morbidity and mortality: When is it not "just a sore throat?" *Am Fam Physician*. 2011;83(1):26, 28.

Ely JE, et al. Diagnosis of ear pain. *Am Fam Physician*. 2008;77(5):621.

Feierabend RH, Shahram MN. Hoarseness in adults. *Am Fam Physician*. 2009;80(4):363-370.

Lockhart P, et al. Antiviral treatment for Bell's palsy (idiopathic facial paralysis). *Cochrane Database Syst Rev*. 2009;4:CD001869.

Lodi G, et al. Interventions for treating oral leukoplakia. *Cochrane Database Syst Rev*. 2006;4:CD001829.

McAllister K, et al. Surgical interventions for the early management of Bell's palsy. *Cochrane Database Syst Rev*. 2011;2:CD007468.

McWilliams CJ, Goldman RD. Update on acute otitis media in children younger than 2 years of age. *Can Fam Physician*. 2011;57(11):1283-1285.

Paradise JL, et al. Developmental outcomes after early or delayed insertion of tympanostomy tubes. *N Engl J Med*. 2005;353:576-586.

Parnes LS, et al. Diagnosis and management of benign paroxysmal positional vertigo (BPPV). *CMAJ*. 2003;169(7):681.

Rosenfeld RM, et al. Clinical practice guideline: Acute otitis externa. *Otolaryngol Head Neck Surg*. 2006;134(4, Suppl):S4-S23.

Salinas RA, et al. Corticosteroids for Bell's palsy (idiopathic facial paralysis). *Cochrane Database Syst Rev*. 2010;3:CD001942.

Schwetschenau E, Kelley DJ. The adult neck mass. *Am Fam Physician*. 2002;66(5):831.

21

Care of the Older Patient

Jason K. Wilbur

CASE 1

An 83-year-old female patient whom you have followed for many years has just been admitted to a nursing home following a short hospitalization. Because of a steady decline in function and lack of family and social support, you and the patient came to the realization that she could no longer safely live alone in her home, and her needs were too great for assisted living. Her medical problems include congestive heart failure, chronic atrial fibrillation, osteoarthritis, and depression. Her current medications are warfarin, furosemide, acetaminophen, calcium carbonate, lisinopril, metoprolol, and fluoxetine. Both the patient and the nursing staff report poor sleep and depressed mood for the last 2 weeks, and the nurses are asking for a sleep aid.

What is the best next step in the management of her insomnia?

A) Add diphenhydramine 50 mg PO HS.
B) Add diazepam 5 mg PO HS.
C) Add amitriptyline 25 mg PO HS.
D) Recommend increased activity during the day, avoidance of naps, warm milk before bed, and waking at the same time each morning.

Discussion

The correct answer is "D." There are no great medicines for promoting sleep in elderly nursing home residents. Given the lack of efficacy data of most hypnotics coupled with the known adverse effects, a trial of good sleep hygiene should be undertaken first. "Good sleep hygiene" generally consists of the following: eliminate daytime naps, encourage daily activities and a set waking time, increase aerobic exercise (but not within a few hours of bedtime), and maintain a quiet, comfortable sleeping environment. Nighttime rituals, such as meditation and warm milk, may help insomnia and are unlikely to cause any harm. If these initial efforts fail, a low dose of a hypnotic (e.g., zolpidem and zaleplon) or trazodone is an appropriate initial choice. Trazodone has fewer anticholinergic and blood pressure effects than other options, such as tricyclics and benzodiazepines, but should still be used with caution while monitoring for adverse effects. Diphenhydramine ("A") has powerful antihistaminic and anticholinergic properties that may result in increased confusion and falls. Diazepam ("B") has an exceptionally long half-life in elderly patients and may cause daytime somnolence. Amitriptyline ("C") is listed by the Centers for Medicare and Medicaid Services (CMS) as a medication to be avoided in nursing home patients due to high potential for severe adverse drug reactions (falls, constipation, etc.).

HELPFUL TIP: There are many potential causes of sleep disturbance in the nursing home. The following are sources of sleep problems that you may want to investigate or treat empirically: pain, anxiety, depression, delirium, dementia, primary sleep disorders (e.g., sleep apnea and restless leg syndrome), environmental issues (e.g., alarms and lights).

* *

The nurses grudgingly accept your recommendation to try sleep hygiene ("Can't we just give her a pill?"), and over the next month your patient's sleep improves, as does her mood. There's one in the win column for the doctor! Unfortunately, she experiences two falls with minor injuries while ambulating in her room. Upon examination, you find normal vital signs, no orthostatic hypotension, and no focal neurological deficits.

Which of the following is the most appropriate next step?

A) Discontinue warfarin.
B) Employ bed and chair alarms.
C) Obtain a computerized tomography (CT) scan of the head.
D) Reduce or discontinue fluoxetine.
E) Restrict activities and prescribe a wheelchair.

Discussion

The correct answer is "D." As often happens in life, there is no great answer here. Falls are usually multifactorial in origin, so simple interventions do not generally solve the problem. SSRIs have been shown (in imperfect studies) to increase the risk of falls in the elderly, so reducing or discontinuing fluoxetine is prudent. She should be monitored for symptoms of depression while her antidepressant therapy is tapered. Answer "A," discontinuing warfarin, may be appropriate if she continues to fall but this action is not likely to reduce her fall risk. Answer "B," the use of bed and chair alarms, is helpful when patients have cognitive impairment and cannot remember to ask for help when getting up; however, these devices can act as tethers to further restrict a patient's movement. Likewise, further restriction of activities and mandatory wheelchair use may lead to deconditioning, loss of muscle strength, and an increased risk of falls. A CT scan of the head may be warranted if the patient sustained a head injury or had an abnormal neurological exam.

* *

Over the next year, you observe a steady decline in your patient's function, with a series of falls despite interventions. Ultimately, your patient has a devastating thromboembolic stroke, which results in right hemiparesis and dysphagia. After a short hospital stay, she returns to the nursing home and undergoes therapy. She continues to have difficulty with her swallowing but is able to tolerate thickened liquids without aspirating. She has a 5% weight loss over the next 2 months, and her nurse reports poor oral intake. Her medications are now warfarin, furosemide, acetaminophen, calcium carbonate, and lisinopril.

In this malnourished, elderly nursing home patient, which of the following interventions or diagnostic studies will most likely lead to improvement in her condition?

A) Admit to the hospital and initiate parenteral feeding.
B) Refer for esophagogastroduodenoscopy (EGD).
C) Screen for depression.
D) Add megestrol acetate.
E) Obtain a complete blood count (CBC).

Discussion

The correct answer is "C." Depression is one of the most common causes of weight loss in the nursing home, and stroke survivors are at high risk for depression. Also, this patient has a history of depression with no current treatment. Consider using a screening tool, such as the Geriatric Depression Scale. A positive screen requires further investigation. Now that she is bedridden, falls are not as much of an issue, so an SSRI may be appropriate. Answer "A" is incorrect. We are not sure of the patient's wishes regarding intravenous (IV) nutrition, and more conservative measures should be instituted before considering parenteral nutrition. Answer "B" is incorrect. While an EGD may be important at some point, proceeding to EGD immediately is premature. Answer "D," megestrol acetate, has been reported to improve food intake in patients with cancer cachexia, but its value in the nursing home is questionable, and it may be associated with an increased risk of mortality. Answer "E" is also incorrect. Evidence of chronic infection or anemia could be found on a CBC, but no signs or symptoms of infection (besides weight loss) are present.

HELPFUL TIP: The initial evaluation of a nursing home patient with weight loss should focus on medication review, gastrointestinal (GI) symptoms, dental and mouth problems, swallowing dysfunction, ability to feed oneself, and psychiatric disorders (e.g., depression, dementia, or psychosis). Hyperthyroidism, hyperparathyroidism, malignancy, and chronic infection should be considered as causes of weight loss (albeit less likely). Factors associated with aging, such as decreased olfaction, taste, and salivation (and nursing home food), may decrease the enjoyment of eating.

* *

You diagnose depression and initiate treatment. Also, you encourage the nursing staff to observe your patient while eating and assist her if necessary. You add a daily multiple vitamin. Her mood improves slightly and her weight stabilizes. However, over the next 6 months, your patient becomes more withdrawn and spends most of her time in bed. Because of her stroke, she is not very mobile, and she requires assistance with transfers and movement in bed. Ultimately, she develops a skin ulcer on her sacrum. Nursing staff reports a sacral pressure ulcer measuring 3 × 2 cm. There appears to be some interruption of the epidermis, like an abrasion.

According to conventional staging criteria, what stage is this pressure ulcer?

A) Stage I.
B) Stage II.
C) Stage III.
D) Stage IV.

Discussion

The correct answer is "B." Pressure ulcers (in older parlance, decubitus ulcers, pressure sores, or bed sores) are caused by unrelieved pressure resulting in damage to underlying tissue. Anatomic areas of concern in bed-bound patients include sacrum, coccyx, heels, and occiput. Chair-bound patients are more likely to develop ulcers over the ischial tuberosities. Risk factors for pressure ulcers include advancing age, immobility, moisture (e.g., urinary or fecal incontinence), malnutrition, and decreased sensory perception. Ulcers are staged by clinical appearance (see Table 21–1).

* *

Because of miscommunication within the nursing home staff, the ulcer goes untended over the weekend. An alarmed nurse calls you to report full-thickness skin loss.

You arrange to visit the patient in the evening . . . here comes another "above and beyond" award.

In the meantime, you prescribe what treatment?

A) Foam pad with occluding dressing (e.g., Allevyn).
B) Wet-to-dry dressing.
C) Topical antibiotics.
D) Transparent, occlusive dressing (e.g., Tegaderm).
E) Chemical enzyme debridement (e.g., Accuzyme).

Discussion

The correct answer is "A." In treating pressure ulcers, there are several principles to follow: relieve pressure, protect the wound and surrounding skin from further trauma, maintain a clean wound bed, provide a moist wound environment, eliminate dead space, control exudates, ensure adequate nutrition, and diagnose and treat infection. Your patient's ulcer has worsened and is now Stage III. Without further information, foam dressing is a safe choice for initial treatment of a Stage III ulcer. Foam pads are useful for deeper wounds with moderate exudate and may also protect the wound from further pressure. In most cases, the wound should be kept moist, so wet-to-dry

Table 21–1 PRESSURE ULCER STAGES

Stage I	Stage II	Stage III	Stage IV	Unstageable
Nonblanchable erythema Intact skin Changes in skin temperature, consistency, or sensation	Partial- thickness skin loss Epidermis and/or dermis Presents as abrasion, blister, or shallow crater	Full- thickness skin loss Damage or necrosis of subcutaneous tissues, extending to underlying fascia Presents as deep crater	Full- thickness skin loss Extensive destruction, tissue necrosis, or damage to muscle, bone or supporting structures	Ulcer covered in eschar and depth unknown

dressings are not appropriate. If moist gauze packing is used, it should be kept moist with intermittent reapplication of saline or changed before drying. From the nurse's report, there is no evidence of necrosis, excessive drainage, or infection, so debridement and antibiotics may not be helpful at this time. A transparent, occlusive dressing is used for Stage II ulcers, but is insufficient for Stage III or IV. In addition to dressing the wound, you should employ the following measures: repositioning every 1–2 hours, pressure-relieving mattress and cushions, and optimizing nutrition. Consultation with a wound care specialist or a surgeon may be necessary if these measures fail.

HELPFUL TIP: There is evidence of benefit from electrical stimulation of pressure ulcers, but there is minimal supporting evidence for the use of other adjunctive therapies (ultrasound, hyperbaric oxygen, ultraviolet light, vasodilators, vacuum devices, etc.).

HELPFUL TIP: To prevent pressure ulcers, schedule regular and frequent repositioning for bed and chair-bound individuals. Turn at least every 2–4 hours on a pressure-reducing mattress or every 2 hours on a nonpressure-reducing mattress. Also, maintain the head of the bed ≤30 degrees if possible to reduce pressure on the sacral area.

Which of the following statements is NOT true about the evaluation and treatment of pressure ulcers?

A) A pressure ulcer covered by eschar cannot be staged until the eschar is removed.
B) If a pressure ulcer shows no signs of healing over 2 weeks, one should reevaluate wound management strategies and reexamine factors affecting the wound.
C) One should consider osteomyelitis or deep soft-tissue infection in a wound that is not healing.
D) Wound cultures should be obtained routinely to target antibiotics toward the organisms found.
E) In an otherwise clean wound that is not healing as expected, one should consider empiric therapy with topical antibiotics.

Discussion

The correct answer is "D." The routine culturing of pressure ulcers is not recommended. Antibiotics are generally not useful since the organisms found are polymicrobial colonizers and not responsible for infection. Obviously, this does not hold true for patients with a true infection, and empiric therapy with topical antibiotics is indicated if a wound shows no improvement with good wound care.

Objectives: Did you learn to . . .

- Manage insomnia in elderly nursing home residents?
- Develop an approach to the problem of falls in nursing home residents?
- Identify nursing home residents at risk for malnutrition?
- Develop a treatment plan for malnutrition in the institutionalized elderly?
- Diagnose, evaluate, and manage pressure ulcers in the nursing home setting?

QUICK QUIZ: VACCINES

A 65-year-old male presents for a routine visit and you recommend pneumococcal vaccination (23-valent polysaccharide vaccine, Pneumovax). Your patient asks what the vaccine is supposed to do.

According to the best available evidence, you are able to say:

A) "This vaccine will reduce your risk of pneumococcal bacteremia."
B) "This vaccine will reduce your risk of pneumococcal pneumonia."
C) "This vaccine will reduce your risk of all types of pneumonia."
D) "This vaccine will reduce your risk of death from influenza."
E) "This vaccine will do all of the above."

Discussion

The correct answer is "A." The 23-valent polysaccharide pneumococcal vaccine has only been shown effective in reducing the risk of pneumococcal bacteremia and meningitis. The vaccine does not appear to reduce the risk of pneumonia in general or even pneumococcal pneumonia in particular. Influenza vaccination decreases the risk of death due to influenza, but pneumococcal vaccination does not.

QUICK QUIZ: HORMONES AND AGING

Noticing advertisements for testosterone treatment to "make you a vital man again," one of your vivacious older female patients asks about testosterone for her husband wondering if it can make him 50 years old again.

Regarding sex hormone changes associated with aging, which of the following is true?

A) Leydig cells in the testes increase with aging.
B) Total testosterone levels increase with aging.
C) Sex hormone binding globulin levels increase with aging.
D) Follicle-stimulating hormone levels are unchanged with aging.
E) Luteinizing hormone levels decrease with aging.

Discussion

The correct answer is "C." Sex hormones in males over age 40 demonstrate declining total testosterone at a rate of 1–2% per year. Simultaneously, sex-hormone binding globulin increases, resulting in a sharper decline in bioavailable testosterone. In response to low testosterone, follicle-stimulating and luteinizing hormone levels increase. Leydig cells (responsible for producing testosterone) decrease in number. Older males with subphysiologic testosterone levels are at increased risk of sexual dysfunction, osteoporosis, diminished lean body mass, and depression. Although controversial, some experts recommend testosterone supplementation in symptomatic males with low serum testosterone. Testosterone supplementation may (notice the word "may") improve strength, lean body mass, depressed mood, bone mineral density, and sexual function in aging males with documented low testosterone levels. Side effects of testosterone supplementation in older males include liver dysfunction, dyslipidemia, erythrocytosis, prostate tissue growth, acne, gynecomastia, and edema.

HELPFUL TIP: Any time you see the word "may," think "may not." They are logical equivalents.

CASE 2

A 79-year-old female patient, well known to you from 5 years of treating her hypertension, presents to your office with concerns about her vision and hearing. Over the last year, she has noticed worsening vision in her left eye. She denies eye pain, tearing, and redness. She wears bifocals and last had an eye exam 3 years ago. At that time, she recalls her eye doctor saying her vision was "stable." Also, her gynecologist recently retired and she would now like you to assume that care.

Which of the following is true regarding common visual problems in older adults?

A) Initial symptoms of macular degeneration include decreased visual acuity and central visual field distortion.
B) Cataracts are less common in the older population than is macular degeneration.
C) Symptoms of open-angle glaucoma are dramatic and manifest early in the disease.
D) Initial symptoms of central retinal artery occlusion include severe pain and sudden loss of vision.
E) If a cataract is detectable on physical exam, it should be removed.

Discussion

The correct answer is "A." By age 65, approximately one person in three has some form of eye disease that results in vision loss. The most common cause of ***blindness*** in older Americans is age-related macular degeneration (AMD). The disease typically presents with loss of vision in the central field with preservation of peripheral vision. Answer "B" is false. Cataracts are more common than is macular degeneration. However, the availability of cataract surgery in the United States has reduced cataract-related vision loss in older Americans so that, even though cataracts are more common, they are less likely than AMD to cause blindness. Worldwide, cataracts are the leading cause of visual impairment. Surgery is indicated when vision loss due to the cataract is interfering with function—not simply because the physician discovers the cataract, so "E" is incorrect. Open-angle glaucoma, the most common form of glaucoma, progresses slowly over time. Significant visual field loss may occur, but is only recognized late in the disease. Central retinal artery occlusion presents with sudden onset of painless monocular blindness. Severe eye pain and loss of vision would be more consistent with acute closed-angle glaucoma.

Which of the following is TRUE of AMD?

A) Among African Americans, AMD is the most common cause of blindness.
B) Risk factors for AMD are similar to those for cardiovascular disease.
C) Risk factors for AMD are similar to those for cataracts.
D) Only nonexudative ("dry") AMD is amenable to treatment with laser photocoagulation.
E) AMD only affects peripheral vision.

Discussion

The correct answer is "B." Risk factors for AMD include age, hypertension, smoking, and previous history of cardiovascular disease. Also, blue eye color and family history appear to predispose persons to AMD. Answer "A" is incorrect. Among African Americans, glaucoma—not AMD—is the most common cause of blindness. Answers "C" and "D" are incorrect. AMD is divided into nonexudative ("dry") and exudative ("wet") AMD. The exudative type is far less common but causes most of the severe vision loss due to AMD. Also, certain patients with exudative AMD benefit from laser photocoagulation, whereas those with nonexudative AMD do not. Finally, "E" is incorrect since AMD causes central visual field deficits.

* *

Your patient performs poorly on a Snellen eye chart visual acuity test, and you decide to refer her to a local ophthalmologist. She then complains that she is less socially active in the last year. Her son thinks she is depressed because she talks on the phone with him less than she did a year ago. Your patient thinks these problems are related to a loss of hearing.

Regarding presbycusis (age-related hearing loss), which of the following is true?

A) Presbycusis usually results in unilateral hearing loss.
B) Presbycusis usually results in low-frequency hearing loss.
C) Presbycusis usually results in loss of speech discrimination.
D) Presbycusis usually results in major depression.
E) Sensorineural presbycusis does not respond to hearing aid use.

Discussion

The correct answer is "C." Presbycusis is present in one-third of patients over 65. Presbycusis typically presents with bilateral high-frequency hearing loss and loss of speech discrimination; patients complain of difficulty understanding rapid speech, foreign accents, and conversation in noisy areas. Types of presbycusis include conductive, sensorineural, mixed, and central hearing loss. While some patients may experience depression with hearing loss, the majority do not. Hearing aids are underutilized in presbycusis but are potentially beneficial for most types of hearing loss, including sensorineural hearing loss. Other devices, such as a portable amplifier with microphone and earpiece (e.g., PocketTalker™), can be used to improve hearing function, especially for one-on-one conversations.

> HELPFUL TIP: Hearing loss, and sensory impairments in general, can be confused with cognitive impairment or an affective disorder. Hearing aids are useful for most cases of presbycusis, but if speech discrimination is <50%, results with hearing aids may be poor.

* *

Your patient asks if medications can cause hearing loss.

Which of the following drugs is NOT associated with sensorineural hearing loss?

A) Ibuprofen.
B) Aminoglycosides.
C) Furosemide.
D) Magnesium salicylate.
E) Acetaminophen.

Discussion

The correct answer is "E." All of these drugs except for acetaminophen can cause hearing loss. Cisplatin, aminoglycoside antibiotics, and loop diuretics have been associated with hearing loss, as have salicylates (e.g., aspirin) and some of the other NSAIDs (e.g., ibuprofen and diflunisal) and chloroquine. This list is obviously not exhaustive.

* *

Your patient (remember she's 79) asks, "Do I have to keep getting mammograms and Pap smears?" She relates a history of normal annual mammograms and Pap smears for the past 20 years. She had a hysterectomy for uterine fibromas and has been monogamous with her husband for 55 years. Her sister died of breast cancer.

Consistent with current guidelines, you recommend:

A) Continue Pap smears and pelvic exams yearly.
B) Discontinue mammography but perform clinical breast exams every 2 years.
C) Discontinue pelvic exams but continue Pap smears.
D) Discontinue Pap smears but continue mammography at 1–2 year intervals.
E) Discontinue all screening tests/exams.

Discussion

The correct answer is "D." Screening decisions in the elderly should be individualized, and the patient's overall health status must be considered. This patient has very little risk of cervical, endometrial, or vaginal cancer (status posthysterectomy for a benign condition, low-risk sexual behavior, and a history of normal exams); therefore, it is reasonable to discontinue Pap smears. Annual pelvic examination is more controversial, with the American Cancer Society (ACS) recommending it as a screening measure for ovarian cancer and the US Preventive Services Task Force (USPSTF) recommending against it. Early detection of breast cancer may result in decreased morbidity and mortality. Screening for breast cancer continues to be recommended for women with a 5–10 years life expectancy, but the optimal interval in older women is unknown. Healthy older women with risk factors, such as this patient, may receive even greater benefit from screening for breast cancer.

* *

Your patient is an overweight white female with no history of bone fracture. She has never had a bone mineral density test and asks if she should have one. You are unaware of any risk factors in her other than Caucasian race and postmenopause status.

What do you tell her?

A) "You are not at risk for osteoporosis and should not be screened."
B) "All women over age 65 should be screened for osteoporosis regardless of risk."
C) "Take 1000 mg of calcium per day to prevent osteoporosis."
D) "Due to your risk factors, you should start a bisphosphonate, vitamin D, and calcium supplementation."
E) "Alcohol use will help decrease your risk of osteoporosis."

Discussion

The correct answer is "B." The USPSTF currently recommends bone densitometry screening for all women age 65 years and older. The National Osteoporosis Foundation recommends bone densitometry for postmenopausal females with one or more of the following risk factors: family history of osteoporosis, personal history of low trauma fracture, current smoking, or low body weight (<127 lbs.). Additional risk factors for osteoporosis include female sex, Caucasian or Asian races, alcohol abuse (thus, "E" is wrong), sedentary lifestyle, and poor intake or absorption of calcium and vitamin D. Smoking is associated with osteoporosis. Diabetes, once thought to protect against osteoporosis, may actually increase the risk of falls and fractures in older adults. The preferred method for measuring bone density is dual-energy radiographic absorptiometry (DEXA). All postmenopausal women should consume 1200 mg of elemental calcium per day in divided doses. The optimal amount of vitamin D is 400–800 IU/day. Weight-bearing exercises also strengthen bone. Bisphosphonates are indicated for treatment of osteoporosis and should not be used without a diagnosis (so "D" is incorrect).

HELPFUL TIP: Supplementing vitamin D is probably more important than supplementing calcium. Calcium supplementation has not consistently demonstrated fracture risk reduction. However, many elderly Americans are vitamin D deficient, and correction of the deficiency results in reduced fracture risk. Given the low risk of adverse effects with daily vitamin D (up to 1000 IU/day), empiric supplementation is justifiable. Finally, 1000 mg (not 1500 mg) of calcium is probably plenty. Additional calcium has been linked to an elevated risk of CAD/MI and no change in fracture risk. Calcium and vitamin D are clearly beneficial in those with osteoporosis, however.

* *

Next, your patient asks whether any of her medications put her at risk for osteoporosis.

Which of the following is LEAST likely to increase the risk of osteoporosis?

A) Glucocorticoids.
B) Anticonvulsants.
C) Sulfonylureas.
D) Loop diuretics.
E) Proton-pump inhibitors.

Discussion

The correct answer is "C." Sulfonylureas do not have a direct effect on bone mineralization. Glucocorticoids and anticonvulsants are known to increase bone turnover, resulting in increased risk of osteoporosis. Loop diuretics cause renal calcium wasting. There is an association between proton-pump inhibitor use and osteoporosis, possibly through reduced calcium absorption or direct effects on bone metabolism. Additionally, heparin, methotrexate, cyclosporin, and gonadotropin-releasing hormone agonists may increase the risk of osteoporosis. Excessive amounts of levothyroxine can cause increased bone turnover. Thiazide diuretics are protective.

* *

Your patient asks what causes osteoporosis.

Although most osteoporosis in women is primary (idiopathic), which of the following cause(s) secondary osteoporosis?

A) Hypoparathyroidism.
B) Multiple myeloma.
C) Estrogen use.
D) Hyperlipidemia.
E) All of the above.

Discussion

The correct answer is "B." About 70% of women have no identifiable cause for osteoporosis and therefore are diagnosed with primary (idiopathic) osteoporosis. Common causes of secondary osteoporosis include chronic corticosteroid use, alcoholism, GI disorders, hyperthyroidism, **hyper**parathyroidism (so, "A" is wrong), multiple myeloma, and primary renal diseases. Hyperlipidemia is not known to be associated with osteoporosis. Estrogen increases bone mineral density.

* *

You encourage appropriate vitamin D and calcium intake as well as weight-bearing exercises. You plan to obtain a DEXA scan.

Using DEXA scan results, osteoporosis is defined as:

A) A T-score of 2.5 standard deviations or more below the mean of a healthy young adult (≤ -2.5).
B) A T-score from 1.0 up to 2.5 standard deviations below the mean of a healthy young adult (−1.0 up to −2.5).
C) A Z-score of 2.5 standard deviations or more below the mean of a healthy young adult (≥ -2.5).
D) A Z-score from 1.0 up to 2.5 standard deviations below the mean of a healthy young adult (−1.0 up to −2.5).
E) None of the above.

Discussion

The correct answer is "A." The T-score compares the patient's bone mineral density to that of young, healthy women (for female patients; male normative data is used for males). Osteoporosis is defined as a T-score of 2.5 standard deviations or more below the mean (≤ -2.5). Osteopenia is defined as a T-score from 1.0 up to 2.5 standard deviations below the mean (−1.0 to −2.5). Answer "C" is incorrect. The Z-score compares bone mineral density to that of age-matched controls. Therefore, it does not reflect the bone loss from baseline in a young healthy female, and it is not used for diagnosis. Answer "D" is incorrect for the same reason.

If you find that your patient has osteoporosis, you may consider using all of the following drugs to treat her osteoporosis EXCEPT:

A) Bisphosphonates (e.g., alendronate and risedronate).
B) Estrogens.
C) Progesterone (e.g., Provera and Depo-Provera).

D) Vitamin D and calcium.
E) Calcitonin.

Discussion

The correct answer is "C." Progesterones are not indicated for the treatment or prevention of osteoporosis. In fact, in young, healthy, premenopausal women, they are associated with a decrease in bone mineral density. This is because they suppress estrogen production (such as with Depo-Provera). All of the other options are acceptable choices and have FDA approval for the treatment of osteoporosis.

* *

She returns to discuss her test results, and her bone density is very low with her hip T-score −3.2. You diagnose her with osteoporosis. "Are my bones like Swiss cheese?" she asks. *No*, you think. *Swiss cheese has more calcium*.

Given that she is otherwise relatively healthy, what is the most appropriate initial therapy for her osteoporosis?

A) Alendronate (Fosamax) 70 mg PO weekly.
B) Estrogen (e.g., Premarin) 0.625 mg PO daily.
C) Teriparatide (Forteo) 20 μg SC daily for 5 years.
D) Zoledronic acid (Reclast) 5 mg IV every 3 months.
E) None of the above. What's the point anyway? Her bones are half dust.

Discussion

The correct answer is "A." Bisphosphonates are the treatment of choice for osteoporosis. Alendronate, risedronate, and zoledronic acid have all been shown to reduce the risk of vertebral and hip fractures in persons with osteoporosis. Ibandronate only appears to lower vertebral fracture risk; therefore, it should not be your first choice. Side effects of bisphosphonates include hypocalcemia (more likely with IV administration and in patients with vitamin D deficiency), nausea, esophagitis, osteonecrosis of the jaw (usually at higher doses, such as those used to treat cancer), and atypical femur fractures. Although you might be tempted to choose "D," zoledronic acid, due to this patient's more severe osteoporosis, there is no clear evidence that zoledronic acid is more effective than oral bisphosphonates. The IV route should be reserved for when the patient has failed oral bisphosphonate therapy for some reason—usually due to upper GI disease or side effects. Zoledronic acid can cause a "flu-like" illness, with diffuse myalgias and arthralgias for days after the infusion. "B" is incorrect as the safety data for bisphosphonates is superior to that for estrogen. "C" is incorrect for two reasons: teriparatide is not first-line therapy and administration should be for 2 years rather than 5. Teriparatide is a recombinant parathyroid hormone that must be administered by daily injection and carries the potential risk of osteosarcoma, which is the reason its use is limited to 2 years. Teriparatide is effective at increasing bone density and reducing fracture risk, but the data is not nearly as robust as the data for bisphosphonates.

HELPFUL (MAYBE) TIP: It seems as though more than 5 years of a bisphosphonate *may* increase atypical femur fracture risk (thought to be due to the suppression of osteoclast activity and reduced ability of bone to remodel). Therefore, a drug holiday is likely warranted. Additionally, many patients maintain bone density after stopping a bisphosphonate after 5 years of therapy—at least for a few years. There are not clear guidelines on this yet. Consider getting a DEXA scan a couple of years after stopping the bisphosphonate. If it shows bone loss, consider restarting the bisphosphonate.

HELPFUL TIP: News flash! Denosumab (Prolia) is a RANKL inhibitor that was approved by the FDA for treatment of postmenopausal osteoporosis in 2011. It appears to be effective in reducing fracture risk (vertebral and hip). It also appears well tolerated. However, it interacts with RANKL in the immune system, and the long-term effects on infection and carcinogenesis are unknown, so stay tuned...

* *

Before she leaves the office, you present your patient with literature on living wills and durable power of attorney for health care (DPOA-HC).

Which of the following is CORRECT regarding advance health-care planning?

A) The Joint Commission requires that patients be asked about their advance directives on admission to the hospital.

B) A DPOA-HC can override a patient's decision regarding treatment.
C) Once the patient has signed a living will, no further changes can be made regarding treatment decisions.
D) A DPOA-HC must be a family member or blood relative.

Discussion
The correct answer is "A." The Joint Commission requires that patients be asked about their advance directives on admission to the hospital. Advance directives can take many forms but are usually manifest in one of two ways: through a living will or a DPOA-HC. The purpose of a living will is to instruct health-care decision making in future events when the patient may not be able to communicate his or her wishes. These documents often contain brief clinical scenarios with patient preferences for life-sustaining measures. In contrast, a DPOA-HC is not as limited and can address situations not foreseen in a living will. If the patient becomes unable to participate in health-care decision making, then the DPOA-HC is instructed to exercise substituted judgment, using the patient's previously stated health-care preferences, to help direct future care. The DPOA-HC is appointed by the patient and can be a family member or another adult. The DPOA-HC cannot override a patient's decision in health-care matters, as such an action would violate patient autonomy.

> HELPFUL TIP: Although advance directives should be addressed with all patients, it is of particular importance to discuss them in the setting of chronic illness, life-threatening illness, advancing age, and with any deterioration in health status. A patient can change advance care plans whenever he or she wishes, as these decisions may change over time depending on goals of care.

Objectives: Did you learn to . . .

- Identify and implement appropriate preventive health services for older females?
- Diagnose and manage common vision problems in older persons?
- Identify and manage common hearing problems in older persons?
- Discuss issues related to breast and gynecologic cancer screening?
- Define appropriate criteria for osteoporosis screening and identify risk factors?
- Recognize the important and complementary roles of DPOA and advance directives?

QUICK QUIZ: GERIATRIC PREVENTIVE CARE

Which of the following statements is INCORRECT regarding preventive health in older adults?

A) Although the optimal interval for vision screening is undetermined, many professional organizations recommend vision and glaucoma screening every 1–2 years in persons over age 65.
B) In women at high risk for breast cancer, tamoxifen reduces the risk of cancer by almost 50%.
C) The ACS and American College of Obstetrics and Gynecology (ACOG) recommend screening ultrasound for ovarian cancer in all women over the age of 60.
D) Although Pap smears are not generally recommended for elderly women, the distribution of cervical cancer cases is bimodal, with peaks at 35–39 years and 60–64 years.

Discussion
The correct answer is "C." In fact, ACOG, the USPSTF, and the American College of Physicians specifically recommend against ultrasound screening for ovarian cancer in asymptomatic women. All other statements are correct.

> HELPFUL TIP: ACOG recommends transvaginal ultrasound to look for ovarian cancer in women with 2 weeks or more of unexplained urinary frequency or urgency, pelvic or abdominal pain, early satiety or difficulty eating and bloating. It is unclear if these guidelines will be beneficial or harmful (unnecessary surgery, etc.).

CASE 3

An 82-year-old male patient presents to your office for confusion. His wife reports that he was in his usual state of health until 3 days ago. At that time, he developed abdominal pain and felt feverish. He then began to have a dry, hacking cough. On examination, his temperature is 100.3°F and blood pressure is 118/56. He is pale and lethargic but in no acute distress. He is oriented to person only. Other than mild upper abdominal tenderness, there are no additional findings on exam. This patient appears to have a new onset of confusion. You suspect delirium.

Which of the following is true with regard to delirium and dementia?

A) In delirium it is rare to find an underlying medical cause.
B) A primary feature of delirium is inattention.
C) Dementia is characterized by a fluctuating course.
D) The diagnosis of delirium in the elderly requires that the patient has underlying dementia.

Discussion

The correct answer is "B." The Diagnostic and Statistical Manual of Mental Disorders (DSM-IV) provides the diagnostic criteria for delirium. A diagnosis of delirium requires the following criteria: disturbance of consciousness with reduced ability to focus attention; disorientation, memory deficit, or another change in cognition that cannot be accounted for by a preexisting dementia; acute onset with fluctuating course (often changing throughout the day); and evidence that the disturbance is caused by an underlying medical condition or drug use. Not all signs and symptoms of delirium are present in every patient with delirium. Delirium can be confused with dementia, depression, or psychosis. Patients with delirium may present as agitated, psychotic, somnolent, or withdrawn. Dementia is typically more chronic in nature with an insidious onset. Dementia progresses over time and usually cannot be reversed. Often delirium is treatable or reversible if the underlying medical condition is identified. Patients with dementia usually have intact attention, whereas patients with delirium have markedly impaired attention. Patients with dementia have "poverty of thought," which implies decreased content of their thoughts. Patients with delirium may have a rich content to their thoughts, but the thoughts are disordered.

HELPFUL TIP: Delirium may be either hypoactive or hyperactive or both, all in the same patient. Many patients with delirium are not even identified due to their hypoactive state (these aren't the ones screaming obscenities and yanking IV lines). Elderly patients are more susceptible to delirium, and delirium is sometimes the only identifiable symptom in an elder with an acute illness (but, contrary to what we were taught, NOT from a simple urinary tract infection (UTI) without fever).

* *

With further history from the patient's wife, you find that he has coronary artery disease, diabetes mellitus type 2, hypertension, and benign prostatic hyperplasia.

Which of the following is the most useful question to elicit risk factors for delirium?

A) "Does the patient have any drug allergies?"
B) "Does the patient use tobacco?"
C) "Does the patient use alcohol?"
D) "Does the patient have edema?"
E) "Does the patient use acetaminophen?"

Discussion

The correct answer is "C." Studies have consistently identified the following risk factors for delirium: advancing age, preexisting dementia, underlying structural brain disease other than dementia, uncorrected impairment in vision or hearing, multiple chronic illnesses, polypharmacy, the use of physical restraints, history of alcohol abuse, male gender, and functional impairment.

While hypoxia (due to myocardial infarction, pulmonary embolus, or any other source) may lead to delirium, tobacco use alone does not predispose a patient to develop delirium. In isolation, knowledge about edema, acetaminophen use, or drug allergies is less helpful. Questioning about alcohol use will help to identify patients who have a tendency to overuse alcohol, putting themselves at risk for delirium.

HELPFUL TIP: Delirium is characterized by impaired consciousness, whereas dementia is characterized by impaired cognition. However, preexisting dementia greatly increases the risk of delirium, and simply moving a patient with dementia to a new environment can precipitate delirium.

The appropriate evaluation of the patient with delirium includes which of the following?

A) Evaluation of metabolic causes such as electrolytes and glucose.
B) Evaluation for infection such as UTI and pneumonia.
C) Evaluation of a patient's medications.
D) Evaluation of oxygen saturation.
E) All of the above.

Discussion

The correct answer is "E." Causes of delirium are protean, often acting together in a multifactorial manner, and are best considered by a systematic approach. Metabolic causes include electrolyte disturbances (don't forget calcium), hypoglycemia, and hypoxia. Numerous infections may lead to delirium. Neurologic causes include head trauma, meningitis, and vasculitis. Many medications cause delirium, including anticholinergics, antidepressants, sedative–hypnotics, and steroids. Dehydration and prerenal azotemia may lead to delirium. Alcohol intoxication or withdrawal may precipitate delirium as well. See Table 21–2.

* *

You reach for the "shotgun," and order a bunch of tests. The chest radiograph shows a left lower lobe consolidation. The abdominal film shows a nonspecific bowel gas pattern. The white blood cell (WBC) count is 12,700/mm^3, blood urea nitrogen 36 mg/dL, creatinine 1.5 mg/dL, and glucose 150 mg/dL. The remainder of the blood counts and chemistries are normal. With the exception of trace ketones, the urinalysis is within normal limits. Cultures will not be available for at least 24 hours. The ECG shows normal sinus rhythm. With the available information, you decide to admit this patient for treatment of delirium due to pneumonia and dehydration.

You are called in the middle of the night for agitated behavior and noncompliance with nursing care. The patient has pulled out his IV and struck a nurse.

Table 21–2 CAUSES OF DELIRIUM, "WHHHHIMP" MNEMONIC

- Wernicke encephalopathy
- Hypoperfusion
- Hypoglycemia
- Hypertensive encephalopathy
- Hypoxia
- Infection or intracranial bleed
- Meningitis or encephalitis
- Poisons or medications

You appropriately prescribe which of the following interventions?

A) Administer haloperidol 0.5 mg PO.
B) Administer haloperidol 1 mg IV.
C) Apply physical restraints.
D) Administer morphine 5 mg IV.

Discussion

The correct answer is "A." Most of the time, delirium DOES NOT require any pharmacologic treatment. However, this patient is at risk of harming himself and others due to his agitated delirium, so some action must be taken. Agitated delirium causes physiologic and psychologic stress on the patient, results in interference with medical care, and portends a poorer prognosis. The incidence of delirium in hospitalized patients of all ages is 30%, and the incidence in postoperative patients may approach 50%. Agitated delirium should be treated quickly, and haloperidol is the treatment of choice. In older patients, drug clearance decreases, so low doses of antipsychotic medication should be administered initially. ("Start low and go slow.") Increasing doses of oral haloperidol can be given every 30 minutes if the patient continues to have agitation. Answer "B" is incorrect because IV haloperidol is associated with a greater degree of QT prolongation; PO or IM haloperidol is preferred. Answer "C" is incorrect; physical restraints may lead to patient injury and may worsen delirium. Restraints should only be applied when absolutely necessary and for as short a duration as possible. Answer "D" is incorrect because we have no reason to believe the patient is in pain, and administering narcotics could worsen his delirium. However, pain can certainly result in agitation, so keep it in mind.

* *

You reflect on the fact that primary prevention of delirium is probably more effective than secondary prevention. For this patient, delirium must now be treated, but you try to avoid this complication in your hospitalized older patients.

You know that research has shown a reduction in delirium in hospitalized older patients when which of the following strategies is employed?

A) Increased sedative medication use for sleep-deprived patients.
B) Early mobilization for immobilized patients.
C) Cholinesterase inhibitor (e.g., donepezil) therapy for cognitively impaired patients.
D) Physical restraints for combative patients.
E) Music therapy for depressed patients.

Discussion

The correct answer is "B." Identifying risk factors and targeting interventions to reduce or eliminate risk factors can prevent delirium. Because one patient may have numerous risk factors for delirium and because delirium is usually a multifactorial syndrome, a multicomponent intervention strategy is warranted.

An often-cited study by Inouye et al. (1999) demonstrated the effectiveness of this strategy. In the study, sleep-deprived patients received a warm drink, relaxing music, and back massage at bedtime. Unit-wide noise reduction was implemented. Early ambulation and active range-of-motion exercises were employed for bed-bound patients. All patients were encouraged to ambulate. Cognitively impaired patients received orienting stimuli and cognitively stimulating activities. Patients with hearing and visual impairments received portable amplifying devices and visual aids, respectively. Investigators used a protocol for early recognition and treatment of dehydration. There was no specific therapy for depression or combativeness.

Which of the following statements about delirium is true?

A) Bed rails and restraints are effective in preventing injury in the patient with delirium.
B) Atypical antipsychotics (e.g., olanzapine and risperidone) can be used to treat delirium.
C) Diphenhydramine is a good choice for a sleep aid in patients who are prone to developing delirium.
D) A feeding tube (e.g., Dobhoff tube) should be used in the patient who is not eating in order to prevent delirium.
E) None of the above is true.

Discussion

The correct answer is "B." Atypical antipsychotics can be used in the treatment of delirium, but nonpharmacologic methods (e.g., bedside sitter and redirection) should be used first. Answer "A" is incorrect because bed rails and restraints actually increase the risk of injury in the patient with delirium. Answer "C" is incorrect. Diphenhydramine is actually a particularly poor choice because of its anticholinergic side effects, which can exacerbate or cause delirium. A short-acting sedative agent (e.g., zolpidem) or trazodone would be better. Answer "D" is incorrect, as anyone who has done inpatient work knows: the feeding tube and the Foley are often the first to get yanked!

HELPFUL TIP: Ethical dilemmas abound in the treatment of delirium. Atypical antipsychotic use in patients with dementia is associated with increased mortality. Older antipsychotics pose a greater risk for extrapyramidal symptoms when compared with atypicals and may have the same mortality risk. By definition, agitated, patients with delirium cannot provide informed consent, so "implied consent" is usually substituted to use drug therapy for patients with delirium at risk for self-injury and to stabilize critically ill patients with delirium.

Objectives: Did you learn to . . .

- Define delirium?
- Describe the signs and symptoms of delirium?
- Distinguish delirium from dementia?
- Identify causes and risk factors for delirium?
- Treat and prevent delirium?

CASE 4

In the early morning hours, a 78-year-old female presents to the emergency department complaining of right buttock and hip pain. Several hours before her arrival, she fell in the bathroom of her daughter's home. She recalls standing on a floor mat, leaning her head back to drink a glass of water, and then hitting the ground. She denies loss of consciousness. Her daughter was at the scene quickly and found the patient awake, alert, and moving all extremities. Her vital signs are normal. Other than right hip tenderness, her examination is unremarkable.

Which of the following is most likely to assist you in determining the cause of her fall?

A) CT scan of the head.
B) ECG.
C) Additional history.
D) Serum chemistry profile.
E) CBC.

Discussion

The correct answer is "C." If there's an option for "more history," it's usually the right answer. History is one of the most important factors in determining the etiology of a fall. Ten percent of falls in older persons can result in serious injury, such as a hip fracture or subdural hematoma—both of which can be deadly. Falls in elderly patients are typically multifactorial in nature. Randomized clinical trials demonstrate a reduction in the occurrence of falls in community-dwelling elders when health-care personnel engage in a multifactorial risk assessment with targeted management. Such an approach requires a thorough history.

All of the following are risk factors for falls in elderly EXCEPT:

A) Use of four or more medications.
B) Orthostatic hypotension.
C) Attempting tai chi, for which good balance is required.
D) Environmental hazards (e.g., poor lighting or uneven walking surfaces).

Discussion

The correct answer is "C." In fact, doing tai chi has been shown to reduce the risk of falls in the elderly. All of the others listed increase the risk of falling. Additional risk factors for falls include history of a fall in the last year, impaired balance and gait, poor vision (acuity <20/60), decreased muscle strength, and syncope or arrhythmia. Still more risk factors: poor lighting, lack of grab bars and handrails, cluttered floor, restraint use, and improper bed height.

During your examination, which of the following physical maneuvers is most likely to assist you in evaluating the risk of future falls?

A) Get-up-and-go test.
B) Test for pulsus paradoxus.
C) Osler maneuver.
D) Lumbar spine flexibility test.
E) Test for nystagmus.

Discussion

The correct answer is "A." The "Timed Get-Up-and-Go-Test" is a commonly used method of assessing disability and fall risk in geriatric assessment. From a seated position, the patient is instructed to stand up, walk 3 m (approximately 10 ft), turn around, and return to her chair. An adult with no disability should be able to complete this test in <10 seconds. Increasingly longer time to perform the test is associated with increasing fall risk. While performing the test, assess the patient's sitting balance, transition from sitting to standing, gait, and steadiness and quickness with turning. While potentially useful in the evaluation, the other tests listed are not directly associated with fall risk.

* *

After a thorough history, you perform a complete workup, including ECG, radiology studies, and appropriate laboratory tests. You find that the fall was caused by environmental factors (poor lighting and a loose throw rug) rather than an organic cause intrinsic to the patient. Fortunately, x-ray of her hip is negative for fracture. The patient asks how exercise might help her avoid future falls.

Which of the following is the best answer?

A) Physical therapist supervision is essential to have an effective fall prevention program.
B) In elderly patients, the effect of exercise on falling is unknown.
C) Strength training has a greater effect than balance training on reducing fall risk.
D) Unsupervised balance and strength training is effective in reducing fall risk.
E) Group exercise is more effective than exercising alone to prevent falls.

Discussion

The correct answer is "D." There is no particular type of exercise that seems to prevent falls to a greater degree than any other type of exercise. Strength, balance, and gait training all appear to be important. Exercise programs have been shown to benefit elders at risk for falls. Although initial instruction by a therapist may be helpful, a physical therapist need not supervise all exercises. Patients are able to perform exercises targeted toward fall prevention at home, and they do not need to be part of an exercise group. A meta-analysis of the Frailty and Injuries: Cooperative Studies of Intervention Techniques (FICSIT) trials found that combined balance and strength training reduces the risk of falls in community-dwelling elders.

> HELPFUL TIP: Peripheral sensory disturbance is a common finding in the elderly and may increase the risk of falling. A common cause of peripheral neuropathy is vitamin B12 deficiency. Elevated blood levels of methylmalonic acid and homocysteine are more sensitive for detecting vitamin B12 deficiency than low blood levels of the vitamin.

* *

You recommend strength and balance exercises to the patient, but she is worried and says, "My heart's too old for exercise."

You assure her that light exercises are safe and then review normal age-related cardiovascular changes, which include:

A) Reduced ventricular compliance.
B) Reduced maximal heart rate.
C) Reduced response to sympathetic nervous stimulation.
D) Increased atrial filling.
E) All of the above.

Discussion

The correct answer is "E." Even in the healthy elderly without signs of vascular disease, there are important changes in the cardiovascular system. Maximum cardiac output is reduced, mostly through reduced maximal heart rate; thus the equation:

$$\text{Estimated maximal heart rate} = 220 - \text{age}$$

Additionally, there is reduced response to sympathetic stimulation, with less chronotropic and inotropic response to stress. Reduced ventricular compliance results in increased atrial filling volume and pressure, increased left atrial size, and increased dependence on atrial contraction for ventricular filling. However, endurance training may improve cardiac output, and active older adults have a higher cardiac output compared with sedentary persons of the same age.

> HELPFUL TIP: Hip fractures in the elderly are often caused by falls. In general, the sooner that a fractured hip is repaired, the better the outcome. Ideally, a hip should be repaired within the first 24 hours after the injury.

* *

Because of her right hip pain, you consider giving the patient an ambulatory device for temporary use. She has good upper extremity strength, can bear some weight on the right, but needs improved stability.

Which of the following devices would be most appropriate in this setting?

A) Wheeled walker.
B) Forearm crutches.
C) Walk cane (hemi-walker).
D) Imperial walker.
E) Multiple-legged cane (quad cane).

Discussion

The correct answer is "E." Ambulatory devices are employed with the following goals: improve mobility, decrease the risk of falling, and relieve discomfort associated with acute or chronic musculoskeletal and neurologic conditions. An inappropriately selected device can increase energy expenditure and the risk for falls. Canes widen a patient's base, resulting in increased stability. They are typically used for balance, not weight bearing. Multiple-legged canes—called "quad canes" because of the presence of four tips—provide a more stable base and some weight bearing, when compared with standard, single-tipped canes. Walk canes are useful for patients who require full weight bearing on one arm, as in a stroke survivor with loss of lower extremity function. Crutches, either forearm or axillary, are used for patients who cannot bear any weight on one leg.

Walkers can support a patient's weight, provide lateral stability, and expand a patient's support base. Standard walkers, those with four rubber tips, provide the greatest support and are helpful in cases of ataxia. Front-wheeled walkers are useful for patients with a fast gait, such as a festinating gait in Parkinsonism. Also, a front-wheeled walker is easier to manipulate than a standard walker. Four-wheeled walkers should be used when the patient requires some increased stability but does not need as much weight bearing as a standard walker would provide. Patients with mild-to-moderate Parkinson disease may benefit from four-wheeled walkers. In this case, the patient requires only improved stability and slight assistance with bearing weight. Of the available choices, the multiple-legged cane is the best option. A single-tipped cane may have been a reasonable choice as well. If you chose answer "D," you—like one of the editors—are a *Star Wars* nerd.

* *

Unfortunately, you do not have access to a multiple-legged cane for your patient. But you do have a supply of adjustable single-tipped aluminum canes available.

If you were to provide her with a cane, what method would you use to fit the cane?

A) Allow the patient to fit the cane length to her comfort level.
B) Select a device with a length equal to the distance from the floor to the greater trochanter of the femur.
C) Fit the cane length so that the handle comes to rest at the patient's waist.
D) Select a device with a length equal to the distance from the floor to the fingertips with the arm relaxed.

Discussion

The correct answer is "B." You should fit a cane for a patient by selecting a device that reaches from the floor to the greater trochanter of the femur. Another option is to fit the cane so that it reaches the flexor crease of the wrist when the arm is extended to the side. A properly fitted ambulatory device should be comfortable, allowing the patient to stand erect without excessive forward flexion of the spine. Excessive forward flexion occurs when the device is too short and can result in increased risk of falling. Also, to obtain maximum efficiency from the upper extremities, the device should not be too long. The usual recommendation is to have a device fitted so that the elbow is flexed at 15–30% when the cane is in use. This is done by measuring as noted above.

Objectives: Did you learn to . . .

- Recognize the morbidity associated with falls in older people?
- Evaluate causes and risks of falls in this population?
- Implement appropriate interventions for falling patients?
- Assess gait abnormalities that may lead to falls?
- Select ambulatory devices for appropriate patients?

QUICK QUIZ: ASSISTIVE DEVICES

If a patient is having difficulty walking due to left-sided leg weakness after a recent stroke, in which hand should a cane be used?

A) Left hand.
B) Right hand.
C) Either hand.
D) No cane should be prescribed; a wheelchair is preferred.

Discussion

The correct answer is "B." Whenever a cane is used to support lower leg function limited by weakness or pain, the cane should be used in the hand *contralateral* to the affected side (left side weak, right hand gets the cane). This enables the patient to maintain normal arm swing while advancing the cane and the affected leg at the same time to reduce the weight-bearing forces on the affected limb during the step.

CASE 5

A 69 year old female with no complaints presents to you office with her two daughters. Further history from her daughters reveals that the patient was widowed 4 years ago, now lives alone, and has experienced memory loss over the last 2 years. One daughter has taken over the patient's checkbook and is responsible for paying the bills. She has noticed that her mother often wears the same clothes and bathes infrequently—new habits for her. The past medical history includes hypothyroidism and hypertension. Family history is significant for depression and memory problems in the patient's mother prior to her death from "old age." The patient takes chlorthalidone, levothyroxine, and acetaminophen as needed.

Physical examination reveals a thin, elderly female in no distress. She is alert but does not correctly identify the year. She describes her mood as "happy" most of the time. The remainder of the exam is unremarkable. You suspect dementia.

Which of the following is true regarding the diagnosis of dementia?

A) The diagnosis is rarely missed in the primary-care setting.
B) To diagnose dementia, impairment in executive function must be present.
C) To diagnose dementia, impairment in memory must be present.
D) Alzheimer disease (AD) is a diagnosis of exclusion.
E) Neuroimaging is essential in the diagnosis of dementia.

Discussion

The correct answer is "C." One of the necessary components in order to make a diagnosis of dementia is memory impairment. Answer "A" is incorrect. In contrast to delirium and depression, the onset of dementia is insidious. Symptoms often go unrecognized for months to years prior to diagnosis. Although the patient may complain of confusion or memory loss, family members are more likely to provide the chief complaint and history. During the initial phases of a dementing illness, patients and family members may attribute cognitive changes to normal aging. In early cognitive impairment, memory symptoms may wax and wane. However, symptoms of dementia can be differentiated from occasional normal lapses based on their increasing severity. For example, it is normal to forget an acquaintance's name, but clearly abnormal to forget a spouse's name. Answer "B" is incorrect. Many patients with dementia have impaired executive functioning (e.g., judgment, reasoning, and planning), but the presence of impaired executive functioning is not a requirement. Answer "D" is incorrect, as AD is diagnosed by a specific set of clinical criteria. DSM-IV provides diagnostic criteria for dementia and AD, making AD a diagnosis of inclusion rather than exclusion. Answer "E" is incorrect. Dementia is a clinical diagnosis and does not require neuroimaging for confirmation. Experts and professional medical associations differ in their recommendations regarding the use of neuroimaging in dementia. In general, neuroimaging is recommended if dementia occurs in the following scenarios: onset before age 65, sudden onset, presence of focal neurologic signs, and suspicion of normal pressure hydrocephalus (NPH).

* *

You use several office assessment tools to further characterize the memory loss. She scores 23/30 on the Folstein Mini-Mental State Exam, missing orientation and recall items. Clock drawing is grossly abnormal. Her Geriatric Depression Scale is 3 positive responses out of 15 (positive screen is 5/15 or greater). She performs all basic activities of daily living (ADLs) independently, but has voluntarily given up driving and control of her finances.

Regarding assessment tools used in the evaluation of memory loss, which of the following statements is most accurate?

A) The Mini-Mental State Exam (MMSE) evaluates executive function and visual-spatial skills.
B) Formal neuropsychological testing offers no benefit over the MMSE for detecting dementia.
C) The use of a screening tool for depression is not helpful in the evaluation of memory loss.
D) Clock drawing evaluates executive function and visual-spatial skills.

Discussion

The correct answer is "D." Clock drawing can be used to evaluate executive function as well as visual-spatial skills. **Clock drawing is a simple test that takes 1 minute or less to perform.** The patient is asked to draw a clock face and set the hands to 2:50 or 11:10. This test requires planning and visual-spatial ability on the part of the patient—two areas that are incompletely evaluated by the MMSE. A normal clock does not rule out dementia, but an abnormal clock is suggestive of cognitive impairment. There are several scoring systems, and the sensitivity and specificity for dementia are as high as 87% and 82%, respectively.

"A" and "B" are incorrect. The MMSE is a 30-point scale, with the cutoff for dementia between 24 and 26. The MMSE can be performed in a few minutes and tests memory, orientation, language, construction, and concentration. The MMSE does not test prosody (expressive and receptive inflection of vocalization) or executive function and, as a result, has poor sensitivity for early cognitive impairment in some individuals. Performance on the MMSE is strongly correlated with education; therefore, there may be false-positives in undereducated patients and false-negatives in highly educated individuals. Compared with the MMSE, formal neuropsychological testing assesses a broader array of cognitive functions, and it identifies behavioral abnormalities and assesses mood disorders. It can also help to differentiate between types of dementia. In general, neuropsychological testing is the most sensitive and specific cognitive assessment tool, but it is time consuming and requires a high level of expertise to administer and interpret.

Answer "C" is incorrect because depression may cause memory problems, especially in the elderly, and depression screening should be included in the workup of memory concerns. Depression often coexists with dementia, and treatment of depression may improve memory problems.

* *

So far, you have collected the following information on this patient: MMSE score 23/30, impairment in driving and managing finances, disorientation to time, but intact abilities to cook, clean, and care for herself.

Using conventional staging for AD, how would you categorize this patient's dementia?

A) Mild.
B) Moderate.
C) Severe.
D) Terminal.
E) Insufficient information to determine the stage.

Discussion

The correct answer is "A."

- Mild AD symptoms include impaired memory, mild personality changes, and mild disorientation. (MMSE 19–24)
- Moderate AD symptoms include aphasia, apraxia, insomnia, and increasing confusion. (MMSE 10–19)
- Severe AD symptoms include severe memory loss, motor impairment, and loss of some basic ADLs (e.g., urinary incontinence and feeding difficulties). (MMSE <10)
- Symptoms of terminal AD include immobility, dysphagia, and increasing susceptibility to infections.

Which of the following findings would most likely cause you to search for a diagnosis other than AD in a patient presenting with memory impairment?

A) Paranoid behavior.
B) Apraxia.
C) Bradykinesia and rigidity.
D) Aphasia and personality changes.

Discussion

The correct answer is "C." Bradykinesia and rigidity are features of Parkinsonism, which, in the setting of memory loss, should prompt consideration of Lewy body dementia or Parkinson disease. Paranoid behavior, delusions, and hallucinations can all occur with more severe AD. Aphasia, apraxia, and personality changes typically occur later in AD but can be initial complaints in atypical presentations of AD.

In order to diagnose dementia, impairment in memory must be present. Additionally, a patient must display at least one of the following cognitive disturbances: aphasia (language disturbance), apraxia (impaired motor abilities despite intact motor function), agnosia (impaired ability to identify objects despite intact sensation), and disturbance in executive function (e.g., planning, judgment, and insight). Finally, the diagnostic criteria for dementia require that these cognitive disturbances result in functional impairments that represent a significant change from a previous level of functioning.

* *

Although you strongly suspect AD in this patient, you consider other types of dementia as well. Suppose this patient presented with urinary incontinence and ataxia in addition to her current findings.

Which of the following diagnoses would be most likely?

A) Creutzfeldt–Jakob disease.
B) Lewy body dementia.

C) Normal pressure hydrocephalus (NPH).
D) Pick disease.
E) Brain rot.

Discussion

The correct answer is "C." NPH classically presents with dementia, gait ataxia, and urinary incontinence. When detected early, it responds to ventriculoperitoneal shunting and is thus a reversible cause of dementia. However, the dementia is rarely fully reversible. Gait abnormalities typically occur first and are the most likely to improve with removal of cerebrospinal fluid (CSF). The diagnosis of NPH is supported by findings on brain MRI, and it is confirmed by symptom improvement after CSF removal. Incidentally, NPH is a misnomer since intermittent CSF pressure elevations have a pathophysiologic role in the disease. If you chose "E," brain rot, you may suffer from it, but this patient does not. Keep reading to learn why the other foils are wrong.

* *

You've got this patient stuck in your head (perhaps with superglue?). On morning rounds in the hospital, your colleague asks your opinion on a patient with frontotemporal dementia (FTD).

You think it unlikely that your patient has FTD because she does not have:

A) Depression.
B) Disinhibition.
C) Hemiplegia.
D) Rapidly progressing dementia.
E) Tremors and hallucinations.

Discussion

The correct answer is "B." FTDs (including Pick disease) constitute a heterogeneous group of neurodegenerative disorders that have the common pathologic finding of cortical degeneration in frontal areas of the brain. Typical features of these dementias include an insidious onset and a slowly progressive course. Patients have impairments in judgment and insight. They are disinhibited and socially inappropriate. Patients may present with anxiety, depression, delusions, or emotional indifference. Answer "A" is incorrect. Depression frequently coexists with many types of dementia but does not define one particular type. Answer "C" is incorrect; the presence of hemiplegia in a patient with dementia should bring to mind vascular causes. Answer "D" is incorrect because rapidly progressing dementia is the hallmark of prion disease, such as Creutzfeldt–Jakob disease. Answer "E" is incorrect as tremors, hallucinations, and memory loss are consistent with Lewy body dementia (named for its characteristic pathological finding—the presence of Lewy bodies in the brain stem and cortex). Clinical features consist of cognitive impairment, detailed visual hallucinations, fluctuation in alertness, and motor symptoms of Parkinsonism.

HELPFUL TIP: AD is the most common form of dementia, encompassing about 60% of patients with dementia. Vascular and Lewy body dementias account for about 15–30%. In many cases, dementia has more than a single cause. AD and vascular dementias frequently coexist—an entity commonly referred to as "mixed dementia."

* *

The elevator is stuck on your way back from making your rounds, giving you more time to consider dementia.

Which of the following is NOT consistent with the diagnosis of vascular dementia?

A) Diabetes.
B) Tobacco use.
C) Diffuse slowing or normal electroencephalogram (EEG).
D) Normal brain MRI.

Discussion

The correct answer is "D." A normal MRI essentially rules out vascular dementia. Features suggestive of vascular dementia include a stepwise deterioration in cognitive function, onset of cognitive impairment with stroke, infarcts and white matter changes on neuroimaging, and focal neurologic findings on examination. There are no well-defined criteria for clinically diagnosing vascular dementia, and available rating scales have poor predictive value when compared with autopsy as the diagnostic standard. A history of vascular risk factors, such as diabetes, hypertension, and smoking, supports the diagnosis.

* *

Finally back in your office with coffee in hand, you decide to evaluate for reversible causes for this patient's dementia, and you consider ordering laboratory tests.

Which of the following lab tests is NOT indicated in the initial evaluation for reversible causes of dementia?

A) Cyanocobalamin (vitamin B12).
B) Liver enzymes.
C) CBC.
D) CSF analysis.
E) Thyroid function tests.

Discussion

The correct answer is "D." When evaluating a newly diagnosed case of dementia, one must consider infectious, metabolic, toxic, and inflammatory etiologies. Therefore, the minimal required laboratory tests should include CBC, serum glucose and electrolytes, vitamin B12, and renal, liver, and thyroid function tests. Further laboratory tests should be obtained as clinical suspicion indicates. In the appropriate patient, one might obtain urinalysis, urine toxicology screen, HIV antibody assay, and CSF analysis. Because of the extremely low incidence of neurosyphilis, routine testing for syphilis is no longer required but should be considered in the appropriate setting. Neuroimaging is not a required part of every workup but may be helpful in some patients. See Table 21–3.

Table 21–3 LABORATORY EVALUATION OF DEMENTIA

Required Minimum Testing
- Complete blood count
- Serum glucose and electrolytes
- Vitamin B12
- Renal function tests
- Liver function tests
- Thyroid function tests

Testing Based on Clinical Suspicion
- Neuroimaging (recommended for all patients by some societies)
- Urinalysis
- Urine toxicology screen
- HIV antigen/antibody assay
- CSF analysis
- RPR or VDRL

* *

Blood chemistries, blood counts, thyroid hormone levels, vitamin B12 level, and liver enzymes are in the normal range. A noncontrast CT scan of the brain shows nonspecific "age-related" changes. The patient and her family return to discuss the test results. You begin to educate them about AD and dementia in general. The two daughters are concerned that other family members may be at risk for developing AD.

Which of the following is the strongest risk factor for developing AD?

A) Age.
B) Apolipoprotein E 4 (APOE 4) allele.
C) Family history.
D) Head trauma.
E) Low educational level.

Discussion

The correct answer is "A." As with many diseases, age is the greatest risk factor for developing AD. Among persons 65–69 years old, the incidence of AD is 1%. In persons 85 years and older, the incidence rises to 8%. All of the other answer options are associated with an increased risk of AD but not to the same degree as age.

Family history is another factor strongly associated with developing AD. By age 90, almost half of persons with first-degree relatives with AD develop the disease. There are genetic risk factors as well. Mutations on chromosomes 1, 14, and 21 are known risk factors for AD. Trisomy 21 is a risk factor for developing AD at an earlier age (often by age 50). APOE 4 allele increases risk and decreases age-of-onset of AD in a dose-related fashion, with the greatest risk present in persons homozygous for APOE 4.

Other potential risk factors include a history of head trauma, lower educational achievement, female gender, and depression. Postmenopausal estrogens may actually increase the risk of dementia. Hypertension, diabetes, and hyperlipidemia are associated with dementia, and controlling these diseases might reduce the risk of developing dementia in the future, but the evidence is not strong. Increased physical, mental, and social activities may reduce cognitive decline in later years.

The patient and family ask about medications to treat AD. Which of the following statements is TRUE?

A) All studies show that vitamin E supplementation improves cognition and prevents further neuron loss in AD.
B) Ginkgo biloba and cholinesterase inhibitors have a synergistic effect, improving cognition in AD.
C) Cholinesterase inhibitors do not prevent neuron loss in AD.
D) Cholinesterase inhibitors maintain cognition at baseline levels for 2 years after initiation of therapy; after that time, patients decline slowly.

Discussion

The correct answer is "C." Cholinesterase inhibitors do not prevent neuron loss. Results with vitamin E have been inconsistent, and some studies have found a slightly **higher** risk of death in those on high-dose vitamin E ($\geq$400 IU/day), primarily in those with coronary artery disease. Given the low cost and potential benefits of vitamin E, it may still be reasonable to use in combination with a cholinesterase inhibitor in AD at a dose of $<$400 IU/day if the patient or family is so inclined. There is no strong evidence to support the use of ginkgo biloba in AD.

As of December 2011, there are just two classes of drugs available to treat AD. Cholinesterase inhibitors (e.g., donepezil, rivastigmine, galantamine, and tacrine) represent the larger class of available pharmacotherapy used to treat mild-to-moderate AD. Studies suggest that decline may stabilize for 3–6 months after which there is steady loss of cognition. By 9–12 months, there is no difference in decline between those on therapy and those on placebo. The other class has only one medication, memantine, which is an N-methyl D-aspartate (NMDA) antagonist used to treat moderate-to-severe AD. NMDA antagonists work differently from cholinesterase inhibitors, and so the two types of drugs can be prescribed in combination. However, there seems to be no benefit to combining these drugs.

> HELPFUL TIP: All of the cholinesterase inhibitors have similar efficacy. Tacrine is known to cause hepatotoxicity and is rarely used. The choice of cholinesterase inhibitor depends on cost, patient acceptance, and physician experience.

You decide to start the patient on a cholinesterase inhibitor.

In your discussion about the medication, you tell the patient and her family:

A) "These drugs are indicated for treating all types of dementia."
B) "These drugs offer no benefit in moderate to severe dementia."
C) "These drugs are proven to reverse memory loss."
D) "These drugs are proven to reduce mortality."
E) None of the above.

Discussion

The correct answer is "E." There is no shortage of controversy when it comes to medications for dementia. One thing is certain: there is evidence that cognitive loss and progressive behavioral problems can be slowed with cholinesterase inhibitors in any stage of dementia. However, whether these changes are clinically significant is arguable. While statistically significant, the changes with drugs are clinically meaningless. There is no change to ADLs, time to nursing home placement, etc. Answer "A" is incorrect. Mostly, these drugs are used in AD. Their use in Lewy body and vascular dementia is off-label but may be worth a try; there is some data to support cholinesterase inhibitors for these patients. However, there is no evidence to support their use in FTDs (e.g., Pick disease). Patients with FTDs should be treated symptomatically (with antipsychotics, a controlled, low-stimulus environment, etc.). Answer "B" is not true. Most studies of cognitive effects of cholinesterase inhibitors have occurred in mild-to-moderate dementia (MMSE 10–24). While there may not be any effect of these drugs on cognition in severe, end-stage dementia, there may be some benefit in patient behavior and function. Answer "C" and "D" are incorrect. Compared with placebo, cholinesterase inhibitors are found to delay further cognitive and functional decline but neither reverse dementia nor affect mortality. In cholinesterase inhibitor studies of mild-to-moderate dementia, there is typically a 3-point difference on the MMSE between treatment and placebo groups at 6 months. This finding is due to a loss of thinking abilities in the placebo group and a delay in that loss in the treatment group.

> **HELPFUL TIP:** Not every confused elderly person should be put on a cholinesterase inhibitor. Consider the diagnosis, severity of disease, and the goals for the patient.

* *

One month after starting your cholinesterase inhibitor of choice, the patient returns concerned about a possible side effect.

All of the following are well-recognized side effects of cholinesterase inhibitors EXCEPT:

A) Tachycardia.
B) Nausea, vomiting, and diarrhea.
C) Anorexia.
D) Exacerbation of asthma and COPD.

Discussion

The correct answer is "A." All of the above except for tachycardia are well-documented side effects of the cholinesterase inhibitors. In fact, they have a "vagotonic" action, which can cause bradycardia and syncope and worsen cardiac conduction abnormalities. To minimize adverse events, the dose of cholinesterase inhibitor should be increased only after the patient has been on a stable dose for 4–6 weeks.

The side effects of cholinesterase inhibitors are symptoms often seen in nursing home patients (e.g., falls due to bradycardia and anorexia). If your patient is losing weight and not eating, consider discontinuing the cholinesterase inhibitor and see if she improves.

* *

One year later, the patient returns with her daughter, with whom she now lives. The daughter reports disturbing symptoms that occur nightly. The patient wakes up in the middle of the night and wanders the house, becoming confused and agitated. With a subtle nod toward her mother, the daughter states, "I just can't take much more of this."

After inquiring about pain and any changes in health status and finding none, your initial recommendation is to:

A) Employ soft restraints only during the night.
B) Consider environmental changes including more daytime structured activities through an adult day care center.
C) Initiate an antipsychotic before bedtime.
D) Initiate a sedative–hypnotic before bedtime.

Discussion

The correct answer is "B." Treating behavioral issues in patients with AD can be very challenging. Further history must explore the possibility of pain-related agitation, decline in comorbid conditions or new health conditions, such as occult infection, and any medication changes that may be playing a role. If a treatable cause is not identified, then environmental change is the best initial recommendation. Adding structured daytime activities may facilitate a better sleep wake cycle. Adult day care programs exist that specialize in day care for elderly people including patients with dementia. Adult day care can provide structured activities during the day, along with respite for the daughter who is obviously asking for extra support. Although medications are sometimes needed, answers "C" and "D" are incorrect for initial treatment in this case. Once environmental changes have failed or there are other immediate health risks involved, then medications may be necessary. Antipsychotics currently offer the only drug treatment for behavioral symptoms in dementia; however, there are no great choices. Haloperidol, risperidone, and olanzapine are used most often. See Table 21–4 for selected medications used to treat behavioral symptoms in dementia. Sedatives, such as benzodiazepines, often result in paradoxical agitation in elderly patients with dementia. Answer "A" is incorrect. Restraints should be avoided in most cases, even soft restraints. Although they are sometimes required to prevent harm to the patient or caretakers, restraints are known to result in worsened agitation and an increased risk of fall and injury.

> **HELPFUL TIP:** When patients with Lewy body dementia receive antipsychotic medication for hallucinations, Parkinsonian features become much more pronounced. If possible, avoid antipsychotics in these patients.

* *

Haloperidol, or "vitamin H," nightly has resolved the agitation. Although you may have increased your patient's risk of dying (as seems to occur when

Table 21–4 MEDICATION MANAGEMENT FOR BEHAVIORAL SYMPTOMS OF DEMENTIA

Behavioral Subtype	Acute Management	Long-Term Management
Psychosis	Conventional High Potency Antipsychotic (CHAP)[a]	Risperidone, CHAP
Anxiety	Benzodiazepines	Buspirone
Insomnia	Trazodone	Trazodone
Sundowning	Trazodone; consider CHAP, risperidone, olanzapine	Trazodone; consider CHAP, risperidone, olanzapine
Aggression, severe	CHAP, risperidone	Divalproex, risperidone, CHAP
Aggression, mild	Trazodone	Divalproex, SSRIs, trazodone, buspirone

[a] CHAP includes haloperidol, perphenazine, and fluphenazine. For elderly patients with dementia, typical doses should be about one quarter of the usual dose (e.g., risperidone 0.25 mg, olanzapine 2.5 mg, or quetiapine 25 mg, and haloperidol 0.25–0.5 mg).

antipsychotics are used in dementia), her daughter is thrilled with the result. Three months later she returns with concerns about depression. The patient spontaneously cries several times per day, her appetite is poor, and she has no desire to leave the house or even get dressed most days.

Since a pill worked last time, her daughter wants to know what antidepressant is most effective for depression in patients with dementia?

A) Citalopram.
B) Mirtazapine.
C) Sertraline.
D) None of the above.

Discussion

The correct answer is "D." There are very few quality studies available to guide treatment of depression in patients with dementia. The available evidence shows no difference between antidepressant therapy and placebo. The diagnosis of depression in a patient with dementia is complicated, since dementia causes apathy, sleep disturbance, appetite loss, and social withdrawal. If depression is suspected in a patient with dementia, a prudent approach would be to employ nonpharmacologic therapy and then provide an empiric trial of an antidepressant.

* *

Over time, as the patient's dementia progresses, you reevaluate end-of-life issues and advance directives. With the support of her family, the patient decides not to have cardiopulmonary resuscitation.

In end-stage AD, which of the following is correct?

A) Malnutrition is the most common cause of death in patients with severe dementia.
B) Hospitalization for pneumonia in patients with severe dementia improves morbidity and mortality.
C) In severe dementia, gastrostomy tube feeding prevents aspiration.
D) To increase comfort, dehydrated patients with severe dementia should receive IV hydration.
E) In advanced AD, treatment of infections with oral and IV antibiotics is equally efficacious.

Discussion

The correct answer is "E." Hospitalization for demented patients with pneumonia is a wash. The number of patients saved by the use of IV antibiotics is offset by an increase in death and functional deterioration as a result of the hospitalization. Thus, on balance, oral and IV antibiotics are equally efficacious in the treatment of infections in these patients; therefore, severely homebound patients with dementia or nursing home residents should be treated in their usual environment rather than hospitalized if the family agrees. Answer "A" is incorrect. The majority of patients with dementia die of infection, not malnutrition. Answer "B" is incorrect as noted above. Answer "C" is incorrect. Even in moderate-to-severe AD, feeding tubes can be useful in the acute setting. But the tube should be removed and natural feeding resumed as soon as the acute event passes. **Permanent gastrostomy tube feeding is not recommended in**

patients with severe or terminal dementia. Tube feeding does not prolong life, prevent aspiration, or promote weight gain in advanced dementia. Although many patients with advanced dementia are malnourished and dehydrated, these conditions do not appear to cause discomfort.

> HELPFUL TIP: Remember the caregivers! Ask about their health and mood. Twenty-five percent of caregivers to the elderly are depressed, while older people caring for their disabled spouses have a 63% higher chance of dying than noncaregivers of the same age.

Objectives: Did you learn to . . .

- Identify symptoms, signs, and diagnostic criteria for dementia?
- Describe different types of dementia and how they are diagnosed?
- Evaluate the patient with dementia, considering the potential causes of dementia?
- Describe potential benefits and limitations of current pharmacologic therapy for AD?
- Describe the natural course of AD?
- Manage a patient with end-stage AD?

CASE 6

A 71-year-old male whom you have known since starting your practice recently suffered a stroke, resulting in language deficits and right hemiparesis. His medical history is significant for hypertension, hyperlipidemia, ulcer requiring partial gastrectomy (remote), and coronary artery disease. He quit tobacco and alcohol 5 years ago. He is retired and widowed. After a 3-day hospitalization, he appears stable enough for discharge. His medications include aspirin, atenolol, lisinopril, and atorvastatin. Prior to entering a nursing home to receive skilled nursing care and therapies, the patient wants to know who will pay for the services. He has Medicare parts A and B.

You are able to assure him:

A) Medicare will cover all expenses indefinitely regardless of personal financial resources.
B) Medicaid will cover **all** of the expenses for the first 100 days of skilled care regardless of personal financial resources.
C) Medicare will cover **part** of the expenses for the first 100 days of skilled care regardless of personal financial resources.
D) Medicare requires a hospital stay of 7 days or longer prior to entering a nursing home for skilled care.
E) Medicaid and Medicare do not cover nursing home expenses under any circumstances.

Discussion

The correct answer is "C." Medicare Part A, which provides some health care for patients 65 years and older if they qualify for Social Security benefits, will pay all costs for skilled care for the first 20 days and part of the costs thereafter up to a total of 100 days per calendar year. This Medicare benefit includes rehabilitation (e.g., physical therapy, occupational therapy, and speech therapy) and skilled nursing care (e.g., nursing home, skilled care facility, and rehabilitation hospital) after a hospital stay of at least 3 days. This benefit is contingent upon the patient having an appropriate diagnosis and rehabilitation potential, and continuing to show improvement during the time the benefit is in place. Medicare does not provide extended nursing home coverage. Medicaid will provide extended nursing home care if a person's assets and income are below a certain threshold, which varies from state to state. Note: Although Medicare Part B will pay for physician visits to nursing home patients, Medicare does not pay for nursing or other care directly related to permanently living in a nursing home.

* *

Although he received fairly intensive physical, occupational, and speech therapies, your patient does not regain much function. He has only minimal movement in the right arm and complains of pain in the right shoulder. A radiograph of the right shoulder shows degenerative changes. Despite maximal doses of acetaminophen administered regularly, your patient continues to complain of shoulder pain. You involve physical therapists in his care to reduce the risk of chronic dislocation of the shoulder.

In order to control his pain, which of the following is the most appropriate to add as a scheduled, and presumably chronic, medication?

A) Acetaminophen.
B) Oxycodone.
C) Gabapentin.

D) Aspirin.
E) Naproxen.

Discussion

The correct answer is "A." Acetaminophen is the safest analgesic of those listed. It may provide sufficient pain relief. If it does not, then another medication may be added, possibly a narcotic in this patient. Answer "B" is incorrect as a first step as narcotics can cause confusion, sedation, urinary retention and falls, and they have been associated with an increased mortality risk in the elderly. However, this patient has a history of an ulcer, and a narcotic analgesic may be a reasonable medication to add after acetaminophen. Answer "C" is incorrect. Gabapentin is indicated for postherpetic neuralgia and is more useful for neuropathic pain (although not very useful there either; TCAs are better). "D" and "E" are incorrect. Aspirin and NSAIDs-like naproxen must be used with caution in the elderly due to increased risks of silent GI bleeding, fatal GI bleeding, and kidney injury. NSAIDs are typically not first-line agents for arthritis pain in this age group and probably offer no greater pain relief than acetaminophen. Nonpharmacologic modalities should be employed as well, including massage, exercises, and physical therapy.

* *

A nurse calls to report that your patient has developed lethargy, decreased appetite, and a temperature of 37.8°C. Your first thought is, "So? That's not a fever."

And then you realize that:

A) An elevated temperature in older persons is most often due to changes in basal body temperature regulation.
B) Oral antibiotics will not be sufficient to treat this infection.
C) Antibiotics will not be necessary to treat this condition.
D) Absence of significant fever in the elderly does not rule out serious bacterial infections.

Discussion

The correct answer is "D." Older persons, especially frail elders and nursing home patients, often have lower basal body temperatures compared with younger persons and may not mount as great a febrile reaction to infection. A temperature >38.1°C in a frail elder is most likely associated with a serious bacterial or viral infection. Absence of significant fever does not rule out serious bacterial infections. "C" is incorrect. With the available information, it is difficult to say with any certainty if the patient has an infection treatable with antibiotics. If he did, oral antibiotics are often appropriate in the nursing home setting, even when treating pneumonia.

* *

With a decline in his function and a mildly elevated temperature, you plan to evaluate this patient for infection. According to the nursing staff, there are no other residents with apparent infections. Your patient has not developed any focal symptoms (e.g., cough, dysuria, diarrhea, and site-specific pain).

Which of the following tests will be LEAST helpful?

A) CBC.
B) Urinalysis and microscopic exam of the urine.
C) Stool culture.
D) Chest radiograph.
E) Blood oxygen saturation (pulse oximetry).

Discussion

The correct answer is "C." He is not having diarrhea so a stool culture is not likely to be of benefit. This is not a black-or-white area, but there are some principles and expert opinions to follow. First, know that the most common infections in nursing home residents originate in the urinary tract, respiratory tract, skin, soft tissue, and GI tract. Patient and family wishes regarding care must be known prior to initiating an evaluation, therapy, or hospital transfer. While the elderly may have a serious infection with only slight or even no leukocytosis, a normal WBC count on CBC will reduce suspicion for serious bacterial infection. Even without specific urinary symptoms, urinalysis is recommended because of the high incidence of UTI in this population (but remember that asymptomatic bacteriuria is also common in this setting). Blood oxygen saturation below the normal range (<90% on room air) may indicate serious respiratory illness; in the setting of hypoxia, a chest radiograph is recommended. If the infection is isolated to one resident who does not have GI symptoms, stool culture is unlikely to help.

Regarding infectious diseases in nursing home settings, which of the following is correct?

A) If the influenza vaccine is administered within 24 hours of an outbreak, patients require no further prophylaxis.
B) All residents who are carriers of methicillin-resistant *Staphylococcus aureus* (MRSA) must be treated with appropriate antibiotics.
C) Most cases of bacteremia are caused by infected skin ulcers.
D) New residents should receive a two-step tuberculin skin test, unless positive on the first test.
E) All residents who are carriers of *Clostridium difficile* must be treated with appropriate antibiotics.

Discussion

The correct answer is "D." The incidence of tuberculosis is relatively high in the older population, as is mortality from the disease. Institutionalized elders should be screened for tuberculosis with the two-step tuberculin skin test. A two-step test involves repeating the tuberculin skin test 1–3 weeks after an initial negative test ($<$10 mm induration). Anergy testing is no longer recommended. The test is positive if the induration is 10 mm or more.

Answer "A" is incorrect. In a nursing home, an influenza outbreak can have devastating results, with a mortality rate up to 30%. In the event of an outbreak, even residents who received the vaccine should receive antiviral prophylaxis (see Chapter 8 for more). Only about 50% of nursing home residents will develop an adequate antibody response to the influenza vaccine, and that response takes up to 2 weeks after administration to develop.

Answers "B" and "E" are incorrect. Residents who are carriers of MRSA or *C. difficile* will not benefit from eradication if they are not infected. In addition, they may return to a carrier state quickly after antibiotic treatment; therefore, antibiotic treatment of these carrier states is not recommended. Answer "C" is incorrect because UTIs are the most common cause of bacteremia in nursing home residents.

HELPFUL TIP: In elderly nursing home residents, a positive response to tuberculin skin testing is most often due to reactivation of old disease. Risk factors associated with reactivation of tuberculosis include chronic steroid use, diabetes, malignancy, malnutrition, renal failure, and chronic institutionalization.

HELPFUL TIP: A recent addition to the influenza prevention armamentarium is the high-dose influenza vaccine (e.g., Fluzone-HD) that has four times the usual dose of antigen and was approved for adults $\geq$65 years by the FDA in 2009. Seroconversion rates are higher for patients receiving the higher dose vaccine, but it has not shown a morbidity or mortality benefit. The cost is higher than that of the other options, side effects are similar, and its role is not well established.

* *

Over the next year, the patient has increasing difficulty with cognition. He begins to experience urinary incontinence several times per day, necessitating the use of a pad. A midstream clean-catch urinalysis shows bacteria and WBCs (2–4 WBC/hpf) but is negative for glucose and nitrites. His postvoid residual bladder volume is 80 cc.

Which of the following is true regarding the potential cause of and therapeutic intervention for urinary incontinence in this patient?

A) The most likely cause is obstruction from the benign prostatplasia, and an alpha-blocker will improve the incontinence.
B) The most likely cause is immobility, and scheduled voiding is indicated.
C) The most likely cause is detrusor hyperactivity, and an indwelling catheter is indicated.
D) The most likely cause is stress incontinence, and pelvic floor muscle strengthening (Kegel exercises) is indicated.
E) The most likely cause is bacteriuria, and antibiotics will improve the incontinence.

Discussion

The correct answer is "B." Urinary incontinence is incredibly frequent in nursing home residents, with a rate of up to 50%. As with many other geriatric syndromes, incontinence is often multifactorial or the result of decreased function. A frequent cause of urinary incontinence in nursing home residents is immobility due to severe physical impairment, dementia, or both. In this setting, the initial treatment of choice is prompted voiding every 2 hours when the patient is awake. Also, fluid and caffeine intake should be monitored and adjusted to reduce urine output without causing dehydration.

Answer "A" is incorrect. Although there is no information about the patient's prostate size, he has a relatively normal postvoid residual volume, making overflow incontinence from outlet obstruction less likely. Answer "C" is incorrect—or at least the diagnosis of detrusor hyperactivity cannot be made on the basis of current information. The patient has not been fully evaluated with urodynamic tests, so it is difficult to determine whether his incontinence is stress-type or urge-type. If he has urge-type incontinence due to detrusor hyperactivity, an indwelling bladder catheter is not appropriate. Detrusor hyperactivity can often be treated successfully with pharmacotherapy.

Answer "D" is also not likely. Stress incontinence is less common in men than women, and urine loss is typically associated with increased abdominal pressure (e.g., coughing, sneezing, and lifting). Finally, "E" is incorrect. The presence of bacteria in the urine is a common finding in nursing home patients. In general, bacteriuria without symptoms—other than incontinence—should not be treated. Studies have demonstrated little or no improvement in incontinence after treating asymptomatic bacteriuria.

> HELPFUL TIP: When urinary incontinence is due to obstruction or detrusor **hypo**reflexia, intermittent bladder catheterization should be employed and chronic indwelling catheters avoided. Appropriate indications for chronic indwelling bladder catheters in the nursing home include comfort care of the terminally ill, presence of skin wounds contaminated by incontinent urine, and urine retention not practically managed with intermittent catheterization.

* *

Although his urinary incontinence improves, your patient develops difficulty with loose stools and occasional fecal incontinence. The stools are quite watery with no blood or melena. Aside from occasionally abdominal cramping, he feels well. He has no new neurologic symptoms.

Which of the following is the most likely cause of fecal incontinence in this situation?

A) Infectious diarrhea.
B) Ulcerative colitis.
C) Decreased anal sphincter tone.
D) Fecal impaction.

Discussion

The correct answer is "D." In nursing home residents with limited physical mobility, overflow incontinence due to fecal impaction is most likely. Nursing home patients are often taking medications that contribute to constipation as well. Even with a stool softener and/or a laxative, constipation may still result. A fecal impaction can be treated with an enema, stool softeners, laxatives, and dietary changes, but sometimes requires manual disimpaction. Decreased sphincter tone may occur as a result of neurologic insult, but this patient was previously continent of stool. Although infection might be causing incontinence, there are no other symptoms of infection. The onset of inflammatory bowel disease is usually seen in younger populations, often with blood in the stools, making ulcerative colitis less likely.

* *

As a result of your patient reporting physical abuse of another patient by the nursing staff, an investigation is under way in the nursing home.

Reflecting on elder abuse and neglect, you realize which of the following is true?

A) Up to 75% of nursing aides in nursing homes have seen or heard of a resident being abused or neglected.
B) A "dependent elder" is defined as anyone living in a nursing home.
C) Approximately 70% of elder abuse and neglect occurs in nursing homes.
D) There is a universally accepted definition of elder abuse and neglect, which is codified in federal law.
E) Elder abuse is widely defined as "purposeful physical harm of anyone over the age of 65 years."

Discussion

The correct answer is "A." In some studies, high rates of mistreatment have been found in nursing homes, with up to 75% of nursing aides witnessing or hearing about acts of abuse. However, it is not known whether nursing home residents are at greater risk than community-dwelling dependent elders. Answer "B" is incorrect. The definition of "dependent elder" is not consistent, and may apply to elders who are cognitively impaired, physically debilitated, or financially dependent. Nursing home residents are frequently dependent; however, living in a nursing home itself is not sufficient to establish that a person is a dependent elder. Answers "C" and "D" are incorrect. The study of elder abuse and neglect (also referred to as elder mistreatment) suffers from lack of a universally accepted definition, variations in laws between states, and inherent difficulties in obtaining accurate reports of abuse. Therefore, attempts to determine the incidence of elder abuse and neglect have resulted in wide variations. Answer "E" is incorrect. Elder abuse may include physical harm, sexual abuse, psychological abuse, neglect, or financial exploitation. Although all states now have laws addressing elder mistreatment, those laws vary between states, and health-care providers are encouraged to know the law in their area.

HELPFUL TIP: Risk factors for elder mistreatment include older age, cognitive impairment, substance abuse, low socioeconomic standing, minority status, and caregiver stress (probably the most important).

* *

As your patient's cognitive impairment progresses, he becomes more withdrawn and uncooperative with nursing care, such as bathing. A nurse calls to ask, "Shouldn't he be on risperidone or something to improve his behavior?"

According to the Omnibus Budget Reconciliation Act of 1987 (OBRA), antipsychotic medication is indicated for demented patients with:

A) Repetitive, bothersome behavior (e.g., name calling).
B) Continuous crying out and screaming.
C) Uncooperative behavior (e.g., refusing to eat and bath).
D) All of the above.

Discussion

The correct answer is "B." One goal of OBRA was to decrease the inappropriate use of antipsychotic medications in nursing home residents. In patients with dementia, antipsychotic medications may be appropriately administered in the following settings: agitated, belligerent acts that present a danger to the patient or other residents; psychotic symptoms (delusions, hallucinations, paranoia); and continuous crying out and screaming (lasting 24 hours or longer). Attempts to redirect the patient should always be employed first. You should also attempt to uncover occult causes of agitation, such as infection or pain. Once behavior control is attained, assess whether the antipsychotic can be reduced in dose or discontinued. According to OBRA, **inappropriate** indications for antipsychotic medication include restlessness, uncooperative behavior, poor self-care, and repetitive, and bothersome actions.

Objectives: Did you learn to . . .

- Describe some common Medicare/Medicaid reimbursement issues for nursing home care?
- Manage chronic pain in the nursing home?
- Describe an appropriate evaluation for the nursing home resident with fever?
- Recognize infectious disease issues commonly presenting in the nursing home?
- Develop an appropriate strategy for the evaluation and management of urinary and fecal incontinence in nursing home residents?
- Recognize the impact of elder abuse and neglect?
- Implement appropriate measures for agitated behavior in the nursing home?

QUICK QUIZ: GERIATRIC PHARMACOTHERAPY

Which of the following is true about drug therapy in the elderly?

A) GI absorption is substantially decreased in the elderly.
B) Sedative–hypnotic drugs should be given an 8-week trial without interruption for anxiety in the elderly.
C) Mirtazapine (Remeron) causes anorexia and weight loss in the elderly.
D) Compared with young adults, the volume of distribution of fat-soluble drugs is increased in the elderly.

Discussion

The correct answer is "D." The volume of distribution of fat-soluble drugs is relatively increased in the elderly due to a loss of muscle mass and proportionately more fat mass. Therefore, fat-soluble drugs, like diazepam, have a greater relative volume of distribution, while water-soluble drugs, like alcohols, will have a relatively smaller volume of distribution. Answer "A" is incorrect because drug absorption does not change substantially with aging. Sedative–hypnotic drugs should be used only for short-term therapy of 2–4 weeks because of the risk of falls and other adverse effects; this is true for both community-dwelling elders and those in nursing homes. Answer "C" is incorrect because mirtazapine can actually increase appetite and lead to weight gain in the elderly. For this reason, it can be useful in patients who are depressed and not eating well.

HELPFUL TIP: Although hepatic drug metabolism does not change substantially with age, drugs tend to have decreased elimination in the elderly as a result of decreased renal function. For these reasons, the half-life of many sedative–hypnotic drugs is substantially increased in the elderly.

CASE 7

Your next patient is an 83-year-old male familiar to your clinic, who presents for routine care. He has hypertension, hyperlipidemia, and osteoarthritis. He has been widowed for 10 years and continues to live independently in an apartment in the same town as his daughter. He stopped smoking 30 years ago, but continues to drink alcohol. He denies any problems related to his drinking, but you inquire anyway and ask specifically how much he drinks. His routine includes three shots of whiskey per day. He says he likes drinking one shot before his daily walk and the other two shots after he returns. He finds the routine very motivating and keeps him in shape.

In regard to his drinking behavior, you are aware that:

A) Older adults accumulate significantly lower blood alcohol levels than younger adults due to decreased absorption.
B) Drinking three shots per day should not be any concern as long as his liver function tests are normal.
C) Alcohol consumption can reduce the availability of nutrients such as zinc, vitamins A, B1, B2, B6, B12, and folate.
D) The lifetime prevalence of alcoholism for men age ≥65 is less than 5%, but should still be screened for routinely.
E) The standard screening CAGE questionnaire for drinking problem behavior has not been validated in older adults.

Discussion

The correct answer is "C." Alcohol consumption can reduce the availability of nutrients such as vitamins A, B1, B2, B6, B12, zinc, and folate. Alcoholic patients often present with malnutrition, poor self-care, and alcohol-related illnesses such as anemia, peptic ulcer disease, diabetes, hypertension, liver disease, neuropathy, and mental status changes. Checking for deficiencies may be warranted in this situation depending on your patient's other dietary intake. Answer "A" is incorrect. Older adults accumulate significantly higher blood alcohol levels than younger adults. A young adult's blood alcohol level will be approximately 0.03% after "one drink" (1.5 ounces of distilled liquor, five ounces of wine, or 12 ounces of beer), while in a 75-year-old, the level may rise as high as 0.08% that is the legal limit for intoxication in many states. **Answer "B" is incorrect. Drinking behavior should be questioned regardless of liver function tests. Further evaluation of potentially harmful drinking behavior** (≥2 drinks/day for women, or ≥3 drinks/day for men) is recommended. The National Institute on Alcohol Abuse and Alcoholism has identified drinking more than one alcoholic beverage daily as potential drinking problem in older adults. Answer "D" is incorrect. The lifetime prevalence of alcoholism for men age ≥65 is higher, approximately 14% for men and 1.5% for women age ≥ 65. Denial of the problem is more frequent in older patients, and impairments in functioning related to alcohol use may not be recognized until serious complications arise. Answer "E" is incorrect. Diagnosis of alcohol abuse and dependence in older adults is challenging. Brief screening tools such as the CAGE questionnaire (Table 21–5) have been validated in the older population and could be used in this situation. A positive response to any CAGE questions suggests

Table 21-5 CAGE SCREENING TOOL FOR PROBLEM DRINKING

C: Have you ever felt you should **C**ut down?
A: Does others' criticism of your drinking **A**nnoy you?
G: Have you ever felt **G**uilty about your drinking?
E: Have you ever had an "**E**ye opener" to steady your nerves or get rid of a hangover?

Positive response to any suggests drinking problem; questionnaire has been validated in older population.

drinking problem. In this case, your patient denies any drinking problems and his CAGE screen is negative.

* *

You advise him to cut back to 1 drink per day or less and plan to follow up. As you review the patient's basic ADLs and instrumental activities of daily living (IADLs), he is independent in all basic ADLs and most IADLs. He walks daily, eats three small meals per day and maintains a steady weight around 180 lbs (BMI = 25 kg/m^2). He manages his own finances, prepares his own meals, but usually has his daughter do the grocery shopping for his convenience. When you ask about transportation, he reports that he mostly drives to get around town to the golf club, social events, and the post office when needed. He denies any vision or hearing problems.

In order to keep him healthy, safe, and functional, you appropriately recommend:

A) Indoor walking only.
B) Weight loss.
C) Periodic screening for hearing impairment.
D) Restricted driving.

Discussion

The correct answer is "C." As of 2011, the USPSTF was in the midst of updating its 1996 recommendation, which was to perform rudimentary office screening for hearing loss in older adults. The Institute of Medicine recommends audiometric testing once each during ages 40–59, 60–74, and 75 and over. In this case, asking about hearing difficulty and testing with a whispered-voice out of the field of vision periodically is a reasonable approach for hearing screening. Answer "A" is incorrect. Daily exercise including walking indoors or outdoors in safe environments (weather permitting) should be encouraged in all age groups. Answer "B" is incorrect. His current weight is adequate, and he is at risk for malnutrition if he has drinking problem, so he does not need to lose weight. Answer "D" is incorrect. Safety is a concern due to the increasing number of older drivers, their high crash rate per mile driven, and their increased likelihood of serious injury and death. However, most seniors prefer automobile transportation to keep active in the community and should continue to drive. In this case, without specific concerns, there is no need to recommend restricted driving.

HELPFUL TIP: If you are concerned about driving safety, ask direct questions about any recent driving problems, such as minor accidents, traffic violations, getting lost, or difficulty with parking. The legal requirements about physician reporting of unsafe older drivers vary from state to state, but the AMA has published a great guide, available online and updated in 2010, called "Physician's Guide to Assessing and Counseling Older Drivers" (http://www.ama-assn.org/ama/pub/category/10791.html) It covers the law in each state.

* *

One month later, your patient's daughter calls to inform you that he fell and broke his left hip while vacationing with the family in California. He had total hip arthroplasty (THA) and is still in the hospital recovering. Now they are trying to make arrangements to bring him home. The discharge planner has identified a local nursing home that can provide rehabilitation, but some of the family would like for him to return to his apartment.

In regard to recovery after hip surgery, you inform the daughter that:

A) Rehabilitation after hospital discharge results in better outcomes for patients with hip fracture.
B) Rehabilitation can only be provided inpatient at a hospital or nursing home, not at home.
C) Surgical repair in elderly patients should be delayed if possible (>72 hours after injury) to reduce 1-year mortality and other complications.
D) Early mobilization after hip surgery is recommended in younger patients, but in older patients weight bearing is usually delayed at least 5 days after surgery to allow proper healing.

Discussion

The correct answer is "A." Studies show that rehabilitation immediately after hospital discharge appears to result in superior outcomes for patients with hip fracture or stroke. Answer "B" is incorrect. Rehabilitation can be provided in either inpatient (i.e., hospital or skilled nursing facility) or outpatient settings (clinic, day hospital or home). For inpatient care, patients must be able to participate in rehabilitation that includes a minimum of 3 hours of therapy 5 days per week. Care usually involves an interdisciplinary team including nurses and various therapists. Home-based services can provide part-time or intermittent therapy as prescribed by a physician. Answer "C" is incorrect. Early surgical repair (<24 hours after fracture) is ideal and has been shown to reduce 1-year mortality and complications such as pressure ulcers and delirium. Delay for medically unstable patients may be necessary. Answer "D" is incorrect. Early mobilization is the standard of care for both hip and knee arthroplasty in younger and older adults. Weight bearing often begins on the second postoperative day.

* *

Your patient and his daughter agree that rehabilitation locally sounds like the best plan.

The goals of rehabilitation include:

A) Restore function.
B) Help patients compensate for and adapt to functional losses.
C) Prevent secondary complications.
D) Maximize potential for participation in social, leisure, or work roles.
E) All of the above.

Discussion

The correct answer is "E." These are all goals of rehabilitation.

* *

The patient returns to the local nursing home for inpatient rehabilitation. Despite wonderful progress with physical therapy, he is unable to ambulate without using a cane. He is frustrated that he cannot walk on his own, and is concerned that all this walking and exercise is going to damage the recently surgically repaired hip joint.

You can tell him that:

A) He does not need to restrict his activity because the hip prosthesis is well designed for bending, walking, and climbing stairs.
B) His frustration is likely a major depressive disorder and will require medication treatment.
C) He should continue the exercises because the advantages outweigh the low risks of surgical failure.
D) He should not expect full recovery even with exercise, because nearly every patient requires an assistive device to walk after THA.

Discussion

The correct answer is "C." Whether correction is with screws, partial repair or complete joint replacement, early weight bearing is usually tolerable with low rates of surgical failure and helps to counteract the poor outcomes clearly associated with prolonged inactivity. As noted in a previous question, early mobilization and continued exercise are the keys to preventing further decline and loss of function. Answer "A" is incorrect. After THA, patients should avoid certain motions such as bending over to tie shoes and crossing legs when seated. Often times a raised toilet seat is also recommended to reduce the load placed on the hip prosthesis in extreme flexion. Walking and general range of motion exercises should be encouraged as tolerated. Answer "B" is incorrect. Depression is not uncommon after a disabling injury such as hip fracture. However, this patient's frustration may or may not reflect clinical depression and should be further evaluated before starting medication. Answer "D" is incorrect. Although hip fractures carry approximately 5% in-hospital mortality and approximately 25% in the year following fracture, about 75% of survivors recover to prior level of function. Up to 50% of these patients require an assistive device, but certainly not everyone.

> HELPFUL TIP: Repair using an anterior approach as opposed to the traditional posterior/lateral approach reduces recovery time and generally allows complete mobility (including crossing legs, etc.) with a lower risk of dislocation.

* *

After 2 more weeks, your patient is now functioning well enough to return home. He can transfer independently and ambulates with a cane for support. Prior to discharge, the rehabilitation team would like to assess his home environment.

The occupational therapy practitioner on the team:

A) Provides a comprehensive assessment wherever the patient is employed based on his/her occupation, which does not typically include the home environment.
B) May provide training for specific adaptive equipment for patients to enhance performance in everyday activities and promote independence.
C) Is a skilled professional who has completed an occupational therapy training program after completion of high school.
D) Is licensed to write prescriptions in most states, primarily for pain control.

Discussion

The correct answer is "B." Occupational therapists (OTs) provide training for specific adaptive equipment to enhance performance in everyday activities and promote independence. They also provide guidance to family members and caregivers if needed. Answer "A" is incorrect. OTs provide home or job-site assessment, regardless of employment status or occupation. Answer "C" is incorrect. OTs are skilled professionals whose education includes the study of human growth and development with an emphasis on the social, emotional, and physiological effects of illness and injury. One must have a bachelors, masters, or doctoral degree to enter the field of occupational therapy. There are also occupational therapy assistants who generally earn an associate degree and practice under the supervision of a trained OT. Answer "D" is incorrect since OTs do not have license to prescribe medications.

Objectives: Did you learn to . . .

- Identify and screen for drinking problem in the older patient?
- Promote early rehabilitation after hip fracture repair?
- Describe some aspects of rehabilitative services?

CASE 8

A 68-year-old male arrives at your clinic to establish care. He admits that he does not visit the doctor regularly, but he feels his health has been pretty good since he changed his "bad habits." He did not bring any records, but he knows he has heart disease and high blood pressure. His bad habits included smoking about 1 pack per day for 40 years, but he proudly states he quit "cold turkey" after a heart attack at age 63. As far as health-care maintenance, he did have a colonoscopy 5 years ago at his wife's request, and he remembers his last PSA was normal, but he does not recall any type of screening for abdominal aortic aneurysm (AAA).

The USPSTF recommends one-time AAA screening:

A) For all men age 65–74 years.
B) For all men age 65–74 years who have smoked >100 cigarettes in their lifetime.
C) For all men age 55–64 years who have smoked ≥1 pack of cigarettes per day for 10 years or more.
D) For all men age ≥75 if life expectancy >10 years.
E) All smokers ≥55, regardless of gender.

Discussion

The correct answer is "B." The USPSTF and a consortium of leading professional organizations recommend one-time AAA screening with abdominal ultrasonography for all men age 65–74 years who have ever smoked (defined as >100 lifetime cigarettes). Answers "A" and "C" are incorrect. The USPTF currently does NOT recommend screening men who have never smoked (<100 cigarettes in a lifetime). The American College of Cardiology/American Heart Association (ACC/AHA) guidelines advise screening men older than 60 years who have a strong family history (parents or siblings) of AAA, but family history is not explicitly considered in the USPSTF guidelines. Answer "D" is incorrect. The evidence in men older than age 75 years and in women does not support AAA screening, and neither of the above guidelines recommends routine screening in those groups.

* *

At the next visit, your patient returns with copies of his medical records, which you have also received and reviewed. He is up to date on his immunizations, colonoscopy, and PSA, but there is no record of AAA screening. He agrees to have the screening ultrasound since the test sounds easy but questions why screening for AAA is necessary.

You inform him that:

A) AAA occurs in approximately 1 in 20 older men who have ever smoked.
B) Rupture of an AAA has a morality rate of 50%.
C) AAA ruptures cause approximately 1000 deaths per year in the United States.
D) Treatment for AAA includes open surgical repair, endovascular repair, or surveillance if AAA is <6 cm.

Discussion

The correct answer is "A." AAA is a common condition, occurring in approximately 1 in 20 older men who have ever smoked. Answer "B" is incorrect. Rupture of an AAA is associated with an even higher mortality rate of 80%, hence the importance of screening. Answer "C" is incorrect. Epidemiologic studies indicate that AAA ruptures cause approximately 10,000–15,000 deaths per year in the United States. Answer "D" is incorrect. Treatment of AAA is based on the aneurysm size, rate of expansion, and symptoms. Asymptomatic patients with aneurysms ≥5.5 cm in diameter should undergo repair, not surveillance. Surveillance for medium-sized aneurysms 4.0–5.4 cm is by ultrasound or CT every 6–12 months and every 2–3 years for aneurysms 3.0 4.0 cm. Earlier repair in men with AAA ≥5.0 or women with AAA ≥4.5 cm may be indicated if rate of increase is ≥0.5 cm in 6 months. AAA repair options include open surgical repair or endovascular repair, but the benefits of endovascular repair are still under investigation. Currently, the ACC/AHA guidelines recommend surgical repair for most patients.

* *

The ultrasound shows minimal atherosclerotic disease of the abdominal aorta. Two years later, the patient returns for follow-up at the prompting of his daughter who has been noticing that he complains about his knees hurting all the time. He has never been interested in surgery, but he would like to try something different. When asked about his pain on a scale of zero to ten (zero meaning no pain and ten meaning the worst pain possible), he reports pain around 2/10 most days, and up to 6/10 after moderate activity. He uses acetaminophen sometimes but does not want to get addicted to pain medicine.

In addition to increasing his dose of acetaminophen, you suggest a topical analgesic such as:

A) The 5% lidocaine patch because it can be applied conveniently anywhere on the body to provide additional knee pain control.
B) The 5% lidocaine patch because it acts locally where applied without achieving clinically significant serum drug levels.
C) Capsaicin cream because it can be applied topically once per day for effective pain control.
D) Capsaicin cream because it only takes 1–2 days to acheive a clinical effect.

Discussion

The correct answer is "B." Older adults are less likely to be adequately treated for pain compared with younger adults. Acetaminophen remains the best choice for first-line therapy of mild-to-moderate pain due to its tolerability. Topical agents such as the lidocaine patch or capsaicin can also provide localized pain control. Topical agents can be very useful pain therapy because they penetrate the skin to act on peripheral nerves and soft tissue directly underlying the application site. These topical agents lack systemic absorption and have limited potential for any clinically significant systemic effect or drug–drug interactions that often is an issue in elderly patients on multiple medications. Answer "A" is incorrect. The lidocaine patch must be applied directly over the painful area for best results. Answer "C" and "D" are incorrect. Capsaicin cream is dosed on a regular schedule every 6 hours to acheive maximal effect, which generally takes 2–4 weeks. Of note, patients frequently have trouble obtaining the lidocaine patch because of limited insurance coverage and high costs. Some patients have success with topical lidocaine ointment or cream instead.

* *

After making some recommendations, you see the patient 1 month later for a follow-up visit. He reports improved pain control. Today he picked up a coupon at the local drug store for an arthritis pill that contains chondroitin. He wants to know if this might help his knee pain.

You discuss the current evidence and inform him that:

A) Large-scale trials indicate significant symptomatic benefit in osteoarthritis with the use of chondroitin supplements.

B) For patients with severe osteoarthritis only, a clinically relevant benefit is likely and the use of chondroitin should be encouraged.
C) Chondroitin is a large macromolecule that is poorly digested and is potentially unsafe in older patients with any stomach problems.
D) The combination of chondroitin and glucosamine is the most popular supplement sold over-the-counter for joint pain in the United States.

Discussion

The correct answer is "D." The combination of chondroitin and glucosamine is the most popular supplement sold over-the-counter for joint pain in the United States. However, scientific evidence is lacking to support the use of chondroitin to prevent or reduce joint pain associated with osteoarthritis. Answer "A" is incorrect. In a systematic review of 20 trials that compared the effects of chondroitin with placebo or no treatment in patients with hip or knee osteoarthritis, chondroitin had minimal or no effect on joint pain. Answer "B" is incorrect. For patients with advanced osteoarthritis, a clinically relevant benefit is unlikely. Answer "C" is incorrect. Chondroitin is a large macromolecule, and only 12–13% of ingested chondroitin is absorbed into the blood stream. However, multiple studies have found no evidence to suggest that chondroitin is unsafe (except to the sharks that provide the cartilage to make the supplement–they are rapidly becoming extinct).

* *

Now that your patient has seen you for a few years, he feels more comfortable in discussing other health concerns... like constipation. He usually has a bowel movement (BM) every 2–3 days, but sometimes he gets hard stools that require excessive straining. His wife tells him to eat more fiber, but he wants to know what else he can do to help "keep regular."

Which of the following statements is true about constipation?

A) The prevalence of self-reported constipation decreases with aging.
B) Patients should be encouraged to defecate before meals when the colonic activity is the greatest.
C) Fiber is a safe, inexpensive approach to improve stool consistency and accelerate colon transit time.

Table 21–6 ROME CRITERIA FOR FUNCTIONAL CONSTIPATION

Two or more of the following should be present for at least 12 weeks out of the preceding 12 months:
- Straining for greater than 25% of defecations
- Lumpy or hard stools for greater than 25% of defecations
- Sensation of incomplete evacuation for greater than 25% of defecations
- Less than three defecations per week
- Manual evacuation or assistance to facilitate defecation

D) Increased caloric intake correlates well with constipation in the elderly.

Discussion

The correct answer is "C." Fiber is a safe, inexpensive approach to improve stool consistency and accelerate colon transit time. Increasing fiber is a good first-line approach and should be encouraged. The daily recommended fiber intake is 20–35 g. Answer "A" is incorrect because the prevalence of self-reported constipation increases with aging—up to 45% of frail elderly individuals report constipation as a health issue. It is not uncommon for patients and physicians to have different clinical definitions of constipation so further history is helpful to clarify what the patient means by "constipation." The Rome Criteria offers a consensus definition of constipation used in clinical trials as outlined in Table 21–6 and may be helpful to further characterize constipation. Answer "B" is incorrect. Patients should be encouraged to defecate first thing in the morning or 30 minutes AFTER meals when colonic activity is the greatest, and to take advantage of the gastrocolic reflex. Answer "D" is incorrect. Decreased (not increased) caloric intake correlates well with constipation in the elderly. Constipation in the presence of weight loss, rectal bleeding, and/or iron deficiency anemia should prompt further examination of the colon to exclude cancer.

* *

You rule out secondary causes of constipation and decide that your patient likely has primary transit constipation. You first provide nonpharmacologic recommendations to promote regular bowel habits, including dietary changes and increased exercise.

Which of the following options would be the *best* pharmacologic approach to use on a *daily basis* in order to help this patient with his constipation?

A) Fiber: psyllium (Metamucil), oat bran, or methylcellulose (Citrucel).
B) Stool softener: docusate calcium (Surfak) or docusate sodium (Colace).
C) Stimulant laxative: senna (Senokot), castor oil, or bisacodyl (Dulcolax).
D) Enema: tap water, sodium bisphosphonate, or soap enema.
E) Prokinetic agent: tegaserod (Zelnorm) a 5HT4 agonist.

Discussion

The correct answer is "A." Primary causes of constipation fall into three categories: (1) normal transit constipation, (2) slow transit constipation, and (3) anorectal dysfunction. There is no evidence-based guideline for the preferred order of using different types of laxatives. Supplemental fiber helps improve stool form and frequency and is a good first step. Psyllium also has the benefit of reducing lipids and improving glucose control in diabetics. Answer "B" is incorrect. While stool softeners are commonly prescribed and may be helpful, they are less effective than other options including psyllium. Answer "C" is incorrect. Stimulant laxatives, when used in recommended doses, are unlikely to harm the colon if used for short duration. However, stimulant laxatives may cause electrolyte imbalance or abdominal pain. Answer "D" is incorrect. Enemas should only be used in acute situations and with caution due to the risk of colonic perforation. Large-volume enemas can result in hyponatremia, while enemas containing phosphate can lead to hyperphosphatemia and renal failure, especially in patients with renal insufficiency. Answer "D" is incorrect. Prokinetic agents stimulate propulsion along the GI tract. The 5HT4 agonist tegaserod (Zelnorm) improves symptoms of constipation but is associated with adverse cardiovascular events and is available only under restricted use.

> HELPFUL TIP: There are many secondary causes of constipation, most commonly medications and coexistent medical conditions such as diabetes, hypothyroidism, scleroderma, and amyloidosis.

Objectives: Did you learn to . . .

- Screen for AAA?
- Provide the safe and effective treatment for osteoarthritis pain?
- Identify and treat constipation in the older patient?

BIBLIOGRAPHY

Allman RM, et al. Pressure ulcer risk factors among hospitalized patients with activity limitation. *JAMA*. 1995;273(11):856-870.

American College of Physicians/American Academy of Family Physicians. Current pharmacologic treatment of dementia: A clinical practice guideline from the ACP/AAFP. *Ann Intern Med*. 2008;148(5):370-378.

American Medical Association/National Highway Traffic Administration/US Department of Transportation; 2010. "Physician's Guide to Assessing and Counseling Older Drivers." Available at: http://www.ama-assn.org/ama/pub/physician-resources/public-health/promoting-healthy-lifestyles/geriatric-health/older-driver-safety/assessing-counseling-older-drivers.page, Accessed September 15, 2011.

American Psychiatric Association. *Diagnostic and Statistical Manual of Mental Disorders (DSM-IV)*. 4th ed. Washington, DC: American Psychiatric Association; 1994.

Barnes A. Legal issues in geriatric medicine and gerontology. In: Hazzard WR, Blass JP, Ettinger WH Jr, et al. eds. *Principles of Geriatric Medicine and Gerontology*. 4th ed. New York, NY: McGraw-Hill; 1999:545-556.

Bentley DW, et al. Practice guidelines for evaluation of fever and infection in long-term care facilities. *Clin Infect Dis*. 2000;31:640-653.

Bergstrom N, et al. Treatment of pressure ulcers. Clinical Practice guidelines No. 15. Rockville (MD): US Department of Health and Human Services, Public Health Service, Agency for Health Care Policy and Research. Dec. 1994. AHCPR Pub. No. 95–0653. (At press time, a new guideline was under review but not yet published.)

Bradley SM, Hernandez CR. Geriatric assistive devices. *Am Fam Physician*. 2011;84(4):405-411.

Geldmacher DS. Alzheimer's disease: Current pharmacotherapy in the context of patient and family needs. *J Am Geriatr Soc*. 2003;51(5):S289-S295.

Gruenewald DA, Matsumoto AM. Testosterone supplementation therapy for older men: Potential benefits and risks. *J Am Geriatr Soc*. 2003;51:101-115.

Inouye SK, et al. A multicomponent intervention to prevent delirium in hospitalized older patients. *N Engl J Med*. 1999;340:669-676.

Loue S. Elder abuse and neglect in medicine and law: The need for reform. *J Leg Med*. 2001;22:159-209.

Mehr DR, Tatum PE. Primary prevention of diseases in old age. *Clin Geriatr Med*. 2002;18(3):407-430.

Panel on Prevention of Falls in Older Persons, American Geriatrics Society and British Geriatrics Society. Updated AGS/BGS clinical practice guideline for prevention of falls in older persons. *J Am Geriatr Soc.* 2011;59(1):148-157.

Pergolizzi J, et al. Opiods and the management of chronic severe pain in the elderly. *Pain Pract.* 2008;8(4):287-313.

Pham CB, Dickman RL. Minimizing adverse drug events in older patients. *Am Fam Physician.* 2007;76(12):1837-1844.

Podsiadlo D, Richardson S. The timed "Up & Go": A test of basic functional mobility for frail elderly persons. *J Am Geriatr Soc.* 1991;39(2):142-148.

Ross GW, Bowen JD. The diagnosis and differential diagnosis of dementia. *Med Clin North Am.* 2002;86(3):455-476.

Schwartz RS, Buchner DM. Exercise in the elderly: Physiologic and functional effects. In: Hazzard

Tariot PN. Medical management of advanced dementia. *J Am Geriatr Soc.* 2003;51(5):S305-S313.

The American Occupational Therapy Association. Available at: http://www.aota.org/featured/area6/index.asp, Accessed November 22, 2007.

US Preventive Services Task Force. Screening for abdominal aortic aneurysm: Recommendation statement. *Ann Intern Med.* 2005;142:198-202

Watson YI, et al. Clock completion: An objective screening test for dementia. *J Am Geriatr Soc.* 1993;41(11):1235-1240.

Wuillen DA. Common causes of vision loss in elderly patients. *Am Fam Physician.* 1999;60(1):99-108.

Zoorob R, et al. Cancer screening guidelines. *Am Fam Physician.* 2001;63(6):1101-1111.

22

Care of the Surgical Patient

Mark A. Graber

CASE 1

You are covering the emergency department (ED) on a Saturday night. While this next scenario will never happen, just pretend. You see an intoxicated gentleman who was in a bar fight, which he lost. He then decided to beat up the only thing he could to prove his manliness. He punched a window putting his hand and arm through the glass. His parents did not believe in immunizations, so he has never had a primary tetanus series.

Exam reveals a puncture wound over the second metacarpophalangeal (MCP) joint on the right hand caused during the fight. There are also puncture wounds further up the arm caused when he hit the window. He cannot adduct his thumb or oppose it with his ring finger. The rest of his neurovascular exam is intact. The puncture wounds that are on the proximal forearm appear contaminated with foreign material

Which of the following is the most appropriate management option for the laceration over his second MCP joint?

A) Antibiotics for 5 days, leave the wound open to drain.
B) Closure with nylon suture and antibiotics for 5 days.
C) Closure with silk suture and antibiotics for 5 days.
D) Orthopedic consult to explore the joint capsule.

Discussion

The correct answer is "D." This is the classic "clenched fist" injury that occurs when a clenched fist hits a mouth and/or tooth. While it looks benign, these injuries have a high likelihood of getting infected, especially if the joint capsule is penetrated. Copious irrigation and exploration of the joint capsule are indicated.

> HELPFUL TIP: Use a syringe with a 30-gauge needle and methylene blue to enter the joint capsule. If there is resistance when you try to inject methylene blue, the joint capsule has not been violated. If the methylene blue flows freely from the syringe and into the wound, it is likely that the joint capsule has been penetrated and operative irrigation and repair are indicated.

* *

The wound is cleansed and explored. No foreign body is found on exploration, radiograph, or ultrasound. You are deciding what to do with the wounds further up his arm since the patient cannot oppose his thumb and ring finger.

Inability to oppose the thumb is associated with:

A) Median nerve injury.
B) Radial nerve injury.
C) Ulnar nerve injury.
D) All of the above.

Discussion

The correct answer is "A." Testing for nerve damage to the hand should be undertaken with any significant hand, wrist, or lower arm laceration. Here's how to do it: (1) radial nerve–check wrist and finger extension, (2) ulnar nerve–check interosseous muscles and finger abduction/adduction, and (3) median nerve–check thumb to fifth finger opposition.

* *

Even though the patient grew up in a family that did not believe in immunizations, the patient now prefers not to die of lockjaw and wants a tetanus immunization.

The BEST regimen for this patient is:

A) Tetanus immune globulin followed by a tetanus toxoid at the same time.
B) Tetanus immune globulin followed by a tetanus toxoid in 2 weeks
C) Tetanus toxoid now followed by a second booster in 2 weeks
D) Tetanus toxoid now followed by a second booster in 2 months.

Discussion

The correct answer is "A." In a patient who has not had a primary series and who likely has a contaminated wound, tetanus immune globulin should be given with simultaneous administration of tetanus toxoid (at a different site from the immune globulin). If the patient has had a primary series, tetanus booster is indicated if it has been 10 years since the last booster **or** the patient has a suspect wound and it has been over 5 years since the last immunization.

HELPFUL TIP: Tdap (tetanus, diphtheria, and pertussis) should be given once during the teen years even if the patient has already received a Td booster. **There is no need to wait for 5 years since the last vaccine** (http://www.nlm.nih.gov/medlineplus/druginfo/meds/a607027.html). Other indications for Tdap include health-care workers with direct patient contact, age 19–64 (these patients should get one dose of Tdap), those with close contact with an infant less than 12 months of age (including caregivers age 65 and over).

HELPFUL TIP: For those between 19 and 65 years of age **who are exposed to pertussis but have not had a Tdap,** you can give the Tdap at any time. It is best to wait 2 years since the last Td but not necessary.

Objectives: Did you learn to . . .

- Perform a neurologic exam of the hand for radial, median, and ulnar nerve injury?
- Manage tetanus boosters/Tdap boosters/tetanus immune globulin in patients with a potentially contaminated injury?
- Evaluate and manage a "clenched fist" injury and joint space violation?

QUICK QUIZ: PAIN CONTROL

Which of the following drugs will give you the most rapid pain control when given intravenously (IV)?

A) Fentanyl (Sublimaze).
B) Hydromorphone (Dilaudid).
C) Meperidine (Demerol).
D) Morphine.

Discussion

The correct answer is "A." Fentanyl has a peak effect at 3–5 minutes. This is followed by meperidine at 5–7 minutes, morphine at 20 minutes, and hydromorphone at 15–30 minutes. Thus, to get rapid control of pain, fentanyl is the preferred agent. Meperidine is the least preferred agent because of drug interactions (MAO inhibitors, SSRIs) and toxic metabolites (normeperidine that can cause agitation and seizures).

CASE 2

You get a call from one of your patients with diabetes that he is having difficulty urinating and quite a bit of pain in the perineal area. He has not felt well for several days and was running a low-grade fever. He went to his chiropractor 2 days ago when he only had pain and swelling, and the chiropractor adjusted his . . . well, we won't go there . . . . He is now noting that his temperature is higher (he doesn't have a thermometer but is feeling warm). You suggest that he presents to your office.

Exam reveals an obese male who is waddling into the office because of pain in his scrotal area. Vitals: blood pressure 150/100, pulse 112, respirations 20, and temperature 39.0°C. Other significant findings include a swollen scrotum that is bright red and tender to touch. You do not have extended laboratory access in your office, but a urine dipstick is negative for blood and leukocyte esterase. His blood sugar, which is usually fairly well controlled, is 320 mg/dL.

Your next step for this patient will be which of the following?

A) Start the patient on nafcillin for *Staphylococcus aureus* and *Streptococcus* coverage and follow up with the patient in the morning.
B) Refer the patient to a surgeon on an emergent basis.
C) Begin amoxicillin/clavulanate and follow up with the patient in the morning.
D) Start an IV and give a single dose of ceftriaxone followed by oral amoxicillin/clavulanate for 10–14 days.

Discussion
The correct answer is "B." This likely represents Fournier gangrene. The erythematous, swollen scrotum along with the symptoms of fever, tachycardia, and elevated blood sugar make Fournier gangrene the most likely diagnosis. The treatment is emergent and surgical. For this reason, antibiotics are inappropriate as a sole therapy. Answer "A" is incorrect because the patient needs broad-spectrum coverage with antibiotics including anaerobic coverage.

Fournier gangrene can best be described as:

A) Necrotizing fasciitis.
B) Necrotizing cellulitis.
C) Caused by aerobic bacteria.
D) Secondary to streptococci.

Discussion
The correct answer is "A." Fournier gangrene is a form of necrotizing fasciitis. This is termed "Type I" necrotizing fasciitis and is caused by mixed aerobic and anaerobic bacterial. "B" is incorrect. Necrotizing cellulitis is isolated from the superficial skin; Fournier gangrene involves deep tissues including the fascia. "C" is incorrect because, as noted above, Fournier gangrene is caused by mixed aerobic and anaerobic bacteria. Finally, "D" is incorrect. **There is necrotizing fasciitis secondary to streptococci** (see below); however, it is a different infection from the organisms that cause Fournier gangrene.

Which of the following is *NOT* a risk factor for Fournier gangrene?

A) Diabetes.
B) Immunosuppression.
C) Varicella infection.
D) End-stage renal disease.

Discussion
The correct answer is "C." All the other options are risk factors for Fournier gangrene. Varicella infection **is** a risk factor for **type II necrotizing fasciitis**, which is a different entity. Type II necrotizing fasciitis is caused by group A *Streptococcus*. Generally, patients with type II necrotizing fasciitis are not diabetic or otherwise immunocompromised. Other risk factors for type II necrotizing fasciitis include IV drug use, penetrating trauma, and blunt trauma.

* *

The surgeon evaluates the patient and asks for your opinion on the antibiotic regimen (don't write letters... we already know this will never happen).

What do you recommend for this patient with necrotizing fasciitis?

A) Penicillin and clindamycin.
B) Clindamycin and metronidazole.
C) Cefotaxime and metronidazole.
D) Ticarcillin/clavulanate (Timentin) **or** ampicillin/sulbactam (Unasyn) plus metronidazole.
E) C or D.

Discussion
The correct answer is "E." As noted above, Fournier gangrene is a mix of aerobic and anaerobic bacteria. The first two choices ("A" and "B") will cover anaerobes and some gram-positive organisms. However, gram-negative coverage is lacking. More broad-spectrum antimicrobial coverage is needed in this situation.

HELPFUL TIP: IVIG has been used in necrotizing fasciitis caused by *Clostridium* species as well as in those with streptococcal fasciitis. While there is a suggestion of benefit, the data are incomplete and more study is warranted. Hyperbaric oxygen has also been used but suffers from the same lack of data.

* *

The patient has a wide excision of necrotic tissue. After surgery, he becomes hypotensive and tachycardic (blood pressure 90/50, pulse 128), and his serum lactate is 8 mg/dL.

What is the most appropriate next step in his management?

A) Start IV dopamine to stabilize his blood pressure.
B) Start IV norepinephrine to stabilize his blood pressure.
C) Start IV saline to stabilize his blood pressure.
D) Start IV albumin to stabilize his blood pressure.

Discussion

The correct answer is "C." This patient is likely hypovolemic secondary to third spacing and/or is in septic shock and needs volume. The lactate of 8 mg/dL suggests that he has hypoperfusion with poor tissue oxygenation (although it could also be secondary to necrotic tissue). Just giving dopamine (or other vasopressors) will not increase peripheral circulation and, in fact, may decrease tissue oxygenation by increasing vascular tone and decreasing perfusion. Albumin has not been shown to have any advantage over crystalloids in almost any circumstance—post paracentesis of >5 L is the exception. Mortality of necrotizing fasciitis approaches 30% even with the best care.

HELPFUL TIP: The thinking about sepsis has changed dramatically in the past several years. Pressors are out. Fluid is in. It is clear that fluid reverses tissue hypoperfusion and tissue hypoxia much more than pressors. The septic patient should get an infusion of normal saline until the serum lactate begins to drop (or you have reached a central venous pressure (CVP) of 8–10 cm water). In general, the septic patient with a serum lactate of >4 mg/dL needs a central line (for CVP monitoring) and intensive care unit (ICU) care.

Objectives: Did you learn to . . .

- Diagnose and treat Fournier gangrene?
- Differentiate between types of necrotizing fascitis?
- Prescribe appropriate fluids and pressors in septic shock?

QUICK QUIZ: CA-MRSA

Which of the following regimens is appropriate for the treatment of *community acquired* methicillin-resistant *S. aureus* (CA-MRSA)?

A) Amoxicillin/clavulanate (Augmentin) plus rifampin.
B) Cephalexin (Keflex).
C) Doxycycline or TMP/SMX (e.g., Bactrim and Septra).
D) Erythromycin plus rifampin.
E) All of the above.

Discussion

The correct answer is "C." The treatment of MRSA is abscess drainage (if an abscess is present) and antibiotics. Doxycycline 100 mg BID **or** TMP/SMX-DS **two tablets** BID are considered appropriate treatments of CA-MRSA. Note that this is a different organism than is hospital-acquired MRSA, which generally requires vancomycin due to greater resistance to a wider array of antimicrobials. Some would add rifampin to these regimens. However, rifampin alone is not advisable because of rapid development of resistance.

HELPFUL TIP: **Vancomycin is not a great drug for treating *Staphylococcus*.** In fact, inpatient mortality rates are higher in patients with methicillin sensitive *Staphylococcal* infections treated with vancomycin than with other antibiotics. So, if you have a sensitive organism (methicillin sensitive *S. aureus*), change antibiotics to something other than vancomycin, such as nafcillin or ampicillin/clavulanate . . . or whatever the susceptibilities indicate.

QUICK QUIZ: ANTIBIOTIC COVERAGE

Which of the following organisms *is/are not generally* covered by TMP/SMX?

A) *S. aureus.*
B) Streptococcal species.
C) *Escherichia coli.*
D) Enterococcus.
E) B and D.

Discussion

The correct answer is "E." Neither *Streptococcus* species nor enterococcus species are sensitive to TMP/SMX. This has implications for the treatment of MRSA. Cellulitis (one of the manifestations of MRSA) can be from either staphylococcal or streptococcal species. So, unless you are confident that you have MRSA (abscess formation, etc.), TMP/SMX is not a great choice for cellulitis. Some would use a combination of TMP/SMX + cephalexin that covers both MRSA and streptococcal species. Yes, we know that some *E. coli* are resistant. But most are still sensitive.

CASE 3

You are working in a rural ED when you get a call that a 62-year-old farmer has been trapped between a tractor and a silo while loading silage. It seems to have pinned his legs and pelvis, but from the waist up he is fine. Nonetheless, the ambulance crew places the patient in a collar and on a backboard and transports him to the ED.

The patient is in significant pain from his lower extremities and pelvis (of course, since he is a stoic farmer, he denies this and just wants to go back to planting corn). His blood pressure is initially 105/65 with a pulse of 115. Primary survey is unremarkable, although he is still boarded and collared.

Which of the following most clearly reflects the best approach to this patient's pain?

A) Use IV meperidine (Demerol) for pain control.
B) Use IV morphine for pain control.
C) Use IV fentanyl (Sublimaze) for pain control.
D) Pain medications are contraindicated at this point given the patient's overall condition.
E) Since he's so tough, just offer him some useless platitudes like "no pain, no gain."

Discussion

The correct answer is "C." Fentanyl generally has a negligible affect on blood pressure (although one should never say "never"). Both morphine and meperidine tend to drop a patient's blood pressure, so they are relatively contraindicated in this patient with a marginal blood pressure or hypotension. Those who chose "D" or "E" have been hanging around old-time surgeons too long. It is unconscionable to withhold pain medication.

* *

Further exam shows that the patient's pelvis is unstable. As you recall, a fractured pelvis can lead to significant blood loss.

***In the short term*, what is the best way to approach this?**

A) Pressors (e.g., dopamine) plus fluids.
B) Pelvic binder.
C) Fluids (normal saline).
D) Activated factor VIIa (NovoSeven).
E) Embolization by interventional radiology (45-minute delay).

Discussion

The correct answer is "B." A pelvic binder will significantly reduce bleeding in an unstable pelvis fracture. "A" is incorrect because in trauma dopamine is not indicated when the problem is hypovolemia (see above). In fact, pressors increase mortality in hypovolemic shock. "C" is incorrect. While normal saline is a good choice for resuscitation fluids, we want to tamponade the bleeding and not just chase our tails with fluids. "D" is incorrect. Recombinant activated factor VIIa has not been shown to improve outcomes after trauma (J Trauma. 2010;69:353–359). Additionally, it has a number of adverse effects including increased thromboembolic phenomenon (PE, deep venous thrombosis [DVT], etc.). Finally, interventional radiology will likely be needed at some point. They are quite good at stopping bleeding vessels. However, the delay time during which you are watching the patient bleed is unacceptable.

> **HELPFUL TIP:** Tranexamic acid, a drug that prevents fibrinolysis, has been shown to (marginally) reduce mortality from bleeding in trauma patients without any downside. The dose is 1 g IV over 10 minutes followed by 1 g over the next 8 hours. It should be started within the first hour. Consider this as a temporizer if you have an actively bleeding patient.

* *

You appropriately place a pelvic binder that tamponades the bleeding. The patient's blood pressure stabilizes. You now turn to other issues. This patient will clearly need a Foley catheter.

Relative contraindications to placement of a Foley catheter include which of the following?

A) Blood at the urethral meatus.
B) Gross hematuria.
C) High-riding prostate.
D) Gross blood from the rectum.
E) A and C.

Discussion

The correct answer is "E." Both blood at the meatus and a "high riding prostate" (ever wonder what it is riding on?) signify the possible disruption of the urethra. Thus, since one does not want to place the catheter in the wrong place, like the peritoneal space, catheterization is relatively contraindicated. "B," gross hematuria, can be from the kidney and is not a contraindication to catheterization.

* *

You find blood at the urethral meatus. The patient complains that he really needs to void.

Your options at this point include which of the following?

A) Urethrogram to document an intact urethra.
B) Performance of suprapubic cystotomy using ultrasound guidance.
C) Use a coudé catheter to catheterize the urethra.
D) Placement of a bladder catheter via the urethra but using a wire guide (such as with a central line).
E) A and B.

Discussion

The correct answer is "E." One could perform a urethrogram using a water soluble dye (e.g., Gastrografin) to document the urethra is intact and if so place a standard Foley. One could also do a suprapubic cystotomy using ultrasound guidance. "C" and "D" are both incorrect. A coudé catheter is used to bypass a stricture (prostate or otherwise) and would be no safer than a regular catheter in this patient. Likewise, a wire could end up anywhere and should not be used in this case.

> HELPFUL TIP: If you feel uncomfortable doing a formal cystotomy, a central line with balloon placed into the bladder can be used as a temporizing solution.

* *

You now turn your attention to his leg. He is complaining of severe leg pain that seems out of proportion to the degree of injury. The calf is tender (no, we are not talking veal here . . .) with increased pain on passive stretch.

Which of the following is true?

A) Since the patient has excellent pulses, a compartment syndrome is not likely.
B) Compartment syndrome is defined as compartment pressures of $>$15 mm Hg.
C) Compartment syndrome is only associated with significant crush injuries or fractures.
D) Pain out of proportion to the injury is a red flag for compartment syndrome.

Discussion

The correct answer is "D." Pain out of proportion to the injury is a red flag for compartment syndrome. "A" is incorrect because pulses can be maintained until there is significant increase in compartment pressures and significant injury to muscle and nerves. "B" is incorrect because it is difficult to define a specific compartment pressure cutoff for compartment syndrome. Some patients tolerate higher pressures and others cannot tolerate 30 mm Hg (normal compartment pressure is zero). However, when the pressure gets above 20–30 mm Hg, strong consideration should be given to the presence of compartment syndrome. "C" is incorrect. Compartment syndrome can be due to a number of factors including electrical injury, excessive muscle use, tetany, and reperfusion after ischemia.

> HELPFUL TIP: Traditionally, we are taught the "5 Ps" of compartment syndrome: pulselessness, paresthesia, pallor, pain, and paralysis. But this is misleading. Pain may be the only symptom. By the time the others are present, there may be significant disruption of vascular supply and extensive injury.

* *

You decide that it is likely that this patient has a compartment syndrome.

Which of the following labs will be the most helpful in treating this patient?

A) CBC.
B) Urinalysis and microscopic exam.
C) Glucose.
D) Sodium.
E) PT/PTT.

Discussion
The correct answer is "B." One of the major complications of compartment syndrome is rhabdomyolysis, which will manifest itself as a urine dipstick positive for blood but with a negative microscopic exam for red blood cells. The positive dipstick is picking up myoglobin in the urine. This can be confirmed by a serum CPK. CBC, glucose, sodium, and coagulation studies may be appropriate depending on the clinical situation but are not useful in establishing the presence of myoglobinuria.

HELPFUL TIP: Myoglobin can be measured in the urine. However, many laboratories have stopped doing this test favoring the positive dipstick/negative microscopic exam approach. Additionally, **there can be false-negative dipstick findings.** Thus, check a CPK as well if rhabdomyolysis is a consideration.

* *

The patient has a positive dipstick for blood with no red blood cells on microscopic exam (presumptive myoglobinuria). A follow-up serum CPK is 32,000 IU/L. You make the diagnosis of rhabdomyolysis and decide to check additional laboratories.

Which of the following would be typically found in rhabdomyolysis?

A) Elevated calcium, decreased phosphate.
B) Decreased potassium, elevated phosphate.
C) Elevated phosphate, decreased calcium.
D) Any of the above combinations may be seen.

Discussion
The correct answer is "C." In addition to an elevated CPK, other laboratory findings in rhabdomyolysis include hyperphosphatemia, hyperkalemia, hypocalcemia, hyperuricemia, and hypoalbuminemia. **Hypocalcemia** is the most common laboratory abnormality, being present in approximately 70% of patients.

The most common adverse consequence and greatest danger of rhabdomyolysis is:

A) Disseminated intravascular coagulation.
B) Acute renal failure.
C) Seizure from hypocalcemia.
D) Acute gout from hyperuricemia.
E) Cardiac arrhythmia from hyperkalemia.

Discussion
The correct answer is "B." Myoglobin precipitates in the renal tubules causing acute renal failure. "A," DIC, can occur but is rare. "C," seizures from hypocalcemia, have not been reported in this condition nor has "D," gout. The potassium elevation from rhabdomyolysis generally does not reach a level sufficient to cause arrhythmias.

The primary treatment of rhabdomyolysis is:

A) Mannitol infusion.
B) Saline infusion.
C) Furosemide.
D) Dialysis.
E) Oral hydration.

Discussion
The correct answer is "B." The most important treatment of rhabdomyolysis is saline infusion with alkalinization of the urine. "A," mannitol, can be used to increase urine flow, but this treatment is secondary to good hydration and urine alkalinization. "C," furosemide, is not used in rhabdomyolysis. Loop diuretics will actually acidify the urine and are contraindicated. "D," dialysis, is what we are trying to avoid using saline. "E," oral hydration, will not achieve the high volumes of fluid needed to treat this condition.

HELPFUL TIP: In patients with rhabdomyolysis, try to maintain urine output of 200–300 cc/hr for an adult. Alkalinize the urine using sodium bicarbonate. Remember that in order to alkalinize the urine, you have to maintain an adequate serum potassium level otherwise the body will reabsorb potassium in exchange for hydrogen ions causing urine acidification.

* *

The patient achieves good urine output after you institute saline.

What treatment are you going to suggest for the underlying compartment syndrome?

A) Fasciotomy.
B) Immobilization and traction.
C) Hot packs and elevation of the affected limb.
D) Ice and elevation of the affected limb.

Discussion

The correct answer is "A." The treatment of compartment syndrome is fasciotomy. A rapid surgical or orthopedic consultation is critical in the treatment of compartment syndrome.

* *

The patient does well and everyone is happy.

Objectives: Did you learn to . . .

- Treat acute traumatic pain?
- Recognize and treat pelvic trauma and intrapelvic hemorrhage?
- Describe contraindications to bladder catheter placement?
- Recognize manifestations of compartment syndrome and understand that compartment syndrome can be present with pain alone?
- Identify patients at risk for compartment syndrome and rhabdomyolysis?
- Manage compartment syndrome?
- Diagnose and treat rhabdomyolysis?

CASE 4

A 60-year-old female presents to your office for severe abdominal pain. She reports that she developed vague left lower quadrant abdominal pain yesterday. This morning she awoke from her sleep with severe, diffuse abdominal pain, anorexia, and vomiting.

On examination she is lying very still. Temperature is 38.4°C, pulse 106, respirations 16, blood pressure 100/62. She has dry mucous membranes. Her abdomen has diminished bowel sounds and is rigid with involuntary guarding and rebound tenderness greatest in the left lower quadrant. On pelvic examination, she is exquisitely tender on the left with a palpable mass. **There is no cervical motion tenderness.** There are no masses on rectal examination, and her stool is negative for occult blood.

Laboratory tests include a negative urine pregnancy (she's 60 after all—but can you be too careful?!), WBC 25,500/mm^3, HCT 32%, platelets 450,000/mm^3, Na 142 mEq/L, K 3.2 mEq/L, BUN 24 mg/dL, and Cr 1.0 mg/dL. Abdominal x-ray demonstrates free air under the diaphragm.

Based on the information available, the most likely diagnosis in this patient is:

A) Diverticulitis.
B) Pelvic inflammatory disease (PID).
C) Appendicitis.
D) Ovarian torsion.
E) Abdominal aortic aneurysm.

Discussion

The correct answer is "A." The most likely cause of this patient's symptoms is diverticulitis. "B," PID, is unlikely in a 60-year-old female. Also, the clinical presentation and pelvic exam findings (gradually worsening pain, no cervical motion tenderness) are more consistent with diverticulitis than PID. "C," appendicitis, is unlikely because the pain is present on the **left** side as opposed to the right side as one would expect with appendicitis. "D," ovarian torsion, is unlikely in a postmenopausal female unless there is a malignancy. Additionally, the pain of ovarian torsion should have a sudden onset, should be colicky rather than constant, and there should be no peritoneal signs (at least until the ovary is necrosed). "E," abdominal aortic aneurysm, is unlikely because of the exam findings here: there is no pulsatile mass, the patient is normotensive, there is fever, and you can palpate a left lower quadrant mass. However, in older patients presenting with abdominal pain, you must always keep the diagnosis of abdominal aortic aneurysm in mind.

> HELPFUL TIP: A palpable aorta need not be present on abdominal exam for there to be an aortic aneurysm with dissection. Also, pulses are often maintained and symmetrical early on. Maintain a high degree of suspicion.

Which of the following is the true of diverticulosis?

A) The majority of patients with this disease will develop symptoms at some time.
B) The condition is associated with a high malignant potential.
C) The condition has peak incidence of occurrence in sixth, seventh, and eighth decades of life.
D) The condition primarily affects the ascending colon.

Discussion

The correct answer is "C." Diverticu**losis** is an acquired disease that peaks in the sixth, seventh, and eighth decades with about 50% of octogenarians having the condition. "A" is incorrect. Most are **asymptomatic** with only 10–20% going on to develop symptomatic diverticu**litis**. Acute diverticulitis has a variety of presentations. Peridiverticular inflammation occurs when a fecalith becomes entrapped in a diverticular wall resulting in a localized, contained, microperforation. Pain is typically acute and located in the left lower quadrant. Examination may reveal only a mildly tender abdomen without any masses. Peridiverticular abscess and phlegmon result in worsening left lower quadrant abdominal pain, and often a mass is palpable.

HELPFUL TIP: Epiploic appendagitis (not appendicitis, yes it is spelled correctly) can mimic both appendicitis and diverticulitis. It generally will present similarly to appendicitis but on the left. It occurs mostly in people in their 30s. It occurs when there is torsion or infarction of an epiploic appendage on the peritoneal aspect ("outside") of the colon. Diagnosis is by CT scan and It generally resolves on its own.

While you are waiting for the local surgeon to arrive, which of the following is the LEAST important part of appropriate preoperative management?

A) Maintaining the patient in an NPO state.
B) Administration of antibiotics to cover gram-negative bacteria.
C) Administration of antibiotics to cover gram-positive bacteria.
D) Administration of antibiotics to cover obligate anaerobic bacteria.
E) IV fluids.

Discussion

The correct answer is "C." The treatment of gram-positive organisms is the least important part of treatment for this patient. Initial treatment of perforated diverticuli should include fluid replacement and electrolyte correction. A urinary catheter can be placed in order to monitor fluid balance if appropriate. Empiric antibiotic therapy should be provided based on the most likely pathogens. Perforations of the appendix, diverticuli, and other parts of the colon account for more than 80% of the causes of acute bacterial peritonitis. Distal small bowel and colonic perforations should include coverage for gram-negative bacteria, such as *E. coli*, and obligate anaerobe pathogens, such as *B. fragilis*. Examples of possible regimens include single-agent treatment with second-generation cephalosporin versus an aminoglycoside with metronidazole or ampicillin/sulbactam. A number of antibiotic combinations are appropriate.

* *

The patient undergoes surgery with a partial bowel resection and primary reanastomosis. Two months following your patient's surgery, she presents complaining of abdominal pain. The pain is crampy and intermittent. Further history reveals a 24-hour history of vomiting, abdominal bloating, and low-grade fever. She reports her last bowel movement was 2 days ago and denies any flatus over the last 24 hours. On examination, her temperature is 37.1°C, pulse 105, respirations 12, and blood pressure 158/60. Her abdomen is slightly distended, diffusely tender to palpation without rebound or guarding, and has hyperactive bowel sounds. On flat plate and upright views of the abdomen, there are dilated loops of small bowel and multiple air fluid levels.

Which of the following is true regarding this patient's current disease process?

A) She most likely has a closed-loop small bowel obstruction.
B) She most likely has an extramural source of obstruction.
C) Dilated loops of bowel are defined as bowel loops >5 cm in diameter on plain film.
D) Both partial and complete bowel obstructions reveal no colonic gas on plain film.

Discussion

The correct answer is "B." This patient most likely has an external source of obstruction. Bowel obstructions are divided into two classes: mechanical and functional (also known as pseudoobstruction, ileus, or neurogenic obstruction). Mechanical obstructions are further classified by both their location and etiology. Possible etiologies include intraluminal bodies (e.g., gallstone ileus or foreign body), intramural lesions (e.g., tumor or intussusception), and extramural lesions (e.g., adhesions).

Obstructions can further be divided into open- and closed loop. Open-loop obstructions have an outlet for gas and secretion relief (e.g., vomiting); whereas closed-loop obstructions block both inflow and outflow to an area. Closed-loop obstructions, like bowel torsion or volvulus, cause acute, severe abdominal pain.

Bowel obstruction presents with crampy, intermittent abdominal pain, vomiting, distention, and obstipation. History often includes previous abdominal surgery. Depending on the degree of obstruction and its duration, there may be hyperactive bowel sounds, high-pitched bowel sounds, or decreased/absent bowel sounds. An upright abdominal plain film or lateral recumbent abdominal film confirms diagnosis with findings of dilated loops of small bowel (bowel >3 cm in diameter) on the flat plate and air fluid levels on the upright or decubitus film. **CT scan is more sensitive for obstruction than are plain films and will often reveal the source of the obstruction.** However, CT should be reserved for patients in whom the diagnosis is unclear. Patients with a complete small bowel obstruction will lack air in the colon on plain film. However, remember that air can be introduced into the rectum during a rectal exam.

Which of the following cause ileus?

A) Burns.
B) Spinal cord injury.
C) Hypokalemia.
D) Pneumonia.
E) All of the above can cause an ileus.

Discussion

The correct answer is "E." All of the above can cause an ileus. Additional causes include peritonitis, pancreatitis, uremia, and narcotics.

HELPFUL TIP: Adynamic ileus with colonic distension (AKA acute colonic pseudoobstruction) is also known as "Ogilvie syndrome." It may respond to neostigmine 2 mg IV. Remember that cholinergics such as neostigmine may cause increased salivation, lacrimation, respiratory secretions, and muscle weakness leading to possible death. Proper dosing is important for avoiding these adverse effects.

* *

You diagnose small bowel obstruction, which you believe is most likely related to adhesion formation after hemicolectomy.

Which of the following is INCORRECT regarding the management of bowel obstruction?

A) Initial treatment orders should include NPO, nasogastric (NG) decompression, IV fluid resuscitation, and electrolyte replacement as needed.
B) This patient should undergo emergent surgical intervention.
C) If she has fever or leukocytosis, she should undergo surgical intervention.
D) If she requires surgery, broad-spectrum antibiotics to cover anaerobes and gram-negative aerobes should be administered perioperatively.

Discussion

The correct answer is "B." Peritoneal adhesions account for more than half of all small bowel obstructions. Up to 80% of episodes of small bowel obstruction caused by adhesions resolve without surgical intervention. Initial treatment includes restricting oral intake, IV fluid resuscitation with normal saline, and electrolyte correction. The goal is to prevent small bowel strangulation. Patients can be safely observed if there is no evidence of strangulation. Indications of strangulation include rapidly progressing abdominal pain or distention, development of peritoneal findings, fever, diminished urine output, leukocytosis, hyperamylasemia, metabolic acidosis, and persistent obstruction. **Complete** bowel obstruction should always be treated surgically. Also, patients with de novo obstruction, (e.g., no history of laparotomy), usually require surgical intervention. If surgery is necessary, broad-spectrum antibiotics that cover anaerobes and gram-negative aerobes should be administered perioperatively to reduce wound infection and abdominal sepsis rates.

HELPFUL TIP: Although an NG tube is traditionally used in small bowel obstruction, the use is optional. An NG tube is indicated to help alleviate vomiting, distention, etc. but does not hasten the resolution of the SBO.

HELPFUL TIP: Remember that patient-controlled analgesia is the most effective modality for treating pain in the postoperative patient and in many other conditions (e.g., pancreatitis and acute chest syndrome). Side effects of narcotics may include urinary retention in addition to constipation or respiratory depression.

FINAL HELPFUL TIP There is no reason to restrict the diet in diverticu**losis**. If anything, nuts, popcorn, and corn **reduce** the incidence of diverticulitis (JAMA. 2008;300:907-914).

Objectives: Did you learn to . . .

- Assess abdominal pain and recognize an acute abdomen?
- Provide appropriate perioperative management for gastrointestinal (GI) surgery?
- Identify and treat small bowel obstruction after abdominal surgery?

CASE 5

Mr. and Ms. Biggs have always been "big boned." They have decided that weight reduction surgery is the thing for them. However, they are concerned that, for the first time in their lives, they may not be big enough.

Which of the following is NOT a necessary condition for weight loss surgery?

A) BMI >40 kg/m^2 regardless of the presence of weight-related disease.
B) BMI >35 kg/m^2 regardless of the presence of weight-related disease.
C) BMI >35 kg/m^2 plus other weight-related disease such as sleep apnea, diabetes, severe joint disease, or weight-related cardiomyopathy.
D) Failure to control weight with diet and other medical interventions.

Discussion

The correct answer is "B." A BMI of >40 kg/m^2 alone is considered an appropriate weight for surgical intervention **in the absence of other comorbidities.** As noted above, a BMI of >35 kg/m^2 with weight-related comorbidities is considered an indication for bariatric surgery. "D" is worthy of comment. Most weight control drugs are fairly useless. However, failure of medical therapy is considered a necessary condition for bariatric surgery, as is an acceptable operative risk.

* *

Much to their chagrin, they do meet the criteria for weight loss surgery. There are several surgeons in town who perform different techniques including a Roux-en-Y and laparoscopic banding.

Which of the following is NOT true?

A) Roux-en-Y is associated with greater weight loss at 1 year.
B) Laparoscopic banding is associated with a greater need for **recurrent surgery** compared with Roux-en-Y.
C) Mortality is higher with Roux-en-Y and there are more hospital admissions for complications.
D) Vertical banded gastroplasty leads to sustained weight loss and few complications.

Discussion

The correct answer is "D." Vertical banded gastroplasty does not lead to sustained weight loss and has many complications including disruption of the staple line, GERD, vomiting, and erosion of the band into the stomach. For this reason, it has (or should have) fallen out of favor. The rest are true. Roux-en-Y results in the best weight loss and requires fewer recurrent surgeries when compared with laparoscopic banding. However, the mortality rate is higher (0.06% vs. 0.17%) for Roux-en-Y and there are more perioperative complications. It also requires longer hospital stays.

* *

Mr. and Ms. Biggs are wondering if this is worth the trouble at all.

You can tell them that:

A) Although they may lose weight, weight loss surgery does nothing for their underlying diabetes, hypercholesterolemia, and coronary artery disease (CAD).
B) There is no psychological or quality-of-life benefit to weight loss surgery: they will have the same existential crisis before and after the surgery.
C) NSAIDs are relatively contraindicated after weight loss surgery.
D) Dumping syndrome is more common after laparoscopic banding than with Roux-en-Y.
E) There is rarely a need for supplemental vitamins after bariatric surgery.

Discussion

The correct answer is "C." The rate of gastric ulcers from NSAIDs is higher after bariatric surgery. The rest are not true. Weight loss does improve cholesterol, CAD, DM, etc., so "A" is incorrect. Additionally, there is both a psychological and quality-of-life benefit ("B"). Finally, dumping syndrome is commonly seen after a Roux-en-Y but not with laparoscopic banding ("D") and most patients will need supplemental vitamins ("E"). Vitamin deficiencies after bariatric surgery are common, especially folic acid, and deficiencies are more of a concern with Roux-en-Y procedures. However, supplementation is recommended for all postbariatric surgery patients.

HELPFUL TIP: Cholelithiasis is also common after bariatric surgery, especially Roux-en-Y, and occurs as a result of rapid weight loss.

* *

After their operations, they return to see you. Mr. Biggs (who opted for the Roux-en-Y procedure and who is changing his name to Mr. Little) complains of recurrent postprandial colicky abdominal pain, diaphoresis, nausea, diarrhea, and tachycardia. His wife, who went for the laparoscopic banding, has no such symptoms. You make the diagnosis of "dumping syndrome."

Your advice is to:

A) Start an anticholinergic to reduce stomach emptying.
B) Increase the content of simple sugars to quickly raise the blood sugar with meals.
C) Increase the size of feedings a bit in order to increase the amount of food available for digestion.
D) Separate solid from liquid intake for at least 30 minutes (no beer with that pizza!).
E) None of the above.

Discussion

The correct answer is "D." Separating liquid from solid intake by 30 minutes may help to reduce dumping syndrome. The others are incorrect. While theoretically plausible, anticholinergics have not been shown to be of benefit in dumping syndrome (nor has octreotide). Additionally, small, frequent meals **devoid of simple sugars** are the way to go. The symptoms seem to be related to the rapid transit of simple sugars into the bowel. Smaller volume meals without simple sugars mitigate the problem.

Objectives: Did you learn to . . .

- Recognize the indications for bariatric surgery?
- Describe some different techniques for bariatric surgery and their pros and cons?
- Provide long-term management of the bariatric surgery patient and dumping syndrome?

CASE 6

A 24-year-old male presents to your clinic with a 5-day history of rectal bleeding. For several years, he has had hard stools but has developed rectal bleeding in the last few days. In addition, he has severe, intermittent, crampy abdominal pain that he thinks is due to constipation. He reports a mild fever.

On examination, temperature is 37.9°C, pulse 95, respirations 12, and blood pressure 108/78. His abdomen is nontender with no guarding or rebound tenderness. Anoscopy reveals gross blood and two internal hemorrhoids.

Regarding hemorrhoids in general, which of the following is true?

A) Patients with hemorrhoids most commonly complain of perianal burning, itching, swelling, and pain.
B) A Grade III hemorrhoid can be reduced manually.
C) If a patient under the age of 50 with rectal bleeding is found to have hemorrhoid on examination, further studies are not indicated.
D) Because they are above the dentate line, **strangulated** internal hemorrhoids are not painful.

Discussion

The correct answer is "B." Grade III hemorrhoids can be reduced manually. Hemorrhoids are normal vascular structures in the anal canal; however, the venules can become engorged and symptoms such as pain, bleeding, and itching may result. Two types of hemorrhoids exist: external hemorrhoids derived from the inferior hemorrhoidal plexus below the dentate line and internal hemorrhoids derived from the anal cushions above the dentate line. Internal hemorrhoids occur on the left lateral, right anterior, and right posterior anal walls and are classified into Grades I–IV. Grade I hemorrhoids slide below the dentate with straining but not through the anus. Grade II hemorrhoids protrude the anus but spontaneously reduce, whereas Grade III hemorrhoids must be manually reduced. Grade IV internal hemorrhoids cannot be reduced. "A" is incorrect because most patients with symptomatic hemorrhoids present with painless rectal bleeding. "C" is incorrect. You should consider further evaluation (e.g., flexible sigmoidoscopy and colonoscopy) in patients under the age of 50 presenting with rectal bleeding, even if hemorrhoids are present and are the likely source of bleeding. In patients older than 50 with rectal bleeding, a full colonoscopy is routinely recommended to rule out any cancerous process. "D" is incorrect. Although most internal hemorrhoids do not cause pain, **strangulated** internal hemorrhoids are very painful and can become necrotic and gangrenous, requiring emergent surgery. Note that **strangulated** is different from **thrombosed**.

Which of the following would you NOT consider as a treatment of this patient's hemorrhoids?

A) Psyllium.
B) Dicyclomine.
C) Warm sitz baths.
D) Short course of topical hydrocortisone.
E) Increased water intake.

Discussion

The correct answer is "B." Dicyclomine (Bentyl, Antispas) is not indicated. Dicyclomine is an anticholinergic and will contribute to constipation—exactly what you want to avoid in hemorrhoids. "A" and "E" are the primary modes of treatment. Psyllium, as well as a diet high in fiber and water, will reduce straining and thus reduces intra-abdominal pressure. "C," warm baths or showers (40°C), have been shown to reduce anal canal pressures. "D," a short course of topical hydrocortisone (e.g., Anusol HC), may be of benefit. Long-term topical steroids are contraindicated. Finally, good hygiene and analgesia should be prescribed as needed.

HELPFUL TIP: Most symptomatic hemorrhoids respond to conservative measures and surgery should not be performed unless conservative measures fail or other indications exist (e.g., strangulation).

Which of the following is true about treating hemorrhoids surgically?

A) Irritable bowel syndrome is a relative contraindication to hemorrhoid surgery.
B) It is best to ligate all hemorrhoids in a single office visit.
C) Band ligation results in sloughing of hemorrhoid in about 1–2 weeks.
D) Following excision, thrombosed external hemorrhoids should be closed to prevent bleeding.

Discussion

The correct answer is "C." Rubber-band ligation generally results in the sloughing of the hemorrhoid in 1–2 weeks. "A" is incorrect. Inflammatory bowel disease (IBD)—not irritable bowel syndrome—is a relative contraindication to the surgical treatment of hemorrhoids. Other contraindications to office-based hemorrhoidectomy procedures include bleeding diathesis, pregnancy and the period immediately postpartum, anorectal fissures, active anorectal infections, AIDS or other immunodeficient states, portal hypertension, rectal wall prolapse, and anorectal tumors. Complications of hemorrhoidectomy include pain, significant bleeding with sloughing, thrombosis of external hemorrhoids, and very rarely sepsis with pelvic cellulitis. "B" is incorrect. Although evidence is scarce, standard of care dictates that only one hemorrhoid be ligated in a single office visit (due to concerns about excessive tissue necrosis). "D" is incorrect. Patients who present with external hemorrhoids that are painful, tender, swollen, with bluish discoloration have thrombosis. If the patient presents within 48 hours of thrombosis, the thrombus should be expressed. It is important **not** to close the hemorrhoid once the clot is expressed. In fact, a small ellipse of the hemorrhoid should be removed to facilitate continued drainage and prevent reaccumulation of clot.

* *

You prescribe conservative treatment of your patient's hemorrhoids, and since he does not return for his next scheduled appointment, you assume he is doing well. You see him again 6 months later. He reports that he had indeed healed. Although he still takes psyllium, he began having painful bowel movements with blood-streaked stool 2 days ago. Upon examination of the anus, you find a fissure.

All of the following findings would lead you to consider Crohn disease EXCEPT:

A) Posterior midline fissure.
B) Painless fissure.
C) Multiple fissures.
D) Nonhealing fissure.

Discussion
The correct answer is "A." The posterior (dorsal) midline is where solitary fissures, unrelated to IBD, are typically located. Fissures in any other location should raise suspicion for Crohn disease. "B," "C," and "D" are also suggestive of Crohn disease.

In a patient with an uncomplicated, initial anal fissure, what do you recommend for *first-line* therapy?

A) Lord dilation.
B) Botulinum toxin injections.
C) Topical nitroglycerin.
D) Oral psyllium.
E) Oral nifedipine.

Discussion
The correct answer is "D." All of the options are employed for treating anal fissures. However, in patients with an uncomplicated, initial anal fissure, it seems prudent to initiate conservative therapy (e.g., psyllium, dietary fiber, water, and warm soaks) prior to proceeding to more invasive measures. Most fissures will respond to conservative measures. Generally, healing takes 2–4 weeks. In addition to the treatments listed, topical diltiazem and topical nifedipine are also used as have various surgical approaches. Lord dilation deserves special mention as a relatively arcane procedure for stretching the anal sphincter muscle (under anesthesia, we hope!).

* *

You note that this patient's fissure is deep, ulcerating, and located at the left lateral aspect of the anus. Given this examination, you are concerned about Crohn disease. You briefly consider what you know about IBD.

Which of the following is true of IBD?

A) Ulcerative colitis is primarily a diagnosis of young males.
B) Crohn disease can be isolated from colonic disease.
C) Ulcerative colitis is generally associated with deep colonic ulcerations and transmural inflammation while those of Crohn disease are more superficial.
D) Crohn disease is more common in blacks, while ulcerative colitis is more common in whites.

Discussion
The correct answer is "B." Crohn disease can be isolated from the colon. "A" is incorrect because ulcerative colitis is evenly distributed between men and women with a similar incidence in each. "C" is incorrect. Crohn disease is associated with deeper ulcerations and transmural inflammation leading to fistulae and strictures, etc. "D" is incorrect. In general, IBD is more common in whites than nonwhites. See Chapter 7 for more questions about Crohn disease.

Objectives: Did you learn to . . .

- Characterize hemorrhoids based on location?
- Grade internal hemorrhoids based on severity?
- Manage hemorrhoids with conservative and surgical treatment?
- Treat an uncomplicated anal fissure?
- Recognize anal fissures as potential signs of Crohn disease?

CASE 7

A 58-year-old female presents to your clinic for a lump found on routine breast self-exam. Her older sister died from breast cancer, and she is very concerned about the possibility of breast cancer in herself. She never misses her monthly breast exam and notes she has never felt this lump before. She first noticed the lump 2 weeks ago, and it has not changed in size or consistency since that time. She has had yearly mammograms since age 40 that have always been normal. She denies any weight loss or fatigue and reports being postmenopausal for the last 5 years. She previously took combination hormone replacement therapy, which she discontinued last year.

On examination, her breasts appear symmetrical with no skin abnormalities. The nipples are symmetric in size, shape, and color without retraction or discharge. You palpate a small, pea-sized thickening in upper outer quadrant of the right breast. This is the lump that she noticed 2 weeks ago. It is fixed to the deep aspect of the chest wall, so you have a hard time delineating whether the borders are smooth.

Regarding breast lumps, which one of the following is FALSE?

A) Abnormal screening mammography is the most common presentation of breast carcinoma.
B) Cysts are more common in premenopausal women than postmenopausal women.
C) A history of fibroadenoma is associated with an increased risk of breast cancer.
D) A radiographic oil cyst is pathognomonic for fat necrosis.

Discussion

The correct answer is "A." The most common presentation of breast carcinoma is a breast lump felt by the patient. Breast masses can be cysts, fibroadenomas, thickened areas with fibrocystic change, fat necrosis, and carcinoma. "B" is true. Cysts primarily present when women are premenopausal and are uncommon in the postmenopausal state, unless the woman is taking hormone replacement. Cysts are well demarcated, mobile, and firm. The diagnosis is confirmed with aspiration of nonbloody fluid followed by complete resolution of the mass. Fibroadenomas occur between the ages of 20–50 and are described as firm, rubbery, and mobile. They can be confirmed by characteristic findings on ultrasound and fine needle aspiration (FNA) if necessary. "C" is also true. While historically believed to be entirely benign, fibroadenomas are associated with a small but significant increased risk for breast cancer. "D" is true. A radiographic oil cyst (a circumscribed mass of mixed soft-tissue density and fat with a rim that is often calcified) is due to fat necrosis, which occurs in areas of the breast that have been subject to trauma, surgery, infection, or radiation therapy. About half of the time, fat necrosis has no precipitant. Oil cysts are most common in the superficial aspects of pendulous breasts of obese women. When an oil cyst is seen radiographically, no further workup is needed.

* *

Your patient is concerned about her family history of breast cancer. She asks about genetic testing.

You are able to tell her that the BRCA 1 gene is associated with which of the following?

A) Breast cancer.
B) Uterine cancer.
C) Ovarian cancer.
D) A and B.
E) A and C.

Discussion

The correct answer is "E." The BRCA (**BR**east **CA**ncer) 1 and 2 genes are related to familial breast cancer, and BRCA 1 is also associated with an increased risk of ovarian cancer. They are not associated with uterine cancer. The usefulness of testing for these genes in primary care is questionable, and they **cannot** be relied upon for general screening or diagnostic purposes.

* *

You are suspicious that this patient's mass may be cancer, and you order **mammography and ultrasound.** However, these studies show no mass. When your patient returns to discuss her test results, you examine her again. The mass is still palpable.

The next best step in management of this patient is:

A) Breast exam and mammogram every 6 months.
B) Breast exam and mammogram every 3 months.
C) Referral to a surgeon to consider excisional biopsy.
D) Ultrasound-guided biopsy.
E) Return to normal screening.

Discussion

The correct answer is "C." A palpable mass that is suspicious for cancer **cannot** be ignored even in the presence of negative radiologic studies. No other option is acceptable, nor would any other option be defensible if this patient were to develop overt breast cancer. "D" would be a viable option if a mass were identified on ultrasound, but none was.

* *

When making diagnostic decisions regarding breast masses, age matters.

Which of the following is NOT TRUE about how a diagnostic evaluation should proceed?

A) In women <40 years of age, lesions that appear benign on ultrasound may be followed simply by a repeat examination in 3 months.
B) In women >40 years of age, lesions that appear benign on ultrasound and cytological analysis need no follow-up.

C) In women >40 years of age where a lesion is palpated but not seen on mammogram or ultrasound, excision should follow if clinical suspicion dictates.
D) In women >40 years of age who have a palpable lesion and desire definitive removal, no further testing is necessary prior to excisional biopsy.

Discussion

The correct answer is "B." Women over the age 40 should be followed up in 3 months even with negative cytology. Clinical diagnosis of carcinoma has accuracy of 60–85%. Extent of workup, however, is driven by clinical suspicion. Radiologic studies should be ordered as indicated. A needle biopsy either by FNA or core needle biopsy is the next step in evaluation of solid tumor masses. Needle diagnosis offers the advantages of being simple, quick, inexpensive, relatively noninvasive, highly available, and an accurate way of diagnosing atypical cells.

Because of the risk for carcinoma, algorithms for workup of solid tumors differ between women <40 versus those 40 and older. Women <40 who desire observation should be evaluated by ultrasound and/or FNA. If either is suspicious, surgical excision should be performed. If there is a negative FNA, the patient can be followed up in 3 months.

In women 40 years of age or older, palpable masses should further be evaluated by ultrasound and mammography. If the lesion cannot be identified radiologically, it should be removed by excision if clinical suspicion dictates. If the lesion appears benign by radiography, it can be followed by FNA. Those with atypia on FNA should be referred for excision. If the lesion appears benign both radiologically and cytologically, it still warrants further follow-up in 3 months by clinical exam. "D" is correct. All women with a palpable breast mass who desire an excisional biopsy can proceed directly to definitive removal, regardless of age.

* *

You perform an FNA, which the cytopathologist reads as "probable malignancy." You recall from previous visits that the patient's older sister had breast cancer. Additionally, your patient went through menopause at age 53, and used hormone replacement therapy for 5 years. You obtain further history, including a history of menarche at 14 years of age and the fact that the patient has never been pregnant.

Which of these factors DOES NOT contribute to an increased risk of breast cancer in THIS patient?

A) Her nulliparity.
B) Her age at menarche.
C) Her family history.
D) Her age at menopause.
E) Her history of hormone replacement.

Discussion

The correct answer is "B." The risk of breast cancer is roughly associated with the lifetime exposure to estrogen. This patient's age at menarche is in the mid-to-late age range and is thus **not** a risk factor for breast cancer. Younger age at menarche (e.g., 10 years old) is associated with an increased risk of breast cancer. Nulliparity and greater age at first pregnancy are associated with an increased risk, as is greater age at menopause. A history of a first-degree relative with breast cancer is a strong risk factor. Finally, as demonstrated in the Women's Health Initiative, estrogen/progesterone replacement therapy (HRT) is associated with an increased risk of breast cancer.

* *

While you wait for definitive pathology results, you consider the different types of breast cancer that this patient might have.

Regarding various types of breast cancer, all of the following are true EXCEPT:

A) Cystosarcoma phyllodes tumors are not always malignant.
B) Infiltrating lobular carcinoma is the most common histological type of invasive breast carcinoma.
C) Paget disease of the breast clinically appears eczematous.
D) Sarcomas, lymphomas, melanomas, and angiosarcomas are all possible causes of cancer in the breast.

Discussion

The correct answer is "B." Infiltrating **ductal** (not lobular) carcinoma is the most common histological type of invasive breast cancer. Invasive breast carcinoma includes a wide variety of histological diseases. Infiltrating **ductal** carcinoma accounts for 65–80% of breast cancers, whereas infiltrating **lobular** carcinoma is the second most frequent, accounting for 10% of breast cancers. "A" is true. Cystosarcoma phyllodes tumors, which have a clinical presentation similar to fibroadenomas but are more rapidly growing, may be either malignant or benign. Yet the malignant nature of cystosarcoma phyllodes is sometimes difficult to determine on cytology, and the lesions may require a wide excision. "C," Paget disease of the breast, is a rare form of breast cancer with eczematous changes of the nipple, including itching, erythema, and nipple discharge. "D" is true as well. Many other malignancies may occur in the breast, including sarcomas, lymphomas, melanomas, and angiosarcomas.

* *

The pathology results are final and show infiltrating ductal carcinoma. Your patient will see a breast surgeon next week. As you await the results of surgery, you consider her prognosis.

All of the following are favorable prognostic indicators in breast cancer EXCEPT:

A) Hormone receptor negative.
B) Absence of axillary nodal involvement.
C) Low-grade tumor.
D) Pure tubular, mucinous, or medullary histological types.
E) Tumor size <1 cm.

Discussion

The correct answer is "A." Patients whose tumors are hormone receptor **negative** have worse outcomes than do patients whose tumors are hormone receptor positive. "B," absence of axillary nodal involvement, is obviously a better prognostic factor than the presence of nodal involvement. In fact, axillary lymph node status is the single most important predictor of overall survival in breast cancer. "C," low tumor grade, is also a good prognostic factor. "D," patients with a single cell type, have a better prognosis as well. "E" is true. A very useful predictor of tumor behavior is tumor size, and tumor size <1 cm is a positive prognostic sign.

HELPFUL TIP: Tumors can be either estrogen or progesterone receptor positive or negative. Tumors that are positive for estrogen and/or progesterone receptors are the most likely to respond to hormonal therapy (e.g., tamoxifen).

HELPFUL (BUT DISTURBING) TIP: It turns out that approximately 20% of women who undergo breast conserving surgery for breast cancer need repeat surgery. And, 15% of those with positive margins did not go for re-excision. Disturbing with major implications for informed consent. (JAMA. 2012;307:467).

Objectives: Did you learn to . . .

- Generate a differential diagnoses for breast masses?
- Evaluate a patient with a breast mass?
- Identify risk factors for breast cancer?
- Describe several types of breast cancers?
- Describe factors that are used to establish prognosis in breast cancer?

QUICK QUIZ: BREAST CANCER RISK

A 50-year-old female presents for a routine physical. She wants to know her risk of developing breast cancer. You want to give her a more accurate picture, and you decide to use the Gail Model.

When taking her history, you must ask about which of the following?

A) Number of first-degree relatives with breast cancer, current age, age at menopause, number of breast biopsies, and age at first live birth.
B) Number of first-degree relatives with breast cancer, current age, age at menopause, and number of children.
C) Number of first-degree relatives with breast cancer, current age, age at first menstrual period, and number of children.
D) Number of first-degree relatives with breast cancer, current age, age at first menstrual period, number of breast biopsies, and age at first live birth.

Discussion

The correct answer is "D." The Gail Model is a computer program that estimates a woman's chance of developing breast cancer. Factors that affect the score include the number of first-degree relatives with breast cancer, current age, age of first menstrual period, number of breast biopsies, and age at first live birth, race and history of atypia in a biopsy. This tool may be useful in patients who are candidates for tamoxifen for breast cancer prophylaxis. **However, the Gail score is much better at predicting the likelihood of breast cancer in populations than in any individual. So, realize that it has limitations.** The National Cancer Institute maintains a Web site for the Gail Model calculation, located at http://bcra.nci.nih.gov/brc/q1.htm.

CASE 8

An orthopedic colleague asks you to consult on a 64-year-old male prior to an elective total hip replacement. The surgery is scheduled for 3 months from now. The patient is a smoker with diabetes mellitus type 2 and has recently had a cardiac catheterization that showed significant, but nonbypassable, coronary disease. He is asymptomatic and is able to walk stairs without dyspnea or chest pain. The surgeon would like some preoperative recommendations.

You would recommend all of the following EXCEPT:

A) The patient should stop smoking 4 weeks before surgery.
B) The patient should have preoperative and postoperative beta-blockers if the pulmonary status allows it.
C) The patient should have a chest radiograph done.
D) The patient should have his hemoglobin/hematocrit drawn.
E) The patient should have his creatinine measured.

Discussion

The correct answer is "A." Paradoxically, unless patients stop smoking 8 weeks or more before surgery, the risk of adverse pulmonary outcomes is increased. The cause of this phenomenon remains unclear but may occur because the cilia are able to mobilize material in the lungs. "B" is true. The use of pre-, intra-, and postoperative beta-blockers is well supported for patients with CAD. One of the most serious intraoperative events is a myocardial infarction. Beta-blockers have been shown in multiple studies to reduce this risk and to improve outcomes if the patient has an elevated risk for a myocardial infarction. **Note, however, that a beta-blocker should be started well in advance of the surgery and not just on the day of surgery.** It is critical to assure that the patient is on a stable dose of a beta-blocker at the time of surgery. Starting the beta-blocker too close to surgery may increase the risk of stroke, likely secondary to intraoperative hypotension. While "C," "D," and "E" are true, a lot of other routine preoperative assessments are not supported in the literature. See Tables 22–1 and 22–2 for the appropriate workup of the preoperative patient.

Which of the following is effective for the prevention of postoperative DVT?

A) Early mobilization.
B) Enoxaparin 30 mg subcutaneously every 12 hours.
C) Enoxaparin 40 mg subcutaneously every 24 hours.
D) Heparin 5000 Units subcutaneously every 12 hours.
E) All of the above.

Table 22–1 PREOPERATIVE STUDIES AND THEIR INDICATIONS

Tests	Indications
Bun/Creatinine	Over 60; history of renal, cardiac, or vascular disease
CBC/H&H	Possible hematologic or infectious process; significant blood loss predicted
Coagulation studies	Stigmata liver disease, history of coagulopathy, possible DIC, anticoagulation, alcohol abuse
ECG/CXR	As indicated by history and physical (e.g., exacerbation of pulmonary disease with cough)
Electrolytes	Diuretic use, history of renal or cardiac disease, possible dehydration by history or physical
Glucose	Diabetics, obese patients, undergoing vascular procedures, other reason for increased glucose (e.g., steroids)
Liver enzymes	History of liver disease or stigmata of liver disease
Urine beta-hCG	If indicated by history
Urinalysis	Pregnancy, diabetes, urologic surgery, symptomatic patients

Table 22–2 MAYO CLINIC PREOPERATIVE GUIDELINES

Age in Years	Studies Indicated
Age <40	No routine preoperative evaluation required
Age 40–59	ECG, creatinine, and glucose
Age 60 or older	ECG, chest radiograph, CBC, creatinine, glucose

Discussion

The correct answer is "E." All of the modalities listed above can prevent the development of DVT. Aspirin and low-dose warfarin (target INR 1.5) are also effective but less than heparin or enoxaparin. Intermittent leg compression may also be used.

> HELPFUL TIP: **Recent data suggests that graded compression stockings are marginally beneficial at best for DVT prevention and may lead to increased skin breakdown, etc.** For this reason, intermittent pneumatic compression is preferred (Ann Surg. 2010;251:393, The Lancet. 2009;373:1958).

* *

The patient undergoes his hip replacement, and his postoperative ECG is normal. Four hours after surgery, he develops mild respiratory distress, a fever, and cough. On chest x-ray, there is a right lower lobe infiltrate. There is no evidence of fluid overload.

Which of the following is the most likely cause of this patient's fever and infiltrate?

A) *Pneumococcus*.
B) Gram-negative organisms.
C) Atelectasis.
D) Aspiration pneumonitis.
E) Aspiration pneumonia.

Discussion

The correct answer is "D." In the hours after surgery, an aspiration **pneumonitis** would be the most likely cause of this patient's current findings. Aspiration pneumonitis occurs when there is aspiration of gastric contents with a pH of less than 2.5. In order for aspiration pneumonitis to develop, the volume of aspirate needs to be at least 1–4 mL/kg of stomach contents. Aspiration pneumonitis develops over a matter of hours. In contrast, pneumococcal and gram-negative pneumonias generally develop several days after surgery (unless a subclinical pneumonia was present at the time of surgery). Aspiration **pneumonia** is caused by anaerobes and mixed flora and develops slowly over days to a week. Atelectasis warrants special mention. **Atelectasis does not cause fever.** Both atelectasis and fever occur frequently in the postoperative period, but their occurrence together is most likely due to chance. The old adage about atelectasis and fever has been shown to be untrue. Thus, in the postsurgical patient with fever, look for another cause besides atelectasis.

Of the following, which generally IS NOT a cause of postoperative fever in the first 48 hours?

A) Malignant hyperthermia.
B) Surgical "trauma" (e.g., cutting through muscle).
C) Wound infection.
D) Hyperthyroidism.
E) Drug fever.

Discussion

The correct answer is "C." Wound infections generally are not found in the first 48 hours after surgery. All of the rest can be found either immediately after surgery (malignant hyperthermia, hyperthyroidism, drug fever, etc.) or soon thereafter (fever from surgical trauma secondary to the release of cytokines). Table 22–3 summarizes the time course and causes of postoperative fever.

* *

The patient's chest radiograph is consistent with aspiration pneumonitis (infiltrate in the right lower lobe... yes, lower lobe is more common).

Which of the following is NOT TRUE with regard to aspiration pneumonitis?

A) It can progress to ARDS.
B) Patients with aspiration pneumonitis present with fever, dyspnea, bronchospasm, and hypoxia.
C) It should be treated with antibiotics that cover for anaerobes.
D) It tends to resolve in about 7 days.

Discussion

The correct answer is "C." Aspiration **pneumonitis** is a chemical process that is unrelated to infection. Thus,

Table 22–3 CAUSES OF POSTOPERATIVE FEVER

Immediate (within hours of surgery):
- Drugs or blood products: Generally hypotension, rash, etc.
- Trauma from surgery or before surgery: Evident from history
- Malignant hyperthermia: Within 30 minutes of anesthesia induction **but** may be hours out

Acute (first week after surgery):
- Nosocomial infections or extension of a preoperative infection
- *Clostridium difficile* infection
- Intubation
- Aspiration
- UTI: Especially if chronic indwelling or urologic manipulation
- Surgical site infection generally >1 week if cause fever but may occur in 1st week. **But** group A *Strep* and *Clostridium* may occur within hours of surgery.
- Also: Pancreatitis, alcohol withdrawal, PE, MI, thrombophlebitis, gout

Subacute (1–4 weeks after surgery):
- IV and central catheter site infections
- Antibiotic associated diarrhea, including *C. difficile* infection
- Drug fever: Beta-lactams, sulfa, heparin, etc.
- DVT, PE, fat emboli from long bones, liposuction, acute chest syndrome (SSA)

aspiration pneumonitis does not need to be treated with antibiotics at all (although it usually is as a practical matter—since it is difficult to differentiate from pneumonia). The rest of the options are true.

HELPFUL TIP: The term "aspiration pneumonia" is used differently in the different parts of the literature. This leads to some confusion. Some use the term to include all pneumonias caused by aspiration. Many of the cases included in this definition are caused by many of the same organisms that cause community-acquired pneumonia, including *pneumococcus* and *Haemophilus influenzae*. These patients tend to have a fever and infiltrate, etc., which develop within 2 days of the aspiration. For these patients, the appropriate antibiotics should include agents to cover hospital-acquired organisms, especially gram-negative organisms, including *Pseudomonas*.

Other groups may define aspiration pneumonia as anaerobic infections that result from aspiration. These patients have a more indolent course, with onset of symptoms over days to weeks. Generally, these patients have purulent sputum, with lower lobe involvement most common. The upper lobes may be involved if the patient aspirates while recumbent. These patients may have a polymicrobial infection including *Peptostreptococcus, Fusobacterium, Bacteroides*, and *Prevotella*. These patients should be treated with antibiotics such as clindamycin, ampicillin/sulbactam, or amoxicillin/clavulanate (avoid metronidazole as a single agent due to high failure rate).

So, when you read the literature about aspiration pneumonia, be sure you know which definition the authors are using, because the description of the disease and the treatments vary.

* *

You treat the patient with fluids and tracheal suction. However, he remains febrile and tachycardic at about 128 bpm. There is no evidence of dehydration at this point and he seems euvolemic.

Which of the following would be the most appropriate first step in the treatment of tachycardia in *this* postsurgical patient?

A) Oral or rectal aspirin.
B) Oral or rectal acetaminophen.
C) IV beta-blockers.
D) IV fluids.

Discussion

The correct answer is "B." The **initial** treatment of this patient is acetaminophen. Reducing the fever and metabolic stress will result in a reduction in the heart rate. "A" is not the best choice since this patient is postsurgical. Giving aspirin, an antiplatelet agent, may result in increased postoperative bleeding. "C," IV beta-blockers, can be used and would be appropriate if the patient was having ischemic symptoms and needed an immediate reduction in pulse. "D," IV fluid, is incorrect in this patient who is already well hydrated (as stipulated in the question). Note that IV fluids **are** appropriate in postoperative tachycardia if the patient is dehydrated.

* *

The patient's pulmonary status has improved. The surgeon notices that the patient has hyperkalemia and thrombocytopenia. The patient is on a number of drugs postoperatively. She is wondering which of these drugs is causing the problem.

You let her know that the most likely cause is:

A) Beta-blockers.
B) Albuterol.
C) Aspirin.
D) Morphine.
E) Heparin.

Discussion

The correct answer is "E." Heparin can cause both hyperkalemia and thrombocytopenia (HITTS, heparin-induced thrombocytopenia thrombosis syndrome). Hyperkalemia is caused by heparin's ability to block the aldosterone system and usually requires prolonged heparin use (although in diabetics and those with renal failure it may occur more rapidly because of poor reserve). Thrombocytopenia is caused by the development of antiplatelet antibodies and occurs 5–10 days after the start of heparin therapy and is associated with thromboembolic phenomenon. Platelets can get as low as 30,000/μL. Stop the heparin and anticoagulate with a nonheparin agent (e.g., bivalirudin). A nonimmune-mediated thrombocytopenia also occurs in up to 20% of individuals who receive heparin. This occurs within the first 4 days of heparin administration with a nadir of 100,000 platelets per microliter and there are no clinical consequences.

"A," beta-blockers, should cause neither hyperkalemia nor thrombocytopenia. "B," albuterol, can cause **hypokalemia** (as can other catecholamines) by driving potassium intracellularly. However, albuterol does not cause **hyperkalemia** or thrombocytopenia. Likewise, "D" is incorrect because morphine is not associated with hyperkalemia or thrombocytopenia.

HELPFUL TIP: Heparin can also cause a postoperative fever.

* *

After you stop the patient's heparin, the thrombocytopenia and hyperkalemia begin to resolve. You start the patient on intermittent leg compression.

Which of the following is TRUE about the use of heparin in patients with a history of heparin-induced thrombocytopenia?

A) The use of low-molecular-weight heparin is contraindicated in patients with a history of heparin-induced thrombocytopenia.
B) Heparin can be reintroduced once the patient is treated with steroids.
C) The use of lepirudin and argatroban are contraindicated in the treatment of heparin-induced thrombocytopenia.
D) Heparin can be used during cardiopulmonary bypass despite a previous history of a thrombocytopenic reaction to heparin.
E) None of the above.

Discussion

The correct answer is "D." Heparin can be used during cardiopulmonary bypass despite a previous history of heparin-induced thrombocytopenia. The theory is that the development of enough antibodies to reproduce thrombocytopenia takes several days and patients will generally be on cardiopulmonary bypass for only a matter of hours. Thus, heparin can be used during cardiopulmonary bypass even if there is a history of prior heparin-induced thrombocytopenia. "A" is incorrect. Low-molecular-weight heparins, including fondaparinux and danaparoid, have been used successfully in patients with a history of heparin-induced thrombocytopenia. Danaparoid is preferred but is no longer available in the United States. "C" is incorrect. In fact, the treatment of patients who need anticoagulation after heparin-induced thrombocytopenia includes lepirudin and argatroban. These two agents are direct thrombin inhibitors that do not cross-react with heparin.

HELPFUL TIP: Drugs that raise the gastric pH (H_2 blockers, proton pump inhibitors) increase the risk of postoperative pneumonia (and *Clostridium difficile*). Normally, the acid pH of the stomach prevents colonization with pathogenic bacteria. This defense is compromised when the stomach pH rises. Thus, infection with aspiration is more likely.

Objectives: Did you learn to . . .

- Perform a preoperative medical evaluation?
- Generate a differential diagnosis for postoperative fever?
- Diagnose and treat aspiration pneumonitis?
- Recognize some complications of heparin use?
- Employ appropriate DVT prophylaxis measures?
- Manage a patient with heparin-induced thrombocytopenia?

QUICK QUIZ: GENERAL ANESTHESIA FOR SURGERY

Regarding anesthesia evaluation both preoperatively and intraoperatively, which one of the following is NOT TRUE?

A) Therapeutic beta-blockade should be administered preoperatively in vascular surgery patients who have underlying cardiac disease in order to reduce perioperative and long-term risks of cardiac events.
B) Minimum potassium before proceeding with elective coronary artery bypass graft (CABG) surgery should be 3.5 mEq/L.
C) American Society of Anesthesiologists (ASA) Class IV designation includes patients who have well-controlled major systemic disease.
D) Risks of anesthesia include allergic drug reactions, failure to intubate and provide adequate oxygenation and ventilation, nerve damage, and malignant hyperthermia.

Discussion

The correct answer is "C." ASA Class IV includes patients who have a systemic disease that is life threatening and **not** well controlled. All the other options are true. "A" is true but the beta-blocker should be started well in advance of the surgery and the patient should be on a stable dose at the time of the surgery. Starting the beta-blocker at the time of the surgery worsens outcomes as noted above. "B" is a correct statement. There are increased perioperative arrhythmias and need for cardiac resuscitation in patients with serum potassium levels <3.5 mEq/L. "D" is also a correct statement. Anesthesia risks include allergic drug reactions, failure to intubate and provide adequate oxygenation and ventilation, nerve damage, and malignant hyperthermia, among others. Mortality rate from anesthesia is surmised to be about 1–2 per 10,000 patients. The ASA classification system is outlined in the Table 22–4.

CASE 9

A 60-year-old male patient of yours is planning to undergo CABG. After you perform a physical exam and laboratory tests, you discuss his case with the surgeon. She asks if you will help to manage him postoperatively, and you agree. She then asks if you are aware of his risk of arrhythmia during the postoperative period.

You correctly reply:

A) "His risk for atrial fibrillation is less than it would be if he were undergoing valve replacement simultaneously with CABG."
B) "Of the potential arrhythmias, he is most likely to encounter bradycardia, which is the most common post-op.
C) "Nonsustained ventricular tachycardia is highly unlikely in this setting."

Table 22–4 ASA PHYSICAL STATUS CLASSIFICATION

Class	Description	Risk of Operative Mortality
Class I	Healthy person	<0.1%
Class II	Patient with mild systemic disease	0.5%
Class III	Patient with severe systemic disease that is controlled	4.4%
Class IV	Patient with severe systemic disease that is uncontrolled and a threat to life	23.5%
Class V	Patient who is unlikely to survive for 24 hours, with or without surgery	50.8%

D) "Keep his potassium low, around 3.0 mEq/L, and he will be less likely to experience tachyarrhythmias."

Discussion

The correct answer is "A." With CABG, the risk of postoperative atrial flutter or fibrillation is around 30%. That risk almost doubles when valve replacement is accomplished simultaneously with CABG. "B" is incorrect because bradyarrhythmias occur less frequently than tachyarrhythmias. "C" is incorrect. Nonsustained ventricular tachycardia is extremely common in the immediate postoperative period. "D" is also incorrect. Plasma potassium levels <3.5 mEq/L are associated with an increased risk of tachyarrhythmias.

Objectives: Did you learn to . . .

- Identify factors that may reduce mortality rates in patients undergoing CABG?

CASE 10

A 15-year-old male presents to your office with a 3-day history of diarrhea and right lower quadrant abdominal pain. He has tenderness in the right lower quadrant with guarding and rebound. He remains afebrile and has been hungry, scarfing down 5 waffles for breakfast (but less than his usual 6 . . .). The patient has no other significant history. You decide that this patient might have appendicitis, so you draw some labs. The white blood cell count is normal ($7500/mm^3$), as is the urinalysis.

Which of the following is true about appendicitis?

A) A normal white count effectively rules out the diagnosis of appendicitis.
B) The majority of patients with appendicitis present with fever.
C) The absence of anorexia effectively rules out appendicitis.
D) A fecalith is found on radiograph in the majority of patients with appendicitis.
E) None of the above.

Discussion

The correct answer is "E." None of the above is true. Taking these in order, 10% of patients with appendicitis have a normal white count, a minority of patients with appendicitis present with fever (15% in one study), only 75% of patients with appendicitis complain of anorexia, and a radiographic fecalith is found in only a small minority of patients.

Which of the following is *specific* for appendicitis?

A) Obturator sign.
B) Psoas sign.
C) Rovsing sign.
D) Tenderness at McBurney point.
E) None of the above is specific for appendicitis.

Discussion

The correct answer is "E." None of the above is specific for appendicitis. An obturator sign is present if there is pain on internal and external rotation of the hip. The obturator sign can be seen with any pelvic abscess that is in contact with the hip area, but is more commonly seen with a retrocecal abscess. The psoas sign is pain on use of the psoas muscle (e.g., lifting the leg at the hip), and it can be seen with any inflammatory process that is in contact with the psoas muscle, including a psoas abscess. Rovsing sign is when pain increases in an area of peritonitis when the abdomen is palpated elsewhere. For example, in a patient with appendicitis, right lower quadrant pain will be increased with palpation of the **left** lower quadrant. This is indicative of peritonitis in the area that has increased pain, but it is not specific for appendicitis. Tenderness at McBurney point can be seen in a number of processes including appendicitis, ileitis, any process in the cecum, and urinary tract infection.

Which of the following is true about the treatment of pain in the acute abdomen?

A) Early treatment with morphine will obscure the proper diagnosis.
B) Treatment with pain medication invalidates informed consent.
C) Early treatment of pain with morphine is safe except in children.
D) Ketorolac is preferred for patients who may undergo a surgical procedure.
E) None of the above is true.

Discussion

The correct answer is "E." None of the above is correct. Early treatment of pain in the acute abdomen actually **improves** diagnostic accuracy in both children and adults. Ketorolac is not a good choice because of its antiplatelet effects, which increase the risk of bleeding intraoperatively. Pain medication does not inherently invalidate informed consent (but obviously can if the patient is hardly arousable).

* *

Although you have thought a lot about his potential problem, you have not actually done anything more for the 15-year-old with abdominal pain!

The test most likely to help you arrive at a diagnosis in this patient is:

A) Erythrocyte sedimentation rate (ESR).
B) C-reactive protein (CRP).
C) Abdominal ultrasound.
D) Abdominal CT scan.
E) Colonoscopy.

Discussion

The correct answer is "D." The test most likely to be helpful in arriving at a diagnosis in this patient is a CT scan of the abdomen looking at the appendix. "A" and "B" are incorrect. Both the CRP and the ESR are nonspecific markers of inflammation and are not helpful in the diagnosis of appendicitis. "C," an ultrasound, can be used. However, it is not as sensitive as a CT scan. Ultrasound can be useful in the female patient in whom other diagnoses need to be ruled out, such as ovarian pathology. But, when looking specifically at the appendix, CT is preferable. "E," colonoscopy, is not particularly useful in the diagnosis of appendicitis but could be used for other purposes such as looking for IBD once appendicitis is ruled out by CT.

> HELPFUL TIP: **Not all patients with potential appendicitis need a CT scan. Those with obvious appendicitis should go directly to the OR.** CT should only be used in patients in whom the clinical diagnosis is equivocal. **There is some long-term risk from radiation exposure, so CT should not be done without a good indication.**

If this patient's CT scan is positive for appendicitis, the likelihood that he will have a normal appendix removed at appendectomy is:

A) 0%.
B) 10%.
C) 20%.
D) 30%.
E) 50%.

Discussion

The correct answer is "B." With the advent of CT scanning, the false positive rate (of taking normal patients to the OR) has improved, but perhaps not as much as you would think. The negative laparotomy rate is still about 10%. The negative laparotomy rate has gone down in men and the young but has increased in the elderly and in women. There is evidence that CT scanning changes the treatment plan in more than half of cases of suspected appendicitis. The sensitivity of CT for appendicitis is 91–98%, but the specificity is as low as 75% depending on the radiologist and the population tested (range 75–93%).

In general, which of the following is true about appendicitis?

A) Pain is in the right upper quadrant in the majority of pregnant women with appendicitis.
B) Atypical presentations are more common in the elderly patient than in other groups.
C) Patients with a retrocecal appendix generally present with well-localized tenderness and signs of peritoneal irritation.
D) All of the above.

Discussion

The correct answer is "B." Symptoms tend to be atypical in the elderly. In fact, elderly patients may have appendicitis with a normal white count, poorly localized pain, and absence of fever. So, maintain a high index of suspicion. "A" is incorrect. Despite classic teaching, patients who are pregnant tend to have "typical" symptoms with right lower quadrant pain. This is especially true in the first half of pregnancy. Certainly the appendix *can* be displaced cephalad, but the majority will still have right lower quadrant pain. "C" is incorrect. Patients with retrocecal appendicitis will commonly complain of a dull ache. However, signs of peritoneal irritation may be minimal or absent.

> HELPFUL TIP: Some patients have recurrent appendicitis. These patients will present with multiple episodes of "typical" appendicitis, which resolve during observation. When the appendix is finally removed, it is frequently scarred down.

Objectives: Did you learn to . . .

- Describe the findings in acute appendicitis?
- Diagnose appendicitis and determine how ancillary tests are best used in the patient presenting with signs and symptoms of appendicitis?
- Manage a patient with appendicitis?

CASE 11

A 72-year-old male presents to your office for a 3-month history of episodic abdominal pain. It is primarily located in the epigastric region and radiates to the back. It occurs both during the night and day and lasts about 1 hour. His past medical history is significant for a 5-year history of diabetes. He takes glyburide, atorvastatin, and aspirin. He has no previous surgical history. You order an ultrasound. The ultrasound reveals a normal aorta, but the technician notes several stones in the gallbladder.

You are concerned that this patient may have symptomatic cholelithiasis.

Which of the following is true of his risk for gallstones?

A) This patient has an increased risk of cholesterol stones because he is diabetic.
B) This patient's risk of gallstones would have peaked in his fourth decade of life.
C) This patient's risk of gallstones is increased because of his atorvastatin use.
D) This patient's risk for cholesterol stones is lower because of his advanced age.
E) This patient's risk of gallstones is increased because he's male.

Discussion

The correct answer is "A." Patients with diabetes have an increased risk of gallstones when compared with the general population. Other associations include female gender (not male, so "E" is wrong), family history, obesity, and certain medical illnesses including hyperlipidemia, cystic fibrosis, short bowel syndrome, parenteral nutrition, hemolytic anemia (e.g., sickle cell), and history of terminal ileum resection. "B" is incorrect because the risk of gallstones increases linearly with age. "C" is incorrect. Atorvastatin and other "statins" are not associated with an increased risk of gallstone formation, but clofibrate and other fibrates are. "D" is also incorrect. Cholecystectomy rates for symptomatic gallstones increase after the fourth decade of life, and increasing age is associated with an increased risk.

Which of the following statements is FALSE regarding the evaluation of the gallbladder?

A) Ultrasound will find pericolic fluid in only 50% of patients with cholecystitis.
B) A HIDA scan can be positive (e.g., no tracer in the duodenum) in the absence of cholecystitis.
C) ERCP has an attendant risk of pancreatitis.
D) The absence of disease on ultrasound effectively rules out gallbladder disease.

Discussion

The correct answer is "D." While ultrasound is highly sensitive for stones (95% or greater), it will miss some. "A" is a correct statement as are "B" and "C." A HIDA (hepatic iminodiacetic acid) scan can not only be abnormal (e.g., no tracer in the duodenum) in cholecystitis but also in any other condition in which the common duct is blocked including a common duct stone or tumor. Additionally, if there is liver disease (which may prevent the uptake of HIDA into the gallbladder), a full gallbladder, gallbladder dysfunction, or spasm of the sphincter of Oddi, one can have a false positive scan (e.g., no tracer in the duodenum).

> HELPFUL TIP: CT is not a very sensitive study for gallstones. Ultrasound is the study of choice for diagnosing gallstones (sensitivity is 25% for CT vs. 95% for ultrasound).

Regarding different types of gallstones, all of the following are true EXCEPT:

A) Cholesterol stones are associated with obesity and hyperlipidemia.
B) Black pigment stones are associated with cirrhosis.
C) Brown pigment stones are associated with liver fluke infection.
D) Blue pigment stones are associated with being an avid fan of the St. Louis Blues hockey team and/or the movie Avatar.

Discussion

The correct answer is "D." While we have noticed that beer-swilling hockey fans might be prone to developing gallstones, there are no studies that show this.

Besides, blue pigment stones do not exist. All the other options are true. Stone types include cholesterol, black pigment, and brown pigment stones. Cholesterol stones are associated with advancing age (due to decreased synthesis of bile salts from cholesterol), hyperlipidemia, diabetes, obesity, and living in the Western Hemisphere. Black pigment stones contain calcium bilirubinate, calcium carbonate, and calcium phosphonate. They are associated with hemolytic diseases, Crohn disease, ileal resection, cirrhosis, and total parental nutrition (TPN). Brown stones are observed more often in East Asia and are associated with liver fluke infection.

* *

You refer the patient to your favorite surgical consultant, Dr. Hugh Jeego, for evaluation of cholecystectomy. However, before his surgery appointment, you see him again in the ED. He presents with fever, nausea, vomiting, and anorexia for the last 48 hours. His exam is significant for temperature 38.9°C, mild tachycardia and tachypnea, and a normal blood pressure. He is tender in the right upper quadrant and has an associated Murphy sign. He has no jaundice or palpable right upper quadrant mass. Laboratory values include WBC 14,800/mm^3, ALT 58 IU/L, AST 64 IU/L, alkaline phosphatase 45 IU/L, total bilirubin 1.5 mg/dL (mildly elevated liver enzymes and bilirubin), amylase 95 IU/L, and lipase 52 IU/L (normal amylase and lipase).

At this point in time, your working diagnosis is:

A) Acalculous cholecystitis.
B) Acute calculous cholecystitis.
C) Pancreatitis.
D) Ascending cholangitis.
E) Myocardial infarction.

Discussion

The correct answer is "B." The clinical presentation, exam, and laboratory data point toward acute cholecystitis. "A" is incorrect because **acalculous** cholecystitis occurs more often in critically ill hospitalized patients, and you already know that this patient has stones, so his cholecystitis is by definition **calculous** in nature. There must be no gallstones detected on ultrasound to diagnose acalculous cholecystitis. "C" is incorrect. His pancreatic enzymes are normal (although one can certainly have pancreatitis with a normal amylase and lipase). "D" is incorrect. Patients with ascending cholangitis usually have markedly elevated transaminases and an obstructive laboratory pattern (e.g., elevated bilirubin, alkaline phosphatase, and pancreatic enzymes). "E" is very unlikely in this patient who has findings more consistent with intra-abdominal pathology, but you should always consider cardiac (and other thoracic organ) etiologies in older patients presenting with abdominal complaints.

Regarding the differential diagnosis of complicated cholelithiasis, which of the following is true?

A) Empyema of the gallbladder is primarily a disease of the elderly and carries a high mortality rate due to associated gram-positive sepsis.
B) Emphysematous cholecystitis occurs primarily in elderly diabetics as a late complication of miliary tuberculosis (TB).
C) The most common consequence of gallbladder perforation is generalized peritonitis.
D) The triad of Charcot (jaundice, fever, and right upper quadrant pain) is associated with cholangitis.

Discussion

The correct answer is "D." The classic triad of Charcot (jaundice, fever, and right upper quadrant pain) is associated with cholangitis, but it is **not** seen in the majority of cases, probably due to early detection of cholangitis. Nonetheless, it can be helpful if present. "A" is incorrect because patients generally develop a gram-**negative** sepsis. "B" is incorrect because emphysematous cholecystitis is not a complication of miliary TB, but it can occur with anaerobic cholecystitis. Miliary TB rarely affects the gall bladder. "C" is incorrect. The most common consequence of gallbladder perforation is a localized, walled off abscess. Additionally, a cholecystenteric fistula may form between the gallbladder and the duodenum or jejunum. Stones can then pass into the bowel. Stones larger than 2 cm in diameter are likely to lodge in the terminal ileum, a process termed gallstone ileus.

Generally, patients with cholecystitis typically have a prior history of biliary colic. Pain with acute cholecystitis is similar to that of cholelithiasis except is more often severe, longer lasting (>24 hours), and associated with anorexia, nausea, vomiting, fever, elevated white count (12,000–15,000), right upper quadrant guarding, and a positive Murphy sign (arresting inspiration when palpating the gallbladder). **But, Murphy sign is only 65% sensitive (less in the elderly). Additionally, 38% with confirmed cholecystitis have neither leukocytosis nor fever.** About 15% of the time there is associated jaundice and 20% of the time there is a palpable mass in the right upper quadrant. Biliary pancreatitis can occur when there is blockage of the ampulla of Vater, and cholangitis occurs when there is ductal stone obstruction and biliary infection. Emphysematous cholecystitis occurs primarily in elderly male diabetics: gas-producing bacteria, most commonly *C. perfringens*, result in gas in the gallbladder and cause a severe sepsis.

* *

Given the physical findings, leukocytosis, and mild elevation of transaminases, you conclude that this patient has cholecystitis.

Which of the following should *NOT* be considered in the management of this disease?

A) Initial treatment includes hospitalization with IV fluid resuscitation.
B) Possible antibiotic regimens include a third-generation cephalosporin +/− metronidazole, ticarcillin–clavulanate, and fluoroquinolone + metronidazole.
C) Most episodes of cholecystitis are caused by a single organism with enterococcus predominating.
D) If early cholecystectomy is not chosen as treatment, it should be performed late (at least 6 weeks after diagnosis).

Discussion

The correct answer is "C." This answer is incorrect for two reasons. First, just over 50% of episodes of cholecystitis are sterile; as a matter of course they are treated with antibiotics because of our inability to determine which are infected. Second, while enterococcus is frequently encountered, it is rarely a solitary pathogen and does not require specific targeted antimicrobial therapy. The initial treatment of cholecystitis includes hospitalization and IV fluid resuscitation. Definitive therapy for cholecystitis is cholecystectomy. Controversy surrounds whether cholecystectomy should be performed acutely or be delayed. Generally, shorter hospitalizations and better outcomes are found with early cholecystectomy.

Objectives: Did you learn to . . .

- Identify risk factors for gallstones?
- Recognize complications of gall bladder disease?
- Manage a patient with symptomatic gallstones and cholecystitis?

CASE 12

A 28-year-old white male who was the restrained front passenger of a vehicle traveling in excess of 60 mph is brought to the ED via ambulance. The driver of the vehicle was found dead at the scene. Ambulance personnel report it took 5–10 minutes to extricate the patient. On arrival, he is mumbling incoherently. He is initially able to give his name, but he is slurring his words. He denies any medical problems, medications, or allergies. Vitals signs include temperature 35.5°C, pulse 148, respirations 35, blood pressure 65/30, and oxygen saturation 81% on 100% oxygen by face mask. On exam, he is in severe respiratory distress. Lung sounds are absent on the right and diminished on the left. Heart sounds are muffled.

You determine that this patient needs immediate treatment of a pneumothorax.

Which of the following is most appropriate at this time?

A) Perform needle decompression on the left.
B) Perform needle decompression on the right.
C) Place a chest tube on the left.
D) Place a chest tube on the right.
E) Perform a chest radiograph and act on the basis of the results.

Discussion

The correct answer is "B." The combination of hypotension, hypoxia, and absent breath sounds suggests a tension pneumothorax. Immediate decompression of the affected hemithorax should be performed by placing a large-bore (14- or 16-gauge) needle through the chest wall to relieve intrathoracic pressure. Traditionally, this was accomplished by placing a needle in the second intercostal space at the midclavicular line. However, due to high risk of mediastinal vascular injuries, current practices recommend placing the needle in the traditional location for chest tube—that is the fifth or sixth intercostal spaces at the midaxillary line. Of particular note is "E." Tension pneumothorax **should never** be diagnosed on a chest radiograph.

It is a true emergency that requires treatment on the basis of clinical exam.

> **HELPFUL (AND UNFORTUNATE) TIP**
> Given the epidemic of obesity in the United States, a simple needle may not be long enough to reach the pleura (yes, really, it has been studied). Have a backup such as a longer, pigtail, catheter.

* *

His vital signs and oxygen saturation improve with needle decompression. You place a chest tube and give boluses of normal saline through two peripheral IVs. Then, the patient is placed in external fixation device for his femur fracture. Operating room fixation is deferred secondary to unstable medical status. He is admitted to the ICU on a respirator with C-collar following negative FAST examination (Focused Assessment with Sonography for Trauma, a sonographic evaluation to rule out fluid in perihepatic, perisplenic, pelvic, and pericardial spaces).

Repeat chest x-ray in the ICU shows the endotracheal (ET) tube and chest tube in appropriate positions. Several rib fractures are noted. There are "fluffy infiltrates" in the left chest that were not present on initial trauma chest series.

Which of the following is true of pulmonary contusions?

A) They occur in less than 25% of patients with **significant** blunt trauma to the chest.
B) Treatment includes aggressive IV steroid and fluid administration.
C) The condition starts to resolve in 48–72 hours.
D) Treatment includes appropriate antibiotics.

Discussion

The correct answer is "C." Pulmonary contusions begin to resolve in 48–72 hours. However, 2–3 weeks may be required for complete resolution. "A" is incorrect. Pulmonary contusions occur in up to 70% of trauma patients with **significant** blunt chest trauma. It is usually, but not always, associated with fractured ribs. There may also be a flail segment noted. Chest x-ray changes are usually evident within 1 hour post-trauma but may not appear for up to 6–7 hours. Pulmonary contusions result in a ventilation–perfusion mismatch, hypoxemia, and an increased A-a gradient. If a patient is able to maintain oxygenation and ventilation, intubation is not required. "B" and "D" are incorrect. Treatment currently only involves intubation as necessary, observation, and tincture of time.

* *

You elect to proceed with pulmonary artery catheter placement due to the severity of this patient's condition. Overnight he begins to decompensate. The nurse pages you with his vital signs and Swan–Ganz readings: temperature 37.0, pulse 100, respirations 20 (ventilator set at 14), blood pressure 82/30, PCWP 24 mm Hg (normal 5–15), cardiac index 2.0 L/min/m^2 (normal 2.5–3.5), SVR 2000 dyne-sec/cm^2 (normal 1000–1500), and oxygen delivery of 700 mL/min (normal 900–1200).

What is the cause of shock at this time?

A) Hypovolemic shock.
B) Neurogenic shock.
C) Cardiogenic shock.
D) Septic shock.

Discussion

The correct answer is "C." This patient appears to be in cardiogenic shock (elevated pulmonary capillary wedge pressure, decreased cardiac index). Cardiogenic shock may be caused by myocardial failure, valve failure, dysrhythmias, and tamponade. Treatment is directed at the underlying disorder. See Table 22–5 for more on the categories of shock.

> **HELPFUL TIP (OR NOTE OF CAUTION)**
> There is no good evidence to support the use of Swan–Ganz catheters in seriously ill patients. In fact, all of the evidence suggests **worse** outcomes with Swan–Ganz monitoring than without (from sepsis, thrombosis, etc.). Be very circumspect before electing to use Swan–Ganz catheters.

* *

Part of the injuries sustained by this patient includes burns to the abdomen and back.

Table 22–5 SURGERY: CATEGORIZATION OF SHOCK BY PHYSIOLOGIC PARAMETERS

Type of Shock	Systemic Vascular Resistance	Pulmonary Capillary Wedge Pressure	Oxygen Consumption (Based on Venous Gas)	Cardiac Output
Hypovolemic	Increased	Decreased	Decreased	Decreased
Cardiogenic	Increased	Increased	Decreased	Decreased
Distributive (sepsis, neurogenic)	Decreased	Decreased or normal	Increased	Increased
Obstructive (PE, vena caval obstruction, tension pneumothorax)	Increased	Low left, high right	Decreased	Decreased

Which of the following is FALSE regarding burn wound management in general?

A) The Parkland formula for fluid resuscitation calls for 2–4 mL/kg/% body surface area burned with half of the volume in the first 8 hours and the other half over the next 16 hours.
B) Escharotomy should be performed on all partial-thickness burns.
C) Patients with chemical burns should be treated first with tap water irrigation.
D) Prevention of wound infection via topical antimicrobial agents, such as silver sulfadiazine cream, or via silver-coated dressings is the standard of care.

Discussion

The correct answer is "B." Escharotomy is not necessary unless there is a full-thickness wound that is circumferential and compromising vascular supply. The thinking about this is changing and some suggest escharotomy of all **full-thickness** burns. "A" is a correct statement about the Parkland formula. "C" is also correct **with the addendum that any particulate matter should be brushed off prior to irrigation. Water may activate some substances such as sodium hydroxide.** "D" is also a correct statement although thinking is changing. Silver delays wound healing and bacitracin is being used with increasing frequency.

HELPFUL TIP: Fluids are required for adults with $>$15% total body surface area (TBSA) burns (second or third degree) and $>$10% for children aged 10 years and under. For adults the "Rule of 9's" is used to determine TBSA affected. Body surface area is estimated as follows: the head, each arm, front of each leg, and back of each leg count for 9% BSA each; the front and back of the trunk each count for 18%; the remaining 1% BSA is accounted for by the genitalia. TBSA affected in children and adolescents should be based on age-specific charts. Both affected and unaffected BSA should be calculated to assure accurate estimation.

HELPFUL TIP: The Parkland formula was designed to assure adequate hydration in burn patients as reflected by urine output (in the patient with functioning kidneys, of course). Adjust fluids appropriately to maintain adequate hydration without inducing congestive heart failure.

Which of the following is TRUE regarding fluid administration in burn and dehydrated patients?

A) A peripheral line will deliver fluid more rapidly than a central line of an equivalent gauge.
B) Albumin is the fluid of choice in the treatment of burns and should be considered for all patients with significant fluid deficits
C) D5 $^1/_2$ normal saline is the preferred fluid for fluid **resuscitation** in patients **other than burn patients.**
D) All of the above are true.

Discussion

The correct answer is "A." A peripheral line will deliver fluid more rapidly than a central line of an equivalent gauge, according to Poiseuille law (flow is directly proportional to tube radius and inversely proportional to tube length). The **shorter** the catheter, the more quickly fluid is delivered (think of a short traffic jam as opposed to a longer one on the same sized road). "B" is incorrect. Albumin is not helpful and may increase adverse outcomes in trauma. "C" is also incorrect. Normal saline—or lactated Ringer's if you are a surgeon—are the fluids of choice for resuscitation. Remember that lactated Ringer's is actually slightly hypotonic and thus may worsen cerebral edema. There is no evidence favoring lactated Ringer's over normal saline.

Objectives: Did you learn to . . .

- Approach a trauma patient with an understanding of advanced trauma life support principles?
- Identify and manage a patient with a tension pneumothorax?
- Describe various types of shock and how they are differentiated?
- Treat a patient in shock?
- Manage a patient with significant burns?

QUICK QUIZ: SURGERY

Carbonized particles in the nasal cavity and/or posterior pharynx in a burn patient should suggest:

A) The need for excision of the perichondrium in the nose to prevent underlying cartilage injury from avascular necrosis.
B) Inhalational injury to the lungs.
C) Ingestion of a large amount of particulate matter.
D) The need to check carboxyhemoglobin levels.
E) B and D.

Discussion

The correct answer is "E." Carbonaceous material in the nares or oropharynx should suggest the possibility of an inhalation injury. Given that this is related to the inhalation of combusted material, a carboxyhemoglobin level should be considered.

CASE 13

A 48-year-old female arrives at the ED via ambulance after witnesses saw her vomiting large volumes of blood in a local convenience store before collapsing to the floor. She is barely communicating and cannot provide any history. Ambulance personnel have placed two large-bore IVs and started normal saline boluses. Just as your start your initial evaluation, she has a large volume hematemesis. You are concerned about her depressed mental status and the severity of her illness and decide to intubate her. After intubation, the chest wall rises symmetrically and the lungs sound clear. Her heart sounds are distant, and she is tachycardic (pulse 120). Her blood pressure is 80/40 mm Hg. Her oxygen saturation is 78%.

The standard of care in detecting esophageal intubation is:

A) Auscultation.
B) Radiograph.
C) End-tidal CO_2.
D) Oxygen saturation.
E) Direct laryngoscopy.

Discussion

The correct answer is "C." The standard of care is the end-tidal CO_2. All of the others are notoriously unreliable. However, they all should be done. If you think you hear breath sounds but the oxygen saturation is not rising and end-tidal CO_2 is low, you are probably in the esophagus.

The end-tidal CO_2 can be falsely negative (detecting no CO_2) in which of the following situations?

A) Ingestion of carbonated soft drinks (or "pop" as we call it in the Midwest).
B) Intubation in the posterior pharynx above the cords.
C) Nasotracheal intubation.
D) During cardiac arrest.

Discussion

The correct answer is "D." The end-tidal CO_2 requires that there should be gas exchange in the lungs. If there is no gas exchange, the CO_2 will be low. This may be the case during cardiac arrest. "A" can actually cause a **false positive**. Carbon dioxide in the stomach will give a positive end-tidal CO_2 with an esophageal intubation. The same is true of "B." If the patient is breathing spontaneously, the CO_2 will be elevated even when the ET tube is above the cords. "C," nasotracheal intubation, should have no effect on end-tidal CO_2.

* *

You order laboratory studies that include a CBC, basic metabolic profile, liver chemistries, amylase, lipase, and coagulation studies. In addition, you type and cross for six units of packed red blood cells. The nurses have already contacted the gastroenterologist on-call, and she is on her way. You decide to perform NG lavage.

Which of the following is FALSE regarding NG lavage?

A) NG lavage may be negative even in the presence of an upper GI bleed.
B) NG lavage should not be attempted in obtunded patients until they are intubated.
C) Iced fluid should not be used to lavage patients with an upper GI bleed.
D) The placement of an NG tube is contraindicated in patients who may have variceal bleeding.

Discussion

The correct answer is "D." Varices **are not** a contraindication to the use of an NG tube. Studies suggest that an NG tube does not increase bleeding. Both "A" and "B" are true statements. Lavage **should not** be done in patients who are obtunded or otherwise unable to protect their own airway unless they are intubated. **In fact, if the patient has obvious blood in the vomitus, NG lavage is not necessary unless it is to clear stomach contents in order to perform endoscopy or to prevent vomiting. It adds nothing to the management of the patient with an upper GI bleed except confirming the diagnosis.** Remember that false-negative NG aspirates occur with intermittent bleeding and bleeding beyond the ligament of Treitz. "C" is also a true statement. Iced lavage fluid should not be used in patients with a GI bleed. The cooler temperature that results from the ice inhibits hemostasis and can increase bleeding.

HELPFUL TIP: Contraindications to gastric lavage include known ingestion of hydrocarbons and caustic agents, such as alkalis and acids.

* *

While your nurse is performing the warm water lavage (although why lavage is being done is a separate question since as noted above it does not add anything to this patient's care), you perform a secondary physical examination on the patient. Her most obvious finding is a markedly jaundiced state. Other pertinent findings include a 6 cm scalp laceration, which continues to actively bleed, moderate ascites, and lower extremity edema. After lavage with nearly 5 L of isotonic fluid, the patient's aspirate continues to be bloody. At this point, her vitals are remaining steady but have shown no sign of improvement. Initial emergent labs have returned: Na 142 mEq/L, K 3.2 mEq/L, Cl 106 mEq/L, CO_2 18 mEq/L, BUN 40 mg/dL, Cr 0.8 mg/dL, glucose 110 mg/dL, WBC 7000/mm^3, Hb 9.8 g/dL, HCT 29%, Plt 62,000/mm^3, INR 3.0, PTT 48, albumin 2.4 g/dL, AST 76 IU/L, ALT 39 IU/L, Bili 3.5 mg/dL, amylase 210 IU/L, and lipase 24 IU/dL. The gastroenterologist is still 5–10 minutes away.

In considering what to do next, which of the following would be most appropriate?

A) Address presence of platelet dysfunction by transfusing with a 10-pack of platelets.
B) In order to accurately assess degree of volume depletion, place a CVP catheter or Swan–Ganz catheter and bladder catheter.
C) Regardless of the gastroenterologist, central line placement should be priority at this time because fluid resuscitation is the primary concern.
D) Emergent gastric tamponade should be attempted with a Foley catheter.
E) None of the above is a great idea right about now.

Discussion

The correct answer is "E." None of the above is a particularly good idea right about now. Looking at them one by one, "A" is not necessary since a platelet count of 62,000 is adequate for hemostasis (although you would not be faulted for giving platelets). A platelet count of <50,000 is considered an indication for platelet transfusion in an actively bleeding patient. "B" and "C" are not good ideas because coagulopathy (INR 3.0) is a **relative** contraindication to central line placement. It can be done but is not needed at this point. Recall from above that peripheral catheters will deliver more fluid more rapidly when compared with central catheters. Thus, two large-bore, peripheral IVs are the access of choice. "D" is incorrect because gastric tamponade with a Foley is like trying to stop a leak in the Hoover dam with putty: it won't work. You may want to give vitamin K and fresh frozen plasma to reverse her coagulopathy, however.

Effective methods for controlling upper GI variceal bleeding that improve outcomes include all of the following EXCEPT:

A) Variceal ligation.
B) Sclerotherapy.
C) TIPS (transjugular intrahepatic portosystemic shunt) procedure.
D) Vasopressin.

Discussion

The correct answer is "D." Vasopressin, while achieving initial control of bleeding in up to 60% of patients, has essentially **no** effect on rebleeding and **no effect on mortality**. This may be because ischemia of the splanchnic bed and other areas caused by vasopressin outweighs any benefit. In more bad news, octreotide also does not have any effect on mortality unless combined with variceal ligation. Variceal ligation and sclerotherapy both reduce mortality. Additionally, a TIPS procedure has been shown to effectively stop bleeding by reducing portal pressures. It also reduces **acute** mortality. Data is conflicting on long-term outcomes but encephalopathy is more of a problem after TIPS.

HELPFUL TIP: An elevated BUN can be indirect evidence of a GI bleed in patients with liver disease. The digestion of blood leads to the elevated BUN.

* *

You consider a central line.

Which of the following techniques is associated with the highest rate of infection?

A) External jugular.
B) Internal jugular.
C) Femoral vein.
D) Subclavian vein.

Discussion

The correct answer is "C." Infection is more likely with cannulation of the femoral vein. This makes intuitive sense given its location. Subclavian veins have a higher risk of complication such as arterial injury, hemothorax, pneumothorax, and lung injury. Thoracic duct injury is most common with left internal jugular cannulation. **Note that ultrasound guidance of central lines is rapidly becoming the standard of care.**

* *

The gastroenterologist arrives and you explain the situation. Vitals at this time include a temperature of 36.8°C, pulse 105, respirations 14 (ventilator dependent), blood pressure 85/40, and oxygen saturation of 92%. The gastroenterologist plans to attempt endoscopy with sclerotherapy, but would like to have the general surgeons available for backup in case emergent operative intervention becomes necessary. As you prepare to contact the surgeon, you recall risk stratification for cirrhotic patients is via the Child–Pugh classification system.

Which of the following is FALSE regarding the Child–Pugh scoring system?

A) The Child–Pugh scoring system can be used to predict the risk of variceal bleeding.
B) The five criteria used in the Child–Pugh classification are ascites, encephalopathy, albumin, bilirubin, and INR.
C) The Child–Pugh scoring system can be used to determine if the patient with a deep hepatic encephalopathy will wake up.
D) A patient with a serum bilirubin of 3.5 mg/dL may have the exact same Child–Pugh score as a patient with a serum bilirubin of 25 mg/dL.

Discussion

The correct answer is "C." The Child–Pugh scoring system does not predict the course of hepatic encephalopathy. The other statements are correct. The Child–Pugh classification includes evaluation of ascites, history of encephalopathy, albumin, bilirubin, and INR. "A" is correct because the Child–Pugh score can be used to predict the risk of variceal bleeding as well as the surgical risk and the overall mortality in patients with liver disease. "D" is correct since there is a ceiling to the Child–Pugh scoring system for each parameter, and the same score is given for all bilirubin levels above 3 mg/dL.

HELPFUL TIP: In severely ill patients, a history of encephalopathy may not be obtainable. This is OK. Severely ill patients can still be a

Table 22-6 CHILD–PUGH CLASSIFICATION

Points assigned	1	2	3
Encephalopathy	None	Low grade	High grade
Ascites	None	Slight	Moderate-large
Bilirubin	1–2 mg/dL	2–3 mg/dL	>3 mg/dL
Albumin	>3.5 g/dL	2.8–3.5 g/dL	<2.8 g/dL
INR	<1.7	1.8–2.3	>2.3

Child–Pugh Class C (the worst class) even with a "1" for hepatic encephalopathy.

Further discussion: The Child–Pugh classification as a global battery of tests can help to more accurately assess degree of cirrhosis, need for transplant (minimum score of 7), mortality rate from variceal bleed, and outcomes after surgery and TIPS, and outcomes with a hepatoma (Table 22–6).

Class A is defined as having 5–6 points, Class B is 7–9 points, and Class C is 10–15 points. The 1- and 2-year survival in patients with Class C disease is 45% alive at 1 year and 35% alive at 2 years.

Class A patients have an operative mortality of 1%, while Class B and C have operative mortalities of 3–10% and 30–50%, respectively. In patients with hepatomas, no Class B or C patients survived 3–5 years following resection, although about 40% of Class A patients survive for 5 years.

HELPFUL TIP: An easier system is the Model for End-Stage Liver Disease (MELD) score. This takes into account serum bilirubin, INR, and serum creatinine. It has done away with some of the subjective judgments required by the Child–Pugh score including judging how much ascites is present and the severity of the encephalopathy. A number of calculators are available; here's one: http://www.mayoclinic.org/meld/mayomodel6.html.

Objectives: Did you learn to . . .

- Manage a patient with a massive upper GI bleed?
- Determine if an ET tube has been placed correctly?
- Recognize the uses and limitations of gastric lavage?
- Recognize the uses and limitations of central line placement and Swan–Ganz catheter placement?
- Evaluate a patient with liver disease, using the Child–Pugh and MELD scores?

QUICK QUIZ: INTUBATION

Which of the following IS NOT a contraindication to a nasotracheal intubation?

A) Patient is not breathing.
B) Patient is anticoagulated or has had TPA.
C) Midface trauma.
D) History of a septoplasty.

Discussion

The correct answer is "D." All of the rest are contraindications to nasotracheal intubation. Specifically, it is not possible to do a nasotracheal intubation in a nonbreathing patient. Patients who are anticoagulated may bleed profusely after a nasotracheal intubation, and midface trauma suggests the possibility that the tube could end up in the brain. **Although the standard of care, two studies have failed to show a difference between CNS complications with orotracheal versus nasotracheal intubation. Nonetheless, avoid nasotracheal intubation in midface trauma, except as a last resort, or you will get dinged if there is a complication.**

CASE 14

You are seeing a 33-year-old resident at a large university hospital setting where medical care is provided freely to him. He is about to complete his Internal Medicine residency and wants to "get his money's worth" of free procedures before he leaves. He has scheduled a full afternoon of procedures with you, including toenail removal, excision of a mole on his neck, and a stylish new cartilage ear piercing for his new job as a cruise ship doctor.

He has had trouble with recurrent pain and inflammation on his left great toe at the medial side. On exam you identify onychocryptosis (ingrown nail). He has tried soaks, growing past the skin, and regular paring—all without success.

Regarding nail removal in this patient, which one of the following is FALSE?

A) The great toe is the most commonly affected toe for onychocryptosis.
B) If the patient chooses partial nail removal, about 25% of the nail should be removed on the affected side.
C) Phenol should be placed for no longer than 10 seconds to the germinal tissue to prevent necrosis.
D) When removing the nail, an upward twist of the hand to the medial side should be performed.

Discussion
The correct answer is "C." Phenol can be left in place for 3 minutes. Ingrown toenails almost exclusively affect the great toe on either the medial or lateral side. Partial or full nail removal should be implemented when conservative measures have failed. Besides ingrown nails (onychocryptosis), onychomycosis (fungal infection of the nail), recurrent paronychia (nail fold inflammation), and onychogryposis (deformed, curved nail) are all indications for partial or full nail removal. If recurrent ingrown nails have occurred, germinal tissue can be ablated with phenol on a cotton swab held in place for 3 minutes, and afterward the phenol should be neutralized with alcohol.

* *

Next, he complains about a small regular mole on his neck that he repeatedly cuts while shaving. He would like to have it removed in whatever way you deem best. The lesion is raised above the skin. Although it is mildly irregular in appearance from the repeated trauma of shaving, there is no evidence of atypia.

Which of the following is *NOT* a correct statement regarding removal of this lesion?

A) Curettage or shave biopsy would be ideal for this sort of lesion.
B) If sutures are required, 6-O nylon would be ideal in this location.
C) If a punch biopsy is performed, skin should be held taught perpendicular to the angle of the mandible (the natural skin lines of the neck).
D) In this location, both shave and punch techniques require closure by suture approximation.

Discussion
The correct answer is "D." Various types of skin lesion removal exist: punch biopsy, shave biopsy, curettage, and elliptical excisional biopsy. Punch biopsy involves taking a full-thickness sample in skin areas (except for the eyelids, lips, or penis). Skin should be help taught perpendicular to the natural skin tension lines, and punch instrument is rotated through the skin. The site is closed with either a single interrupted or vertical mattress suture. Shave biopsy is indicated for removal of elevated skin lesions, while complete thickness removal is unnecessary. Shave should be made from both lateral edges into center to avoid cutting too deep. No suturing is necessary. Curettage entails a method of removing lesions that also does not require full-thickness sampling. A Fox dermal curettage is used to scrape away unwanted tissue followed by electrical or chemical cautery for hemostasis. Finally, elliptical excision is used when full dermal thickness excision is necessary. Contraindications to skin biopsy include infection at the site or coagulopathy.

* *

Finally, your patient is a little embarrassed to be seen at the mall getting his ear pierced, and asks if you could pierce it for him. He is considering a standard lobe pierce versus an auricular cartilage piercing.

Which of the following is true in regard to counseling and technique?

A) Eczema at the site is a contraindication to piercing.
B) Auricular cartilage piercing should only be performed by a trained physician.
C) Ears should be pierced from the posterior to anterior site.
D) Ear piercing involves boring a 20-gauge needle to the marked site.
E) Ear piercing is contraindicated in nerds.

Discussion
The correct answer is "A." Eczema in the area is a contraindication to piercing. Other contraindications

include infection, previous keloid formation, immunodeficiency, and coagulopathy. Auricular cartilage piercing is prone to infection and generally least advisable—although it certainly is popular. All of the other options are incorrect. "E" deserves special mention, as "nerds" can be made "hipsters" simply by piercing their ears. A corollary to this is that any male with a gray ponytail should avoid piercings. It won't make them look younger and hip.

> HELPFUL TIP: Auricular cartilage piercing is prone to infection with destruction of the cartilage. *Pseudomonas* is a common pathogen and oral fluoroquinolones are indicated as treatment.

Objectives: Did you learn to . . .

- Describe techniques and indications for toenail removal?
- Describe various skin biopsy techniques?
- Identify contraindications to ear piercing?

QUICK QUIZ: DOC, IS THAT A HOSE IN MY CHEST?

What statement represents *correct* chest tube management?

A) A tube that shows no water fluctuations when placed on "water seal" should have wall suction increased to attempt to reopen.
B) Initial postoperative setting of a chest tube is most often –100 cm H_2O.
C) Unless there is major injury to the lung, continuous bubbling of the water seal chamber most likely represents an apparatus leakage.
D) If a purse string was placed during initial placement of the chest tube, tightly tying the purse string when pulling the chest tube is enough to prevent pneumothorax.

Discussion

The correct answer is "C." Continued bubbling in the water seal chamber suggests that there is a leak in the system. Theoretically, once the pleura are drained of air, there should be no further bubbling. Air leakage is seen as air bubbles that increase with increased intrathoracic pressure (e.g., cough, Valsalva maneuver, and positive pressure ventilation). Continuous air leakage may be due to a large tear in the lung parenchyma, bronchopleural fistula, or an apparatus leak. "A" is incorrect. A tube that is nonfunctional should be removed. Increasing the suction will not reopen it. "B" is incorrect as well. Initial suction should be – 20 cm H_2O. "D" is incorrect because an occlusive dressing, such as petrolatum gauze, should be placed over the former chest tube site once the tube is removed.

A chest tube can be removed when the following criteria are met: fluid drainage is less than 150 cc/day, the lung is fully expanded on chest x-ray, and no air leak is present. Typically, chest tubes are first placed to "water seal" for 6–24 hours to see if the patient will tolerate having the tube removed.

CASE 15

John is a 63-year-old male who presents to your office for a physical exam. As part of the exam, you do a rectal exam and stool guaiac. The guaiac is heme positive. On colonoscopy, he is noted to have biopsy-proven colon cancer.

Regarding colon cancer, what is the most likely type of cancer you will find?

A) Squamous cell carcinoma.
B) Adenocarcinoma.
C) Clear cell carcinoma.
D) Lymphoma.

Discussion

The correct answer is "B." Adenocarcinoma represents the overwhelming majority of colon cancers. Other histologic types of colon cancer include adenosquamous, poorly differentiated cancers with neuroendocrine aspects, small cell carcinomas (of neuroendocrine origin), and others.

* *

John has the perennial question that only theologians can answer: "Why me?" In this case, however, we can help to provide some insight.

Which of the following is *NOT* considered a risk factor for colon cancer?

A) Familial polyposis.
B) Alcohol use.

C) Obesity.
D) Inflammatory Bowel Disease.
E) Chronic constipation.

Discussion
The correct answer is "E." Chronic constipation is not a risk factor for colon cancer. Other risk factors include acromegaly, diabetes mellitus, and being African American, among others. In fact, African Americans have the highest risk for colon cancer of any ethnic group with a 20% increase in mortality when compared with whites.

* *

John is justifiably worried about the possibility of colon cancer in his offspring. Unfortunately, none of his offspring exercise (which reduces colon cancer risk) and they are avowed carnivores eschewing fruit, vegetables, and anything with fiber (which **may** reduce colon cancer risk, although the data is conflicting).

Which of the following has been shown to reduce cancer risk and takes so little effort that even John's slothful offspring may partake?

A) Metformin.
B) Aspirin.
C) Antioxidants.
D) Vitamin B6 but not other antioxidants.
E) B and C.

Discussion
The correct answer is "B." Aspirin and other NSAIDs have been shown to reduce the risk of colon cancer. Unfortunately, the rest of the answers are incorrect and none have been found to reduce the risk of colon cancer

* *

It is time to stage John cancer. The Duke's Classification system is no longer used for colon cancer and has been replaced with the more standardized TMN system.

Which of the following is *the most common* first site of metastasis of colon cancer?

A) Lungs.
B) Liver.
C) Bone.
D) Brain.

Discussion
The correct answer is "B." The liver is the most common first site of colon cancer metastases, which arrive via the portal system. Colon cancer can also metastasize to the lungs, bone, lymph nodes and brain (uncommon). Intraperitoneal spread may also occur.

While tumor markers for colon cancer are not used in staging disease, the presence of which of these markers suggests a poor prognosis if it remains elevated after surgical resection of the tumor?

A) Carcinoembryonic antigen (CEA).
B) Beta-hCG.
C) CA-195.
D) VIP.

Discussion
The correct answer is "A." The presence of CEA after resection of a colon cancer is a poor prognostic factor. This should be obvious: there is still tumor present. Beta-hCG is elevated in testicular cancer; CA-195 is a marker for ovarian cancer (although it is also expressed by colon cancer cells). VIP is either the patient who everyone swarms over and nobody can please *or* vasoactive intestinal peptide, which is found with some pancreatic adenocarcinomas and carcinoid tumors.

HELPFUL TIP: While 5-HIAA sounds like an acronym for some new government initiative, it is a marker of carcinoid tumor activity.

* *

John undergoes surgery and by some fluke (or error) ends up with a total colectomy and ileostomy.

Which of the following is NOT true of ileostomy care?

A) Fluid output tends to be relatively high with an ileostomy requiring increased fluid intake to prevent dehydration.
B) Since the diameter of the ileostomy is limited, avoiding large amounts of nondigestible fiber helps to prevent bezoar formation.
C) Time-release drugs are usually OK because most of the digestion and absorption occur before the colon anyway.

D) Proteolytic enzymes are present in the effluent and may lead to skin breakdown.

Discussion

The correct answer is "C." Time-release medications should be **avoided,** since absorption often takes place in the colon. All of the rest are correct.

> HELPFUL TIP: Loperamide can be used to reduce output in short bowel syndrome (including in those with an ostomy) as long as bacterial overgrowth is not an issue.

* *

John does well and has a happy and long life, although his children remain slugs and he supports them well into their 40s.

Objectives: Did you learn to . . .

- Describe some tumor markers for various cancers?
- Define various histologic types of colon cancers and the pattern of metastasizing?
- Recognize risk factors for colon cancer and ways to reduce the risk of colon cancer?
- Manage ostomies?

BIBLIOGRAPHY

American College of Surgeons. *Advanced Trauma Life Support for Doctors: Student Course Manual*. 8th ed. American College of Surgeons; 2008.

Cameron JL. *Current Surgical Therapy*. 9th ed. St. Louis, MO: Mosby, Inc.; 2007.

Graber MA, et al. *The Family Practice Handbook*. 5th ed. Philadelphia, PA: W.B. Saunders Company; 2006.

Lawrence PF. *Essentials of General Surgery*. 4th ed. Philadelphia, PA: Lippincott Williams & Wilkins; 2005.

Marino PL, et al. *The ICU Book*. 3rd ed. Philadelphia, PA: Lippincott Williams & Wilkins; 2006.

Mulholland MW, et al. *Greenfield's Surgery: Scientific Principles and Practice*. 4th ed. Philadelphia, PA: Lippincott Williams & Wilkins; 2006.

Pfenninger JL, Fowler GC. *Procedures for Primary Care Physicians*. 3rd ed. St. Louis, MO: Mosby, Inc.; 2011.

Scott-Conner CEH, Dawson DL. *Operative Anatomy*. 2nd ed. Philadelphia, PA: Lippincott Williams & Wilkins; 2003.

Townsend CM, et al. *Sabiston's Textbook of Surgery*. 18th ed. Philadelphia, PA: W.B. Saunders Company; 2008.

23

Psychiatry

Mark A. Graber, Jason K. Wilbur, and Benjamin Shepherd

CASE 1

You are seeing a 48-year-old female who presents with a 3-month history of low mood, low energy, poor concentration, and irritability. She has lost interest in most things she had enjoyed and has also noticed a 20-pound weight gain. She has been having frequent headaches, has been short tempered, and has noticed that it is hard to wake up in the morning. She reports no thoughts of suicide but has wondered if death would be a relief. She says she has felt restless for a while and feels that she is a bad person. Her mother suffered from depression. She does not consume alcohol or any other substances. She is divorced and has no children.

You think that this patient may meet criteria for a depressive disorder.

Which of the following is NOT a criterion for the diagnosis of *major* depressive disorder (MDD)?

A) Low mood.
B) Presence of suicidal ideation.
C) Decreased appetite.
D) Anhedonia.
E) Irritability.

Discussion

The correct answer is "E." The presence of irritability, while often seen with depressive disorders, is not used to make the diagnosis. All of the other options listed are part of the criteria set forth in the *Diagnostic and Statistical Manual of Mental Disorders*, 4th ed. (DSM-IV). Special emphasis is placed on the presence of depressed mood and decreased interest, one of which must be present in order to diagnose MDD. The criteria for the diagnosis of a major depressive episode are listed below.

Criteria for Major Depression: Two weeks or more of depressed mood **or** loss of interest or anhedonia **AND** four of the following: (1) significant change in weight or appetite; (2) insomnia or hypersomnia; (3) psychomotor agitation or retardation; (4) fatigue or loss of energy; (5) feeling worthless or excessive guilt; (6) poor concentration; and (7) recurrent thoughts of death, suicidal ideation, attempt, or plan.

HELPFUL TIP: Several mnemonics have been developed to help clinicians remember the DSM-IV criteria and two of these are "SIG-ECAPS" and "SPACE DIGS." **S**leep, **I**nterest, **G**uilt, **E**nergy, **C**oncentration, **A**ppetite, **P**sychomotor changes, **S**uicidality.

Which one of this patient's symptoms is considered a symptom of *atypical* depression?

A) Hypersomnia.
B) Low mood.
C) Anhedonia.
D) Psychomotor retardation.
E) Irritability.

Discussion
The correct answer is "A." The typical vegetative symptoms of depression include poor sleep or insomnia, reduced appetite, and decreased libido. Patients with **atypical depression** have hyperphagia, hypersomnolence, and mood reactivity among other symptoms.

* *

You begin to explain the nature of depression to this patient.

Which of the following epidemiological statements is NOT true?

A) The average American has about a 16% chance of developing depression over his or her lifetime.
B) About 7% of Americans suffer depression each year.
C) Women are five times as likely to suffer depression as are men.
D) The incidence of depression is increasing in younger cohorts.
E) Divorced people are more likely to be depressed.

Discussion
The correct answer is "C." Depression is a chronic illness that often begins early in life and is recurrent with significant morbidity and mortality. The lifetime prevalence of MDD is 16% with 6.6% of adults suffering from MDD in any given year. Women are **twice** (not five times) as likely to have depression, as are men. The rate becomes equal in the elderly with elderly men being at a higher risk of suicide than elderly women. Being divorced is a risk factor for depression.

> HELPFUL TIP: Anxiety, not meeting the level of an anxiety disorder, frequently accompanies depression (70%). However, 60% of people with a lifetime diagnosis of MDD have had a **diagnosable anxiety disorder.**

* *

This patient's situation is not unusual for your practice.

What is the prevalence of MDD in primary care patients?

A) 1–2%.
B) 5–10%.
C) 25–30%.
D) 45–50%.
E) 100% (seems like everyone... even the clinic staff).

Discussion
The correct answer is "B." About 5–10% of primary care patients meet criteria for MDD and about twice of that (10–20%) many have "minor" depression. If you answered "E," you work in a sad, sad place. Hire a clown to work the front desk.

Which of these epidemiological statements about depression in primary care is true?

A) Most depressed patients (about 80%) seek mental health care from primary care physicians.
B) Only about 50% of the patients with depression are recognized by their primary care physician.
C) Only about half of the patients diagnosed with MDD receive adequate treatment.
D) The United States Preventive Task Force (USPTF) recommends **against** screening unless support services are already in place.
E) All of the above.

Discussion
The correct answer is "E." All are correct. In 2009, USPTF changed their recommendation to advise against screening for depression unless **"staff-assisted depression care supports are in place to assure accurate diagnosis, effective treatment, and follow-up."** One reason for lack of diagnosis of depression in primary care is that depression often presents with somatic complaints. Another is that the spectrum of disease in primary care offices is less severe leading to fewer diagnoses.

> HELPFUL TIP: There are several brief self-rating depression scales that can be used for screening (e.g., Beck Depression Inventory, Primary Care Evaluation of Mental Disorders, Patient Health Questionnaire, and Zung Depression Scale). A two-patient question screen may be as effective for screening as these more extensive scales. Simply ask:
>
> - Over the past 2 weeks, have you often felt down, blue or in the dumps?

- Over the past 2 weeks, have you lost interest in most activities or things that used to bring you pleasure?

A positive answer to either of those two questions should prompt a more thorough evaluation of depression. A negative answer to both effectively rules out depression in most patients.

* *

You realize that it is also important to focus on the social history in patients with depression.

Which of the following is associated with a DECREASED risk of depression?

A) Unemployment.
B) Poverty.
C) Being unmarried.
D) Family history.
E) Being Black.

Discussion

The correct answer is "E." Factors associated with an increased risk of depression include **female gender** (2× risk), unemployment, poverty, being unmarried (single or divorced), having a family history of depression, a recent childbirth or pregnancy, medical comorbidities, lack of social support, and substance use. Protective factors include marriage, Black race, and being retired (so retired is when we are supposed to have fun!).

* *

You believe that your patient is suffering from an episode of major depression, and you decide to initiate treatment with an antidepressant.

Following the first episode of depression, what is her risk of relapse?

A) <1%.
B) 25%.
C) 50%.
D) 75%.
E) >99%.

Discussion

The correct answer is "C." The incidence of relapse following the first episode of depression is roughly 50%; this can be reduced by two-thirds by continuing antidepressant medications chronically. Following the second episode, the risk of relapse is roughly 75%, climbing up to 90% after the third episode. In order to reduce the risk of relapse, most authorities recommend antidepressant therapy for 6–12 months after remission of symptoms in patients with their first episode of depression. Some patients probably benefit from indefinite medical therapy, including those with a severe first episode (e.g., significant suicide attempt), patients with a psychotic depression, patients with three or more episodes, elderly patients with their first episode of depression, and possibly those with a strong family history of depression.

* *

You choose a serotonin reuptake inhibitor (SSRI) and tell your patient to contact you if she suffers from adverse effects.

Which of the following is NOT a typical adverse effect of SSRIs?

A) Nausea.
B) Headaches.
C) Restlessness.
D) Insomnia.
E) Urinary retention.

Discussion

The correct answer is "E." Urinary retention is not seen with SSRIs, but the other four options are typical of SSRIs. The anticholinergic effect of urinary retention is typical of the tricyclic antidepressants (TCAs). Sexual dysfunction and GI problems are commonly seen with SSRIs. Akasthisia and dystonic reactions can (rarely) be seen with SSRIs as well.

* *

Your patient returns to see you 2 weeks after starting her SSRI and reports that she has not noticed any benefit from the medication.

Which of the following statements is most accurate?

A) The antidepressant is not going to work, so she should switch medicines to one of the same class.
B) The antidepressant is not going to work, so she should switch medicines to another antidepressant from a different class.
C) It is too early to judge the efficacy of the antidepressant at this point.

D) She's probably suffering a paradoxical reaction of increased depression with her medication.
E) Going up on the dose is not an option at this time.

Discussion
The correct answer is "C." Antidepressants begin to exert their **biological** effects immediately with increases in neurotransmitters, but the effects on mood are not apparent for about 2–4 weeks. As such, it is premature to abandon this medication. Increasing the dose **or** giving it at least 4–6 weeks total at the current dose would be the best options.

* *

You increase the medication dose, and the patient returns to see you in another 2 weeks. This time, she is feeling better and more energetic. People at work are beginning to notice her improved attitude, and her sleep has become more refreshing now. She wants to know how long she should stay on the medication.

The correct answer is:

A) At least 1 month.
B) At least 2 months.
C) At least 4–6 months.
D) At least 2 years.
E) Forever.

Discussion
The correct answer is "C." Different organizations recommend different durations of treatment but the shortest recommended course is 4–6 months, with most authorities treating for 6–12 months after recovery.

Objectives: Did you learn to . . .

- Diagnose MDD?
- Appreciate the epidemiology and natural history of depression?
- Recognize features of atypical depression?
- Initiate treatment of depression?
- Identify adverse effects of SSRIs?

CASE 2

You are assessing a 45-year-old professional male who has a history of MDD in his early 20s but has fully recovered since then. He recently suffered an uncomplicated anterior wall myocardial infarction (MI). His wife mentions that she thinks he is depressed. He is tired all the time, has poor sleep, a poor appetite, and he has been irritable. He has also been tearful and blames himself for his MI (too many "pounder" burgers . . . with cheese and bacon). He is willing to consider the diagnosis of depression because he remembers having suffered from it before. He also knows a history of MDD puts him at risk of medical illnesses.

Which of the following illnesses is more prevalent in patients with MDD?

A) Coronary heart disease.
B) Cerebrovascular disease.
C) Diabetes mellitus.
D) Osteoporosis.
E) All of the above are more prevalent in depressed patients.

Discussion
The correct answer is "E." **It is unclear if patients with depression are more likely to have these illnesses as a result of the depression or the reverse; patients with these illnesses are more likely to be depressed.** Depressed patients have an average of 3.4 more chronic medical conditions than nondepressed patients. At least two studies have now linked a lifetime history of MDD to an increased risk (1.2–3 times) of early menopause (of course, that would be a bit strange in our patient, a male).

* *

You know that some of this patient's symptoms could be secondary to his medical illness.

Which one of the following symptoms, if present, is the *most specific* for depression?

A) Sleep problems.
B) Appetite difficulties.
C) Psychomotor agitation.
D) Low energy.
E) Excessive preoccupation with death.

Discussion
The correct answer is "E." In the mnemonic "SPACE DIGS," the last four letters stand for symptoms that are more specific for depression and more independent of somatic illnesses. These symptoms are **D**epressed mood, loss of **I**nterests, inappropriate **G**uilt, and thoughts of **S**uicide ("DIGS"). The presence of any of these symptoms should lead you to suspect depression.

> **HELPFUL TIP:** While depression can often be precipitated by a stressor, it can also arise with no precipitating factor, and the response to treatment is independent of whether it is "reactive" (identifiable stressor present) or "endogenous" (no identifiable stressor).

Which of the following statements is NOT true about depression post-MI?

A) Major depression is an independent risk factor for post-MI mortality.
B) Minor depression is an independent risk factor for post-MI mortality.
C) Minor depression is more prevalent than major depression post-MI.
D) Treating depression improves cardiac outcomes in post-MI patients.
E) Approximately half of the people who sustain an MI have symptoms of depression afterward.

Discussion

The correct answer is "D." In the post-MI period, major depression prevalence is almost 20%, and minor depression is about 27%. Concurrent major depression elevates mortality risk after MI by a factor of 3.5, which is the same degree of risk as congestive heart failure (CHF). Patients with a mood disturbance (e.g., minor depression) also have a higher mortality rate. While treatment of depression has been shown to improve some medical outcomes (e.g., HbA_{1c} levels in diabetics), this is not the case in cardiovascular disease. Treatment of depression does not change mortality or morbidity after an MI (but may increase quality of life).

> **HELPFUL TIP:** Patients suffering strokes also have an elevated risk of depression with approximately one-third of post-stroke patients meeting criteria for MDD; there is a similar correlation of depressive symptoms to stroke mortality.

* *

You decide to recommend treatment to this patient.

Which of the following therapies is the LEAST desirable choice for treating his depression?

A) Bupropion (Wellbutrin).
B) Cognitive Behavioral Therapy.
C) Nortriptyline.
D) Paroxetine (Paxil).
E) Sertraline (Zoloft).

Discussion

The correct answer is "C." TCAs should be avoided in patients with cardiovascular disease because of their arrhythmogenic potential (e.g., torsades de pointes). Remember that SNRIs and citalopram (Celexa) can also prolong the QT interval. Bupropion and cognitive behavioral therapy (CBT) are also reasonable choices.

> **HELPFUL TIP:** Consider a baseline ECG in all patients for whom you are considering tricyclics to evaluate the QT interval. If the QT is prolonged at baseline, it predisposes patients to tricyclic-induced arrhythmias.

Objectives: Did you learn to . . .

- Diagnose depression occurring with an acute medical illness?
- Recognize the impact of depression on other medical conditions?
- Treat a post-MI patient with depression?

QUICK QUIZ: PSYCHIATRIC DIAGNOSIS

A 44-year-old patient of yours has come to see you multiple times for low mood. She does not have trouble with energy, sleep, concentration, or appetite. Basically, she tells you, "I've been depressed for as long as I can remember." You have tried treating her with two different SSRIs, but she had trouble with side effects and did not notice much improvement in her mood.

Which of the following is the best diagnosis for this patient?

A) Adjustment disorder.
B) Bipolar effective disorder.
C) Dysthymia.
D) MDD.
E) Premenstrual dysphoric disorder.

Discussion

The correct answer is "C." Dysthymia is best conceptualized as long-term, low-level depressive symptoms that do not meet criteria for MDD. Dysthymic symptoms include depressed mood most days for at least 2 years and two or more of the following six symptoms: appetite change, sleep disturbance, low energy or fatigue, low self-esteem, concentration difficulties, and hopelessness. In order to diagnose dysthymia, the person cannot be free of the symptoms for >2 months during the first 2 years. Treatment is the same as for depression with primary care efficacy studies showing response to SSRIs and psychotherapy. Many people with dysthymia may also experience one or more episodes of MDD in their lifetime.

CASE 3

A 34-year-old female presents to your clinic for treatment of depression. She reports a lifelong history of low-level depressive symptoms that have worsened over the past 6 months since she lost her job (don't worry—this is a different case than the previous one). She also suffers from inadequately controlled diabetes mellitus (HbA_{1c} 9.0%) and has been diagnosed with a personality disorder in the past. She drinks 3–4 beers everyday (hmm . . . multiply by 2 just to be safe) and has been arrested for driving while intoxicated twice. On questioning, you realize she has a moderately severe level of depression. She is not suicidal so you decide to initiate treatment as an outpatient with close follow-up.

Which of these factors does NOT contribute to a poor outcome when treating depression?

A) Chronic depressive symptoms.
B) Female gender.
C) Personality disorder.
D) Comorbid medical conditions.
E) Alcoholism.

Discussion

The correct answer is "B." Even though females are twice as likely to get depressed as males, gender does not seem to influence treatment response. The presence of any of the other factors listed reduces the chance of a successful response to treatment.

* *

In choosing an antidepressant for this patient, you would like to use one with a high success rate (as opposed to other patients who you might treat with one that doesn't work or a placebo—what?). However, you know that the success rates for most antidepressants are fairly similar.

What are the chances of this patient *failing to respond* to the first antidepressant chosen?

A) <1%.
B) 10–20%.
C) 30–40%.
D) 60–70%.
E) 90–95%.

Discussion

The correct answer is "C." Studies have consistently shown an antidepressant response rate of somewhere between 60% and 70% with 30–40% failing to respond, regardless of what antidepressant is tried. When unpublished studies are included, the failure rate for SSRIs approaches 50%.

> HELPFUL TIP: Fifty percent of patients who do not respond to an initial SSRI will respond to another drug in the same class. So, changing to another SSRI is reasonable in a patient who has failed one SSRI. Is this observed effect due to differences between drugs, pharmacodynamics, or just longer treatment? No one knows.

* *

When you spin your Random Depression Therapy Wheel that your occultist friend gave you for your birthday, it lands on venlafaxine (Effexor). So, you start your patient on that drug. Ten days later, she calls you just to say that the new medicine seems no better and her sleep is even worse. She started taking the medication in the morning because she thought it might be interfering with her sleep. She tends to lie in bed for 2 hours before falling asleep.

In addition to recommending good sleep hygiene and increased exercise, you prescribe:

A) Trazodone.
B) Zolpidem.
C) Lorazepam.
D) Phenobarbital.
E) Two shots of whiskey QHS.

Discussion

The correct answer is "A." Trazodone is often added to help with insomnia and boost serotonergic activity. For depression, it is preferred to benzodiazepines unless anxiety is a significant issue. Phenobarbital should be avoided. Zolpidem might be a consideration (Hey, I don't remember driving the car in my underwear and baking two pans of lasagna last night, but oh well.), but trazodone is preferred in patients with depression.

HELPFUL TIP: Indications for psychiatric referral for depression include:

- Failure of medical treatment.
- Imminent suicidality.
- Severe depression for which hospitalization is thought to be necessary.
- Diagnostic clarification or treatment recommendation.
- Comorbidities that make treatment response less likely.
- Patient requests referral.

* *

You add trazodone 50 mg HS PRN and titrate up to the maximum dose of venlafaxine, and your patient's symptoms are now coming under control. When you see her next, she describes a 20-minute episode of chest tightness, dyspnea, diaphoresis, and extreme anxiety. You believe that she suffered a panic attack. You wonder if you should alter your diagnosis.

In which of the following disorders do panic attacks NOT occur?

A) Panic disorder.
B) MDD.
C) Generalized anxiety disorder.
D) Social phobia.
E) None of the above.

Discussion

The correct answer is "E." Panic attacks are a cluster of symptoms signifying anxiety and are not a disorder by themselves. As such, they can be part of any effective syndrome and are frequently seen in a variety of syndromes including those mentioned above. The presence of a single panic attack in a person with a depressive disorder should not necessarily lead to a new diagnosis.

Objectives: Did you learn to . . .

- Identify risk factors for a poor outcome when treating depression?
- Assess the likelihood of a successful outcome in a patient with depression?
- Generate alternative methods for treating resistant depression?

CASE 4

A 41-year-old female comes to your office complaining of difficulty trusting people, irritability, low mood, and recurrent nightmares. Her symptoms started following the death of her parents in a house fire when she was a teenager. She has never been able to forgive herself for surviving while her parents died. She has not been able to form close relationships, and she is seeking help because of renewed nightmares. They were common in the first 2 years following the incident but had faded away until recently. Continuing news reports of terrorist activities and bombings have brought all of this back to the forefront again. She sometimes wakes up in a fright after dreaming that her own house is on fire. She is afraid to go near any bright lights or fireworks displays. When she is forced to be in the presence of fires, she frequently notices palpitations, dyspnea, and a sense of doom.

What is the patient's primary diagnosis?

A) MDD.
B) Generalized anxiety disorder.
C) Panic disorder.
D) Posttraumatic stress disorder (PTSD).
E) Dysthymia.

Discussion

The correct answer is "D." The patient's symptoms are characteristic of PTSD, which arises after one has been exposed to a situation in which one's life or "physical integrity" is in danger.

Which of the following is NOT necessary for a diagnosis of PTSD?

A) The patient needs to experience, witness, or be confronted by a potentially life-threatening event, or an event threatening the physical integrity of the patient or others.
B) The patient must respond with intense fear, horror, or helplessness.

C) Symptoms have to be present for more than a month.
D) The patient must be involved in combat.
E) The patient must meet a specified number of symptoms.

Discussion
The correct answer is "D." Although PTSD is common among military veterans (and was previously known by terms like "shell shock" and "battle fatigue"), there is no specified criterion that the patient must have been in combat. To meet criteria for PTSD, the patient must have been exposed to an event that is threatening to the integrity or life of the patient or another. Such events are as varied as combat, rape, assault, cancer, or an intensive care unit stay (or, one could hypothesize, taking the boards . . .). The patient then has recurrent intense fear, helplessness, or horror **that lasts for >1 month.** Symptoms occurring within 4 weeks of the event and lasting for at least 2 days but less than a month can qualify for the diagnosis of acute stress disorder.

Which of the following is *NOT* a part of PTSD?

A) Nightmares.
B) Flashbacks.
C) Hypervigilance.
D) Fear of death.
E) Difficulty maintaining relationships.

Discussion
The correct answer is "D." Fear of death is not a criterion. Symptoms of PTSD are divided into three clusters. To meet the symptom criteria for PTSD, the patient needs one symptom from the first cluster, three from the second, and two from the third.

The **first cluster** involves reexperiencing a previous traumatic experience (e.g., flashbacks, nightmares, and psychological distress in response to triggers that evoke the experience).

The **second cluster** involves avoidance of stimuli associated with the trauma (people, places, events); a numbing of general responsiveness (markedly diminished interest or participation in significant activities, feeling of detachment or estrangement from others, restricted range of affect, a sense of a foreshortened future).

The **third cluster** involves persistent symptoms of increased arousal, such as difficulty falling or staying asleep, irritability or outbursts of anger, difficulty concentrating, hypervigilance, or an exaggerated startle response

Which of the following is true of treatment for PTSD?

A) There is no effective treatment.
B) There are no FDA-approved medications.
C) Most patients experience spontaneous remission.
D) Though treatment is often effective, most patients do not achieve cure.
E) Atypical antipsychotics have no role in treatment.

Discussion
The correct answer is "D." Symptom improvement, but not cure, is the norm. SSRIs are the first-line drugs followed by SNRIs. There is no good efficacy data for TCAs, atypical antipsychotics, monoamine oxidase inhibitors (MAOIs), or other drugs. Prazosin may help with sleep and nightmares but the studies are small . . . like minuscule, like 12 patients (really). Psychotherapy can be helpful and benzodiazepine use should be limited because of the high risk of dependency in this population and the lack of efficacy as monotherapy.

Objectives: Did you learn to . . .

- Recognize risk factors for PTSD?
- Diagnose PTSD?
- Treat PTSD?

CASE 5

A 29-year-old female presents to you for a second opinion, bringing a large stack of medical records with her. In fact, she says that this is more like a "fourth or fifth opinion" (lucky you). She heard from a friend of a friend that you are the smartest doctor around and could determine what is wrong with her. Although you find many negative diagnostic studies in her record, she is sure that her many symptoms must have some physical cause. Over the last few years, she has had chronic headaches, multiple joint pains, and intermittent abdominal and chest pains. She has diarrhea and bloating on occasions, but upper endoscopy, colonoscopy, CT scans, and other studies have not revealed an etiology. She reports severe anxiety that has worsened with the onset of "seizures" in the last year (and you note that brain MRI, EEG, and neurological exam at the time did not support a seizure disorder). Additionally, she complains of some vague weakness and numbness and thinks that she might have had a stroke. Finally, she complains of pain with sexual intercourse. Nothing she does improves any of these symptoms. Further review of her records shows a variety of diagnoses from different physicians: "chronic pain syndrome," "chronic fatigue," "fibromyalgia," "irritable bowel syndrome," "premenstrual syndrome," and others.

Which of the following is the most likely primary diagnosis?

A) Hypochondriasis.
B) Somatization disorder.
C) Generalized anxiety disorder.
D) Factitious disorder.
E) Conversion disorder.

Discussion

The correct answer is "B." Typically, patients with unexplained symptoms see many doctors, have numerous tests, and often undergo a variety of procedures. At the outset, it is important to consider a primary psychiatric disorder, but a thorough and appropriate evaluation into possible organic causes should be completed before a psychiatric diagnosis is reached. Many times, patients with unexplained symptoms will ultimately be diagnosed with a **somatoFORM** disorder (of which "A," "B," and "E" are all types).

This patient presents with somatization disorder, which by definition must have:

- Four pain symptoms,
- Two gastrointestinal symptoms,
- One sexual symptom,
- One pseudoneurological symptom.

Also, in order to diagnose somatization disorder

- the complaints must have started before age 30,
- have no identifiable organic basis,
- and not be intentionally feigned.

"A" is incorrect. **Hypochondriasis** is characterized by a **preoccupation that one has some sort of serious disease** based on misinterpretation of bodily cues. "C" is incorrect because anxiety is present but totally overshadowed by the somatic complaints. "D," **factitious disorder,** is diagnosed in patients who intentionally produce symptoms (e.g., overdosing on insulin, injecting feces into the bloodstream) to assume the "sick role." "E" is incorrect. With **conversion disorder,** patients present with sudden onset of anatomically implausible neurological symptoms (e.g., whole-body numbness and bilateral deafness). Conversion disorder is, by definition, not under conscious control. If it is under conscious control, the diagnosis is "malingering" (really . . . that is a diagnosis).

* *

You believe that this patient has somatization disorder.

You begin by saying:

A) "Relax. This is all in your head."
B) "Your pain isn't real. But your psychiatric illness is. It's called somatization disorder."
C) "You have a number of symptoms that are very real but cannot be explained by our investigations. The evidence suggests that you do not have any life-threatening illnesses. You have a well-defined disorder, and other patients have similar problems."
D) "You have a lot of very serious symptoms. But my physical exam is inconsistent with your complaints. Basically, I don't believe a word your saying. The sooner that you admit to falsifying these symptoms, the sooner I can start helping you."
E) "I have a specialist to refer you to in Outer Mongolia . . . take your time getting back."

Discussion

The correct answer is "C." In patients with somatization disorder, it is best to use an honest but gentle approach. Most patients feel better if they have a name for an illness, but using the term "somatization disorder" may actually be detrimental. It is important to affirm the patient's symptoms (these are real problems) and to try to find some common language to use to describe what he or she is feeling. Patients may not be receptive to your interpretation initially, but repeating the discussion at subsequent visits and focusing on normal diagnostic tests may help them accept the diagnosis.

* *

Next, you discuss a plan of action with this patient.

You recommend:

A) A multidisciplinary approach, utilizing many different specialty services.
B) Starting an SSRI.
C) Starting electroconvulsive therapy (ECT).
D) Monthly visits with you and limited diagnostic testing and specialty consultation.
E) Referral for exploratory laparotomy.

Discussion

The correct answer is "D." It is best to have patients with somatization disorder establish regular clinic visits, typically with one provider. Unscheduled visits to the emergency department should be discouraged unless first discussed with the primary provider. Patients should be allowed to discuss all of their complaints, and a physical exam should be performed at every office visit. These measures will let the patients know that their concerns are being taken seriously. Lab tests, radiographs, and consultations should be limited, with the clinician using his or her best judgment as to when such diagnostic tests are indicated. "B" and "C" are incorrect as SSRIs and ECT are not accepted therapy for somatization disorder. But, you could probably prescribe an atypical antipsychotic or benzodiazepine (neither of which work) but will sedate the patient enough that she won't bother you any more.

> HELPFUL TIP: In patients who are willing to be referred to psychiatry, individual psychotherapy, CBT, and group therapy may be beneficial.

Objectives: Did you learn to . . .

- Recognize and describe various somatoform disorders?
- Generate an appropriate plan for a patient with somatization disorder?

CASE 6

A 21-year-old college student presents to your office for evaluation. She is complaining of feeling stressed out. She is taking classes full-time and is also in one of the military reserve units at the college. One weekend a month, she must attend drill that involves handling weapons. Although she did not have problems handling the weapons initially, she now gets very emotional and upset when she thinks about having to use them at the next drill weekend. She is nervous and is afraid that she might accidentally fire a weapon. She knows that her fears are silly and she has been telling herself to "just get over it." Last weekend, while at drill, she suddenly felt that she was going to have a heart attack. She developed tightness in her chest, her heart was racing, and she felt unable to breathe. Although the symptoms eventually abated, the episode made her even more alarmed, and now she is worried that it will happen again and she will have a heart attack. She comes to see if you can help.

Which of the following is UNNECESSARY for the initial workup?

A) Take more medical, psychiatric, and family history.
B) Order an echocardiogram.
C) Perform a physical exam.
D) Order thyroid function tests.
E) Perform a mental status exam.

Discussion

The correct answer is "B." Given the information you have so far, an echocardiogram is not indicated and is rarely used as part of a primary workup. When it comes to test questions, never say no to more history (unless you are supposed to be managing a patient's airway). A complete history and physical exam are essential in the evaluation of this new patient. Thyroid abnormalities can be a cause of some of these symptoms, including palpitations and chest tightness.

* *

She has no prior psychiatric history, but her mother is taking medication for depression. While taking her social history, you ask questions regarding substance abuse.

Use of which of the following substances might explain her symptoms?

A) Nicotine.
B) Alcohol.
C) Caffeine.
D) Herbal weight loss medication.
E) Any of the above.

Discussion

The correct answer is "E." Many substances can cause symptoms like this patient has. These include stimulants, such as caffeine and nicotine, and some herbal weight loss products containing ephedra (*Ma Huang*). Withdrawal from hypnotics like alcohol can also lead to similar symptoms.

* *

She does not smoke, doesn't drink alcohol (you can tell she's not a Hawkeye . . . no tailgating?!), and drinks coffee on weekday mornings before class. Her physical exam is normal. Her mental status exam is remarkable for a neutral mood, a restricted and anxious affect, but no suicidal thoughts and no psychotic symptoms. The laboratory tests you order are normal. You are leaning toward a psychiatric diagnosis at this point, specifically an anxiety disorder.

Which of the following is NOT an anxiety disorder?

A) Panic disorder.
B) Obsessive–compulsive disorder.
C) PTSD.
D) Generalized anxiety disorder.
E) Delirium.

Discussion
The correct answer is "E." Delirium, while it may present with features similar to an anxiety disorder, is a cognitive disorder. Anxiety disorders are the most common form of mental illness in the United States, affecting about 19.1 million people or 13% of the adult population. They include options "A" through "D" as well as social anxiety disorder (social phobia), specific phobias, acute stress disorder, anxiety disorder not otherwise specified, and anxiety disorders that are judged to be secondary to a medical condition or a substance.

* *

Of the listed anxiety disorders, you think she has developed panic disorder and that she has been having panic attacks.

Which of the following is NOT a typical symptom of a panic attack?

A) Palpitations.
B) Diaphoresis.
C) Syncope.
D) Dyspnea.
E) Dizziness.

Discussion
The correct answer is "C." The symptoms of a panic attack are those associated with an activation of the "fight-or-flee response," or the overactivation of the sympathetic nervous system. Typical symptoms include palpitations, sweating, trembling, dyspnea, a sense of smothering, fear of dying, chest pain, nausea, dizziness, numbness and tingling, and derealization or depersonalization. (At this point, we'd like to ask Mother Nature how chest pain helps us when facing a saber-toothed tiger.) It would be rare for a patient to actually lose consciousness from a panic attack (though they may feel they might), and actual syncope should force one to look for an alternate diagnosis.

> **HELPFUL TIP:** Hyperventilation can cause cerebral vasoconstriction and secondary cerebral hypoxia resulting in syncope. However, this is pretty unusual.

* *

To make your diagnosis of panic disorder, the patient needs to meet certain criteria set forth by DSM-IV.

Which of these is NOT a criterion for panic disorder?

A) Recurrent and unexpected panic attacks.
B) At least 1 month of worry about having more attacks.
C) Worry about the implication of the attack or its consequences (dying, "going crazy," etc.).
D) Change in behavior related to the attacks.
E) Predictable panic attacks that occur in response to cues.

Discussion
The correct answer is "E." The criteria for panic disorder do not include predictable panic attacks in response to cues. After patients have had repeated panic attacks, they often develop phobic avoidance of places, objects, or events associated with their symptoms (e.g., agoraphobia). This is a symptom that indicates very severe panic disorder. Patients often scout out routes of escape before going to places that might provoke an attack.

> **HELPFUL TIP:** The vast majority of patients with panic disorder present with somatic complaints rather than cognitive or mood symptoms. Patients are often misdiagnosed initially. Consider panic attacks in patients presenting with the appropriate somatic symptoms. And never rule out a physical diagnosis (e.g., PSVT) without an appropriate workup.

* *

Your patient is worried that these attacks will keep occurring.

How would you best describe the prognosis for panic disorder?

A) It is easily curable in most patients.
B) There is no effective treatment of it.
C) Most patients do not improve over time.
D) It is a recurrent or chronic illness.
E) None of the above.

Discussion

The correct answer is "D." Panic disorder is a recurrent or chronic disease in most patients. "A" and "C" are incorrect. Although panic disorder is not easily curable, almost all patients will improve over time, but very few attain complete remission even with medical treatment. Relapse is common.

* *

The patient is, of course, very concerned about future panic attacks. She asks what to do when another occurs.

You advise her to do all of the following EXCEPT:

A) Move to a quiet area.
B) Slow down her breathing.
C) Reassure herself that she is not dying.
D) Breathe into a brown paper bag.
E) Avoid stimulants like caffeine or nicotine.

Discussion

The correct answer is "D." All of the other options are reasonable recommendations for a patient suffering from panic attacks. Although commonly observed in popular lore, breathing into a paper bag is not recommended. Breathing into a brown paper bag can have the opposite effect of that intended—the patient may continue hyperventilating with CO_2 building up, which may contribute to more panic symptoms. Educating the patient on hyperventilation and helping her consciously slow her breathing may help abort the panic attack. Quiet rooms and reassurance can also help.

* *

You begin to discuss treatment options with this patient.

Which of the following is NOT an effective treatment of panic disorder?

A) Benzodiazepines such as clonazepam (Klonopin).
B) Bupropion (Wellbutrin).
C) Psychotherapy such as CBT.
D) SSRIs such as fluoxetine (Prozac).
E) TCAs such as imipramine.

Discussion

The correct answer is "B." Bupropion does not work for anxiety disorders. Among effective medications, no class has proven superior, and medication choice is based on safety, adverse effect profile, tolerability, comorbid illnesses, history of substance use, cost, etc. SSRIs are frequently considered first line. Psychotherapy has been found to be as effective as medications for the treatment of mild-to-moderate panic disorder and can be used in combination with medications for more severe cases.

* *

As you decide on the medication and dosage, you remember an article you just read in a journal on common mistakes made by physicians treating panic disorder in the community.

Which of these is NOT one of the common mistakes made in the treatment of panic disorder?

A) Starting the SSRI too high.
B) Not achieving a high enough target dose.
C) Underutilization of benzodiazepines.
D) Too rapid a titration.
E) Often using medications not proven to work with panic disorder.

Discussion

The correct answer is "C." Far from being underutilized, **benzodiazepines are often overprescribed.** While effective for panic disorder, problems with tolerance, dependence, and abuse limit benzodiazepines as long-term agents for panic disorder. Patients with panic disorder are extremely sensitive to medication side effects and are likely to suffer from jitteriness and restlessness if started at a too high dose of an SSRI. In order to reduce the chances of precipitating jitteriness and restlessness, a lower dose of SSRI (about half the starting dose used to treat depression) is usually recommended. The same problems can occur with rapidly increasing doses of SSRIs, so "start low and go slow," increasing the dose every 2–4 weeks to reach the maximum allowable dose.

> HELPFUL TIP: If using benzodiazepines for panic attacks or panic disorder, use longer half-life agents such as clonazepam or diazepam. Shorter half-life drugs can be prescribed for aborting panic attacks if needed. Taper benzodiazepines as soon as possible. Avoid them in patients with severe personality disorders and substance abuse.

* *

Your patient says, "I know another female in the reserve who has something similar, but I've never noticed the guys to have a problem. Is this just something that happens to women?" You tell her a bit about gender differences in anxiety disorders.

Which of these is *NOT* true about the gender ratio of the following anxiety disorders?

A) Generalized anxiety disorder affects more women than men in a 2:1 ratio.
B) Obsessive–compulsive disorder affects men and women equally.
C) PTSD affects men more than women in a 2:1 ratio.
D) Social anxiety disorder affects men and women equally.

Discussion

The correct answer is "C." Many effective illnesses (mood and anxiety disorders) including depression and some anxiety disorders are biologically sexist: women are more likely to be affected than men. All of the options listed are correct except "C," which inverts the true ratio.

Objectives: Did you learn to . . .

- Evaluate patients with anxiety symptoms?
- Recognize panic attacks and diagnose panic disorder?
- Initiate treatment of panic disorder?
- Describe some epidemiologic issues with anxiety disorders?

CASE 7

You have a 34-year-old male patient who has started sustained-release bupropion (Wellbutrin SR) 150 mg BID for depression. He reports partial but not total resolution in his symptoms. He also thinks that the medication is causing some side effects.

Which of the following is the most likely adverse effect attributable to this medication?

A) Insomnia.
B) Sexual dysfunction.
C) Weight gain.
D) QT prolongation.
E) Increased smoking.

Discussion

The correct answer is "A." Bupropion is associated with vivid dreams and insomnia. Taking the second dose no later than 4 PM can help reduce the likelihood of this side effect. Unlike most other antidepressants, bupropion is not associated with sexual dysfunction or weight gain. In fact, it has been associated with weight loss in the short term, and patients who quit smoking are less likely to gain weight if they are taking it. Bupropion can cause dry mouth and nausea, which are usually self-limited. It does not cause QT prolongation, unlike TCAs. Bupropion appears to curb the cravings for nicotine. It lowers the seizure threshold and should be avoided in patients with epilepsy.

* *

This patient is relatively healthy and takes no other medications, giving you a wide number of options for treatment. In other words, you did not have to think too hard before starting bupropion.

In which of the following disease states would bupropion be contraindicated?

A) Hypertension.
B) Severe depression.
C) Bulimia nervosa (BN).
D) Bipolar depression.
E) Borderline personality disorder.

Discussion

The correct answer is "C." Bupropion is contraindicated in patients with anorexia nervosa (AN) or BN (an increased risk of seizures is found in both diseases) or a current or past seizure disorder. Additionally, bupropion must be avoided in patients taking MAOIs. It is as effective as the other antidepressants, and it can be used in bipolar disorder and severe depression.

* *

You decide to switch his medication from bupropion to citalopram (Celexa).

Which is the best way to accomplish this switch?

A) Stop the bupropion immediately and then wait for 2 weeks before starting citalopram.
B) Taper the bupropion over 2 weeks to avoid a discontinuation syndrome, and then start the citalopram.
C) Start citalopram immediately, and then taper the bupropion over several days.
D) Start citalopram now; then taper off the bupropion a couple of weeks later if he is doing well.

Discussion

The correct answer is "C." Unlike SSRIs that can cause a serotonin withdrawal syndrome, bupropion can be discontinued with a minimal taper. A brief taper may avoid a sudden rebound of depressive symptoms, while the new agent is started. "A" is incorrect. Bupropion can be taken with an SSRI. However, "D" is less desirable, as it is preferable to stop the bupropion rather than continuing it indefinitely while taking another medication. A single effective agent is generally preferred.

Objectives: Did you learn to . . .

- Use bupropion appropriately?
- Identify adverse effects of bupropion?
- Recommend strategies to transition from bupropion to another antidepressant?

QUICK QUIZ: PSYCHIATRIC DIAGNOSIS

A 22-year-old college student who moved to your town from Lagos, Nigeria, last month is referred to you by his academic advisor for concerns that he may be depressed. Although he speaks English well, he does not know anyone in town. His family is still in Lagos, and he does not anticipate returning to see them anytime soon. He has not made many friends yet. He enjoys watching soccer in his spare time (which, of course, nobody in the United States appreciates, but that is another matter . . .), but he is not sleeping well, and he feels quite homesick.

Which of the following is the most appropriate diagnosis at this time?

A) MDD.
B) Adjustment disorder.
C) Bipolar affective disorder.
D) Dysthymia.
E) Footballer's withdrawal syndrome.

Discussion

The correct answer is "B." Adjustment disorder is the development of emotional or behavioral symptoms in response to identifiable stressor(s) occurring within 3 months of the onset of the stressor(s). The symptoms or behaviors must be clinically significant, such that either the patient's distress is in excess of what would be expected from exposure to the stressor, or there should be impairment in social or occupational/academic functioning. The patient's symptoms cannot be due to bereavement (a separate diagnosis). Once the stressor (or its consequences) is terminated, the symptoms should resolve within 6 months. Treatment depends on the level of distress and can range from supportive care to active intervention with medications, therapy, or hospitalization.

CASE 8

An 85-year-old woman is brought to the emergency department by her daughters because she has been acting strangely lately. Her house is a mess, even though for most of her life she has been quite fastidious. She has been calling her daughters at odd hours of the night, upset, and insisting that her youngest daughter is stealing her money. During the day, she goes outside of her house in her nightgown and housecoat, again quite unlike her usual customs. Four months ago, her husband of 58 years was diagnosed with a brain tumor. His condition has deteriorated quite rapidly, and he is now in a nursing home, and does not recognize his wife or daughters. Because of these events, the daughters have attributed your patient's odd behavior to the stress she is under. But as her symptoms have continued to worsen, they are now quite concerned and decide they must bring her in for evaluation.

In the emergency department, the patient is dressed in her housecoat and slippers and appears disheveled. She is lying on a cart, but she keeps trying to get up and leave. She is angry at her two daughters who are with her, and she is uncooperative with the physical exam. When you ask her about what has been happening, she appears distrusting, and her answers do not make sense.

Which of the following diagnoses is LEAST likely at this point in time?

A) Delirium.
B) Dementia.
C) Bereavement.

D) Psychotic depression.
E) Alcohol abuse

Discussion
The correct answer is "C." Although your patient's husband is gravely ill and she is grieving, her symptoms are more severe than what is expected for bereavement. Bereavement is a normal process, but it does not include severe impairment in social or occupational functioning, nor does it include paranoid delusions or other psychotic symptoms. All of the other diagnoses listed could result in the severity of symptoms described in this case.

Which of the following tests is indicated in the evaluation of this patient's behavior changes?

A) Chest x-ray.
B) Urinalysis.
C) CBC.
D) B-12 levels.
E) All of the above.

Discussion
The correct answer is "E." A thorough medical workup is warranted in the patient with "mental status changes" (e.g., delirium and new onset psychotic symptoms). Several medical problems—infection, hypoxia, MI, to name a few—can cause the symptoms the patient is experiencing and must be ruled out.

* *

Her workup does not reveal an organic cause for her altered mental state. You are now suspecting that she has psychotic depression.

All of the following are appropriate management options at this time EXCEPT:

A) Discharge with referral for outpatient psychotherapy.
B) Admission to a psychiatric unit.
C) ECT.
D) Psychiatric consultation.

Discussion
The correct answer is "A." Psychotherapy is not an appropriate single therapy for psychotic depression—especially in this patient, whose symptoms are so severe. "B" is appropriate, as the patient may benefit from hospitalization. "C" is appropriate as well. ECT is effective in treating psychotic depression and is often indicated if safety is of immediate concern or an early response is needed. "D" is appropriate. In general, patients with psychotic depression should be referred to a psychiatrist.

* *

You determine that your patient's symptoms are severe enough for hospitalization. Her daughters agree, but the patient is adamantly opposed and insists on returning to her home.

How would you proceed?

A) Call hospital security and make plans to hospitalize her. After all, she appears quite ill and cannot care for herself. When she is well, she will understand that it was the right plan.
B) Discharge her home, asking her daughters to take turns staying with her until she is better.
C) Follow state-dictated protocol to attempt to obtain a legal order for hospitalization against her will.
D) Follow national protocol (New World Order Directive 55.12.A) to attempt to obtain a legal order for hospitalization against her will.
E) Make a medical determination that she is not competent, allowing you to hospitalize her despite her objection.

Discussion
The correct answer is "C." Each state has its own laws that govern how an involuntary hospitalization process is conducted. If the patient poses an imminent threat to himself or others, the law generally allows involuntary hospitalization for a brief period of time until a court hearing is held. Involuntary hospitalization is also allowed if the patient is unable to care for herself and she is suffering from a mental illness that renders her incapable of making health-care decisions. "D" is incorrect. There are no national laws governing involuntary hospitalization (and the New World Order is a paranoid delusion of some extremists . . . or maybe we just want you to believe that). "B" is incorrect. Because of the severity of this patient's symptoms, it would be inappropriate to simply discharge her to the care of her daughters.

* *

You have admitted the patient under a 72-hour hold, and you are discussing treatment options with the psychiatrist, who thinks that ECT might be appropriate. You are concerned about cognitive problems in this patient.

All of the following are associated with an increased risk of memory loss with ECT EXCEPT:

A) Concomitant lithium use.
B) Bilateral electrode placement.
C) High stimulus doses.
D) History of seizure disorder.

Discussion

The correct answer is "D." Seizure disorder is not associated with an increased risk of memory loss with ECT. ECT is known to cause transient problems with memory loss. This usually manifests with the patient having trouble remembering events that occur around the time of the ECT (remember that the patient is basically being treated by inducing seizure-like activity). Most of the memory complaints completely resolve within a few months of completing ECT. However, some situations may increase the risk of memory loss, including concomitant lithium use, bilateral electrode placement (unilateral is safer), and a higher stimulus dose.

* *

In further discussions with the patient and her family, you try to explain ECT and dispel some myths.

All of the following are potential complications or adverse effects of ECT EXCEPT:

A) Delirium.
B) Nonsustained ventricular tachycardia.
C) Headache.
D) Dementia.
E) Fatigue.

Discussion

The correct answer is "D." Although transient memory loss and even delirium can occur after ECT, it does not cause dementia. A number of cardiac rhythm disturbances can occur and are more likely in patients with cardiac disease. However, these are self-limited and generally minor (e.g., premature ventricular contractions, atrial premature complexes, and nonsustained ventricular tachycardia). Headache and fatigue are common after ECT.

Objectives: Did you learn to . . .

- Recognize abnormal behavior and generate an appropriate differential diagnosis?
- Evaluate a patient with new cognitive and behavioral problems?
- Determine when involuntary hospitalization is appropriate and how it might be undertaken?
- Discuss potential adverse effects of ECT?

QUICK QUIZ: PSYCHIATRIC DIAGNOSIS

A 47-year-old female presents to your clinic in tears, requesting your help. She cannot stop crying, her sleep is poor, and she feels terribly lonely. She tells you that last week her mother had a stroke. She survived, but is now in a nursing home and suffering from Broca aphasia. Your patient describes her mother as her "best friend." She has not had trouble with depression or other mental illness in the past.

Which of the following is the most likely diagnosis?

A) Bereavement.
B) Adjustment disorder.
C) MDD.
D) Bipolar effective disorder.
E) Dysthymia.

Discussion

The correct answer is "A." Bereavement is a natural reaction to the loss of a loved one. Some of the symptoms may mimic those of a depression and making the diagnosis can be complicated. The duration and expression of bereavement also differs among different cultural groups and subgroups, further complicating the diagnostic process. Generally, a diagnosis of MDD is not given unless the symptoms of depression are present 2 months after the loss.

CASE 9

You get a call from a patient complaining of "not feeling well and getting worse" over the past 3 days. She has had electrical shock sensations in her upper extremities and head and also complains of dizziness and malaise. She takes no medications since she stopped her paroxetine (Paxil) a few days ago.

Which of the following is the most likely diagnosis?

A) Influenza.
B) Bupropion discontinuation syndrome.

C) SSRI discontinuation syndrome.
D) Serotonin syndrome.
E) Hypertensive crisis.

Discussion
The correct answer is "C." OK. We already told you above that bupropion does not have a discontinuation syndrome. So you all got this one right, yes? A discontinuation syndrome (also known as withdrawal syndrome) has been associated with SSRIs when they are suddenly stopped or doses are missed or reduced. This is especially common with paroxetine. The symptoms described above are typical of the discontinuation syndrome, particularly the paresthesias that patients often describe as an "electric shock" (Table 23–1).

Which of the options below is INCORRECT information to give the patient over the telephone?
A) Symptoms usually begin within a few days of stopping the SSRI.
B) The symptoms rarely last longer for 2 weeks and are self-limited.
C) Restarting the medication takes about 2 weeks to relieve symptoms.
D) The longer the patient has been on the medication, the more likely the risk of a discontinuation syndrome.

Table 23–1 SYMPTOMS OF SSRI DISCONTINUATION SYNDROME

Somatic symptoms
- Disequilibrium (e.g., dizziness, vertigo, ataxia, and tremor)
- Gastrointestinal symptoms (e.g., nausea, vomiting, and anorexia)
- Flu-like symptoms (e.g., fatigue, lethargy, myalgias, chills, and headache)
- Sensory disturbances (e.g., paresthesias and sensations of electric shock)
- Sleep disturbances (e.g., insomnia and vivid dreams)

Psychological problems
- Anxiety/agitation
- Crying spells
- Irritability
- Overactivity
- Depersonalization
- Decreased concentration/slowed thinking
- Confusion and memory problems

Discussion
The correct answer is "C" (which is not true). Symptoms can be noticeable in some patients with just one missed dose (especially with paroxetine [Paxil]) but typically develop within 2 days of medication discontinuation. The syndrome is uncomfortable but usually self-limited, lasting <2 weeks. Restarting the medication will lead to cessation of symptoms within 24 hours in virtually all cases. The risk of discontinuation increases with length of therapy, particularly when the patient has been on an SSRI longer than 7 weeks.

Which SSRI is LEAST likely to cause a discontinuation syndrome?
A) Fluoxetine.
B) Sertraline.
C) Paroxetine.
D) Citalopram.
E) Fluvoxamine.

Discussion
The correct answer is "A." The risk of withdrawal increases with **shorter** half-lives. The half-life of fluoxetine is about 4–6 days, while its active metabolite, norfluoxetine has a half-life up to 16 days, making it highly unlikely that fluoxetine would cause a discontinuation syndrome in most patients, as it effectively acts as its own taper. Fluvoxamine (with a half-life of 15 hours) and paroxetine (21 hours) have the shortest half-lives and are most likely to cause the discontinuation syndrome. To minimize the risk of withdrawal syndrome, taper off SSRIs when stopping them.

HELPFUL TIP: Discontinuation syndrome is likely a hyposerotonergic state; therefore, all serotonergic agents can cause a serotonin withdrawal. These agents include SSRIs, MAOIs, TCAs, serotonin–norepinephrine reuptake inhibitors (SNRIs), and mirtazapine (Remeron)... but not bupropion (is that horse dead or should we beat it some more?).

* *

Your patient restarts her SSRI and feels better. She has questions about antidepressants in general, wondering if she is taking the right one. As you start to discuss benefits and risks of different medications, you remind yourself about some important issues. For example, all SSRIs are not the same.

Which SSRI has the most anticholinergic activity?

A) Fluoxetine.
B) Paroxetine.
C) Sertraline.
D) Citalopram.
E) Escitalopram.

Discussion

The correct answer is "B." With the exception of paroxetine, SSRIs do not possess appreciable anticholinergic activity.

Which of the following SSRIs is LEAST likely to have drug–drug interactions?

A) Fluoxetine.
B) Paroxetine.
C) Citalopram.
D) Sertraline.
E) Fluvoxamine.

Discussion

The correct answer is "C." Citalopram and its stereoisomer, escitalopram, have relatively clean profiles with no major interactions with any of the cytochrome P450 enzymes. Sertraline is also an attractive option if drug–drug interactions are a concern. The other three have significant drug–drug interactions that have clinical importance.

Mirtazapine (Remeron) is commonly associated with the following side effects EXCEPT:

A) Sedation.
B) Weight gain.
C) Dizziness.
D) Lycanthropy.
E) Increased triglycerides.

Discussion

The correct answer is "D." Lycanthropy is, of course, the ability to transform into a werewolf. Although close in behavior to antisocial personality disorder, lycanthropy is not caused by mirtazapine but rather by the bite of another lycanthrope. Mirtazapine is a potent antihistamine, and an α1-adrenergic agonist, potentially leading to orthostatic hypotension. Sedation is present in over 50% of patients taking the drug, while weight gain is reported in as many as 12%. It can also lead to increased triglycerides. Paradoxically, the side effect of sedation lessens with increasing doses. It is a great antidepressant for patients who have lost their appetite, lost weight or have insomnia. Typical doses range from 15 to 60 mg/day.

Which of the following antidepressants has a black box warning about hepatic failure?

A) Nefazodone (Serzone).
B) Bupropion.
C) Paroxetine (Paxil).
D) Nortriptyline.
E) Phenelzine (Nardil).

Discussion

The correct answer is "A." Nefazodone is a 5HT-2A receptor antagonist and is an effective antidepressant with sedative properties. It has significant inhibitory effects on CYP3A4 and has several significant drug interactions as a result. In the recent past, several cases of hepatic failure have been reported with this drug, leading to a black box warning on the package insert and limiting its clinical use. None of the other antidepressants listed have had such problems.

Venlafaxine has been noted to typically cause all of the following side effects EXCEPT:

A) Increased blood pressure.
B) Dizziness.
C) Dry mouth.
D) Weight gain.
E) Sexual disturbance.

Discussion

The correct answer is "D." Venlafaxine and duloxetine (Cymbalta) block both norepinephrine and serotonin reuptake inhibitors and have minimal activity on the cholinergic, histaminergic, and alpha-receptors. There is a dose-related increase in blood pressure, with a mean elevation of 10–15 mm Hg in diastolic pressure at doses of 300 mg or greater in up to 10% of patients. There is a slight increase in pulse, as well. "D" is not true. In fact, weight loss is a common complaint. Venlafaxine generally has the same side effect profile as the SSRIs, potentially causing sexual dysfunction, dizziness, and dry mouth. Patients can have a significant withdrawal from venlafaxine and should be tapered off of it slowly.

HELPFUL (AND SCARY) TIP: Venlafaxine (Effexor) and duloxetine (Cymbalta) are toxic in overdose and now cause as many deaths as TCAs (at least in England). They cause QT and QRS prolongation in overdose. Treatment is the same as the treatment of TCA overdose (bicarbonate, etc.), although data is limited.

* *

You decide to switch the patient to fluoxetine and she does well.

Objectives: Did you learn to . . .

- Identify SSRI discontinuation syndrome?
- Recognize important antidepressant interactions?
- Describe adverse effects of various antidepressants?

QUICK QUIZ: MAOIS

You are seeing a new patient with a history of recurrent major depression. Many years ago a different physician put him on phenelzine (Nardil), which you recognize as having potentially serious food and drug interactions. You are considering switching him to an SSRI.

How long after an MAOI is discontinued can an SSRI be started?

A) 1 day.
B) 3 days.
C) 7 days.
D) 14 days.
E) SSRIs and MAOIs can be given together.

Discussion

The correct answer is "D." Because of significant drug–drug interactions (see next question), SSRIs should not be started until 2 weeks after discontinuation of an MAOI.

QUICK QUIZ: MAOIS

What is the drug–drug interaction of concern with SSRIs and MAOIs?

A) Serotonin syndrome.
B) Tyramine crisis.
C) Anticholinergic crisis.
D) Hypertensive crisis.
E) Stevens–Johnson syndrome.

Discussion

The correct answer is "A." Serotonin syndrome is caused by an excess of serotonin and can be caused by drug–drug interactions involving serotonergic agents including SSRIs, buspirone, meperidine, dextromethorphan, litium, tramadol, and triptans among others. It is characterized by muscle rigidity, hyperreflexia, hyperthermia, confusion and agitation among other symptoms. It can be fatal. As a result, the concurrent use of an SSRI and MAOI is absolutely CONTRAINDICATED. Hypertensive crisis occurs when foods containing tyramine (e.g., aged cheese and cured meats) interact with MAOIs to release catecholamines, causing hypertension, headaches, nausea, and diaphoresis. In severe cases, it can lead to strokes or death. Stevens–Johnson syndrome is an autoimmune dermatological disorder that leads to desquamation of mucosal surfaces and is not associated with antidepressant use (although it can be seen with other drugs).

HELPFUL TIP(S): Linezolid is absolutely contraindicated with MAOIs. It is a serotonergic drug. Among the foods that cause a hypertensive crisis with an MAOI are banana peels (but not the banana . . . we are not sure who figured this one out . . . Yum, banana peels), draught beer (boo) but not bottled beer (yes!), and kimchi.

CASE 10

A 43-year-old man who you started on citalopram 4 weeks ago returns for a follow-up visit. He feels better but complains of delayed ejaculation. You consider changing him to an antidepressant that is less likely to cause sexual dysfunction.

Which of the following would you AVOID?

A) Nefazodone.
B) Bupropion.
C) Mirtazapine.
D) Trazodone.
E) Nortriptyline.

Discussion

The correct answer is "E." Sexual dysfunction is a common side effect of most psychotropics. There are few controlled data to guide us as to how to approach this issue, but sildenafil (Viagra) is effective in antidepressant-induced sexual dysfunction. Of the options given, nortriptyline—and other TCAs—are more frequently associated with sexual dysfunction.

> HELPFUL TIP: St. John wort, which may be effective in mild-to-moderate depression, is a known inducer of the P450 enzyme, reducing the efficacy of oral contraceptives. It has also been associated with decreased efficacy of antiretrovirals, cyclosporine, digoxin, theophylline, and warfarin.

* *

This patient is also having sleep difficulties and asks what herbal therapy he might be able to use.

Which of the following is an herbal alternative to benzodiazepines for anxiety and insomnia?

A) Valerian.
B) St. John wort.
C) Saw palmetto.
D) Ginseng.
E) Ginkgo.

Discussion

The correct answer is "A." Valerian (*Valeriana officinalis*) has been touted to have anxiolytic properties, similar to benzodiazepines, and its mechanism of action is thought to be similar (e.g., inhibition of GABA). It appears to be safe and has the same drug interactions and contraindications as benzodiazepines. The other options are not known to affect sleep to a significant degree.

> HELPFUL TIP: Kava-kava is advertised as an anxiolytic but should generally be avoided. Kava-kava (*Piper methysticum*) has been reported to cause liver damage, in some cases leading to liver transplant or eventual death.

Objectives: Did you learn to . . .

- Develop an approach to the problem of sexual dysfunction with antidepressants?
- Recognize herbal therapies that might be employed in treating symptoms of depression?

CASE 11

You are seeing a 28-year-old patient whose first child you delivered a month ago. She comes to your clinic with her son for his 1-month well child check. You observe that she seems tired and is less animated than usual. She is gentle with her infant, but her face doesn't seem to light up with the glow that you often see with new mothers. You know . . . the glow of terror, sleeplessness and anxiety? That's the one.

Which of the following best explains your observations?

A) Sleep deprivation.
B) Marital discord at home.
C) Postpartum depression.
D) Thyroid dysfunction.
E) Any of the above.

Discussion

The correct answer is "E." Your patient's symptoms could be due to any of these problems and more, including, difficulty with role adjustment and anemia.

* *

You want to gather more information to see if there is a pathological process underlying her behavior.

You would do all of the following EXCEPT:

A) Ask her to fill out an Edinburgh Postnatal Depression Scale (EPDS).
B) Order thyroid function tests.
C) Order a sleep study.
D) Ask more questions about how things are at home and how she is coping.
E) Ask about a previous history of depression.

Discussion

The correct answer is "C." In this case, there are many other more likely problems than a primary sleep disorder, and a sleep study is unlikely to be helpful (plus as those of us who have had infants know, your sleep is naturally disordered). The EPDS is a validated self-rated scale that is useful for detecting postpartum depression. Hypothyroidism can always mimic depression and might need to be ruled out. A thorough history is always essential.

The incidence of postpartum depression is about:

A) 1%.
B) 10%.
C) 30%.
D) 50%.

Discussion

The correct answer is "B." About 7 in 10 women suffer from "baby blues," postpartum symptoms that can manifest as mood swings, anxiety, fatigue, and sadness occurring within a few days of delivery and lasting only a week or so. However, postpartum depression affects up to 10% of women, and symptoms can appear anywhere from weeks to months after birth. The diagnosis is often missed because many mothers are ashamed to admit feeling unhappy at a time when they think (and society tells them) that they should be happy. Physicians may focus on the infant's physical health and miss assessing the mother–baby interaction

* *

In obtaining more history, you realize that this patient was having some troubles with depression even during her pregnancy.

When is the most common time for pregnancy-related depression to occur?

A) At conception.
B) First trimester.
C) Second trimester.
D) Third trimester.
E) Postpartum.

Discussion

The correct answer is "D." A large epidemiological study from the United Kingdom followed pregnant women prospectively throughout the course of their pregnancies and found that the **incidence of depression was actually higher in the third trimester than it was in the postpartum period**. This suggests the need for the physician to begin to inquire about symptoms earlier.

HELPFUL TIP: Repeat after me... "Pregnancy does not treat depression." For some reason, it had been assumed that a woman's depression would abate during pregnancy. Studies in the last couple of years have disproved this myth.

* *

If you had been aware of her depression earlier and wanted to prescribe an antidepressant during her pregnancy, you would have been cautious, prescribing a Pregnancy Safety Category B drug.

Which of the following antidepressants is Category B in pregnancy?

A) Fluoxetine.
B) Bupropion.
C) Nortriptyline.
D) Mirtazapine.
E) None of the above.

Discussion

The correct answer is "E." None of the above, and no antidepressant, is category B for pregnancy. All the drugs listed are category C.

Risks associated with SSRI use during pregnancy include all of the following EXCEPT:

A) Irritability of the neonate.
B) Preterm delivery.
C) Low birth weight.
D) Persistent pulmonary hypertension.
E) Tetralogy of Fallot.

Discussion

The correct answer is "E." A number of adverse effects have been associated with SSRI use in pregnancy, including neonatal irritability, low birth weight, and preterm labor. A recent meta-analysis of studies examining neonatal outcomes when women took antidepressants during pregnancy showed that infants exposed to SSRIs during the second half of pregnancy (i.e., after 20 weeks gestation) had an increased risk (approximately 1% absolute risk) of developing persistent pulmonary hypertension, a potentially life-threatening condition, after birth. (*BMJ*. 2012 Jan 12;344:d8012. http://dx.doi.org/10.1136/bmj.d8012) SSRIs have not been linked to development of Tetralogy of Fallot.

If you had decided to prescribe an antidepressant medication for her during pregnancy, which one of the following would have been LEAST desirable?

A) Fluoxetine.
B) Paroxetine.
C) Sertraline.

D) Nortriptyline.
E) Citalopram.

Discussion
The correct answer is "B." Although no antidepressant medication has been shown to be risk free when used during pregnancy, paroxetine is the only antidepressant medication listed that is Category D in pregnancy, due to the increased incidence of cardiac anomalies (mainly atrial and ventricular septal defects) in infants who were exposed in utero.

* *

You start her fluoxetine and offer to watch her baby for a few days, and everyone is happy!

Objectives: Did you learn to . . .

- Recognize the high incidence of depression and depressive symptoms in the postpartum period?
- Diagnose postpartum depression?
- Treat depression in the pregnant and postpartum patient?

CASE 12

A couple you have known for some time brings in their 7-year-old son, Jimbo, to your clinic because his behavior has changed over the past month. His school performance has worsened, and he has started to get into fights at school. He is not eating as well and is having frequent nightmares. He now has frequent headaches and stomachaches and clings to his mother when it is time to go to school. The parents cannot understand what is going on and report no antecedent trauma.

Which of the following is the most likely diagnosis?

A) MDD.
B) PTSD.
C) Adjustment disorder.
D) Bereavement.
E) Normal childhood difficulties expected with being named Jimbo.

Discussion
The correct answer is "A." Up to 3% of children and 8% of adolescents suffer from depression. DSM-IV criteria are the same as in the adult, except **irritability can be substituted for the depressed mood requirement** in children. PTSD is unlikely as there is no antecedent trauma. Adjustment disorder is not likely since there have been no major changes in the child's regimen, and bereavement is not likely since there have been no losses in the child's life. The patient's symptoms are clearly not part of normal childhood, even if his name is Jimbo.

HELPFUL TIP: Of course bullying at school and other social problems need to be investigated as part of this child's evaluation and any other child presenting with symptoms of depression.

Which of the following is NOT true about depression in children?

A) Abuse or neglect increases the risk of depression.
B) Having a depressed parent increases the risk of being a depressed child.
C) The clinical course is roughly the same as in adults
D) "Masked" symptoms, such as abdominal pain, are more common in children than the typical symptoms of depression, such as sleep disturbance.
E) Male and female children are equally affected by depression.

Discussion
The correct answer is "D." Although clinicians should be aware of age-appropriate manifestations (see Table 23–2), symptoms of depression are similar in children and adults. In fact, typical symptoms of depression are more common in children than are

Table 23–2 COMMON MANIFESTATIONS OF DEPRESSION IN CHILDREN

- Increased irritability, anger, or hostility
- Being bored
- Reckless behavior
- Outbursts of shouting, complaining, unexplained irritability, or crying
- Poor school performance
- Fear of death
- Alcohol or substance abuse
- Frequent nonspecific physical complaints such as headaches, muscle aches, stomachaches, or fatigue

Depression in Children and Adolescents, National Institutes of Health Publication No. 00–4744 (http://www.nimh.nih.gov/publicat/depchildresfact.cfm).

"masked" symptoms such as stomachaches and fear of leaving home.

* *

You tell the family about Jimbo's prognosis.

Which of the following statements regarding prognosis is *FALSE*?

A) Childhood MDD confers a two- to fourfold increase in risk for adult MDD.
B) 25% of adolescents with MDD develop substance abuse disorders.
C) Almost half of children with MDD will attempt suicide sometime in their life.
D) Roughly 20% of adolescents have suffered at least one episode of MDD by 18, while 65% report transient symptoms of depression.
E) After the initial episode, only 10% will suffer a relapse.

Discussion

The correct answer is "E." Between half and two-thirds (**not** 10%) will have a recurrence within 5 years after resolution of their first episode. The other options are all true. In children and adolescents, the mean depression episode length is 7–9 months with remission typically occurring over 1.5–2 years.

HELPFUL TIP: The risk of suicide is very high among depressed youths. It is the third leading cause of death in the 15–24 year age group, and children with MDD have a four- to fivefold higher lifetime incidence of suicide attempts than nondepressed children. Twenty percent of adolescents have suicide ideation each year, and 5–8% attempt suicide each year.

* *

You recommend treatment for Jimbo.

Which of the following therapies has NOT shown efficacy in childhood depression in randomized controlled trials?

A) Fluoxetine.
B) Sertraline.
C) CBT.
D) Venlafaxine.
E) Interpersonal therapy.

Discussion

The correct answer is "D." In fact, the makers of venlafaxine sent out a "Dear Doctor" letter suggesting that venlafaxine not be used in children under 18 because it lacks efficacy data, and it has an increased incidence of emotional lability. The bottom line is that fluoxetine is probably the SSRI of choice in children, followed by sertraline. **However, the NNT is 10 to benefit one child.** Avoid paroxetine since it may be associated with a higher suicide risk. TCAs should be avoided because of lack of efficacy and potential suicide risk. CBT and interpersonal therapy have been shown to be effective in children and adolescents.

HELPFUL TIP(S): As you would expect, therapy plus an antidepressant are more effective than either modality alone. Adverse effects of medication in children are similar to those in adults and include insomnia, fatigue, headaches, and nervousness.

Objectives: Did you learn to . . .

- Increase your awareness of childhood depression?
- Diagnose depression in children?
- Describe the natural history of depression in children?
- Generate an appropriate treatment plan for children with depression?

CASE 13

Tommy is a 9-year-old male who has been having difficulty with his behavior since he started first grade. He is often fidgety and squirming in his chair and has difficulty remaining in his seat. He talks out of turn, is often "on the go," and is not liked by the other kids because he intrudes into games and has a hard time waiting his turn. He is the product of an uncomplicated pregnancy and has no significant past medical history.

What is the most likely diagnosis?

A) Attention-deficit/hyperactivity disorder (ADHD).
B) Adjustment disorder.
C) Oppositional defiant disorder (ODD).
D) Conduct disorder (CD).
E) Nonverbal learning disorder.

Discussion

The correct answer is "A." The symptoms of ADHD are listed below. "B," adjustment disorder, is unlikely since there is no history of a significant life event. ODD and CD are characterized by aggressive behavior and a disregard for rules and adults. These are not given as part of Tommy's history. Nonverbal learning disorder presents with school performance problems and may be associated with ADHD but would not be directly responsible for this patient's hyperactivity.

For the diagnosis of ADHD, patients must meet one of the following criteria:

1) At least six symptoms of inattention for at least 6 months that is maladaptive and inconsistent with level of development
   - Careless mistakes, poor attention to details
   - Cannot sustain attention
   - Does not seem to listen
   - Poor follow through on tasks
   - Difficulties with organization
   - Avoids or dislikes tasks that require sustained attention
   - Often loses things required for a task (notebooks, pens, etc.)
   - Easily distracted from a task
2) Six or more of the following hyperactive–impulsive symptoms for 6 months, which is maladaptive and inconsistent with level of development.

   Hyperactivity symptoms
   - Fidgets or squirms in seat
   - Leaves seat in classroom at inappropriate times
   - Hyperactivity in inappropriate settings
   - Cannot play or relax quietly
   - Always in motion
   - Talks too much

   Impulsivity symptoms
   - Blurts out answer before questions completed
   - Trouble waiting for turn in games, school, etc.
   - Interrupts others (verbally, in games, etc.)

   Additionally, the following are required:
   - Must be present before age of 7 years!
   - Impairment in two settings (home, work, school, worship, etc.)
   - Clinically significant impairment in social, academic, or occupational spheres
   - Symptoms are not due to another problem (developmental delay, personality disorder, mood disorder, etc.)

Which of the following is FALSE about ADHD?

A) It affects 3–7% of children.
B) There are genetic and environmental influences on the risk of developing ADHD.
C) Males are more likely to have ADHD than females.
D) The incidence of ADHD has increased over the years.
E) Comorbid disorders are not common.

Discussion

The correct answer is "E." ADHD affects 3–7% of children and its incidence has almost doubled over the past decade. Heritability is 70%, similar to that for schizophrenia and bipolar disorder. Alcohol and tobacco exposure in utero have both been linked to at least a twofold increase in risk. Males are three to six times more likely to be diagnosed with ADHD than females. Comorbid disorders are very common in ADHD with CD, ODD, depression, anxiety, learning disabilities, and developmental delay being the most frequent.

Which of the following is NOT TRUE of the prognosis and treatment of Tommy's ADHD?

A) The natural history of ADHD is that one-third of children will outgrow the symptoms, one-third will have the same frequency and intensity of symptoms, and one-third will have residual symptoms, which are subclinical.
B) Tommy has a 70–80% chance of responding to stimulants.
C) If Tommy is treated with stimulants, his risk of drug abuse is halved.
D) Tommy is at increased risk of getting into accidents.
E) Behavior therapy is effective for reducing ADHD symptoms.

Discussion

The correct answer is "E." Unfortunately, intensive behavior therapy has been shown to be ineffective. The breakdown of the prognosis for children with ADHD symptoms is that roughly one-third will experience complete symptom resolution, one-third will get some improvement, and one-third will remain ill with the disorder. Stimulants, which are first-line therapy, will work in 70–80% of the patients. If a patient does not respond to the first stimulant, he still has a 70–80% chance of responding to a second stimulant. Children treated with stimulants are half as likely to abuse substances as those who were not treated. Children with ADHD are at risk for impulsive behavior and risk-taking, which leads to substance abuse, accidents, etc.

* *

You decide to start Tommy on methylphenidate.

Which of the following is NOT true about treatment with methylphenidate?

A) It improves handwriting.
B) Optimal dosing is 0.6–1 mg/kg/day.
C) It can cause reduced growth.
D) Short-term memory is not affected.
E) Tommy might get along better with his classmates.

Discussion

The correct answer is "D." In fact, stimulants improve short-term memory in patients with ADHD. The rest are true. Do you think this is why doctors have notoriously bad handwriting? Maybe we all need stimulants... Stimulants have a widespread effect on multiple domains, some of which are listed in Table 23–3.

Table 23–3 STIMULANT EFFECTS

Effects of stimulants on motor response.
- Reduce activity to normal
- Decrease excessive talking, noise, and disruption in the classroom
- Improve handwriting
- Improve fine motor control

Effects of stimulants on social skills.
- Reduce off-task behavior in classroom
- Improve ability to play and work independently
- Decrease intensity of behavior
- Reduce bossiness with peers
- Reduce verbal and physical aggression
- Improve (but not normalize) peer social status
- Reduce noncompliance, defiance, and oppositional behavior with adults
- Parents and teachers become less controlling and more positive

Effects of stimulants on cognitive ability.
- Improve ability to sustain attention, especially in boring tasks (like this one)
- Reduce distractibility
- Improve short-term memory
- Reduce impulsivity
- Increase amount of academic work completed
- Increase accuracy of academic work

Side effects
- Lack of appetite
- Decreased growth, especially initially
- Insomnia
- Headaches and stomachaches
- Irritability
- Tachycardia or blood pressure increase (rare)
- Muscle tics or switches (rare)
- Psychosis or delirium (rare)

* *

Tommy's father is happy with his son's response to methylphenidate and wonders if he too would benefit from a similar medication. He recalls being in trouble ever since in grade school for talking "out of turn" and always being put in detention. He was always restless and fidgety but this has improved as he ages. He has a hard time at work sitting through meetings, as he tends to daydream, and he has numerous fights with his wife because she accuses him of not listening to her. He has been unable to get promoted because he cannot pass the exams he has to take, but he thinks that he is smart enough. He says that he just cannot concentrate.

Which of the statements below would NOT be consistent with an adult presenting with ADHD?

A) Adults present with the same core symptoms as children but in a different fashion.
B) Adults are less likely to have overt hyperactivity symptoms compared with children.
C) Adults often present when their children are diagnosed.
D) Adults are less likely to smoke than same-age persons without ADHD.
E) Adults often seek professions that allow them to use their symptoms to their advantage.

Discussion

The correct answer is "D." Adults present differently than children, but have the same core symptoms of hyperactivity, inattention, and impulsivity. Many adults are diagnosed with ADHD only when their children have been diagnosed or when increasing difficulty at work or at home leads them to seek help. Often,

Table 23–4 PRESENTATIONS OF ADHD SYMPTOMS IN CHILDREN AND ADULTS

Children	Adults
Hyperactive child: squirms, cannot stay in his seat, and constantly on the go	Hyperactive adult: has subjective inner restlessness and trouble relaxing
Impulsive child: blurts out answers, interrupts others, and talks incessantly	Impulsive adult: speeding tickets, car crashes, impatient, smokes more, higher divorce rate, higher substance use rate, and overeating
Inattentive child: does not follow through, is forgetful, does not listen. Fewer enter college and graduate, compared with children their age without ADHD	Inattentive adult: often late for appointments, forgets anniversaries, has difficulty with work meetings; problems with focusing, planning, organizing, and completing tasks at home and at work; advances more slowly at work than peers; misplaces keys, glasses, and other items; may forget to pay bills, pick up the kids on time, etc.

comorbidities drive them to seek help, and the primary diagnosis of ADHD is made only incidentally. Adults typically present seeking help for their inattention and concentration difficulties, as overt hyperactivity lessens with age. Some adults compensate by taking part in careers that reward their intellectual curiosity, endless energy, and desire for change (like emergency medicine, for example?). Table 23–4 compares adult and child presentations of ADHD.

HELPFUL TIP: Remember that adults may have residual symptoms, which do not meet full criteria for ADHD at the time of evaluation. **A clear history of symptoms starting in childhood before age 7 must be present to diagnose an adult with ADHD. There is no such thing as "Adult Onset ADHD."** Confirmation of the history can be obtained from collateral sources, including old school reports and family members. Think about other diagnoses such as anxiety disorder and depression in patients who think they have "adult onset ADHD."

* *

You decide to treat Tommy's father with a medication. He would prefer not to have a stimulant, and he asks if there are other options for treatment.

Which of the following medications would you recommend?

A) Fluoxetine.
B) Bupropion.
C) Mirtazapine.
D) Phenelzine.
E) Risperidone.

Discussion

The correct answer is "B." In addition to stimulants, which are also first-line agents in adults, there are a variety of medications that can be used to treat ADHD, although most studies are undertaken in children and most of these medications are not FDA-approved for treating ADHD. Second-line agents include the antidepressants bupropion, desipramine, imipramine, and nortriptyline. The alpha-blockers guanfacine and clonidine are also used, mostly as an adjunct in children with concomitant conduct disorder or sleep problems. Remember that a history of substance abuse or psychotic disorder is almost always a contraindication to stimulant use.

HELPFUL TIP: Stimulants do not cause cardiac problems and seem to be safe in both children and adults (*JAMA.* 2011;306:2673, *JAMA.* 2011;306:2723, *N Engl J Med.* 2011;365:1896).

HELPFUL TIP: Atomoxetine (Strattera) is a nonstimulant drug approved for ADHD (it is a selective norepinephrine reuptake inhibitor) and the only drug approved for adult ADHD. It is not a controlled prescription, having no apparent abuse potential. Its place in therapy is not yet well defined but might be used in those with a drug abuse history, etc. Maximum efficacy of atomoxetine is achieved in a few weeks, and it has a similar side effect profile to the stimulants.

Objectives: Did you learn to . . .

- Recognize childhood and adult presentation of ADHD?
- Prescribe efficacious treatments of ADHD?
- Recognize side effects and advantages of various medications for ADHD?

CASE 14

A gentleman calls your office because he is concerned that his wife of 2 years is acting strangely. She has not slept for most of the past week, staying up at night cleaning the house, and calling random people in the phonebook. She even went out and spent $3000 on a dress that left nothing to the imagination and was seen kissing another man. You ask him to bring his wife in as soon as possible.

That afternoon you find a provocatively dressed 30-year-old female sitting in your office and laughing giddily as her husband gives most of the intelligible history. She keeps reaching over to touch you on the leg as you interview her. You find her hard to understand because she talks so fast. You manage to catch something about "winning Miss America."

What is the most likely diagnosis?

A) Mania.
B) Psychosis.
C) Agitated depression.
D) Anxiety disorder.
E) ADHD.

Discussion

The correct answer is "A." Mania is the correct diagnosis. None of the other conditions can fully explain the abnormal elevation in mood and the subsequent behavior changes. Patients with **bipolar I disorder** must have had at least one episode of mania: a distinct period of abnormally and persistently elevated, expansive, or irritable mood, lasting at least 1 week (or any duration if hospitalization is necessary). In addition, there must be at least three of the following symptoms concurrently: (1) inflated self-esteem or grandiosity, (2) decreased need for sleep, (3) more talkative than usual, (4) flight of ideas or racing thoughts, (5) distractibility, (6) increased goal-directed activity or psychomotor agitation, and (7) excessive involvement in pleasurable activities that have a high risk for negative consequences/impulsivity (spending, spree, risky sexual indiscretions, etc.). The episode must cause impairment in occupational or social functioning and cannot be substance induced.

Patients with **bipolar II disorder** have had at least one episode of hypomania: a distinct period of persistently elevated, expansive, or irritable mood, lasting for at least 4 days, which is clearly distinct from the usual, nondepressed mood. During the hypomanic episode, at least three of the manic symptoms listed above must be present, although the episode is not severe enough to cause marked impairment in occupational or social functioning, require hospitalization, or include psychotic symptoms.

HELPFUL TIP: Although patients with bipolar disorders often have depressive episodes as well as manic or hypomanic episodes, depression is not required for the diagnosis of bipolar disorder ("So why is it called bipolar," you ask? Well, who are you to question tradition?).

Regarding the epidemiology of bipolar illness, which of the following is FALSE?

A) The prevalence of bipolar 1 is about 1.5%.
B) Many patients are misdiagnosed initially with depression.
C) Untreated suicide rate is almost 20%.
D) Women are twice as likely to be affected as men.
E) Suicide risk is highest in the depressed or mixed state.

Discussion

The correct answer is "D." Unlike depression, bipolar illness affects males and females equally. Bipolar 1 affects about 1.5% of the population, while bipolar 2 affects about double that number. Untreated, nearly 20% will commit suicide—a rate about 20 times that of the general population. Risk is highest in depressed states or the mixed states (both mania and depression present at the same time). Bipolar disorder typically has its onset in early adulthood, although it can begin in childhood or adolescence. Depression is present 20–30% of the time, even with ongoing maintenance treatment. Over half of bipolar patients are initially misdiagnosed with depression, and the average patient is only accurately diagnosed after 5 years of symptoms.

HELPFUL TIP: Up to 50% of people with bipolar disorder have concomitant alcohol abuse or dependence.

You want to start a medication for this patient.

Which of the following would NOT be an appropriate treatment choice for her mania?

A) Lithium.
B) Olanzapine.
C) Divalproex.
D) Carbamazepine.
E) Buspirone.

Discussion
The correct answer is "E." Buspirone is not effective in the treatment of bipolar disorder. Lithium was the first medication approved for treatment of bipolar mania and depression. It reduces the incidence of recurrence of mania, hypomania, and depression by about two-thirds. Lithium has a significant antisuicide effect with an estimated eight- to ninefold reduction in risk. It is dosed at nighttime or twice daily. Lithium has a narrow therapeutic window, and there are numerous drug–drug interactions.

Both divalproex and olanzapine have FDA approval for treatment of acute mania and appear to be somewhat effective in the prevention of recurrent episodes. However, only lithium and lamotrigine (Lamictal) are FDA-approved for bipolar treatment and maintenance. Carbamazepine is a second-line agent that is also effective, but side effects limit its use.

* *

You decide to start lithium.

Which of the following is a well-recognized side effect of lithium?

A) Diabetes.
B) Hypothyroidism.
C) Immunosuppression.
D) Abnormal hair growth.

Discussion
The correct answer is "B." Patients who take lithium should have their thyroid function monitored. Also, lithium can affect renal function and electrolyte levels, so check serum electrolytes periodically. As lithium has a narrow therapeutic window, serum lithium levels should be measured as well, with a goal of 0.6–1.0 mEq/L.

Which of the following drugs or drug classes do NOT alter lithium levels?

A) NSAIDs
B) Diuretics.
C) ACE inhibitors.
D) ARBs.
E) Narcotics.

Discussion
The correct answer is "E." Lithium is cleared by the kidney. Anything that can cause a change in renal function can affect lithium levels. NSAIDs, diuretics, ACE inhibitors, and ARBs can all affect renal function.

Objectives: Did you learn to . . .

- Recognize and diagnose bipolar disorder?
- Initiate treatment of bipolar disorder?
- Describe some potential adverse effects of treatment of bipolar disorder?

CASE 15

A 20-year-old white female gymnast presents to you because she has missed her period for 6 months. She feels cold all the time and has noticed that when she crosses her legs, she gets pins-and-needles sensations down her leg. She had a stress fracture of her right tibia 5 years ago but denies any other medical history. She denies being sexually active and the review of systems is positive for frequent heartburn, constipation, and fatigue.

Which of the following diagnoses would NOT be in your differential?

A) Pregnancy.
B) Hyperthyroidism.
C) Malignancy.
D) Anorexia nervosa (AN).

E) All of the above should be included in the differential.

Discussion

The correct answer is "E." All the answers should be part of a reasonably broad differential diagnosis in this young woman. In patients presenting with weight loss and a possible eating disorder, you should eliminate medical causes of weight loss, using history, physical exam, and appropriate labs. Despite her denial of sexual activity, a pregnancy test is a necessary part of the evaluation, since pregnancy is the most common cause of amenorrhea in this population. Hyperthyroidism and malignancy can present with vague complaints similar to this patient's. Likewise, AN can give rise to this patient's constellation of symptoms.

* *

As you take more history, you realize that this patient is a very finicky eater. She is a strict vegan (So? What is wrong with that?) and restricts her calories to <1000/day in order to stay in shape. She is 5 ft 3 in tall and weighs only 100 pounds, but she thinks she is overweight.

Which of these additional findings would you expect on physical exam?

A) Bradycardia.
B) Hypertension.
C) Adnexal mass.
D) Clonus.
E) Proptosis.

Discussion

The correct answer is "A." Common physical findings in weight loss, and specifically AN, include emaciation, sunken cheeks, hypotension, bradycardia, lanugo, mottled teeth, and dry or yellow skin. Peripheral edema may develop during weight gain or when laxative or diuretic abuse is stopped. Murmurs can occasionally be auscultated.

Patients with AN may present with:

A) Paresthesias.
B) Cold intolerance.
C) Constipation.
D) Fatigue.
E) All of the above.

Discussion

The correct answer is "E." All of the above are symptoms of AN. These are common symptoms seen in starvation. "A" is not intuitive but is true. Loss of fat allows for greater exposure of superficial nerves, so the act of crossing the legs or sitting down on a hard chair can cause paresthesias.

HELPFUL TIP: Patients with AN rarely have insight into the illness and often deny that weight loss is a problem. These patients are often perfectionists and overachievers who are sensitive to criticism and come from families with conflict. Weight loss is a method of control and is seen as a significant achievement.

HELPFUL TIP: The word "anorexia" in AN is a misnomer, as loss of appetite is exceedingly rare in this illness. Patients are hungry but voluntarily restrict their caloric intake. The initial weight loss may be precipitated by appetite loss caused by depression, medical illness, dieting, or stressful life event.

Which would be an expected laboratory finding in this patient?

A) Leukocytosis.
B) Hyperkalemia.
C) Increased amylase.
D) Decreased cholesterol.
E) Erythrocytosis.

Discussion

The correct answer is "C." Amylase may be increased as a result of purging behavior (and thus salivary stimulation). "A" and "E" are incorrect. Leukopenia, not leukocytosis, with a mild, normochromic, normocytic anemia is a common hematologic finding, although the CBC may be normal. "B" is incorrect. There is usually whole-body depletion of potassium, zinc, magnesium, and phosphate (from vomiting and inadequate intake). "D" is also incorrect, as cholesterol is often elevated (as are BUN and liver enzymes). This cholesterol elevation is neither intuitive nor well understood but is observed to occur in patients with AN. See Table 23–5 for more medical complications of AN.

Table 23-5 SELECTED MEDICAL COMPLICATIONS OF ANOREXIA NERVOSA

Neurologic	Seizures Peripheral neuropathy Cortical atrophy Cognitive impairment
Cardiovascular	Bradycardia Orthostatic hypotension Heart failure ECG changes: low voltage, nonspecific ST segment changes, QT prolongation
Endocrine	Amenorrhea Low T3, T4 and TSH (transient central hypothyroidism)- previously called "euthyroid sick syndrome". Osteopenia/osteoporosis Growth retardation
Fluids and electrolytes	Dehydration Metabolic alkalosis Hypokalemia Hypomagnesemia Hypocalcemia
Gastrointestinal	Elevated liver enzymes Constipation Esophagitis Mallory–Weiss tears Parotid gland hypertrophy
Dermatologic	Lanugo Brittle nails and hair Acrocyanosis Dry, scaly skin
Hematologic	Bone marrow suppression

* *

In order to increase your patient's motivation to comply with medical recommendations, you describe some of the adverse effects of excessively low weight.

All of the following abnormal findings will resolve when an adequate body weight is regained EXCEPT:

A) Bradycardia.
B) Muscle wasting.
C) Osteoporosis.
D) Infertility.

Discussion

The correct answer is "C." Patients with AN are usually young and therefore experience some of their lowest weights at the same time they are expected to reach peak bone mass. If a patient becomes osteopenic or osteoporotic when she is young, she will remain so as she ages (sans treatment). Return to good nutrition will not add bone mass that has been lost. All of the other physical changes listed should return to normal with return to a normal weight.

Which of the following is the most appropriate next step in the management of this patient?

A) Tell her to stop gymnastics, withdraw from classes, and go to live with her mother.
B) Start an antidepressant.
C) Admit her to the hospital.
D) Consult psychiatry and nutrition specialists.

Discussion

The correct answer is "D." This patient is most likely to benefit from a coordinated plan involving a multidisciplinary team, including primary care, psychiatry, and nutrition. "A" is incorrect, as it is a dramatic reaction that does not address the patient's primary problem, and the patient is unlikely to comply with it. "B" is incorrect. An antidepressant may be helpful in patients with a clearly defined depressive or anxiety disorder. However, the use of antidepressant therapy for AN has not been successful, and certain antidepressants are associated with weight loss. "C," hospitalization, is not likely to be beneficial at this point. The utility of hospitalization has been difficult to determine in AN. Commonly accepted reasons for hospital admission include the following: severe low weight (70–75 % of ideal body weight), severe bradycardia (<40 bpm) or cardiac arrhythmia, marked symptomatic hypotension or syncope, acute psychiatric emergency (threatened suicide), significant dehydration or electrolyte disturbances, acute food refusal, and failed intensive outpatient therapy.

* *

While you plan to involve psychiatric and nutritional services, you continue your discussion of eating disorders with this patient.

Which of the following is NOT TRUE about the epidemiology of eating disorders?

A) At least 90% of eating disorder patients are female.
B) Rates are higher in industrialized, Western nations.

C) A family history of depression increases the risk of females developing eating disorders.
D) Male wrestlers have a higher risk of eating disorders than the average male.
E) Mortality rates in AN are similar to the general population.

Discussion

The correct answer is "E." AN is characterized by a high mortality, one of the highest of psychiatric illnesses. It must be taken very seriously. Up to 10% of hospitalized patients die from direct effects of starvation, refeeding syndrome, suicide, or electrolyte imbalance leading to cardiac arrhythmias. At least 90% of eating disorder patients are female with prevalence rates higher in certain groups, such as models, actresses, athletes, and dancers. Western, industrialized societies endorse thinness and dieting as an ideal for women, resulting in higher rates of eating disorders. Despite having a normal body weight, **over 40% of 9- and 10-year-old American girls believe they are overweight** and consider dieting as an option! Eating disorders are distinctly uncommon in poorer countries where starvation is widespread, and there is no cultural endorsement of thinness. "C" is true. A family history of depression or obesity increases risk of an eating disorder by two- to fivefold, with a family history of depression alone increasing the risk about fivefold. "D" is also true. In males, wrestlers have a higher prevalence of eating disorders because of weight requirements in their sport. In men, body shape and not necessarily absolute body weight is the typical focus of concern.

> HELPFUL TIP: There are two subtypes of AN: restrictive and binge/purge. Therefore, a patient who binges and purges (through forced emesis, laxatives, etc.) does not necessarily have bulimia.

> HELPFUL TIP: Comorbidities are prevalent in eating disorder patients and include MDD (50–75%), anxiety disorders, obsessive–compulsive disorder, and substance abuse. Personality disorders are also prevalent with the anxious, sensitive, rigid, and perfectionistic types predominating (Cluster C).

* *

In your discussions of eating disorders, your patient asks about bulimia and how you distinguish between AN and bulimia.

Which of the following is NOT TRUE when comparing patients with AN and BN?

A) BN is more prevalent than AN.
B) BN patients are more likely to be normal weight than AN patients.
C) The prognosis for AN is better than that for BN.
D) BN patients are more likely to have esophageal tears.
E) Medications are effective in BN but not in AN.

Discussion

The correct answer is "C." BN has a better prognosis than AN, with only 20% of patients still meeting diagnostic criteria 5–10 years after initial presentation. BN is more common than AN, with the prevalence increasing just like it has with AN. "B" is true. Patients with BN are usually close to normal weight. However, they show several stigmata: loss of dental enamel and chipped teeth with cavities; enlarged parotid salivary glands with elevated serum amylase from repeated vomiting episodes; menstrual irregularities; bradycardia, hypotension; and decreased metabolic rate. Rare complications include esophageal tears from frequent vomiting or gastric rupture due to gastric dilatation secondary to binging. "E" is true. Treatment of BN involves the same principles as AN. Fluoxetine is the first-line drug with a target dose of 60 mg being shown to be effective in trials. Other SSRIs are second line. Third-line agents include TCAs, MAOIs, and trazodone. These agents reduce binge eating and bulimic symptoms whether patients are depressed or not.

> HELPFUL TIP: The mean age of onset of eating disorders is 17 years, with very rare onset in women older than 40 (although recurrence can occur in this population).

Objectives: Did you learn to . . .

- Evaluate a young person with a suspected eating disorder?
- Diagnose AN?
- Recognize medical complications of eating disorders?

- Distinguish between AN and BN?
- Initiate appropriate treatment and referral for a patient with an eating disorder?

QUICK QUIZ: EATING DISORDERS

In order to be diagnosed with BN according to DSM-IV, a patient must meet all of the following criteria EXCEPT:

A) Recurrent purging via self-induced vomiting.
B) Recurrent binge eating.
C) Symptoms are present at least twice per week for at least 3 months.
D) Self-evaluation is unduly influenced by body shape and weight.

Discussion

The correct answer is "A." For the diagnosis of BN, self-induced vomiting need not be present. Rather, some sort of compensatory behavior must be present during bulimic episodes. This behavior might include vomiting, but is not limited to vomiting, and may also include laxative or diuretic use, fasting, or excessive exercise. "B," "C," and "D" are required for the diagnosis of BN. BN affects about 1–3% females (usually white) and 0.1–0.3% males. Comorbidities of depression, anxiety, substance abuse, and personality disorders are also common. Dramatic, unstable personality traits (cluster B) predominate in this illness unlike the sensitive, rigid (Cluster C) personality traits in AN.

QUICK QUIZ: EATING DISORDERS (OR, HOLD THE PIE FOR NOW, PLEASE)

A previously healthy 17-year-old female is hospitalized for AN. She has her weight rapidly restored with intravenous fluids and a 3000 kcal/day diet. She rapidly gains 10 pounds in her first 2 days (so gaining 10 pounds in 2 days sounds like a good thing?) and seems to be doing well. However, when you round the next morning, she is nonresponsive. Physical exam reveals evidence of JVD, pulmonary rales, and lower extremity edema.

What is the most likely cause of this patient's apparent CHF?

A) Previously undiagnosed heart disease.
B) Refeeding syndrome.
C) Suicide attempt by SSRI overdose.
D) MI.

Discussion

The correct answer is "B." The scenario described fits with the clinical picture caused by refeeding syndrome. Refeeding syndrome occurs when rapid expansion of the circulating volume overwhelms the cardiovascular system's ability to adapt, leading to CHF. It also involves changes in electrolytes and glucose. It typically occurs in malnourished patients. Prevention involves careful monitoring of electrolytes including magnesium, phosphorus, potassium, and calcium, while advancing caloric intake in a small, linear fashion and keeping track of volume status. "A" and "D" are incorrect as the patient is unlikely to have significant heart disease given her age and gender.

HELPFUL TABLE: There is no case for this table but editors hate it when there is no "call out" for a table. So, see Table 23–6 for warning signs that an agitated patient may become violent. See Table 23–7 for ways to calm the agitated patient (although in the editors' experience nothing beats IM haloperidol and IM lorazepam).

Table 23–6 WARNING SIGNS THAT AN AGITATED PATIENT MAY BECOME VIOLENT

Hyperactivity: pacing or other increase in psychomotor activity
Loud, angry, or profane speech
Increased muscle tension, manifested by clenched jaw, fist, rigid posture, gripping chair, sitting on chair edge, etc.
Intoxication
Suspicious, angry, or irritable affect
Breathlessness, tachycardia, diaphoresis, pupillary dilation, visibly palpitating temporal arteries
Uncooperativeness with requests
Door slamming, chair toppling, or other form of property destruction
Grabbing objects that could be potential weapons
Verbal or physical threats
The clinician's response to the patient: if you feel anxious, take it seriously and be alert to possible danger

Table 23–7 TECHNIQUES TO CALM THE AGITATED PATIENT

Remove the patient to a quiet and nonstimulating environment
Keep a distance from the patient and avoid physical contact
Identify exits and alarms
Maintain nonthreatening demeanor and stance
Keep your hands at your side where they are easily visible
While maintaining steady eye contact, speak in a steady but authoritative voice, using the patient's name with each sentence
Avoid sudden jerky movements and remain calm
Have familiar faces nearby if possible
Show the patient concern but tell him that violence is not acceptable and you are willing to work with him if he calms down
There is strength in numbers. Have other personnel nearby to help if necessary
Call for help from police or security if needed. A backup system, which has been tested, should be in place
Consider antipsychotics, such as haloperidol (available in oral and parenteral forms) and risperidol (available in liquid). A benzodiazepine may be used as an adjunct, but should **not** be used alone
Mechanical restraints may be employed if absolutely necessary
Remember to figure out **why** the patient is agitated (e.g., take history, perform mental status exam, and order appropriate tests)

QUICK QUIZ: PHYSICIAN HEAL THYSELF?

Which of the following is true about physicians' risk of suicide compared to the general population?

A) Female physicians have a risk of successful suicide equal to male physicians.
B) Physicians are more likely to be depressed than the general population.
C) Female physicians are more likely to attempt suicide than the general female population.
D) Medical students and residents are less likely to be depressed than the general population.

Table 23–8 FACTORS AFFECTING SUICIDE RISK

Risk factors
- Living alone (particularly first year alone)
- Loss of spouse or separation
- Alcohol use
- Having access to a gun or lethal means
- Loss of activity, job, property, or capabilities
- Mild/minimal cognitive impairment
- Paranoia
- Hopelessness
- Anxiety
- Older white male
- Personal or family history of suicide attempt or completion
- Urban dweller

Protective factors
- Effective treatment of mental and physical disorders
- Social and family support
- Coping skills
- Resilience
- Religious faith
- Lack of access to lethal means

Discussion

The correct answer is "A." In the general population, women have two to four times more suicide attempts than men, while men are four times more likely than women to be successful. However, among physicians, the rate of successful suicide in men and women is equivalent (we didn't study all of that pharmacology for nothing!). This occurs despite the fact that female physicians have fewer attempts than the general female population. Physicians have roughly the same rate of depression as the general population, while medical students and residents have higher rates than the general population (15–30% vs. 16% in the general population). Other factors affecting suicide risk (in addition to being a physician) are noted in Table 23–8.

QUICK QUIZ: SUICIDE RISK

You have a colleague who is depressed and has transient thoughts of suicide.

Which of the following would suggest that he should be hospitalized today?

A) He thinks about suicide only infrequently.
B) He has not formulated a plan to commit suicide.

C) He has updated his will within the past few days.
D) He is willing to follow up in clinic tomorrow.
E) He has given away his guns.

Discussion

The correct answer is "C." If a person admits to suicidal ideation, ask the following questions to assess his level of risk and to determine whether or not he should be hospitalized.

- How often does he think about suicide?
- Does he have a concrete plan? And if so, is it plausible?
- Is he giving away treasured belongings, updating his will, making final plans, etc.?
- Is he in danger of acting on his thoughts?
- Why has he not attempted suicide yet? What keeps him from doing it?
- Does he have access to harmful means (e.g., guns and drugs)?

QUICK QUIZ: PSYCHOTROPIC DRUGS

Which of these antidepressants can be administered once weekly?

A) Paroxetine (Paxil).
B) Buspirone (Wellbutrin).
C) Fluoxetine (Prozac).
D) Escitalopram (Lexapro).
E) Venlafaxine (Effexor-SR).

Discussion

The correct answer is "C." Fluoxetine has a long enough half-life that it can be administered once a week. You don't need to prescribe the "long acting" fluoxetine. Any fluoxetine can be dosed once weekly.

CASE 16

You are on call and have been paged to see a 21-year-old female who has just overdosed on a handful of acetaminophen because her boyfriend left her after their most recent fight. She has had similar overdoses three times in the past (they fight a lot). According to a friend, she has a history of tumultuous relationships. In the emergency department, she is combative and yelling, "I'm so angry that I'm still alive!" She has a blood alcohol level of 106 mg/dL. There are scars on her arms from cutting.

What is the most likely primary diagnosis?

A) Antisocial personality disorder.
B) Bipolar effective disorder.
C) MDD.
D) Borderline personality disorder.
E) Somatization disorder.

Discussion

The correct answer is "D." This patient's history is consistent with a diagnosis of borderline personality disorder. Persons with borderline personality disorder often have stormy relationships, characterized by extremes of emotional intensity (e.g., "love–hate" relationships). You might also consider depression as a diagnosis here, but the history does not support MDD. However, concomitant depression is common in patients with borderline personality disorder. "A," "B," and "E" are not supported by the clinical presentation. Borderline personality disorder is mostly a diagnosis of females (over 90%). Characteristics are listed in Table 23–9.

HELPFUL TIP: A personality disorder is an enduring pattern of relating to the world in ways that are inflexible, ineffective, and markedly different from cultural norms. Personality disorders cause distress or functional impairment and start by adolescence in most people. The prevalence rate of personality disorders varies widely across studies, with borderline personality disorder being the most prevalent of all.

Table 23–9 CHARACTERISTICS OF BORDERLINE PERSONALITY DISORDER

- Fears of abandonment
- Unstable and intense relationships
- Unstable sense of self
- Impulsivity
- Suicidal behavior, threats or gestures or self-mutilation. (Cutting is often a feature of borderline personality disorder.)
- Significant mood reactivity
- Chronic feelings of emptiness
- Intense anger outbursts
- Transient stress-related paranoid ideation or dissociation

* *

Your patient's boyfriend storms into the emergency department and demands to see her. He has "love" and "hate" tattooed on his knuckles. The nurse recognizes him immediately as a frequent visitor. Apparently, he has been in the emergency department on multiple occasions for injuries sustained from fights. Your patient pulls you aside to tell you that she is afraid of him, saying, "I just worry when he gets mad. He went to jail for beating and raping his last girlfriend." The nurse also informs you that he is suspected of stealing narcotics from a pharmacy in town. You call security.

Which of the following personality disorders is most likely in this man?

A) Paranoid personality disorder.
B) Histrionic personality disorder.
C) Schizotypal personality disorder.
D) Antisocial personality disorder.
E) Imajerk personality disorder.

Discussion

The correct answer is "D." antisocial personality disorder is primarily seen in males, and of the options given, it is the only personality disorder that really fits. Antisocial personality disorder is quite prevalent in prison populations. "A" and "C" are incorrect because these are Cluster A disorders, which are characterized by strange rather than violent behavior. "B" is incorrect. Histrionic personality disorder shows attention-seeking and seductive behavior. Although patients with antisocial personality disorder can be charming, they also use violence and threats to achieve their purposes. "E" is incorrect because it does not exist as a disorder—it's a joke (I'm-a-jerk, get it?)—although if it did exist, this patient would be a prime example. Characteristics of antisocial personality disorder are listed in Table 23–10.

Table 23–10 CHARACTERISTICS OF ANTISOCIAL PERSONALITY DISORDER

- Recurrent criminality
- Deceitfulness shown by repeated lying, use of aliases, or conning others
- Impulsivity
- Irritability and aggression
- Reckless disregard for safety
- Consistent irresponsibility, failing to fulfill financial obligations or work
- Lack of remorse
- Childhood conduct disorder and person now at least 18

Besides borderline personality disorder, which other personality disorder increases the risk of *completed suicide* the most?

A) Paranoid personality disorder.
B) Histrionic personality disorder.
C) Schizotypal personality disorder.
D) Avoidant personality disorder.
E) Antisocial personality disorder.

Discussion

The correct answer is "E." Along with borderline personality disorder, antisocial personality disorder is the other personality disorder most likely to be seen in completed suicides.

Considering the current psychiatric diagnosis classification system, under what axis will you classify this patient and her boyfriend in terms of their personality disorders?

A) Axis I.
B) Axis II.
C) Axis III.
D) Axis IV.
E) Axis of Evil.

Discussion

The correct answer is "B." The current psychiatric classification system is listed in Table 23–11.

HELPFUL TIP: Impulsivity is a risk for completed suicide. Even though patients may not want to die, an impulsively taken overdose or other suicide attempt may inadvertently lead to death. This is why patients with borderline personality disorder and antisocial personality disorder have a high risk of completed suicide.

* *

You have a frank discussion with your female patient about suicide.

Table 23–11 CURRENT PSYCHIATRIC CLASSIFICATION SYSTEM

Axis I: Major psychiatric disorders (e.g., depression and schizophrenia)

Axis II: Personality disorders and developmental delay

- Cluster A: "the **weird** cluster"—patients are aloof, act strange, and prefer to be alone. Paranoid, schizoid, and schizotypal personality disorders are included here.
- Cluster B: "the **wild** cluster"—patients have significant problems with mood lability, impulsivity, or are preoccupied with being admired for their sexuality or intelligence. Borderline, antisocial, histrionic, and narcissistic personality disorders are included here.
- Cluster C: "the **whiny** cluster"—patients are clingy, sensitive, and rigid. Avoidant, dependent, and obsessive–compulsive personality disorders are included here.

Axis III: General medical conditions potentially relevant to understanding the psychiatric disorders.

Axis IV: Psychosocial and environmental factors that may contribute to the patients' distress (e.g., homelessness and recent divorce).

Axis V: Global Assessment of Function, a 0–100-point scale for assessing the individual's overall level of functioning in the physician's judgment.

Which of the following is NOT TRUE about suicide in the general population?

A) Medical diagnoses can increase the risk of suicide.
B) Over 90% of people who commit suicide have a mental or substance abuse disorder.
C) Older Americans are at higher risk of suicide.
D) The rate of successful suicides has increased over the years.
E) Suicide is one of the top 10 causes of death in the United States.

Discussion

The correct answer is "D." The rate of successful suicide has actually stayed stable over time. "A" is a correct statement. Medical diagnoses can be risk factors for suicide, especially chronic pain, chronic illness, terminal illness, or recent surgery. Older Americans commit suicide at a rate four times than that of the general population with a peak incidence at age 75 for men and 60 for women. "E" is also correct. Suicide is the seventh leading cause of death in the United

Table 23–12 MNEMONICS FOR SUICIDE RISK ASSESSMENT

NO HOPE	SAD PERSONS
No framework for meaning (Reading Nietzsche and being an existentialist?)	**S**ex—male
Overt change in clinical condition	**A**ge—older
Hostile interpersonal environment	**D**epression
Out of hospital recently	**P**revious attempt
Predisposing personality factors	**E**thanol abuse
Excuses for dying to help others	**R**ational thought loss
	Social support lacking
	Organized plan
	No spouse
	Sickness

States and the third leading cause of death in those aged 15–24. There are two mnemonics that are useful for assessing suicide risk: "NO HOPE" and "SAD PERSONS" (see Table 23–12).

HELPFUL TIP: Seventy-five percent of older Americans who commit suicide have seen their primary care physician within the preceding 4 weeks and 39% within the same week. Up to half of successful suicides have made a prior attempt.

Objectives: Did you learn to . . .

- Identify borderline and antisocial personality disorders?
- Classify personality disorders?
- Assess suicide risk?

CASE 17

A 21-year-old man presents to your clinic because his girlfriend dragged him in. He just started his first year in college but quit 2 days ago because he feels that "they are all out to get me." ("If he's talking about the IRS, he's probably right," you think to yourself.) He has not been sleeping because he thinks he might be murdered in his sleep. He tells you that the FBI has bugged your office and, therefore, does not want to answer your questions.

Which of the following would you NOT expect to find on mental status exam?

A) Delusions.
B) Hallucinations.
C) Lack of insight.
D) Decreased psychomotor activity.
E) Poverty of speech.

Discussion

The correct answer is "D." The patient described is acutely psychotic. You would expect him to have increased psychomotor activity. All of the other options would also be anticipated findings in this patient. Common symptoms of psychosis include delusions, hallucinations, psychomotor agitation, flight of ideas, nonsensical speech and behavior, lack of insight into one's behavior, and lack of judgment. Note that "poverty of speech" refers to brief, empty replys to questions and not to content which may be quite fanciful.

All of the following are potential causes of this patient's psychosis EXCEPT:

A) Substance abuse.
B) Alcohol withdrawal.
C) Bipolar disorder.
D) Bereavement.
E) Schizophrenia.

Discussion

The correct answer is "D." Bereavement may result in mild delusions and sometimes hallucinations regarding the bereaved subject (Hey? Is that mom back from the dead?), but it should not cause overt psychosis. Moreover, there is nothing in the history here to support a diagnosis of bereavement. The remaining options are potential cause of psychosis, and they are listed along with other potential causes in Table 23–13.

Table 23–13 CAUSES OF PSYCHOSIS AND DELIRIUM: A PARTIAL LIST

Potentially life-threatening causes:
- Meningitis or encephalitis
- Hypoxemia
- Hypertensive encephalopathy
- Wernicke encephalopathy
- Intracranial bleed
- Drug withdrawal, intoxication, or reaction to prescribed drugs

Other medical causes:
- Metabolic disorders (e.g., hyperglycemia and hyponatremia)
- Neurologic disorders
- Nutritional deficiencies (e.g., pellagra, beriberi, and pernicious anemia)
- Industrial exposure to toxins

Psychiatric causes:
- Schizophrenia or schizophreniform disorders
- Brief psychotic disorder
- Mood disorders including bipolar disorder and psychotic depression
- Schizoaffective disorder
- Dementia
- Delirium
- Delusional disorder

HELPFUL TIP: Psychosis is a symptom and not a diagnosis and should prompt a search for an etiology. Some of the causes are potentially life threatening.

* *

The patient relaxes and becomes cooperative, and you are able to obtain a history and perform a physical exam. He denies drug use or medical illnesses. Your patient worries that he is going "crazy" and admits that he has been having these symptoms "for a while" but did not want to tell anybody, for fear of being institutionalized. Your physical exam and labs are unremarkable.

Which of the following diagnoses is the most likely cause of this patient's psychosis?

A) Schizophrenia.
B) Psychotic depression.
C) Delirium.
D) Drug intoxication.
E) Dementia.

Discussion

The correct answer is "A." Schizophrenia is a heterogeneous group of disorders characterized by the following: positive symptoms (delusions, hallucinations, disorganized behavior, disorganized speech); negative symptoms (poverty of speech, anhedonia, effective flattening, avolition, asociality); mood symptoms (dysphoria, suicidal thoughts, hopelessness); and cognitive symptoms (attention and memory deficits and difficulty with abstract thinking). It is the most common of the psychotic disorders. A negative laboratory evaluation and physical exam make drug intoxication unlikely, while this patient's ability to converse with you and give a history makes delirium and dementia unlikely. Psychotic depression is unusual in young people, but rather is more commonly seen in older patients with severe depression.

Which of the following is NOT TRUE about schizophrenia?

A) Nearly 50% attempt suicide with a 10% success rate.
B) Lifetime prevalence is 1% worldwide, consistent across cultures.
C) Schizophrenia is a disease of late adolescence or early adulthood.
D) Men are more likely to be affected than women.
E) Risk of relapse is at least 50% after successful treatment in patients who do not remain on antipsychotic maintenance therapy.

Discussion

The correct answer is "D." Schizophrenia has a worldwide prevalence of about 1%, which is true for all cultures, countries, and both genders. It generally begins in late adolescence or early adulthood, and onset after age 50 is rare and should prompt the search for other etiologies to explain the psychosis. Men have a slightly earlier age of onset (early 20s) than women (late 20s), but men and women are affected equally by the illness. The course is variable with some patients having exacerbations and remissions (although full remissions are rare), while others remain chronically ill. About half of the patients who develop schizophrenia have a family history of schizophrenia. Suicide attempts are common, usually the result of depression or a response to command hallucinations, paranoid delusions, or agitation. Nearly 50% will attempt suicide, while about 10% will be successful. After successful treatment of the first episode, about 50% will relapse if not on maintenance medication.

Which of the following medication options is the proper treatment choice?

A) Olanzapine (Zyprexa).
B) Risperidone (Risperdal).
C) Haloperidol (Haldol).
D) Aripiprazole (Abilify).
E) Any of the above.

Discussion

The correct answer is "E." All of the antipsychotics listed are first-line treatment choices for schizophrenia. Most psychiatrists have replaced older "typical" agents like haloperidol with newer "atypical" agents (e.g., risperidone and olanzapine) because of better tolerability and possibly increased benefit for negative symptoms. Although, the newer agents are significantly more expensive than the older agents, more generics are becoming available. Also, many "atypicals" cause significant weight gain, and some have been linked to new onset diabetes. Of the newer agents, aripiprazole (Abilify) and ziprasidone (Geodon) are less associated with weight gain and diabetes.

Which of the following IS TRUE of the course of schizophrenia?

A) Positive symptoms usually occur first.
B) Negative symptoms are easier to treat than positive symptoms.
C) Negative symptoms often look like depression.
D) Schizophrenia is not typically associated with brain changes.
E) Family therapy is not helpful in this illness.

Discussion

The correct answer is "C." Negative symptoms often precede the development of the positive symptoms by many years, are often nonspecific, and can be mistaken for depression. A typical history is that of a normal young man who begins to fail classes and avoid his old friends as he gets to the end of high school. This is often mistaken for teenage rebellion, depression, or drug use until the onset of positive psychotic symptoms of hallucinations or delusions several years later. "B" is incorrect. Negative symptoms are chronic and are resistant to treatment with all currently available antipsychotics. Antipsychotic drugs modulate dopamine and/or serotonin and are much better at treating positive symptoms. "D" is not true, as brain imaging may reveal enlargement of cerebral ventricles and decreased brain volume. However, these findings are neither sensitive nor specific enough to have much value in diagnosis. "E" is incorrect. A large body of literature supports the fact that family therapy, especially directed at support and psychoeducation, reduces the risk of relapse. Recent evidence indicates that individual CBT can also be effective.

Objectives: Did you learn to . . .

- Recognize psychosis and its causative diagnoses?
- Treat psychosis?
- Recognize schizophrenia and understand its epidemiology and prognosis?

CASE 18

A 33-year-old factory worker comes to your clinic complaining of sleep difficulty since he moved to the "graveyard shift." He complains of falling asleep at work and having difficulty sleeping during the day.

Which of the following is the most likely diagnosis?

A) Narcolepsy.
B) Circadian rhythm sleep disorder.
C) Obstructive sleep apnea.
D) Primary insomnia.

Discussion

The correct answer is "B." This patient suffers (as do most residents and a significant number of physicians) from a circadian rhythm sleep disorder, which is defined as a sleep disruption leading to excessive sleepiness when the patient wishes to be awake or insomnia when the patient wishes to be asleep. It occurs as a result of a mismatch between the biological circadian rhythm and the person's environment. He does not give a history consistent with narcolepsy or obstructive sleep apnea, and primary insomnia is a diagnosis of exclusion.

* *

He asks your advice on how to treat his sleeplessness.

What would be the best advice to offer at this time?

A) Have him sleep at work (we do!).
B) Have him take naps throughout the day.
C) Tell him to quit his job.
D) Recommend bright light at night before going to work.
E) Prescribe stimulants for when he is at work.

Discussion

The correct answer is "D." This patient's circadian rhythm disturbance might also be called a "phase-advance" type sleep disorder (early sleep onset with insomnia at the desired sleep period). Such problems respond best to bright light in the evening to keep one awake during the time the individual would usually be asleep. Light boxes are available commercially and should provide white light at 2500 lux or more. The light should be fairly close to the patient's eyes, and a bit off to the side. The other options are not likely to be helpful if this patient wants to keep his job.

If this patient wished to use a nutritional or herbal supplement, which of the following would you recommend?

A) Melatonin.
B) Kava-kava.
C) Ginkgo.
D) Ginseng.
E) St. John wort.

Discussion

The correct answer is "A." There is some evidence to suggest that melatonin can help with circadian rhythm disorders. (It is an FDA-approved "orphan drug" for this indication.) Melatonin should be taken at the time of day the patient wants to sleep. In this case, you should advise him to take it in the morning. The doses used for circadian rhythm disturbances are much less than the dose used for primary insomnia, typically 0.5 mg or less, compared with 3 mg. The other herbal supplements have no evidence for use in sleep disturbances except for kava-kava that is too dangerous to recommend.

Which of the following is NOT a delayed sleep phase type of circadian rhythm sleep disorder?

A) Readaptation to day work from night work.
B) West-to-east jet lag.
C) East-to-west jet lag.
D) All of the above are delayed sleep phase disorders.

Discussion

The correct answer is "C." Delayed sleep phase involves a persistent pattern of late sleep onset and late morning awakening. This is exemplified by the average teenager during summer vacation (just try to get him to mow the lawn before noon!). West-to-east jet lag and readapting to day shift after working night shift also cause similar problems. "C" does not cause a delayed sleep phase disturbance. East-to-west jet lag causes the opposite problem, advancing sleep phase so that persons are sleepy early in the evening but then awake early in the morning. A potentially effective treatment of delayed sleep phase would include prescribing a bright light in the morning and melatonin in the afternoon.

Objectives: Did you learn to . . .

- Recognize circadian rhythm disorders?
- Recommend treatment of circadian rhythm disorders?

QUICK QUIZ: YOU WILL FORGET IT WITHOUT REPETITION

A 70-year-old man presents with memory loss that has been progressive over the years. He often has fluctuating attention and is rigid with bradykinesia. He frequently experiences visual hallucinations.

Which of the following is the most likely diagnosis?

A) Alzheimer disease.
B) Dementia with Lewy bodies (DLB).
C) Parkinson disease.
D) Vascular dementia.
E) Frontotemporal dementia.

Discussion

The correct answer is "B." DLB shares many features in common with Parkinson disease. These features include parkinsonian motor symptoms, such as bradykinesia, rigidity, and tremor. Both Parkinson disease and DLB are characterized histologically by the presence of Lewy bodies. However, in DLB, Lewy bodies are diffusely spread in the cortical regions and brainstem, whereas in Parkinson disease, Lewy bodies are primarily present in the subcortical nuclei. Fluctuating cognition that resembles delirium, visual hallucinations, and an exquisite sensitivity to the adverse effects of neuroleptics all characterize DLB. There is a lack of response of dopaminergic agents with DLB but cholinesterase inhibitors offer a modest benefit.

QUICK QUIZ: DEMENTIA

A 65-year-old man with a history of hypertension, diabetes, and peripheral vascular disease has been noted to have abrupt deterioration in his cognitive ability following an episode of disorientation and word-finding difficulty 1 month ago.

Which of the following is the most likely diagnosis?

A) Alzheimer disease
B) DLB.
C) Parkinson disease.
D) Vascular dementia.
E) Frontotemporal dementia.

Discussion

The correct answer is "D." Vascular dementia (previously known as multiinfarct dementia) is caused by vascular disease and, next to Alzheimer disease and Lewy body dementias, is one of the most common causes of dementia. It classically presents with an abrupt onset followed by step-wise deterioration of cognitive function. Medical comorbidities are common, including diabetes, hypertension, and obesity. Evidence of vascular disease is usually present on clinical exam with focal neurological signs, such as are seen after a stroke involving motor areas. Imaging typically shows infarctions of periventricular and deep subcortical white matter, presenting as white matter hyperintensities on T_2 weighted MRI. Treatment includes modifying vascular risk factors.

CASE 19

A 37-year-old female patient returns to see you for follow-up of depression. You last saw her 4 weeks ago, and at that time she was experiencing her third relapse of recurrent major depression. She had been in remission for 3 years before, and until 2 years ago she had been taking sertraline 150 mg daily, a regimen that she had found effective during an 18-month course of treatment. At her visit last month, you assessed her symptoms with the Patient Health Questionnaire-9 (PHQ-9), and her score at that time was 21. You reinstituted sertraline at 50 mg daily for 2 weeks and then 100 mg daily, which she is currently taking. At her visit today, her PHQ-9 score is 17. She denies having thoughts of death or suicide.

Which of the following options is LEAST appropriate to recommend to your patient at this time?

A) Continue sertraline 100 mg daily and return for follow-up in 1 month.

B) Continue sertraline 100 mg daily, add weekly CBT, and return for follow-up in 1 month.
C) Increase sertraline to 150 mg daily and return for follow-up in 1 month.
D) Stop the sertraline and start citalopram 20 mg daily and return for follow-up in 1 month.
E) Continue sertraline 100 mg daily and add bupropion SR 150 mg BID, return for follow-up in 1 month.

Discussion

The correct answer is "D." At the current visit, the patient has been taking sertraline for 1 month and has been at the present dose for 2 weeks. It can take up to 6–8 weeks for an antidepressant medication to reach its full effect, so it is reasonable to maintain the medication at its present dose and reassess in 1 month. However, options "B," "C," and "E" are reasonable as well. Combination treatment with CBT and an antidepressant medication has been shown to be more effective for treating depression than either treatment strategy alone. You can also consider the addition of an augmentation agent (burpproprione, T3, or a second generation antipsychotic). Since she has had a partial response to the current regimen, adding an augmentation agent is a reasonable option. Switching to a new antidepressant at this time is not indicated.

Which of the following statements is NOT true regarding the PHQ-9?

A) The PHQ-9 is a clinician-administered questionnaire to evaluate for symptoms of major depression.
B) It takes 3–5 minutes to complete the PHQ-9.
C) A score of 10 or more on the PHQ-9 is a positive screen.
D) The PHQ-9 can be used to screen for depression as well as to monitor symptom severity over time.
E) The PHQ-9 does **NOT** assess for suicide risk.

Discussion

The correct answer is "A." The PHQ-9 is a patient-administered, nine-item questionnaire that takes 3–5 minutes to complete. It can be used to screen for major depression as well as to monitor symptom severity over time. A score >10 is considered a positive screen, while a score <5 is considered to be negative or in remission. The maximum score is 30. While the PHQ-9 does ask about the presence of "thoughts of death or dying," it does not assess whether someone is at low or high risk for suicide attempt.

* *

Despite increasing the dose of sertraline, your patient's depression does not improve. She's been watching a lot of TV (no wonder she's depressed) and seen adds for medications to augment traditional antidepressant therapy. She says, "I think I need one of those new wonder drugs, Doc."

Which of the following have gained FDA approval as add-on therapy for depression?

A) Aripiprazole.
B) Haloperidol.
C) Olanzapine.
D) Quetiapine.
E) All of the above.

Discussion

The correct answer is "A." Aripiprazole (Abilify) has been approved by the FDA as add-on therapy for depression to be used in conjunction with traditional antidepressant therapy. Other antipsychotics have been used to treat depression, but as of 2012, aripiprazole is the only one with an FDA-approved indication for add-on therapy. Olanzapine is marketed as a combination pill (fluoxetine/olanzapine) for treatment of resistant depression, but is not FDA-approved as add-on therapy alone. The benefits of adding aripiprazole to a traditional antidepressant appear marginal (a statistically significant 3-point difference on a 60-point scale when compared with placebo); it's expensive; and sizable minority of patients develops akathisia or restlessness. And remember that statistically significant does not necessary mean clinically significant. For aripiprazole, the number needed to treat to achieve this small reduction in depressive symptoms is 10. On the bright side, aripiprazole is less associated with weight gain compared with other atypical antipsychotics.

Objectives: Did you learn to . . .

- Develop strategies to treat resistant depression?
- Describe a widely used depression assessment tool, the PHQ-9?

The world of psychiatry is consonantly moving. See the table below for some newer psychiatric drugs.

SOME NEWER PSYCHIATRIC DRUGS

Name	Indication
VYvanse (lisdexamfetamine)	ADHD
Pristiq (desvenlafaxine)	Depression
Savela (Milnacipran)	Depression, fibromyalgia
VIIbryd (Vilazadone)	Depression
Saphris (asenapine)	Schizophrenia, Bipolar Types 1 and 2

BIBLIOGRAPHY

Ables AZ, Nagubilli R. Prevention, recognition, and management of serotonin syndrome. *Am Fam Physician.* 2010;8:1139-1142.

American Psychiatric Association. *Practice Guideline for the Treatment of Patients with Major Depressive Disorder*, 3rd ed., 2010. Available at: http://psychiatryonline.org/content.aspx?bookid=28&sectionid=1667485.

Diagnostic and Statistical Manual of Mental Disorders. 4th ed., Text Revision. Washington, DC: American Psychiatric Association; 2000.

Glick ID, et al. Mid-term and long-term efficacy and effectiveness of antipsychotic medications for schizophrenia: A data-driven, personalized clinical approach. *J Clin Psychiatry.* 2011;72:1616-1627.

Hendin H, et al. Confronting depression and suicide in physicians: A consensus statement. *JAMA.* 2003;289: 3161-3166.

Khan A, et al. Suicide rates in clinical trials of SSRIs, other antidepressants, and placebo: Analysis of FDA reports. *Am J Psychiatry.* 2003;160:790-792.

Rader R, et al. Current strategies in the diagnosis and treatment of childhood attention-deficit/hyperactivity disorder. *Am Fam Physician.* 2009;79:657-665.

Rush AJ, et al. Acute and longer-term outcomes in depressed outpatients requiring one or several treatment steps: A STAR*D report. *Am J Psychiatry.* 2006; 163:1905.

Schatzberg AF, et al. Antidepressant discontinuation syndrome: Consensus panel recommendations for clinical management and additional research. *J Clin Psychiatry.* 2006;67(Suppl 4):27-30.

Stahl SM. *Essential Psychopharmacology of Depression and Bipolar Disorder.* Cambridge: Cambridge University Press; 2001.

Uncapher H, Arean PA. Physicians are less willing to treat suicidal ideation in older patients. *J Am Geriatr Soc.* 2000;48:188-192.

Wagner KD, et al. Efficacy of sertraline in the treatment of children and adolescents with major depressive disorder: Two randomized controlled trials. *JAMA.* 2003;290:1033-1041.

Wheeler BW, et al. The population impact on incidence of suicide and non-fatal self harm of regulatory action against the use of selective serotonin reuptake inhibitors in under 18s in the United Kingdom: Ecological study. *BMJ.* 2008;336:542.

24 Nutrition and Herbal Medicine

Philip Gregory and Mark A. Graber

CASE 1

A 59-year-old male presents for follow-up. He is well known to you, receiving chronic anticoagulation with warfarin for a mechanical aortic valve. His protime and INR have been in the therapeutic range for years. When asked, he denies taking any other medications. He has had no new medical problems and is feeling well.

Today his INR is 6.2 (therapeutic range 2.5–3.5). You inquire about dietary changes, focusing on foods rich in vitamin K.

Which of the following is true regarding vitamin K?

A) Vitamin K is a water-soluble vitamin.
B) Broccoli and olive oil are good sources of vitamin K.
C) Vitamin K deficiency results in a hypercoagulable state.
D) Warfarin reduces the absorption of vitamin K.
E) Vegetarians are at risk for developing vitamin K deficiency.

Discussion

The correct answer is "B." Vitamin K is a fat-soluble vitamin present in leafy green vegetables such as spinach and cabbage and in other foods such as milk, butter, bacon, and vegetable oils. Olive oil and broccoli are particularly rich in vitamin K. Therefore, vegetarians are not at high risk for developing vitamin K deficiency. Vitamin K deficiency causes a **hypo**coagulable state resulting in a reduction in clotting factors and elevated prothrombin time and INR, leading to poor clotting ability and hemorrhage. Warfarin does act on vitamin K, but by reducing conversion of vitamin K to its active form rather than reducing absorption.

You would be more likely to suspect vitamin K deficiency in this patient if he also suffered from which of the following conditions?

A) Crohn disease.
B) Irritable bowel syndrome.
C) Hepatitis C.
D) Coronary artery disease (CAD).
E) All of the above.

Discussion

The correct answer is "A." Vitamin K deficiency can occur with chronic small bowel disease, after small bowel resection, and with use of broad-spectrum antibiotics. Microorganisms in the bowel synthesize vitamin K, and use of broad-spectrum antibiotics reduces the numbers of these organisms. The majority of vitamin K is absorbed in the distal small bowel, and any disease affecting this area—including Crohn disease and celiac diseases—can reduce the absorption of the vitamin. Irritable bowel syndrome is a functional disease not associated with impaired absorption.

* *

Upon more direct questioning, the patient denies any changes in his diet but admits to recently starting a vitamin therapy program. He has no clue what he is actually taking and calls his wife to find out what the products contain (it was Miracle Mega Man something . . .). Meanwhile, you suspect that he is taking excessive doses of vitamins that may affect his INR.

Large doses of which of the following vitamins are most likely to result in an increased INR in patients taking warfarin?

A) Vitamin A.
B) Vitamin C.
C) Vitamin D.
D) Vitamin E.
E) Zinc.

Discussion

The correct answer is "D." Large doses of Vitamin E (>400 mg/day) can interfere with vitamin K metabolism and platelet function, resulting in increased prothrombin time and therefore increased INR in some patients. In patients taking warfarin, starting a high-dose vitamin E supplement should be done cautiously. Extra monitoring of INR and/or warfarin dose adjustments may be needed. See Table 24–1 for more on supplements that can affect the INR.

The other options are unlikely to affect the INR. Vitamin A consumed in quantities exceeding 10 times the Recommended Daily Allowance (RDA) for several months may cause alopecia, ataxia, glossitis, and hepatotoxicity. Vitamin C is usually well tolerated but large doses can cause nausea, diarrhea, and abdominal pain. Excessive intake of vitamin D may cause hypercalcemia, hypercalciuria, nausea, vomiting, myalgia, and bone demineralization. Zinc toxicity manifests as anemia, loss of sense of smell and taste, and depressed immune function.

Table 24–1 COMMON VITAMINS AND HERBALS THAT INTERACT WITH WARFARIN (PARTIAL LIST)

Warfarin Interaction	Vitamin/Herbal
↑ INR and risk of bleeding	Danshen Dong quai Fish oil Garlic Ginkgo Policosanol Vitamin E
↓ INR and risk of bleeding	Coenzyme Q10 St. John wort Vitamin K

HELPFUL TIP: Compared with water-soluble vitamins (A and C), fat-soluble vitamins (A, D, E, and K) are more likely to accumulate, resulting in toxicity.

(VERY) HELPFUL TIP: Vitamin K can be useful in patients with a hard to control INR. Start a vitamin K supplement of 100–200 μg/day. This will help to eliminate diet-dependent INR fluctuations (*Pharmacotherapy.* 2005; 25:1746-1751, *Curr Opin Hematol.* 2008 Sep; 15(5):504-508).

* *

The patient learns that the vitamin therapy he currently takes has large amounts of vitamins E, but no vitamin K. You counsel him to discontinue this supplement, hold a dose of warfarin, and then continue on the same dose. You ask him to come back next week for another prothrombin time/INR. Before leaving, he asks about taking a multivitamin.

From available evidence, you are able to tell him:

A) "Most multivitamins do not contain enough vitamin E to cause a problem."
B) "Multivitamins should be standard preventive medicine and have a well-described role in improving health."
C) "Iron supplements are recommended for middle-aged males."
D) "Folic acid and B vitamins should be taken by everyone to reduce homocysteine."

Discussion

The correct answer is "A." Most multiple vitamins contain less than 400 IU of vitamin E and usually will not cause a problem. A fairly well-balanced North American diet provides the necessary nutrients to avoid vitamin deficiency syndromes. Supplementation with multivitamins is usually not necessary unless there are dietary intake deficiencies related to an unbalanced diet.

Taking a multivitamin generally has **not** been linked to improved health status (*Arch Intern Med.* 2009;169:294, *J Am Geriatr Soc.* 2007;55:35-42).

Average adult males generally have adequate iron stores and should not receive supplemental iron due to the potential for exacerbating undiagnosed iron storage disease. **While folate, vitamin B6, and vitamin B12 lower serum homocysteine levels, there is no evidence that this intervention is helpful in reducing disease burden or improving health** (*JAMA*. 2008;300:795, *JAMA*. 2010;303:2486).

Regarding vitamin and mineral supplementation, all of the following are true EXCEPT:

A) Folate supplementation during pregnancy is recommended to decrease the risk of neural tube defects.
B) Calcium and vitamin D supplementation in postmenopausal females is recommended to reduce the risk of osteoporosis and fractures.
C) Vitamin D supplementation in elderly patients may reduce the risk of falling.
D) Vitamin E supplementation in elderly patients may reduce the risk of cardiovascular disease.

Discussion

The correct answer (and false statement) is "D." "A" has plenty of evidence to back it up. Folate supplementation is universally recommended during the prenatal period and should be started even before pregnancy actually occurs. "B" is widely recommended, although the evidence for calcium reducing fracture risk is weak. As for "C," one meta-analysis has concluded that vitamin D supplementation in older adults is associated with decreased fall risk (Bischoff-Ferrari, et al., *JAMA*. 2004). "D" is a false statement since vitamin E supplementation has not been shown to reduce the risk of cardiovascular disease and may be associated with an increased risk of all-cause mortality at doses >400 IU/day as well as with an increase in prostate cancer in men (*JAMA*. 2011;306:1549).

HELPFUL TIP: In general, daily multiple vitamins do not contain large enough doses of vitamins to result in toxicity.

HELPFUL TIP: Coenzyme Q has been shown to be effective for statin-induced myopathic pain in small trials (*Am J Cardiol*. 2007;99:1409-1412). However, not all trials are positive. Co-Q has also been used as an orphan drug for several mitochondrial diseases and is likely effective in these disorders.

Objectives: Did you learn to . . .

- Describe symptoms, signs, and causes of vitamin K deficiency?
- Identify common vitamins and herbals that interact with warfarin?
- Recognize symptoms of fat-soluble vitamin toxicities?
- Identify benefits, risks, and limitations of vitamin supplementation?

QUICK QUIZ: SUPPLEMENTS TO BREAST MILK

A 6-month-old male infant presents for routine health exam and immunizations. His mother is a strict vegan and has been nursing him exclusively. She has not introduced any foods and she wants to keep breastfeeding him primarily for at least the next 6 months . . . or until his friends start to tease him, she jokes (you hope). She takes no medicines and no supplements of any kind.

This breastfed patient should have supplementation of all of the following EXCEPT:

A) Vitamin B12.
B) Vitamin C.
C) Vitamin D.
D) Iron.

Discussion

The correct answer is "B." Children breastfed by strict vegan mothers should have vitamin B12 supplementation. Vitamin D is now recommended for all breastfed infants. Iron is recommended in all breastfed infants 6 months of age or older who are not eating iron-fortified foods. Vitamin C supplementation is not required. There are a variety of liquid multiple vitamins to choose from (e.g., Poly-Vi-Sol®).

CASE 2

A 34-year-old female presents to your office with concerns about weight gain. She has gained over

100 pounds since she graduated from high school. She tearfully reveals that the weight gain has come despite "not eating much." She walks for exercise, but is unable to quantify her walking.

She denies chronic illnesses. Her only surgery was a tubal ligation after her last child. She smokes 10 cigarettes per day and is unwilling to quit due to fears of further weight gain. She drinks alcohol once or twice per week, never consuming more than three beers. The review of systems is positive for a dry cough, bilateral knee pain, and fatigue.

On physical examination, you find an afebrile female with an elevated blood pressure (142/94 mm Hg). She is 5 ft, 3 in tall and weighs 231 pounds. Her body mass index (BMI) is 41 kg/m^2. You find trace pitting edema at the ankles bilaterally. There is increased pigmentation in the folds of the neck and the knuckles. The remainder of the exam is unremarkable.

The patient realizes that she is overweight and asks, "How bad am I?"

Regarding definition and classification of obesity, which of the following is true?

A) Obesity is defined as BMI $\geq$25 kg/m^2.
B) Severe obesity is defined as BMI >30 kg/m^2.
C) Underweight is defined as BMI <20 kg/m^2.
D) Obesity is defined as BMI $\geq$30 kg/m^2.
E) Malnourished supermodel status is defined as BMI <30 kg/m^2.

Discussion

The correct answer is "D." Obesity is defined by BMI $\geq$30 kg/m^2; therefore, only "D" is correct. See Table 24–2 for definitions of weight status by BMI.

BMI calculation:

$$\text{BMI (kg/m}^2) = \text{weight (kg)}/[\text{height (m)}]^2.$$

Table 24–2 DEFINITION OF WEIGHT STATUS BY BMI

Weight Status		BMI (kg/m^2)
Underweight		<18.5
Normal		18.5–24.9
Overweight		25.0–29.9
Obese	Class I	30.0–34.9
	Class II	35.0–39.9
Extremely obese	Class III	$\geq$40.0

Example: weight = 110 pounds (50 kg), height = 59 inches (1.5 m), therefore

$$\text{BMI} = 50/(1.5)^2 = 22.2 \text{ kg/m}^2$$

HELPFUL TIP: In American adults, the combined prevalence of obesity and overweight (BMI $\geq$25 kg/m^2) is 60% for men and 51% for women. Now that's what we call an epidemic!

HELPFUL (BUT UNFORTUNATE) TIP: If WHO criteria for obesity were used in the United States (based on percentage of body fat), even more individuals in the United States would qualify as obese (*Obstet Gynecol.* 2010 May;115:982).

* *

You ask her about medications, focusing on those related to obesity.

All of the following drugs are associated with weight gain and an increased risk of obesity EXCEPT:

A) Olanzapine.
B) Metformin.
C) Amitriptyline.
D) Valproic acid.
E) Glipizide.

Discussion

The correct answer is "B." Metformin may help patients with diabetes lose or maintain weight and, therefore, is not associated with worsening obesity. See Table 24–3 for a more complete list of medications associated with weight gain.

Which of the following is the most appropriate next step in the evaluation of this patient's weight gain?

A) Refer for a sleep study.
B) Check urinary free cortisol level.
C) Draw blood for thyroid-stimulating hormone level.
D) Evaluation for adrenal adenoma causing Cushing disease.

Table 24–3 DRUGS ASSOCIATED WITH WEIGHT GAIN (NOT AN EXHAUSTIVE LIST)

Class	Specific Agents
Alpha-blockers	Prazosin, doxazosin, terazosin
Anticonvulsants	Valproate, carbamazepine, gabapentin
Antidepressants	Tricyclics (e.g., amitriptyline) and monamine oxidase inhibitors Selective serotonin reuptake inhibitors (SSRIs) in some patients
Antihistamines	Cyproheptadine, diphenhydramine
Antipsychotics	Olanzapine, thioridazine, haloperidol, risperidone
Beta-blockers	Propranolol, metoprolol, atenolol
Diabetes drugs	Insulin, sulfonylureas, thiazolidinediones
Steroid hormones	Corticosteroids, oral contraceptives, estrogen, progesterone, testosterone

Discussion

The correct answer is "C." Because of her obesity, this patient is also at risk for sleep apnea, diabetes, hypertension, and hyperlipidemia. These concerns will need to be addressed. However, her chief complaint is weight gain. Although in most overweight patients a cause for weight gain is not found, the physician is obligated to search for potentially treatable causes of weight gain, including hypothyroidism. The symptoms of hypothyroidism are often nonspecific and include weight gain and fatigue.

> HELPFUL TIP: Complications of obesity include heart disease, type 2 diabetes, hypertension, stroke, hyperlipidemia, gallbladder disease, reduced fertility, increased risk of certain cancers (prostate, colon, breast, endometrial), and emotional distress.

The finding of acanthosis nigricans in this patient raises concern for which of the following diseases?

A) Skin cancer.
B) Diabetes.
C) Hemochromatosis.
D) Colon cancer.
E) Hypertriglyceridemia

Discussion

The correct answer is "B." Acanthosis nigricans, classically described as velvety hyperpigmentation in skin creases (axilla, back, neck, flexor aspects of arms), is associated with a number of diseases. Acanthosis nigricans occurs in insulin-resistance syndromes, commonly in patients with type 2 diabetes. It is also associated with other endocrine abnormalities, including Cushing disease and hypothyroidism. Acanthosis nigricans can be an external sign of internal malignancy, most commonly gastrointestinal (GI) cancers. However, this patient is at lower risk of colon cancer than diabetes given her age, weight gain, and lack of other signs and symptoms of cancer. Hemochromatosis, hypertriglyceridemia, and skin cancer are not directly associated with acanthosis nigricans.

* *

She wonders what diet she should use to lose weight.

You let her know that the most effective diet is:

A) Low carbohydrate ("Atkins").
B) Low fat ("Ornish").
C) Low glycemic load diet ("Zone diet").
D) Portion restriction such as Weight Watchers.
E) Any diet that you can stick to.

Discussion

The correct answer is "E." Any diet you can stick to that limits calories seems to work. There does not seem to be any advantage to one diet over another (except for making the proprietors wealthy; *JAMA*. 2005;293:43-53). For example, Weight Watchers may have a bit better success because of peer pressure, weekly meetings, motivational techniques, etc. (*BMJ*. 2011;343:d6500). But any diet that you can stick to will work.

* *

She is wondering about her level of physical activity and is afraid that her obesity will decrease her ability to become functionally fit with exercise.

Your response to this is that:

A) Gluttony and sloth go together, so give up the exercise.

B) One cannot improve one's physical performance without weight loss.
C) Dante did not know what he was talking about. It is TV and sloth that go together.
D) Exercise is beneficial for fitness regardless of whether or not one loses weight.

Discussion

The correct answer is "D." Losing weight is notoriously hard to do. Thankfully, exercise, in and of itself, increases functional capacity regardless of weight loss (*N Engl J Med.* 2011 Mar 31;364:1218). Obviously, patients do better if they both exercise and lose weight. But sticking to an exercise regimen is still helpful. With regard to the others, there was no evidence-based medicine or TV during the time of Dante, so we will never know.

HELPFUL TIP: A low-glycemic index diet (oat bran, whole oats, beans, rice, lentils, nuts, etc.) can lower HbA_{1c} in type 2 diabetics when compared with a high whole grain carbohydrate diet (brown rice, whole wheat foods, etc.) Psyllium (Metamucil and others) will do the same (*JAMA.* 2008 Dec 17;300:2742).

* *

You find that the patient's thyroid function is normal. After consultation with a nutritionist and a prescription for exercise, she returns 3 months later. Her weight is 222 pounds. Tearfully, she tells you that she barely eats and needs something more to help her lose weight.

Which of the following is the most appropriate next step?

A) Prescribe L-thyroxine.
B) Refer to surgery for gastric bypass.
C) Prescribe sibutramine
D) Prescribe orlistat (Xenical, Alli)
E) Prescribe paroxetine (Paxil).

Discussion

The correct answer is "D." Drug therapy is considered appropriate as an add-on to lifestyle management for people with a BMI of 30 kg/m^2 or greater, or a BMI of 27 kg/m^2 or more who already have a comorbid condition such as diabetes, hypertension, or hyperlipidemia. Of the choices listed, orlistat is the most appropriate (more below). "A" is incorrect, as obesity alone is not an indication for L-thyroxine. "B" is incorrect since surgery is not yet indicated in this patient. See Chapter 22 for a discussion of indications, etc., for gastric bypass surgery. Some of you may have chosen "C." However, the manufacturer of sibutramine voluntarily removed it from the market in the United States in 2011 at the request of the FDA because of cardiovascular side effects. "E" is incorrect because paroxetine may be associated with weight gain and is not indicated for obesity.

Which of the following weight loss drugs results in GI side effects in up to 40% of patients using it?

A) Orlistat (Alli, Xenical).
B) Sibutramine (Meridia, Reductil).
C) Phentermine (Adipex-P, Ionamin).
D) Leptin.

Discussion

The correct answer is "A." Orlistat is a lipase inhibitor that functions in the intestines and prevents the absorption of about 30% of dietary fats. Because of its mechanism of action, orlistat is associated with GI side effects in 40% of patients taking the drug. The most bothersome potential adverse events include fecal incontinence and abdominal pain. Orlistat should be taken with meals. The prescription dose is 120 mg three times per day. Weight loss is modest: 3–4 kg over 1 year compared with placebo. As you already know, sibutramine is off the market. Phentermine is a sympathomimetic and causes hypertension, tachycardia, etc. It should only be used for 12 weeks. Leptin has been used successfully but is not FDA approved for weight loss.

HELPFUL TIP: The OTC dose of orlistat (Alli) is half the dose of the prescription strength. However, it is equally effective (or ineffective!) at this lower dose.

* *

You initiate a medication to help her lose weight and refer her to a weight loss program that focuses on overall lifestyle modification. When she returns in 3 months, her weight is 235 pounds, and she is very frustrated.

You appropriately recommend which of the following?

A) Adding a second drug for weight loss.
B) Referral to psychiatry.
C) Referral to bariatric surgery.
D) Referral to plastic surgery.
E) Referral to "The Biggest Loser" TV program.

Discussion

The correct answer is "C." This patient now meets accepted indications for bariatric surgery. See Chapter 22 for more information about weight loss surgery.

> HELPFUL TIP: Drug therapy and surgery are no substitute for basic lifestyle modifications, including an appropriately calorie-restricted diet and regular aerobic exercise. These lifestyle approaches should be continued during drug treatment and after surgery.

Objectives: Did you learn to . . .

- Define normal weight, overweight, and obesity?
- Appropriately evaluate the obese patient?
- Recognize goals and methods of treating obesity?
- Recognize cholelithiasis as a complication of bariatric surgery?
- Recognize complications that occur as a result of obesity?

QUICK QUIZ: VITAMIN DEFICIENCIES

A 63-year-old male presents to the office after his daughter came home for the holidays and found him confused. At first she thought he was drunk, but after a day without alcohol, the confusion persisted ("Eh? Maybe it is withdrawal...how could you write such a vague case?" you ask. Our response: "It is our prerogative as author/editors. We will stipulate the confusion isn't from alcohol withdrawal.") According to the daughter, the patient drinks about half of a bottle of vodka per day and has done so for years (Hawkeye Vodka is the Iowa favorite... $12.00/1.75 L). Although the patient is not able to give much of a coherent history, you are able to determine that he has developed shortness of breath and leg edema. His appetite has been poor for "a long time" and he may have lost some weight although he is not sure.

Physical examination reveals a malnourished, disoriented male who appears older than his stated age and is disheveled. He is mildly tachycardic, but his other vital signs are normal. He has bibasilar crackles on lung exam, 2+ pedal edema, hepatomegaly, and spider telangiectasias.

What is your first action to take with this patient?

A) Administer D50 intravenous (IV).
B) Administer thiamine IV.
C) Administer vitamin B12 IM.
D) Administer niacin orally.
E) Administer folate orally.

Discussion

The correct answer is "B." This patient almost certainly has thiamine (vitamin B1) deficiency and appears to be symptomatic. In the United States, thiamine deficiency is most often seen in malnourished alcoholics. Early symptoms of thiamine deficiency are vague—anorexia, fatigue, and irritability. Thiamine deficient patients may progress to beriberi (wet or dry), possessing symptoms of heart failure and/or neuropathy (motor and sensory). Other possible manifestations of thiamine deficiency include Wernicke encephalopathy (ataxia, occular motor abnormalities [e.g., gaze paralysis], mental status changes, dietary deficiency) and Wernicke–Korsakoff syndrome (Wernicke syndrome plus additional memory loss and confabulations). **Note that most patients do not have all of the findings. Most have a partial syndrome.** Treatment is to administer thiamine IV and then to continue oral supplementation.

> HELPFUL TIP: The dosage of thiamine administered for treatment and prevention of Wernicke encephalopathy differs. For prevention of Wernicke encephalopathy, give thiamine 100 mg daily. For treatment of Wernicke encephalopathy, give thiamine 500 mg IV three times for 2 days followed by 500 mg IV daily for 5 more days (although recommendations vary and no randomized trials support one regimen over another).

HELPFUL TIP: Other micronutrient deficiencies that occur in alcoholic patients include niacin deficiency resulting in pellagra (dermatitis, diarrhea, and dementia); folate deficiency resulting in macrocytic anemia; vitamin B12 deficiency (generally due to problems with GI absorption rather than as a direct effect of alcoholism) resulting in anemia, neuropathy, and dementia. A multivitamin is certainly reasonable in this patient population.

CASE 3

A 58-year old postmenopausal female presents to your office with concerns about osteoporosis. A review of her medical history shows a bone density T-score of −1.8 from 2 years ago, suggesting moderate osteopenia. Medical history is also significant for mild untreated hyperlipidemia with total cholesterol of 210 mg/dL, LDL 140 mg/dL and HDL 45 mg/dL, and triglycerides 125 mg/dL. She had a partial thyroidectomy 15 years ago and currently takes levothyroxine 88 μg/day.

Based on the evidence, which of the following supplements is most appropriate for this patient?

A) Calcium.
B) Calcium plus vitamin D.
C) Vitamin D.
D) Ipriflavone.

Discussion

The correct answer is "B." Postmenopausal women should take 1200 mg/day of **elemental** calcium with total of diet plus supplements not exceeding 2000 mg of elemental calcium per day. Vitamin D is also appropriate and many women do not get enough. As supplements go, vitamin D may be more important than calcium.

The calcium dose for adolescents is 1300 mg of elemental calcium per day and the dose of calcium for women to age 50 and men to age 70 is 1000 mg of elemental calcium per day. Beyond these ages, the recommendation is 1,200 mg/day of elemental calcium. In terms of vitamin D, recommended doses are 400 IU/day for infants, 600 IU/day for ages 1–70, and 800 IU/day in those over age 70 (Institute of Medicine, 2011).

The guideline also concludes that there is not any good evidence for vitamin D beyond its use for bone health. Of course, all of us are familiar with the literature that suggests vitamin D reduces falls and increases muscle strength in the elderly (*Osteoporos Int.* 2009;20:315-322, *BMJ.* 2009;339:b32692) and may be helpful for some chronic pain patients (*J Am Geriatr Soc.* 2008;56:785). We are not sure how the board will deal with this on the test. But there's the info.

Ipriflavone is a semisynthetic isoflavone produced from soy isoflavones. There is evidence that it can prevent bone mineral density loss when used with calcium in postmenopausal women, but it has not been shown to reduce fracture rates. There are also concerns that it might cause lymphocytopenia in some patients.

* *

You counsel her to take 1200 mg of elemental calcium per day.

In order to improve GI absorption of calcium, you recommend:

A) Taking 1200 mg at one time with a meal.
B) Taking 1200 mg at one time an hour before eating.
C) Taking 1200 mg in three divided doses with meals.
D) Taking 1200 mg at in three divided doses on an empty stomach.
E) Taking 1200 mg with her levothyroxine.

Discussion

The correct answer is "C." Calcium is best absorbed when taken with food. Theoretically, GI absorption of calcium is limited, and for that reason divided dosing in 500–600 mg aliquots is recommended. Patients should take levothyroxine separately from their calcium. If taken together, calcium reduces levothyroxine absorption. This is also true of iron and levothyroxine.

HELPFUL (AND IMPORTANT) TIP: Why not higher doses of calcium? Calcium supplementation can cause an increase in cardiovascular disease (or at least most of the data is leaning this way). Additionally, higher doses are probably not of any additional benefit (*BMJ.* 2011;342:d2040, *BMJ.* 2011;342:d1473).

* *

She then asks you about her cholesterol levels and whether taking soy would be helpful. A friend told her that older women should take soy to prevent heart disease, breast cancer, and osteoporosis.

Which of the following is appropriate to tell this patient?

A) Soy isoflavone supplements are preferred for reducing lipid levels.
B) Dietary soy protein is not associated with a reduced risk of developing heart disease in Western women.
C) Soy protein is as effective as a statin for lowering cholesterol.
D) Soy isoflavones are an acceptable alternative to calcium and vitamin D for preventing osteoporosis.

Discussion

The correct answer is "B." Soy protein can modestly reduce lipid levels in some patients but has been shown not to affect important outcomes such as heart attack or death in Western women. Soy isoflavone supplements have not been shown to reduce lipid levels. Soy protein is not nearly as effective as are statin drugs (e.g., atorvastatin and simvastatin). Soy protein or soy isoflavone supplements are not an appropriate alternative to calcium and vitamin D.

* *

Your patient is hoping you can settle a bet. She asks about her younger sister who is going through "the change" and started taking black cohosh. Her sister swears the black cohosh helps her hot flashes, but your patient thinks it's "all in her head."

Regarding the use of black cohosh for the treatment of perimenopausal vasomotor symptoms, you tell her:

A) Black cohosh is equivalent to hormone replacement therapy.
B) Black cohosh is equivalent to placebo.
C) Black cohosh is not good for vasomotor symptoms but does promote liver health.
D) Black cohosh is only effective when taken as part of a multibotanical supplement.

Discussion

The correct answer is "B." Most studies of black cohosh are negative (e.g., *Menopause*. 2008;15:51). This does not mean patients should not to try it. And in fact, one specific preparation (Remifemin, Phytopharmica/Enzymatic Therapy) is possibly effective. "C" is of special note since black cohosh has been associated with hepatotoxicity—far from liver health.

HELPFUL TIP: Soy protein integrated into the diet is not harmful and is acceptable for women who want to try it. But it should not replace proven therapies. See Table 24–4 for an overview of soy benefits.

Table 24–4 OVERVIEW OF THE EFFECTIVENESS OF SOY

Condition	Effectiveness Data	Comment/Recommendation
Breast cancer	Higher intake of soy in the diet is associated with decreased risk of breast cancer. But most research limited to Asian populations. May not apply to Western populations. No clinical trials.	Unknown benefits in Western populations. Data are not strong enough to recommend dietary soy for this use.
Hyperlipidemia/ Cardiovascular disease	Consuming soy protein in place of other protein sources might modestly reduce lipid levels. Does not apply to soy isoflavone supplements. No evidence that eating soy improves outcomes such as death or heart attack. Population research shows no decreased risk of these outcomes in Western women.	Substituting dietary soy for other proteins is acceptable, but only modest benefit expected; not an alternative to mortality- or cardiovascular event-reducing therapies such as statins.
Osteoporosis	Consuming dietary soy protein might improve bone mineral density in postmenopausal women and possibly reduce fracture risk; however, not all evidence is consistent.	There is possible benefit to adding soy protein to the diet, but benefit is likely to be modest at best. Soy is not a substitute to calcium and vitamin D.

HELPFUL TIP: While other herbal products like phytoestrogens, wild yam, primrose oil, and vitamin E claim efficacy in treating menopausal symptoms, rigorously designed clinical trials performed to date have not confirmed their efficacy.

Which of the following natural products could be recommended for lowering LDL cholesterol?

A) Fish oil.
B) Psyllium.
C) Garlic.
D) Policosanol.
E) All of the above.

Discussion

The correct answer is "B." Taking a psyllium supplement (e.g., Metamucil) 10–12 g daily can modestly reduce total cholesterol by up to 14% and LDL by up to 10%. Fish oil is effective for lowering triglycerides, but not total cholesterol or LDL cholesterol. Garlic was long considered effective for modest reduction in cholesterol, but the most recent evidence shows that garlic does not significantly reduce cholesterol in most people (*Arch Intern Med.* 2007;167:346-353). Similarly, policosanol was once considered effective for reducing cholesterol, but evidence is inconsistent. The most reliable evidence shows that it is ineffective.

What percentage of Americans uses alternative therapies?

A) 10%.
B) 20%.
C) 30%.
D) 40%.
E) 60%.

Discussion

The correct answer is "D." Thirty-eight percent of adults and 12% of children use complementary or alternative therapy (Barnes, et al. 2007). Only 40% of patients informed their physicians of their use of these therapies. Examples of unconventional therapies used include:

Relaxation	Self-help groups
Chiropractic	Biofeedback
Massage	Energy healing
Imagery	Hypnosis
Homeopathy	Spiritual healing
Lifestyle diets	Acupuncture
Herbal medicine	Exercise
Megavitamins	Prayer
Coining	Cupping

* *

At least 15 million patients take prescription medications along with their alternative medications, sometimes with adverse outcomes.

Which of these is *NOT* a reason that patients claim when using alternative therapies?

A) They believe they are safer than medications.
B) Conventional medicine is too technical or impersonal.
C) Prescription medicines are too expensive.
D) Cultural practices.
E) They didn't like the shark in Jaws and therefore use shark cartilage in an attempt to rid the oceans of sharks.

Discussion

The correct answer is "E." Many patients use alternative therapies including herbals for various reasons, some of which are listed above. Other reasons cited include perceived physician apathy, difficulty with physician access, fear of medication side effects, belief that medications lack efficacy, and the fact that they are not "natural." Many patients do not inform their physicians about their use of these products, mistakenly believing that "natural" means safe. As for "E," unfortunately there is a large demand for shark cartilage including its use as chondroitin sulfate. Shark populations have been severely stressed as a result. Up to 100 million sharks per year are killed for their fins and cartilage.

What is the current status of the regulation of "natural" therapies?

A) The FDA does not have a regulatory role with regard to natural therapies.

B) Natural products have to be proven safe and effective in order to be marketed in the United States.
C) Natural therapies are regulated by the Department of Health and Human Services.
D) As long as they contain the ingredients claimed, natural therapies can be marketed in the United States.
E) Natural therapies are regulated by Pan, the Greek god of nature.

Discussion

The correct answer is "A." The FDA has no regulatory role with regard to natural therapies. They are classified as dietary supplements and not medications. All of the rest are incorrect. "B" is incorrect because natural therapies need **not** be proven safe and effective in order to be marketed (witness the use of ephedra). "D" is incorrect. There is no quality control on "natural" therapies in the United States. Products may contain varying amounts of the advertised therapy or, in some cases, none at all. In fact, there are data suggesting that **most** products for sale do not contain what they advertise and in other cases, contain prescription drugs such as warfarin, steroids, alprazolam, and diethylstilbestrol.

HELPFUL TIP: The FDA can remove natural therapy products if it can show that they are hazardous. This is a slow and laborious process as evidenced by how long it took to remove ephedra from the US market.

HELPFUL TIP: Patients using herbals should be warned that the products may not contain what they claim and that they should take the products at their own risk.

A partial list of unsafe alternative remedies is as follows:

- Hepatotoxicity: Chaparral, germander, life foot
- Carcinogenic: Borage, calamus, coltsfoot, comfrey, life root, sassafras
- Miscellaneous toxicity: Ma Huang, licorice, poke root

HELPFUL TIP: The role of omega 3 fatty acid in CAD is controversial. The best studies show no benefit in those with pre-existing CAD or stroke. The role in primary prevention is less well established. *BMJ*. 2010 Nov 29;341:c6273. (http://dx.doi.org/10.1136/bmj.c6273). Omega-3 may have some minor benefit in treating depression and ADHD but the jury is still out: the effect size, if it exists, is small.

Ginkgo has some antiplatelet effect and is touted for helping with vascular disease and dementia (although proof is lacking). *JAMA*. 2009 Dec 23/30;302:2663.

HELPFUL TIP: Valerian root has benzodiazepine-like effects and works to reduce sleep latency.

Grapefruit juice interacts with multiple medications. Which of the following IS NOT affected by grapefruit juice?

A) Tacrolimus.
B) Itraconazole/Ketoconazole.
C) Benzodiazepines.
D) Clopidogrel.
E) Aspirin.

Discussion

The correct answer is "E." All of the other drugs interact with grapefruit juice. Grapefruit juice is a potent CYP3A4 inhibitor and can interact with numerous medications including some calcium channel blockers, carbamazepine, those listed above, benzodiazepines, amiodarone, atorvastatin, lovistatin, simivastatin and others. This underscores the importance of knowing what "alternative" medications your patient might be using.

Which of the following herbs has been touted as being effective for memory problems and peripheral circulatory problems?

A) *Ginkgo biloba*.
B) **S-Adenosylmethionine** (SAM-e).
C) *Ma Huang*.

D) Glucosamine.
E) None of the above.

Discussion

The correct answer is "A." *Ginkgo biloba* is one of the most popular herbal products and is promoted for mild memory loss, dementia, and peripheral circulatory disorders. **As noted above, it is ineffective.** Ginkgo can have antiplatelet effects so should be used with caution or not at all in patients taking aspirin. Side effects include GI disturbances, headaches, and dizziness. "B," SAM-e, is used for arthritis and depression and has been shown to be "likely effective." "C," *Ma Huang*, is ephedra and is used to increase energy and promote weight loss. "D," glucosamine, has NOT been shown to be effective for osteoarthritis. Most of the data is of poor quality.

Which herbal product has aldosterone-like properties and can cause a pseudohyperaldosteronism?

A) *Ma Huang.*
B) Ginseng.
C) Licorice.
D) Melatonin.
E) None of the above.

Discussion

The correct answer is "C." Licorice (*Glycyrrhiza* spp.) has aldosterone-like effects and can lead to fluid retention, hypertension, and hypokalemia. Thus, it should not be combined with other potassium-wasting drugs such as nonpotassium sparing diuretics. It is also contraindicated in patients with severe liver disease and in pregnant patients (may induce premature labor).

Which of the following diseases is NOT supposedly treated by SAM-e?

A) Depression.
B) Fibromyalgia.
C) Cirrhosis.
D) Osteoarthritis.
E) The urge to watch grade B monster movies from the 1950s.

Discussion

The correct answer is "E." SAM-e is "likely effective" in treating depression and osteoarthritis. It is "possibly effective" in treating fibromyalgia, and there is insufficient evidence to rate its use in cirrhosis. SAM-e is contraindicated in bipolar patients as it can induce mania. SAM-e can possibly interact with antidepressants, including MAOIs, leading to serotonin syndrome. GI disturbance is the only notable side effect.

Which of these is useful in the treatment of migraine headaches?

A) St. John wort.
B) Valerian.
C) Ginger.
D) Feverfew.
E) Saw palmetto.

Discussion

The correct answer is "D." Feverfew is "possibly effective" in treating migraine headaches (*Neurology.* 2012 April 24;78(17):1346–1353). "A," St. John wort, is useful for depression. **However, there are major interactions between St. John's wort and other multiple drugs including cyclosporine, nevirapine, and digoxin among others.** "B," valerian root, is useful for insomnia. Ginger is used for nausea and seems to be effective (*Am J Obstet Gynecol.* 2006 Jan;194:95–99). Saw Palmetto is used for benign prostatic hypertrophy but is ineffective (*JAMA.* 2011 Sep 28;306:1344).

Which of these is NOT potentially useful for women with pregnancy-related nausea and vomiting?

A) Ginger.
B) Acupressure.
C) Vitamin B6.
D) Doxylamine.
E) Black cohosh.

Discussion

The correct answer is "E." Ginger is "possibly effective" in treating nausea and vomiting in pregnancy, postoperative vomiting, and vertigo. Vitamin B6 (pyridoxine) and doxylamine, an antihistamine, have been shown singly and together to be safe and effective in pregnancy-related nausea and vomiting. Acupressure has no known adverse effects, and there is some suggestion of efficacy. **Black cohosh can stimulate uterine contractions and has no known efficacy for nausea and vomiting in pregnancy and so is contraindicated in pregnancy.**

Objectives: Did you learn to . . .

- Describe the prevalence of alternative therapy use?
- Appreciate the various indications for various herbal products and the evidence base for them?
- Recognize herbs considered safe and those considered unsafe?
- Recognize problematic drug interactions with a variety of alternative therapies?

QUICK QUIZ

One of your patients who often uses complementary and alternative medicine comes into your office with several days of rhinorrhea, sore throat, and ear pain. Your exam reveals a viral upper respiratory infection. He asks you to recommend an alternative cure.

Which of these are touted as alternative remedies for the common cold?

A) Echinacea.
B) Zinc.
C) Vitamin C.
D) All of the above.
E) None of the above.

Discussion

The correct answer is "D." The three choices listed above have the reputation of helping alleviate the symptoms of the common cold. The efficacy of all of these is questionable, however. Some zinc has been removed from the market in the United States because of permanent loss of sense of taste and smell.

CASE 4

A 17-year-old male patient of yours comes to your office for a sports preparticipation physical. He is a little smaller than most of his classmates and has heard that creatine supplementation can help him increase muscle mass and improve his performance.

Which of the following is *NOT* true about creatine?

A) Creatine exists primarily in skeletal muscle.
B) It causes weight gain by increasing muscle mass.
C) It is ineffective in boosting performance in aerobic exercise.
D) It can lead to increased creatinine levels in patients with normal renal function.

Discussion

The correct answer is "B." Creatine monohydrate is a naturally occurring protein in the body that exists primarily in skeletal muscle. High levels of creatine are thought to enhance the ability to renew ATP for short burst of energy. It appears to be effective for enhancing muscle performance during repeated bouts of **brief**, high-intensity exercise but ineffective for other types of exercise. It does not improve performance in aerobic exercise nor does it benefit older adults seeking to build muscle mass. It also does not appear effective for increasing endurance or for improving performance in highly trained athletes, but its use is widespread among athletes, both amateur and professional. It causes weight gain by increasing water retention and not by affecting muscle mass. Creatine can cause elevated creatinine levels in patients with normal renal function as creatine is metabolized to creatinine. Complicating this is the fact that creatine has been linked to renal dysfunction in some cases.

Which of these is *NOT* a disease that creatine is purported to treat?

A) Heart failure.
B) Neuromuscular disease.
C) Mitochondrial cytopathies.
D) Muscular dystrophies.
E) Diabetes.

Discussion

The correct answer is "E." Creatine is also promoted for CHF, neuromuscular diseases, mitochondrial cytopathies, and various muscular dystrophies. Oral creatine may improve exercise tolerance **in patients with CHF** but has no effect on ejection fraction. IV creatine seems to improve ejection fraction temporarily. When used orally, it seems to **marginally** improve muscle strength and daily-life activity in adults and children with various muscular dystrophies in the **short term.** There is no evidence of its efficacy in the treatment of diabetes. It appears to be safe when used orally and in appropriate doses, though high doses raise the concern of adverse hepatic, renal, or cardiac function. Side effects include GI pain, nausea, and diarrhea, while college athletes taking it frequently complain of muscle cramping.

QUICK QUIZ

A 51-year-old female patient of yours with knee osteoarthritis comes to your office because she has seen commercials on TV advertising a product containing glucosamine and chondroitin sulfate, which was touted as being effective for osteoarthritis. She has been using naproxen with symptom relief but has had heartburn and is worried about the potential for bleeding. Moreover, she likes the idea of using something "natural." She asks for your advice.

Which of the following is true about the use of glucosamine sulfate and/or chondroitin sulfate for osteoarthritis?

A) The combination is more effective than either product alone.
B) Glucosamine is effective in improving symptoms of osteoarthritis.
C) Glucosamine may lower blood sugars.
D) Chondroitin can help patients with coagulation disorders.
E) Chondroitin is "possibly effective" in osteoarthritis.

Discussion

The correct answer is "E." Glucosamine sulfate is a glycoprotein that occurs naturally in the body but is available commercially as a synthetic product or from marine exoskeletons. It is not effective in osteoarthritis. Side effects are generally mild and GI in nature including nausea, heartburn, diarrhea, and constipation.

Patients at risk for diabetes, hyperlipidemia, and hypertension should use this product cautiously as glucosamine can increase both blood glucose and insulin levels. It can increase blood sugars by impeding glucose-induced insulin secretion and impairing the insulin-induced glucose uptake by skeletal muscle.

Chondroitin sulfate is a glycosaminoglycan made from animal and fish cartilage. It is "possibly effective" in osteoarthritis, although there are both positive and negative studies. It is a minor component of the low molecular weight heparin, danaparoid, so there is the concern of possible anticoagulant activity. This has not been shown in studies but because of this concern, it should be used with caution (or not at all) in patients on antiplatelet or anticoagulant agents or those with bleeding disorders. It is generally well tolerated but can cause epigastric pain and nausea in some patients. Chondroitin dosing is typically 200–400 mg two to three times daily. Although chondroitin sulfate and glucosamine sulfate are frequently sold together in combination products, no evidence supports the notion that both are better than either alone.

QUICK QUIZ: A BLOODY HERB

A 51-year-old patient of yours is about to have a scheduled cholecystectomy. He is in otherwise good health and is taking the following herbs and supplements.

Which would you recommend he stop before surgery because of association with prolonged bleeding time?

A) Valerian.
B) Ginseng.
C) Vitamin B complex.
D) Echinacea.
E) Ginkgo.

Discussion

The correct answer is "E." Ginkgo is the only one above that has been associated with a prolonged bleeding time. Thus, it should be stopped prior to planned surgery. Other herbal products that have antiplatelet effects include garlic, feverfew, and fish oil.

BIBLIOGRAPHY

Barnes PM, et al. *CDC National Health Statistics Report #12.* Complementary and Alternative Medicine Use Among Adults and Children: United States; 2007.

Calcium and vitamin D supplementation: Who needs it? Pharmacist's Letter/Prescriber's Letter 2011;27(1): 270102.

DeMaria EJ. Bariatric surgery for morbid obesity. *N Eng J Med.* 2007;356:2176-2183.

Fletcher RH, Fairfield KM. Vitamins for chronic disease prevention in adults. *JAMA.* 2002;287:3127.

Gartner LM, et al. Breastfeeding and the use of human milk. *Pediatrics.* 2005;115:496.

Holick MF, et al. Evaluation, treatment, and prevention of vitamin D deficiency: An endocrine society clinical practice guideline. *J Clin Endocrinol Metab*. 2011;96: 1911-1930. Epub 2011 Jun 6.

Institute of Medicine. *Dietary Reference Intakes for Calcium and Vitamin D*. Washington, DC: The National Academies Press; 2011.

Jellin J, Gregory P, eds. *Natural Medicines Comprehensive Database*. Stockton, CA: Therapeutic Research Faculty; 2011.

Newton KM, et al. Treatment of vasomotor symptoms of menopause with black cohosh, multibotanicals, soy, hormone therapy, or placebo: A randomized trial. *Ann Intern Med*. 2006;145:869-879.

North American Menopause Society. Management of osteoporosis in postmenopausal women: 2006 position statement of The North American Menopause Society. *Menopause*. 2006;13:340-367.

Vitamin D and Calcium: Systematic Review of Health Outcomes, Structured Abstract. Agency for Healthcare Research and Quality, Rockville, MD. Available at: http://www.ahrq.gov/clinic/tp/vitadcaltp.htm.

25

Substance Use Disorders

Dustin DeYoung and Mark A. Graber

CASE 1

A 45-year-old male presents to your clinic to establish care for his chronic back and leg pain. He denies any other medical conditions. He reports being injured at work approximately 5 years ago, at which time he was started on oxycodone. He reports being on a stable dose for the last few years. He appears slightly drowsy during the appointment, has small pupils, and is having moderate difficulty describing his injury and previous treatments. He reports his mood as okay, but becomes irritable when you begin to ask specifics about his injury. He has not been able to keep a job for the last year because "everyone fires me." He states that he needs the oxycodone to function and that he ran out of his medication 1 week ago. He does report occasional alcohol use, although he states the he knows not to mix alcohol with his oxycodone.

What is the most likely explanation of the patient's current presentation?

A) Opioid withdrawal.
B) Opioid intoxication.
C) Uncontrolled pain.
D) Alcohol intoxication.
E) Alcohol withdrawal.

Discussion

The correct answer is "B." The patient presents with pupillary constriction, drowsiness, impairment in attention and memory, psychological changes (dysphoria/irritability), and impairment in functioning (not able to keep a job). All of these findings are included in the diagnostic criteria for opioid intoxication. "A" is incorrect and will be discussed later in this case. "C" is incorrect because patient would not display above symptoms with significant pain. "D" could be correct because acute alcohol intoxication is characterized by slurred speech and impairments in memory and judgment; however, the patient did not have an unsteady gait or nystagmus, but he does have miosis. "E" is incorrect as the patient was not hypertensive, febrile, diaphoretic, and did not have tremors or vomiting.

The criteria for opioid intoxication include: (1) Recent use of an opioid with clinically significant maladaptive behavior or psychological changes (euphoria followed by apathy, dysphoria, psychomotor agitation or retardation, impaired judgment, or impaired social or occupational functioning) that develops during, or shortly after, opioid use. (2) Pupillary constriction and one or more of the following signs: drowsiness or coma, slurred speech, and impairment in attention or memory. (3) The symptoms are not due to a general medical condition or another mental disorder.

> HELPFUL TIP: Although true as a general rule, not all opiates are always associated with miosis. Exceptions include morphine, meperidine, pentazocine, diphenoxylate/atropine (Lomotil), and propoxyphene.

* *

You are hesitant to prescribe this medication and thus you offer him alternatives for pain control, including a referral to physical therapy, NSAIDs, and a TENS unit. He says he has tried them all and none of them work. He gets upset and walks out of your office. Two days later, while you are covering an emergency room (ER) shift, the same male presents to the ER for severe, uncontrolled pain. He is vomiting, complains of muscle aches and diarrhea, his pupils are dilated, and he is febrile.

What is the most likely explanation for the patient's current presentation?

A) Opioid withdrawal.
B) Opioid intoxication.
C) Uncontrolled pain.
D) Alcohol intoxication.
E) Alcohol withdrawal.

Discussion

The correct answer is "A." The criterion for opioid withdrawal is cessation (or reduction in) opioid use that has been heavy or prolonged (several weeks or longer) or administration of an opioid antagonist after opioid use with three or more of the following developing within minutes to several days after the above: dysphoric mood, nausea or vomiting, muscle aches, lacrimation or rhinorrhea, pupillary dilation, piloerection, or sweating, diarrhea, yawning, fever, or insomnia.

* *

The patient is transferred to a substance abuse treatment center voluntarily. Based on the available resources in your community, you decide on buprenorphine induction and maintenance treatment.

All of the following are true of buprenorphine EXCEPT:

A) Buprenorphine should be administered prior to withdrawal symptoms.
B) Typical first dose of buprenorphine is 4 mg, with a maximum first day dose of 8 mg.
C) Buprenorphine monotherapy, without naloxone, should be used for patients addicted to long-acting opioids (such as methadone or sustained-release morphine).
D) Continue to increase buprenorphine on subsequent days by the total dose of the previous day plus an additional 4 mg dose, until withdrawal symptoms are relieved.
E) Nearly all patients will stabilize on 16–24 mg daily.

Discussion

The correct answer, and false statement, is "A." Buprenorphine should usually start 12–24 hours after the last use of short-acting opioids (such as heroin or oxycodone) when patients are exhibiting early signs of withdrawal. For longer-acting opioids, waiting for 24–48 hours may be needed. The first day dose should be 4 mg, and patients should be monitored for withdrawal symptoms for 2–4 hours, with the opportunity to administer an additional dose. Monotherapy (i.e., without naloxone) is appropriate for patients on long-acting opioids for the first 1–2 days to avoid any possibility that naloxone will cause withdrawal effects, but then these patients should be transferred to combination therapy. Nearly all patients will stabilize on 16–24 mg daily; however, some may require doses up to 32 mg daily, which is the maximum.

HELPFUL TIP: Advantages of buprenorphine over methadone are that it can be dispensed at a physician's office (with an appropriate DEA waiver), unlike methadone, which can only be dispensed at designated treatment centers; and because of its partial agonist action, buprenorphine has a "ceiling effect" with regard to overdose. Methadone produces increasing respiratory suppression with increasing doses.

HELPFUL (IF DEPRESSING) TIP: Unintentional opioid overdoses have quadrupled between 2000 and 2010. This rise corresponds to an increased prescribing of opioids for chronic noncancer pain. If you choose to treat chronic pain with an opioid, select patients carefully and monitor them closely.

HELPFUL TIP: Suboxone is a combination of buprenorphine and naloxone. In order to prescribe it, a physician needs a special "X" DEA number.

Objectives: Did you learn to . . .

- Define opioid intoxication and withdrawal?
- Describe the use of buprenorphine to manage opioid dependence?

CASE 2

A 70-year-old female is brought into the clinic by her daughter due to concerns about her mother's sleeplessness, isolation, weight loss, falls, and anxiety over the past year. In addition, since the patient has been staying at her daughter's home the past 3 days, she began vomiting, hallucinating, perspiring profusely, and wanting to return to her own home. The patient has no history of medical problems. She is disheveled, confused, diaphoretic, and tremulous. Her blood pressure is 162/110 mm Hg, pulse is 120, and temperature is 38.5°C. She blames her symptoms on being unable to have a cigarette. She also blames her daughter's nagging. When asked about alcohol use, the patient says she has had a cocktail every evening since she retired from her job last year, and that this helps her to sleep.

Which of the following best describes the patient's current clinical condition?

A) Alcohol withdrawal.
B) Alcohol intoxication.
C) Alcohol tolerance.
D) Alcohol abuse.
E) Alcohol dependence.

Discussion

The correct answer is "A." The patient presents tachycardic, hypertensive, and febrile, with diaphoresis, tremors, vomiting, and hallucinations. All of these findings are included in the diagnostic criteria for alcohol withdrawal. "B" is incorrect. Acute intoxication is characterized by slurred speech, unsteady gait, nystagmus, and impaired memory and judgment. "C," "D," and "E" are incorrect and are discussed later in this case.

The criteria for alcohol withdrawal include: (1) The patient has stopped or reduced a previously heavy alcohol intake **and** (2) **two** of the following within hours or days: Autonomic hyperactivity (hypertension, sweating, tachycardia, etc.), hand tremor, insomnia, nausea or vomiting, hallucinations, agitation, anxiety, or grand mal seizures. Additionally, one must have significant impairment in functioning with the withdrawal **and** no other illness causing the symptoms.

Which class of drugs would you choose to treat the symptoms of alcohol withdrawal?

A) Benzodiazepines.
B) Antipsychotics.
C) Antibiotics.
D) Alcohol.
E) Phenytoin.

Discussion

The correct answer is "A." The treatment of choice is metabolic support and the tapering use of benzodiazepines to decrease physical distress and to prevent major withdrawal (delirium tremens, DT) from occurring. Thiamine, folate, magnesium, and other vitamin supplements are often given prophylactically, although they are generally unnecessary. However, they are like chicken soup for your cold; they might help and they won't hurt. "D" is incorrect. Although alcohol will work to prevent withdrawal, it has a fairly short half-life, and you generally do not want to endorse the use of alcohol in a patient with an alcohol use problem.

> HELPFUL TIP: The traditional "banana bag" with multivitamins is unnecessary. Oral vitamin supplements are just as effective and less expensive. The only exception is thiamine which you may want to give IV or IM.

What would be the best approach to evaluating this patient for alcoholism?

A) Ask her the average amount she drinks.
B) Ask her how often she drinks.
C) Ask her how frequently she gets drunk.
D) Ask what her family and friends say about her drinking.
E) Order a complete laboratory workup.

Discussion

The correct answer is "D." The defense mechanism of denial is so strongly evident in alcoholism that the best approach is to explore how alcohol affects her life, rather than direct questions about drinking behavior. Information from family and friends may provide a more accurate account of the problem. Laboratory workups cannot be relied upon to make the diagnosis. The CAGE questionnaire is a very brief and useful screening tool, employed effectively in the primary care setting. A positive answer to two or more questions is very sensitive and specific for an alcohol use disorder. It consists of asking the patient the following four questions:

Have you ever

C: felt that you should **Cut Down** on your drinking?

A: been **Annoyed** that people criticized your drinking?

G: felt bad or **Guilty** about your drinking?

E: taken a drink first thing in the morning (**Eye Opener**) to get rid of a hangover or steady your nerves?

> HELPFUL TIP: Asking the question "How many times in the past year have you had 5 or more drinks in a day (for men) or 4 or more drinks (for women) in a day?" is a useful screen for frequency of heavy drinking. A positive screen is one or more incidents of heavy drinking. If you have a positive screen, ask about usual frequency and quantity of alcohol consumed to help determine the presence or absence of alcohol abuse or dependence. This question alone has about an 82% sensitivity for detecting an alcohol use disorder. Sensitivity for the CAGE ranges from about 75% to 95%, but the CAGE may miss nondependent alcohol use disorders (e.g., binge drinking).

> HELPFUL TIP: Unfortunately, you cannot always trust the family's history either. They may be enabling the alcohol addiction or unaware of it.

* *

Upon further questioning, you begin to uncover a long history of heavy drinking—seems that there was more than just a nightcap.

Which of the following statements about this patient's situation is true?

A) Cerebellar degeneration is uncommon.
B) She is at risk for developing peripheral neuropathy.
C) Alcoholic "fatty liver" is irreversible.
D) She is at decreased or normal risk for heart disease.
E) Immune function should remain relatively intact.

Discussion

The correct answer is "B." Peripheral neuropathy can be seen in 10% of heavy drinkers as a result of vitamin deficiencies and the direct impact alcohol has on nerve function. "A" is incorrect because cerebellar degeneration—suggested by ataxia and nystagmus—does occur as a result of alcohol overuse. "C" is incorrect because alcoholic "fatty liver" will reverse with abstinence from alcohol. "D" is incorrect. **Heavy** drinking raises blood pressure and levels of triglycerides, increasing risk of myocardial infarction. Finally, "E" is incorrect. Heavy drinking lowers the white blood cell count and interferes with specific aspects of the immune system; for example, it compromises T-cell function.

* *

This patient reports to you that she has needed to drink increasing amounts of alcohol to help her fall asleep.

The need for increasing amounts of alcohol is an example of:

A) Intoxication.
B) Dependence.
C) Tolerance.
D) Relapse.
E) Abuse.

Discussion

The correct answer is "C." Tolerance is defined as the need for increasing amounts of a drug to achieve the same, or diminishing effect, for the use of the same amount of a drug. "A" is incorrect. Intoxication is a characteristic syndrome of maladaptive behavior or psychological changes that occurs with substance use, is drug-specific, and reverses when the drug use is discontinued. "D" is incorrect. Relapse involves restarting use of the drug after being abstinent for a while.

The criteria for substance abuse and dependence include:

A) **Dependence:** Substance use with impairment or distress with at least three of the following within 1 year: tolerance; withdrawal; need for increasing amounts of substance; unable to cut down; significant time spent obtaining, consuming, or recovering from substance use; persistent use despite knowledge of adverse effects.

B) **Substance abuse:** Substance use with impairment or distress with one of the following within 1 year: substance use impairs functioning at job school or home; use in hazardous circumstances (e.g., alcohol when driving); recurrent legal problems; continued use despite having persistent or recurring interpersonal problems.

Which of the following lab test results are you most likely to find in this patient?

A) Microcytic anemia.
B) Low ferritin.
C) Decreased serum triglycerides.
D) Hyperglycemia.
E) Increased gamma-glutamyltransferase (GGT).

Discussion

The correct answer is "E." Elevated GGT is considered to be the most sensitive (but not specific . . . it is an inducible enzyme and can be induced by a number of medications) indicator of alcohol intake and is often present along with elevation of the alanine and aspartate transaminases (ALT and AST). The classic AST:ALT ratio in active alcohol abusers is 2:1. Remember, however, that these laboratory findings are **not specific** for alcohol use and can be caused by medications and other illnesses. The other answers are incorrect. Patients with alcoholism typically have **macrocytic anemia**, **elevated** serum triglycerides, and **hypoglycemia**. Ferritin is often **increased** in active alcohol users in the absence of iron overload. Additionally, the transferrin saturation may be elevated because alcohol inhibits transferrin synthesis.

* *

You have ordered liver function tests, but the results will not be available until the next day.

Which of the following medications would be indicated to prevent DT in a patient with *hepatic impairment*?

A) Alprazolam (Xanax).
B) Chlordiazepoxide (Librium).
C) Diazepam (Valium).
D) Lorazepam (Ativan).
E) Clonazepam (Klonopin).

Discussion

The correct answer is "D." Benzodiazepines that are metabolized by the cytochrome P450 system will build up in the presence of liver disease, so using those with intermediate half-lives and no active metabolites is essential. Only lorazepam, oxazepam, and temazepam meet these criteria. "B" is incorrect. Although chlordiazepoxide is often used to prevent symptoms of alcohol withdrawal, it is hepatically metabolized and has an exceptionally long half-life and, therefore, should be avoided in patients with liver problems. Alprazolam is too short acting to use in this situation.

* *

You are considering whether or not this patient has DT.

Which of the following is true of DT?

A) The majority of patients with alcohol withdrawal develop DT if not treated.
B) Auditory hallucinations are more common than visual hallucinations in DT.
C) Symptoms of DT could easily be confused for dementia.
D) Her last drink would need to be about 1 week ago for her to have DT.
E) Autonomic instability is present in DT.

Discussion

The correct answer is "E." Autonomic instability with elevated pulse, blood pressure, and fever are common in DT. "A" is incorrect. Minor withdrawal symptoms are quite common, but DT develops in only 3–5% of patients undergoing alcohol withdrawal. "B" is incorrect. Visual hallucinations are **common** in DT; auditory hallucinations are less likely. "C" is incorrect. Withdrawal **delirium** typically presents acutely over a matter of hours or days, whereas, in **dementia**, the cognitive decline is over a course of months to years. Additionally, autonomic instability is not a feature of early dementia (OK, maybe in Shy–Drager syndrome although cognition is usually well preserved—just like our patient's liver). Finally, "D" is incorrect because the risk for DT usually peaks 72 hours after the last drink.

Which medication would be the best choice for DT in a patient who is vomiting profusely and who has no IV access?

A) Diazepam (Valium).
B) Alprazolam (Xanax).
C) Chlordiazepoxide (Librium).

D) Lorazepam (Ativan).
E) Clonazepam (Klonopin)

Discussion

The correct answer is "D." Lorazepam is absorbed well intramuscularly. This makes it a good choice for the vomiting patient. Diazepam **is erratically** absorbed IM and thus should not be used in patients without an IV.

> HELPFUL TIP: The IV form of lorazepam can also be administered sublingually to speed absorption.

DT carries a fatality rate of:

A) <1%.
B) 5%.
C) 10%.
D) 25%.
E) 50%.

Discussion

The correct answer is "B." Prior to modern treatment, the mortality reached up to almost 40% per episode. The rest are incorrect.

Which of the following does NOT predispose to developing DT?

A) Prior episodes of DT.
B) Pneumonia.
C) Gastrointestinal (GI) bleed.
D) Female gender.
E) Hepatic failure.

Discussion

The correct answer is "D." Female gender does not predispose an individual to DT but the other options do.

Which of the following is NOT a complication of alcoholism?

A) Dementia.
B) Pancreatitis.
C) Hypermagnesemia.
D) Megaloblastic anemia.
E) Marchiafava–Bignami disease.

Discussion

The correct answer is "C." All of the above, with the exception of hypermagnesemia, are associated with alcohol abuse. A few merit special comment. Alcoholic dementia may be related to direct effects of alcohol on the brain or to nutritional deficiencies. **Hypo**magnesemia is a complication of alcoholism. Hypomagnesemia may decrease the response to thiamine administration. **Marchiafava–Bignami** disease is demyelination and/or necrosis of the corpus callosum and the adjacent white matter. It presents with dementia, dysarthria, spasticity, and inability to ambulate. It can occasionally be seen in nondrinkers as well.

> HELPFUL TIP: Elderly patients with alcohol problems often go unrecognized. Have a high index of suspicion in patients with signs and symptoms such as labile hypertension, insomnia, legal or marital problems, frequent falls and injuries, headaches or blackouts, and vague GI complaints.

Which of the following is FALSE about alcohol use disorders?

A) Most patients who develop alcohol disorders do so by their mid-20s.
B) The lifetime prevalence of alcoholism is between 14% and 24%.
C) Alcoholism is frequently comorbid with other psychiatric illnesses.
D) Alcohol abuse is five times more frequent in males than in females.
E) About 30% of patients with alcohol abuse meet the DSM-IV criteria for major depressive disorder.

Discussion

The correct answer is "A." Most people who develop alcohol use disorders do so by their late 30s, **not** their late 20s. The rest are correct statements. Especially noteworthy is "C." Half of all people with alcohol abuse have a comorbid Axis I diagnosis. For example, about 50–60% of people with bipolar illness have problems with alcohol abuse or dependence. "E" is a correct statement as well. **Although over 80% of patients with alcohol use disorders complain of depressive symptoms, only 30% meet criteria for**

major depressive disorder. A useful way to approach patients who complain of depression along with their alcohol abuse is to obtain a longitudinal history to see which came first. If it is impossible to tease out, as is often the case, observe for 1–3 weeks off alcohol. If depression is still present without alcohol use, it is prudent to treat with an antidepressant. Be careful when treating alcohol abusers with antidepressants: active substance use severely reduces the efficacy of these drugs.

HELPFUL TIP: Substance use rates are highest between ages 18 and 25. A lot of this is experimentation that will end as the individual matures. Some, of course, will go on to chronic abuse.

HELPFUL (AND IMPORTANT) TIP: The best way to deal with alcohol withdrawal is using PRN doses of IV diazepam. True DTs may require up to 500 mg of IV diazepam in 24 hours (yes, you read that right... 500 mg... my personal best is 70 mg IV over 1 hour (well, not for myself, of course). Give 5–10 mg of diazepam IV every 5–10 minutes until the patient is sedated. Diazepam is long enough acting that once a patient's symptoms are controlled, they often will not need a second dose of drug. But treat them IV PRN for symptoms. The traditional "Librium taper" requires more drug and more time in the hospital. **Phenytoin is ineffective for the prevention of alcohol related seizures.**

Objectives: Did you learn to...

- Recognize signs and symptoms of alcohol withdrawal?
- Describe diagnostic criteria for alcohol withdrawal?
- Identify adverse effects of heavy alcohol use?
- Differentiate between substance abuse and dependence?
- Treat alcohol withdrawal?
- Appreciate how denial of the illness plays a role in the assessment of substance abuse?
- Identify laboratory abnormalities observed in alcohol abuse and understand the limitations of laboratory studies?

QUICK QUIZ: NIGHTMARE IN MARGARITAVILLE

A 50-year-old divorced Caucasian male presents to your clinic in an agitated state, complaining of nausea, vomiting, and double vision. He smells of alcohol, has gross bilateral hand tremors, and is disheveled. He is picking at his shirtsleeves and is oriented to name only. On physical exam, he has lateral nystagmus and an ataxic gait. Vital signs include: blood pressure 160/92 mm Hg, pulse 100, and respirations 20. Labs are drawn, and his GGT is moderately elevated.

Which of the following is the most likely cause of his symptoms?

A) Wernicke encephalopathy.
B) Normal pressure hydrocephalus.
C) Dementia.
D) Stroke.
E) Alcohol withdrawal.

Discussion

The correct answer is "A." Wernicke encephalopathy is the result of thiamine deficiency and can occur in alcoholics and other patients with poor nutrition. See the next question for a description of the clinical findings. Note that several symptoms of Wernicke encephalopathy can mimic withdrawal (agitation, etc.). However, as noted in the question, this patient is still intoxicated.

QUICK QUIZ: WERNICKE ENCEPHALOPATHY

The triad of Wernicke encephalopathy includes all of the following EXCEPT:

A) Ataxia.
B) Oculomotor dysfunction.
C) Incontinence.
D) Encephalopathy.

Discussion

The correct answer is "C." Wernicke encephalopathy may present with the classic triad of ataxia, encephalopathy (confusion), and oculomotor dysfunction (nystagmus, lateral rectus palsy, etc.). However, the majority of patients presents with an incomplete syndrome and may be missing ophthalmoplegia, ataxia, or encephalopathy. If you choose "B," maybe you were thinking of normal pressure hydrocephalus, which presents with dementia, incontinence, and ataxia.

QUICK QUIZ: JUST SAY NO

What is the most abused illicit substance in the United States?

A) Marijuana.
B) Cocaine.
C) Methamphetamine.
D) Heroin.
E) LSD.

Discussion

The correct answer is "A." Marijuana is by far the most common illicit substance used, outstripping the use of all other illicit substances combined.

CASE 3

A 28-year-old married, pregnant patient and her mother are presenting for a follow-up appointment. At the appointment today, the patient's mother shares that her daughter has been drinking alcohol during her pregnancy. The daughter is very annoyed when confronted with her use of alcohol and will not give specific information about it, but she does admit to drinking. She does not agree to quit during her pregnancy or to be referred for substance abuse evaluation.You discuss some of the effects alcohol might have on the developing fetus, including fetal alcohol syndrome (FAS). The diagnosis of FAS requires specific manifestations in three areas.

They are:

A) At least two facial anomalies, retardation of growth below the 20th percentile, and little motor activity.
B) At least two facial anomalies, retardation of growth below the 10th percentile, and central nervous system (CNS) problems that may include tremulousness, hyperactivity, attentional deficits, or mental impairment.
C) At least three facial anomalies, retardation of growth below the 20th percentile, and poor sucking reflexes.
D) Small size, hyperactivity, and one generalized facial anomaly.

Discussion

The correct answer is "B." The diagnosis of FAS requires in utero exposure to alcohol and at least two facial anomalies, retardation of growth below the 10th percentile, and CNS problems that may include tremulousness, hyperactivity, attentional deficits, or mental impairment. The other options are incorrect. See Figure 25–1.

> HELPFUL TIP: The rate of FAS is 10–50% among the children of women who abused alcohol during pregnancy. **FAS is the leading cause of mental retardation in the Western Hemisphere.** Children with this disorder have an average IQ of 68–70.

Symptoms and signs of FAS may be detected at what point after birth?

A) Within 12 hours.
B) After the first week.
C) At 1 month.
D) At 3 months
E) After 1 year.

Discussion

The correct answer is "A." Soon after birth, the neonate may display symptoms of withdrawal, including tremulousness, inconsolability, vomiting, and poor feeding. The characteristic cluster of facial/physical malformations include short palpebral fissure, a short upturned nose, a hypoplastic upper lip, and a diminished philtrum, and are evident within 12 hours of birth. Other principal features are CNS dysfunction, growth deficiency at birth, joint and limb abnormalities, and heart defects.

* *

In addition to FAS, you discuss some of the potential problems seen with more limited in utero exposure to alcohol.

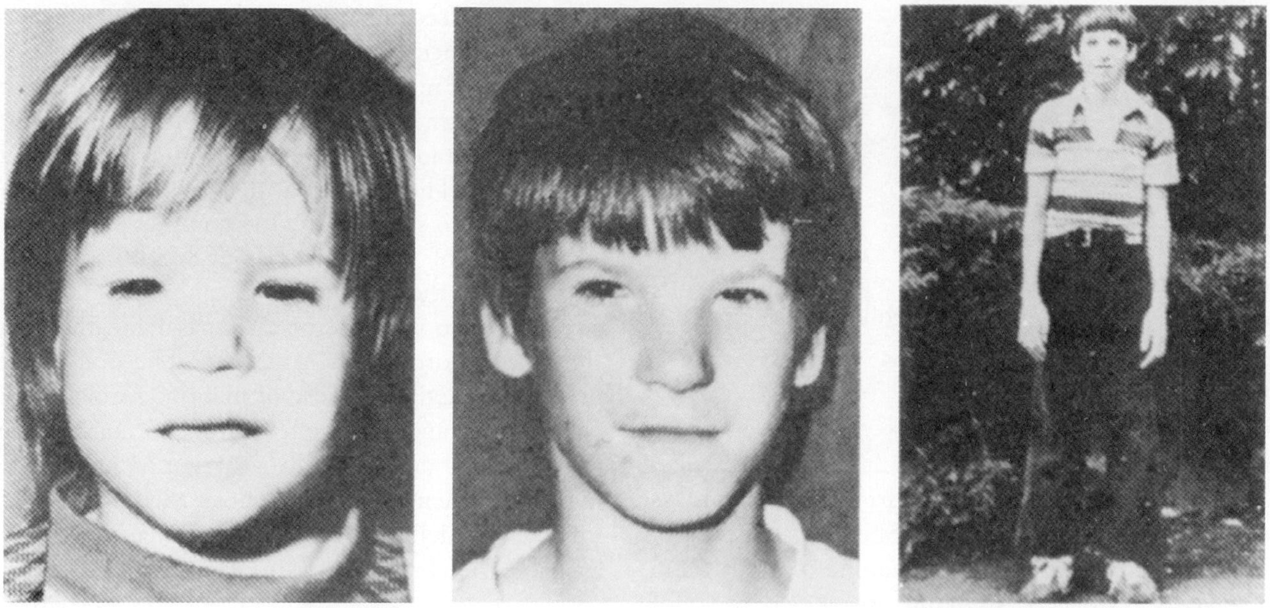

A B C

Figure 25–1 **Fetal alcohol syndrome. A. At 2 1/2 years. B, C. At 12 years. Note persistence of short palpebral fissures, epicanthal folds, flat midface, hypoplastic philtrum, and thin upper vermilion border. This individual also has the short, lean prepubertal stature characteristic of young males with fetal alcohol syndrome. (Reproduced from Streissguth AP, Clarren SK, Jones KL. Natural history of the fetal alcohol syndrome: A 10-year follow-up of eleven patients. *Lancet.* 1985;326:85–91, with permission from Elsevier.)**

What are the criteria for fetal alcohol effects (FAE)?

A) Small size, prematurity, hyperactivity, learning disabilities.
B) Inability to complete tasks, very active, very excitable.
C) Facial malformations, heart defects, hyperactivity.
D) Growth deficiency at <10th percentile, learning disabilities.
E) Congenital cardiac anomalies, growth deficiency at <10th percentile, facial malformations.

Discussion

The correct answer is "A." Knowledge continues to grow regarding the more subtle effects of maternal drinking, such as that seen with "social" alcohol use. FAE can occur with even moderate drinking during pregnancy. The abnormalities commonly observed with FAE include small size, prematurity, hyperactivity, and learning disabilities.

In which stage of pregnancy does the teratogenic action of alcohol cause facial malformations?

A) During the embryonic phase, at the eighth week after conception.
B) During the third week of pregnancy.
C) During the late first trimester.
D) During the second trimester.
E) During the third trimester.

Discussion

The correct answer is "B." **Facial malformations occur with the use of alcohol during the third week.** Organs and limbs appear most susceptible to the effects of alcohol during the embryonic phase, which is completed by the eighth week of conception, a time when most women are first confirming pregnancy. Alcohol exposure during any stage of development may effect brain development or function.

* *

You are able to convince this patient to reduce and eventually eliminate her use of alcohol; she delivers a healthy-appearing newborn whom she names "Harley" after the motorcycle.

HELPFUL TIP: Never name your child after a motorcycle (Harley), a Western land formation (e.g., Sierra, Cheyenne, or Cody) or a gun (Wesson or Remington). It is a sure bet that if

> you do they will have neurologic problems (at least that is our experience). Now, if you name your kid after a brand of whiskey (like the singer Pink did), no telling how far he'll go!

Objectives: Did you learn to . . .

- Identify problem drinking in a pregnant patient?
- Approach a patient with alcohol abuse in pregnancy?
- Describe the findings of FAE and FAS?

CASE 4

A 60-year-old female presents to your office and is determined to stop smoking. She has a history of schizophrenia treated with clozapine (Clozaril) and a 43-year history of smoking up to two packs of cigarettes per day. She asks you what is available to help her stop. You tell her that nicotine replacement therapy (NRT), bupropion (Zyban), and varenicline (Chantix) are currently approved to aid patients who want to stop smoking.

You want to offer her a NRT that is easy to use, has few side effects, and provides steady blood levels of nicotine over the whole day.

Which do you choose?

A) Nicotine patch.
B) Nicotine gum.
C) Nicotine nasal spray.
D) Nicotine inhaler.
E) Nicotine suppositories.

Discussion

The correct answer is "A." There are benefits and drawbacks to each of the smoking cessation aids. Like other NRT, the nicotine patch is available without prescription. It is applied to the skin daily and provides a steady release of nicotine through the skin. For a patient with a heavy, long smoking history, begin with the 21 mg patch and taper to the 7 mg patch over a 3-month time frame. Some of the drawbacks of the patch include slower release of nicotine, the potential for skin irritation, insomnia, and vivid dreams. Some of these side effects can be reduced by having the patient rotate application sites daily (to avoid skin irritation) and removing the patch before bedtime. Nicotine gum is an ion-exchange resin that releases nicotine for absorption through the buccal mucosa with only 30% bioavailability in the rest of the GI tract. Side effects include mouth and throat soreness, jaw fatigue, hiccups, and undesirable taste. There are advantages of nicotine gum: it involves an active coping mechanism (chewing, placing the gum in one's mouth, etc.) and is more likely than the patch to delay weight gain. The nasal spray delivers 0.5 mg nicotine per dose and is sprayed one to two times per hour for a maximum of 5 sprays per hour and 40 sprays per day. Most of the nicotine nasal spray side effects are attributable to its route of use—nasal and throat irritation, rhinorrhea, sneezing, etc. The oral inhaler provides an active delivery of nicotine similar to the nasal inhaler, and its side effects are also a consequence of its route of delivery—throat irritation and coughing. There are no nicotine suppositories—thankfully! Finally, varenicline, a nicotine receptor agonist, is also available to help with smoking cessation.

Which of the following is the most significant side effect of varenicline (Chantix)?

A) Desire to commit violence or commit suicide.
B) Desire to watch endless reruns of Godzilla movies
C) Leukocytosis.
D) Urinary retention.

Discussion

The correct answer is "A." There is an FDA warning about the possibility of suicidal or homicidal ideation. This is not good, especially in someone who already has a psychiatric disorder. Other common side effects include flatulence (really), nausea, headache, and insomnia.

* *

Although this patient does not mind spending $6–7 per day on cigarettes, she does not want to pay a lot for something to help her quit (Why is this, you ask? So do we . . .).

Which smoking cessation aid is the most expensive?

A) Nicotine patch.
B) Nicotine gum.
C) Nicotine nasal spray.
D) Nicotine inhaler.
E) Varenicline.

Discussion

The correct answer is "E." Varenicline costs approximately $130 per month. The nicotine products are less expensive in the range of $60–80 per month. Of course, some health insurance programs will support smoking cessation aids.

* *

"I tried those things, Doc, and nicotine didn't work and varenicline made me shoot my boyfriend in the leg. Isn't there something else?"

Which of the following medications might you also prescribe to aid this patient in smoking cessation?

A) Naloxone.
B) Metoprolol.
C) Haloperidol.
D) Bupropion.

Discussion
The correct answer is "D." Bupropion is marketed as the antidepressant Wellbutrin and the smoking cessation aid Zyban. It reduces the symptoms of nicotine withdrawal by blocking dopamine in the brain's reward center, and this mechanism is thought to result in reduced nicotine craving. Studies have shown that people who use bupropion doubled their chances of quitting smoking. Its effect appears to be additive to that of NRT. Its effect on smoking cessation is independent of its antidepressant effect, as shown by its equal efficacy in depressed and nondepressed patients. One of the advantages of bupropion is its ability to prevent the weight gain that occurs in most people when they stop smoking. Bupropion should be started at a dose of 150 mg daily for 3 days then increasing to 150 mg twice daily, if the patient is tolerating the drug. The patient should be advised to stop smoking during the second week of treatment.

* *

This patient wonders whether, at age 60 and with an 86-pack-year history, there is even any reason to quit.

How long does it take to reduce the risk of having a heart attack by half after one stops smoking?

A) 24 hours.
B) 6 months.
C) 1 year.
D) 10 years.
E) 15 years.

Discussion
The correct answer is "C." Twenty minutes after quitting smoking, blood pressure drops and the temperature of hands and feet increases to normal. After 24 hours, the risk of heart attack begins to decrease. At 1 year, the chance of having a heart attack is cut in half. After 5 years, stroke risk is reduced to that of a nonsmoker. After 10 years, the risk of dying from lung cancer is about half that of a person who continues to smoke. After 15 years, the risk of coronary heart disease approaches that of a nonsmoker.

* *

Your patient expresses concern that she will fail in this attempt to quit smoking, as she has in the past.

On average, how many attempts to quit smoking are made before a person succeeds?

A) 2.
B) 6.
C) 10.
D) 16.

Discussion
The correct answer is "B." It takes an average of six attempts at quitting before success.

> HELPFUL (AND UNFORTUNATE) TIP: None of these cessation aids have a great track record of success. You can find numbers all over the board. With nicotine aids, something like 15% of patients will be tobacco free at 1 year. (A study in 2011 showed **no difference** in long-term abstinence rates between users of nicotine aids and those who quit on their own [*Tob Control* doi:10.1136/tobaccocontrol-2011–050129].) With bupropion, the number is closer to 23%. Varenicline also has about a 23% 1-year abstinence rate. Counseling may increase the success rate, and all smokers should be urged to quit at every appointment.

* *

This patient has been on clozapine (Clozaril) for control of her psychosis.

The combination of clozapine and bupropion should be used with caution because:

A) Both may lower the seizure threshold.
B) Both may cause hypertension.
C) Bupropion may interfere with the metabolism of clozapine.
D) Severe GI symptoms could occur.
E) A psychotic episode could be precipitated.

Discussion

The correct answer is "A." Both drugs may lower the seizure threshold. Hypertension should not be a concern. Bupropion does not interfere with the metabolism of clozapine, cause severe GI symptoms, or precipitate psychotic episodes.

* *

After all of your discussion, the patient wants to quit "cold turkey." You gently explain that going from 40 cigarettes per day to zero might be hard on her.

All of the following are symptoms of nicotine withdrawal EXCEPT:

A) Increased appetite.
B) Dysphoria.
C) Tachycardia.
D) Insomnia.
E) Irritability.

Discussion

The correct answer is "C." Nicotine withdrawal is actually associated with **decreased** heart rate. In addition to the above, trouble concentrating and restlessness are also common symptoms.

HELPFUL TIP: Cystine, an herbal derivative, is effective in smoking cessation (placebo 2.4% vs. cystine 8%). It is less expensive than varenicline and varenicline is actually a derivative of cystine (*N Engl J Med.* 2011; 365:1193).

HELPFUL TIP: Other measures that are effective in helping a patient quit are automated cell phone messages (*Lancet.* 2011;378:49), intensive interaction (nurse phone calls, bedside teaching after an MI, etc.) (*CMAJ.* 2009; 180:1297), and paying patients to quit (*N Engl J Med.* 2009;360:699). Additionally, public policies such as taxes on cigarettes and banning smoking indoors have demonstrated effectiveness at increasing quitting rates.

Objectives: Did you learn to . . .

- Employ pharmacotherapy in the treatment of tobacco addiction?
- Enumerate the physiological advantages of smoking cessation at any age?
- Recognize signs and symptoms of nicotine withdrawal?

QUICK QUIZ: ALL IN THE FAMILY

A known risk factor for substance abuse is being the child of an alcoholic.

Which of the following characteristics is NOT true of the children of alcoholics?

A) They experience earlier onset of problem drinking.
B) They experience earlier pregnancies (well, not the males . . .).
C) They have less stable family involvement.
D) They experience poor academic and social performance in school.
E) They have more antisocial behavior.

Discussion

The correct answer is "B." There is no data to suggest early pregnancy as a characteristic. Twin, adoption, and half-sibling studies and studies of familial versus nonfamilial alcoholism indicate that children of alcoholics have four times the risk for developing alcoholism. They also have worse school performance, more antisocial behavior, and less stable family situations.

CASE 5

A 35-year-old intoxicated female presents to your office requesting to be started on disulfiram (Antabuse). She is otherwise healthy and recently has begun to drink in response to the death of her sister. Before this, she was a teetotaler.

Disulfiram acts by inhibiting:

A) Lactic dehydrogenase.
B) Gastric dehydrogenase.
C) Aldehyde dehydrogenase.
D) Dopamine beta-hydroxylase.
E) Alcohol dehydrogenase.

Discussion

The correct answer is "C." Disulfiram inhibits aldehyde dehydrogenase, the enzyme that catalyzes the oxidation of acetaldehyde to acetic acid. If alcohol is ingested after inhibition of this enzyme, blood acetaldehyde levels rise, resulting in the characteristic symptoms of the disulfiram–ethanol interaction (keep reading for more on this exciting topic).

Disulfiram should not be administered until the patient has been abstinent from alcohol for how long?

A) 4 hours.
B) 12 hours.
C) 24 hours.
D) 48 hours.
E) 72 hours.

Discussion

The correct answer is "B." A minimum of 12 hours should have elapsed before giving disulfiram to avoid the disulfiram–alcohol reaction. Of course, this depends on how much they were drinking. Remember, we are in a college town here...

HELPFUL TIP: Disulfiram is absorbed slowly from the GI tract and is eliminated slowly; therefore, **a patient should wait at least 1 week after stopping disulfiram before returning to drinking.**

If the patient consumes alcohol while taking disulfiram, which of the following is *most likely to occur?*

A) Respiratory depression.
B) Hypertension.
C) Nausea and vomiting.
D) Cardiovascular collapse.
E) Convulsions.

Discussion

The correct answer is "C." The disulfiram–ethanol interaction generally includes flushing of the skin, nausea, vomiting, palpitations, hypotension, sweating, blurred vision, and dizziness. Rarely, in more severe reactions, respiratory depression, cardiovascular collapse, convulsions, and death may occur. The severity of the reaction is typically dose related and depends on the amount of alcohol ingested.

Common side effects of disulfiram include which of the following?

A) Hypotension.
B) Peripheral neuropathy.
C) Insomnia.
D) Nausea.
E) Depression.

Discussion

The correct answer is "B." Drowsiness, hepatotoxicity, rashes, hypertension, peripheral neuropathy, metallic after-taste, and optic neuritis may occur with disulfiram use. These effects are independent of alcohol ingestion.

HELPFUL TIP: Multiple cases of hepatitis have been reported with usage of disulfiram, and baseline liver enzymes should be obtained prior to starting disulfiram and then approximately 2 weeks after initiation of treatment. Occasionally, a rash may occur early on. The rash can be treated with antihistamines and the drug can be continued.

* *

After a discussion, the patient thinks that disulfiram is the "one thing that might work." She tries it, but at follow-up, she is not having much success. She continues to drink heavily and (thankfully) has been noncompliant with taking disulfiram regularly. She reports strong craving for alcohol.

At this point, as an alternative to disulfiram, you decide to prescribe:

A) Naltrexone (Revia).
B) Naloxone (Narcan).
C) Nortriptyline.
D) Nitroprusside.

Discussion

The correct answer is "A." Naltrexone is FDA-approved for the treatment of alcoholism. As an opioid antagonist, it blocks the euphoric effects of alcohol. Topiramate (Topamax) and baclofen can also be used to decrease the craving for alcohol. However, they are not FDA-approved for this indication. None of the other drugs listed are used to treat alcohol abuse and dependence.

* *

This patient seems to recall something about using camel paws to treat alcoholism. You very perceptively realize she means Campral (acamprosate).

Which of the following is true about acamprosate?

A) It is contraindicated in those with renal impairment/renal failure.
B) At 1 year, acamprosate is no better than placebo in preventing relapse of alcoholism.
C) The combination of acamprosate and naltrexone is no more effective than either alone.
D) Drug reps will tell you that all of these medications are great and that you should prescribe them.
E) All of the above.

Discussion

The correct answer is "E." All of the above are true. Unfortunately, at 1 year none of these drugs are significantly better than placebo. How do they get past the FDA, you ask? So do we . . .

Which of the following is true about acamprosate?

A) Patients receiving opioid maintenance therapy or opioids for pain will need higher levels of opioid medication.
B) It is contraindicated in those with liver impairment/liver failure.
C) Patients who require detoxification can be continued safely on acamprosate.
D) All of the above.

Discussion

The correct answer is "C." Acamprosate does not interact with benzodiazepines or other medications used in medical detoxification and thus can be continued safely if a patient starts drinking and then requires detoxification. Acamprosate is not metabolized by the liver and can be used safely even in patients with severe liver disease, whereas naltrexone and disulfiram are contraindicated. Those receiving opioids for acute or chronic pain or receiving opioid maintenance treatment can use acamprosate because it does not affect these medications.

HELPFUL TIP: Other medications that have been used to treat alcoholism include topiramate, baclofen, ondansetron and SSRIs. Topiramate has the best data and ondansetron is only effective in early onset alcoholism in those who have a specific gene for 5-HT transporter.

HELPFUL TIP: In case we didn't make the point clear above, disulfiram (Antabuse), naltrexone (Revia), and acamprosate (Campral) are not particularly effective drugs in the long term, with success rates no greater than placebo.

Objectives: Did you learn to . . .

- Describe the mechanism of action of disulfiram?
- Recognize side effects of disulfiram?
- Describe the alcohol–disulfiram reaction?
- Prescribe other medical therapies for alcohol use disorders?

CASE 6

A 25-year-old comatose female presents to the ER with pinpoint pupils and respiratory depression.

Which of the following is the most likely cause of coma?

A) Blood alcohol level of 200 mg/dL.
B) Cocaine overdose.
C) Methadone overdose.
D) Benzodiazepine withdrawal.
E) Phencyclidine (PCP) intoxication.

Discussion

The correct answer is "C." The classic "triad" of opioid overdose consists of coma, respiratory depression, and pinpoint pupils (miosis). Certain patients may have atypical presentations, and the triad may not always be present in opioid overdose. Miosis is particularly variable, often not being seen in those with meperidine and propoxyphene overdoses; and coingestions, such as sympathomimetics and anticholinergics, can also prevent miosis. "A" is incorrect. A patient with a blood alcohol level of 200 mg/dL would likely be ataxic; but alcoholic coma typically occurs at blood levels >400 mg/dL and depends on the level of tolerance. Stimulant overdose would not likely present with somnolence. Alcohol and PCP intoxication would more likely present with nystagmus and not constricted pupils.

* *

You treat her with naloxone and she wakes up (spitting mad, agitated, and in withdrawal).

What is the minimum amount of time that you should observe a patient who has overdosed on methadone?

A) 1 hours.
B) 4 hours.
C) 12 hours.
D) 36 hours.
E) 72 hours.

Discussion
The correct answer is "D." Methadone has a long half-life (up to 60 hours), and therefore a patient who has overdosed on methadone should be monitored for at least 36–48 hours.

How many doses of naloxone (Narcan) 0.4 mg would most likely be needed in a patient with an overdose of a large quantity of methadone?

A) 1.
B) 2.
C) 3.
D) 4.
E) >5.

Discussion
The correct answer is "E." Naloxone hydrochloride, a pure opioid antagonist, reverses the CNS effects of opioid overdose. An initial IV dose of 0.4 mg reverses symptoms within 2 minutes. However, the half-life in adults is 30–90 minutes. Thus, multiple doses of naloxone may be needed, and patients need to be observed even if they respond symptomatically to a dose of naloxone.

* *

Through eyewitness history, you are able to determine that this patient did indeed overdose on an opioid.

Which of the following would most likely be FALSE concerning this patient?

A) Hyperthermia would be present.
B) Cardiac arrhythmias such as bradycardia can be present.
C) Pulmonary edema can be present.
D) Track marks might be present.

Discussion
The correct answer is "A." Hypothermia would be more likely with opioid intoxication. "B" is true; the patient can become bradycardic. "C" is true. Patients can develop noncardiogenic pulmonary edema as a result of heroin and other opioids. This is likely due to prolonged hypoxemia, although the mechanism isn't entirely clear. "D" would be true of a patient injecting drugs, as is often the case with opioid abusers.

* *

You discover that the patient has been on a methadone maintenance program, but then she lapsed and overdosed on a combination of methadone and heroin. Her urine drug screen returns positive for opioids.

What would be the next most appropriate course of action?

A) Detoxify the patient off methadone as an outpatient.
B) Contact the authorities to have the patient arrested.
C) Contact the patient's methadone maintenance clinic for dose increase.
D) Notify the patient of her positive urine drug screen and let her know you are not surprised by the result, as methadone is metabolized to heroin.
E) Have the patient committed to a substance abuse treatment facility.

Discussion
The correct answer is "C." The fact that this patient has relapsed into heroin use may mean that her methadone dose is too low for maintenance. This can lead to additional heroin use. The rest are incorrect. "A" would be dangerous. "B" is not necessary. "E" would be ineffective for a patient not interested in quitting (but is often used anyway as desperate measure). "D" is of particular note. Methadone is metabolized to morphine and not heroin.

HELPFUL TIP: High-dose methadone can lead to QT prolongation and torsades de pointes.

Methadone is typically prescribed for opioid maintenance therapy:

A) Once daily.
B) Twice daily.
C) Three times daily.
D) Three times weekly.
E) Once monthly.

Discussion

The correct answer is "A." Methadone has an elimination half-life of up to 60 hours (range 15–60 hours). Thus, once daily dosing is appropriate for the treatment of narcotic addiction. The advantage here is that the medication can be given under direct observation.

> HELPFUL TIP: Methadone should be dosed every 6–8 hours if being used for pain control. It may not reach a steady state for 3–5 days. Remember that you do not need a special DEA license to prescribe methadone for pain, only for addiction. And it may be a reasonable analgesic in the properly selected patient.

* *

After regaining consciousness, the patient informs you that she is 20 weeks pregnant.

Regarding pregnancy and usage of opioids, which of the following would most likely have the best outcome?

A) Continuing the patient on methadone.
B) Withdrawing the patient from all opioids in the first trimester (too late for this one).
C) Withdrawing the patient from all opioids in the second trimester.
D) Withdrawing the patient from all opioids in the third trimester.

Discussion

The correct answer is "A." Opioid withdrawal in a pregnant woman can cause fetal distress and low birth weight. Methadone is currently the standard of care in the United States for the treatment of opioid addiction in pregnant women. Methadone maintenance has multiple advantages, including longer durations of maternal drug abstinence, better obstetrical care, reductions in fetal illicit drug exposure, and enhanced neonatal outcomes (e.g., increased fetal growth, reduced fetal mortality, and decreased risk of preeclampsia).

Objectives: Did you learn to . . .

- Recognize symptoms and signs of overdose with opioids and other illicit drugs?
- Use methadone for opioid addiction?
- Treat a pregnant patient with opioid addiction?

CASE 7

A 40-year-old female is admitted through the ER, arriving via ambulance from a smaller hospital. The local physician called to report that her friends said that she had "shot up a lot of meth." She is known to use her son's Ritalin prescription on a regular basis. She appears frightened and anxious. She is uncommunicative, rocking back and forth on the exam table, and picking at her skin trying to remove imaginary bugs. She becomes angry easily and lashes out at staff in the emergency department.

A *reasonable* differential diagnosis for this patient would include all of the following EXCEPT:

A) Schizophrenia.
B) Drug-induced psychosis.
C) PCP, hallucinogen, or cocaine intoxication.
D) Diabetes.
E) DT.

Discussion

The correct answer is "D." Just checking to see if you're awake. Though hypoglycemic patients can certainly become confused, diabetes is least likely to be causing these symptoms. Although there is a history of amphetamine use, the other options should not be eliminated out of hand. There may be more than one substance involved (of course, we never see that sort of thing in Iowa . . . no, never).

* *

The urine drug screen is positive for amphetamines.

The following are all symptoms of amphetamine use EXCEPT:

A) Tachycardia
B) Hypertension.
C) Perspiration or chills.
D) Weight gain.
E) Psychomotor agitation.

Discussion

The correct answer is "D." Weight loss, not weight gain, can be anticipated in the amphetamine user. All of the other symptoms can be seen as a result of amphetamine use. Symptoms can progress to confusion, arrhythmias, seizures, dystonias, or coma.

HELPFUL TIP: Stimulant use can cause coronary artery occlusion and severe hypertension. Myocardial infarction with stimulant use should be treated like any other MI. Hypertension should be treated with alpha and beta-blockers.

HELPFUL TIP: Chronic methamphetamine use is associated with widespread dental caries and gingival disease that can result in loss of many, or even all, teeth. "Meth mouth," as this is commonly called, is probably due to prolonged periods of poor dental hygiene, xerostomia, high calorie food and drink, and tooth grinding.

Which of the following does NOT address the needs of this patient during withdrawal?

A) Provide a secure environment.
B) Provide regular meals and snacks.
C) Make sure the patient is awakened if she spends excess time sleeping.
D) Consider giving a benzodiazepine if the patient remains anxious.
E) Provide education as an intervention towards change.

Discussion

The correct answer is "C." Amphetamine withdrawal requires sleep, nutritious food, and a safe place until the unstable state of being has diminished. The patient should be allowed to sleep. Stimulant abusers often stay up for a week or more at a time and then "crash" or sleep for days during withdrawal. Antipsychotic medications and benzodiazepines may be administered if needed.

Objectives: Did you learn to . . .

- Recognize the signs and symptoms of amphetamine intoxication?
- Appropriately treat a patient with amphetamine intoxication and withdrawal?

CASE 8

A 15-year-old male is brought into the ER by his neighbor who found the boy passed out in his backyard with a bag full of glue nearby. He had difficulty rousing the boy. Currently, the patient is lethargic with slurred speech and difficulty walking. When his parents arrive, they are shocked, as their son has been a "good kid." They had no idea he was using any drugs. Of course, he bought lots of tubes of "model glue" but they never did see any completed models. . . .

The signs and symptoms of inhalant use include all of the following EXCEPT:

A) Dizziness.
B) Slurred speech.
C) Unsteady gait.
D) Smell of solvents or glue.
E) Dilated pupils

Discussion

The correct answer is "E." Inhalant intoxication is identified by impaired judgment, impaired social interaction, and aggressive behavior often leading to altercations. Higher doses can lead to lethargy, psychomotor retardation, stupor, or coma. Dilated pupils are seen in anticholinergic toxicity and other drugs (e.g., sympathomimetics) but not with inhalants.

All of the following are considered inhalants used by abusers EXCEPT:

A) Kerosene.
B) Cleaning solvent.
C) Gasoline.
D) Spray paint.
E) Glue.

Discussion

The correct answer is "A." Kerosene is not volatile enough to be abusable. The rest can be abused by inhalation.

HELPFUL TIP: The acute intoxicant effect of volatiles generally lasts about 30 minutes. Gasoline is an exception; in the case of gasoline, the intoxication can last for up to 6 hours.

Withdrawal from inhalants has been described and includes all of the following features EXCEPT:

A) Onset of symptoms 24–48 hours after use has stopped.
B) Transient illusions.
C) Diaphoresis.
D) Confusion.
E) Intense hunger.

Discussion
The correct answer is "E." Intense hunger is not a sign of withdrawal. In fact, the patient may be nauseated. All of the other options are correct.

All of the following can result from chronic solvent or hydrocarbon inhalation EXCEPT:

A) Chronic brain injury.
B) Muscle weakness.
C) CNS microhemorrhages and secondary seizures.
D) Erythrocytosis.
E) Liver and renal damage.

Discussion
The correct answer is "D." Solvents and hydrocarbons can cause all of the effects noted above except for erythrocytosis. In fact, one can see bone marrow suppression as a result of chronic inhalant use.

Risk factors for inhalant abuse include all of the following demographic factors EXCEPT:

A) Female.
B) Age 13–15.
C) Low socioeconomic state.
D) Native American.
E) Poor school performance.

Discussion
The correct answer is "A." Males, not females, are more likely to abuse inhalants. Inhalant users tend to be of lower socioeconomic status, younger (age 13–15), and have difficulty in school. There is an increased incidence of inhalant abuse among Native Americans.

> **HELPFUL TIP:** "Sniffing" is when fumes are inhaled directly from a source container or the substance is placed into a bag and inhaled from the bag. "Huffing" is when the substance is placed on a rag and then inhaled with the rag placed over the nose and mouth. Gotta know the lingo.

Objectives: Did you learn to . . .

- Identify some types of inhalants abused?
- Recognize the symptoms of inhalant abuse?
- Describe the demographics of inhalant abuse?

CASE 9

A 40-year-old male who has been smoking marijuana daily for the past 20 years would like to quit his marijuana habit. He wants to apply for a new job, and a drug screen is part of the application process. He makes an appointment with you to discuss what he can expect when he quits and how long will it be until his drug screen is negative.

All of the following are symptoms of marijuana intoxication EXCEPT:

A) Euphoria.
B) Sensation of slowed time.
C) Increased mental alertness.
D) Increased appetite.
E) Dry mouth.

Discussion
The correct answer is "C." Marijuana intoxication decreases mental alertness, although it can reportedly enhance the senses. When inhaled, intoxication peaks after 10–30 minutes and last about 3 hours.

How long can marijuana (THC) be detected in the urine?

A) 30 days if used regularly; 2–7 days if used occasionally.
B) 2 weeks.
C) 1 week for females; 2 weeks for males.
D) 24–48 hours.
E) It cannot be detected in urine samples.

Discussion
The correct answer is "A." This patient will have to stop smoking marijuana for a minimum of 30 days before applying for the job, if he wants to assure his urine drug screen will be negative. The drug can be present in hair samples for an extended period of time—anywhere from 1 to 6 months.

Which of these is NOT one of the touted benefits of marijuana?

A) Pain reliever.
B) Anxiolytic.
C) Antiemetic.
D) Appetite stimulator.
E) Antidepressant.

Discussion
The correct answer is "E." In fact, the use of marijuana has been shown to actually worsen depression. Marijuana has been used to treat pain, nausea, anorexia, glaucoma, etc.

HELPFUL TIP: There may be an association between marijuana use and schizophrenia (see *Lancet*. 2007 Jul 28;370:319). However, causality has not been proven and other studies take exception to the results of this study.

Objectives: Did you learn to . . .

- Recognize the symptoms of marijuana intoxication?
- Anticipate effects of marijuana use?

QUICK QUIZ: DUDE, WHAT WAS IN THAT POT?

A 20-year-old male is brought by the police into the emergency department because of severe agitation after smoking what he thought was crack cocaine. He exhibits slurred speech, ataxia, circumoral numbness, and horizontal nystagmus.

Which of the following substances is most likely causing his symptoms?

A) Cannabis (THC).
B) Heroin.
C) Methamphetamine.
D) PCP.
E) Nicotine.

Discussion
The correct is "D." PCP (also called "angel dust") intoxication is characterized by agitation, impulsiveness, nystagmus, hypertension, tachycardia, numbness, ataxia, and perceptual distortions. Intoxication begins 5 minutes after use and peaks in 30 minutes. PCP-induced psychosis is the most common PCP-induced disorder and may mimic a schizophrenic psychotic episode. PCP may be added to other drugs unbeknownst to the user.

HELPFUL TIP: A few words on designer drugs.
Ecstasy, also known as MDMA (or 3,4-methylenedioxymethamphetamine), produces sensations of euphoria, intimacy, and disinhibition. Users often use pacifiers because ecstasy can cause bruxism (Didn't you wonder why all of those teens are sucking on candy pacifiers? Just to look cool?) MDMA can cause seizures, liver disease, and hyperthermia among other side effects.
K2 (also known as "spice" and "chill x") is a synthetic cannabinoid that is much more potent than marijuana. It is often sold as incense. The users then inhale the smoke. Side effects include tachycardia, memory lapses, paranoia, and hallucinations.
Bath salts are a synthetic stimulant. Symptoms are those of a sympathomimetic such as methamphetamine. It is reported that bath salts produce prolonged feelings of suicidality. This is anecdotal, of course.
GHB (AKA "grievous bodily harm," "Georgia home boy," and others). A short-acting drug, it produces both sedation and stimulation (which may cycle rapidly). Patients may be bradycardic and near apneic but when stimulated may become agitated and violent.

QUICK QUIZ: QUICK COUNSELING

Brief intervention for alcohol problems is one of the most clinically effective and cost-effective preventive services from among those recommended by the USPSTF.

All of the following are components for conducting brief interventions EXCEPT:

A) Ask and give feedback on screening results.
B) State recommendations about safe drinking levels and offer advice about change.
C) Assess the patient's readiness to change.

D) Negotiate goals and strategies for change.
E) Follow up annually.

Discussion

The correct answer (and the thing to avoid) is "E." Follow-up should be arranged much sooner than 1 year. The "5 A's" method for brief interventions has substantial research support for its utility in alcohol use disorders across a variety of settings and can be incorporated with motivational strategies in a step-by-step process. The "5 A's" approach is a brief, goal-directed way to more effectively address substance use with patients. Altogether, the "5 A's" may take 1–5 minutes, depending on a provider's clinical setting and roles. These components include **A**sking about use, **A**dvising to cut down/quit, **A**ssessing willingness to quit, **A**ssisting with strategies for abstinence, and **A**rranging follow-up.

BIBLIOGRAPHY

Connors GJ, et al. *Substance Abuse Treatment and the Stages of Change: Selecting and Planning Interventions.* New York, NY: Guilford Press; 2004.

Edwards S, et al. Current and promising pharmacotherapies, and novel research target areas in the treatment of alcohol dependence: A review. *Curr Pharm Des.* 2011;17:1323-1332.

Howard MO, et al. Inhalant use and inhalant use disorders in the United States. *Addict Sci Clin Pract.* 2011;6:18-31.

Johnson BA, et al. Topiramate for treating alcohol dependence: A randomized controlled trial. *JAMA.* 2007;298:1641-1651.

Maisto SA, et al. *Alcohol Use Disorders.* Hogrefe and Huber Publishing; 2007.

National Institute on Drug Abuse. Available at www.nida.nih.gov, Accessed January 12, 2012.

Winslow BT, et al. Methamphetamine abuse. *Am Fam Physician.* 2007;76:1175-1176.

26

Ethics

Janeta F. Tansey and Mark A. Graber

CASE 1

A 54-year-old married female, Charlene, has insulin-dependent diabetes and has seen you for her care for the last 7 years. In the last year, she has developed diabetic retinopathy and neuropathy. To your great frustration, Charlene continues to resist the recommended lifestyle changes required to control her diabetes.

She is a casual, friendly woman known as the "candy lady" in her neighborhood where she lives with her husband of 30 years. She loves children and volunteers at the local elementary school, where she is well known for a quick smile, a reassuring hug, and a piece of candy in her large pockets. In fact, she is noted during most of her appointments to be munching on M&M's—her favorite candy. She has had dietary consults and many education-oriented doctor appointments but says, "I know I shouldn't eat the way I do, but I just don't have the heart to change who I am, even if it does help my eyes and legs. Who I am is about what I eat and do."

You wonder about Charlene's capacity for decision making, given her frank noncompliance with care, even in the setting of serious complications from her diabetes.

All of the following variables are necessary in decision-making capacity (DMC) EXCEPT:

A) Ability to communicate a choice.
B) Voluntary choice.
C) Understanding of the variables involved in the decision.
D) Ability to appreciate the personal impact of choices.
E) Family agreement that the patient is competent.

Discussion
The correct answer is "E." All of the other options are considered important for determining DMC. Certainly family concerns need to be addressed but family agreement has nothing to do with determining a patient's competence. One additional necessary element for DMC is the ability to reason about the options in the setting of personal values.

What is the *most* relevant piece of information in Charlene's account that suggests that her capacity is intact?

A) Therapeutic alliance with you despite noncompliance with treatment recommendations.
B) Integration into community relationships, including a stable marriage and responsibilities in the elementary school.
C) Expression of placing perceived self-identity as a higher priority than control of diabetes and its complications.
D) Awareness that her dietary choices are associated with symptoms of eye disease and neuropathy.
E) Flagrant disregard for medical recommendations by eating candy while at her appointment.

Discussion
The correct answer is "C." While several of these variables are relevant in assessing DMC, the capacity for DMC is typically thought of in a stepwise fashion,

starting with ability to communicate a choice, then basic understanding of the variables, then ability to appreciate the personal impact of choices, and finally the ability to reason about the options while considering personal values. This last step is not only the most complicated but also the most strongly indicative that DMC is intact.

Which of the following is TRUE about DMC?

A) Patients who have been found legally incompetent do not have DMC.
B) A patient's DMC may vary according to the circumstances of the situation.
C) A minor's DMC is not clinically relevant since there is a surrogate who bears the responsibility for decision making.
D) DMC should not be evaluated in cases in which the patient makes an unconventional choice.
E) Patients with psychiatric disease, who are committed to a treatment facility, do not have DMC.

Discussion

The correct answer is "B." DMC is not an all-or-none distinction but can vary widely from case to case or setting to setting. Even patients who have been declared legally incompetent or who have been legally and involuntarily committed may still have a measure of DMC. Moral theory typically urges clinicians to consider the wishes and reasoning of their patients as morally and clinically relevant, regardless of the placement of a legal guardian or the state as a surrogate decision maker. DMC may ultimately be overridden in certain kinds of legal circumstances, but it should not be done lightly as it suggests a fundamental denial of patient autonomy. As a result, many patients with psychiatric illness still have the right to make choices, even with diagnoses such as schizophrenia. Making unconventional choices can sometimes be a marker that DMC is not intact but does not automatically lead one to this conclusion (e.g., Jehovah Witness and blood transfusions; refusing blood is unconventional but DMC may be intact). Finally, though minors technically cannot make many health-care choices, their wishes should be taken into consideration as they are often able to articulate a preference.

* *

Charlene continues to have a slow decline over time but remains in good spirits despite the complications of her uncontrolled diabetes. One day her husband brings her to the emergency department. He had found her in the bathroom, unconscious, and called an ambulance. She has had a stroke and remains unresponsive, on ventilation in the ICU. Her prognosis is poor.

What are appropriate considerations for making a treatment decision about end-of-life care for Charlene?

A) Oral statements to her husband about her end-of-life care.
B) Her husband's wishes for her care as designated health-care proxy.
C) Written advance directives.
D) Oral statements to her physician about her end-of-life care.
E) All of the above.

Discussion

The correct answer is "E." Written advance directives are considered the most binding, although all of these issues are relevant in making end-of-life decisions.

Which of the following statements can be used to describe medical futility?

A) No worthwhile goals of care can be achieved.
B) The likelihood of success is very small.
C) The patient's quality of life is unacceptable.
D) The prospective benefit is not worth the resources required.
E) All of the above.

Discussion

The correct answer is "E." All of the above meanings have been explicitly or implicitly drawn into discussions about medical futility. For this reason, many theorists have objected to the use of the term "futility" as a justification for decisions and urge clinicians to be precise about the concerns that arise in a given patient's clinical situation. Another definition of "futility" is trying to make it through this book and pass the recertification test.

* *

After discussion with her husband, you decide to discontinue ventilation. Charlene dies.

This intervention is appropriately considered:

A) Active, nonvoluntary euthanasia.
B) Physician-assisted suicide.
C) Withholding medical intervention.

D) The principle of double effect.
E) Withdrawing medical intervention.

Discussion
The correct answer is "E." While the answer might seem intuitive to you, many persons (including physicians) do not recognize the differences between these various interventions. Active euthanasia ("A") is when the physician both supplies the means of death and is the final human agent in the events leading to the patient's death (e.g., the physician administers the lethal drug). Whether or not active euthanasia is voluntary, involuntary or nonvoluntary depends on the DMC of the patient. Assisted suicide ("B") occurs when the physician provides the means of death but the patient carries out the act, such as taking an overdose of phenobarbital. Withholding medical intervention ("C") means not initiating care for a disease state such that the disease itself results in death. Withdrawing medical intervention ("E") means discontinuing an intervention that has already been used, although the disease state itself results in death with the intervention's discontinuation. The principle of double effect ("D") is an ethical theory that suggests that if there is an unintended bad outcome (e.g., death) while pursuing an intended purpose (e.g., pain relief), there is diminished moral responsibility for the unintended outcome. This principle is sometimes used to justify the use of high-dose opiates or sedatives in patients with intractable pain, even when the unintended effect is respiratory depression and death.

Which of the following is TRUE about the role of law in life-sustaining interventions?

A) Courts must be involved in decisions after a patient has been declared incompetent.
B) Life-sustaining treatment may be withheld only if patients are terminally ill or permanently unconscious.
C) Physicians may face criminal charges for providing appropriate palliative care and not treating the underlying disease.
D) The most prudent legal advice is to continue treatment in medically futile cases.
E) The law presents few barriers to physicians withholding life-sustaining interventions.

Discussion
The correct answer is "E." Sometimes physicians inappropriately provide treatment to patients who have made their end-of-life choices clear and have stated that they do not want prolongation of life. Respecting the patient's prior wishes will **not** result in legal liability for the physician, but the converse is not true; one can be legally liable for treating a patient who does not want treatment (e.g., transfusing a Jehovah Witness patient who refused transfusion). "A" is incorrect. After a patient is declared incompetent, the courts no longer need to be involved, as a legal surrogate is appointed by the court to make decisions for the patient. "B" is also incorrect as treatment may be withheld at any time at the request of a competent patient.

Objectives: Did you learn to . . .

- Evaluate a patient's DMC?
- Recognize how DMC may vary based on the patient and the clinical setting?
- Identify some ethical issues in end-of-life care?
- Describe medical futility and understand its importance in making ethical decisions?

> HELPFUL TIP: Do "noncompliant" patients make you frustrated and angry? Just internalize the principle of patient autonomy. We can make suggestions, but is up to the patient to decide how to act on our advice. In fact, it is their **right** to do so. Understand this and you will have a lot less heartburn.

QUICK QUIZ: AN ETHICAL DILEMMA

You are seeing George, a 30-year-old, HIV-positive male, for routine care and to assess his HIV status. During your conversation, he mentions that he is in a new relationship, a relationship that he hopes will become long term. They use condoms "some of the time" but have unprotected sex on a regular basis when there is no condom available. When you ask him whether or not he has disclosed his HIV status to his partner, he states that he has not done so and will not do so because of the fear his partner will leave him. He also forbids you to contact his partner to notify her of his HIV status.

Your response in this situation is to:

A) Attempt to convince George to notify his partner of his HIV status.

B) Depending on your state, contact the health department and have them follow up on the patient's sexual contacts.
C) Contact the partner directly and let her know of George's HIV status.
D) Maintain strict confidentiality and do not warn George's partner **nor** report his HIV status regardless of the situation.
E) A, B, and C.

Discussions

The correct answer is "E." "A" is clearly correct. Anything we can do to convince George that it is critical he notify his partner of his HIV status (short of coercion) should be done. "B" is correct but may vary by state. As of this writing, all 50 states and most territories have confidential, name-based reporting for HIV. However, patients can still be tested anonymously which precludes reporting. This can circumvent reporting laws. For this same reason, "D" is incorrect. There are mandatory reporter laws on the books. "C" is also correct. Although this is somewhat controversial and there are conflicting duties (the patient's autonomy and confidentiality vs. the duty to warn the partner), we have a duty to protect the patient's partner. In cases of a direct threat to a known individual, we have a duty to warn the individual. A more clear-cut case would be if George were threatening to shoot his partner and storms out of the office with a gun. While this is a more immediate example, the same principle holds. Clearly, we must not take the breaking of patient confidentiality lightly. And, we must inform the patient of our course of action. You may want to set a time frame for George to notify his partner with the understanding that if he does not do so, you must.

Alternatively, if all we know is that George is HIV positive and have no knowledge of his partner(s), we cannot publicize George's HIV status in order to "protect the public." But if we have a specific name of an ongoing sexual partner, we have a duty to warn that individual which competes with our duty to George.

CASE 2

Robert, a 27-year-old married nurse from your hospital, is referred to your emergency department for an urgent evaluation by his supervisor. In the past 2 weeks, he has been noted to be increasingly distressed while at work, with occasional tearfulness, distractibility, and irritability.

During the initial assessment, Robert reveals that there is a specific reason that he has been so preoccupied. He indicates that 2 weeks ago he was jailed for operating a vehicle while intoxicated and that he feels ashamed. He is afraid that his coworkers have read about it in the newspaper, although no one on his floor has indicated that this is the case. This is his first legal infraction of any kind and he describes it as humiliating.

On further questioning, Robert indicates that he uses alcohol regularly. While it has not overtly affected his work as far as he can tell, it has caused significant marital strife. He reports that his pattern is to stop by the bar on the way home from work to "relax and let go of the hospital stuff that I worry about." He typically drinks three beers and then drives home, where he continues to drink beer throughout the evening. He notes that his wife and kids complain that he is emotionally absent and even irritable with them, but he says that his family simply doesn't understand the stress of the workplace and his need to "forget about it for a few hours." He and his wife have started arguing lately about his alcohol use, especially since the driving charge. He takes special exception to her stating that he is an "alcoholic."

As you take the history, Robert begins to be more guarded in his responses and more restricted in his affect. Suddenly, he blurts out, "I don't think I'm an alcoholic, but I don't want you to put anything in my record about any of this stuff! And I want you to tell my supervisor that there are some personal problems going on at home and that I'll be fine in a few days."

Which of the following statements is TRUE about your obligation with regard to documentation in the chart?

A) You are obligated to document the visit as it occurred so far as the medical facts are concerned, including the concern about alcohol abuse.
B) You can enter incorrect information into the chart in order to protect the patient.
C) You are under no obligation to document anything said and can withhold information from the chart at the patient's request.
D) Hospital administration or legal counsel should be involved if information is going to be purposefully left out of the chart.

Discussion
The correct answer is "A." The ethical principles of beneficence, nonmaleficence, and justice drive the decision here. A patient may legitimately ask for nonactive medical problems (e.g., distant history of sexual abuse) to be withheld from current documentation of an active problem (e.g., allergic rhinitis). However, a patient **cannot** legitimately ask to have information withheld from the record if that information is pertinent to an ongoing condition currently being evaluated and treated. In this case, Robert is receiving care simply by virtue of being seen in the emergency department and disclosing the chief complaint and its associated variables. It is important for you to be forthcoming in explaining why the information may not be withheld from the medical record and also in reassuring him that nonrelevant medical information will be omitted from the record if he feels that this is necessary. For example, the specifics of the argument with a wife need not be detailed beyond the comment that there is nonviolent marital conflict over the patient's alcohol use—important because it supports an alcohol abuse disorder. Furthermore, many institutions have specific policies on managing sensitive medical information and there may be a formal mechanism for increasing the security of the patient's medical record.

Why is protection of confidentiality important in medical practice?

A) It shows respect for patient autonomy.
B) It helps prevent stigmatization and discrimination against patients based on private medical issues.
C) It helps solidify trust within the physician–patient relationship.
D) It helps establish a boundary between the physician–patient relationship and the rest of the medical system.
E) All of the above.

Discussion
The correct answer is "E." The physician–patient relationship is a long-honored tradition in medicine that is increasingly fragile in a medical system with numerous competing obligations. Nevertheless, it is prudent to remember the aspect of the Hippocratic Oath, which states, "What I may see or hear in the course of the treatment... which on no account one must spread abroad, I will keep to myself, holding such things shameful to be spoken about." This is not only important to the tradition of medicine itself but also to the physician–patient relationship. There is no doubt that loss of confidentiality may cause harm to the patient when others are in possession of confidential medical information. Such harms may be as overt as denying medical coverage for certain genetic conditions or as subtle as devaluing a person seen waiting to see the psychiatrist.

Which of the following are legally protected exceptions to the rule of maintaining patient confidentiality?

A) Reporting tuberculosis to public officials without patient consent.
B) Warning a third party at risk of imminent and serious bodily harm from the patient without patient consent.
C) Reporting a patient's alcohol abuse to a work supervisor without the patient's consent.
D) A and B.
E) All of the above.

Discussion
The correct answer is "D." Under current national and state laws, physicians are mandatory reporters of some infectious diseases and of intent to harm another. In most other cases, provision of medical information without the patient's written consent is not legally protected, although there may be cases in which it is felt to be morally justifiable. Physicians need to weigh violations of patient confidentiality very carefully, even when legally sanctioned. Ethicists typically agree that if a physician is going to compromise a patient's confidentiality for an overwhelming moral obligation that, in respect for patient autonomy, the patient needs to be notified. In many situations in which a physician hopes to communicate confidential information to a third party even when the patient is unwilling, a process of education and negotiation with the patient occurs such that respect for autonomy is acknowledged while simultaneously making the patient aware of competing moral obligations.

> HELPFUL TIP: Having a faxed, e-mailed, or mailed report containing a patient's confidential medical information misdirected to an unintended recipient is *not* legally protected. Be cautious about transmission of patient information.

Which of the following interferes with protecting patient confidentiality in the medical structure?

A) Involvement of managed care organizations in patient care and medical payments.
B) Electronic records and transmissions.
C) Group practices and/or teaching hospitals with multiple care providers.
D) A and B.
E) All of the above.

Discussion

The correct answer is "E." While individual physicians and patients continue to prize the tradition of respect for confidentiality, the multiple players in healthcare make it nearly impossible to restrict all information to the dyad of physician and patient. Insurance companies will not provide payment without, at least, information about the diagnosis, and notably, insurance companies are not legally bound by the same legal and ethical codes of conduct regarding patient privacy. Electronic records and transmissions by e-mail, cellular phones, faxes, and other means are much more easily accessed by the curious or unintended recipients who have no reason to have confidential information. Open waiting rooms and multiple providers of care mean that larger and larger numbers of the community are aware that a patient is being seen in certain clinics for certain purposes. While patient records are not often considered a confidentiality issue, the reality is that once information is in written form, it is more difficult to control who might, either now or in the future, have access to the details of the report. For this reason, some physicians try to err on documenting only that which is considered absolutely necessary to patient care, although the distinction between the "absolutely necessary" and unnecessary can be a difficult line to draw in the sand, especially without the ability to appreciate how multiple variables may play out in the patient's future medical care.

* *

Robert is asking you to be deliberately deceptive with the supervisor. You disagree with this.

Which of the following is FALSE?

A) Trust in the physician–patient relationship depends on allowing the patient to make such a directive about communication with outside persons.
B) A physician who establishes a precedent for deception may be expected to practice deception in a future situation in which the harms greatly outweigh the benefits.
C) A physician who deceives may undermine general trust in the profession.
D) B and C.
E) All of the above.

Discussion

The correct answer is "A." Another way of phrasing the question is, "What drives a physician to be honest even when what the patient really wants is not honesty?" Will the patient trust you more if you are deceptive for him? Will this help him (aside from allowing him to keep his job)?

The physician–patient relationship is generally not considered an adequate reason to lie to a third party about the nature of a patient's illness and treatment. There has been concern that a physician who deceives a third party, even in the immediate interest of the patient's confidentiality or other concerns, establishes himself or herself as a physician who may not be trustworthy in other matters. A patient may not consider this at the time a deception is requested. These kinds of ripple effects from the decisions of an individual physician can affect the profession in general, ultimately producing fears that physicians will take the self-serving path rather than the higher moral ground.

* *

You tell Robert that he has alcohol dependence and then provide education about the diagnosis and treatment options. You recommend outpatient treatment in Alcoholics Anonymous (AA) and a chemical dependency program. Robert agrees, more for the sake of his family stability than because of any true insight into the severity of his problem. You then arrange for follow-up with one of your partners (you've been selected as a contestant on the next *Survivor* and get to escape to a tropical island).

At the next appointment, Robert meets his new physician, Dr. Pincus. At this appointment, Robert indicates that he did attend two AA meetings but was very uncomfortable with the aspect of the 12-step program that requires acknowledging a "higher power." Robert indicates that he is an atheist and secular humanist, believing that the locus of self-control comes from within the individual human spirit (or perhaps a bottle of bourbon—depends on his mood). He has refused to continue in AA due to his rejection of its theistic foundation. He has had no further legal problems and reports that work is still going fine, with diminished irritability once he resolved in his mind that his coworkers were unaware of his previous driving violation. However, he continues to drink six to nine alcoholic beverages per night and admits that he occasionally needs a shot of whisky in the morning to "make sure I don't lose it with all the work stress" (this is where his self-control theory really comes together). He also works a night shift about once per week and does use approximately the same amount of alcohol before beginning the night shift, although he denies being intoxicated while on the job on these nights ("six beers just get me started"). He doesn't think this is a problem because "things are quiet at night and everyone just helps each other keep the patients comfortable." He reports that his family is satisfied with the decrease in consumption and that he considers the matter of alcohol abuse resolved.

Dr. Pincus has had her own problems with alcohol in the past. She has had a rocky course over the past many years but found AA to be very helpful. She has become very active in her Jewish synagogue and community, where she receives support and is accountable to her friends. Her own alcohol history has been marked by difficulty with alcohol bingeing, such that when she starts to drink, she drinks to intoxication. Only with aggressive honesty at a professional-group AA as well as a substance abuse protocol through the state board of medical examiners does she feel that she's been able to remain completely abstinent for the last 4 years.

* *

Dr. Pincus is considering revealing to Robert some of her own struggles as a health-care professional with a substance abuse disorder. She believes that this will help him reevaluate the role of AA in sobriety and the importance of very tight control of alcohol consumption to prevent relapsing illness.

Self-disclosure is best described as involving the ethical issues of:

A) Deception and nondisclosure.
B) Privacy and boundaries.
C) Informed consent.
D) Impaired colleagues.
E) Autonomy.

Discussion

The correct answer is "B." There are explicit and implicit boundaries that exist between a physician's private experiences and the physician–patient relationship. One of these boundaries has to do with preventing physician needs and private matters from encroaching into the visit in a way that is not therapeutic to the patient and does not respect the physician's boundaries. While it would appear that Dr. Pincus has therapeutic reasons—for Robert, not for herself—for crossing the boundary of self-disclosure, both physician motivation for self-disclosure and the immediate and potential effects of the self-disclosure need to be weighed very seriously before private matters are revealed. If there is even a potential of harm, crossing the boundary in this way should be considered a violation of professional norms.

How could Dr. Pincus appropriately respond to Robert's refusal to participate in AA on the basis of his religious impulse?

A) "AA is still shown the best intervention for preventing relapsing alcohol use. I hope you can go and get something out of it without acknowledging your acceptance of the 'higher power' explicitly."
B) "AA has important group support from others who understand how difficult it is to stop using alcohol. It is not meant to be religious, but rather a community of care."
C) "I have found both AA and a theistic worldview to be very helpful in understanding my own powerlessness to control some of my behaviors. Would it be helpful to you to hear more about this?"
D) "I understand how the religious aspect of AA is inconsistent with your own philosophy. Would you be willing to investigate nonreligious group meetings for alcohol abusers?"
E) "AA's 'higher power' can be understood as yourself and is not intended as a theistic conception."

Discussion

The correct answer is "D." AA is an example of a prescribed treatment that involves an active religious component. AA's first step involves acknowledgment of a higher power, traditionally invoking a specific monotheistic conception of the divine as a necessity to surrendering the illusion of control. **In the interest of respecting a patient's religious rights in a diverse community and of optimizing treatment options, it would be disrespectful and ineffective to have the patient participate in AA, while ignoring the first step of the program and the foundational**

philosophy of AA. While there are fewer studies about the efficacy of nonreligious alcohol treatment groups, it is appropriate to respect Robert's beliefs by investigating nonreligious alternatives. **As to option "A," the Cochrane database concludes, "No experimental studies unequivocally demonstrated the effectiveness of AA."**

Whether or not self-disclosure of one's own religious beliefs is appropriate is an important question. As mentioned in the Discussion in the question above, it is very important for the physician to measure the intent of the disclosure. Also, physicians need to be exquisitely sensitive to the power differential that exists between a physician and a patient such that strong individual viewpoints might become threatening or coercive in the physician–patient relationship. In certain religious traditions, sharing one's faith is an important step, demonstrating courage and integrity; nevertheless, physicians should be strongly cautioned to pay heed to the virtue of practical wisdom and the unique circumstances of the medical relationship that makes proselytizing most often inappropriate. A better strategy, if a physician feels that a patient might be seeking additional spiritual or philosophical direction, is to ask open-ended questions and then make an appropriate referral to pastoral care or a spiritual counselor who will be sensitive to the issues the patient has raised as relevant.

Which of the following is true about intervening with an "impaired colleague," like Robert?

A) Impairment should be reported only to a state licensing board if the colleague's patients are placed at known and documentable risk.
B) Because alcohol abuse is a confidential matter, it is inappropriate for a treating physician to report a colleague's impairment to a licensing board.
C) Removing a colleague from direct patient care and increasing supervision during patient care are reasonable first-step interventions for a colleague who is actively engaged in substance **treatment** (e.g., a report has already been made).
D) It is preferable to contact a state licensing board directly as opposed to discussing the matter with the patient or institutional administration. This protects both the reporter and the colleague from unnecessary negative repercussions.
E) None of the above.

Discussion

The correct answer is "C." Legal statutes on reporting impaired colleagues vary from state to state, with some state laws making physicians mandatory reporters of impaired physician colleagues, while others simply recommend reporting. Furthermore, state laws are even less prescriptive with regard to nonphysician health professionals with impairments. Any impairment should be treated seriously, preferably with support from the institution's administration. It is imperative to protect patients from harm. While reporting the impaired colleague may result in anger and disappointment from the colleague or even supervisors who are reluctant to tackle such a difficult question, physicians should consider the needs of vulnerable patients and the patients' rights to adequate care.

Confidentiality adds an additional ethical dimension when an impaired colleague reveals his or her impairment to his treating physician. In an effort to respect patient autonomy, physicians will often urge impaired colleagues to report themselves as well as voluntarily engage in treatment protocols. Many states have less-restrictive policies for treatment and monitoring for impaired colleagues who self-report. If a physician intends to report her patient's impairment without the consent of the patient, the physician is obligated to be truthful with the colleague about her intentions and rationale for reporting.

A colleague may be impaired in her practice by which of the following?

A) Substance use.
B) Major depression.
C) Dementia.
D) Deficits knowledge.
E) All of the above.

Discussion

The correct answer is "E." Any one of these, whether acute or chronic, does not automatically imply global impairment in medical practice. However, each may have many implications for a colleague's medical practice. Special attention should be given to the colleague's actual and possible consequences in practice, given her specific job requirements and compensatory skills/supports, while assessing the presence and degree of impairment. One might say that dementia is OK in physicians working for insurance companies (or at least it seems so!!).

Objectives: Did you learn to . . .

- Identify what items are required for inclusion in the medical record?
- Recognize the importance of patient confidentiality and understand when confidentiality might be broken in order to fulfill other ethical obligations?
- Recognize obstacles to protecting patient confidentiality?
- Describe the importance of individual and societal trust in individual physicians and the medical profession as a whole?
- Describe the ethical principles involved in self-disclosure?
- Identify an impaired colleague and determine how to best intervene?

CASE 3

Anne is a 19-year-old single female presenting for her first prenatal visit. She is G1P0, and roughly 10 weeks' gestation by last menstrual period. She is new to your practice. Anne has had no medical care at this facility and no physician appointments since childhood. In recollecting the past medical history, Anne reveals that she has had several first-degree female relatives who have been diagnosed with breast and/or ovarian cancer: her mother, two maternal aunts, and a maternal grandmother. A great aunt also died young of unknown causes. Anne is unsure of the workup that they had, but there was significant morbidity and mortality as a result of the illnesses. Anne only recently became aware of this family history when her mother and aunts were diagnosed in the last 5 years. When you ask if she has discussed genetic risks for breast cancer, Anne looks at you blankly and replies, "No."

Anne has been in a stable relationship with her boyfriend, Jordan, since they were juniors in high school. They cohabitate and are engaged to be married, but have not set a wedding date. Anne has completed high school and has been working in telemarketing while applying to art schools. The pregnancy was not planned, but she and Jordan are thrilled, even if "a little nervous," about having a baby.

You are concerned about the BRCA1 and 2 genes. In families with a high incidence of breast and ovarian cancer, mutations in BRCA1 are associated with an 85% lifetime risk of developing breast cancer and a 50% risk of ovarian cancer.

You wonder if this is the best time to bring up genetic concerns with Anne, given Anne's concurrent transition with an unplanned pregnancy.

Which of the following is/are true about disclosure?

A) Nondisclosure is not justifiable due to fears that a patient will be distressed by the information, unless disclosure might cause death (e.g., suicide at hearing a diagnosis of cancer).
B) Regardless of the consequences, nondisclosure could be considered deception and would be morally wrong on the basis of this intrinsic feature.
C) Disclosure is important because it respects patient autonomy and optimizes a patient's ability to make an informed choice.
D) Nondisclosure may be a sign of paternalism rather than beneficence.
E) All of the above.

Discussion

The correct answer is "E." There are a variety of moral theories used to comment on whether or not deception or nondisclosure is morally appropriate. Most theorists rely on the principle of respect for patient autonomy, such that a person who has incomplete information is not able to act freely in making a choice for herself. "Consequentialism" is also a commonly used moral theory, suggesting that it is not the intrinsic nature of the act itself but the consequences that follow determine whether the act is good or evil (as in "the end justifies the means"). In virtue ethics, by comparison, the nature and motivation of the act are very important as a reflection of the physician's character and habits. In virtue ethics, deception is morally blameworthy because it is comparable to lying. In virtue ethics, motivation is also an important issue to judge the goodness of the action. Answers "B" and "C" both make reference, at least in part, to virtue theory.

Which of the following is FALSE about testing for genetic conditions?

A) Informed consent for genetic testing should be taken more seriously and formally than other kinds of blood testing, such as obtaining a hemogram.

B) Physicians should ask patients what they would do with the different possible outcomes of the genetic test before the test is performed.
C) Physicians should make a recommendation regarding genetic testing guided by evidence-based medicine and the patient's specific narrative and values.
D) Physicians should urge patients to disclose positive results to relatives or spouses if the information is pertinent medically or emotionally to these third parties.
E) Physicians should never disclose genetic information to a third party without the consent of the patient.

Discussion

The correct answer is "E." Genetic testing differs from other blood tests because of multiple actual and potential risks, including personal effects on the patient and her family, as well as discrimination by employers or insurers. There is a shortage of formally trained genetic counselors, and patients rely on their physicians to not only help guide their decision making about whether or not to perform the test, but what to do with the information obtained. Because such testing has profound medical and/or psychosocial effects on the patient and family, a discussion about disclosure should happen both before and after the test is obtained.

Confidentiality is important for many reasons, not only in establishing and maintaining a good physician–patient relationship and respecting patient autonomy but also because of the potential discriminations and misuses of genetic information in today's culture. However, when the risk of harm to another related person is high and the patient refuses to disclose important genetic information, there may be adequate cause to break confidentiality in order to prevent serious harm to the third party; therefore, "E" is a false statement.

HELPFUL TIP: Many diagnostic and screening tests (e.g., HIV antibody, PSA, and biopsies) should be approached in this way, assuring that the patient has a clear understanding of the implications of the test, including further diagnostic testing, therapies, and prognosis.

* *

You decide to disclose the possibility of genetic risk factors to Anne at the first prenatal visit and also discuss the risk of passing genes to the fetus. Anne seems overwhelmed and asks to bring Jordan to the next visit to discuss this further. When Anne returns with her fiancé, you discuss your concerns about the BRCA1 and 2 genes and why Anne's family history is suspicious. Jordan says: "I think you should be tested right away, Anne. This would totally change our future." Anne replies: "What are you saying? Will you leave me if I have the gene? I can't raise this baby by myself!"

Which of the following statements are appropriate to consider in promoting the patient's best interests?

A) Patients are vulnerable.
B) Physicians have expertise that patients lack.
C) Patients rely on their physicians.
D) Physicians and patients often agree on what constitutes a patient's best interests, although they may differ in the way they plan to meet those interests.
E) All of the above.

Discussion

The correct answer is "E." The nature of a relationship between a physician and a patient may have as many permutations as there are individuals. However, it is important to appreciate the position of the patient and the need that has pushed her to seek care. Patients are vulnerable in many ways, and the vulnerability is enhanced by limited access to technologic and scientific information. When external variables, such as Jordan's comment and Anne's response, come into play, physicians should pay attention to this narrative and take some responsibility for establishing and maintaining a supportive network even outside of the office. This is particularly important as physicians give patients information about difficult choices. While physicians and patients may often be able to negotiate a mutually acceptable alternative, an active dialogue is important. Supports and advocates who are familiar with the patient's values and wishes can be an important adjunct to medical decision making, as long as there is no material or psychological conflict of interests. Physicians should not adopt a completely hands-off policy in decision making; rather, physicians should pay attention to supporting the patient with real options and evidence-based variables in a noncoercive, empowering relationship.

* *

Anne decides not to have the test, but to have an elective abortion "just in case I passed on a gene to the baby." For the sake of argument, you are philosophically opposed to elective abortions in this scenario, but you would consider abortion an appropriate intervention if the fetus tests positive for the gene by chorionic villus sampling.

What is the best ethical option for you at this point?

A) Explain that you are personally uncomfortable with abortion, but in deference to Anne's legal rights, you will make a referral to another physician who is willing to provide the elective abortion.
B) Refuse to perform or make a referral for the abortion.
C) Refer to a "pro-life" counseling agency.
D) Tell Anne, for reasons that you do not feel comfortable disclosing, you will no longer be able to care for her.
E) Perform the elective abortion, despite personal convictions, out of respect for the law, and patient autonomy.

Discussion

The correct answer is "A." Abortion is a fiercely contentious topic in the United States. Under the 1973 *Roe v. Wade* decision and in subsequent rulings such as *Planned Parenthood v. Casey*, the Supreme Court has affirmed a woman's legal right to abort a fetus. Physicians have responsibilities that should transcend views about a physician's own moral values, such as ensuring that informed consent is practiced and that the patient has medical care available. Informed consent requires a physician to provide the necessary information about the various medical choices available and to assess the patient's emotional needs. Coercion and failure to disclose clinically relevant information is inappropriate; for example, a referral to a pro-life group without informing the patient of the counseling center's perspective (when known) is a form of manipulation and failure to disclose. Abandoning the patient without a simple explanation is disrespectful, although the physician should be careful not to coerce her in other ways while revealing personal values/beliefs.

Physicians should note that in some states there have been rulings requiring physicians to participate in elective abortions if working in a public aid clinic or in an area with limited physician resources where transfer of care is not an option. Some physicians or institutions (such as Catholic hospitals with clear policies influenced by theological statements) have practiced conscientious objection and been subject to discipline of various forms, including legal sanction. Physicians should be mindful of competing moral values, seeking support and professional guidance in difficult moral and legal cases such that they can act with integrity and purpose in their roles as physicians and moral agents.

* *

Three years later, Anne is seen in a new clinic. She had the abortion. Anne is now an art student and is married to Jordan. Since her last clinic visit, Anne has had a prophylactic mastectomy following a positive test for the BRCA1 gene. She has also had an elective tubal ligation. Anne wants to consider in vitro fertilization (IVF) and has a friend, Jessica, who is willing to donate ova. They put 18 embryos into cold storage, using Jessica's ova and Jordan's sperm. Anne has 6 embryos implanted, with the result of two fetuses that are carried to term. Anne decides that she does not want any more children and contacts the lab to discard the remaining embryos, eliminating storage costs. The lab agrees and sells the embryos to a private lab, where stem cell research is under way.

What is NOT true about stored tissue samples?

A) The embryos are considered Anne's property only as long as she claims them.
B) Samples used for research purposes are potentially identifiable by third parties as belonging to Jessica and Jordan.
C) Tissue samples may be used only for their initial intended purpose, after which time they must be destroyed.
D) Third parties, such as research labs, upon discovering genetic anomalies in tissue samples, have no legal obligation to find and inform Anne, Jordan, and/or Jessica.
E) Embryos sold to a private lab may be used to establish germ lines via destruction of the embryo.

Discussion

The correct answer is "C." At the time of publication, there is ongoing discussion about how to regulate use of tissue samples. While it might seem that this is an ethical question far removed from the purview of the family physician, patients in family practice clinics are very frequently targeted for various research protocols due to their regular follow-up and easy accessibility.

Patients donating tissue samples often give little thought to what happens to those tissues after they are obtained. In many cases, tissues are banked indefinitely after the initial research is conducted, with various identifiers linked to the tissue potentially including the donor's gender, geographic location, educational level, family history, or other private information. While efforts are made to respect the privacy of the donor, it has been established that there are ways to track down the donor using even the limited identification information associated with the stored sample. Such means are especially facilitated by the wide availability of personal information via the Internet.

* *

Tissue samples may be collected for one purpose, but later used for another. Tissue samples are very important in research and are often the limiting factor for studies, but should informed consent include asking donors for permission for each and every lab test run on the tissue sample? At what point, if any, does the tissue sample become the sole property of the lab? In the example of embryos, discarded embryos are sometimes sold to private labs; parents using IVF technology are often unaware that such embryos may be used to establish a stem cell line from which genetically identical embryos can be created using nuclear transfers. Such stem cell lines are highly lucrative for research purposes, and there has been discussion, for example, of whether parents should be compensated in some manner when a lab sells their discarded embryos or a research facility develops a product using the embryonic stem cells.

> HELPFUL TIP: Family physicians should continue to serve as advocates for their patients. You can do so by investigating the policies and procedures of research groups prior to allowing access to patients and by taking some responsibility for the informed consent process when patients are volunteering to participate in research.

Which of the following are concerns about the consequences of human somatic cell nuclear transfer, commonly called human cloning in the lay literature?

A) Will cloning result in increased miscarriages and deformed fetuses, due to limitations of current technology to perform nuclear transfer?
B) Will cloning result in a culture preoccupied with "designer babies?"
C) Will cloning result in a culture that devalues persons with disabilities?
D) Will cloning increase reproductive options for same-sex couples, diminishing value of traditional settings for reproduction?
E) All of the above.

Discussion

The correct answer is "E." All the above choices have been raised as concerns, although there are many more arguments on both sides of the discussion about the relative risks and benefits.

Objectives: Did you learn to . . .

- Describe the ethical issues regarding disclosure?
- Appreciate the many competing interests involved in genetic testing?
- Identify patient and physician factors that affect the patient–physician relationship?
- Find an ethical and acceptable way to disagree with a patient and continue to assure that patient's healthcare?

BIBLIOGRAPHY

American Medical Association. Code of Medical Ethics, updated 2003. Available at http://www.ama-assn.org/ama/pub/category/2503.html.

Beauchamp TL, Childress JF. *Principles of Biomedical Ethics.* 4th ed. New York, NY: Oxford University Press; 1994.

Campbell A, et al. *Medical Ethics.* 3rd ed. South Melbourne, Australia: Oxford University Press; 2001.

Lo B. *Resolving Ethical Dilemmas: A Guide for Clinicians.* 2nd ed. Philadelphia, PA: Lippincott Williams & Wilkins; 2000.

Smith HL, Churchill LR. *Professional Ethics and Primary Care Medicine.* Durham, NC: Duke University Press; 1986.

27

End-of-Life Care

Michelle Weckmann

CASE 1

A 75-year-old male patient is admitted to the hospital for a congestive heart failure (CHF) exacerbation. This is his second admission for CHF within the last 6 months. His nurse asks if he is an appropriate candidate for hospice care.

Which of the following would qualify your patient for the Medicare hospice benefit?

A) His cardiac ejection fraction is 20%, and he is dyspneic with moderate exertion (NYHA class II heart failure).
B) He agrees to a do not resuscitate (DNR) status in the event of cardiorespiratory failure.
C) He needs assistance with ambulation.
D) His implanted cardiac defibrillator (ICD) has fired once in the past year.
E) He has had escalating cardiac hospitalizations despite optimal medical management.

Discussion

The correct answer is "E." Medicare is attempting to make hospice easier for physicians and patients to access. These are the infamous "death panels" that we keep hearing about. If your patient has a terminal disease with declining function, worsening symptoms, worsening laboratory tests, or escalating hospitalizations, he or she probably qualifies for hospice. "A," a low cardiac ejection fraction (typically <20%), is a recommended criterion for heart disease **but must be accompanied by dyspnea at rest** (class IV heart failure). "B" is incorrect. Despite popular belief, a hospice patient need not agree to a DNR status; however, hospice agencies are permitted to have different admission criteria and some require a DNR status for admission. Check with your local hospice agencies. Regardless, you should have a frank discussion with the patient about the role of aggressive resuscitation and the goals of hospice care. "C" is also incorrect. While a decline in functional status is a strong indication of worsening prognosis, it is not automatically a criterion. Most patients with heart failure need assistance with at least four activities of daily living (ADLs) before having a prognosis of <6 months. "D" is incorrect. Patients with ICDs are eligible for hospice, and whether or not it has fired does not impact enrollment decisions. It is important to talk about the ICD, ideally before a patient approaches the final weeks/days of life. Many patients choose to have it disabled once they enroll in hospice. If an ICD is not disabled, it is important that the hospice staff be aware of it and know what to do as it will fire when the patient dies and that can be distressing for both the patient and the family.

> HELPFUL TIP: As opposed to an ICD, a pacemaker does not cause distress (shocks) during the dying process; however, if the patient's cardiac rhythm is completely dependent on the pacemaker, then the pacemaker is considered to be life prolonging.

> HELPFUL TIP: Although prognosis may be the most difficult task a physician faces, an attempt at prognosis in patients with a terminal

illness may help them. The simple question "would you be surprised if this patient died in the next year?" is a good screening tool and has been shown to be a reasonably accurate way to predict who might benefit from a hospice referral.

* *

You think that your patient may be appropriate for hospice and decide that a palliative medicine consult might be useful to address his goals of care, review symptom management, and discuss hospice.

Which statement accurately reflects how palliative medicine is different from hospice?

A) Only palliative medicine affirms life and attempts to help patients live as fully as possible.
B) Palliative medicine offers treatments including aggressive medical treatments such as radiation therapy, intravenous (IV) fluids, or interventional radiologic procedures, while hospice does not.
C) Palliative medicine is performed by a physician only, while hospice care involves an entire team of providers.
D) Both palliative medicine consults and hospice care are reimbursed through the Medicare hospice benefit.
E) Palliative care can be offered at any time during a life-limiting illness, even if a patient is still actively seeking a cure.

Discussion

The correct answer is "E." Palliative care is specialized medical care for people with serious illnesses focused on providing patients with relief from the symptoms, pain, and stress of a serious illness—whatever the diagnosis. The goal is to improve quality of life for both the patient and the family. Palliative care is provided by a team of doctors, nurses, and other specialists who work with a patient's primary team to provide an extra layer of support. Palliative care is appropriate at any age in a serious illness and can be provided together with curative treatment. Hospice care is a type of palliative care, which occurs during the final months of someone's life when cure is no longer possible. "A" is incorrect because both hospice and palliative care strive to make life meaningful and comfortable for patients. "B" is incorrect. Since the goal of both hospice and palliative care is to prevent and relieve suffering, any of these modalities may be used if appropriate. In fact, **any intervention** can be considered palliative if the intention is to relieve distressing symptoms associated with the fatal disease (such as a hip-pinning for pain control after a pathologic fractures). There are no restrictions prohibiting a hospice agency from providing "aggressive" interventions designed to relieve pain and suffering. "C" is incorrect because both hospice and palliative medicine are built on the concept of a team providing care to the patient and family. Hospice care is directed by the primary physician. "D" is incorrect because palliative medicine services are typically billed as inpatient consult services and are reimbursed by Medicare Part A.

Which of the following is TRUE regarding the Medicare home-hospice benefit?

A) The Medicare hospice benefit requires all care related to the primary admitting illness to be covered by the **hospice agency** including physician fees, as long as the physician is not employed by the hospice program.
B) The hospice benefit, similar to the Medicare home care benefit, requires that the patient be homebound.
C) Respite care within an acute hospital setting is provided for up to 5 days every 6 months.
D) Hospice entry requires that the patient cannot live alone (must have an on-site primary caregiver).
E) A flat per diem rate is paid to the licensed hospice program regardless of the level of services provided.

Discussion

The correct answer is "A." The Medicare hospice benefit requires all care related to the primary admitting illness to be covered by the hospice agency: Think of it as capitated care. However, Medicare affords individual hospice agencies wide latitude in determining what modalities they use to treat the symptoms of a particular illness. For example, one agency might allow blood transfusions for the relief of dyspnea, while another agency only covers the use of medications such as morphine or lorazepam for dyspnea. If necessary for acute symptom management, Medicare also covers acute hospitalizations related to the primary illness. "B" is incorrect. A hospice patient does not need to be homebound. Respite care can be offered as frequently as needed, which makes "C" incorrect. The Medicare hospice benefit provides respite care. This can last up to five nights at a time. The respite care needs to be provided in a setting where there is a registered nurse available continuously, and the patient must come from a home setting (including assisted living). This can be used if the caregiver needs a vacation or is otherwise unable to care for the patient. "D" is incorrect because Medicare does not require that the patient have a primary caregiver in the home to receive the hospice benefit; however, an individual hospice agency may require a primary caregiver be identified before enrolling a patient. "E" is incorrect because Medicare pays the hospice organization a stratified per diem rate depending on the level of care the patient requires.

* *

After meeting with the palliative care team, your patient's family inquires more about hospice care. They ask what other services are covered.

The Medicare hospice benefit includes coverage for all of the following expenses EXCEPT:

A) Medications related to symptom management.
B) Social work visits.
C) Home health aid services.
D) Room and board for a patient living in a nursing home.
E) Bereavement services.

Discussion

The correct answer is "D." All of the other options listed are services covered under the Medicare hospice benefit. A patient living in a nursing home **is eligible** for hospice care, but the cost of room and board for the nursing home is not paid by the hospice benefit. In some special circumstances, nursing home care will be paid for a short duration (e.g., when a hospice patient uses the five-night respite care benefit or if the patient is admitted to a nursing home for management of a distressing symptom that cannot be controlled in the home setting).

* *

A few months go by and your patient has again been hospitalized. You now believe that he has fewer than 6 months to live. The local hospice medical director reviews the case and agrees. The patient is dyspneic at rest and, requires 24-hour oxygen by nasal cannula, and his cardiac ejection fraction has decreased to 15%. He wishes to avoid further hospitalization and has elected to have a DNR status. His family wants to know what you can do when he becomes severely dyspneic.

Which of the following is appropriate palliative treatment of severe dyspnea in this patient?

A) Intubation and ventilation.
B) Morphine.
C) Scopolamine.
D) Buspirone.
E) Hyperventilating into a paper bag.

Discussion

The correct answer is "B." Morphine and other opioids are indicated for palliation of dyspnea in cardiac failure. Despite concerns about opioids worsening respiratory function in end-stage heart failure, studies have concluded that oral morphine improves dyspnea in this patient population and does not cause respiratory failure or hasten death. This is supported by recommendations from the American College of Cardiology and the American Heart Association. If you choose "A," his ghost will be back to haunt you. This patient has chosen a far less aggressive stance toward life-prolonging measures, and his wishes should be honored. "C" is incorrect. Scopolamine is used to reduce pharyngeal secretions (resulting in sonorous respirations) but is not likely to relieve dyspnea in this patient. "D" is incorrect. While anxiety and dyspnea often occur together and exacerbate each other, buspirone (BuSpar) is a weak anxiolytic and has no direct effect on dyspnea. Low-dose lorazepam would be a reasonable alternative if you felt his dyspnea was complicated by anxiety. And "E" is just plain wrong—although still not as bad a choice as "A."

> HELPFUL TIP: Benzodiazepines may be used in combination with narcotics for added relief of dyspnea and anxiety. The patient should be monitored for excessive sedation and respiratory depression.

Objectives: Did you learn to . . .

- Identify appropriate patients for end-of-life care, particularly for the Medicare hospice benefit?
- Describe the features of the Medicare hospice benefit?

- Treat patients with dyspnea related to end-stage cardiac disease?

QUICK QUIZ: PAIN RELIEF

A 30-year-old male patient you have known for several years was diagnosed with metastatic melanoma several months ago. He presents now with intermittent, severe headaches associated with nausea. A head CT scan performed last week showed three metastatic foci with surrounding edema. He currently takes maximum doses of acetaminophen and large doses of morphine.

What is the best treatment option to help relieve his headache and nausea?

A) Neurosurgical intervention.
B) Dexamethasone.
C) Sumatriptan.
D) Ibuprofen.
E) Increased morphine doses.

Discussion

The correct answer is "B." Corticosteroids are the preferred therapy for headaches due to increased intracranial pressure from edema, as is presumably the case here. Whole brain or stereotactic radiation therapy, alone or in combination with corticosteroids, may also be used as palliative therapy for multiple brain metastases. "A" is incorrect because neurosurgical consultation for craniotomy should be reserved for patients who fail other interventions or who present with rapidly worsening symptoms. "C" and "D" are incorrect. Sumatriptan and ibuprofen should not be used to treat increased intracranial pressure. "E," increased morphine doses, may be required, but corticosteroids are typically used first.

CASE 2

A 74-year-old female was diagnosed with adenocarcinoma of the colon 3 years prior to beginning hospice care. She has known metastases to her liver and pelvis. She complains of a cramping pain in her abdomen and a "deep pain" in her groin. She is currently receiving morphine 10 mg PO every 4 hours (except when asleep) and acetaminophen 650 mg PO TID. She says that her pain is 4 out of 10 on a numeric pain scale. Her past medical history includes hemorrhage secondary to a gastric ulcer 4 years ago (*Helicobacter pylori* negative on biopsy).

Which of the following strategies is the best next step for improving this patient's pain control?

A) Start gabapentin to treat the neuropathic aspect of her pain.
B) Add a strong nonsteroidal anti-inflammatory drug (NSAID) such as ketorolac (Toradol) to her current regimen.
C) Add scheduled tramadol to try to decrease her morphine use.
D) Start a long-acting morphine (e.g., MS Contin) at a dose 20% higher than her current morphine use.
E) Maximize the dose of acetaminophen to 1000 mg every 4 hours.

Discussion

The correct answer is "D." The patient is taking short-acting opioids around the clock, which can lead to "chasing the pain" (not to be confused with "chasing the dragon" that is inhaling heroin smoke, which leads to a leukoencephalopathy.... you never know.... it could be on the test!). Patients often receive much better pain control when they are maintained on a long-acting opioid. It is common practice to increase the dose of opioids by 15–25% when a patient's pain is only partially controlled. It is then recommended to have the breakthrough dose equivalent to 10% of her 24-hour use. "A" is incorrect since her pain is better described as visceral or somatic rather than neuropathic. Gabapentin is an OK choice for neuropathic pain (TCAs are betters) but will likely not be effective for this patient. "B" is incorrect. Ketorolac is the NSAID with the highest rate of renal disease and gastrointestinal (GI) bleeds and is contraindicated in a patient who has had a GI bleed. If you were to add an NSAID, ibuprofen would be a better choice, and GI protection with a PPI would be advisable for this patient. "C" is incorrect. Tramadol is a nonnarcotic that is much less efficacious than morphine, and it is not likely to benefit a patient with severe pain from her cancer and metastases. Tramadol also has a number of troubling side effects such as an increased risk of seizures and serotonin syndrome. "E" is incorrect because the current recommended daily maximum dose of acetaminophen for elderly patients is 3000 mg (don't blame us... blame the FDA), and the frequency suggested in "E" would far exceed this amount.

* *

When determining what medications are appropriate for treating pain, it helps to know what type of pain the patient has.

Cancer is known to cause which type(s) of pain?

A) Neuropathic pain.
B) Visceral pain.
C) Soft tissue/bony pain.
D) Pain from increased intracranial pressure.
E) All of the above are types of pain.

Discussion

The correct answer is "E." Physiologic pain is separated into four categories: soft tissue or bony pain (also called somatic pain), neuropathic pain, visceral pain, and the pain of increased intracranial pressure. An example of somatic pain is the musculoskeletal pain (e.g., sports injuries and fractures) that everyone experiences at some point. Neuropathic pain is generally described as burning and results from nerve damage, inflammation, and compression. Visceral pain includes pain from capsular distention (e.g., liver enlargement from metastases, and colicky pain from the colon). Depending on where a metastasis or primary tumor is located, it may cause somatic pain (e.g., bone tumors), neuropathic pain (e.g., Pancoast tumor), visceral pain, or a headache from increased intracranial pressure.

HELPFUL TIP: Avoid using meperidine (Demerol). It has toxic metabolites that may cause agitation and seizures. Meperidine can also interact with a number of drugs to cause serotonin syndrome.

* *

You decide to increase her morphine dose.

Which of the following statements is TRUE?

A) IV morphine is 10 times more potent than oral morphine.
B) Naloxone should be given if a patient near death demonstrates confusion, decreased responsiveness, a slowed respiratory rate, or cool extremities.
C) Patients exhibiting a local rash or intense pruritus at the site of IV morphine administration must be considered allergic and given an alternate narcotic.
D) Tolerance to morphine does not occur in patients with cancer, so any increased analgesic need is due solely to unmet pain.
E) Renal and hepatic insufficiency both contribute to the accumulation of morphine and its metabolites.

Discussion

The correct answer is "E." "A" is incorrect. IV morphine is about three times as potent as oral morphine. "B" is incorrect. Patients who are within several days or hours of death often exhibit pallor, peripheral vasoconstriction, apneic episodes, and obtundation as part of the physiologic process of dying. Counseling the family and the dying patient is preferable to administering naloxone, which can cause abrupt opioid withdrawal and significant distress and discomfort to the patient (again... don't make her ghost haunt you). "C" is also incorrect. Local histamine release is a known effect of IV morphine administration. Histamine-mediated skin changes proximal to the IV infusion site of morphine do not represent a contraindication to future morphine use. In fact, antihistamines (e.g., diphenhydramine) can be used to counter morphine-related histamine effects, such as rash, itching, and hypotension. "D" is incorrect. All patients can develop tolerance to the effects of morphine. Of course, in patients with terminal cancer, increasing opioid requirements are often entirely due to increasing pain. And even if your dying patient develops morphine tolerance, you still need to treat the pain. Finally, "E" is correct. Patients with renal and hepatic insufficiency can accumulate metabolites of morphine, some of which are helpful in pain control and others of which may have an antianalgesic effect. These patients often need **lower** doses of opioids. If a patient is actively dying and has evidence of renal failure, opioid doses can often be decreased significantly without a worsening of pain control. Fentanyl and methadone are considered the safest opioids in renal failure.

HELPFUL TIP: Start patients on a regimen to prevent constipation when initiating opioids. Think about the bowel regimen each time you increase the opioid dose. It will save you and your patient a lot of grief in the long run.

HELPFUL TIP: For patients whose pain cannot be controlled with typical treatments, low-dose ketamine, infusion or oral, can control pain without causing dissociation.

Which of the following statements is NOT accurate regarding the appropriate use of opioids in end-of-life situations?

A) At times, delirium can be improved with opioid dosage reduction and/or the addition of opioid-sparing analgesics (e.g., acetaminophen).
B) If oral morphine cannot be swallowed, then either an enteral feeding tube or a parenteral route (IM/IV/subcutaneous) must be used.
C) Dosage conversion from one opioid to another is affected by the type of opioid used and the route of administration.
D) Transdermal opioid delivery products are expensive, have a slow onset of action, and have erratic absorption.
E) There is no preestablished ceiling dosage for opioids, and you may increase the opioid dose until adverse side effects occur.

Discussion

The correct answer (and the false statement) is "B." Concentrated oral morphine solutions (20 mg/mL) can be given in small amounts to patients who are unable to swallow. While it was previously thought that morphine elixir worked by absorption through the buccal mucosa, it is now believed to trickle down the throat to be absorbed through the gastric mucosa. Since concentrated morphine elixir is effective in patients who cannot swallow, feeding tubes or parenteral routes of administration are unnecessary. "A" is true. Delirium is a common and disturbing finding toward the end of life, and it is sometimes precipitated or exaggerated by opioids. On the flip side, untreated pain can cause delirium, and the delirium may improve when opioid doses are escalated. In these situations, it can be helpful to rotate opioids because the lack of cross-tolerance means that the dose can often be decreased while maintaining the same level of pain control. Acetaminophen is the safest opioid-sparing analgesic, and its adjuvant action may allow for opioid dosage reduction without a loss of overall analgesia. In the appropriate patient, NSAIDs may also be used. "C" is true. When a patient chronically taking one opioid switches to another, a dose adjustment calculation must be made. You cannot switch milligram for milligram. Also, some authorities recommend that after the calculation, you slightly reduce the dose of the new narcotic due to incomplete cross-tolerance. (refer to narcotic dose conversion charts available in numerous pharmaceutical texts and handbooks.) "D" is true. The transdermal fentanyl patches, though convenient, have fluctuating bioavailability over the three days that each patch is worn, and breakthrough doses of an alternative opioid should be available. The fentanyl patches are expensive and initially have a slow onset until a steady state is achieved. For this reason, a fentanyl patch should never be used alone as an initial treatment of acute pain. "E" is true. Because of the extraordinarily wide dosage range of opioids, the ceiling dosage cannot be calculated or assumed. Rather, analgesic requirements allow for continual increase unless adverse side effects clearly undermine the use of the drug.

HELPFUL TIP: There is no consistent relationship between blood levels of morphine and analgesic effects. This is because of tolerance, individual variability in drug effect, etc. Thus, there is no single "right" dose. You should titrate morphine to the desired effect while watching for side effects.

* *

You increase the morphine dose considerably over a 2-week period and your patient begins having escalating pain and muscle twitching.

Which statement is true about opioid-induced hyperalgesia (OIH)?

A) Patients with OIH always become delirious.
B) When a patient has OIH, the pain does not change when the opioid dose is increased.
C) The pain in OIH is described as a worsening of the original pain being treated.
D) OIH needs to be differentiated from worsening underlying disease and pseudotolerance.

Discussion

The correct answer is "D." Before we presume that a patient has OIH, we need to ensure that the increase in pain is not due to further disease progression. We also need to consider additional increased pain resulting from increased activity or other exacerbation (such as trips to x-ray). Additional features that can help distinguish OIH from increased pain include the development of muscle twitching, presence of allodynia (pain elicited from ordinarily nonpainful stimuli, such as stroking skin with cotton), and development of seizures or delirium. However, not all patients with OIH become delirious, making "A" incorrect. The key feature of OIH is that the pain increases as the dose of the opioid is increased and will decrease when the dose is decreased. We are not certain why OIH occurs but several mechanisms have been proposed. "C" is incorrect as well. OIH typically produces diffuse pain, less defined in quality and extending beyond the preexisting pain distribution.

* *

You are concerned about OIH and you decide to rotate to methadone.

Which of the following statements is FALSE regarding the use of methadone?

A) Methadone can be legally prescribed for pain and addiction by a physician with a current schedule II DEA license.
B) Methadone is more easily absorbed by those with bowel problems than is sustained-release morphine.
C) The half-life of methadone is 22 hours.
D) Methadone may be useful for neuropathic pain because it inhibits receptors in the dorsal horn of the spine.
E) Methadone is primarily excreted in the stool and thus drug dosages do not need to be modified in those with mild to moderate renal disease.

Discussion

The correct answer (and false statement) is "A." Methadone **can** be prescribed for pain control by physicians with a schedule II DEA license but **cannot** be prescribed for opiate withdrawal or maintenance without a special license. "B" and "C" are true. Methadone has a long half-life, and sustained-release preparations are not needed. Sustained-release morphine may pass unabsorbed in patients with short gut or dysfunctional gut, whereas methadone would be absorbed. "D" is true; methadone may be especially useful in treating neuropathic pain. "E" is also true. Methadone is primarily excreted into the GI tract. Patients with liver disease should have doses adjusted. However, those with renal disease may tolerate "normal" doses since renal excretion is a minor part of methadone elimination.

HELPFUL TIP: Since methadone interacts at the NMDA receptors, it is the opioid of choice for neuropathic pain, which is often poorly responsive to other opioids. Additionally, methadone is the only **long-acting** opioid that comes in a liquid form and can be given buccally or in an enteral tube. Methadone can be dosed every 8–12 hours with many pain patients requiring Q 8 hours dosing. Remember that methadone prolongs the QT in high doses and can cause torsades de pointes.

Which of the following is TRUE regarding the use of the fentanyl patch?

A) The fentanyl patch is not as effective on the skin of cachectic patients due to lack of subcutaneous fat.
B) The fentanyl patch can be titrated upward in dosage every 24 hours in patients with escalating pain.
C) Alternative analgesics should be continued for 12 hours after fentanyl patch placement.
D) Fentanyl will cease to be absorbed from subcutaneous tissue into the blood immediately after patch removal.

Discussion

The correct answer is "C." A previously administered opioid should not be discontinued immediately upon placing the first fentanyl patch because of the delayed time to onset of pain relief. Patients typically need their previous pain medication continued for at least 12 hours after placement of the fentanyl patch. "A" is incorrect since there is no evidence to support the prevailing wisdom that a normal amount of subcutaneous fat is necessary. "B" is incorrect because the delayed action of the patch requires that dosage adjustment occurs every 48–72 hours. "D" is incorrect because fentanyl continues to be delivered up to 12 hours after patch removal.

HELPFUL TIP: An opioid-naive patient should never be started on a fentanyl patch. A patient needs to be taking an oral morphine equivalent of at least 25 mg in 24 hours before the lowest dose (12.5 μg) fentanyl patch can be applied.

* *

As time goes on, the patient has other concerns including constipation, weight loss of 20 pounds over 2 months, sleeplessness, nausea, and anxiety. In addition, she expresses how her loss of functional abilities is a hardship for her and her adult daughter who serves as her primary caregiver. Her guilt for losing her health is a continual source of frustration and anger.

What is true regarding her social and emotional pain?

A) It will not affect the patient's analgesic requirements.
B) It will likely complicate treatment adherence.
C) Active treatment of emotional sources of pain should occur after the physical source has been addressed and treated.
D) Prophylactic antidepressants in patients within 6 months of death decrease the probability of developing depression.

Discussion

The correct answer is "B." Adherence, always an issue, is especially compromised in those dying patients whose social, spiritual, and emotional problems are not effectively addressed. Similarly, analgesic control of somatic pain is complicated when social, emotional, and spiritual sources of pain exacerbate the patient's response and perception to her somatic pain. Concurrent treatment of all sources of pain is necessary. Antidepressant therapy in dying patients who do not have clinical depression offers no prophylaxis against the development of depression.

* *

You estimate your patient's life expectancy to be 2 months or less. Her frailty has progressed to the point where she is bedbound and utterly dependent for all her ADLs. You have made some adjustments, and she is now taking the following medications:

Hydromorphone (Dilaudid) 20 mg PO Q 4 hours
Acetaminophen 1000 mg PO TID
Sorbitol 30 cc PO TID
Metoclopramide 20 mg PO TID

You want to consolidate her medications.

Which of the following is the most appropriate medication adjustment to make at this time?

A) Hydromorphone → scheduled **controlled** release morphine.
B) Hydromorphone → scheduled **immediate** release morphine.
C) Hydromorphone → scheduled controlled release morphine and immediate release morphine as needed.
D) Acetaminophen → immediate release morphine.
E) Acetaminophen → nortriptyline.

Discussion

The correct answer is "C." A patient who has reached a stable dose of short-acting narcotic, such as hydromorphone, should subsequently be switched to a long-acting narcotic agent. An immediate release medication should be available for acute pain or "breakthrough" pain. There is no reason to change the acetaminophen. Nortriptyline is sometimes useful as an adjuvant medication and is particularly helpful when treating neuropathic pain.

* *

The hospice nurse calls you. Your patient is at home and has become restless with slow respirations (6/minute) along with paroxysmal coughing and gagging with a large amount of secretions.

The following are all appropriate orders for this patient EXCEPT:

A) A subcutaneous infusion pump and syringe to provide medications and, if necessary, fluids.
B) Lorazepam 1–2 mg PO or SL Q 1 hour PRN.
C) Scopolamine transdermal patches changed every 3 days.
D) Midazolam 0.4–4 mg SC Q 1 hour PRN.
E) Naloxone 2 mg SC Q 2 hours PRN.

Discussion

The correct answer is "E." Naloxone is a potent opioid receptor antagonist. Although the sudden change in the patient's status could be partly due to narcotic accumulation, the risks of naloxone antagonism are great and include severe pain, cardiac arrhythmias, and seizures (remember, you don't want that ghost haunting you). Withholding or reducing the next dose of opioids is a safer approach. "A" is correct. A subcutaneous infusion pump may allow effective administration of medications and fluids in patients who cannot tolerate oral administration. The use of hydration at the end of life is debatable. Withholding of fluids and nutrition has strong merit, but the evidence is not compelling enough to declare that fluid infusion is futile and possibly harmful in this setting. In addition, dehydration is a common cause of delirium at the end of life and her confusion may improve with gentle hydration. It is more important to review the patient's goals and only administer fluids if that is consistent with her goals. "C" is correct. Scopolamine patches have been shown to decrease oral/pulmonary secretions that lead to the "death rattle" in the final days and hours of life. Such treatment benefits the patient and her grieving family and friends. "B" and "D" may also be useful. Benzodiazepines have the potential to reduce anxiety, agitation, and insomnia; however, any benzodiazepine can worsen confusion and cause delirium. In addition, benzodiazepines with an extended half-life (e.g., diazepam and chlordiazepoxide) should generally be avoided because of the potential for toxic accumulation.

> HELPFUL TIP: When using scopolamine patches to control secretions at the end of life, you can apply up to three patches at a time; however, if a patient is still aware and alert, using more than one patch can cause delirium. An alternative for secretion control in a patient able to take oral medications is glycopyrrolate (Robinul), an anticholinergic that does not cross the blood–brain barrier as readily as atropine and scopolamine.

Objectives: Did you learn to . . .

- Define major physiologic pain categories?
- Describe the pharmacology of pain control?
- Prescribe narcotic pain medications and adjuvant therapies?
- Identify emotional, social, and spiritual symptoms and recognize how they can affect pain management?

QUICK QUIZ: THE SUBCUTANEOUS ROUTE

Regarding the subcutaneous administration of fluids and medications, which of the following is true?

A) Not more than 500 cc of saline per day can be given by hypodermoclysis (subcutaneous administration).
B) Only medication with low lipid solubility can be delivered via subcutaneous administration.
C) Most drugs used in end-of-life care can be given subcutaneously.
D) In general, subcutaneous administration dosage conversion is closer to oral dosage than to IV dosage.

Discussion

The correct answer is "C." The subcutaneous route can be quite effective. Adverse events such as local irritation, pulmonary edema, and local edema are often less frequent with subcutaneous administration when compared with IV administration. In general, most drugs used in end-of-life care can be given subcutaneously. "A" is incorrect. Evidence demonstrates that up to 3000 cc of crystalloid solution can be given subcutaneously in a 24-hour period with limited adverse effects. Experience suggests that even greater volumes can be given. "B" is incorrect. Lipid solubility is not a clinically relevant aspect of bioavailability during subcutaneous administration. "D" is also not true. Subcutaneous doses are generally very close to, but lower than, the IV dose of a drug. As with IV administration, the onset of action is more rapid than with enteral dosing.

CASE 3

You assume care for the 84-year-old father of one of your patients. He has severe dementia, which has caused him to require nursing home care for the last 5 years. He has stable heart failure due to ischemic cardiomyopathy. He requires full assistance to eat, which the staff members spend an hour doing at each meal. He has lost 20 pounds in the last 6 months (BMI now is 21). A facility nurse calls you worried about his weight.

What would be the best recommendation for weight gain in this patient?

A) Megestrol.
B) Nutritional supplements.
C) Dronabinol.
D) Mirtazapine.
E) Feeding tube.

Discussion

The correct answer is "B." The most effective means to maintain weight in elderly patients with dementia is hand feeding, which is expensive and often problematic in nursing homes with limited staff. When hand feeding is not effective, nutritional supplements are the least invasive alternative with minimal side effects and have been shown to be modestly effective in promoting weight gain in elderly patients with dementia. "A," megestrol (Megace), is minimally effective in improving appetite and increasing weight in patients with cancer cachexia and weight loss related to AIDS, but there is sparse evidence for use in geriatric patients. Trials are of short duration (1–2 months) using widely varying amounts of megestrol (240–1600/day), and the weight gained is typically not muscle mass. With such poor evidence for benefit but well-known side effects, there is no role for megestrol in this setting. In fact, there is no role for hormones or steroids in the treatment of weight loss in the elderly patient with dementia. "B," dronabinol, is synthetic derivative of cannabis. It increases appetite and improves nausea, but again the studies are small and exploratory in nature and focused mainly on patients with AIDS and cancer. "D" is incorrect. If the patient were depressed and losing weight as a result, mirtazapine might be a reasonable choice since it may stimulate appetite. However, mirtazapine has not been shown to boost appetite in nondepressed subjects (and like the SSRIs does not improve depression in the demented elderly anyway, *Lancet*. 2011;378: 403-411). Some antidepressants, such as SSRIs and bupropion, are associated with **weight loss**. Finally, a feeding tube is invasive with numerous side effects. *While enteric tube feeds may improve caloric intake, they do not extend life, increase weight, or reduce the incidence of pressure sores or aspiration.* Thus, "E" is incorrect.

* *

Your nutrition shakes are not doing the trick. The patient continues to lose weight. To further stage his dementia, you attempt a Folstein Mini Mental Status Exam, but he cannot participate. The nurse reports that he needs assistance with all ADLs, he is incontinent, and he is unable to speak more than six intelligible words (and although you remember a couple of post-call days when you were in the same condition, you say nothing). The nursing staff asks you if the patient is appropriate for hospice care.

Which of the following is TRUE?

A) The life trajectory of terminally demented patients is unclear. Wait until his cardiac disease worsens.
B) He does not yet meet Medicare hospice benefit criteria for dementia.
C) A history from the nursing staff or family regarding the rate of his functional loss is the best predictor of death.
D) The nursing home staff can provide all of the end-of-life services provided by hospice.
E) Presence of a stage 2 pressure ulcer and aspiration risk is sufficient for referral to hospice.

Discussion

The correct answer is "C." Predicting death in patients with dementing illness is difficult which is why it is one of most underutilized diagnoses for referral to hospice care. However, waiting until a more predictable organ system failure occurs is not a reason for delaying a hospice referral, which makes "A" incorrect. "B" is incorrect because he *does* meet criteria for hospice enrollment. The National Hospice and Palliative Care Organization (NHPCO) hospice guidelines for eligibility in dementia include (1) severe dementia (needs assistance with all ADLs, incontinent), (2) unable to speak more than six intelligible words, and (3) either unexplained weight loss or a severe premorbid condition in the past 6 months (i.e., aspiration pneumonia, pyelonephritis, and septicemia). "E" is incorrect. Aspiration risk and stage 2 pressure ulcers are not sufficient for referral to hospice. If the patient had stage 3 or 4 pressure ulcers, he would likely meet NHPCO hospice criteria for severe dementia. It is the extrapolation of the patient's loss of basic functions over time that best predicts death, as in answer "C." Answer "D" is incorrect because while most nursing homes routinely care for dying patients

Table 27–1 CAUSES AND TREATMENT OF NAUSEA AND EMESIS

Type of Nausea	Receptors Causing Nausea	Useful Drug Classes	Examples of Drugs of Choice
V Vestibular	Cholinergic Histaminic	Anticholinergic Antihistaminic	Scopolamine Promethazine
O Obstruction (caused by constipation)	Cholinergic Histaminic 5-HT_3?	Stimulate myenteric plexus	Senna products Prunes
M Dysmotility	Cholinergic Histaminic 5-HT_3?	Prokinetics to stimulate 5-HT_4 receptors	Metoclopramide
I Infection, inflammation	Cholinergic Histaminic 5-HT_3?	Anticholinergic Antihistaminic	Promethazine
T Toxins (stimulating the CTZ in the brain, i.e., opioids)	Dopamine 2 5-HT_3	Antidopaminergic 5-HT_3 antagonist	Prochlorperazine Haloperidol Ondansetron

5-HT_3, 5-hydroxytryptamine (serotonin); CTZ, chemoreceptor trigger zone.

without the assistance of hospice, they are typically not able to offer the full range of services or the end-of-life expertise that hospice offers.

* *

Your patient develops nausea and vomiting and on exam you feel a large abdominal mass. He is still having bowel movements, which are guaiac positive. You inform the family that you suspect he has colon cancer and they elect for no further evaluation but want his symptoms aggressively managed.

Which of the following drugs is the best initial choice for treatment of this patient's nausea and vomiting?

A) Octreotide.
B) Metoclopramide.
C) Diphenhydramine.
D) Ondansetron (Zofran).
E) Aprepitant (Emend).

Discussion

The correct answer is "D." "B" is not correct. Using a pro-peristaltic agent in a patient who may have an obstruction is not a good idea in general. Also, metoclopramide has central antidopaminergic properties and can cause confusion and extrapyramidal side effects. By understanding the pathophysiology of nausea and targeting antiemetics to specific receptors, therapy can be optimized and side effects minimized. An easy way to remember the causes of vomiting is to use the "VOMIT" mnemonic. In Table 27–1, pathophysiologic mechanisms causing nausea are described using the letters of the mnemonic. Blockade of these receptors allows rational, focused therapy.

Using Table 27–1 another reasonable alternative would be promethazine, although promethazine is not a great antiemetic. "A" is incorrect. Octreotide works by slowing the GI, and its main use is found in patients with nausea and vomiting due to malignancy-related intestinal obstruction. However, it does not rapidly treat nausea and is not easily administered (usually continuous IV infusion but can be given subcutaneously). "C" is incorrect because diphenhydramine alone is a weak antiemetic, mostly used for motion sickness, and it can cause confusion, particularly in the elderly. Aprepitant (Emend) is a neurokinin receptor antagonist that is most effective when used with serotonin receptor antagonists; its primary use is in the management of chemotherapy-induced nausea; and it is very expensive.

HELPFUL TIP: When treating chemotherapy-induced nausea, add something to their current regimen. Do not just drop one medication and add another. This is counterintuitive but is considered the approach of choice.

* *

The patient's nausea is ultimately controlled with scheduled low-dose promethazine and metoclopramide (See? Two drugs instead of a large dose of one . . . .). He is continuing to lose weight and has been coughing after eating. He spikes a fever and you suspect he has developed aspiration pneumonia.

Which is true regarding the use of antibiotics in patients with terminal dementia?

A) Antibiotic use is considered the standard of care and should be initiated without discussing with the family.
B) Antibiotics can prolong patients' life but the treatment can cause increased pain, depression, anxiety, and depression.
C) Antibiotics given in a controlled setting such as a nursing home, where compliance can be ensured, leads to less antibiotic resistance.
D) Parenteral or intramuscular antibiotics are more successful at treating aspiration pneumonia in patients with dementia.

Discussion

The correct answer is "B." The previous prevailing belief of carte blanche use is being challenged. Currently, antibiotic use is very common in nursing homes, and a majority of nursing home residents will receive antibiotics in the 2 weeks before their death. Most of those antibiotics will be given intravenously, which increases patient discomfort. "A" is incorrect because antibiotic use in patients with dementia (specifically in patients with dementia who are hospice appropriate) should always be discussed with the surrogate decision maker, and antibiotic use should be based on an informed choice and the patient's wishes/goals. While antibiotics have been shown to prolong life in patients with dementia, they do so with the cost of increasing discomfort, making "B" the correct answer. Families need this information when deciding if antibiotics should be used. "C" is incorrect because nursing homes have been shown to harbor drug-resistant bacteria, likely due in part to the frequent use of antibiotics in these patients. Oral antibiotics have been shown to be as effective as other more invasive administration routes in patients with dementia, making "D" incorrect.

* *

The patient is enrolled in hospice and 3 weeks later you are called by the nursing home nurse who reports an acute condition change. You go to see the patient and he is unresponsive, breathing is labored, and his feet are mottled.

All of the following can be signs of impending death EXCEPT:

A) Cheyne–Stokes breathing.
B) Fever.
C) Cyanosis and mottling.
D) Aldosterone escape phenomenon with increased urinary output.
E) Talking to someone who is already dead (and not via medium at Coney Island).

Discussion

The correct answer is "D." Most dying patients have a decrease in urinary output prior to death. The other answers describe changes that are commonly seen in patients who are actively dying. Respiratory changes in the active dying phase include Cheyne–Stokes breathing, terminal secretions (the "death rattle"), and periods of apnea. Dying is often accompanied by decreased circulation, which can result in cool extremities and mottling (the skin turning blue and patchy particularly in the fingers and toes). It is not uncommon for a dying patient to have a fever in the last 24–48 hours of life, typically thought to be secondary to aspiration pneumonia or urosepsis. It is not uncommon for someone who is dying to talk about going on a journey or talk about seeing someone who is dead. This is typically believed to be part of the normal dying process and in the absence of other symptoms should not be confused with delirium or psychosis.

HELPFUL (OR AT LEAST INTERESTING) TIP: A visit from Oscar the (therapy) cat in a Rhode Island nursing home has proved to be a very accurate predictor of imminent death (really) (*N Engl J Med.* 2007;357:328). Presumably, Oscar is reacting to the lack of patient movement or the smell of ketones, etc. Then again, Oscar could be the Angel of Death in a wolf's (well, cat's) clothing.

HELPFUL TIP: Delirium is very common (up to 85%) in the last few days of life. If the symptoms are distressing to the patient or family, it is best treated with an antipsychotic such as haloperidol.

* *

You need to call the son to tell him of his father's decline.

Which of the following should you say when giving the son an update?

A) "There have been some changes in your father's condition. I think you should go to see him. Call me if you have any questions after you have seen your dad."
B) "Good news, your dad will soon be out of his misery and released from this mortal coil."
C) "I'm afraid I have some bad news for you regarding your dad. Would you like to talk over the phone or meet at my office later today to discuss it?"
D) "Your dad is dying. If you want to see him alive again you had better go today."
E) Don't call at all. Ask the nurse to inform the son of his father's condition while you duck out quietly.

Discussion

The correct answer is "C." It gives a warning shot and allows the person receiving the bad news some control by allowing him to determine how and where he wants to receive the bad news. "A" avoids giving the bad news at all. "B" is inappropriately flippant and uses euphemisms. "D" is inappropriately blunt and just inappropriate (believe it or not, we are very caring doctors. It is just that we have amused ourselves [and you] with this book). "E" avoids having the discussion at all and is only appropriate, if for some reason you will be unable to reach the son in a timely fashion. Besides, you will be forever after known to the nurses as "Dr. Wuss." A common format for giving bad news is to use the SPIKES six-step protocol in Table 27–2.

HELPFUL TIP: When giving bad news, do not use phrases such as, "I'm afraid there is nothing more we can do for you." This leaves patients and family feeling abandoned. It is better to be more specific to say, "I am afraid that I don't have any treatments that will cure your cancer, but there is still a lot I can offer to help to keep you comfortable in the time you have left." This assures the patient and the family that there is still something to be done and that you will not abandon them.

Table 27–2 A MNEMONIC FOR GIVING BAD NEWS

S Setting. An inappropriate setting can make it difficult to give bad news effectively. Make sure the physical setting is as conducive as possible by trying to ensure privacy, involving significant others, sitting down, connecting with the patient (eye contact, hand holding), ensuring enough time, and minimizing interruptions.

P Patient's perception. Ask what the patient's (or family's) knowledge and understanding of the current medical illness is.

I Invitation. Ask what information the patient wants to receive. Some patients do not want to hear bad news themselves, and in this case it can be helpful to ask if there is someone else with whom you should speak.

K Knowledge. Give the medical facts in a straightforward manner using vocabulary and language appropriate to the patient's level. Avoid medical jargon and do not be excessively blunt (i.e., avoid saying things such as "you have very bad cancer and unless you do something, you will die"). Give the information in small chunks and frequently assess what the patient has understood. When possible start off with a warning shot (i.e., "Unfortunately, I have some bad news for you").

E Exploring/empathy/emotion. A patient's emotional reaction can vary and is often hard for a physician to experience. An empathetic response can be helpful. This can be fostered by allowing silence after breaking the bad news and watching and listening for the emotion. When you have identified the emotion, it can be helpful to name it and determine what caused it. Then make an empathetic statement such as "I'm sorry. I know this isn't what you wanted to hear."

S Strategy/summary. After the emotions have been addressed, it is helpful to review what has been said and agree on a plan. Consider asking the patient if he wants to discuss treatment options at this time or wait until a future meeting. Receiving bad news can be overwhelming, and patients often forget the details of what is said. It is important to have clear, well-defined, timely follow-up such as "Go home and talk with your family, I will see you (and your family) back tomorrow at 9 AM, and we can discuss specific treatment options and answer questions at that time."

Data from Baile WF, Buckman R, Lenzi R, et al. SPIKES-A six-step protocol for delivering bad news: application to the patient with cancer. *The Oncologist.* 2000;5:302–311.

* *

Breaking bad news is difficult in person and can be more difficult over the phone.

Which suggestion below is NOT recommended when breaking bad news over the phone?

A) Take time to prepare what you are going to say and find a quiet place to make the call
B) If no one answers the phone, it is OK to leave a message or voicemail detailing the bad news.
C) Identify yourself and avoid answering any direct questions until you are sure of the identity of the person to whom you are talking.
D) Ask if the person is alone.
E) Speak clearly and slowly, allow time for questions; be empathetic.

Discussion

The correct answer is "B." When breaking bad news over the phone, steps similar to breaking bad news in person should be used. You should obtain the full name, address, and phone number(s) of the person(s) you are calling. If you are not calling the patient, try to establish from the chart and nursing staff the relationship of the contact to the patient. Additionally, it can be helpful to write down the key information you need and review what you will say and find a quiet area with a phone. Don't delay in making the call. When you do call, clearly identify yourself and ensure you are able to speak with the person closest to the patient (ideally, the health-care proxy or the contact person indicated in the chart). Avoid responding to any direct question until you have verified the identity of the person to whom you are speaking. Not only is it morally risky but it also violates HIPPA. Ask if the contact person is alone. Do not give death notification to minor children. If you do not have a prior relationship with the person you are speaking to, ask what they know about the patient's condition. Provide a warning shot. Never deliver the news of death to an answering machine or voice mail. Instead, leave specific contact information. Allow time for questions; be empathetic and ask if you can contact anyone for them. Assess their emotional reaction and follow up as indicated.

HELPFUL TIP: When you need to inform a family that a patient has died, words like "dead" or "died" should be used; avoid euphemisms such as "expired," "passed away," or "didn't make it" (also, "kicked the bucket," "bit the bullet," "bought the farm," and so on), which can be misinterpreted.

Objectives: Did you learn to . . .

- Generate a management plan for a patient with weight loss due to a terminal disease?
- Describe criteria for hospice admission in patients with severe dementia?
- Identify and treat causes of nausea and vomiting at the end of life?
- Identify signs of the active dying process?
- Recognize the proper steps for breaking bad news?

HELPFUL TIP: Beware of Oscar the cat.

BIBLIOGRAPHY

Adler ED, et al. Palliative care in the treatment of advanced heart failure. *Circulation*. 2009;120:2597-2606.

Baile WF, et al. SPIKES—A six-step protocol for delivering bad news: Application to the patient with cancer. *Oncologist*. 2000;5:302-311.

Bannister K, Dickenson AH. Opioid hyperalgesia. *Curr Opin Support Palliat Care*. 2010;4:1-5.

Bharadwaj P, Ward KT. Ethical considerations of patients with pacemakers. *Am Fam Physician*. 2008;78:398-399.

Center to Advance Palliative Care. http://www.capc.org/tools-for-palliative-care-programs/marketing/public-opinion-research/2011-public-opinion-research-on-palliative-care.pdf, 2011.

Cervo FA, et al. To PEG or not to PEG: A review of evidence for placing feeding tubes in advanced dementia and the decision-making process. *Geriatrics*. 2006;61:30-35.

Clemens KE, Klaschik E. Dyspnoea associated with anxiety–symptomatic therapy with opioids in combination with lorazepam and its effect on ventilation in palliative care patients. *Support Care Cancer: Official Journal of the Multinational Association of Supportive Care in Cancer*. 2011;19:2027-2033.

Coyne PJ, et al. Nebulized fentanyl citrate improves patients' perception of breathing, respiratory rate, and oxygen saturation in dyspnea. *J Pain Symptom Manage*. 2002;23:157-160.

D'Agata E, Mitchell SL. Patterns of antimicrobial use among nursing home residents with advanced dementia. *Arch Intern Med*. 2008;168:357-362.

Donner B, et al. Direct conversion from oral morphine to transdermal fentanyl: A multicenter study in patients with cancer pain. *Pain*. 1996;64:527-534.

Fox CB, et al. Megestrol acetate and mirtazapine for the treatment of unplanned weight loss in the elderly. *Pharmacotherapy*. 2009;29:383-397.

Givens JL, et al. Survival and comfort after treatment of pneumonia in advanced dementia. *Arch Intern Med*. 2010;170:1102-1107.

Jacox A, et al. *Management of Cancer Pain.* Clinical Practice Guideline No. 9 N. 94–0592. Vol 8: AHCPR Publication; 1994.

Johnson MJ, Oxberry SG. The management of dyspnoea in chronic heart failure. *Curr Opin Support Palliat Care.* 2010;4:63-68.

Lampert R, et al. HRS expert consensus statement on the management of Cardiovascular Implantable Electronic Devices (CIEDs) in patients nearing end of life or requesting withdrawal of therapy. *Heart Rhythm.* 2010;7:1008-1026.

Mannix K. Palliation of nausea and vomiting. In: PS, ed. *Oxford Textbook of Palliative Medicine.* 2nd ed. New York, NY: Oxford University Press; 1998:489-499.

Moss AH, et al. Prognostic significance of the "surprise" question in cancer patients. *J Palliat Med.* 2010;13:837-840.

Murtagh FE, et al. The use of opioid analgesia in end-stage renal disease patients managed without dialysis: Recommendations for practice. *J Pain Palliat Care Pharmacother.* 2007;21:5-16.

Pattison M, Romer AL. Improving care through the end of life: Launching a primary care clinic-based program. *J Palliat Med.* 2001;4:249-254.

Reuben DB, et al. The effects of megestrol acetate suspension for elderly patients with reduced appetite after hospitalization: A phase II randomized clinical trial. *J Am Geriatr Soc.* 2005;53:970-975.

Sampson EL, et al. Enteral tube feeding for older people with advanced dementia. *Cochrane Database Syst Rev.* 2009;(2):CD007209.

Silverman SM. Opioid induced hyperalgesia: Clinical implications for the pain practitioner. *Pain Physician.* 2009;12:679-684.

Vandekieft G. Breaking bad news. *Am Fam Physician.* 2001;64(12):1975-1978.

van der Steen JT, et al. Treatment strategy and risk of functional decline and mortality after nursing-home acquired lower respiratory tract infection: Two prospective studies in residents with dementia. *Int J Geriatr Psychiatry.* 2007;22:1013-1019.

Walsh G. Hypodermoclysis: An alternate method for rehydration in long-term care. *J Infus Nurs.* 2005;28:123-129.

Yeh SS, et al. Pharmacological treatment of geriatric cachexia: Evidence and safety in perspective. *J Am Med Dir Assoc.* 2007;8:363-377.

28

Evidence-Based Medicine

Mark A. Graber

Yeah, we don't like numbers either. But they are at the end of the chapter for those you who want to learn 2×2 tables, etc. We do like evidence-based medicine (EBM) though, and it will be on the exam so here goes. . . .

Table 28–1 is here for reference. You may want to refer to it as you work your way through the chapter.

CASE 1

Research published in a well-respected medical journal studied screening for lung cancer using a new method. The researchers reported that patients who were screened and had lung cancer detected lived longer after diagnosis than people who were not screened.

Which is true?

A) This shows that screening is effective at prolonging survival.
B) This may be an example of lead-time bias.
C) This may be an example of verification bias.
D) Well-respected medical journals (and board review books) are always right.

Discussion

The correct answer is "B." This may be an example of lead-time bias. Screening is intended to diagnose disease earlier than without screening, hopefully allowing for interventions that prevent or slow the progression of the disease. Without screening, the disease may be discovered only after symptoms develop when it may be too late to intervene. Screening, however, can also give the appearance of longer survival, even though in reality no additional life has been gained. This is called lead-time bias. Here's an example. Mr. X has the test, is diagnosed with disease, receives treatment, and dies 5 years later. Mr. Y is in the control group, develops symptoms 4 years later and dies one year after that. They have both lived for 5 years after the screening study. Mr. X and Mr. Y both die at age 65 of the same disease. Did Mr. X have more survival time or just more "disease time?" This lead-time bias may be avoided by using age-specific mortality rates rather than survival time from diagnosis. Answer "C," verification bias, occurs when you are looking at a new diagnostic modality, and patients with a negative test result (for the new test) are not evaluated with the gold standard test. For example, verification bias could occur in a study where people with a negative cardiac stress test do not proceed to a cardiac catheterization. This underestimates the prevalence of disease in the population studied (we don't really know about those who didn't have a cath) and overestimates the value of the stress test (seemingly, all patients with cardiac disease were picked up by the stress test . . . but only because we didn't look far enough). See Table 28–2 for more types of bias found in studies.

* *

As part of a quality control study, the hemoglobin A_{1c} values of patients with diabetes at two clinics are compared. In a study of 4000 patients, it is found that the mean hemoglobin A_{1c} value in group 1 is 7.4% and the mean hemoglobin A_{1c} value in group 2 is 7.6%.

Table 28–1 USEFUL EQUATIONS

Sensitivity: True Positives/(true positives + false negatives)

Specificity: True Negatives/(true negatives + false positives)

False Positive Rate: 1 – specificity

False Negative Rate: 1 – sensitivity

Positive Predictive Value: True Positive/(true positive + false positive)

Negative Predictive Value: True Negative/(true negative + false negative)

The authors did the correct statistical test and found a *p*-value of 0.04 for this comparison.

Based on this information, you conclude:

A) Group 1 is significantly different from group 2: Reject the null hypothesis.
B) Group 1 is not significantly different from group 2: Don't reject the null hypothesis.
C) Group 1 is not significantly different from group 2: Reject the null hypothesis.
D) Group 1 is significantly different from group 2: Don't reject the null hypothesis.

Discussion

The correct answer is "A." To answer this question, you have to know what the usual cutoff for significance is for a *p*-value, and you also have to know what a null hypothesis is. A null hypothesis is the hypothesis that there is not a significant difference between two groups being compared to each other. By setting up null hypotheses in this way, we can then search for proof that the null hypothesis is incorrect. Tests of significance are a method of looking for evidence that a null hypothesis is incorrect. The *p*-value gives you the probability that the results of the study occurred by chance alone. A *p*-value of 0.04 means that if the study results were untrue, we would expect to see these results only 4% of the time by chance alone and not related to the treatment. By convention, a *p*-value of 0.05 or smaller is considered statistically significant. Thus, when you have a *p*-value of less than 0.05, you have evidence that the null hypothesis is false and can therefore reject it.

HELPFUL TIP: **A type I** error occurs when a difference is found when none is present. For example, a *p*-value of 0.05 is considered

Table 28–2 SOME COMMON TYPES OF BIASES SEEN IN STUDIES

Type of Bias	Effect
Selection bias	Occurs when subjects selected for the study do not represent the population. This is avoided by having large, representative samples.
Confounding bias	Occurs when two or more factors are associated with the outcome and only the one being studied is accounted for (i.e., being a Cubs fan is associated with annoying behavior, but being a Cubs fan is also associated with public intoxication that is also associated with annoying behavior; therefore, if we don't account for the drunkenness—the confounding variable—we may wrongly say being a Cubs fan *causes* annoying behavior . . . of course, this may also be true . . .).
Length time bias (**not** lead time)	Occurs because screening tests are more likely to find slow-growing tumors rather than those that are rapidly growing. This can bias results in favor of screening because more slow-growing cancers with a good prognosis will be found with a screening test.
Compliance bias	Occurs because study volunteers and persons willing to undergo screening tests are more likely to be compliant. Compliant patients have better outcomes.
Performance bias	This occurs when care provided to the experiment and control groups differs substantially—other than the intervention. It is avoided by blinding. Patients and doctors tend to behave differently if they know they are being studied. An example of this is estrogen for heart disease. Case–control studies suggested estrogen was protective, but it didn't pan out in randomized, controlled trials. The purported affect was due to something else; maybe the women on estrogen exercised more, maybe they had better diets, maybe they smoked less. Randomized, blinded trials protect against this bias.

statistically different. What this means, however, is that 5% of the time, the same conclusion would be produced by chance alone. By contrast, a *p*-value of 0.005 means that there is only a 0.5% chance that the conclusion is mistaken and occurred by chance.

HELPFUL TIP: **A type II error** occurs when a study fails to show a difference where one exists. This may occur because there are not enough subjects in a study or when there is measurement error. For example, in a (real) study of lorazepam versus diazepam for seizures, twice as many patients had their seizures stop with lorazepam. However, the conclusion of the study was that there was no difference between the two drugs. This is only because there were not enough subjects for this to reach statistical significance. Including another 100 subjects would have made this reach statistical significance. Remember this by "Type **II** error is **too** few patients."

Objectives: Did you learn to . . .

- Recognize forms of bias in research studies?
- Define *p*-value and null hypothesis?
- Describe the significance of *p*-value and type I error?
- Recognize a type II error?

CASE 2

The number of falls that occurred in 9 Boston nursing homes in November 2004–April 2005 was reported as: 127, 104, 103, 81, 86, 117, 89, 97, and 95.

What is the median number of falls among the nursing home residents?

A) 89.
B) 103.
C) 97.
D) 117.
E) 96.

Discussion

The correct answer is "C." Data are most commonly investigated at its center—where the observations have a tendency to cluster (i.e., measures of central tendency). Three common measures of central tendency are mean, median, and mode (see the following examples). To calculate the median in a set of data with "n" observations, where "n" is odd, the median is the middle value $(n+1)/2$; in our case, since there are 9 observations, the mean is $(9+1)/2 = 5$). If "n" was even, the median is the average of the two middle values, that is, the average of observations $(n/2)$ and $(n/2)+1$. To find the median in our sample, first rank the observations:

$$81, 86, 89, 95, 97, 103, 104, 117, 127$$

Then take the number of observations and add one because there is an odd number of observations and divide by 2 ($[n+1]/2$ or $[9+1]/2 = 5$). The fifth ranked number of falls, the median, is 97.

What is the mean of falls among the nursing home residents, rounded to the nearest whole number?

A) 89.
B) 100.
C) 97.
D) 101.
E) 98.

Discussion

The correct answer is "B." In a set of data with "n" observations, find the mean by summing the total observations and divide by "n": $(81+86+89+95+97+103+104+117+127)/\,9 = 99.89$.

HELPFUL TIP: The mean is sensitive to extreme observations (e.g., if there are data points 1, 1, 1, 1, 1, and 100, the mean is 21 even though the majority of observations are "1"). When outliers like this occur or when the data are not symmetrically distributed, the median may be the best measure of central tendency.

What is the mode of falls among the nursing home residents?

A) 89.
B) 99.89.
C) 117.
D) 101.
E) Unable to solve the problem with data provided.

Discussion

The correct answer is "E." **The mode of a sample is the observation that occurs most frequently.** In the data provided, there is no unique mode because all the observations occur only once. However, if you were checking daily fall rates in one nursing home and they were 1, 2, 3, 3, 2, 3, 2, 3 the mode would be 3 (since this is the observation that occurs most frequently).

> HELPFUL TIP: If the data distribution is symmetric (e.g., normally distributed), then it is a unimodal distribution. Data may have more than one mode (i.e., bimodal and trimodal).

> HELPFUL TIP: Subgroup analyses (you know, the "our drug worked in women over 60" pitch) can **only** be used to generate a hypothesis. This is called the **"derivation set."** Before accepting it into practice, a second study of that subgroup, called the **"validation set"** must be done. This is always true. Don't let them tell you otherwise.

Objectives: Did you learn to...

- Calculate the mean, mode, and median in a data set with an odd number of data points?
- Apply these measures of central tendency to the analysis of data?

QUICK QUIZ: FEELING SENSITIVE ABOUT SOMETHING SPECIFIC?

Which of the following statements is true?

A) Specificity is the most important test characteristic when trying to find a very dangerous disease.
B) As sensitivity increases, specificity decreases.
C) Specificity need not be considered as long as a test is sensitive enough.
D) As sensitivity increases, specificity increases.

Discussion

The correct answer is "B." As sensitivity increases, specificity decreases. This makes intuitive sense. The more cases you detect, the more false positives you will have. Ideally, we would like to have a diagnostic screening test with both high sensitivity and high specificity. In reality, there is an inherent trade-off between sensitivity and specificity—as sensitivity increases, specificity decreases and vice versa. "A" is **incorrect**. Generally, when it is very dangerous not to detect disease, it is important to have a highly sensitive test (one that will find "all" cases) with an acceptable specificity. "C" is **incorrect**. This is why we do both an ELISA and a Western blot when trying to detect HIV. The ELISA is very sensitive (will pick up the great majority of HIV cases) but is not very specific (will categorize a lot of patients who **do not have the disease** as positive). The Western blot is more specific and will filter the true positives from the false positives found on the screening test (the ELISA).

QUICK QUIZ: ALL THAT GLITTERS...

You are having a meaningful discussion with an industry representative (yeah, right). OK, let's recalibrate: You are being sold a package of goods by an industry representative. She says that if their test for Dread Disease is positive, the likelihood ratio of the disease being present is 3.

Your response to this is:

A) "Great! The disease is 3 times more likely to be present if the test is positive."
B) "Not so great! A likelihood ratio of 3 is pretty much worthless in differentiating between those who are ill and those who are not."
C) "What is this likelihood ratio stuff anyway?"
D) "What happened to my free lunch?"

Discussion

The correct answer is "B." In a situation in which the pretest probability of a disease is between 30% and 70%, a likelihood ratio can meaningfully **reduce** the possibility of disease presence **only** if it is <0.1. In a situation in which the pretest probability of a disease is between 30% and 70%, a likelihood ratio can meaningfully **increase** the possibility of disease presence **only** if it is over 10. So, a likelihood ratio of 3 is more or less useless.

Draw some lines on this and you will see what we mean (Figure 28–1).

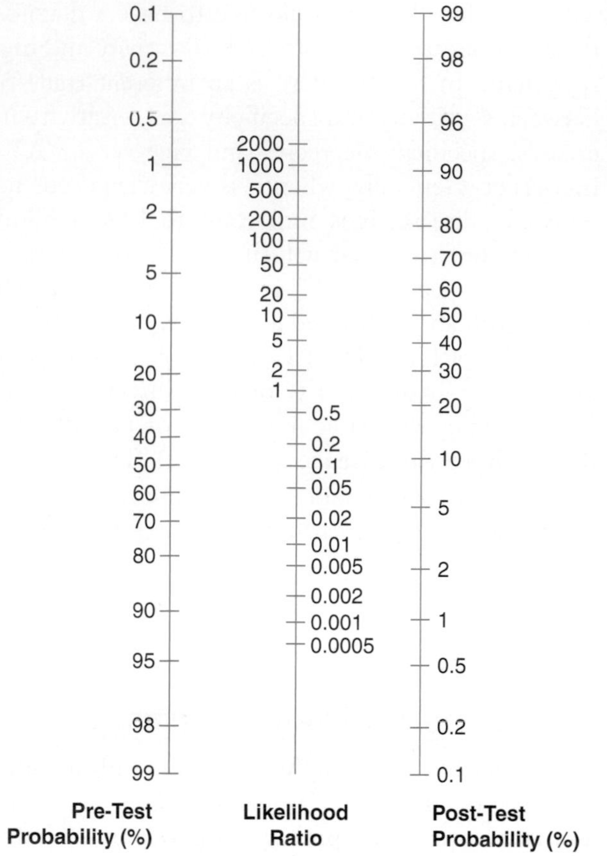

Figure 28–1 **Reproduced from the Centre for Evidence-Based Medicine. Available at http://www.cebm.net**

* *

One common and debilitating complication of diabetes is neuropathy. In a study of patients with diabetes, one group had routine therapy and an experimental group had intensive therapy. The first group, routine therapy, had 10% of patients develop neuropathy. The second group, intensive therapy, had 2% of patients develop neuropathy (as all of you know, intensive therapy doesn't really work in type 2 diabetics, so let's just pretend . . . it is just like the tooth fairy).

Using the data above, how many patients with diabetes need to be treated with intensive therapy to prevent the development of one case of neuropathy?

A) 10.
B) 11.
C) 8.
D) 12.5.
E) 25.5.

Discussion

The correct answer is "D." The question is really asking, "What is the number needed to treat (NNT)?" In this question, the absolute risk reduction is 8% (10% in control group vs. 2% in the treated group). The NNT is the number of patients who need to be treated to prevent one adverse outcome. To calculate this, we need to know a few other terms:

ARR = **A**bsolute **R**isk **R**eduction = control group event rate (CER) – experimental group event rate (EER).

NNT = 1/ARR (in percent . . . . e.g., 8% = 0.08 and 20% = 0.20)

Using the values given above, ARR = 10 – 2% = 8% and NNT = 1/0.08 = 12.5.

* *

The anticlotting properties of aspirin are well studied. In a trial studying the long-term outcome of stroke patients, 1% of patients on long-term aspirin therapy developed new onset of strokes and 50% of patients without aspirin therapy developed new strokes.

Using the data above, how many stroke patients need to be treated with aspirin therapy to prevent one new stroke (what is the NNT)?

A) 2.
B) 8.
C) 10.
D) 12.
E) 25.

Discussion

The correct answer is "A." Again, the NNT is the number of patients who need to be treated to prevent one adverse outcome. NNT = 1/ARR, where ARR = CER – EER. Using the values given above, 50 – 1% = 49% = ARR and NNT = 1/0.49 = 2.

* *

In a pharmaceutical study, Group A is the placebo group and Group B is the group that received the actual new drug. Data were gathered on Groups A and B and confidence intervals (CI) were calculated. Side effect rates were calculated as a percentage of each group.

Using the 95% CI, which of the following group comparisons are statistically significantly different?

A) Group A CI 30–46% and Group B CI 44–88%.
B) Group A CI 10–30% and Group B CI 44–88%.
C) Group A CI 0.1–0.3% and Group B CI 0.2–0.4%.
D) Group A CI 88–90% and Group B CI 88–90%.
E) None of the above is statistically significant.

Discussion

The correct answer is "B." The CI is a range of possible high to low values of data. The true mean is likely to be in the specified range. So, for example, if the relative risk (RR) of an adverse outcome is 2 and the CI is −2 to 10 (usually identified by "95% CI −2–10"), this means that there may be up to 10 times the risk of an adverse outcome **or** 2 times **less** a risk of an adverse outcome. In general, the larger the study group, the more narrow the CI. When you have a large study, you are more likely to get closer to the true value.

"B" is correct because when comparing the CI between two groups, there is no overlap. When there is an overlap of CI, as in the other options, the groups are not statistically significantly different. For example, in answer "A" the true mean value of Group A could lie anywhere between 30% and 46% (it could be 45%), and the true mean value of Group B could lie anywhere between 44% and 88% (it could also be 45%); therefore, the groups have no statistically significant difference.

HELPFUL TIP: CI are usually given as "CI 95%," meaning that there is a 95% probability that the true mean value will be within the CI. When looking at CI for RR, relative benefit, odds ratio, etc., remember that if the CI 95% crosses "1," there is no difference between the groups. Thus, RR 4.2 CI 95% 0.8–10 is consistent with a 0.8 times risk or a 10 times risk (or benefit). However, since the CI 95% crosses "1," there is no real difference between the groups.

HELPFUL TIP: Confidence intervals are useful when determining the magnitude of a treatment effect. For example, if a RR has CI 95% 1.2–1.4, this means there is a small difference (0.2–0.4 times) between the two groups, even though it is statistically significant. **Something that is statistically significant may not be clinically significant.** On the other hand, if the RR has a CI 95% 10–20, this is a major difference between the groups. This means that one group has a 10–20 times greater risk (or benefit depending on what is being studies) than does the other group.

* *

In a clinical trial testing a new provider order entry (POE) technology at a university hospital, relative and absolute risk reduction is discussed. A group of family practice residents at the hospital used the traditional hand-written orders during their intern year and averaged seven medication errors per year. In the FP residents' second year, POE was instituted (which alerted physicians to medication errors before finalization of orders) and the group's medication errors dropped to an average of four per year.

Which of the following is true?

A) The RR reduction is 43% and the absolute risk reduction is 3 in medication errors.
B) The RR reduction is 57% and the absolute risk reduction is 3 in medication errors.
C) The RR reduction is 43% and the absolute risk reduction is 4 in medication errors.
D) The RR reduction is 57% and the absolute risk reduction is 4 in medication errors.
E) The RR reduction cannot be calculated with the information given and the absolute risk reduction is 3 in medication errors.

Discussion

The correct answer is "A." POE compared with no POE (the control group) results in a 43% relative decrease in the risk of a medication error—from seven to four errors per year (3/7 = 43%). The difference in the number of medication errors before and after POE is three errors (7 − 4 = 3), which is the absolute reduction in the risk of a medication error.

CASE 3

Mr. Handsome Q. Drugrep has come to tell you all about HappyLuckyGolden Drug (HLGD) that is newly indicated for the treatment of the Dreadful Yucks. As a primary care doctor, you are concerned about better treatment of this disease. Current standard treatment involves ChemoRAdical Pharmacotherapy (CRAP). Cure rates with CRAP are only about 10%. Mr. Drugrep has a study that shows

HLGD has a 12% cure rate versus placebo. He's very excited and expects HLGD to be the new standard of care.

To his argument, you appropriately respond:

A) "Wow. HLGD is clearly superior to CRAP."
B) "Hmm. HLGD is statistically no different from CRAP."
C) "Wow. HLGD is clearly superior to placebo."
D) "Do you have free samples of HLGD? Where's lunch?"
E) "I need more information before I can make an informed decision."

Discussion

The correct answer is "E." You need more information. Before coming to market, a drug manufacturer must demonstrate safety and efficacy of a drug. The new drug may or may not be compared with another currently available treatment. Without a study comparing HLGD to CRAP, you cannot say anything about how these drugs compare, even if HLGD looks better versus placebo. Additionally, "C" is incorrect because the placebo results have not been given.

* *

You ask Mr. Drugrep for more information. He proudly tells you the drug study involved 10,000 subjects with the Dreadful Yucks, randomly assigned to placebo (5000) or HLGD (5000). All of the subjects completed the trial. At the end of 1 year, 400 subjects on placebo (8%) were cured and 600 subjects on HLGD (12%) were cured.

He correctly tells you that:

A) The NNT is 10,000.
B) The number needed to harm (NNH) is 10,000.
C) The relative benefit of HLGD versus placebo is 50% greater cure rate.
D) The absolute benefit of HLGD versus placebo is 50% greater cure rate.

Discussion

The correct answer is "C." When looking at drug studies, benefit is often stated as "relative benefit" or relative risk reduction. In this question, 600/5000 patients benefit from HLGD and 400/5000 benefit from placebo; thus, 200 more patients are cured with HLGD, $200/400 = 0.5 = 50\%$ relative benefit of the drug. The absolute benefit is only 4% (12% cure with HLGD vs. 8% cure with placebo). For the NNT in this example, think about the previously given equation: $NNT = 1/ARR$, where $ARR = CER - EER$. The control group, the placebo, had a risk reduction of 8% (92% still had disease); and the experiment group had a risk reduction of 12% (88% still had disease). So, the ARR $=12 - 8\% = 4\%$, and NNT $= 1/0.04 = 25$. NNH cannot be calculated with the information available since the adverse event rate is not known.

In real life, there are often more dramatic examples of how relative and absolute risks differ. It may be stated that there is a 50% reduction in complications of diabetes using Drug A versus placebo. However, when translated into patients, this could be 1/1000 complications of diabetes in the drug group versus 2/1000 complications of diabetes in the placebo group. This is a 50% relative decrease in adverse outcomes but in fact may be clinically meaningless. The **absolute** risk reduction is 1/1000 or 0.1%! This ploy is often used to make drug studies look good. Thus, anytime you are looking at a new drug, ask for the **absolute** risk reduction **and** the NNT and the NNH.

* *

Mr. Drugrep tells you that the adverse event rate for HLGD is only 1%. Aren't you impressed? But he frowns a little when you want to know the NNH.

To calculate NNH, you ask him for:

A) The types of adverse events that occurred in the treatment group.
B) The number of adverse events that occurred in the control group.
C) The percentage of adverse events with standard treatment.
D) The cure rate in the treatment group.

Discussion

The correct answer is "B." **Adverse effects** of a drug will often be reported as an absolute number, and here it is 1%. So, the conclusion you are given by the pharmaceutical industry may be **50% reduction in disease and only a 1% risk of side effects of the drug.** Both of these statements are true, but it's an "apples and oranges" comparison. We prefer comparing apples-to-apples (or corn-to-corn in Iowa). In order to directly compare benefits and harms, we need to know the NNT and the NNH.

Let's say that when you ask Mr. Drugrep, he tells you that the adverse event rate in the placebo group was 0.5%. Here's the calculation: NNH = 1/ARI, where ARI (absolute risk **increase**) = risk in experiment group – risk in control group.

Using the numbers in this question: ARI = 1 – 0.5 = 0.5; NNH = 1/0.5 = 2.

So, for HLGD, the NNT is 25 and the NNH is 2. By the way, the adverse event in question is disfiguring, painful ear hair growth. You will have to treat 25 patients with HLGD to cure one case of the Dreadful Yucks; but with every two patients you treat, one will have an adverse event. Demand NNT and NNH: how many patients who take the drug will benefit and how many will be harmed?

Objectives: Did you learn to . . .

- Employ CI in the analysis of data?
- Analyze data using risk reduction and relative benefit?
- Understand the importance of absolute risk reduction, NNH, and NNT when clinically applying data from a study?

CASE 4

Mounting paperwork and electronic medical record hassles have played role in your decision to make a career change. You have found a nice academic job with a research focus—minimal patient care, 10 weeks of vacation, no paperwork (just like us!). Your work centers on reducing the risk of stroke in patients who have survived one stroke.

This is an example of which category of prevention?

A) Primary prevention.
B) Secondary prevention.
C) Tertiary prevention.
D) Quaternary prevention.

Discussion

The correct answer is "C." The idea behind **primary prevention**, a big interest in primary care, is to prevent a disease from occurring at all by removing its cause (i.e., influenza vaccine to prevent illness from influenza). Primary prevention may occur in the health-care setting but is often in the domain of public health. **Secondary prevention** detects disease at an early stage so that intervention can prevent progression (i.e., Pap smears detecting dysplasia prior to cancer declaring itself). Your new job will be to study **tertiary prevention**: the reduction in complications and mortality due to disease after it is recognized. The line between secondary and tertiary prevention can be blurry: some would consider preventing another stroke "secondary" prevention and preventing stroke complications (e.g., muscle atrophy and pressure ulcer) "tertiary" prevention. There is no such thing as quaternary prevention.

* *

In between day trading and coffee breaks, you plan to study two groups of patients (A and B) to see if variable XYZ makes any difference in death or recurrent stroke. There is no randomization and no interventions. You are just reviewing records to see how each group did. Subjects in Group A had a stroke and then had another stroke or died a year later. Subjects in Group B had a stroke but were alive with no recurrent stroke at the time of the study. You assess the presence of XYZ in each group.

This type of study is called a:

A) Prospective study.
B) Case–control study.
C) Cohort study.
D) Randomized, controlled study.

Discussion

The correct answer is "B." A case–control study, like this one, will look at select subjects who are categorized based on outcome and try to find associations with certain variables. Case–control studies do not follow subjects over time and therefore are not prospective. Cohort studies look at groups starting at time zero and following them for a specified amount of time to find an association between a variable and an outcome. The variable in question is not under the researcher's control. An example of a cohort study might be one looking at the association between two different diets (e.g., high-protein vs. high-carbohydrate) and the development of type 2 diabetes. The highest quality evidence is produced by a randomized, double-blind, controlled trial, in which the researcher has control over exposure to a variable and studies its effect on an outcome. In general, the strength of trial design goes: experimental study > cohort study > case–control study > cross-sectional study. Unfortunately, it is not possible to design randomized controlled studies for all conditions. So, a well-done cohort study may be the best we can do.

* *

You are concerned about numerous confounding variables in your study population.

Never fear! Your trusty statistician recommends the following in order to minimize confounding:

A) Multivariate analysis.
B) Careful calculation of *p*-values.
C) Matched controls and cases.
D) A and B.
E) A and C.

Discussion

The correct answer is "E." Confounders can be a serious threat to any study. Confounders result from extrinsic factors—things that may affect the outcome and are also associated with the variable but are not accounted for in the study. As an example, a study may find an association between long-haul truck driving and lung cancer. If tobacco use was not accounted for in this study, the results of the study would be meaningless. Tobacco is a confounder. It is always advisable to look at a study with an eye for what confounder might be missing. Confounding can be limited by a study design that anticipates confounders and matches controls and cases ("C"). It is important to note that if you match your control and cases on a variable, you can no longer study that variable as a potential cause of the outcome. For example, if you match cases and controls on county of residence among the truck drivers, you can no longer explore county of residence as risk factor for lung cancer. Also, multivariate analysis ("A") is a statistical method that allows for adjustment of known confounders. "B" is incorrect because *p*-value has nothing to do with confounding but will tell you whether the results should be considered significant or not.

* *

When you review the literature, you find that there are a number of small studies looking at the effect of intervention XYZ on stroke victims. You even find a meta-analysis.

If this is a well-done meta-analysis, you should find all of the following EXCEPT:

A) Statistically confirmed heterogeneity between the included studies.
B) A thorough search for all valid studies.
C) An evaluation of whether estimates change with varying assumptions.
D) The exclusion of poor-quality studies.
E) The studies included measure the same underlying effect.

Discussion

The correct answer is "A." Hopefully, a meta-analysis would confirm *homogeneity* between studies. Although there is controversy regarding the appropriate use of meta-analyses, they are often used to study various outcomes by combining smaller studies. A meta-analysis is a systematic review that combines the results of previous studies to evaluate the magnitude or direction of an effect or to evaluate the effect on a subgroup. All valid studies looking at similar outcomes should be included and poor-quality studies excluded. A number of statistical maneuvers are done with meta-analyses, including an evaluation of whether estimates will change if study assumptions change (called a sensitivity analysis).

Objectives: Did you learn to . . .

- Define different types of prevention?
- Define different study types?
- Identify and account for confounding?
- Describe some characteristics of a meta-analysis?

CASE 5

Uh, oh . . . Here comes the math. This section is important, especially the concepts of positive and negative predictive values (PPV and NPV) and the concept of sensitivity and specificity. You need not do the math if you do not want to (although it is simple). Here is a summary:

Sensitivity: How often the test will pick up the disease if it is there. Sensitivity = true positives/true positives + false negatives. Note that the sum of true positives + false negatives represents all of the people with disease.

Specificity: Specificity is defined as the proportion of patients who do not have the disease and who will test negative for it. Specificity = True negatives/true negatives + false positives. Note that the sum of true negatives + false positives represents all of the people who do not have disease.

* *

A new test, the "reception-o-meter," has been developed that can tell whether a cell phone will have reception in a given area (besides a guy walking around asking "can you hear me now?"). When compared with the gold standard of turning on your cell phone and checking whether you have reception or not, the new test has a sensitivity of 90% (will pick up a signal 90% of the time when there is one) and a specificity

Table 28–3 SAMPLE TABLE

Test	Disease	
	+	–
+	a (true positive)	b (false positive)
–	c (false negative)	d (true negative)
Total	a + c	b + d

of 95% (there are only 5% false positives... 95% of the time when the reception-o-meter says there is a signal, there will actually be one).

So how can you tell if the phone company is pulling a fast one or if this is a good test? You need to know the PPV of the test.

In order to calculate the PPV, you need three pieces of data: the sensitivity of the test (how often the test will pick up the disease if it is there), the specificity of the test (how often you will get a false positive), and the prevalence of the condition, which in this case is the prevalence of having cell phone reception (in other words, the true amount of cell phone reception in a given area).

You are currently in Los Angeles, attending a CME course where the reception for carrier X is 99%. You check your "reception-o-meter" and it says you have coverage. But does this mean you have coverage?

In order to answer this question, you can use Bayes theorem or set up 2×2 tables. Here's the 2×2 table method. Begin by drawing a 2×2 table and filling in what you know. See Tables 28–3 and 28–4.

So this makes it easy.

Sensitivity = a/(a + c),
Specificity = d/(b + d),
PPV = a/(a + b),
NPV = d/(c + d)

If we have 100 phones, the data will look like that above.

Table 28–4

		Actual Reception	
		+	–
Test	+	90 (true positive)	5 (false positive)
Reception	–	10 (false negative)	95 (true negative)
Total		100	100

Table 28–5

After Adding Actual Prevalence			
		Actual Reception	
		+	–
Test	+	8910	5
Reception	–	990	95
Total		9900	100
		(99% prevalence)	

So let's add actual numbers to the table (above). Let's use a population of 10,000. We multiply by the prevalence of reception to get the subpopulation totals. Ninety-nine percent of the population has reception (99% prevalence). So, 99% prevalence × 10,000 = 9900 with reception; 1% × 10,000 = 100 without reception. Once we have these numbers, we simply multiply by the sensitivity and the specificity to get the exact cell numbers as in the table above (9900 × 90% sensitivity = 8910 for cell "a"-true positives); 9900 – 8910 = 990 for cell "c-false negatives)" 100 × 95% specificity = 95 for cell "d"; 100 – 95 = 5 for cell "b"). See Table 28–5.

Once the table is filled in, these numbers can then be used to calculate the PPV, using the equation above. In this case, a/(a + b) = 8910/8915 = 99.9%.

For those who prefer the Bayes theorem method, here's how this approach is done. Bayes theorem shows the relationships between sensitivity, specificity, prevalence, PPV, and NPV. The equation for PPV, derived from Bayes theorem, is shown, as is the calculation based on the numbers from the question.

$$\text{PPV} = \frac{\text{Number of true positives}}{\text{Number of true positives} + \text{Number of false positives}}$$

$$\text{PPV} = \frac{\text{Sensitivity} \times \text{prevalence}}{(\text{Sensitivity} \times \text{prevalence}) + [(1 - \text{specificity}) \times (1 - \text{prevalence})]}$$

$$= \frac{0.9 \times 0.99}{(0.9 \times 0.99) + [0.05 \times 0.01]} = 99.9\%$$

What would the likelihood of not having coverage be if the "reception-o-meter" had said you did not have coverage (what is the NPV)?

A) 95%.
B) 90%.
C) 50%.
D) 9%.
E) None of the above.

Discussion

The correct answer is "D." The question asks for the NPV—the likelihood of not having coverage if the reception-o-meter is negative. This also can be derived from Bayes theorem or calculated using a 2×2 table. For those of you who prefer the Bayes theorem method, the equation for NPV, derived from Bayes theorem, is shown, as is the calculation based on the numbers from the question.

$$\text{NPV} = \frac{\text{Number of true negatives}}{\text{Number of true negatives} + \text{number of false negatives}}$$

$$\text{NPV} = \frac{\text{Specificity} \times (1 - \text{prevalence})}{[\text{Specificity} \times (1 - \text{prevalence})] + (1 - \text{sensitivity})}$$

$$= \frac{0.95 \times 0.01}{(0.95 \times 0.01) + 0.10} = 8.7\% \text{ (which rounds to 9\%).}$$

* *

You are now in rural Russia where you were invited to help with community efforts to fight multidrug resistant tuberculosis. Here cell phone reception is 10% for Carrier Y. You check your "reception-o-meter" and it says you have reception.

What is the likelihood that your cell phone actually will have reception if you try to make a call?

A) 91%
B) 83%
C) 67%
D) 16%
E) None of the above.

Discussion

The correct answer is "C." You can use the 2×2 method or the Bayes theorem methods.

Here's what our 2×2 table looks like. See Table 28–6.

To convert to 10% prevalence, we start with a large baseline population and multiply by the prevalence to get the subpopulation totals (10% prevalence × 10,000 = 1000 with reception; 90% × 10,000 = 9000 without reception). Once we have the subpopulation totals, we multiply by the sensitivity and the specificity to get the exact cell numbers (1000 × 90% sensitivity = 900 for cell "a"; 1000 – 900 = 100 for cell "c" (or alternately 1000 × 10% will get the same result for cell "c"); 9000 × 95% specificity = 8550 for cell "d"; 9000 – 8550 = 450 for cell "b").

These numbers can then be used to calculate the PPV, using the equation above. In this case, a/(a + b) = 900/(900 + 450) = 66.7% (rounds to 67%).

Using Bayes theorem, the equation is as follows.

$$\text{PPV} = \frac{\text{Sensitivity} \times \text{prevalence}}{(\text{Sensitivity} \times \text{prevalence}) + [(1 - \text{specificity}) \times (1 - \text{prevalence})]}$$

$$= \frac{0.9 \times 0.1}{(0.9 \times 0.1) + [0.05 \times 0.9]} = 66.7\%$$

What would the likelihood of having coverage be if the "reception-o-meter" said you did not have coverage?

A) 50%.
B) 40%.
C) 30%.
D) 1%.
E) None of the above.

Discussion

The correct answer is "D." Again, you can use the 2×2 method or Bayes theorem. The 2×2 table for this question is the same as it was for the previous question. However, unlike previously, you are asked for the likelihood of reception if the "reception-o-meter" said there was no reception. In other words,

Table 28–6

Before Adding Actual Prevalence				After Adding Actual Prevalence			
		Actual Reception				Actual Reception	
		+	–			+	–
Test	+	90	5	Test	+	900	450
Reception	–	10	95	Reception	–	100	8550
Total		100	100	Total		1000	9000
		(50% prevalence)				(10% prevalence)	

you have been asked to calculate the false negative rate (FNR) for this scenario. The equation for the FNR is below.

$$FNR = \frac{\text{False negatives}}{\text{False negatives} + \text{true negatives}} \text{ or}$$

$$\frac{c}{c+d} = \frac{100}{100+8550} = 1\%$$

You were not asked to calculate it, but there is also a false positive rate (FPR), which is shown below.

$$EPR = \frac{\text{False positives}}{\text{False positives} + \text{true positives}} \text{ or}$$

$$\frac{b}{a+b} = \frac{450}{450+900} = 33\%$$

* *

Cervical cancer is a disease in which early detection can make a great difference in halting disease progression. One screening procedure for this disease is the Papanicolaou ("Pap") smear. To assess the competency of technicians who read the Pap smear slides, a local lab checked their technician's work against patient records.

A total of 1000 Pap smears were read. Of these, 100 patients had cervical abnormalities based on biopsy (gold standard). Of this group, 75 had abnormal (positive) Pap smears and 25 had negative Pap smears. There were 900 women without disease. Of these 900 women, 200 had positive Pap smears and 700 had negative Pap smears. **Note that these are example numbers only, have no basis in reality, and do not reflect the actual sensitivities and specificities of these tests.**

Using the data above, which of the following is true about this survey of Pap smear technicians?

A) FNR is 20%.
B) FPR is 15%.
C) The sensitivity of the Pap test is 75%.
D) The specificity of the Pap test is 98%.
E) The prevalence of cervical cancer in this sample is 7.5%.

Discussion

The correct answer is "C." The sensitivity of the test is 75%. Setting up the data in a 2×2 table, we are able to answer the question. See Table 28–7.

Table 28–7

Pap Test Result	Cervical Disease	No Cervical Disease
Positive	True positive (TP) = 75	False positive (FP) = 200
Negative	False negative (FN) = 25	True negative (TN) = 700
Total	TP + FN = 100	FP + TN = 900

Sensitivity: Probability that a patient with the disease will have a positive result (e.g., how many patients with the disease are misclassified as not having the disease).

Sensitivity = (TP/(TP + FN))= 75/100 = 0.75 or 75% sensitive.

Specificity: Probability that a patient without the disease will have a negative test (e.g., how many patients without the disease are misclassified as having the disease).

Specificity = (TN/(FP + TN))= 700/900 = 0.777 or about 78% specific.

FNR: Patient has the disease but the test is negative.

FNR = (FN/(TP + FN)) = 25/100 = 25% FNR. Also calculated as 1 − sensitivity.

FPR: The patient has a positive test but does not have the disease.

FPR = (FP/(FP + TN)) = 200/900 = 0.22 or 22% false positive. Also calculated as 1 − specificity.

* *

Prevalence of the disease: The proportion of individuals who have the disease at any point in time = ((TP + FN)/Total population) = 100/1000 = 10% or prevalence of 100 per 1000 people.

Given the above results of the Pap smear screening tests and if the prevalence of cervical abnormalities among women is 10%, then applying Bayes theorem, we find:

A) The PPV is 27%.
B) The NPV is 96%.
C) The PPV is 0.999.
D) Unable to solve the problem with data provided.
E) A and B.

Discussion

The correct answer is "E." The prevalence of a disease is the proportion of individuals who have the disease at a given point in time ((TP + FN)/(Total population) = 0.1 or 10%).

The **PPV** of a test is **the probability that a disease exists given a positive test result** = TP/(TP + FP) or 75/275 = 27%. So, a patient with a positive test result only has a 27% chance of actually having the disease because there are so many false positives.

The **NPV** of a test is the probability of no disease given a negative test result (TN/(FN + TN)) = 700/725 = 96%. So, a patient with a negative test has a 96% chance of **not** having the disease. This is because there are few false negatives compared with the size of the overall population. If, for example, there were 200 false negatives in the same population, the negative predictive value would be only 700/900 = 78%. This is because there are so many false negatives.

* *

Recall that 100 out of 1000 women had positive biopsies and thus had the disease regardless of what the Pap test said.

How does the pretest probability of cervical abnormalities among women compare with the posttest probability?

A) Posttest probability is about three times greater than the pretest probability.
B) Pretest probability is three times greater than the posttest probability.
C) Posttest probability is 10 times greater.
D) Pretest probability is 10 times greater.
E) The pretest and posttest probabilities are equal.

Discussion

The correct answer is "A." The pretest probability is given above as 100/1000 or 10%. We know that 10% of the population has the disease. **The posttest probability is defined as the PPV.** Remember from above the **PPV** of a test is the probability that a disease exists given a positive test result = TP/(TP + FP) or 75/275 = 27%. Comparing the two results, pretest probability of 10% and posttest probability of 27%, we find that the posttest probability is about three times greater than the pretest probability. If answer "E" were correct and the pretest and posttest probabilities were equal, there would be no point in doing the test.

Objectives: Did you learn to . . .

- Define and calculate sensitivity and then apply it to data interpretation?
- Define and calculate specificity and then apply it to data interpretation?
- Calculate positive and negative predictive values?
- Apply Bayes theorem to determine the utility of a test?

BIBLIOGRAPHY

Fletcher RH, et al. *Clinical Epidemiology: The Essentials*. 2nd ed. Baltimore, MD: Williams & Wilkins; 1988.

Friedland DJ, et al. *Evidence-Based Medicine*. New York, NY: McGraw-Hill; 1998.

Gordis L. *Epidemiology*. Philadelphia, PA: WB Saunders Co; 1996.

Pagano M, Gauvreau K. *Principles of Biostatistics*. 2nd ed. Australia: Duxbury Thomson Learning; 2000.

29

Patient-Centered Care

David Bedell and Jason K. Wilbur

Note: This chapter deals with cultural competency and patient safety. Because not all Black patients are from America (and thus are not "African Americans"), the authors have elected to use the term "Black" in this chapter as inclusive of African Americans as well as those individuals who are of African descent but may be from another country. We understand the sensitivity of this terminology and ask your understanding.

CASE 1

You are doing a locum tenens job in Arizona on the Navajo reservation. You are seeing a lot of diabetes and remember that Native Americans, Hispanics, and Blacks all have a greater incidence of diabetes.

Which of the following is TRUE about the age-adjusted incidence of diabetes in adults?

A) All Alaska Native and Native American tribes have a higher incidence of diabetes than non-Hispanic Whites (NHW).
B) Cuban Americans and South Americans have a higher incidence of diabetes than NHW.
C) Mexican Americans and Puerto Ricans have close to 90% higher incidence of diabetes than NHW.
D) Pima Indians in Mexico have the same high incidence of diabetes as the Pima Indians in Arizona.
E) Non-Hispanic Blacks have a lower incidence of diabetes than Hispanics in the United States.

Discussion

The correct answer is "C." Mexican Americans and Puerto Ricans have a higher incidence of diabetes compared with NHW. The other statements are false, and here's how they break down. Although their diabetes incidence is increasing rapidly in 2010, Alaska Natives historically had a 5.5% age-adjusted incidence of diabetes compared with 7.1% for NHW. Cubans and South Americans actually have the same incidence as NHW. The Pima Indians in Mexico whose lifestyle is not sedentary and who eat a more traditional diet actually have a diabetes incidence of about 7%, while those in Arizona have an incidence of 38%. Non-Hispanic Blacks have an incidence higher than those of Hispanics and NHW but not quite as high as the Mexican Americans and Puerto Ricans.

HELPFUL TIP: Ethnic and cultural groups are not uniform from an epidemiological or cultural belief standpoint. Hence, there are often large differences between subgroups. This is complicated further by the fact that we all belong to, and are influenced by, multiple different cultural groups. We're more of a chunky stew than a melting pot.

CASE 2

You are seeing a 57-year-old Navajo male with poorly controlled type 2 diabetes. You are trying to understand why his hemoglobin A_{1c} is so high since he has access to healthcare, medicines, supplies, and an amazing doctor (if you do say so yourself). You remember a lecture on patient-centered medicine where they talked about investigating a person's health problem using both disease and illness models.

The difference between disease and illness is:

A) Disease is the biomedical explanation of the health condition; illness is the patient's experience and understanding of the health condition.
B) Disease is chronic; illness is acute.
C) Diseases have known causes; illnesses do not.
D) Disease is more serious and frequently needs treatment; illness will resolve without medical intervention.
E) Disease versus illness... really? Aren't we just into some phony semantics here?

Discussion

The correct answer is "A." Simply put, "disease" is the way that physicians understand a health problem and "illness" is the way the patient experiences it. The patient-centered model looks not only at the pathophysiology of disease, which is the focus of most of our early medical training, but also at what the patient is experiencing, how it impacts him or her, and what is the larger social–personal context of that health condition. The patient-centered physician weaves back and forth between the disease and illness model, diagnosing and treating both the disease and illness problems of the patient.

* *

You want to focus on your patient's illness in the larger context of his life and avoid just discussing glucose metabolism, diet, exercise, lab results, and medication adherence. (Your usual approach of explaining diabetes and its complications has not improved his control.) You ask him, "What has your experience with diabetes been like?" And he looks at you strangely and answers that it has been tough.

One way to help get an understanding of his beliefs about diabetes would be to:

A) Interview family members or tribal medical personnel to learn about cultural belief systems and understanding of diabetes.
B) Do a literature search on Navajo health beliefs with respect to diabetes and then ask him if ascribes to any of those beliefs.
C) Ask about very specific aspect of his health experience and beliefs in a nonjudgmental way (tighten up your questions so you avoid vague answers).
D) All of the above.

Discussion

The correct answer is "D." Any of these options may help you understand this patient's health beliefs. Community members can be a good source of cultural information. Having a general idea of a cultural belief system makes it easier to ask question about whether those beliefs apply in this case and how. Asking the right questions will help to get more useful information. There are some canned questions that can be of assistance. One example is the series of questions below developed by a psychiatrist-anthropologist named Arthur Kleinman.

- What do you call your problem?
- What do you think caused your problem?
- Why do you think it started when it did?
- What does your sickness do to you? How does it work?
- How severe is it? Will it have a short or long course?
- What do you fear most about your disorder?
- What are the chief problems that your sickness has caused for you?
- What kind of treatment do you think you should receive?
- What are the most important results you hope to receive from the treatment?

HELPFUL TIP: Don't memorize all these health beliefs questions. Focus on the nature of the questions and their simplicity, and you will be able to develop your own method.

* *

Your patient develops severe osteomyelitis of his right leg and is admitted to your in-patient service. He has not responded to several weeks of appropriate IV antibiotics and debridement. The infection is gradually spreading proximally, and a decision has been made with the patient that you will proceed with a below-the-knee amputation. Although you are confident that this is the right clinical decision, you worry about the fact that Native Americans (Navajos reportedly highest in the world), Hispanics, Blacks, and poor people all have higher rates of amputation of limbs even when adjusting for incidence of diabetes. The surgeon you are working with asks you to obtain informed consent from the patient. You have heard that Navajos believe that by talking about something bad happening (i.e., informing them of the risk of a procedure) you make those adverse events more likely to occur.

How do you want to get informed consent from your patient?

A) Just like any other patient explain the benefits and the risk of the procedure.
B) Tell him the benefits but do not talk about the risk.
C) Tell him what percentage chance he has of a good outcome and do not talk about the bad things that are possible.
D) Explain the information to a tribal leader and let the tribal leader decide what to communicate with the patient.
E) Explain the process of informed consent to the patient and allow him to opt out of any part of the process he desires to avoid.

Discussion

The best answer is "E." Using the four guiding principles of medical ethics (autonomy, beneficence, nonmaleficence, and justice) is one way to work through this dilemma. Some would argue for "A" because the patient cannot make an informed decision without knowing the potential risk (autonomy) and "it's the law." However if the patient has traditional Navajo beliefs, proceeding with the full informed consent may deter the patient from undergoing a beneficial or even life-saving procedure, so would conflict with the principles of beneficence and nonmaleficence. "B" and "C" rely on stereotypes without making sure of the patient's beliefs. Asking a tribal leader and/or someone from the tribe who works in medicine is an excellent way of obtaining a cross-cultural perspective; however, ultimately we need to respect the patient's autonomy.

* *

Your patient consents for the surgery with a request that makes you uneasy: he wants to take the amputated limb home with him after the surgery. He gives two reasons why this is important to him: (1) the belief that a body must be whole to "cross over" to the next world and (2) a worry that the body parts could be used to cast spell on him or his family.

Which of the following would you NOT do in responding to his request?

A) Explain to him the potential health hazards of taking an infected limb home.
B) Explore how other people in the community who have had amputations have managed this.
C) Explain to him that you understand his concerns; however, the health risk of him taking the limb home far outweighs any other consideration so the limb will have to be disposed of by standard hospital practice.
D) Allow family members and community leader to participate in the discussion if the patient wishes.
E) Negotiate a way where as much as possible his wishes could be met, personal and public health and safety preserved, and community and hospital regulations followed.

Discussion

The answer is "C." Although hospital policy may limit your options, there is usually enough flexibility to allow you to accommodate the patient's wishes at least to some degree. You can use the LEARN mnemonic (**L**isten, **E**xplain, **A**cknowledge, **R**ecommend, **N**egotiate) to help approach this cultural conflict. First, you **Listen** to the patient's perspective. Often you have to probe with nonjudgmental questions to elucidate this. "B" and "D" can provide some cultural context for both the **Listening** and **N**egotiating phases. "A" would be part of **E**xplaining your perspective. Next you **Acknowledge** both the differences and similarities between the two perspectives. Then you **R**ecommend a plan hopefully where you and the patient both get what you want. Finally, as in "E," you may need to **N**egotiate.

Objectives: Did you learn to . . .

- Describe some differences in diabetes prevalence among different ethnic groups?
- Define the terms "disease" and "illness?"
- Explore a patient's personal and cultural reasons for nonadherence to traditional medical advice?
- Develop some tools for providing care to patients who have health beliefs that diverge from those of traditional Western medicine?

CASE 3

A young couple that just immigrated to your town from Bosnia comes to your clinic because they are expecting their first baby. The wife is 23 years old, in her first trimester, and without any medical problems. Your scheduler knows that many Bosnians are Muslim and has heard that female Muslims are supposed to avoid male physicians.

When making the appointment for this patient, the scheduler should:

A) Assign her to the first available OB provider.
B) Assign her to the first available female OB provider.
C) Assign her to your only Bosnian-speaking OB provider who is male.
D) Ask if she has a preference as to who she would like to receive care from.
E) Assign her to the OB provider who has the most experience and interest in working with patients from diverse cultures (maybe Dr. Smith since he eats out at a different ethnic restaurant every night).

Discussion

The answer is "D." Although it is true that many, if not most, Muslim women would find it inappropriate to have a male provider this is not universally true. Besides that, we are not even sure this patient is Muslim (about 40% of Bosnians are Muslim according to 2002 estimates). Cultural characteristic and belief systems are generalizations that often accurately describe a population. However, if you assume that is what is true of the group in general is also true for an individual, you are stereotyping and may often come to the wrong conclusion.

HELPFUL TIP: Use your knowledge of a patient's culture as a starting point. Ask about any assumptions or suspicions. Make sure you know how the belief applies in the current context.

* *

When she arrives in your clinic, you realize she speaks no English and her husband speaks only a little. Using his limited English and some hand gestures, you feel that you could conduct an interview with them. Because you completed a course titled "Advanced Life Support for Cultural Competence," you are able to deal with such a situation. Your mind drifts a little, back in time, to that course . . . ah, CME on the beach!

You recall that "cultural competence" is defined as:

A) Learning about multiple cultures.
B) Being able to speak multiple languages.
C) Taking diversity classes.
D) Adopting a set of cultural behaviors and attitudes that enable you to deliver effective medical care to people of different cultures.
E) Hiring staff from a variety of different cultures—preferably all good cooks who will provide some excellent ethnic cuisine.

Discussion

The correct answer is "D." While the other answers are laudable goals, they do not define cultural competency. Cultural competence is a set of behaviors and attitudes that aims to help health-care providers deliver better care to patients from many different cultures.

* *

You rack your brain trying to remember why cultural competence is important to you. You now regret skipping some of the lectures to go snorkeling.

Which of the following is NOT a benefit of achieving cultural competence?

A) It allows efficient use of time and resources.
B) It increases the chance of providing services that are consistent with patient needs.
C) It might improve health outcomes for minority patients.
D) It might improve patient retention.
E) It is less expensive in the long run.

Discussion

The correct answer is "E." Cultural competence allows you to use your time and resources efficiently, increasing the likelihood that you will provide the services your patient actually wants. This can lead to improved health outcomes for your patients and increased patient satisfaction, allowing you to retain more minority patients. Unfortunately, no studies so far show that it can reduce your practice's costs.

* *

Pondering this, you decide to try and provide culturally competent care to this nice couple in front of you.

Which one of the following is NOT a step in providing culturally competent care?

A) Understanding your own culture.
B) Understanding others' cultures.
C) Accepting every cultural practice as equally valid even when against best medical practices.
D) Understanding how your patients' cultural beliefs affect their attitude toward healthcare.
E) Adapting your way of working to provide optimal care.

Discussion

The correct answer is "C." The goal of cultural competence is to provide better healthcare for patients from different cultures. Some of the specific things this goal calls for include:

- Being respectful of cultural differences.
- Learning about other cultures.
- Being aware of the health impact of cultural beliefs and practices.
- Being sensitive to patients' needs.
- Using interpreters when necessary.
- Adapting to provide optimal care.

An easy way to achieve these goals is by using the Berlin and Fowkes' LEARN model described earlier in the chapter. However, this does not mean accepting every culture's practices as equally valid. A case in point would be female genital mutilation which is practiced in some 28 countries. This is clearly unethical.

> HELPFUL TIP: While learning and respecting patients' different cultural beliefs is vital, providing good care does not call for accepting practices that are detrimental to your patient's health. But beware... there are many potential ethical dilemmas that can occur when traditional Western medicine intersects with a culture that has radically different health beliefs. Many cross-cultural medical decisions are not as black and white as we and our patients would like to believe.

* *

Now that you are ready to proceed with caring for your patient, the question of language comes up. Should you use the husband to interpret (he seems to know a bit more English)?

To help guide you, you call your hospital compliance officer who tells you that:

A) It is Federal Law that you must provide an interpreter for patients who need it, at your own cost if necessary.
B) It is Federal Law that patients must provide their own interpreters at their own expense.
C) Most insurance companies reimburse for interpreter services.
D) Using family and staff to translate rarely reflects current practice.
E) There are no privacy concerns when using nonprofessional interpreters.

Discussion

The correct answer is "A." The 2007 census found that more than 55.4 million adults (around 20% of the US population) speak a non-English language at home, while almost 13% of the US population is foreign born. When the health-care professional does not speak the primary language of the patient, loss of important information, misunderstanding of physician instructions, and poor shared decision making can occur. Title VI of the 1964 Civil Rights Act requires health-care professionals to provide translation services for patients who need them, at the physician's cost if necessary. Failure to do so would qualify as discrimination and could be prosecuted. Unfortunately, most insurance companies do not reimburse for these services. Interpreters can be scarce and costly. As a result, many physicians use any help they can get for translation, including staff members and family members who are bilingual (so, "D" is a false statement). This leaves room for error. Using a family member as an interpreter makes it hard for the patient to disclose private information they do not want known by the family. Professional interpreters have been trained and certified, while ad hoc interpreters often have no formal training and can make translation mistakes.

Regarding healthcare, language barriers may result in:

A) Increased risk of intubation for children with asthma.
B) Greater nonadherence to medication regimens.
C) Higher resource use in diagnostic testing.
D) Increased risk of drug complications.
E) All of the above.

Discussion

The correct answer is "E." Language barriers have been associated with worse health status, lower likelihood of having a usual source of medical care, lower likelihood of being given a follow-up appointment after emergency department visit, greater nonadherence to medication regimens, increased risk of drug complications, impaired patient understanding of diagnoses, medication, and follow-up, lower patient satisfaction, longer medical visits, higher resource use in diagnostic testing, increase risk of intubation for children with asthma, greater risk of being assigned more severe psychopathology, and increased risk of leaving the hospital against medical advice.

What is the proper way to use an interpreter?

A) Address all questions to the interpreter while facing the interpreter.
B) Address questions to the patient while looking at the interpreter.
C) Address questions to the patient while facing the patient.
D) Address questions to the interpreter while facing the patient.
E) Have the interpreter get you coffee while you muddle through using gestures.

Discussion

The correct answer is "C." The physician should speak to and look at the patient; in other words, don't speak about the patient in the third person. Remember that nonverbal communication is important even when common languages are not shared. The physician should speak clearly and give the interpreter time to translate questions and answers. The physician should periodically pause and ensure that the patient understands the questions that are being asked. One way to do this is by asking brief, close-ended questions. Failure to look at the patient while asking questions may be interpreted as rude and should be avoided.

* *

You remember from medical school that there was disagreement as to the degree that a medical interpreter should function as a cultural advocate.

Which of the following would be the most effective preencounter instructions for your interpreter to facilitate the best possible communication between you and your patient?

A) "Translate word-for-word all that the patient and I say. You may repeat phrases, but do not rephrase anything."
B) "When clarifying, explaining or culturally translating concepts, make sure that you are transparent (i.e., let the both parties know what you are saying and why)."
C) "Be sure to culturally translate whenever you think it is appropriate."
D) "If the patient doesn't seem to understand, go ahead and explain whatever you think that I mean."
E) "Just make me sound like I know what I'm talking about."

Discussion

The correct answer is "B." Ideally, an interpreter would do an exact translation. However, many concepts do not translate literally or have very different meanings depending on the context that surrounds them. Good interpreters are often aware when the health-care provider and the patient do not have the same understanding of an event, concept, or plan. In this case, the translator should be sure to let each party know exactly what has been communicated. This feedback to each party is important so that the interpreter's moral values don't get projected onto the patient and unduly influence decisions made by the patient. Transparency is thus critical.

* *

You remember that low literacy is associated with poor outcomes.

Which of the following is NOT true?

A) Patients with low literacy have a 50% increased risk of hospitalization.
B) Only half of all patients take medications as directed.
C) Low literacy is a stronger predictor of a person's health than race.
D) Low literacy is only an issue among minorities and immigrants.

Discussion

The correct answer is "D." Poor health literacy skills are a stronger predictor of health status than a person's race, age, income, socioeconomic status, or employment. This relationship holds across different racial and cultural groups. Unfortunately, up to 90 million people in the United States have low-literacy skills and many are ashamed to share this with their physicians. This can lead to "noncompliance" because patients cannot read prescriptions and other instructions. It is not surprising, then, that low-literacy patients have an increased risk of hospitalization. To help combat this problem, the American Medical Association (AMA) Foundation has launched "Ask Me 3" program (http://www.npsf.org/for-healthcare-professionals/programs/ask-me-3/). "Ask Me 3" urges doctors to make sure their patients ask and understand the answers to three simple questions: What is my main problem? What do I need to do? Why is it important for me to do this? Other suggestions to improve communication include (1) asking the patient to repeat instructions back to the physician; (2) using basic, nonmedical language when talking to patients; and (3) allowing patients to talk uninterrupted at the beginning of the visit.

* *

You're interested in doing your part to help decrease problems with health literacy. You recently heard that the American Academy of Pediatrics has an office-based intervention to improve reading capability in young children call "Reach Out and Read."

Which of the following is/are true about reading and "Reach Out and Read?"

A) It is a program of primary prevention of reading problems that is evidence based.
B) Physicians model reading out loud during the well-child visit.
C) Free age- and development-appropriate books are given to children between 6 months and 5 years at their well-child visits.
D) All of the above.

Discussion

The correct answer is "D." Between 10% and 40% of low-income children have no books at home—a depressing and surprising statistic. A quarter of college-educated parents do not read to their young children daily. Reach Out and Read can be summarized by the SAFER mnemonic: **S**how the book early in the visit, **S**hare the book with the child yourself, modeling the reading for the parents, **A**sk the parents about reading, **A**ssess the child's development and the parent–child relationship, give **F**eedback about what you've observed the child do, give **F**eedback about parents' attitudes and interactions with the child, **E**ncourage the parents to read daily to the child, **E**xplain about literacy development, **R**efer to the library and literacy programs, and **R**ecord in the chart what you did. Other than giving a book and briefly reading to the child, you need not do all the activities at each visit. If your clinic is not involved in the program, you can get started at www.reachoutandread.org.

HELPFUL TIP: The National Center for Cultural Competence at Georgetown University has identified six compelling reasons that health-care providers should incorporate cultural competency into their practice. They are:

1. To respond to current and projected demographic changes in the United States.
2. To eliminate long-standing disparities in the health status of people of diverse racial, ethnic, and cultural backgrounds.
3. To improve the quality of services and health outcomes.
4. To meet legislative, regulatory, and accreditation mandates.
5. To gain a competitive edge in the marketplace.
6. To decrease the likelihood of liability/malpractice claims.

Objectives: Did you learn to . . .

- Describe ways in which you inquire about a patient's culturally related health beliefs?
- Define cultural competence and understand its importance?
- List some complications that can occur as a result of language barriers?
- Use interpreter services effectively and appropriately?
- Describe the state of health literacy in the United States and its impact on population health?

CASE 4

You are seeing a 67-year-old Black male for the first time in your clinic. He claims to be healthy but has not seen a physician for over three decades. He says, "Doctors . . . I try to avoid them. My wife made me come today." You tell him you are going to take a history and then perform a physical exam on him. After you are done, you tell him you recommend age-appropriate screening exams for colon and prostate cancer. The patient politely declines both. You try to explain the importance of screening to him.

Which of the following statements about screening is INCORRECT?

A) Prostate cancer is a leading cause of death among Black men.
B) Colon cancer is a leading cause of death among Black men.
C) There is clear evidence that screening for colon cancer reduces mortality in Black men.
D) There is clear evidence that screening for prostate cancer among Black men saves lives.
E) Prostate cancer disproportionately affects Black men.

Discussion

The correct answer is "D." There is no firm evidence that screening for prostate cancer reduces mortality from the disease (see Chapter 16). Prostate cancer is the fifth leading cause of cancer death overall in the United States, and the burden of prostate cancer varies among different racial and ethnic groups. **Black men have about a 60% higher incidence and a 2.4-fold higher mortality rate from prostate cancer compared with White men.** Compared with White men, mortality from prostate cancer is 17% lower in non-White Hispanics and 55% lower in Asian Americans and Pacific Islanders.

* *

Your patient now agrees to colon cancer screening but still declines prostate cancer screening. Your exam also revealed an elevated blood pressure (BP) of 160/90 mm Hg with no abnormal cardiac, lung, or other organ system findings.

Assuming you confirm this elevated BP reading at subsequent visits, which of the following antihypertensives would you recommend?

A) Hydrochlorothiazide.
B) Ramipril.
C) Minoxidil.
D) Atenolol.
E) Losartan.

Discussion

The correct answer is "A." While diuretics are a good choice for most patients with hypertension, they are an especially good choice in Blacks. Diuretics are particularly effective in Blacks, who tend to have extremely salt-sensitive hypertension. Blacks are more likely than other patients with hypertension to have low renin levels, which make them **less likely to respond to ACE inhibitors. Beta-blockers also tend to be less effective in Black patients.** A reasonable second-line therapy in this patient would be a calcium channel blocker.

* *

Your patient agrees to your medication choice, but he wants to know if the research on which you based your choice included Black people. You can confidently say yes, knowing that the ALLHAT trial specifically addressed the issue of generalizability by making sure that about a third of the 33,357 subjects were Black. However, you know this has not always been true in scientific research. In fact, you know that minorities are very underrepresented in research data on which we base our treatment choices.

Which of the following is *NOT* a reason why there are few minorities in research studies?

A) Past history of abuse leading to mistrust of the health-care system.
B) Lack of representation of minorities in the medical profession.
C) Discrimination.
D) Overrepresentation of minorities in lower socioeconomic status.
E) Minorities are more likely to volunteer for studies but are generally excluded.

Discussion

The correct answer is "E." Minorities' contact with the medical system has been fraught with abuse in the past. Possibly the most egregious example of this is the Tuskegee Syphilis Study where Black men with syphilis were recruited for a naturalistic study of the disease in the 1930s. Over 400 Black men with syphilis were recruited with 200 men without syphilis as controls. There was no informed consent, and they were told the lie that spinal taps (done for research) were a form of treatment. It was soon apparent that the death rate among those with syphilis was about twice as high as it was among the controls. When penicillin was found to be effective as a cure for syphilis in the 1940s, the participants were neither informed nor offered treatment, so the naturalistic study could continue.

These and other examples of past mistreatment by the medical community constitute a significant source of distrust for minority patients, who are less likely to participate in research. There have also been overt and subtle discriminatory barriers against minority participation in clinical trials. Minorities are more likely to be poor and undereducated, and research subjects are generally more educated and of higher socioeconomic status. Finally, there is a significant underrepresentation of minorities in the medical profession. For example, even though Blacks comprise 13% of the population, they are only 3.5% of the physician population. All these problems lead to difficulties recruiting minority participants for research trials.

What percentage of Americans belong to a minority group?

A) 15%.
B) 20%.
C) 25%.
D) 36%.
E) 62%.

Discussion

The correct answer is "D." According to the 2010 US Census estimates, 36% of Americans are ethnic minorities, up from 31% in 2000 and 24% in 1990. Yet, only 10% of physicians are from underrepresented minority groups. This is problematic. The lack of minority physicians leads to a discrepancy in health-care access. Data shows minority physicians are more likely to serve minority patients and are more likely to serve in urban, underserved areas (where there tends to be greater concentration of underprivileged patients).

HELPFUL TIP: Black physicians are 5 times more likely to treat Black patients, and Hispanic physicians are 2.5 times more likely to treat Hispanic patients, as compared with non-Black and non-Hispanic physicians, respectively. Minority physicians are also more likely to serve Medicaid patients and those without insurance.

HELPFUL TIP: Patients of all ethnic backgrounds consistently rate their relationships with their physician better when their physician is of the same ethnic background.

Which of the following is NOT true?

A) Patients living in a disadvantaged neighborhood have an increased incidence of coronary artery disease.
B) Patients living in inner city, disadvantaged neighborhoods have an increased incidence of asthma.
C) Patients of the same minority group who are not economically deprived have the same incidence of disease as those who are economically deprived.
D) Very low-income Black children have a higher incidence of asthma than White children of the same social economic status.
E) Patients from disadvantaged neighborhoods not only have a higher risk of developing most cancers but also are less likely to receive aggressive treatment once diagnosed.

Discussion

The correct answer is "C." Patients living in disadvantaged neighborhoods have increased incidences of coronary artery disease, most cancers (lung, colon, cervical), diabetes, arthritis, accidents, adverse birth outcomes, **and** asthma. They also get less care and less aggressive care (except for limb amputations in diabetics) for their ailments and are less likely to have care that adheres to treatment guidelines. Minority patients who are economically well off tend to have better health than poorer members of their ethnic group.

In taking care of Black patients, all of these general principles are helpful to keep in mind EXCEPT:

A) Family relationships are extremely important.
B) Religion often has a role in the patient's life.
C) It is expected that physicians will call patients by their first name.
D) Food is an important part of Black culture.
E) Nonverbal communication is often as important as what is said.

Discussion

The correct answer is "C." Blacks often maintain extended family ties and view healthcare as a family responsibility. Therefore, physicians should consider enlisting the family's help in taking care of an ill family member.

Religion is often an important aspect in Black cultures, and members of the clergy are highly respected in the community. Churches are very helpful for community outreach efforts, and evidence exists that using churches to conduct preventive care services, such as immunizations and screening programs for illnesses, leads to better patient compliance with preventive guidelines. Some patients may view illness as a test of one's faith, and it is prudent for the physician to acknowledge and respect the patient's beliefs and perception of illness to the extent that it influences their seeking or receiving healthcare. Poorer Blacks have little choice but to eat what is available at a low cost. This means our advice to patients to eat a well-balanced diet with fresh fruit, lean meat, and fresh vegetables may be met with a deaf ear. Advising simple changes in diet including substituting fish or chicken for red meat in dishes, eating inexpensive raw vegetables, modifying cooking techniques, and changing to a vegetable-based rather than a meat-based diet may be more likely to meet with success.

Communication is important, with Blacks being particularly attentive to nonverbal aspects of communication such as body language and voice inflection. Respect is also emphasized in the culture, and patients often like to be addressed by their formal titles and not their first names or appellations like "honey" or "sweetie" that are generally condescending. Asking patients permission to call them by their first names is appreciated.

Blacks often prefer information using real-life examples, rather than cold, dry data, or written messages. A nice summary of general principles to keep in mind when taking care of Blacks is found in an article on Preventive Care for African Americans by Witt et al. (2002). They are:

- Gaining trust and understanding the historical distrust of the health-care system.
- Understanding and employing the kinship web in decisions regarding screening and treatment.
- Involving the church in developing and delivering prevention and care messages.
- Asking patients about the meaning of words or phrases.
- Asking patients about the use of alternative medicines and herbs.
- Tailoring messages about prevention to depictions of real-life situations.
- Paying attention to body language and other nonverbal communication.

* *

You have learned in medical school about the importance of behavior change in tackling chronic diseases like hypertension, heart disease, and diabetes, yet are frustrated that you have less success in patients who are poorer or from different racial or ethnic backgrounds.

Which of the following behaviors or attributes is most strongly associated with your patient's health status:

A) How often they exercise.
B) Whether they have health insurance or not.
C) How healthy a diet they eat.
D) Their social economic status (how wealthy they are).
E) How much they smoke.

Discussion

The correct answer is "D." It's like U2 says in their song *God Part II*: "The rich stay healthy; the sick stay poor." Socioeconomic status is a key driver in health status.

HELPFUL TIP: Fresh produce is often not available or quite expensive in low-income neighborhoods. Predominantly White neighborhoods have four times as many supermarkets as predominantly Black and Latino neighborhoods. This makes dietary change especially difficult.

CASE 5

Your next two patients are a couple of Cuban friends who present to your office seeking a family physician to take care of their general health needs. They are both Cuban but while one is White, the other is Black.

Which of the following assumptions is correct?

A) Hispanic people are of one race.
B) Hispanic people can all speak English.
C) Hispanic people share a common language.
D) Hispanic people are not American.
E) Hispanic people all like to be called Latino.

Discussion

The correct answer is "C." The term *Hispanic* denotes an ethnic group who shares in common some cultural practices with Spanish as their primary language. However, they comprise a significantly diverse group who may or may not speak English, may be of any race, hail from different countries of origin, have differing histories, socioeconomic status, and cultural identity. Some feel the term *Hispanic* is derogatory, reflecting their European ancestry, and may prefer the term Latino. Thirteen percent of the overall US population is now "Hispanic," and they are the largest ethnic group in the United States having increased by 58% during the 1990s. Despite the diversity represented within the Latino culture, there exist certain values that are shared. As with many Black cultures, there are strong family ties with families tending to be large and extended. Families serve as the main source of support and often share in decision making. Physicians with a warm bedside manner who demonstrate appropriate respect (especially to the elderly) are appreciated. Immigrants from Latin America may come to the United States for economic or political reasons, and increasingly because of family connections. Hispanics come from a broad spectrum of socioeconomic backgrounds and enter a variety of living conditions in the United States, which has an enormous impact on immigrant and public health.

HELPFUL TIP: Despite alarmist paranoia from some parts of our political spectrum, second-generation Hispanic immigrants are as likely to speak English as were prior waves of immigrants from European countries.

Which of the following is FALSE regarding health issues affecting the Latino community?

A) Infectious diseases are common.
B) Fear of deportation prevents some from seeking healthcare.
C) Lack of insurance can be a potent barrier to accessing healthcare.
D) Moving to the United States can paradoxically raise the risk for habits that lead to illness such as obesity and diabetes.
E) Elderly Latinos have a higher mortality than their White counterparts.

Discussion

The correct answer is "E." Recent immigrants are often prone to infectious diseases due to inadequate housing, sanitation, and/or immunizations. Many reasons exist why patients may not get vaccinated. These include disbelief in the need for the vaccine, being unaware of the vaccine, lack of patient education by a health-care provider, lack of transportation, and financial restrictions.

Immigrating to the United States can result in worse nutrition, obesity, a sedentary lifestyle, and an increase in smoking and risky sexual behavior in Latinas (Hispanic women). This translates, in part, into a twofold increased incidence of diabetes in Latinas. For Latino males, there is an increased risk of drug abuse, alcohol abuse, tobacco use, and driving under the influence. These risks increase the longer the patient lives in the United States.

Latinos often fail to get preventive healthcare. For example, they have a lower rate of screening for diabetes and hypertension than Blacks or Whites. Some avoid presenting for healthcare because they fear being discovered by immigration authorities. Others are hindered by the lack of insurance. Complementary and alternative practices are also common. Even though they are less likely to access healthcare, older Hispanics seem to have a similar or greater life expectancy than same-age Whites in the United States and enjoy lower mortality rates from cardiovascular diseases, cancer, and chronic illnesses. The risk of diabetes, however, is higher. This phenomenon has been described as "selective immigration" and implies a predilection for healthier individuals to immigrate to this country.

* *

You get into a discussion on race with your new Cuban patients, and they point out several things to you that you had not thought of before.

Which of the following is true about race?

A) It is a valid biological construct.
B) It is interchangeable with ethnicity.
C) All members of a certain culture are the same race.
D) It is a purely social construct.

Discussion

The correct answer is "D." Race is a much politicized and emotionally charged topic in the history of the United States. Since the late 18th and early 19th centuries, attempts have been made to validate race as being biologically based to justify discriminatory practices. However, the Human Genome Project demonstrated conclusively that there is **no** biological basis for race. Humans share over 99.9% of their DNA, and one cannot tell a member of one race from another on the basis of genetics. "B" is incorrect. While race and ethnicity are often used interchangeably, they are not necessarily equivalent. Race is an arbitrary social construct that is given to people based on visual appearance, while ethnicity refers to people with a common country of origin, a shared ancestry, or a common history. Culture refers to a specific set of values, beliefs, and customs shared by members of a community. "C" is obviously incorrect. People from the same culture can be of different races so one can have White and Black Hispanics from Cuba, for example.

Which of the following health outcome disparities is FALSE?

A) White Hispanics have a higher incidence of breast and colorectal cancer than Blacks and NHW.
B) Clinicians may order fewer diagnostic tests if they do not understand a patient's description of symptoms.
C) Clinicians may overcompensate by ordering more tests when they do not understand what their patients are saying.
D) Minority children are more likely to be evaluated and reported for suspected abuse even after controlling for likelihood of abusive injury.
E) Blacks have the highest colorectal cancer mortality rates.

Discussion

The correct answer is "A." The **incidence** of colorectal and breast cancer is actually lower in White Hispanics than in other Whites and Blacks. However, this does not always translate into less significant disease. There are significant disparities in health-care quality and outcomes for minorities compared with nonminorities, even when controlling for possible confounding factors such as income, education, and insurance. **So even though Hispanics have a lower incidence of the above-named cancers, they have a similar mortality when compared with non-Hispanics.** All of the rest of the statements are correct. Of particular note, Blacks have the highest colorectal cancer mortality rates. Also, of note is the fact that when toddlers of different races present with similar fractures, minority toddlers are significantly more likely to be reported for suspected abuse, even after controlling for age, insurance status, and likelihood of abuse. This is a reflection of biases and stereotyping.

HELPFUL TIP: Minority patients are significantly less likely to have their pain treated by physicians. Additionally, there are few, if any, pharmacies in poor, inner-city areas that have narcotics available for patients with a prescription. This adversely affects the pain management of minority patients even further.

* *

In general, mortality rates among racial and ethnic minorities are higher for cancer, heart disease, diabetes, stroke, kidney failure, and HIV/AIDS. Minority groups are also disproportionately affected by asthma, lead poisoning, accidents, homicides, and other environmental health concerns. Some minorities experience higher infant mortality rates and are less likely to receive timely prenatal care. There are numerous other examples of health-care disparities that exist between majority and minority groups. These include but are not limited to:

- Infant death rates for Blacks are twice that of Whites.
- Heart disease mortality rates are 40% higher in Blacks as compared with Whites.
- Hispanics are almost twice as likely as Whites to die from diabetes and are more likely to be obese and have high blood pressure than are NHW.
- Blacks are 13% less likely to undergo coronary angioplasty and one-third less likely to undergo bypass surgery than are Whites.
- Only 7% of Black and 2% of Hispanic preschool children hospitalized for asthma are prescribed routine medications to prevent future hospitalizations compared with 21% of White children (not in itself a good reflection on our profession).
- The length of time between an abnormal screening mammogram and follow-up diagnostic testing is more than twice as long for Asian American, Hispanics, and Blacks compared with Whites.
- Minorities are less likely to get immunizations, mammograms, and other preventive care, even when paid for by Medicare.
- There are higher rates of un-insurance and lack of physicians in minority communities, leading to reduced access to primary care.
- Minorities are less likely to get heart catheterizations, CABG, dialysis, lung cancer surgery, and organ transplants.
- Blacks have 55% higher mortality rate and 6-year shorter life expectancy than Whites.
- Several studies show the deleterious effect of discrimination on health outcomes, including increasing the risk of diabetes, hypertension, depression, and preterm birth independent of other risk factors.

HELPFUL TIP: Although perhaps not overtly racist, there is data that suggests that unconscious biases can affect our care of patients. A well-known study in the NEJM in 1999 found that, all things being equal, physicians were **60% less likely** to refer Black women for cardiac catheterization than men and Whites. Hopefully, by being made aware of this unconscious bias, its effect can be mitigated and better care provided to all patients.

Objectives: Did you learn to . . .

- Describe some health disparities based on race, culture, and ethnicity?
- Delineate the differences between the terms race, culture, and ethnicity?

CASE 6

You are on the board of your hospital's therapeutics and safety committee and you have been asked to address the issue of medication. Mrs. X, a 72-year-old patient with diabetes who was hospitalized for an acute myocardial infarction, had died from what seems to be a sudden cardiac event. This was unexpected as she was recovering rather well. One of the nurses on the floor had told her supervisor that Dr Watters, your partner, had written an order for 6 U of insulin but the new nurse, fresh out of nursing school, had misread this as 60 U of insulin and had proceeded to give the poor lady that amount, precipitating the hypoglycemic event that was to lead to her death. The nurse is distressed as she thought she was only following orders. Around your office, Dr Watters' handwriting is a thing of legend: many pharmacists have had to call to double-check his prescriptions on more than one occasion.

Which of the following would have been an effective way to prevent the type of error that occurred?

A) The nurse should have called to confirm the dose of insulin before giving it.
B) Writing out "units" rather than "U."
C) Use of computerized physician order entry.
D) Having a clinical pharmacist as part of the team could have helped catch the error and prevent it from happening.
E) All of the above.

Discussion

The correct answer is "E." It is estimated that between 44,000 and 98,000 deaths annually are attributable to medical errors, most of which are preventable. Though the numbers have been challenged, it is unarguable that medical errors continue to contribute to adverse outcomes in our patients. One of the large contributors to this is medication errors. One of the leading causes of medication errors is the use of potentially dangerous abbreviations and dose designations. The use of "U" as above has been reported in the literature to be very problematic as it can easily be misread as a zero or a four, leading to up to 10-fold overdoses that can often have terrible consequences in patients using insulin.

Which of these would *NOT* be recommended as a way to prevent prescription errors?

A) Computerized order entry systems.
B) A brief notation of the purpose for the prescription.
C) Metric system for all therapies except those like insulin and vitamins that use standard units.
D) Inclusion of age, and when appropriate, weight of the patient.
E) A trailing zero after a decimal.

Discussion

The correct answer is "E." Nurses and pharmacists may not see the decimal point and thus give an order of magnitude higher dose of medication.

Which of these is prohibited by Health Insurance Portability and Accountability Act (HIPAA)?

A) Calling out patients' names in the waiting room.
B) Leaving a message on a patient's answering machine.
C) Releasing health information to a specialist without patient authorization if that information is to be used for purposes of treatment, payment, or health operations.
D) Faxing patient information.
E) None of the above.

Discussion

The correct answer is "E." Since the HIPAA went into effect, many physicians have been confused as to what they can and cannot do under the HIPAA law. Providers can still call out patients' names in the waiting room as long as you do not go into particulars of their presenting complaint in front of other people (e.g., don't say, "Ms. Smith I'm ready to check on your herpes infection" to the whole waiting room). You may leave a message on a patient's machine if the patient has authorized you to do so. You may fax information once you verify the fax number is correct—but you can only fax to persons the patient designates or consents to. If you fax health information to a wrong number, you are responsible and could be violating HIPAA. Finally, HIPAA gives physicians broad leeway in sharing information with other physicians, provided the information is used for treatment, payment, and health-care operations. You must give a notice of your privacy practices to the patients and ask them to sign a form acknowledging receiving the notice or make a good-faith effort to get them to sign it.

Objectives: Did you learn to . . .

- Recognize some causes of medical errors and ways to prevent them?
- Describe elements of the HIPAA law?

BIBLIOGRAPHY

Cultural Competence Compendium: Section IV-Underserved and underrepresented racial, ethnic, and socioeconomic groups. American Medical Association. Available at: http://wwwama-assn.org/ama/pub/category/2661.html.

Diaz VA, Jr. Cultural factors in preventive care: Latinos. *Primary Care; Clinics in Office Practice*. 2002;29(3):503-517.

Institute of Medicine. Unequal treatment: Confronting racial and ethnic disparities in health care. Available at: http://books.nap.edu/books/030908265X/html/.

National Center for Cultural Competence. Available at: www.georgetown.edu/research/gudc/ncc6.html.

Recommendations to Correct Error-Prone Aspects of Prescription Writing, NCCMERP Council Recommendation, adopted September 4, 1996. Available at: www.nccmerp.org.

Rodriguez MA. Cultural and linguistic competence: Improving quality in family violence health care interventions. *Clin Fam Pract*. March 2003.

Witt D, et al. Cultural factors in preventive care: African-Americans. *Primary Care; Clinics in Office Practice*. 2002; 29(3)

Yarnall KSH, et al. Primary care: Is there enough time for prevention? *Am J Public Health*. 2003;93:635-641. Available at: http://www.acgme.org.

30

Final Examination

Mark A. Graber and Jason K. Wilbur

This is your final exam. See how you do . . . .

1) Which of the following IS NOT an *absolute* contraindication to cardiac exercise testing?

A) Unstable angina.
B) Recent pulmonary embolism.
C) Active pericarditis.
D) Left bundle branch block.

See p. 64.

2) Which of the following is the preferred antiplatelet drug for treating chest pain in the emergency department?

A) Aspirin 81 mg PO.
B) Aspirin 325 mg PO.
C) Clopidogrel 75 mg PO.
D) Clopidogrel 300 mg PO.
E) 2B/IIIA glycoprotein inhibitor.

See p. 51.

3) This ECG, shown on page 894, represents an:

A) Inferior wall MI.
B) Anterior wall MI.
C) Inferolateral MI.
D) A normal ECG.

See p. 102.

4) The most appropriate initial treatment of this rhythm in a stable patient, shown on page 895, is:

A) Amiodarone.
B) Adenosine.
C) Diltiazem.
D) Lidocaine.

See p. 71.

5) Which statement is true?

A) An elevated troponin is always indicative of cardiac ischemia/infarct.
B) Troponin rises before CPK and stays elevated for a longer period of time.
C) Pulmonary embolism and renal failure are two causes of an elevated troponin.
D) CPK is overall the most sensitive (but not specific) cardiac marker for cardiac ischemia.

See pp. 49–50.

6) In a patient with coronary artery disease or >20% risk of cardiac disease in the next 10 years, what is the recommended LDL goal?

A) <130 mg/dL.
B) <110 mg/dL.
C) <100 mg/dL.
D) There is no LDL goal if the HDL is >50 mg/dL.

See p. 60.

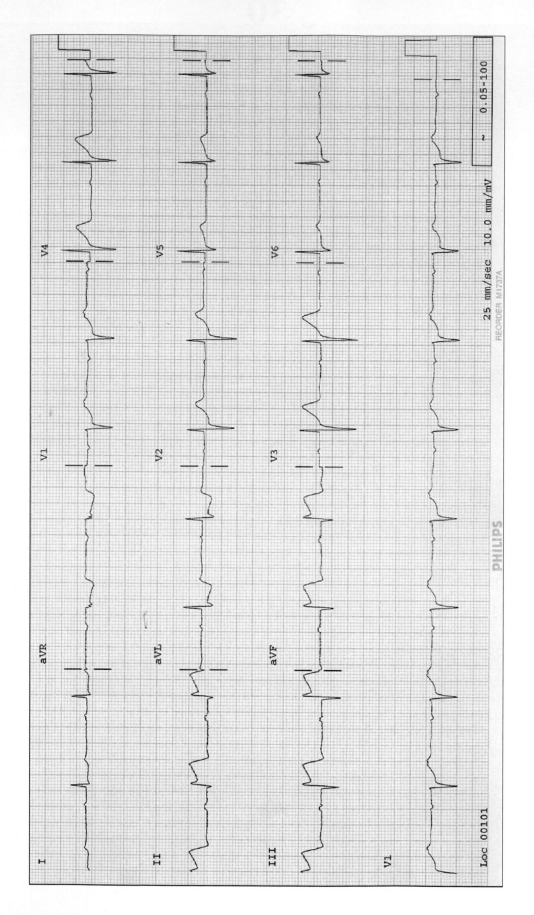

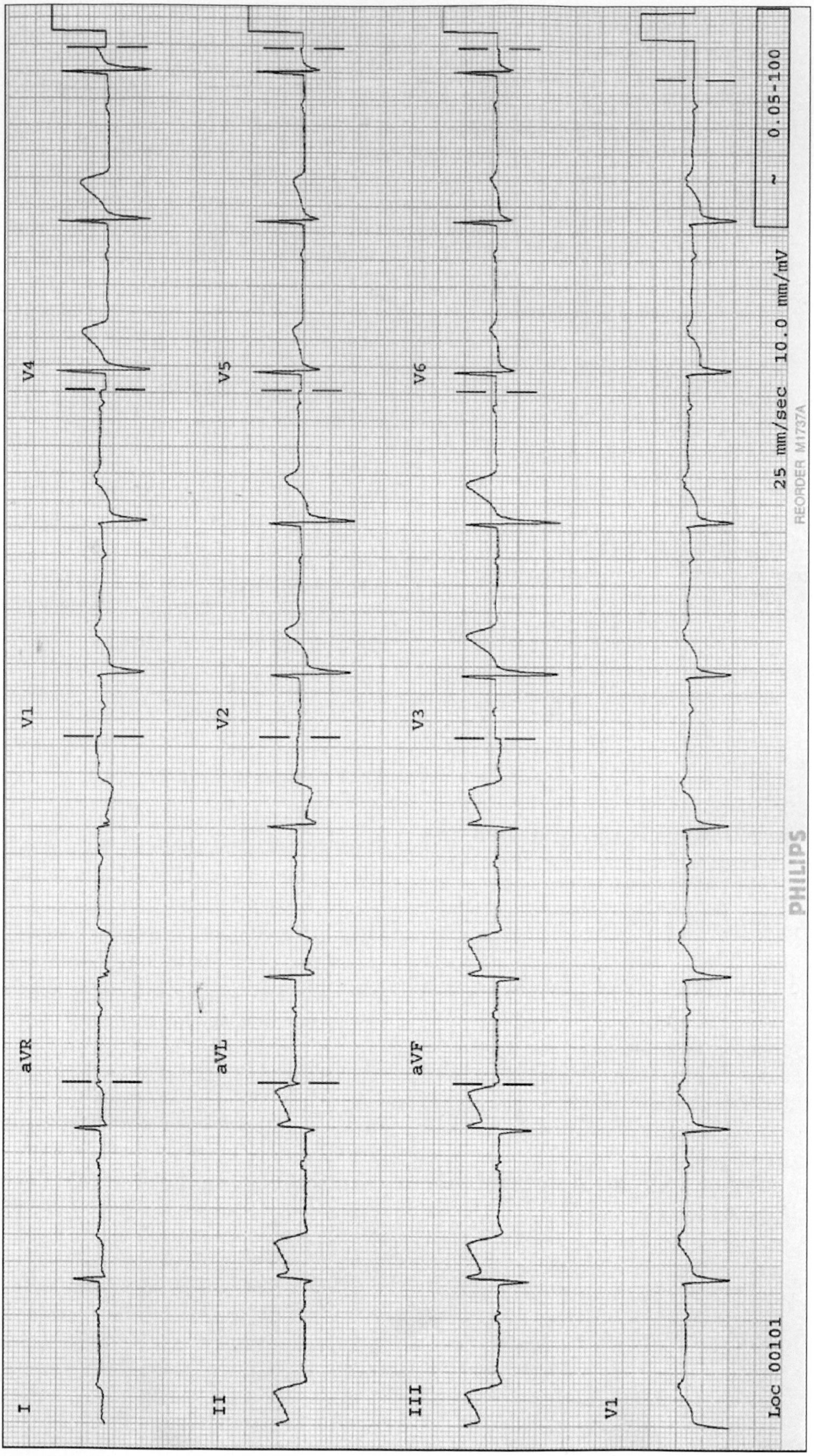

I
aVR
V1
V4
II
aVL
V2
V5
III
aVF
V3
V6
V1
Loc 00101
25 mm/sec 10.0 mm/mV
~ 0.05-100
PHILIPS
REORDER M1737A

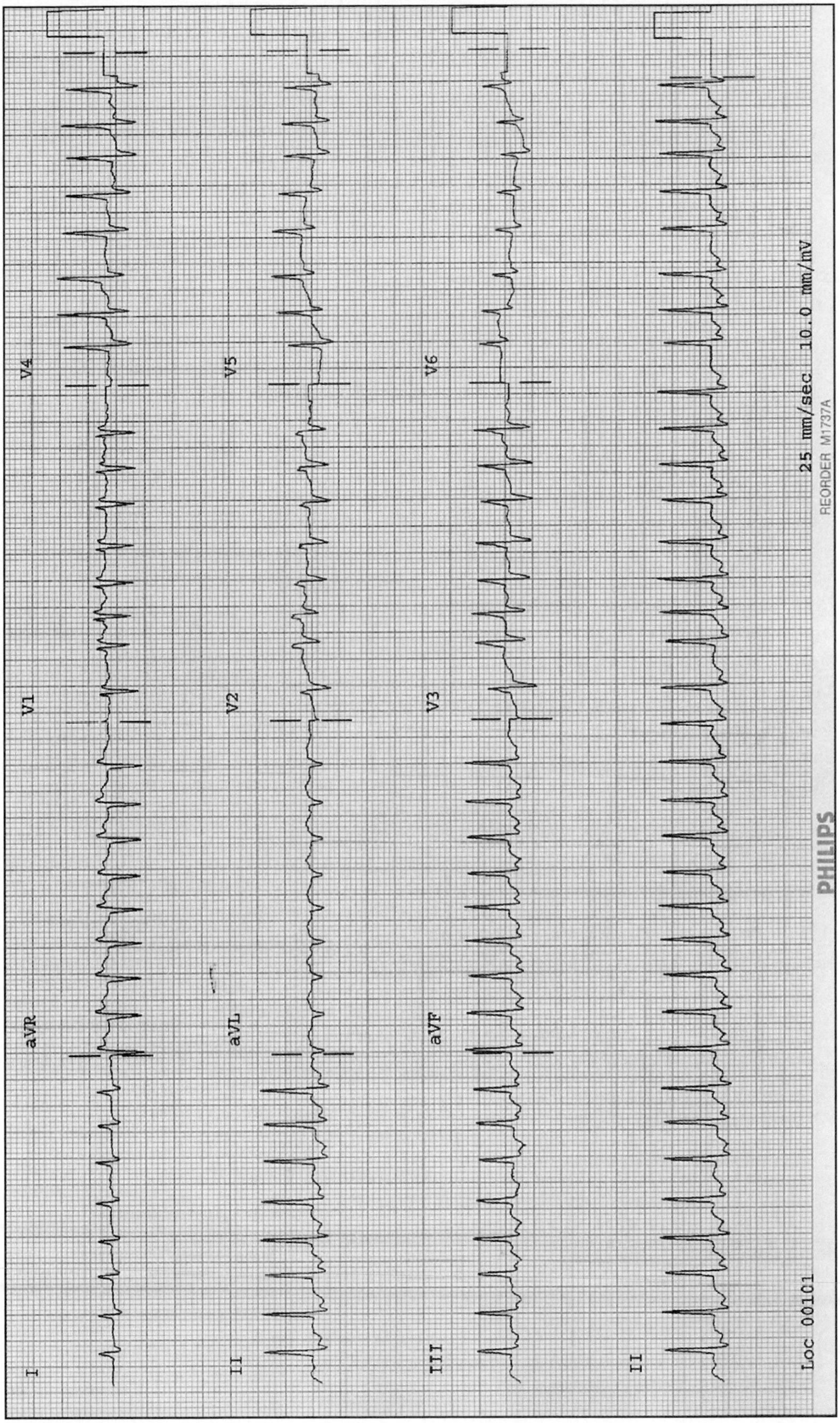
I
aVR
V1
V4
II
aVL
V2
V5
III
aVF
V3
V6
II
Loc 00101
25 mm/sec 10.0 mm/mV
REORDER M1737A
PHILIPS

7) Which of the following IS NOT a contraindication to the use of tPA in MI?

A) Blood pressure of >180/110 mm Hg.
B) Noncompressible vascular puncture (e.g., subclavian line).
C) Major surgery within 3 weeks.
D) Menstrual bleeding.

See p. 54.

8) Which of the following IS NOT a class 1 indication for tPA in a patient with an acute myocardial infarction?

A) Greater than 1 mm ST elevation in 2 or more contiguous leads.
B) Pain for less than 10 hours.
C) Age <75.
D) New complete bundle branch block and typical history suggestive of MI.

See pp. 54–55.

9) Your patient has an elevation of his liver function tests after starting an HMG-CoA reductase inhibitor. When would you consider stopping this patient's HMG-CoA reductase inhibitor?

A) Doubling of LFTs.
B) Tripling of LFTs.
C) Quadrupling of LFTs.
D) Only when there is biopsy evidence of bridging fibrosis.

See p. 60.

10) A CHADS2 score of 2 mandates which of the following options for a patient in atrial fibrillation?

A) Aspirin.
B) Warfarin.
C) Xarelto (*rivaroxaban*) or Pradaxa (*dabigatran*).
D) Either aspirin, warfarin, rivaroxaban, or dabigatran.

See p. 73.

11) Which of the following DOES NOT improve cardiovascular mortality in CHF?

A) Digoxin.
B) Spironolactone.
C) ACE inhibitors.
D) Beta-blockers.

See p. 79.

12) Which statement is true regarding gastric lavage in a patient with a toxic ingestion?

A) Gastric lavage should be done if it has been less than 4 hours after the ingestion.
B) Gastric lavage should be done until the returned material is clear (maximum of 10 liters).
C) Gastric lavage is associated with esophageal injury and aspiration.
D) Gastric lavage is indicated for petroleum distillates within 1 hour of ingestion.

See p. 1.

13) HPV vaccine is indicated for all of the following EXCEPT:

A) 24-year-old female with cervical dysplasia.
B) 39-year-old female who has never been sexually active.
C) 18-year-old female with known HPV.
D) Immunosuppressed 15-year-old female who is HIV positive.

See p. 446.

14) Topical tretinoin (Retin-A) is most effective in what kind of acne?

A) Cystic/nodular.
B) Inflammatory papular.
C) Pustular.
D) Comedonal.

See pp. 595–596.

15) In a study of drug A, 50% of patients in the treatment of arm benefit versus 25% in the placebo group. What is the number needed to treat?

A) 2.
B) 4.
C) 6.
D) 8.

See p. 870.

16) The most common cause of erythema multiforme is:

A) Herpes zoster.
B) Streptococcal pharyngitis.
C) Genital herpes.
D) Rhus exposure ("poison ivy").

See p. 597.

17) "Sensitivity" is best defined as:

A) True positives/(true positives + false negatives).
B) True positives.
C) True positives/(true positives + true negatives).
D) True positives/(true positives + false positives).

See p. 867.

18) Which of the following is true regarding isotretinoin (Accutane)?

A) Women should be on one form of birth control before using this drug.
B) Pregnancy should be avoided for 3 months after discontinuation of this drug.
C) Monthly pregnancy tests should be done on women who are sexually active with men.
D) Isotretinoin may increase the HDL.

See p. 596.

19) In general, what will happen with an innocent flow murmur during a Valsalva maneuver?

A) It gets louder.
B) It gets softer.
C) It is unchanged in volume.
D) The sound becomes more harsh.

See p. 486.

20) What blood level of morphine is the most appropriate when treating pain from a terminal cause?

A) 1 μg/dL.
B) 5 μg/dL.
C) 10 μg/dL.
D) Blood levels are irrelevant in determining the appropriate dose of morphine in the terminally ill.

See p. 856.

21) Which of the following is NOT seen with an anticholinergic overdose?

A) Dry, flushed skin.
B) Miosis.
C) Confusion.
D) Low-grade fever.

See p. 5.

22) Which of the following IS NOT a cause of an elevated anion gap acidosis?

A) Methanol and other ingestions (e.g., salicylate).
B) Diabetic ketoacidosis.
C) Uremia.
D) GI bicarbonate loss.

See p. 8.

23) Reperfusion of extremities in hypothermia can cause all of the following EXCEPT:

A) Acidosis.
B) Hypokalemia.
C) Paradoxical central temperature drop.
D) Arrhythmia.

See p. 23.

24) What is the appropriate course of action after treating a child with croup with inhaled epinephrine?

A) Admission for observation.
B) Admission if room air oxygen saturation is less than or equal to 95%.
C) Observation for 12 hours followed by discharge if stable.
D) Observation for 2 hours followed by discharge if stable.

See p. 44.

25) Which of the following is NOT included in the "drug cocktail" for the unconscious patient?

A) Glucose.
B) Thiamine.
C) Naloxone (Narcan).
D) Flumazenil (Romazicon).

See p. 3.

26) Which of the following is indicated in the child with croup (laryngotracheobronchitis)?

A) Amoxicillin.
B) Azithromycin.
C) Dexamethasone.
D) Oral theophylline.

See p. 44.

27) Which of the following is true?

A) A negative pregnancy test effectively rules out ectopic pregnancy.
B) Absence of an adnexal mass effectively rules out ectopic pregnancy.
C) Every woman of reproductive age with a uterus in the ED with abdominal pain is pregnant until proven otherwise.
D) The hCG should double every 5 days early in a normal pregnancy (e.g., when one is worried about an ectopic pregnancy).

See p. 34.

28) Which of the following is the best drug indicated for dyspnea in the terminally ill patient who wishes to be DNR?

A) Buccal scopolamine.
B) Lorazepam or other benzodiazepine.
C) Morphine or other opiate.
D) Nebulized lidocaine.

See p. 853.

29) What is the one best drug to reduce headache and confusion secondary to CNS tumor with surrounding edema?

A) Acetaminophen.
B) Dexamethasone.
C) Morphine.
D) Sumatriptan.

See p. 616.

30) Ipecac:

A) Should not be used.
B) Can be used if the ingestion may cause mental status changes.
C) Is effective if used within 30 minutes of an ingestion.
D) Is available OTC in American pharmacies.

See p. 1.

31) How frequently should methadone be dosed when used for pain control in the terminally ill?

A) Q 12 hours.
B) Q 8–12 hours.
C) Q 4–6 hours.
D) Methadone should not be used for pain management in the terminally ill.

See p. 857.

32) NSAIDs can cause ulceration in:

A) Stomach.
B) Duodenum.
C) Colon.
D) All of the above.

See p. 257.

33) What is true about the treatment of gastroesophageal reflux disease (GERD)?

A) Treatment of *H. pylori* is effective in curing GERD.
B) Treatment should always start with a proton pump inhibitor.
C) Surgical options (e.g., fundoplication) are often suboptimal with patients still requiring medication.
D) Esomeprazole is vastly superior to omeprazole.

See p. 249.

34) Which of the following is true regarding Barrett esophagus?

A) All patients with GERD should have an endoscopy to stage their disease vis-à-vis Barrett esophagus.
B) Barrett esophagus is a change from the normal columnar epithelium to squamous epithelium.
C) Barrett esophagus is present in >50% of patients with GERD.
D) Barrett esophagus can regress with adequate treatment of GERD.

See pp. 249–250.

35) Which of the following lesions is considered premalignant on colonoscopy?

A) Sessile polyp.
B) Hyperplastic polyp.
C) Tubular adenoma.
D) Pedunculated polyp.

See pp. 259–260.

36) Which of the following histories in a patient with GERD is most concerning for serious underlying disease?

A) Food bolus impaction on two separate occasions.
B) Dysphagia to solids followed in several months with dysphagia to liquids.
C) Reflux of undigested food at night.
D) Halitosis.

See p. 253.

37) Which of the following is an appropriate test of cure for *H. pylori*?

A) Stool antigen test done 1 month after finishing treatment.
B) Serum antibody test done 3 months after finishing treatment.
C) CLO test done 1 week after finishing treatment.
D) Breath urea test done 1 week after finishing treatment.

See p. 254.

38) What is true about a gastric feeding tube in the demented elderly?

A) It increases the patient's quality of life.
B) It should be used as a comfort measure only.
C) It reduces mortality.
D) It does nothing to improve quality of life but can cause complications.

See p. 712.

39) Which of the following is NOT a component of CREST syndrome?

A) Calcinosis.
B) Renal failure.
C) Esophageal dysmotility.
D) Sclerodactyly.

See p. 252.

40) Which of these drugs is indicated for control of an *acute* flare of Crohn disease?

A) Any 5-ASA moiety.
B) Oral prednisone.
C) Sulfasalazine.
D) Thalidomide.

See p. 262.

41) Which of the following is a contraindication to use of sulfasalazine in Crohn disease?

A) Aspirin allergy.
B) Heme positive stools.
C) Fever.
D) Platelet count $<100,000$.

See p. 263.

42) Which of the following is the best screening test for hepatitis C?

A) Quantitative HVC PCR.
B) Hepatitis C antibody.
C) RIBA.
D) Qualitative HVC PCR.

See p. 269.

43) Which of the following is the most specific test for gluten enteropathy (nontropical sprue)?

A) Antiendomysial IgA antibody.
B) Tissue transglutaminase antibody.
C) Antigliadin antibody.
D) Breath hydrogen test.

See p. 266.

44) *C. difficile* colitis has been linked to all of the following EXCEPT:

A) Hospitalization.
B) Use of fluoroquinolones.
C) Use of PPIs.
D) Use of H_2 blockers.

See p. 295.

45) Which of the following is recommended for treating Giardia?

A) Metronidazole.
B) Vancomycin.
C) Ciprofloxacin.
D) Azithromycin.

See pp. 261–262.

46) Which of the following foods DOES NOT contain gluten?

A) Oats.
B) Rye.

C) Rice.
D) Sticky rice.

See p. 267.

47) Which of the following tests is the most sensitive for the diagnosis of bacterial overgrowth syndrome (of the GI tract)?

A) Breath urea test.
B) Breath xylose test.
C) Breath hydrogen test.
D) CLO test.

See p. 266.

48) Which of the following is a relative contraindication to treatment of hepatitis C with interferon?

A) Fever.
B) Severe depression.
C) Severe osteoarthritis.
D) Severe eczema.

See p. 274.

49) Routine prenatal screening in the first trimester includes all of the following EXCEPT:

A) Blood type and antibody screen.
B) Hepatitis B surface antigen.
C) HIV antibody.
D) MSAFP (maternal serum alpha-fetoprotein).
E) Rubella antibody.

See p. 498.

50) A 22-year-old G2P2 female is ready to leave the hospital on postpartum day 2 after NSVD, but she develops lower abdominal pain and fever. She denies urinary symptoms. She reports constipation and moderate lochia. Her temperature is 38.8°C. She had prolonged rupture of membranes and prolonged labor, and the placenta was removed manually. The most appropriate course of action now is:

A) Discharge with acetaminophen for fever and follow up in 2 days.
B) Discharge with amoxicillin and follow up in 2 days.
C) Keep the patient in the hospital and obtain cultures for gonorrhea and chlamydia.
D) Keep the patient in the hospital and start IV gentamicin and clindamycin.
E) Manual exploration of the uterus for retained placenta.

See p. 503.

51) A 21-year-old G0 female presents for a physical exam and her first Pap smear. She has recently started sexual activity and has one lifetime partner. The results of the Pap smear show low-grade squamous intraepithelial lesion (LSIL). In accordance with guidelines, you recommend:

A) Immediate colposcopy.
B) Immediate referral for excisional procedure.
C) Return in 12 months for Pap smear.
D) Return in 3 months for Pap smear.
E) Return in 6 months for colposcopy and Pap smear.

See p. 528.

52) A 48-year-old female presents with menopausal symptoms. She has had a total hysterectomy but her ovaries are intact. She would like to know the benefits and risks of taking estrogen-only hormone replacement therapy. You tell her that estrogen-only HRT is associated with:

A) Decreased risk of breast cancer.
B) Decreased risk of ovarian cancer.
C) Increased risk of colon cancer.
D) Increased risk of osteoporosis.
E) Increased risk of stroke.

See p. 532.

53) A 25-year-old G5P4 female at 26 weeks' gestation presents to labor and deliver with abdominal pain. The pain is sharp or tearing and located in her lower abdomen. She has not had any contractions. She just began to have a little vaginal spotting before she came in. Her pregnancy has been complicated by tobacco use and hypertension. What is the most likely diagnosis?

A) Cervical cancer.
B) Normal labor.
C) Placenta previa.
D) Placental abruption.
E) Uterine rupture.

See p. 499.

54) The USPSTF recommends screening for osteoporosis in:

A) All adults aged 65 and older.
B) All men aged 75 and older.
C) All women aged 65 and older.
D) All women at onset of menopause.
E) Women who smoke at age 50 and older.

See p. 695.

55) A 79-year-old male presents with his wife who complains that he has been more forgetful over the past month. The patient agrees and complains of forgetting where he put things, where the car is parked, and names of acquaintances. Also, he is more irritable and angers easily. He has trouble sleeping, and he has lost 5 pounds. He is healthy and takes no medications. He has poor eye contact, a blunted affect, and poor concentration. His vitals and physical exam are otherwise normal. He can recall three items and draw a clock with no difficulty. The most likely cause of his symptoms is:

A) Delirium due to metastatic carcinoma.
B) Delirium due to underlying systemic infection.
C) Dementia due to Alzheimer disease.
D) Dementia due to stroke.
E) Depression.

See pp. 705–706.

56) You are considering treating a 65-year-old male with supplemental testosterone due to low serum testosterone levels associated with fatigue, muscle weakness, and mild depression. After initiating testosterone, it is most important to check which of the following?

A) Creatinine.
B) Hemoglobin.
C) Potassium.
D) Sodium.

See pp. 567–568.

57) Delirium in the hospitalized elderly patient can be prevented by implementing all of the following interventions upon admission EXCEPT:

A) Assuring patient has access to usual aides (hearing aides, glasses, etc.).
B) Early mobilization.
C) Lorazepam 1 mg QHS.
D) Noise reduction at night.
E) Orientation stimuli.

See p. 701.

58) A 75-year-old male with mild dementia, atrial fibrillation, osteoarthritis, and depression presents after sustaining a fall in his home 1 week ago. His son states, "He is a little banged up but otherwise fine." Your routine evaluation should include all of the following EXCEPT:

A) Asking about potential neglect and abuse.
B) CT scan of the brain.
C) Medication review.
D) Neurological examination.
E) Observation of the patient ambulating.

See p. 702.

59) A 75-year-old female fell and injured her hip. She did not fracture it but has significant pain. She has a remote history of peptic ulcer disease. She takes lisinopril for hypertension and phenytoin for a seizure disorder. Which pain medication will be safest for her to take?

A) Aspirin.
B) Meperidine.
C) Hydrocodone.
D) Piroxicam.
E) Propoxyphene.

See pp. 712–713.

60) An 80-year-old female nursing home resident with dementia recently started refusing medication and slapping at the staff when they try to bathe her. The nurse at the care center calls to request "something for her agitation." As the safest and most effective intervention, you recommend:

A) A behavior log to track when the agitation occurs and what might be causing it.
B) Haloperidol 1 mg IV prior to bathing and medication administration.
C) Haloperidol 1 mg PO BID.
D) Restraints with bathing.
E) Risperdal 0.5 mg PO QHS.

See p. 716.

61) The most appropriate next step for a 60-year-old male with a PSA level 12.5 ng/mL is:

A) 1 month of a fluoroquinolone followed by repeat rectal exam.
B) Referral for prostate biopsy.
C) Repeat PSA in 6–12 months.
D) Transrectal ultrasound of the prostate.

See p. 569.

62) A 33-year-old male with depression had been taking paroxetine 60 mg daily for a year for depression. Due to sexual problems, he decided to try another medication, and his doctor prescribed bupropion. He stopped the paroxetine 1 day and started bupropion the next. He comes in 5 days later feeling dizzy, nauseated, and fatigued. He complains of myalgias and insomnia. These symptoms are most likely due to:

A) Adverse effects of bupropion.
B) Hyperthyroidism.
C) Major depression.
D) Serotonin syndrome.
E) SSRI discontinuation syndrome.

See p. 778.

63) Sudden cardiac death in adolescent athletes is most often due to:

A) Hypertrophic cardiomyopathy.
B) Long QT syndrome.
C) Myocardial infarction.
D) Tetralogy of Fallot.

See p. 484.

64) A 17-year-old female runner with secondary amenorrhea should be further evaluated with all of the following EXCEPT:

A) Assessing calcium intake.
B) MRI of the pituitary.
C) Screening for eating disorders.
D) Urine beta-hCG.

See pp. 483–484.

65) Gynecomastia in an adolescent male occurs as a response to which of following mechanisms?

A) Excessive DHEA.
B) Excessive estrogen compared with testosterone.
C) Excessive growth hormone.
D) Excessive progesterone compared with testosterone.
E) Rapidly developing obesity.

See p. 561.

66) Treatment of a patient in diabetic ketoacidosis includes all of the following EXCEPT:

A) Aggressive volume replacement.
B) Frequent glucose monitoring.
C) Insulin.
D) Potassium.
E) Sodium bicarbonate.

See p. 350.

67) A 30-year-old male presents with difficulty obtaining an erection sufficient for penetration. He has GERD and takes cimetidine. He reports a good relationship with his wife and denies depression. He does not smoke and rarely drinks alcohol. The most appropriate intervention at this time is:

A) To order a testosterone level.
B) To perform cardiac stress testing.
C) To refer him to a urologist.
D) To replace cimetidine with omeprazole.
E) To send him to a psychologist.

See p. 574.

68) A frequent side effect of metformin is:

A) Constipation.
B) Hypoglycemia.
C) Lactic acidosis.
D) Renal failure.
E) Weight loss.

See p. 354.

69) A 40-year-old male presents with generalized weakness for 1 month. He has lost some weight, perhaps 10 pounds. He briefly lost consciousness yesterday while getting out of bed. He denies depression, drug or alcohol use, and any significant medical history. He is hypotensive but not tachycardic. He has orthostatic hypotension as well. Lab tests reveal mild anemia, low sodium,

elevated potassium, and normal TSH, BUN, creatinine, and glucose. He is surprisingly tan. To confirm your presumptive diagnosis, you order:

A) 24-hour urine catecholamines.
B) Free T4 and T3.
C) Plasma metanephrines.
D) Serum cortisol and ACTH.
E) Serum testosterone.

See p. 345.

70) A 62-year-old female presents to the emergency department with a sudden "hole" in her right visual field developing today. She also has a right temporal headache present for the last 2 weeks, shoulder and neck pain for a month, and weight loss of 5 pounds. She is slightly hypertensive and has a prominent tender vessel at the right side of her head. Her CBC is normal but the ESR is 85 mm/hr. What is the most appropriate course of action?

A) Administer IV methylprednisolone and admit for further evaluation.
B) Admit for cardiac monitoring and rule out myocardial infarction.
C) Discharge to home with oral antibiotics.
D) Discharge to home with referral to an ophthalmologist in the next week.
E) Perform a CT scan of the brain and discharge to home if normal.

See p. 374.

71) You find a new and suspicious skin lesion in a patient who has had a liver transplant for hepatitis C. You plan to perform a biopsy. If the skin lesion turns out to be malignant, it will most likely be:

A) Basal cell carcinoma.
B) Distant metastasis from liver cancer.
C) Melanoma.
D) Squamous cell carcinoma.

See p. 584.

72) The fractional excretion of sodium (FENa) is useful for determining:

A) If the patient has true hyponatremia.
B) Whether the patient has oliguric or anuric renal failure.
C) Whether the renal failure is due to acute tubular necrosis or another cause.
D) Whether the renal failure is due to intrinsic renal disease or a prerenal cause.
E) Why the patient has hyponatremia.

See p. 198.

73) The major Jones criteria for rheumatic fever include all of the following EXCEPT:

A) Carditis.
B) Fever.
C) Polyarthritis.
D) Subcutaneous nodules.
E) Sydenham chorea.

See p. 371.

74) A 29-year-old female daycare teacher presents with a severely pruritic rash that started at her wrists and has progressed to the web spaces of her fingers, under her arms, around her waist, and around her nipples. On exam, she has multiple excoriations and few small, erythematous papules. The most appropriate next step is:

A) Biopsy of normal-appearing skin.
B) Biopsy of one of the papules.
C) Empiric treatment with topical clotrimazole.
D) Empiric treatment with topical lindane 1%.
E) Empiric treatment with topical permethrin 5%.

See pp. 305–306.

75) A 60-year-old female with diabetic nephropathy is hospitalized with chest pain and a cardiac catheterization is planned. Which one of the following is the best option to reduce her risk of contrast-induced nephropathy?

A) Administer ketorolac and IV saline.
B) Administer mannitol and IV saline.
C) IV saline alone.
D) Administer n-acetylcysteine.

See p. 180.

76) A 58-year-old man with hypertension, diabetes, heart failure, and chronic kidney disease (stage 4, GFR ~25 mL/min/1.73 m^2) presents for follow-up. His current medications are insulin, aspirin, metoprolol, and lisinopril. His blood pressure is 142/86 mmHg and he has significant

dependent edema. His labs reveal a serum potassium of 5.3 mEq/L. To achieve his blood pressure to goal (<130/80) while avoiding adverse events, the best initial step is:

A) Discontinue lisinopril.
B) Furosemide 20 mg PO QAM.
C) Hydrochlorothiazide 12.5 mg PO QAM.
D) Increase lisinopril.
E) Losartan 25 mg PO daily.

See pp. 207–208.

77) Which of the following is most likely to cause hypokalemia?

A) Excessive use of "lite" salt.
B) Hypoaldosteronism.
C) Hypomagnesemia.
D) Overdose of propranolol.
E) Renal tubular acidosis type 4.

See p. 195.

78) A patient presents with thickened, yellowish, dystrophic toenails. What is the most appropriate next step?

A) Recommend that the patient return for toenail removal.
B) Send nail scrapings for KOH stain and/or fungal culture.
C) Start treatment with a topical antifungal.
D) Start treatment with an oral antifungal.

See p. 585.

79) All of the following are consistent with a diagnosis of syndrome of inappropriate antidiuretic hormone secretion (SIADH) EXCEPT:

A) High urine osmolality.
B) Low plasma osmolality.
C) Low urine sodium.
D) Normal adrenal function.
E) Normal thyroid function.

See p. 202.

80) A 21-year-old male is brought in the emergency department by his girlfriend after he overdosed on aspirin. He took "a bottle, maybe 100 pills or so," but he denies other ingestions. He complains only of nausea. He becomes more somnolent during the evaluation. He is slightly tachycardic and febrile with a normal blood pressure. His blood gas shows: pH 7.38, $PaCO_2$ 20 mm Hg, PaO_2 98 mm Hg, HCO_3 15 mEq/L. His creatinine, CBC, and electrolytes are normal, except for low potassium. What is the best description of this patient's blood gas?

A) Metabolic acidosis and metabolic alkalosis.
B) Metabolic acidosis and respiratory alkalosis.
C) Metabolic alkalosis and respiratory acidosis.
D) Normal blood gas (no acidosis or alkalosis).

See p. 213.

81) A 19-year-old college student presents to the emergency department with fever, headache, myalgias, and confusion. She has had a splenectomy but is otherwise healthy. The exam is notable for somnolence, fever, and nuchal rigidity. Due to her inability to follow directions, the neurological exam is difficult to complete, but it appears to be nonfocal. There are several other seriously ill patients in the ED to triage. Which of the following interventions should not wait an hour and must be done now?

A) Administer ceftriaxone, vancomycin, and dexamethasone.
B) Consult a neurosurgeon.
C) Perform lumbar puncture.
D) Obtain blood cultures.
E) Order CT of the brain.

See p. 296.

82) You perform joint aspiration on a patient with a painful, swollen knee. Microscopic exam of the fluid shows rhomboid-shaped, positively birefringent crystals. Which one of the following is the most likely to alleviate the patient's symptoms?

A) Acetaminophen daily.
B) Allopurinol daily.
C) Ceftriaxone IM.
D) Corticosteroid injection into the knee.

See p. 382.

83) A 23-year-old male with HIV stopped taking all of his medications 3 months ago due to cost. He was feeling fine until 3 weeks ago when he developed a cough. He now has daily fevers (T~101°F), a nonproductive cough, dyspnea on

exertion, fatigue, chills, and tightness in his chest with inspiration. His exam is notable for fever, diaphoresis, bilateral crackles with inspiration, and mild tachypnea. Chest x-ray shows diffuse bilateral interstitial infiltrates. Which of the following is the most likely causative agent for this pulmonary infection?

A) Adenovirus.
B) *Cryptococcus neoformans.*
C) *Mycobacterium tuberculosis.*
D) *Pneumocystis jiroveci* (PCP).
E) *Toxoplasma gondii.*

See pp. 321–322.

84) Which of the following is not useful in the treatment of hepatic encephalopathy?

A) Lactulose.
B) Polyethylene glycol (Golytely).
C) Oral neomycin.
D) Enemas for acute encephalopathy.

See p. 277.

85) An otherwise-healthy 70-year-old female is admitted and started on ceftriaxone and azithromycin for pneumonia. On hospital day 3, her serum creatinine is found to have tripled from admission. She is mildly nauseated and has an erythematous, macular rash on her trunk and arms. Her CBC shows that her white cell count has declined from admission, but she now has a prominent eosinophilia. Urinalysis shows 1+ protein, and urine sediment shows white cell casts and eosinophils. The most appropriate next step is:

A) Add metronidazole to her antibiotic regimen.
B) Bolus with IV 0.9% saline.
C) Consult a nephrologist for possible renal biopsy.
D) Discontinue ceftriaxone and consider an alternative antibiotic.
E) Start furosemide to improve urine output.

See p. 214.

86) Each of the following patients is found to have asymptomatic bacteruria. Which one should be treated with a course of antibiotics?

A) An 88-year-old female nursing home resident.
B) A 20-year-old pregnant patient.
C) A 75-year-old male with an indwelling Foley catheter for BPH.
D) All of the above.

See p. 298.

87) Which of the following will cause a low SAAG ascites?

A) Carcinomatous peritonitis.
B) Portal hypertension.
C) Bud–Chiari syndrome.
D) Cirrhosis.

See p. 275.

88) A patient comes to the emergency department after sustaining a needle stick. She is a nurse who had just finished drawing blood for culture on a patient with AIDS, and somehow she stuck herself through her glove. She bled a little. She washed the area copiously. What is the most appropriate next step?

A) Prescribe antiretrovirals for 4 weeks.
B) Prescribe antiretrovirals for 2 weeks.
C) Reassure the patient as her risk of contracting HIV is negligible.
D) Test her for HIV and treat based on the results.

See p. 329.

89) Which of the following IS NOT useful in the treatment of alcoholic liver disease with portal hypertension?

A) Pentoxifylline (Trental).
B) Nadolol.
C) Isosorbide dinitrate.
D) Cilostazol (Pletal).

See p. 275.

90) Which of the following is generally true in alcohol or toxin-related liver disease?

A) AST is 2× greater than ALT.
B) ALT is 2× greater than AST.
C) Both ALT and AST are elevated to the same degree.
D) The GGT is specific for liver disease and higher than either the ALT or AST.

See p. 282.

91) Appropriate antibiotic treatment of diverticulitis includes all of the following EXCEPT:

A) Ciprofloxacin + metronidazole.
B) Amoxicillin clavulanate.
C) Trimethoprim/Sulfamethoxazole + metronidazole.
D) Clindamycin + metronidazole.

See p. 290.

92) Which of the following is true about the treatment of pancreatitis?

A) Antibiotics should be used in most cases of pancreatitis.
B) Enteral feedings with the feeding tube in the jejunum is the preferred method of nutrition.
C) Pseudocysts must be drained for pancreatitis to resolve.
D) The Ransom criteria can be used at the time of admission to accurately predict mortality.

See p. 285.

93) Which of the following does NOT promote gastric emptying in gastric paresis?

A) Erythromycin.
B) Metoclopramide.
C) Amoxicillin.
D) Cisapride.

See pp. 286–287.

94) The most common cause of pancreatitis in the United States is:

A) Alcohol.
B) Cholelithiasis.
C) Thiazide diuretics.
D) Viruses.

See p. 283.

95) All of the following are causes of nonalcoholic fatty liver disease EXCEPT:

A) Statin use.
B) Hypothyroidism.
C) Diabetes.
D) Obesity.

See p. 280.

96) The most common cause of the development of drug resistance in HIV is:

A) Failure to include zidovudine in the treatment regimen.
B) Failure to initiate treatment until the patient has a known AIDS defining illness.
C) Poor compliance with medications.
D) Failure to include a protease inhibitor in the treatment regimen.

See p. 317.

97) At what $CD4^+$ level should one initiate prophylactic treatment of *Pneumocystis jiroveci* (previously *Pneumocystis carinii*)?

A) $CD4^+ \leq 50$
B) $CD4^+ \leq 75$
C) $CD4^+ \leq 100$
D) $CD4^+ \leq 200$

See p. 324.

98) Which of the following recommendations regarding Pap smear screening in an HIV+ woman is true?

A) No modification is needed in the Pap smear regimen.
B) If the $CD4^+$ count is normal and the patient has two normal Pap smears at 1 year intervals, you can go back to routine screening.
C) If the patient has a $CD4^+$ count of <200, screening should be done Q 6 months regardless of whether or not the patient has had negative Pap smears.
D) Pap smears can be suspended in HIV-positive patients since they will likely die from HIV before they die from cervical cancer.

See p. 327.

99) Which of the following statements best reflects the current thinking about treating influenza?

A) Rimantadine and amantadine are most effective against influenza B.
B) Treatment with oseltamivir (Tamiflu) is highly effective, thus negating the need for influenza vaccine.
C) Oseltamivir must be started within 48 hours of symptom onset to be of any benefit.

D) There is no resistance of influenza A to oseltamivir.

See pp. 292–293.

100) Which of the following patients needs isoniazid treatment?

A) A patient with no risk factors who has a PPD reaction of 5 mm.
B) A patient with recent exposure to TB and a PPD reaction of 5 mm.
C) A health-care worker with a PPD reaction of 5 mm.
D) A health-care worker with a PPD reaction of 10 mm and a positive chest radiograph.

See pp. 300–301.

101) The recommended empirical antibiotic treatment of meningitis in an adult is:

A) Ceftriaxone.
B) Ceftriaxone + vancomycin.
C) Ceftriaxone + ciprofloxacin.
D) Ceftriaxone + TMP/SMX.

See p. 297.

102) The most common bacterial organism causing meningitis in adults is:

A) Pneumococcus.
B) Meningococcus.
C) Haemophilus.
D) Listeria.

See p. 297.

103) All of the following can be used for malaria prophylaxis EXCEPT:

A) Doxycycline.
B) Mefloquine.
C) Azithromycin.
D) Atovaquone/proguanil (Malarone).

See p. 311.

104) Which of the following is true regarding the diagnosis of urolithiasis?

A) Over 90% of patients will have blood in their urine at the time of diagnosis.
B) Urolithiasis may be difficult to differentiate from aortic dissection at the initial time of presentation.
C) Hematuria will reliably differentiate urolithiasis from aortic dissection.
D) A negative "FAST" ultrasound scan is considered the standard and if negative rules out urolithiasis.

See p. 188.

105) Which of the following profiles are you likely to see in a patient with a prerenal cause of elevated creatinine?

A) Urine sodium <20, fractional excretion of sodium <1%.
B) Urine sodium <20, fractional excretion of sodium >2%.
C) Urine sodium >40, fractional excretion of sodium <1%.
D) Urine sodium >40, fractional excretion of sodium >2%.

See pp. 198–199.

106) Aldosterone resistance (such as occurs with diabetic nephropathy) or hypoaldosteronism will present with which of the following?

A) Hypokalemia.
B) Hyperkalemia.
C) Hyperphosphatemia.
D) Hypophosphatemia.

See p. 181.

107) Which of the following regimens IS NOT recommended for treatment of a simple cystitis?

A) Amoxicillin 500 mg PO TID for 3 days.
B) Levofloxacin 250 mg PO daily for 3 days.
C) Nitrofurantoin 100 mg PO TID for 5 days.
D) TMP/SMX 1 PO TID for 3 days.

See p. 31.

108) Which of the following drugs is LEAST LIKELY to slow proteinuria?

A) Enalapril.
B) Losartan.
C) Verapamil.
D) Nifedipine.

See pp. 182–183.

109) The definition of nephrotic syndrome requires all of the following EXCEPT:

A) Hypoalbuminemia.
B) Urine albumin excretion >3 g per day.
C) Edema.
D) Renal biopsy showing appropriate changes.

See p. 192.

110) Which of the following patients should have a carotid endarterectomy based on all current US guidelines?

A) A 60-year-old female with a unilateral symptomatic 70% carotid plaque.
B) A 60-year-old male or female with an asymptomatic 69% carotid plaque.
C) Patient of either gender with bilateral 50% carotid plaque, symptomatic or asymptomatic.
D) None of the above meet current qualification criterion.

See p. 607.

111) If cost were NOT an issue, which of he following drugs/drug combinations would be the ideal regimen for the secondary prevention of stroke?

A) Aspirin + clopidogrel (Plavix).
B) Aspirin + dipyridamole.
C) Aspirin alone.
D) Clopidogrel alone.

See p. 606.

112) Which one of the following entities presents with reflexes preserved?

A) Guillain–Barré.
B) Amyotrophic lateral sclerosis.
C) Charcot–Marie–Tooth disease.
D) Diabetic neuropathy.

See p. 622.

113) Which one of the following agents is most effective for controlling the pain of peripheral neuropathy?

A) Tricyclic antidepressant.
B) Gabapentin or other newer antiepileptic drug (e.g., Topamax).
C) Oxycodone or other narcotic.
D) Carbamazepine or other traditional antiepileptic.

See p. 612.

114) Which of the following drugs IS NOT associated with rebound headaches?

A) Acetaminophen.
B) DHE.
C) Nortriptyline.
D) Sumatriptan.

See p. 617.

115) The risk of having a second seizure after a first febrile seizure is:

A) 2–5%; the same as the rest of the population.
B) 6–10%; slightly higher than the general population.
C) 11–15%; significantly higher than the general population.
D) Unknown.

See p. 636.

116) You determine that a 77-year-old female has Parkinson disease that is interfering with her daily life. The best drug or drug combination to alleviate her symptoms and improve her function is:

A) A COMT inhibitor (e.g., Entacapone).
B) A dopamine agonist (e.g., Requip).
C) Levodopa/carbidopa (e.g., Sinemet).
D) Apomorphine.

See p. 628.

117) The PRESENCE of an RAPD (relative afferent pupillary defect) can be indicative of:

A) Cataracts.
B) Large retinal detachment.
C) Bleed into the anterior chamber.
D) Severe refractive error.

See p. 640.

118) Which of the following patients has an indication for cataract surgery?

A) Vision 20/100 bilaterally in a patient who has no visual complaints or functional impairment.

B) Vision 20/20 OD and 10/100 OS in a patient who can see well enough to do everything she desires.
C) Vision 20/30 OD and 20/30 OS in a patient who is bothered by her inability to quilt
D) Vision unknown in a patient who can carry out all ADLs to her own satisfaction.

See p. 659.

119) All of the following intraocular muscles are innervated by cranial nerve III EXCEPT:

A) Inferior oblique.
B) Inferior rectus.
C) Lateral rectus.
D) Medial rectus.
E) Superior rectus.

See p. 661.

120) Skinnier, "politically correct" Santas are in vogue this year (bearing gifts of celery, no doubt). Your patient is in tizzy: he has played Santa for years without the need for pillows. He wants to keep up his tradition as St. Nick. What can you tell him about weight reduction surgery?

A) "Sorry, even though you may lose weight, it will not help your overall health."
B) "You must have a BMI >40 kg/m^2 before qualifying for bariatric surgery regardless of other underlying conditions."
C) "You must have a BMI of >35 kg/m^2 AND significant reversible disease (HTN, DM) to qualify for bariatric surgery."
D) "The reindeer union says it won't work if Santa's weight is under 300 pounds—they need to keep 8 reindeer working the sleigh at all times."

See p. 735.

121) A 70-year-old male patient complains of severe unilateral visual loss. He has no other symptoms. Here is a picture of his fundus. His diagnosis is:

A) Acute glaucoma.
B) Acute venous disruption.
C) Acute arterial occlusion.
D) Diabetic retinopathy.

See p. 656.

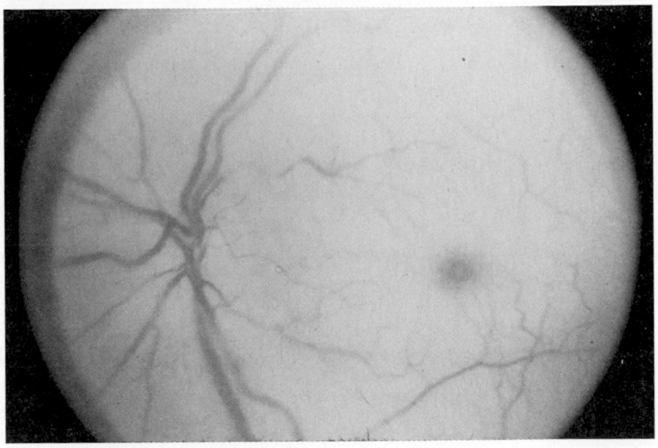

122) What is the general course of rheumatoid arthritis during pregnancy?

A) Worsening during pregnancy.
B) Worsening during pregnancy but only if methotrexate is used.
C) RA may remit during pregnancy and MTX is relatively contraindicated.
D) Morning sickness is worse in those with RA.

See p. 370.

123) A diagnosis of rheumatoid arthritis can be made after symptoms have been present for at least:

A) 15 minutes.
B) 2 weeks.
C) 6 weeks.
D) Duration of symptoms is no longer a criterion for diagnosing RA.

See p. 367.

124) You make a diagnosis of rheumatoid arthritis based on laboratory and clinical criteria. The best time to begin disease-modifying antirheumatic drugs (DMARDs) is:

A) At the time of diagnosis.
B) After failure of 2 NSAIDs.
C) After the failure of prednisone.
D) When complications of rheumatoid arthritis occur.

See pp. 368–369.

125) You are seeing a 57-year-old male in your practice who is complaining of bi-temporal headache. He checked the web and decided that

he has giant cell (temporal) arteritis. The only thing of it is that his ESR is only 30 mm/hr. The CRP is not much more edifying. You appropriately respond to him:

A) "You may still have temporal arteritis since 15% or more will have normal ESR and CRP."
B) "You seem to be displaying drug seeking behavior since you came in to the ER with the same complaint 1 month ago."
C) "You may still have temporal arteritis, but we need to perform a temporal bone biopsy."
D) "You may still have temporal arteritis, but we will need to submit your head to the state lab for formal testing... you don't mind... do you?"

See p. 372.

126) When treating gout, which one of these drugs for gout will be ineffective in those with renal insufficiency?

A) Allopurinol.
B) Probenecid.
C) Prednisone.
D) Colchicine.

See pp. 381–382.

127) In regard to therapy for giant cell arteritis, which of the following statements best describes the appropriate relationship of aspirin, prednisone, and giant cell arteritis?

A) ASA (81 mg/day) can be used as adjunctive therapy for those on prednisone.
B) ASA (325 mg/day) can be used as adjunctive therapy for those on prednisone.
C) High-dose ASA (650 mg/day) can be used in those who do not tolerate prednisone.
D) ASA has no role in the treatment of giant cell arteritis.

See p. 373.

128) The one best, first-line drug treatment of osteoarthritis pain is:

A) Acetaminophen.
B) Celecoxib (Celebrex).
C) Ibuprofen.
D) Naproxen.

See p. 375.

129) The best initial pharmacologic therapy for fibromyalgia pain is:

A) Duloxetine.
B) Ibuprofen.
C) Nortriptyline.
D) Tramadol.

See p. 389.

130) Which of the following should NOT go into the calculus of what antibiotic to use for a patient with community acquired pneumonia?

A) Appearance of infiltrate on chest x-ray (lobar vs. "atypical").
B) Comorbid medical conditions.
C) Likelihood of resistant organisms (based on recent antibiotic use, daycare exposure, etc.).
D) Patient age.

See p. 156.

131) The use of Depo-Provera should be limited to 2 years because of the risk of:

A) Osteoporosis.
B) Breast cancer.
C) Ovarian cancer.
D) Prolonged or permeant amenorrhea.

See pp. 696–697.

132) Bleeding in a nonpregnant, amenorrheic patient in response to a "progesterone challenge" (e.g., medroxyprogesterone given for 10 days and then stopped) indicates that the patient has sufficient endogenous:

A) FSH.
B) LH.
C) Progesterone.
D) Estrogen.

See p. 360.

133) You get the following results on a vaginal wet prep: pH 5.0 and a positive "whiff" test. Wouldn't you know it, the rest of the results got lost. With the information available, the most likely diagnosis is:

A) Vulvovaginal candidiasis.
B) Bacterial vaginosis.

C) Vaginal trichomoniasis.
D) Physiologic vaginal discharge.

See pp. 543–544.

134) When is screening for Group B *Streptococcus* in the pregnant female recommended?

A) 30–32 weeks, gestation.
B) 32–34 weeks, gestation.
C) 35–37 weeks, gestation.
D) Intrapartum only.

See p. 499.

135) Which of the following is the most appropriate treatment of chronic menorrhagia in a 42-year-old female hypertensive smoker?

A) Low androgenic progesterone oral contraceptive.
B) Progesterone IUD (e.g., Mirena and Progestasert).
C) Copper T IUD.
D) Low estrogen oral contraceptive.

See p. 519.

136) You are called to see a partner's patient who is G3P2 at 32 weeks, gestation and is having regular contractions. After monitoring and an exam, you suspect that she is in labor. The SINGLE most important step, and the first step to take, at this point is:

A) Administration of corticosteroids to hasten fetal lung maturation.
B) Administration a tocolytic such as terbutaline.
C) Insertion of a cervical cerclage to delay delivery.
D) Antibiotic therapy (ampicillin) from now until delivery.

See p. 511.

137) This fetal tracing, shown on page 912, is:

A) Reassuring.
B) Worrisome.
C) An indication for immediate C-section.
D) An indication for the addition of Pitocin.

See p. 501.

138) Which of the following must be present to make the diagnosis of pelvic inflammatory disease?

A) Adnexal pain.
B) Elevated WBC count.
C) Elevated CRP.
D) Temperature of >38°C.

See p. 529.

139) A negative fetal fibronectin suggests that:

A) The fetal lungs are immature.
B) There is little likelihood that the patient will deliver within the next 2 weeks.
C) There is an amniotic fluid leak.
D) Is not helpful. A positive fibronectin suggests imminent delivery.

See p. 510.

140) Which of the following is true about tocolytics for premature labor?

A) They are effective at stopping labor and can arrest labor for an average of 1 week.
B) They have very few side effects and should be used routinely in premature labor.
C) Their use is mostly to buy time for antenatal steroids to work for those pregnancies between 24 and 34 weeks.
D) Terbutaline is the only FDA-approved tocolytic.

See p. 511.

141) As you start a patient on fluoxetine for depression, you counsel him about the adverse effects of this class of medications. All of the following are common adverse effects of SSRIs EXCEPT:

A) Anxiety.
B) Diarrhea.
C) Headaches.
D) Hypersexuality.
E) Insomnia.

See p. 778.

142) A 12-month-old female presents to the emergency department after 24 hours of vomiting, diarrhea, and fever. She is lethargic, tachycardic, and hypotensive with poor skin turgor. What is the most appropriate initial method of providing her fluids?

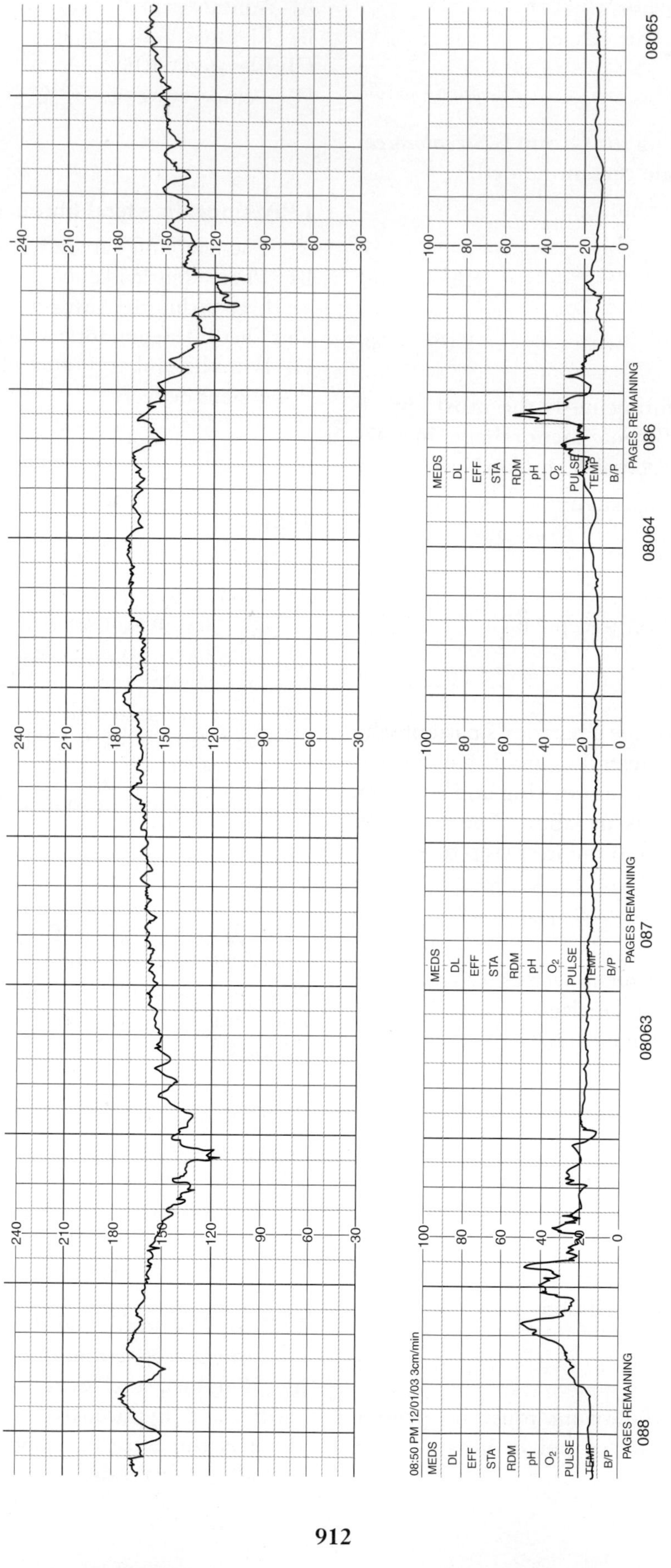
08:50 PM 12/01/03 3cm/min
MEDS
DL
EFF
STA
RDM
pH
O2
PULSE
TEMP
B/P
PAGES REMAINING
088
240
210
180
150
120
90
60
30
100
80
60
40
20
0
PAGES REMAINING
087
08063
PAGES REMAINING
086
08064
08065

A) Half-normal saline, 20 mL/kg bolus.
B) Half-normal saline with 5% dextrose, 10 mL/kg bolus.
C) Normal saline, 100 mL/kg bolus.
D) Normal saline, 20 mL/kg bolus.

See p. 448.

143) A 15-month-old male is brought to the clinic by his parents. Like everyone else at his home, he has had some rhinorrhea and diarrhea in the last week. However, 4 hours ago the patient developed episodes of inconsolable crying accompanied by lying in "the fetal position" for 15–20 minutes at a time. At first his parents were puzzled but not too worried, but these episodes have occurred six to seven times now and he has become more lethargic. Finally, he had a bloody bowel movement, so they decided to bring him in to the office. On exam, he is afebrile, lethargic but arousable, and well hydrated. His abdomen appears benign. What is your leading diagnosis?

A) Cholecystitis.
B) Gastroenteritis.
C) Intussusception.
D) Volvulus.

See p. 451.

144) Which of the following screening tests is recommended universally for all children in the United States?

A) Eye exam at 24 months.
B) Hearing testing at 1 or 2 days old.
C) Hemoglobin at 12 months.
D) Lead level at 12 months.

See p. 461.

145) During a visit for a physical exam, you note that this 33-year-old female has checked "depression" on her health-screening questionnaire. You ask her more about this and find that she has felt that her mood has been depressed for 15 years or more. She generally feels fatigued and has low self-esteem, but she denies suicidal ideation and feelings of guilt and worthlessness. What diagnosis best characterizes her symptoms?

A) Avoidant personality disorder.
B) Borderline personality disorder.
C) Dysthymia.
D) Major depressive disorder.

See p. 767.

146) Which of the following symptoms would be LEAST likely to be due to a panic attack and therefore would prompt further investigation in a patient with known panic disorder?

A) Chest pain.
B) Dyspnea.
C) Palpitations.
D) Syncope.

See p. 772.

147) A 23-year-old male presents with symptoms suggestive of panic attacks, an underlying anxiety disorder, and possibly panic disorder. You refer him for counseling services and recommend starting a medication. Which of the following drugs is LEAST effective for treating panic disorder?

A) Bupropion.
B) Nortriptyline.
C) Sertraline.
D) Venlafaxine.

See p. 773.

148) All of the following are part of the CHADS2 score EXCEPT:

A) Age >65.
B) History of stroke, thromboembolic disease, etc.
C) Diabetes.
D) CHF.

See p. 73.

149) You are watching a really bad grade B movie. Who do you think will win?

A) Mothra.
B) King Ghidorah.
C) Biollante.
D) Godzilla.
E) Mechagodzilla.

Never bet against Godzilla.

Answers

1. *Answer: D.*
2. *Answer: B.*
3. *Answer: A.*
4. *Answer: C.*
5. *Answer: C.*
6. *Answer: C.*
7. *Answer: D.*
8. *Answer: B.*
9. *Answer: B.*
10. *Answer: D.*
11. *Answer: A.*
12. *Answer: C.*
13. *Answer: B.*
14. *Answer: D.*
15. *Answer: B.*
16. *Answer: C.*
17. *Answer: A.*
18. *Answer: C.*
19. *Answer: B.*
20. *Answer: D.*
21. *Answer: B.*
22. *Answer: D.*
23. *Answer: B.*
24. *Answer: D.*
25. *Answer: D.*
26. *Answer: C.*
27. *Answer: C.*
28. *Answer: C.*
29. *Answer: B.*
30. *Answer: A.*
31. *Answer: B.*
32. *Answer: D.*
33. *Answer: C.*
34. *Answer: D.*
35. *Answer: C.*
36. *Answer: B.*
37. *Answer: A.*
38. *Answer: D.*
39. *Answer: B.*
40. *Answer: B.*
41. *Answer: A.*
42. *Answer: B.*
43. *Answer: B.*
44. *Answer: D.*
45. *Answer: A.*
46. *Answer: C.*
47. *Answer: B.*
48. *Answer: B.*
49. *Answer: D.*
50. *Answer: D.*
51. *Answer: C.*
52. *Answer: E.*
53. *Answer: D.*
54. *Answer: C.*
55. *Answer: E.*
56. *Answer: B.*
57. *Answer: C.*
58. *Answer: B.*
59. *Answer: C.*
60. *Answer: A.*
61. *Answer: B.*
62. *Answer: E.*
63. *Answer: A.*
64. *Answer: B.*
65. *Answer: B.*
66. *Answer: E.*
67. *Answer: D.*
68. *Answer: E.*
69. *Answer: D.*
70. *Answer: A.*
71. *Answer: D.*
72. *Answer: D.*
73. *Answer: B.*
74. *Answer: E.*
75. *Answer: C.*
76. *Answer: B.*
77. *Answer: C.*
78. *Answer: B.*
79. *Answer: C.*
80. *Answer: B.*
81. *Answer: A.*
82. *Answer: D.*
83. *Answer: D.*
84. *Answer: B.*
85. *Answer: D.*
86. *Answer: B.*
87. *Answer: A.*
88. *Answer: A.*
89. *Answer: D.*
90. *Answer: A.*
91. *Answer: D.*
92. *Answer: B.*
93. *Answer: C.*
94. *Answer: B.*
95. *Answer: A.*
96. *Answer: C.*
97. *Answer: D.*
98. *Answer: C.*
99. *Answer: C.*
100. *Answer: B.*
101. *Answer: B.*
102. *Answer: A.*
103. *Answer: C.*
104. *Answer: B.*
105. *Answer: A.*
106. *Answer: B.*
107. *Answer: A.*
108. *Answer: D.*
109. *Answer: D.*
110. *Answer: A.*
111. *Answer: B.*
112. *Answer: B.*
113. *Answer: A.*
114. *Answer: C.*
115. *Answer: A.*
116. *Answer: C.*
117. *Answer: B.*
118. *Answer: C.*
119. *Answer: C.*
120. *Answer: C.*
121. *Answer: C.*
122. *Answer: C.*
123. *Answer: D.*
124. *Answer: A.*
125. *Answer: A.*
126. *Answer: B.*
127. *Answer: A.*
128. *Answer: A.*
129. *Answer: C.*
130. *Answer: A.*
131. *Answer: A.*
132. *Answer: D.*
133. *Answer: B.*
134. *Answer: C.*
135. *Answer: B.*
136. *Answer: A.*
137. *Answer: B.*
138. *Answer: A*
139. *Answer: B*
140. *Answer: C.*
141. *Answer: D.*
142. *Answer: D.*
143. *Answer: C.*
144. *Answer: B.*
145. *Answer: C.*
146. *Answer: D.*
147. *Answer: A.*
148. *Answer: A.*
149. *Answer: D.*

Index

Note: Page numbers followed by f and t indicates figure and table respectively.

G

T

U